INFECTIOUS DISEASES IN OBSTETRICS AND GYNECOLOGY

SIXTH EDITION

GILLES R. G. MONIF, MD
Professor of Obstetrics and Gynecology
University of Oklahoma College of Medicine–Tulsa
Tulsa, Oklahoma

AND

DAVID A. BAKER, MD
Professor of Obstetrics and Gynecology
Stony Brook University Medical Center
Stony Brook, New York

informa
healthcare

Notice: Medicine is an ever-changing science. As new research and clinical experience broaden our knowledge, changes in treatment and drug therapy are required. The editors and the publisher of this work have checked with sources believed to be reliable in their efforts to provide drug dosage schedules that are complete and in accord with the standards accepted at the time of publication. However, readers are advised to check the product information sheet included in the package of each drug they plan to administer to be certain that the information contained in these schedules is accurate and that changes have not been made in the recommended dose or in the contraindications for administration. This recommendation is of particular importance in connection with new or infrequently used drugs.

© 2008 IDI Publications

First published in the United Kingdom in 2008 by Informa Healthcare, Telephone House, 69–77 Paul Street, London EC2A 4LQ. Informa Healthcare is a trading division of Informa UK Ltd. Registered Office: 37/41 Mortimer Street, London W1T 3JH. Registered in England and Wales number 1072954.

Tel: +44 (0)20 7017 5000
Fax: +44 (0)20 7017 6699
Website: www.informahealthcare.com

British Library Cataloguing in Publication Data
Infectious diseases in obstetrics and gynecology - 6th ed.
1. Communicable diseases in pregnancy 2. Generative organs, Female - Infection
I. Monif, Gilles R. G. (Gilles Reza G) II. Baker, David A., 1945-618

ISBN-10: 0 415 43948 5
ISBN-13: 978 0 415 43948 0

Distributed in North and South America by
Taylor & Francis
6000 Broken Sound Parkway, NW, (Suite 300)
Boca Raton, FL 33487, USA

Within Continental USA
Tel: 1 (800) 272 7737; Fax: 1 (800) 374 3401
Outside Continental USA
Tel: (561) 994 0555; Fax: (561) 361 6018
Email: orders@crcpress.com

Distributed in the rest of the world by
Thomson Publishing Services
Cheriton House
North Way
Andover, Hampshire SP10 5BE, UK
Tel: +44 (0)1264 332424
Email: tps.tandfsalesorder@thomson.com

Composition by Egerton & Televijay
Printed and bound in India by Nutech Photolithographers

Contents

Contributors

David A. Baker, MD
Professor of Obstetrics and Gynecology,
Stony Brook University Medical Center,
Stony Brook, New York

David S. Bard, MD
Professor of Obstetrics and Gynecology,
University of Arkansas School of Medicine,
Little Rock, Arkansas

Michael S. Burnhill, MD, DMSc
Planned Parenthood Federation of America,
New York, New York

James W. Daly, MD
Former Professor and Chairman of Obstetrics and Gynecology,
University of Missouri College of Medicine,
Columbia, Missouri

Gilbert G. Donders, MD, PhD
Professor of Obstetrics and Gynecology,
Gasthuisbery University,
Leuven, Belgium

Robert J. Fagnant, MD
College Hill Clinic,
Rock Springs, Wyoming

Reinaldo Figueroa, MD
Associate Professor of Clinical Obstetrics and Gynecology,
Stony Brook University Medical Center,
Stony Brook, New York

Stanley Gall, MD
Professor of Obstetrics, Gynecology and Women's Health,
Professor of Public Health and Information Sciences,
University of Louisville,
Louisville, Kentucky

David J. Garry, DO
Associate Professor of Obstetrics and Gynecology,
Albert Einstein College of Medicine of Yeshvia University,
Bronx, New York

Douglas D. Glover, RPh
West Virginia University School of Medicine,
Morgantown, West Virginia

Craig S. Hill, PhD
Senior Scientist, Gen Probe,
San Diego, California

Mahmoud Ismail, MD
Professor of Obstetrics and Gynecology,
University of Chicago School of Medicine,
Chicago, Illinois

Bryan Larsen, PhD
University Research and Biomedical Graduate Studies,
Professor of Microbiology and of Obstetrics and Gynecology,
Des Moines University, Des Moines, Iowa

William J. Ledger, MD
Professor of Obstetrics and Gynecology,
Weill Cornell Medical College of Cornell University,
New York, New York

Mark G. Martens, MD
Professor of Obstetrics and Gynecology,
University of Oklahoma College of Medicine–Tulsa,
Tulsa, Oklahoma

Gilles R. G. Monif, MD
Professor of Obstetrics and Gynecology,
University of Oklahoma College of Medicine–Tulsa,
Tulsa, Oklahoma

J. Patrick O'Leary, MD, FACS
The Isidore Cohn, Jr., M.D. Professor and Chairman,
Louisiana State University School of Medicine,
Department of Surgery, New Orleans, Louisiana

Newton G. Osborne, MD, PhD
Professor of Obstetrics and Gynecology,
Howard University College of Medicine,
Washington, D.C.

Paul Summers, MD
Professor of Obstetrics and Gynecology,
University of Nevada School of Medicine,
Reno, Nevada

Timothy S. Tracy, PhD
Professor and Head,
Department of Experimental and Clinical Pharmacology,
University of Minnesota College of Pharmacy,
Duluth, Minnesota

Steven S. Witkin, PhD
Professor of Immunology,
Director of Division of Immunology and Infectious Diseases,
Weill Cornell Medical College of Cornell University,
New York, New York

Preface to the Sixth Edition

In its conception, *Infectious Diseases in Obstetrics and Gynecology* was created to address an unmet need for a depository of information specially focused on the uniqueness that pregnancy confers, and the special conditions that differentiate the adverse impact of infectious disease entities between men and women.

Books, by virtue of the time required for development may not always be at the immediate cutting edge of diagnostics and therapeutics. The foundation of the editions of *Infectious Diseases in Obstetrics and Gynecology* has been their emphasis on addressing a given disease entity from the organism and disease perspective independently. By understanding the events which combine to produce disease, future advances in diagnostics and therapeutics can readily be integrated into the overall patient healthcare management.

In terms of style the commitment has been to deliver sophisticated information in a pragmatic form so as to better empower and educate those who man the patient–physician frontier. Authors are and have been chosen based upon demonstrated clinical and intellectual abilities. The editorial mandate to each is and has been to write each segment based upon a foundation derived from their patient care experience and its correspondence in the literature. The awards and recognition the book has received speak to the validity of this deviation from a traditional infectious disease book in which each statement is carefully documented. Those authors who contributed to this edition were chosen because of their extensive clinical experience as well as intellect, which enable them to supersede the printed word when it errs.

Gilles R. G. Monif

December 2007

Without art there can be no true science
and without a love of humanity there can be no true art.

This edition is dedicated to my parents who helped forge
and nurture these concepts.

Understanding the Bacteriology of the Female Genital Tract

INTRODUCTION

Compared to our understanding of bacterial diseases of the female genital tract, relatively little is understood about what constitutes and maintains a healthy ecological system within the microbiological flora of the female genital tract. Why is an understanding of normality important? At some future date, therapy may graduate from the eradication of pathogen bacteria causing disease to the promotion of bacteria responsible for vaginal/cervical microbial wellness, and physicians may prevent disease rather than eradicate it through the use of probiotics.

That one microbial species can inhibit a different form of microbe has resulted in the coining of the term "probiotics." A probiotic is the feeding or placing of an organism or product that enhances or maintains a nonpathogenic flora. Gorbach's advice as to what constitutes a probiotic is important to understand that less nonefficacious combinations of organisms or products destroy the perceived validity of the approach of competitive inhibition of pathogenic or potentially pathogenic bacteria: "the purported benefits for any probiotic must pass the highest standard of scientific scrutiny before the claims can be accepted."

The shallowness of our microbiological observations emanate from the inadequacy of sampling technology, failure to quantitate the majority of observations, and the seeming lack of its importance.

Analyses of published studies reveal compromising of microbiological data by inappropriate or suboptimal methods of culturing, failure to use appropriate transport media or enriched media, and/or a lack of stringent adherence to or use of anaerobic technology in the processing and culture of specimens.

The isolation of a given bacteria does not necessarily confer as to its functional significance. The microbial load of a given bacteria appears to govern the relative risk of asymptomatic versus symptomatic infection. A case in point is *Streptococcus pneumoniae*. During the winter months, it is not uncommon for 4% to 5% of the population to have nasal colonization with an encapsulated strain of the bacteria, unassociated with disease. Quantitative studies document the relatively low level of bacterial replication. In contrast, pneumococcal disease is associated with a 5 to 6 log increase in demonstrable organisms. Louis Pasteur put this concept into clear perspective when he asserted that "the mere presence of an organism is insufficient to produce disease." What constitutes a pathogen in a given situation is not only the type of offending organism and its specific virulence, but also the absence of competitive microbial governance.

Insufficient attention in the study of bacterial disease has been given, not to which bacteria is isolated, but rather to what bacteria that are normal inhabitants of a given focus of disease are not present. Bacteria causing overt streptococcal disease, whether it be of the upper respiratory tract or the female genital tract, have few, if any, co-isolates. Similarly, in acute disease due to group A and group B streptococci. With the exception of *Staphyloccus aureus* and *Staphylococcus epidermidis*, when acute disease due to the group A and group B streptococci occurs, few if any other bacterial are concomitantly isolated.

BACTERIOLOGY OF NORMAL FEMALE GENITAL TRACT FLORA

The microbiological flora of the normal female genital tract constitutes a dynamic interplay of microbial and environmental checks and balances.

Disease of the female genital tract can be due to endogenous bacteria such as *Bacteroides/Prevotella* species, *Gardnerella vaginalis*, or the group B streptococcus, or exogenous bacteria such as *Neisseria gonorrhoeae* or the group A streptococcus.

In order to understand abnormality, one must first understand normality: what bacteria are considered the normal inhabitants of the female genital tract.

The number of bacteria recoverable from the lower female genital tract is relatively staggering. The aerobic isolates and their relative prevalence is listed in Table 1; that for anaerobic bacteria is listed in Table 2. The diversity of isolates from one woman to another is not a phenomenon of randomness. When quantitative and inhibition studies are done, a picture of a highly regulated governance is demonstrable.

Once the normal bacterial constituents of the female genital tract are defined, one is confronted with having to explain why apparently commensal bacteria, such as *G. vaginalis*, group B streptococcus, and *Escherichia coli*, are transformed into regional pathogens and produce disease.

Change in the local microbiological environment is one of the principal means by which endogenous bacteria gain the numerical representation necessary for suppression of competitive bacterial inhibitors and production of disease, or for introduction of environmental factors that directly stimulate specific bacteria: quantitative replication. In animal model systems, peritonitis is more frequently induced when blood is injected with the threshold inoculum. Myonecrosis occurs when calcium chloride is implanted into the muscle along with the *Clostridium* species. Salmonellosis can be induced in animals by the administration of an antibiotic that eradicates its competitive inhibitors.

For endogenous bacteria that gain access to the female genital tract, such as *N. gonorrhoeae* or group A streptococcus, an alteration of a natural host defense barrier needs to occur. The

TABLE 1 Prevalence of aerobic (facultative) isolates reported in vaginal flora studies in the published literature

Aerobic isolate	Prevalence in vaginal flora (%)		
	Low	Mean	High
Gram-positive rods			
Diphtheroids	3	40	80
Lactobacilli	18	60	90
Gram-positive cocci			
Staphylococcus aureus	0	2	25
Staphylococcus epidermidis	5	50	95
Streptococcus species			
Alpha-hemolytic	8	20	38
Beta-hemolytic	3	15	22
Nonhemolytic	0	20	32
Group D	2	28	45
Gram-negative rods			
Escherichia coli	3	18	33
Klebsiella and Enterobacter species	0	10	20
Proteus species	0	5	10
Pseudomonas species	0	0.1	3

Source: From Larson (1994).

most common factors are the loss of mucosal integrity, blood alteration of local pH, and mechanical compromise of endocervical mucus. Virulence is constitutive to a given pathogen. The number of organisms in the linear phase of growth determines the amount of enzyme, exotoxin, endotoxin, etc., available for disease production.

WHAT DISEASE HAS TAUGHT US

Studies of bacterial diseases within obstetrics and gynecology have demonstrated several key principles:

1. Monoetiological bacteria produce disease by numerical expansion.
2. Aerobic virulent bacteria can alter the disease spectrum by the recruitment of additional bacteria.
3. Anaerobic bacteria require a low oxidation–reduction potential to allow a single anaerobic bacteria to progress to abscess formation.
4. Anaerobic bacteria can utilize more aerophilic bacteria to collectively produce disease.
5. Changes within the locus of disease can cause autoelimination of inciting and/or contributing organisms.

Monoetiological Pathogens

Monoetiological bacteria are bacteria whose genetic virulence is capable of producing disease without intervention of other bacteria or significant alteration of oxidation–reduction potential. Both exogenous bacteria, i.e., group A streptococci, and endogenous bacteria, i.e., *E. coli*, can do so. What is required is a breach of anatomical barriers to bacterial invasion, such as parturition. In these situations, the bacteria attain access to a site in which no bacteria capable of their inhibition exist in large numbers.

Other monoetiological pathogens require a release from the inhibitory effects of the dominant bacteria locally functioning: the prime aerobic example is *Salmonella typhi*; and prime anaerobic bacteria, *Clostridium difficile*. In both

TABLE 2 Prevalence of anaerobic microorganisms present in cultures of cervical and vaginal specimens obtained from asymptomatic women (selected reports)

Organism	Percentage according to reference[a]				
	A	B	C	D	E
Bacteroides species					
B. bivius[b]	—	21	—	—	—
B. fragilis	17	4	40	12	16
B. melaninogenicus[c]	—	—	—	33	—
Other	40	—	18	46	—
Bifidobacterium species	10	—	—	2	2
Clostridium species					
C. perfringens	3	4	—	—	—
Other	13	2	—	—	—
Any	—	—	—	4	0
Eubacterium species	3	7	—	31	7
Fusobacterium species	—	7	28	13	—
Gaffkya species[d]	—	—	—	2	—
Lactobacillus species	—	10	—	46	52
Peptococcus species[e]					
P. asaccharolyticus	—	48	—	12	—
P. magnus	—	11	—	17	—
P. prevotii	—	17	—	21	—
Other	—	11	—	33	—
Any	7	—	64	65	8
Peptostreptococcus species					
P. anaerobius	—	34	—	15	—
P. intermedius	—	5	—	10	—
P. micros	—	7	—	8	—
P. productus	—	—	—	6	—
Any	33	—	76	35	15
Propionibacterium species	—	2	—	8	0
Veillonella species	27	11	6	4	0

Dashes signify that no specific information was available.
[a]A: Keith et al. (1972); B: DeBoer and Plantema (1988); C: Harris and Brown (1928); D: Thadepalli et al. (1982); E: Tashijian and Coulam (1976).
[b]Prevotella bivia. [c]Prevotella melaninogenicus. [d]Aercoccus species.
[e]Peptostreptococcus species.
Source: Adapted from Larsen and Monif (2001).

cases, antibiotics with a significant spectrum of efficacy for gram-positive anaerobic bacteria release the bacteria from their local inhibitory restraints. Once passed threshold levels of replication, the resultant numerical increase in organisms produces acute disease and exotoxin production respectively.

Synergistic Coupling

Within obstetrical and gynecological bacterial infections, the best example of synergistic coupling is progressive synergistic bacterial gangrene, in which *S. aureus* combines with a microaerophilic streptococcus to produce a disease that neither organism can cause independently.

Immediate Anaerobic Syndrome

Contamination of a hematoma with a single class III anaerobic bacteria and its subsequent conversion into an abscess is the classical example of the immediate anaerobic syndrome. This syndrome occurs when a low oxidation–reduction potential is combined with a bacteria capable of successful replication under such conditions.

The Anaerobic Progression

The anaerobic progression occurs when the environment with a contiguous bacterial flora lowers its oxidation–reduction potential, but does not lower it sufficiently to permit the immediate anaerobic syndrome. Initial replication by aerobic/microaerophilic bacteria within the contiguous flora further lowers the oxidation–reduction potential. In so doing, they promote the growth of more anaerobic bacteria, which, in turn, begin the process of autoelimination of the governing bacteria. Within the anaerobic progression, both selective recruitment and autoelimination occur. The classical example of anaerobic progression is gonococcal salpingitis, in which *N. gonorrhoeae* initiates the first phase of disease and then recruits mixed aerobic/anaerobic bacteria, which results in tissue damage as well as ultimate elimination of *N. gonorrhoeae*. In a sense, the anaerobic progression cures the gonococcal infection, but usually at the price of tissue destruction.

MICROBIAL REGULATORS OF VAGINAL BACTERIAL FLORA

Bacteria reside within the female genital tract by virtue of systems of checks and balances. Anything which disturbs a governing component has the potential to realign the distribution and quantitative distribution of the bacteria present.

Bacteria have the ability to inhibit one another. They do so through the elaboration of a number of antimicrobial byproducts, i.e., bacteriocins, hydrogen peroxide, hemolysins, etc. The effectiveness of the resultant inhibitory substance is a function of bacterial susceptibility to it, its potency, and the number of producing organisms.

Only two bacteria, *Lactobacillus* species and *G. vaginalis*, have been shown to be recoverable as the sole isolate from the female genital tract. What is implied by this fact is that they can individually function as ultimate regulators of the bacterial flora of the female genital tract. The term applied to the ability of one bacterium to suppress the replication of another is called "bacterial interference." The in vitro studies of Chaisilwattana and Monif (1995) have documented the ability of *Lactobacillus* species to inhibit *G. vaginalis*, and conversely, the ability of *G. vaginalis* to inhibit *Lactobacillus* species. The quantitative relationship between these two bacteria is the key to which will govern the bacterial flora. The ability of each to impose bacterial interference on the other when present in high multiplicity has been shown in clinical studies. Carson et al. (1997) identified *Lactobacillus* species in 131 cultures of vaginal specimens. *G. vaginalis* was recovered as a coisolate in only seven cases. In six of the seven cases, the multiplicity of coisolates implied that both organisms existed in low multiplicity within the anaerobic progression. In women with bacterial vaginosis in which *G. vaginalis* isolates predominated at high multiplicity, aerobic *Lactobacillus* species were never isolated.

The absence of aerobic *Lactobacillus* species is a risk marker for an abnormal bacterial flora. A microbiological environment can supersede virulence in the production of disease. For disease to occur, exogenous and endogenous bacteria must possess pathogenic prerequisites and attain replication dominance. Their ability to do so is largely governed by inhibitory or synergistic interrelationships with other bacteria.

SELECTED READING

Bartlett JG, Moon NE, Goldstein PR, et al. Cervical and vaginal bacterial flora: ecologic niches in the female lower genital tract. Am J Obstet Gynecol 1978; 130:658.

Bartlett JG, Onderdonk AB, Drude E, et al. Quantitative bacteriology of the vaginal flora. J Infect Dis 1977; 136:271.

Carson HM, LaPoint PG, Monif GRG. Interrelationships within the bacterial flora of the female genital tract. Infect Dis Obstet Gynecol 1997; 5:305.

Chaisilwattana P, Monif GRG. In vitro ability of the group B streptococci to inhibit gram-positive and gram-variable constituents of the bacterial flora of the female genital tract. Infect Dis Obstet Gynecol 1995; 3:91.

DeBoer JM, Plantema FHF. Ultrastructure of in situ adherence of Mobiluncus to vaginal epithelial cells. Can J Microbiol 1988; 34:757.

De Klerk HC, Cortez JM. Antibiosis among lactobacilli. Nature 1961; 192:340.

Gopplerud CP, Ohm MJ, Galask RP. Anaerobic and aerobic flora of the cervix during pregnancy and the puerperium. Am J Obstet Gynecol 1976; 126:858.

Gorbach SL. Probiotics and gastrointestinal health. Am J Gastroenterol 2000; 95(suppl):S2.

Gorbach SL, Menda KB, Thadepalli H, Keith L. Anaerobic microflora of the cervix of healthy women. Am J Obstet Gynecol 1973; 117:1053.

Harris JW, Brown JH. The bacterial content of the vagina and uterus on the fifth day of the normal puerperium. Bull Johns Hopkins Hosp 1928; 43:190.

Hillier SL, Krohn MA, Rabe LK, et al. The normal flora, H_2O_2 producing lactobacilli, and bacterial vaginosis in pregnant women. Clin Infect Dis 1993; 16(suppl 4):S273.

Holmes KK, Chen KC, Lipinski CM, et al. Vaginal redox potential in bacterial vaginosis (nonspecific vaginitis). J Infect Dis 1985; 152:379.

Keith LG, England D, Barizal F, et al. Microbial flora of the external os of premenopausal cervix. Br J Vener Dis 1972; 48:51.

Larsen B, Galask R. Vaginal microbial flora: composition and influence of host physiology. Ann Intern Med 1982; 96:926.

Larsen B. Microbiology of the female genital tract. In: Pastorck J, ed. Obstetric and Gynecologic Infectious Disease. New York: Raven Press, 1994:11–25.

Larsen B, Monif GRG. Understanding the bacterial flora of the female genital tract. Clin Infect Dis 2001; 32:e69.

Larsen B, Markovetz AJ, Galask RP. Quantitative alterations of the genital microflora of female rats in relation to the estrous cycle. J Infect Dis 1976; 134:486.

Levison ME, Corman LC, Carrington ER, et al. Quantitative microflora of the vagina. Am J Obstet Gynecol 1977; 127:80.

Monif GRG. Semiquantitative bacterial observations with group B streptococcal vulvovaginitis. Infect Dis Obstet Gynecol 1999; 7:227.

Monif GRG, Jordan PA, Thompson JL, et al. Quantitative and qualitative effects of Betadine liquid on the aerobic and anaerobic flora of the female genital tract. Am J Obstet Gynecol 1980; 137:432.

Monif GR, Welkos SL, Baer H. Impact of diverging anaerobic technology on cul-de-sac isolates from patients with endometritis/ salpingitis/peritonitis. Am J Obstet Gynecol 1982; 124:896.

Ohm JM, Galask RP. Bacterial flora of the cervix from 100 prehysterectomy patients. Am J Obstet Gynecol 1975; 122:683.

Pasteur L, Joubert JF. Charbon et septicemic. CRSoc Bio Paris 1877; 85:101.

Redondo-Lopez V, Cook RL, Sobel JD. Emergence of lactobacilli in the control and maintenance of the vaginal bacterial microflora. Rev Infect Dis 1990; 12:856.

Reves R. The bacteriocins. Bacteriol Rev 1965; 29:25.

Roy S, Sharma M, Ayyagari A, Malhotra S. A quantitative study of bacterial vaginosis. Indian J Med Res 1994; 100:172.

Savage DC. Microbial interference between indigenous coisolates yeast and lactobacilli in rodent stomach. J Bacteriol 1969; 98:1278.

Shubair M, Synder IS, Larsen B. Gardnerella vaginalis hemolysin. III. Effects on human leukocytes. Immunol Infect Dis 1993; 3:149.

Tashijian JH, Coulam CB, Washington JA. Vaginal flora in asymptomatic women. Mayo Clin Proc 1976; 51:557.

Thadepalli H, Savage EW Jr, Salem FA. Cyclic changes in cervical microflora and their effect on infections following hysterectomy. Gynecol Obstet Invest 1982; 14:176.

Immunological Defense Mechanisms in the Female Genital Tract

2

Steven S. Witkin

INTRODUCTION

The lower portion of the female genital tract is exposed to numerous microorganisms due to environmental contact, contamination from the rectum and fingers, sexual activity, soiled underclothing, etc. In addition, colonization of the vagina by potentially pathogenic microorganisms is universal. Immune defense mechanisms have evolved to protect women from developing clinical infections as a result of this microbial onslaught. Until recently, studies of female genital tract immunity were limited for the most part to a description of antibody concentrations and isotypes. In the past several years, however, spurred in part by the need to understand factors involved in the heterosexual transmission of the HIV virus, there has been a concerted interest in other female genital tract immune defense mechanisms. The participation of female genital tract epithelial cells in immune defense has also been verified.

The immune system can be subdivided into innate and acquired immunity. Innate immunity is rapid, nonspecific and involves a very limited number of genes (probably <100). It is the initial response to infection and alerts the acquired immune system to the need for initiating a pathogen-specific antibody and/or a cell-mediated immune response. Acquired immunity, in contrast, takes several days to develop, is induced in response to a specific microbe, and recognizes only that microorganism and involves a great number of genes (~10^{15}).

INNATE IMMUNITY

A major component of the innate immune system are the Toll-like receptors (TLRs) present on the surface or endosomal membrane of antigen-presenting cells such as macrophages and dendritic cells as well as epithelial cells and trophoblastic. First identified in *Drosophila* and later in mammals including humans, the TLRs recognize specific molecules on microbial pathogens called pathogens-associated molecular patterns. For example, TLR2 recognizes yeast zymosan, and in combination with TLR1 recognizes triacyl lipopeptides; TLR2-TLR6 heterodimers bind diacyl lipopeptides. TLR3 recognizes double-stranded viral RNA. TLR4 recognizes lipopolysaccharide from gram-negative bacteria, TLR5 recognizes bacterial flagellen, TLR7 and TLR8 recognize viral components and TLR9 recognizes a unique dinucleotide sequence, unmethylated CpG, only present in bacterial DNA. The binding of a specific microbial component to a TLR activates the intracellular pathway, leading to the transcription of proinflammatory cytokines, activation of phagocytic cells, and the triggering of cell-mediated immunity.

An additional mechanism of innate immune system activation of adaptive immunity is provided by the heat shock proteins. Heat shock proteins, also first identified in *Drosophila*, were so named because their intracellular concentration greatly increased the when cells were exposed to elevated temperatures. It later became apparent that any cellular stress, including exposure to infectious agents, resulted in a rapid activation of several heat shock protein genes. According to the so-called "danger hypothesis," the release of heat shock proteins from damaged stressed cells is the initial signal to the immune system that danger is present and immune activation is required. Several different heat shock proteins bind to receptors on antigen-presenting cells, triggering their maturation and the release of proinflammatory cytokines that activate T- and B-lymphocytes. One member of the heat shock protein family, the inducible 70 kDa heat shock protein, has also been shown to directly activate the complement system. This provides another antigen-nonspecific mechanism of combating microbial invaders. Activated complement components are capable of lysing bacterial cells and, by depositing complement component C3 on the bacterial surface, marking these cells for ingestion by phagocytic cells that contain cell surface C3 receptors.

Antimicrobial peptides are also components of innate immunity. They are expressed by phagocytic and epithelial cells and are capable of disrupting the cell membranes of a broad spectrum of gram-positive and gram-negative bacteria, fungi, and enveloped viruses. Under physiological conditions, these peptides have a cationic charge and so bind to anionic moieties on the microbial surface. The most widely studied antimicrobial peptides are the defensins alpha as beta. Additional antimicrobial peptides in humans include cathelicidins, bactericidal/permeability-increasing protein, histatins, lipophilins, and natural killer lysine.

Another innate inhibitor of viruses, bacteria, and fungi is called secretory leukocyte protease inhibitor (SLPI). This protein is a serine protease inhibitor produced by epithelial cells and is present in many body secretions. A recent study has suggested that SLPI blocks the binding of HIV to target cells, thereby inhibiting its transmission.

An innate immune system component that is active in defense against microbial infection and has received much research attention lately is mannose-binding lectin (MBL).

MBL is a plasma protein and a member of the collectin protein family. MBL is defined as a pattern-recognition molecule since it recognizes and binds to mannose, N-acetyl-glucosamine, and fucose-rich carbohydrate patterns on the surface of bacteria, fungi, and viruses. Importantly, MBL does not bind to carbohydrate moieties present in human glycoproteins. Subsequent to MBL binding to a microbial surface, the complement system is activated, and complement components are deposited on the surface of the affected microorganism. This makes the microbe susceptible to opsonization by complement receptor-bearing phagocytic cells. Binding and opsonization of MBL-bound microbes also occur by binding to collectin receptors on macrophages. Additionally, complement activation can also lead directly to microbe killing by the creation of holes in the microbial cell wall. A decreased concentration of circulating MBL in some individuals is due to single nucleotide genetic polymorphisms in the MBL gene, located on chromosome 10. These variations interfere with effective aggregation of the MBL polypeptide chains, resulting in a complex having reduced activity and stability.

ACQUIRED IMMUNITY

In contrast to innate immunity, which is a generalized and nonspecific immune response to infection, acquired immunity is specific for the particular pathogen that is present. Briefly, antigen-presenting cells such as macrophages and dendritic cells engulf the pathogen or pathogen components and break them down into small peptides. The peptides then associate with molecules belonging to either class 1 or class 2 of the major histocompatibility complex (MHC), and the peptide–MHC complexes are transported to the cell surface. T-helper lymphocytes as well as B-lymphocytes have receptors that recognize peptide–MHC complexes on antigen-presenting cells. When a single T-cell binds to the microbial peptide–MHC complex, the cell "learns" to recognize that specific microbial antigen. The activated T-cell than releases the cytokine interleukin (IL)-2, which initiates its rapid multiplication, resulting in a population of antigen-specific cells. The T-cells activate B-lymphocytes, which then also bind to processed antigens. The resulting proliferation of these antigen-specific B-cells results in the formation of an antibody-producing army with specificity for this one microbial antigen. The T-cells also release interferon gamma (IFN-gamma), which activates phagocytic cells to more effectively engulf and process microbes and so create additional T- and B-cells with specificity for other microbial antigens. The net result is the formation of so-called memory T- and B-cells capable of activating an antibody or cell-mediated immune response whenever in the future that specific microbial antigen is recognized.

VAGINAL EPITHELIAL CELLS AND INNATE IMMUNE DEFENSE MECHANISMS

It has become increasingly clear that epithelial cells in the vagina contribute to the local immune defense against microbial pathogens. The vaginal mucosa does not contain many immunocompetent cells, and so the vaginal epithelium is the first line of defense against exogenous microbial pathogens. Vaginal epithelial cells, as well as epithelial cells in the ectocervix and endocervix, have recently been shown to express several TLRs: TLR1, TLR2, TLR3, TLR5, and TLR6. TLR4 is absent from the vagina and ectocervix but has been identified in the endocervix. The capacity of TLRs to recognize the presence of diverse microbial pathogens bestows on the vaginal epithelium the function of sentinel. A microbial invader binds to the TLRs and triggers the epithelial cells to synthesize and release proinflammatory cytokines. This, in turn, summons and activates cells of the acquired immune system to mount a specific immune attack. The cytokines IL-1, IL-6, IL-8, IL-10, IL-12, tumor necrosis factor alpha (TNF-alpha), and macrophage colony stimulating factor have all been detected in vaginal fluids and/or in vaginal epithelial cell culture supernatants. In addition, IFN-gamma and TNF-alpha have been shown to induce the expression of MHC class 2 antigens on vaginal and cervical epithelial cells in vitro. This converts these cells into antigen-presenting cells, enabling them to present microbial antigens for recognition by T-lymphocytes.

SLPI has been identified in the female genital tract and is produced by epithelial cells in the vagina. The ability of SLPI to inhibit microbial growth has already been mentioned. Women with lower genital tract infections such as Trichomonas vaginalis, Neisseria gonorrhoeae, Chlamydia trachomatis, and Candida albicans and with disturbed vaginal flora characteristic of bacterial vaginosis have reduced levels of SLPI in the vagina. Microbe-produced proteases probably degrade SLPI and, thereby, aid the proliferation of these microorganisms. It has been hypothesized that one mechanism whereby vaginal infections function as cofactors for the sexual transmission of HIV is by degradation of SLPI, an inhibitor of HIV binding to target cells.

At least three antimicrobial peptides, beta-defensin-1, intestinal defensin-5, and cathelicidin, have been shown to be expressed by the vaginal epithelial cells. Beta-defensin-1 levels are highest in pregnant women, indicating a hormonal influence on its expression. Similarly, defensin-5 reaches its highest concentration in the vagina during the secretory phase of the menstrual cycle. Synthesis of both defensin-5 and cathelicidin are upregulated by proinflammatory cytokines, suggesting their role in combating infection in the vagina.

The expression of bactericidal/permeability-increasing proteins on the surface of epithelial cells in the ecto- and endocervix has recently been demonstrated, suggesting that this innate immune component may aid in the regulation of bacterial colonization of the genital tract mucosal tissue.

MBL has been identified in vaginal secretions, and a decrease in vaginal concentrations has been associated with susceptibility to recurrent vulvovaginal candidiasis (see below).

Additional components of innate defense produced by vaginal epithelial cells include the antimicrobial compounds lactoferrin and lysozyme.

ANTIBODY PRODUCTION IN THE FEMALE GENITAL TRACT

The female genital tract is a component of the mucosal immune system, which is distinct from systemic circulating immunity. Most of the antibodies present in the female genital tract are produced locally and differ in specificity from antibodies present in the blood. Thus, it is possible for a woman to have antibodies to a genital pathogen in her cervico–vaginal secretions while these antibodies are absent from her serum. This point has clinical implications for antibody testing. For example, in women undergoing in vitro fertilization (IVF), the presence of antibodies to *C. trachomatis* in cervico–vaginal fluids correlates with a poor IVF outcome. In contrast, there is no relation between circulating antichlamydial antibodies and IVF success.

Most of the antibody-producing cells in the female genital tract are located in the endocervix, although antibody-producing cells have also been identified in the ectocervix and the vagina. Polymeric secretory immunoglobulin A (IgA) is the major immunoglobulin produced within the genital tract. IgG antibodies are also present in genital tract secretions and probably consist of a mixture of locally produced antibodies and systemic antibodies that enter the genital tract by transduction in the vagina and the uterus. The concentrations of antibodies produced in the cervix vary throughout the menstrual cycle. Antibody levels are highest during menstruation and lowest during the periovulatory period.

A major question that has been brought into sharp focus by the AIDS epidemic is how to optimally induce local female genital tract immunity as distinct from systemic immunity. Surprisingly, it has recently been demonstrated that the induction of immunity within the nasal cavity appears to be the most effective means for inducing long-lasting immunity in the female genital tract to a wide variety of antigens. By mechanisms still to be delineated, activated antigen-presenting cells and T- and B-lymphocytes in the nasal mucosa apparently preferentially migrate to the mucosa of the female genital tract.

RECURRENT VULVOVAGINAL CANDIDIASIS: AN IMMUNE DISORDER

In most women, the presence of *C. albicans* in the vagina leads to the release of cytokines that activate phagocytic cells to engulf and destroy this microorganism. In addition, production of IFN-gamma inhibits the yeast form of *C. albicans* from germinating into the invasive fungal phenotype. Thus, the immune response to *C. albicans* prevents its proliferation to levels capable of causing clinical symptoms. It can be readily appreciated that interference with proinflammatory cytokine production would leave the individual highly susceptible to developing a clinical *C. albicans* infection, provided of course that subclinical levels of this microorganism are already present. This is precisely what occurs in many women suffering from recurrent vulvovaginal candidiasis.

One mechanism leading to the inhibition of proinflammatory cytokine production is an allergic (immediate hypersensitivity) response. If a woman is allergic to a compound (allergen), she has IgE antibodies that are bound to the surface of basophils and mast cells that recognize this specific allergen. When exposure to the allergen occurs, the allergen binds to these IgE antibodies, triggering the basophils and mast cells to release histamine as well as other inflammatory mediators. The histamine induces macrophages to release high concentrations of prostaglandin E_2 (PGE_2), which inhibits the release of proinflammatory cytokines and blocks phagocytic cell activation. Furthermore, other cytokines, notably IL-4, IL-5, IL-6, and IL-10, are induced under these conditions, which stimulate further production of IgE antibodies.

The induction of allergic responses in the human vagina has been amply demonstrated. Allergens shown to induce a vaginal allergic response include seminal fluid constituents, *C. albicans*, environmental allergens such as rye grass and pollen, and components of contraceptive spermicides or antifungal medications. The seminal fluid allergen in some cases is an intrinsic component present in all seminal fluids. In other cases, it might be an allergen unique to one particular seminal fluid: a medication or food ingested by the male and present in the ejaculate. It is also possible for a male with a genital allergy to transmit both IgE antibodies and allergen to the female during sexual intercourse, resulting in induction of a vaginal allergic response in a nonallergic woman.

C. albicans has several unique properties that enable it to take advantage of localized allergic reactions. This microorganism is able to synergize with histamine to greatly increase the concentration of PGE_2 released by macrophages. Furthermore, PGE_2 stimulates the yeast to hyphae morphogenetic transition of *C. albicans*, increasing its pathogenicity. Recent studies have demonstrated that *C. albicans* possesses an immunosuppressive PGE_2-like molecule that also induces hyphae formation.

C. albicans is present in the vagina of about 20% of women as a commensal microorganism. If a vaginal allergic reaction occurs in a woman harboring this microorganism, the resulting localized immune responses will allow the *Candida* to proliferate and to undergo a transition to the hyphae form. This will result in the clinical symptoms characteristic of vulvovaginal candidiasis. Subsequent antifungal antibiotic treatment will most likely result in an alleviation of symptoms. However, since all current antifungal drugs are fungistatic and not fungicidal, low levels of *Candida* will remain in the vagina. This will leave the woman susceptible to recurrent vulvovaginal *Candidal* infections upon subsequent exposures to an allergen to which she is sensitized. It has been demonstrated using the highly sensitive polymerase chain reaction that women with a history of recurrent vulvovaginal candidiasis harbor *C. albicans* in their vagina even at times when they are free of symptoms. Furthermore, heat shock proteins are present in their vaginal fluids, indicating a persistent perturbation of the vaginal environment of women susceptible to recurrent vulvovaginal infections.

Given that a vaginal allergy renders a woman susceptible to vulvovaginal candidiasis, it seems clear that treatments aimed at alleviating the underlying immune predisposition may be beneficial to ending the cycle of recurrences. Unfortunately, at present, there is no clearly defined treatment that is universally effective. Limited published studies as well as anecdotal evidence suggest several potential protocols that seem to be effective in a variable percentage of patients. If the offending allergen can be identified, then avoidance of exposure usually results in elimination of recurrent symptoms. This may involve the use of a condom in cases of seminal fluid allergy or changes in locally applied contraceptives or medications. In cases of allergic reactions to seminal fluid or to *C. albicans*, successful systemic desensitization has been reported in limited studies. Other treatments have involved blocking the allergic reaction at various stages: use of a mast cell stabilizer (cromolyn sodium) to inhibit histamine release, antihistamines to inhibit histamine binding to lymphoid cells, prostaglandin synthesis inhibitors to interfere with PGE_2 production, etc.

The innate immune system component implicated as a major contributor to anti-*Candida* defense in the genital tract is MBL. Recent analyses of women with a polymorphism in the gene coding for MBL demonstrated a clear association between the variant genotype, greatly reduced MBL vaginal concentrations, and an increased incidence of recurrent vulvovaginal candidiasis. Thus, a genetic alteration in a component of vaginal innate immunity readily influences a woman's susceptibility to infection.

EFFECT OF SEXUAL INTERCOURSE ON VAGINAL IMMUNITY

Spermatozoa are viewed as foreign by the female immune system. Therefore, in order to preserve fertility, mechanisms have evolved to prevent women from developing antisperm immunity. Human seminal fluid has the highest concentration of PGE_2 of any body fluid, and so semen is highly immunosuppressive. In addition, human seminal fluid is a potent inducer of IL-10, an inhibitor of cell-mediated immunity.

While preventing induction of immunity to spermatozoa, the immunosuppressive properties of seminal fluid may aid in the proliferation of pathogens in the vagina. If *C. albicans* is present in the vagina of a woman who then engages in sexual intercourse, the deposition of semen will result in conditions favoring *Candida* proliferation and germination. Similarly, the female's immune response to microorganisms present in the male ejaculate may be inhibited by seminal fluid. Semen-induced immunosuppression may also explain the observation that while antibiotic treatment of male partners does not reduce the incidence of bacterial vaginosis, sexual activity is an established risk factor for this condition.

SELECTED READING

Akira S, Takeda K, Kaisho T. Toll-like receptors: critical proteins linking innate and acquired immunity. Nat Immunol 2001; 2:675–680.

Babovic-Vuksanovic D, Snow K, Ten RM. Mannose-binding lectin (MBL) deficiency. Variant alleles in a midwestern population of the United States. Ann Allergy Asthma Immunol 1999; 82:134–138.

Babula O, Lazdane G, Kroica J, et al. Relation between recurrent vulvovaginal candidiasis, vaginal concentrations of mannose-binding lectin, and a mannose-binding lectin gene polymorphism in Latvian women. Clin Infect Dis 2003; 37:733–737.

Breloer M, Dorner B, More SH, et al. Heat shock proteins as danger signals: eukaryotic Hsp60 enhances and accelerates antigen-specific IFN-gamma production in T cells. Eur J Immunol 2001; 31:2051–2059.

Canny GO, Trifonova RT, Kindelberger DW, et al. Expression and function of bactericidal/permeability-increasing protein in human genital tract epithelial cells. J Infect Dis 2006; 194:498–502.

Cole AM, Ganz T. Human antimicrobial peptides: analysis and application. BioTechniques 2000; 29:822–831.

Draper DL, Landers DV, Krohn MA, et al. Levels of vaginal secretory leukocyte protease inhibitor are decreased in women with lower reproductive tract infections. Am J Obstet Gynecol 2000; 183:1243–1248.

Fazeli A, Bruce C, Anumba DO. Characterization of Toll-like receptors in the female reproductive tract in humans. Human Reprod 2005; 20:1372–1378.

Fichorova RN, Anderson DJ. Differential expression of immunobiological mediators by immortalized human cervical and vaginal epithelial cells. Biol Reprod 1999; 60:508–514.

Giraldo PC, Babula O, Goncalves AK, et al. Mannose-binding lectin gene polymorphism, vulvovaginal candidiasis, and bacterial vaginosis. Obstet Gynecol 2007; 109:1123–1128.

Hancock REW. Cationic peptides: effectors in innate immunity and novel antimicrobials. Lancet 2001; 1:156–164.

Janeway CA Jr, Medzhitov R. Innate immune recognition. Annu Rev Immunol 2002; 20:197–216.

Jeremias J, Mockel S, Witkin SS. Human semen induces interleukin 10 and 70 kDa heat shock protein gene transcription and inhibits interferon-gamma messenger RNA production in peripheral blood mononuclear cells. Mol Hum Reprod 1998; 4:1084–1088.

Kozlowski PA, Williams SB, Lynch RM, et al. Differential induction of mucosal and systemic antibody responses in women after nasal, rectal or vaginal immunization: influence of the menstrual cycle. J Immunol 2002; 169:566–574.

Krieg AM. CpG motifs in bacterial DNA and their immune effects. Annu Rev Immunol 2002; 20:709–760.

Mestecky J, Russell MW. Induction of mucosal immune responses in the human genital tract. FEMS Immunol Medical Microbiol 2000; 27:351–355.

Quayle AJ, Porter EM, Nussbaum AA, et al. Gene expression, immunolocalization, and secretion of human defensins-5 in human female reproductive tract. Am J Pathol 1998; 152:1247–1258.

Wallin RPA, Lundqvist A, More S, et al. Heat-shock proteins as activators of the innate immune system. Trends Immunol 2002; 23:130–135.

Anaerobic Infections

3

INTRODUCTION

Understanding the events that combine to produce polymicrobial anaerobic infection is critical to effective antibiotic selection in obstetrics and gynecology. Polymicrobial infection usually requires polydrug antibiotic regimens.

CLASSIFICATION

Pasteur was the first investigator to demonstrate that microbial metabolism was possible in the absence of air. In 1857, he classified anaerobic bacteria into two groups. The first group he termed "facultative anaerobes," which he defined as bacterial organisms that could grow either with or without air. The second group were designated "obligatory anaerobes." These were bacteria whose growth and viability were irreversibly impaired by air.

Approximately 146 technologic years later, we have not radically altered these basic concepts. The current classification scheme divides bacteria into three classes as shown in Table 1.

Each of these classification schemata is valid only in reference to the time of collection. For example, a strain of *Bacteroides fragilis* isolated from an ovarian abscess six weeks after vaginal hysterectomy will be a Class 3 extremely oxygen sensitive (EOS) organism; however, when recruited from the vaginal flora, it existed as a microaerophilic Class 2 bacteria. Under the environmental selection engendered by disease, the strain becomes a Class 3 (EOS) bacteria. Any breach of anaerobic technique at the time of collection or in the subsequent handling of the specimen would result in loss of the organism. However, once propagated in vitro under strict anaerobic conditions, the strain of *B. fragilis* will regain its original oxygen tolerance and can be handled outside the anaerobic glove box without impairment of viability for up to four to six hours.

SOURCE OF THE BACTERIA

When anaerobic disease occurs, it is primarily due to bacteria derived from the patient's own microbiologic environment. Anaerobic bacteria constitute a significant component of the endogenous flora of our skin and most mucous membranes. In this context, humans are their own reservoir of potentially pathogenic anaerobic bacteria.

PATHOGENESIS

The Anaerobic Progression

In the majority of instances in obstetrics and gynecology, anaerobic disease has its genesis in multiple bacteria whose abilities to replicate at different oxygen levels vary significantly. The catalytic event that takes an endogenous bacterial flora and gives it pathogenicity is an alteration in the oxidation–reduction potential of the microbiological environment. Normal healthy tissue has an oxidation–reduction potential of approximately $+150\,mV$. Iatrogenic lowering of the oxidation–reduction potential often occurs during an operation, when tissue is crushed by clamps, devitalized by loss of blood supply, and/or subjected to microhematoma formation or the development of serous fluid collection.

A given disease can similarly lower the oxidation–reduction potential and thus initiate the anaerobic progression. With the lowering of the oxidation–reduction potential, acidification of the local environment and removal of molecular oxygen, the polymicrobial flora of disease undergoes selective changes. The more aerobic bacteria (which cannot replicate under these progressively adverse conditions) undergo a process of sequential auto-elimination. This process is termed the anaerobic progression (Fig. 1). Abscess formation is the ultimate culmination of the anaerobic progression. From well-developed abscess material, usually only a single genus of bacteria is isolated.

The Immediate Anaerobic Syndrome

The anaerobic progression is the major but not sole pathway to anaerobic disease. The appropriate oxidation–reduction potential can be combined with the right bacterium or bacteria to produce anaerobic infection, i.e., a hematoma contaminated with a major Class 2 anaerobe or iatrogenic or spontaneous penetration of the gastrointestinal tract. In these instances, there is no need for alteration of the microbiological environment to initiate the disease process since it already is present (e.g., feces has the lowest oxidation–reduction potential recognized, $-200\,mV$, and the gastrointestinal anaerobic flora has a 100-fold dominance over its Class I counterpart).

DIAGNOSIS

The diagnosis of polymicrobial (aerobic–anaerobic) disease is usually inferred from the clinical situation. The clinical setting

TABLE I Classification of anaerobic bacteria

Class 1: Bacteria that grow better in the presence of air than in its absence

Class 2: Bacteria that are unable to initiate growth unless the oxidation–reduction potential of the medium is low (the exception being when they are inoculated in large numbers)

Class 3: Bacteria that perish on even transient contact with atmospheric oxygen: EOS (extremely oxygen sensitive) bacteria. These organisms are incapable of surface replication at oxygen concentrations of 0.5%

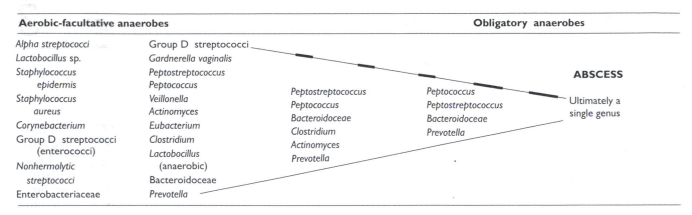

FIGURE 1 The anaerobic progression.

in which disease occurs dictates the presumptive diagnosis (Tables 2 and 3). For example, postpartum endometritis following cesarean section may be due to a monoetiological agent such as the group A beta-hemolytic streptococci; however, in the majority of instances, disease has its genesis in the anaerobic process. Some of the clinical clues that should suggest advanced anaerobic infection include the following:

1. Presence of foul-smelling discharge
2. Failure to achieve the anticipated therapeutic response with the combination of a penicillin and an aminoglycoside in the absence of a surgically amenable focus of infection
3. Failure of bacteria visualized on gram stain to grow from purulent material
4. The development of septic thrombophlebitis

Clinically, the most useful clue is foul-smelling discharge. The odor is caused by the cleavage of –SH groups from amino acids, which occurs only under strict anaerobic conditions. More advanced disease (abscess formation) of the immediate anaerobic syndrome is usually clinically evident.

Specimen Selection
It is very important to avoid contamination of the diagnostic specimen by bacteria inherently present on skin and mucous membranes. Since the anaerobes causing anaerobic disease are derived from the endogenous bacterial flora, it is pointless to collect specimens from a site that requires the sampling vehicle to have contact with an area that has an endogenous bacterial flora.

TABLE 2 Clinical situations commonly associated with polymicrobial infections

Obstetrics	Gynecology
Septic abortion	Pelvic cellulitis
Infected ectopic pregnancy	Cuff abscess or cellulitis
Retained products of conception	Ruptured tubo-ovarian abscess
Post-cesarean section endomyometritis	Postoperative abdominal wound infections
Postpartum endometritis associated with obstetrical trauma	

Specimen Collection
Good anaerobic bacteriology is time consuming and expensive. Therefore, it is important that only specimens that have been appropriately selected and properly collected be submitted for anaerobic culture. A bad specimen will not only give useless or misleading results, it will also prevent the laboratory personnel from devoting sufficient attention to valid specimens.

An appropriate culture for anaerobic progression is normally obtained by aspiration with a needle and syringe. Great care must be taken to exclude air. Even transient contact with molecular oxygen is as lethal as an autoclave for Class 3 anaerobes. In selected instances, e.g., ruptured tubo-ovarian abscess or gangrenous wound infections, it is not possible to obtain a specimen for bacteriological analysis by aspiration. In these circumstances, a fragment of infected tissue constitutes a valid specimen. Any time a cotton swab (even one stored in a tube free of molecular oxygen) is exposed to room air in the course of obtaining a culture sample, the validity of the specimen becomes suspect. Of even greater concern is the necessity to sample an area with an inherent bacterial flora. The only reason to obtain bacteriological cultures in these circumstances is not to identify the constituents of the anaerobic progression but rather to exclude the presence of exogenous aerobic bacteria that may have epidemiological or nosocomial significance, i.e., *Neisseria gonorrhoeae*, group A streptococci, *Listeria monocytogenes*.

TABLE 3 Appropriate specimen for anaerobic cultures in obstetrics and gynecology

Specimen	Technique
Abscess (cuff, ovarian, tubo-ovarian, Bartholin's gland, etc.)	Aspiration
Peritonitis (pelvic inflammatory disease, uterine perforation, etc.)	Aspiration via culdocentesis
Buboes (lymphogranuloma venereum, etc.)	Direct aspiration
Septic abortion, ruptured tubo-ovarian abscess	Tissue
Deep wounds direct aspiration	Tissue

TABLE 4 Differential diagnosis of anaerobic bacteria from the abscess pus based on gram stain morphology

Coccus		*Bacillus*	
Gram-positive	**Gram-negative**	**Gram-positive**	**Gram-negative**
Peptostreptococci: (anaerobic streptococci) pairs and chains	*Veillonella:* pairs or clusters	*Clostridia:* large straight rods (boxcars)	*Bacteroides/Prevotella:* round ends
Peptococci: (anaerobic staphylococci) clusters		*Actinomyces:* filamentous growth	*Fusobacterium:* pointed end or filaments
			Eubacteria: slender rods
			Propionibacteria: (anaerobic corynebacteria) banding, beading, clubbing; V-Y arrangement; Chinese letters

Role of the Gram Stain

Next to the physician's ability to anticipate when the anaerobic progression is functioning, the most important diagnostic tool is the gram stain. When dealing with a well-established abscess, the ocular–cerebral reflex is almost as accurate as an anaerobic diagnostic facility. Whenever you take an anaerobic culture, make a gram stain (Table 4).

THERAPY—GAINESVILLE CLASSIFICATION

When confronted clinically with the anaerobic progression, in the majority of instances, antibiotic selection cannot be guided by bacteriological cultures. The problems with specimen collection, specimen handling, and a dynamic pathogenic flora (the anaerobic progression) are not readily addressed in diagnostic bacteriology laboratories. These problems have led to the creation of the Gainesville Classification. The Gainesville Classification subdivides the polymicrobial flora that function in the anaerobic progression into its first four categories.

The concept of *category designation* must be concurrently used. Category designation equates with the ability to eradicate >94% of the bacteria within that category.

The bulk of clinical isolates belongs to Category IA and IB of the Gainesville Classification (Table 5). Since the majority of the bacterial isolates are susceptible to penicillin and/or its semisynthetic analog, the earlier successes of obstetricians and gynecologists with such simple therapy as ampicillin alone or penicillin and an aminoglycoside is readily understandable.

The effectiveness of antimicrobial therapy for polymicrobial anaerobic disease is influenced by the prevailing oxidation–reduction potential. If the oxidation–reduction potential is not in a critical zone that will sustain the successful replication of pathogenic Class 2 anaerobic bacteria, the ongoing polymicrobial disease can be effectively aborted by the eradication of the majority of the dominant constituents, which are predominantly Class 1 anaerobes. However, once a critical oxidation–reduction potential is achieved, partial eradication of the bacteria present will not abort progression of disease. At this point, it becomes necessary to eradicate all existing anaerobic bacteria in Category IB and Category II.

SURGICAL INTERVENTION

How aggressive the clinician must be surgically is dictated in part by the clinician's understanding of the anaerobic progression and the immediate anaerobic syndrome. In dealing with potentially life-threatening disease, there will be isolated instances where, given a choice between all-encompassing antibiotic coverage and the Bard–Parker blade, one must pre-empt surgical intervention over medical therapy. Retained products of conception in association with thrombophlebitis, an ovarian abscess, and a ruptured tubo-ovarian abscess are examples of situations in which the adverse microbiological environment must be mechanically removed or disrupted to achieve a therapeutic cure. It cannot be stressed too strongly that where there is necrotic tissue or a significant abscess, rarely can a bacteriological cure be achieved with antibiotic therapy alone. However, once a surgically amenable focus of infection has been excluded, a commitment can be made to attaining a nonoperative medical cure.

ANTIBIOTIC SELECTION FOR POLYMICROBIAL ANAEROBIC DISEASE

When dealing with polymicrobial disease, the major therapeutic commitment must be to Categories I, II, and IV if the principal morbid sequelae (septicemia, septic thrombophlebitis, and abscess formation) are to be averted. Confronted with life-threatening polymicrobial disease, the antibiotic selection is that of triple therapy (classically penicillin or ampicillin, clindamycin or metronidazole, and an aminoglycoside) or its equivalent. Triple therapy gives you +++1/2 to ++++ in each category of the Gainesville Classification, thus creating "an antibiotic stone wall." When medical failures occur, they are due to a beta-lactamase, a clindamycin-resistant or aminoglycoside-resistant strain of *Staphylococcus aureus*, a clindamycin-resistant strain of *B. fragilis*, or a multiresistant *Enterobacteriaceae*. Being aerobic bacteria, *S. aureus* and the *Enterobacteriaceae* will be identified by conventional bacteriological cultures. The concept of triple therapy was designed to give obstetricians and gynecologists the ultimate ability to dissect out medically amenable disease from that requiring surgical intervention.

Early in the course of postoperative infectious complications, the clinician usually does not deal with life-threatening disease, but rather with the anaerobic

TABLE 5 Gainesville Classification

Anaerobic bacteria
 Category IB: Anaerobes for which penicillin is the drug of choice for highly effective therapy
 Category II: The nonpenicillin-sensitive anaerobic bacteria which includes most strains of *Bacteroides fragilis* and *Prevotella* spp. (bivia, disens)
Aerobic bacteria
 Category IA: The gram-positive aerobic bacteria
 Category III: The group D streptococci—specifically the enterococci
 Category IV: The gram-negative aerobic rods of the Enterobacteriaceae

progression. The effectiveness of antimicrobial therapy for polymicrobial disease is influenced by the existing oxidation–reduction potential. When that potential is not in a critical zone, anaerobic infection can be effectively dealt with by the eradication of the major constituent of the facilitating bacterial flora in the anaerobic progression. Once a critical oxidation–reduction potential is reached, partial eradication of the bacterial flora present will not abort disease. It becomes necessary to eradicate all bacterial constituents.

The majority of postoperative infectious complications should be treated aggressively with two-drug therapy, which effectively ($+++1/2$ to $++++$) covers two or more categories in the Gainesville Classification. Initial selection of the antimicrobial agents is often dictated by the disease entity per se. No matter what combination of drugs is used, the clinician must be cognizant of the gaps, in terms of the Gainesville Classification, of his or her antibiotic selection. If the anticipated therapeutic response does not develop in 24 to 36 hours, the antibiotics necessary to effectively cover the categorical gaps should be substituted.

SELECTED READING

Bartlett JG, Louis TJ, Gorbach SL, Onderdonk AB. Therapeutic efficacy of 29 antimicrobial regimens in experimental intra-abdominal sepsis. Rev Infect Dis 1981; 3:535.

Bartlett JG, Onderdonk AB, Drude E. Quantitative microbiology of the vaginal flora. J Infect Dis 1977; 136:271.

Brook I. Anaerobic bacteria in suppurative genitourinary infections. J Urol 1989; 141:889.

Carter B, Jones CP, Aleter RL. *Bacteroide* infections in obstetrics and gynecology. Obstet Gynecol 1953; 1:491.

Carter B, Jones CP, Ross RA, Thomas WL. A bacteriologic and clinical study of pyometra. Am J Obstet Gynecol 1951; 62:793.

Chow AW, Marshall JR, Guze LB. Anaerobic infections of the female genital tract: prospects and prospectives. Obstet Gynecol Surv 1975; 30:477.

Dasgupta RK, Rao RS, Rajaram P, Natarajan MK. Anaerobic infections in pregnant women undergoing caesarean section and associated risk factors. Asia Oceania J Obstet Gynaecol 1988; 14:437.

Engelkirk PG, Duben-Engelkirk, J, Dowell VR Jr. Principals and Practice of Clinical Anaerobic Bacteriology. Belmont, Calif: Star Publishing Co., 1992.

Finegold SM, George WL. Anaerobic Infections in Humans. San Diego, CA: Academic Press, Inc., 1989.

Finegold SM, Baron EJ, Wexler HM. A Clinical Guide to Anaerobic Infections. Belmont Calif.: Star Publishing Co., 1991.

Finegold SM, Jousimies-Somer HR, Wexler HM. Current perspectives on anaerobic infections: diagnostic approaches. In: Washington JA II, ed. Laboratory Diagnosis of Infectious Diseases, vol. 7. Infectious Disease Clinics of North America. Philadelphia: WB Saunders Co., 1993:257–275.

Gorbach SL, Bartlett JG. Anaerobic infections. N Engl J Med 1974; 190:1177.

Gorbach SL, Menda KB, Thadepalli H, Keith L. Anaerobic microflora of the cervix in healthy women. Am J Obstet Gynecol 1973; 117:1053.

Hall WL, Sobel AI, Jones CP, Parker RT. Anaerobic postoperative pelvic infections. Obstet Gynecol 1967; 80:1.

Holden J. Collection and transport of clinical specimens for anaerobic culture. In: Isenberg HD, ed. Clinical Microbiology Procedures Handbook. Washington, DC: American Society for Microbiology, 1992:2.2.1–2.2.7.

Holdeman LV, Cato EP, Moore WEC. Anaerobic Laboratory Manual, 4th ed. Blacksburg, VA: Virginia Polytechnic Institute and State University, 1977.

Kirby BD, George WL, Sutter VL, et al. Gram-negative anaerobic bacilli: their role in infection and patterns of susceptibility to antimicrobial agents. I. Little known Bacteroides species. Rev Infect Dis 1983; 5:876.

Ledger WJ. Postoperative pelvic infections. Clin Obstet Gynecol 1969; 12:265.

Ledger WJ. The surgical care of severe infections in obstetric and gynecologic patients. Surg Gynecol Obstet 1973; 136:753.

Ledger WJ. Selection of antimicrobial agents for treatment of infections of the female genital tract. Rev Infect Dis 1983; 5(suppl):98.

Ledger WJ, Normal M, Gee C, Lewis W. Bacteremia in an obstetric/gynecologic service. Am J Obstet Gynecol 1975; 121:205.

Marcoux JA, Zabransky RJ, Washington JA 2nd, et al. Bacteroides bacteremia: a review of 123 cases. Minn Med 1970; 53:1169.

Mason PR, Katzenstein DA, Chimbira TH, Mtimavalye L. Vaginal flora of women admitted to hospital with signs of sepsis following normal delivery, cesarean section or abortion. The Puerperal Sepsis Study Group. Cent Afr J Med 1989; 35:344.

Monif GRG. Anaerobic infections—Parts I and II. Infect Dis Ltrs Obstet Gynecol 1981; 3:31.

Monif GRG. The potential uses of metronidazole in obstetrics and gynecology. In: Finegold SM, ed. First United States Metronidazole Conference. Biomedical Inform Corp, 1983:219.

Monif GRG, Welkos SL. *Bacteroides fragilis* infection in obstetrics. Clin Obstet Gynecol 1976; 19:131.

Monif GRG, Clark P, Baer H, Shuster JE. Susceptibility of anaerobic bacteria and the group D streptococci to the semi-synthetic penicillins: carbenicillin, piperacillin and ticarcillin. Antimicrob Agents Chemother 1979; 14:543.

Pearson HE, Anderson GV. *Bacteroides* infections and pregnancy. Obstet Gynecol 1970; 35:21.

Pearson HE, Anderson GV. Perinatal deaths associated with bacteroides infections. Obstet Gynecol 1967; 30:486.

Snydman DR, Tally FP, Knuppel R, et al. *Bacteroides bivius* and *Bacteroides disiens* in obstetrical patients: clinical findings and antimicrobial susceptibilities. J Antimicrob Chemother 1980; 6:519.

Sweet RL. Anaerobic infections of the female genital tract. Am J Obstet Gynecol 1975; 122:891.

Swenson RM, Michaelson TC, Daly MJ, et al. Anaerobic bacterial infections of the female genital tract. Obstet Gynecol 1973; 42:538.

Thadepalli H, Gorbach SL, Keith L. Anaerobic infections of the female genital tract: bacteriologic and therapeutic aspects. Am J Obstet Gynecol 1973; 117:1034.

Weinstein WM, Onderdonk AB, Bartlett JG, Gorbach SL. Experimental intra-abdominal abscesses in rats: development of an experimental model. Infect Immun 1974; 10:1250.

Weinstein WM, Onderdonk AB, Bartlett JG, et al. Antimicrobial therapy of experimental intraabdominal sepsis. J Infect Dis 1975; 132:282.

Antibiotic Selection in Obstetrics and Gynecology

4

INTRODUCTION

Why Do the Ground Rules Covering Antibiotic Selection in Obstetrics and Gynecology Differ from Those of Internal Medicine?

The internist deals with infectious diseases that are primarily monoetiological: a single organism is responsible for a given set of symptoms. Although the obstetrician/gynecologist also deals with monoetiological disease, the pathogenic spectrum is often different. The principal infectious disease pattern in obstetrics and gynecology is one of polymicrobial infection in which microaerophilic and obligatory anaerobic bacteria frequently function. When the 10 most common bacterial pathogens for the internist and the obstetrician/gynecologist are compared, the degree of overlap is not significant. On the other hand, when bacterial isolates from the intravascular compartment are contrasted, the differences are obvious (Table 1).

Even when the two disciplines are dealing with the same genus of bacteria, the spectrum of disease may diverge significantly (e.g., the group A beta-hemolytic streptococci). In regard to the obstetrician/gynecologist, this means post-IUD-insertion endometritis, postpartum endometritis/peritonitis (puerperal sepsis), or Meleny type I ulcer (necrotizing fasciitis). These are not the typical clinical presentations of the group A beta-hemolytic streptococci for the internist. Nevertheless, the basic ground rules for both disciplines are the same (Table 2).

The dominant cleavage factor between internal medicine and obstetrics and gynecology is the prevalence of polymicrobial infection and the potential for participation by the penicillin-resistant *Bacteroides* and *Prevotella* species.

ANTIBIOTIC SELECTION FOR MONOETIOLOGICAL DISEASE

The rule governing antibiotic selection states that for monoetiological disease, use the drug of choice. When infection is due to group A or B beta-hemolytic streptococci, *Listeria monocytogenes*, *Neisseria gonorrhoeae*, *Mycoplasma hominis*, etc., it is primarily monoetiological disease. Sometimes, monoetiological disease may be due to *Escherichia coli*, *Klebsiella pneumoniae*, *Proteus mirabilis*, *Enterobacter cloacae*, or the gram-positive cocci. The initial antibiotic selection for presumed monoetiological disease must anticipate the probable spectrum of offending organisms for that disease entity and varying susceptibility to antibiotics within a pathogen group in order to select a valid drug of choice.

In those instances of monoetiological disease with a broad spectrum of potential pathogens (e.g., urinary tract infection, chorioamnionitis, primary pneumonia), the rule governing antibiotic selection is best drug for the anticipated spectrum. This may necessitate two-drug therapy when disease is potentially life threatening (e.g., maternal chorioamnionitis with septicemia). In certain instances, monoetiological diseases may be transformed into polymicrobial infection. For example, with acute endometritis/salpingitis/peritonitis due to *N. gonorrhoeae*, when peritonitis is well established, anaerobic superinfection from organisms derived from the vaginal flora may occur. A broader spectrum of coverage would be indicated.

Chorioamnionitis, in its initial phase, is caused by a single organism, usually a facultative anaerobe, such as a motile member of the *Enterobacteriaceae* or the virulent cocci (i.e., the group A beta-hemolytic streptococci or *N. gonorrhoeae*). The divergent antibiotic susceptibility patterns and the potential ramifications of disease, if allowed to evolve, argue

TABLE I Septicemic bacterial isolates (Shands Teaching Hospital)

Frequency of isolates	Medicine	Obstetrics
1	*Staphylococcus aureus* (21%)	Bacteroidaceae (17%)
2	*Escherichia coli* (18%)	*Gardnerella vaginalis* (17.5%)
3	*Pseudomonas* (16%)	Anaerobic streptococci (10.8%)
4	*Klebsiella pneumoniae* (8.7%)	Groups A and B streptococci (10.8%)
5	*Proteus* (7.6%) (indole-positive and -negative)	Enterococci (10.8%)
6	Enterococci (6.4%)	*Escherichia coli* (6.7%)

TABLE 2 Basic ground rules in antibiotic selection

1. The antibiotic or antibiotics selected must be highly effective, if not drug of choice against the presumed etiological agent or agent (drug of choice vs. best fit for potential pathogen spectrum)
2. Antibiotic selection must be done with patient's safety as being a foremost consideration
3. Antibiotic selection must be able to achieve therapeutic concentrations at the site of infection
4. Proper determination of dosage must be calculated to avoid dose-related adverse drug reactions. Adjustments include body weight route of administration, functional status of the principal mode of detoxification, patient's physiological status (i.e., pregnancy, third-space), pooling
5. Consideration should be given to the frequency of administration
6. An anticipated therapeutic response needs to be projected

for the combination of two drugs. Therapy for a gravida involves two biologically unique individuals.

In chorioamnionitis, it is necessary to treat the potential fetal/neonatal as well as the maternal infection. Because of its augmented ability to attain significant levels in amniotic fluid and cord blood, ampicillin is substituted for penicillin. The therapy of choice is the combination of ampicillin and an aminoglycoside, preferably gentamicin. In this instance, fetal considerations modify maternal therapy.

In dealing with presumed monoetiological disease entities whose pathogenic bacterial spectrum includes *Clostridium* species, *Staphylococcus aureus*, group A beta-hemolytic streptococcus, and in very rare cases *E. coli*, reliance on antibiotic therapy may not be sufficient. Evidence of concomitant multisystem involvement should alert the physician about either the presence of a toxin-producing strain of bacteria or an erroneous presumption of bacterial spectrum.

ANTIBIOTIC SELECTION FOR NOSOCOMIAL, MONOETIOLOGICAL DISEASE

Septicemia in intensive care units is usually monomicrobial in etiology; however, the ability to document causation in a clinically meaningful time frame is lacking. Most causes of nosocomial septicemia are aerobic bacteria belonging to Categories V, VI, and VII of the Gainesville Classification (Table 3).

Like the obstetrician/gynecologist confronted with life-threatening disease, the physician in the intensive care unit resorts to "triple therapy":

- Imipenem for Categories I, IV, and V
- Amikacin for Categories IV, V, and VI
- Vancomycin for Categories I and VII

The governing concept of antibiotic selection in obstetrics and gynecology for life-threatening disease is the need to cover the spectrum of potential pathogens with antibiotics encompassing Categories I through IV. The governing concept for internal medicine is best category-fit-for-spectrum encompassing potential pathogens.

ANTIBIOTIC SELECTION FOR POLYMICROBIAL COMMUNITY-ACQUIRED DISEASE

The effectiveness of antimicrobial therapy for polymicrobial infection is significantly influenced by the existing oxidation–reduction potential. When the oxidation–reduction potential is not yet in a critical zone, anaerobic infection can effectively be dealt with by eradicating the major constituent of the facilitating bacterial flora within the anaerobic progression. In this situation, it is not necessary to eradicate each bacterial constituent. However, once a critical oxidation–reduction potential is achieved, partial eradication of the bacteria present will not abort disease.

The presumptive clinical diagnosis usually alerts the physician that he or she is dealing with a polymicrobial infection (Table 4). In dealing with anaerobic polymicrobial infection, antibiotic coverage should be directed at the first four major categories of the Gainesville Classification schemata (Table 3).

TABLE 3 Gainesville Classification

Anaerobic progression portion	Penicillin-sensitive aerobes
Category I A and B	(A) and anaerobes (B)
Category II	Penicillin-resistant anaerobes
Category III	Community-acquired enterococci
Category IV	Community-acquired Enterobacteriaceae
Nosocomial disease portion	Multiresistant
Category V	Enterobacteriaceae
Category VI	Pseudomonas species
Category VII	Methicillin-resistant staphylococci

Although focused on the anaerobic participants in the anaerobic progression, the first four categories of the Gainesville Classification effectively deal with the predominantly aerobic bacteria, which may be involved in obstetrical or gynecological infections. The multidrug-resistant *Klebsiella* and *Pseudomonas* are rarely a problem for the obstetrical or gynecological patient unless the patient has been in the intensive care unit for long periods of time or has been subjected to complex medical care, which biases her for the potential acquisition of nosocomial infection. The aerobic bacteria involved in obstetrical and gynecological infections can usually be effectively dealt with by penicillin or a semisynthetic analog and an aminoglycoside.

When life-threatening polymicrobial infection occurs in a patient without a surgically amenable focus of infection, the first four categories of coverage (Gainesville Classification) need to be instituted. If abscess formation has occurred, surgical intervention is required. It cannot be stressed too strongly that where there is necrotic tissue or abscess, a bacteriologic cure with antibiotic therapy alone can rarely be achieved.

Assuming exclusion of microbiological situations amenable to surgical therapy in which a critical oxidation–reduction potential is present (i.e., ruptured tubo-ovarian abscess, retained products of conception, etc.), triple therapy (penicillin– or ampicillin–clindamycin–aminoglycoside) or an equivalent is indicated for life-threatening disease.

Three $(+++)$ to four $(++++)$ types of coverage must be achieved in each of the therapeutic categories. When dealing with the anaerobic progression, any combination of drugs that gives you at least a $+++$ coverage for the penicillin-sensitive anaerobes and $++$ to $+++$ coverage in the remaining three categories is recommended (Tables 5–7).

TABLE 4 Clinical situations commonly associated with polymicrobial infections

Obstetrics	Gynecology
Septic abortion	Pelvic cellulitis
Infected ectopic pregnancies	Cuff abscess or cellulitis
Retained products of conception	Ruptured tubo-ovarian abscess
	Cul-de-sac abscess
Postcesarean-section endometritis	Postoperative abdominal wound infections
Postpartum endometritis	

TABLE 5 Spectrum of coverage achieved within the Gainesville Classification by antibiotics with Category I designation

Category I antibiotics	Gainesville Classification categories			
	I	II	III	IV
Penicillins				
First generation	++++	–	+++	+–++
Second generation	++++	–	++++	++
Third generation	++++	++–+++	++½	++¼
Fourth generation	++++	++–+++	+++	++½
Fifth generation	++++	+++	++++	+++
Cephalosporins				
First generation	+++	+/–	+	++¼
Second generation	+++	++–+++	+	++½
Third generation	+++	++	+–++	+++¼
Erythromycins	++++	–	+++	+
Vancomycin	++++	–	+++	–
Imipenem/cilastatin	++++	+++	+++	++++

If the first four categories are covered effectively, a relative antibiotic stone wall is created for aerobic/anaerobic polymicrobial infection. This permits the evaluation of current and future antibiotics in terms of delineating the existing gaps. Whenever a given antibiotic is used, the physician must be cognizant of the gaps. If the anticipated therapeutic response does not occur and there is not a surgically amenable or manageable focus of infection, it is imperative to close the gap with appropriate therapy. The system is designed to give obstetricians and gynecologists the ability to dissect out medically amenable disease from that requiring surgical intervention.

ANTIMICROBIAL RESISTANCE

In the future, antibiotic selection will be influenced by the emergence of antimicrobial resistance. This phenomenon and its spread represent the convergence of a variety of factors, which include mutations in common resistance genes, the exchange of genetic information among microorganisms, and the selective pressures engendered by antibiotic utilization both in hospitals and within the community. A number of multiresistant bacterial phenotypes have impacted or have the potential to impact on obstetricians and gynecologists (Table 8).

TABLE 6 Coverage designation within the Gainesville Classification of antibiotics with Category II

Category II antibiotics	Gainesville Classification categories				
	IA	IB	II	III	IV
Clindamycin	+++	+++	+++	–	–
Metronidazole	–	+++	++++	–	–
Imipenem/cilastatin	++++	+++½	+++	+++	++++
Ampicillin/sulbactam	++++	+++½	+++	++++	++–+++
Ticarcillin/clavulanate	+++	+++½	+++	++	++–+++
Piperacillin/tazobactam	++++	+++½	+++	+++	+++

TABLE 7 Coverage within the Gainesville Classification of antibiotics with Category III efficacy

Category III antibiotics	Gainesville Classification categories				
	IA	IB	II	III	IV
Penicillins	++++	++++	–	+++	+
Erythromycins	++++	+++	–	+++	+
Chloramphenicol	++	+++	++++	+++	++
Trimethoprim/sulfamethoxazole	+++	+++	+	+++	++

Multiresistant *N. gonorrhoeae* and *Streptococcus pneumoniae* have become well established in the community. Multiresistance for these bacteria to beta-lactam and non–beta-lactam antibiotics is not the result of common resistance mechanisms or genetic linkage. What happens is the clonal spread of relatively few beta-lactam resistant strains. A small percentage of these bacteria also express resistance to one or more non–beta-lactam antibiotics. When the beta-lactam strains become endemic, switching antibiotic therapy selects for increased antibiotic resistance to non–beta-lactam antibiotics.

The beta-lactam resistance mechanism of *N. gonorrhoeae* involves both chromosomal and plasmid-mediated mechanisms. The mechanism of *S. pneumoniae* beta-lactam resistance involves plasmid-mediated alterations in penicillin-binding proteins of high molecular weight in the cell wall.

Hospital Multiresistant Bacteria

Among gram-positive bacteria, the most common mechanisms for exchange of genetic material involve transformation and transduction, whereas with gram-negative bacteria, conjugation is the most commonly recognized mode of genetic transfer.

Multiresistance, and in particular that to vancomycin, of Enterococcus faecalis is borne on mobile plasmids and transposons. Not all resistance genes that transfer among bacteria are expressed or maintained. The frequent use of vancomycin in the 1990s for therapy of methicillin-resistant *S. aureus*, *Clostridium difficile*, and inline bacteremia caused by coagulase-negative staphylococci was the predominant selective pressure that resulted in the development and spread within hospitals of vancomycin-resistant enterococci. The intensity of use of vancomycin is proportional to resistance levels in bacteria within hospital settings. The selective pressure caused by vancomycin utilization has impacted on *S. aureus* and *S. epidermidis*.

Physicians need to monitor local antibiotic resistance patterns. When confronted with a life-threatening disease within the disease spectrum of a multiresistant bacteria or a 10% resistance to a given potential multiresistant bacteria within a hospital or community, antibiotic selection should conform to "best-fit-for-spectrum" of all significant pathogens.

TABLE 8 Multiresistant bacteria potentially impacting on obstetrics and gynecology

Enterococcus faecalis	Staphylococcus epidermidis
Neisseria gonorrhoeae	Streptococcus pneumoniae
Staphylococcus aureus	

Antibiotics and Pregnancy

Revised by Douglas D. Glover and Timothy S. Tracy /
Revised by Gilles R. G. Monif

5

MATERNAL–FETAL DISTRIBUTION

The transport of drugs is governed by diffusion, surface area available for transfer, lipid solubility, molecular weight, degree of ionization, partition coefficient, and maternal–fetal concentration gradient. The availability of a drug for transport is dependent, in turn, on the binding of the drug to the plasma proteins. Forming a drug–protein complex is contingent upon covalent and ionic bonding between polar and nonpolar groups on the antibiotic and upon the polarity of amino acids available for binding. The unbound fraction in the serum is pharmacologically active and in a state of dynamic equilibrium with the drug present in the extracellular space. As free drug is excreted or metabolized, protein-bound drug is released so as to maintain a relatively constant proportion of free drug. Serum protein levels do not influence the eventual utilization of all of the drug present in the plasma, but rather determine the amount of free drug available at any given moment. Only the unbound drug passes freely across membranes separating biologic compartments. It is this form of the drug that is capable of antimicrobial action. The affinity of plasma proteins for a specific drug is not necessarily indicative of their binding capacity. Certain carrier proteins may have a high affinity for a given drug but a relatively low binding capacity. When the binding sites are saturated, a secondary plasma protein usually participates in the reaction, even though its binding affinity is lower. Different drugs may compete for the same binding site on a protein molecule. The unbound plasma levels will be increased if a drug bound on a protein molecule is displaced by another drug with a greater affinity for that particular binding site. Once the free form of the drug has entered into a given biologic compartment, such as the fetal intravascular space or the amniotic fluid, it is again subjected to the binding ratios of those proteins present. The lack of a significant amount of protein in certain biologic compartments such as the cerebrospinal fluid and amniotic fluid may account for the relative efficiency of certain drugs in eradicating bacteria, despite the low concentrations achieved relative to those in the corresponding vascular compartment. The significance of protein binding is brought into sharp focus when therapy is initiated for the fetus rather than the mother. Because of its protein binding, the distribution of ampicillin is such that it is often the drug of choice in terms of first-line fetal therapeutics.

Recent evidence has demonstrated that placental drug transport may also be regulated by transporters expressed in the placenta, particularly efflux transporters that serve to "pump" drug back to the mother, limiting fetal exposure. Several efflux transporters have been identified in the human placenta with P-glycoprotein (MDR1) being the most studied. Many drugs are transported by the P-glycoprotein transporter, including drugs such as digoxin that are used for in utero treatment. However, transporters from the multidrug resistance–associated protein (MRP) family as well as the breast cancer resistance protein (BCRP/MXR/ABCP) have also been found in human placenta. The MRP transporters appear to prefer organic anion drugs, glutathione conjugates, glucuronate conjugates, urinates, and sulfates. Although less understood, the BCRP transporter appears to transport compounds such as topotecan and mitoxantrone and probably other drugs. Because these transporters pump drug back to the mother from placenta tissue, they can serve a protective role following maternal drug exposure. However, in some cases, in utero drug treatment is desired (e.g., intra-amniotic infection, HIV, or cardiac conditions) and these transporters may limit fetal exposure and thus reduce drug efficacy.

Also, the placenta possesses limited capabilities to metabolize compounds via both oxidative metabolism pathways (e.g., cytochrome P450 enzymes) and drug conjugation pathways (e.g., glucuronosyl transferases or glutathione *S*-transferases). In most cases, metabolism by these pathways results in the production of inactive and more easily excreted metabolites. However, in some cases, reactive or toxic metabolites may be produced. Substantial research in this area has focused on the inducibility of placental oxidative enzymes (e.g., cytochrome P450 1A1) in mothers who smoke during pregnancy. In pregnant women who smoke, placental cytochrome P450 1A1 has been shown to be induced up to 100-fold as compared with the basal state. This is especially important since cigarette smoke contains a number of polycyclic aromatic hydrocarbons that are metabolized to produce reactive metabolites that can be mutagenic or carcinogenic. However, the glutathione *S*-transferase enzymes, which are not induced by cigarette smoking, can conjugate glutathione with these polycyclic aromatic hydrocarbon reactive metabolites. Thus, an imbalance can result in women who smoke, potentially placing the fetus at additional risk.

Although they are not studied extensively, oxidative enzymes such as cytochrome P450 1A1 and conjugative enzymes such as glutathione *S*-transferase and glucuronosyl transferases may also participate in the metabolism of drugs given for in utero treatment of various fetal disorders. Although at the present time, limited research is available regarding the activities of these enzymes in placental tissue toward commonly used drugs, it is reasonable to assume that they would affect maternal–fetal distribution.

Antibiotic Groups Requiring Dosing Adjustments in Pregnancy

Antimicrobial effects of some antibiotic groups depend on drug concentration (Table 1). The expanding intravascular and extracellular compartments associated with progressive pregnancy risk rendering drug efficacy suboptimal. To compensate, a physician can either increase the dosage or shorten the interval between drug administrations.

Antibiotics for the Fetus

The obstetrician is in the unique position of being simultaneously a therapeutician for both the mother and the fetus. The mother and the fetus are biologically unique individuals whose ability to metabolize a drug or be adversely affected by the compound or its degradative derivatives may differ significantly.

Certain antibiotics, which would constitute drug of choice for the nonpregnant female, must be avoided during gestation due to their ability to induce drug embryopathy in the fetus or cause an adverse reaction in the enzymatically immature neonate. The Food and Drug Administration (FDA) has created a scale from A to D, which predicates upon real or theoretical in utero risk to the fetus when the antibiotic is administered for maternal indications (Table 2).

Antibiotic Therapy for Congenital Infection in Utero

Selected organisms that have the ability to traverse the placenta and establish congenital infection in the fetus, are responsive to maternal antimicrobial therapy (Table 3). Chorioamnionitis complicates 1% to 5% of term pregnancies. The incidence of intra-amniotic infection approaches 25% to 40% of cases of preterm labor and is a major contributor to increased maternal and fetal morbidity and mortality. Although chorioamnionitis may result from hematogenous dissemination of systemic disease, most cases are caused by ascending infection from the vagina and are frequently polymicrobial. *Listeria monocytogenes* is a classic example of descending or hematogenous infection whereas *Escherichia coli*, *Bacteroides* species, anaerobic streptococci, and group B streptococcus are commonly associated with ascending intra-amniotic infection. Prolonged labor, membrane rupture of greater than 12 hours, and multiple vaginal examinations may be contributing factors.

Little data exist to guide the clinician as to when to initiate antibiotic therapy or the optimal time frame for delivery. A literature review reveals only two randomized clinical trials

TABLE 1 Congenital infections for which antimicrobial therapy exists

Organism	Drug of choice
Bacteria	
Listeria monocytogenes	Ampicillin
Haemophilus influenzae	Ampicillin
Salmonella typhi	Ampicillin
Spirochetes	
Treponema pallidum	Penicillin
Protozoan	
Toxoplasma gondii	Pyrimethamine and sulfonamides

TABLE 2 Antibiotics contraindicated in pregnancy

Tetracyclines
- In the first trimester, if administered during osseous organogenesis, they may induce thalidomide-like deformities
- In the second and third trimesters, they induce an embryopathy affecting bone growth and primary and permanent dentition
- The old-generation tetracyclines, if administered to a gravida with occult renal compromise or acute pyelonephritis, may induce fulminating hepato-renal decompensation
- The tetracyclines are effective chelators of heavy metals. They are competitive at the osteoblastic level with calcium in the areas of new bone formation. Their presence impedes the incorporation of C14-proline into a cartilage as well as of Ca46 into the organic matrix of bone. This action results in the inhibition of bone growth (Figs. 2 and 3)

Chloramphenicol
- Due to enzymatic immaturity resulting in a relative inability to conjugate compound for bioelimination, free unconjugated drug acts to produce a clinical pattern of cardiopulmonary collapse termed "the gray-baby syndrome"
- As long as the fetus resides in utero, there is no adverse effect resulting from maternal administration of the drug

Quinolones and fluoroquinolones
- Quinolones and fluoroquinolones produce permanent cartilaginous defects in the bones of animal fetuses and growing juveniles

Sulfonamides
- If administered immediately prior to parturition, they can achieve cord levels comparable to those observed in maternal serum. The sulfonamides can displace bilirubin from its albumin carrier. The bilirubin thus freed has the ability to traverse the neonatal blood–brain barrier and occasionally induce kernicterus

Trimethoprim
- These antimicrobial compounds have been shown to be teratogenic in animal model systems. Although there are no data to document teratogenicity for the human fetus, it is best to avoid their use in pregnancy

Metronidazole
- The drug is an excellent mutagen. Data derived from animal model systems have demonstrated oncogenic potential for selected strains. Drug use in pregnancy or during breastfeeding must be carefully evaluated in terms of maternal benefits versus theoretical fetal/neonatal risks

Streptomycin
- It adversely affects subsequent neonatal cochlear function. The effect is dose related

comparing antibiotic regimens and neither was placebo controlled. Gibbs et al., in a randomized trial, enrolled 48 women to receive either ampicillin or gentamicin. The results indicated that intrapartum use of antibiotics was associated with a reduction in neonatal sepsis and pneumonia; but the results did not reach statistical significance. No difference in the incidence of maternal bacteremia was noted. A trend toward a lower incidence of postpartum endomyometritis was noted in those receiving triple antibiotic therapy, but the results did not reach statistical significance. Meta-analysis by Hopkins and Small of these two studies is inconclusive regarding the choice of antibiotic regimens to treat intra-amniotic infection.

The use of antibiotics as an adjunct to tocolysis in the management of preterm labor with intact membranes remains controversial. Data from 13 randomized trials meeting the criteria for a meta-analysis produced variable results, with limited improvement in both prolonging gestation and increasing the birth weight. The efficacy of antibiotic use in

TABLE 3 Unique adverse drug reactions observed with tetracycline administration in pregnancy

First trimester
    Fetal considerations: probable teratogen, with induction of micromelia and other skeletal abnormalities
Second trimester
    Fetal considerations: tetracycline embryopathy, inhibition of bone growth, abnormal formation of deciduous teeth
Third trimester
    Fetal considerations: continued tetracycline embryopathy, deposition within deciduous teeth and bones[a]
    Maternal consequences: hepatic fatty metamorphosis[a]

[a]Associated with IV administration in patients with pyelonephritis or renal impairment.

cases of preterm labor with intact membranes is lacking and fails to show a true benefit from their use.

Untreated asymptomatic bacteriuria appears to play a role in preterm labor and delivery. A meta-analysis of the treatment results of asymptomatic bacteriuria revealed a direct relationship of this entity and preterm birth. A significant benefit of treating asymptomatic bacteriuria in addition to prevention of pyelonephritis has been shown.

An association has been demonstrated between bacterial vaginosis and preterm labor in high-risk populations. However, this association has not been confirmed in low-risk populations with asymptomatic bacterial vaginosis.

The literature does not support routine use of antibiotics as an adjunct to tocolytic agents in the management of a woman with idiopathic preterm labor. There is a consensus, however, that sexually transmitted diseases, group B streptococcus colonization, asymptomatic bacteriuria, and symptomatic bacterial vaginosis should be treated with the appropriate antimicrobial therapy. Eradication of group B streptococcal colonization of the genitourinary tract in pregnancy has been shown to be unsuccessful and treatment is usually delayed until labor. The other infections are best treated at the time they are diagnosed.

ADVERSE DRUG REACTIONS IN PREGNANCY

Antimicrobial therapy in pregnancy assumes the concept that drug action will occur within not one, but two biologically unique individuals. As a general rule, all drugs are more toxic in the fetus than in infants or adults. Antibiotics may have such deleterious effects on the fetus that their very use in pregnancy is openly questioned (Table 2).

Tetracyclines
The tetracyclines have two major effects:

1. They inhibit protein synthesis by interfering with the transfer of amino acids from aminoacyl RNA to polypeptides.
2. They act as efficient chelators of heavy metals, in particular, calcium.

Adverse fetal or maternal effects of tetracycline are mediated by one or both of these mechanisms.

Although the deleterious consequences of the tetracyclines are related to total dosage and duration of administration, the types of adverse drug reactions occurring in pregnancy are such that there is to all intents and purposes no time that is deemed safe for their therapeutic administration. Although there are individual toxicologic variations between the several tetracyclines, for discussion purposes, they are considered a group.

Fetal Considerations
Throughout the three trimesters of gestation, the tetracyclines are contraindicated because of fetal considerations (Table 3). The evidence derived from animal model systems is almost as incriminating as that which existed for thalidomide prior to the massive experiment in human teratology. Administration of a tetracycline during the period of osseous organogenesis in an animal may result in hypoplasia of the anterior limb buds, with micromelia and other skeletal abnormalities. It would be presumptuous to interpret experiments in animals as being directly analogous to that in human. Nevertheless, clinical reports suggest that a relationship exists and that these observations can be extrapolated from rats, rabbits, and chickens and applied to human. Carter and Wilson (1962) reported on a group of 13 mothers who were given large doses of tetracycline in the first 12 weeks of pregnancy, of whom six had malformed babies. Similarly, Woollam and Miller (1963) reported the occurrence of four malformations in the offspring of 37 women who received comparable doses of tetracycline.

Although bone is the major fetal site of tetracycline action, it is not the sole target organ. In teeth, tetracycline enters the developing tooth substance roughly in proportion to the amount of crystalline surface rather than in proportion to the calcium content. Dental injury occurs if tetracycline is administered when the crowns of the deciduous anterior teeth are being formed, which is from mid-pregnancy to about the sixth month of postnatal life. This phenomenon translates as hypoplasia of deciduous teeth and intrinsic staining of the enamel. Both the degree of discoloration and hypoplasia are dose dependent.

Maternal Considerations
There is a well-defined syndrome of fulminating hepatic decompensation described in women treated for pyelonephritis with large intravenous doses of tetracycline. Characteristically, the syndrome occurs during the last trimester of pregnancy. The women have jaundice, severe nausea and vomiting, hematoemesis, abdominal pain, and headaches, and they may lapse into coma. Death is not an unusual outcome. The clinical course of the entity is often indistinguishable from acute fulminating viral hepatitis in pregnancy. Distinction between the two diseases is often on the basis of liver biopsy. Microscopic examination of the liver reveals widespread, small intracytoplasmic triglyceride-rich vacuoles within hepatocytes (Fig. 1). Sheehan (1940), in his original description, termed it "obstetrical acute yellow atrophy"; the condition has subsequently been grouped with acute fatty liver of pregnancy.

It can be shown that the hepatic alterations are dose dependent. Patients with pyelonephritis exhibit a significantly decreased renal clearance of the drug. Upon this

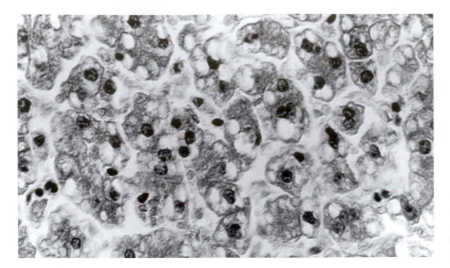

FIGURE 1 Multiple small intracytoplasmic lipid-laden vacuoles within hepatocytes in a patient with evidence of hepatocellular decompensation following 9 g tetra cycline IV (H&E, ×270).

state of compromised renal function is then superimposed the renal toxicity of tetracycline. The adverse effect of tetracycline is manifested by

1. inability of the kidney to concentrate urine and
2. rising serum "bun" and creatinine levels.

Not infrequently, a concomitant feature of tetracycline hepatotoxicity is pancreatitis. Isolated pancreatitis has also been identified when a dose of only 1 to 2 g/day has been administered parenterally.

Chloramphenicol

Chloramphenicol is a very valuable drug. Yet, because of the possibility of fatal drug-induced aplastic anemia, its clinical use should be restricted to potentially life-threatening situations that warrant the risk involved, and then only when the patient is under close hematologic supervision.

Chloramphenicol is capable of traversing the placental barrier. Studies in term infants reveal drug concentrations in the plasma that are between 30% and 80% of maternal concentrations. Despite the ability of chloramphenicol to interfere with the function of messenger RNA, no drug embryopathy has yet been attributed to its administration during gestation.

Once fetal viability is achieved, the existence of an acceptable alternative antibiotic is a relative contraindication to the use of chloramphenicol in the third trimester. Often maternal complications warranting its administration result in fetal death in utero or in premature termination of pregnancy. If premature birth occurs, because of transplacental transfer of the drug, the fetus is exposed to an immediate risk from an adverse drug reaction. As long as the integrity of the maternofetal placental circulation is maintained, the fetus is capable of drug equilibrium with the maternal host, and its capability to eliminate the drug and its metabolic products is not challenged.

The major mechanisms for the elimination of chloramphenicol from the body are

1. inactivation through conjugation with glucuronic acid and
2. excretion by (*i*) glomerular filtration of free chloramphenicol and (*ii*) tubular excretion of the glucuronic acid conjugate.

Neonates, especially premature infants, when receiving large doses of the drug, have developed a clinical pattern, which is termed the "gray-baby syndrome." Clinical deterioration due to chloramphenicol toxicity usually begins four days after therapy has started. Onset of toxicity can be influenced by the relative fetal immaturity or increasing drug dosage, or both. In the first 24 hours, the infant vomits, suffers from irregular and rapid respiration, shows abdominal distention, and refuses to suck. Within the next 12 to 24 hours, the characteristic ashen discoloration (from which the syndrome derives its name), hypothermia, and flaccidity develop. These signs are followed shortly by neonatal demise secondary to what has been interpreted as cardiovascular collapse. No characteristic pathologic changes attributable to the use of chloramphenicol are demonstrable in any organ system, including the hematopoietic system.

Chloramphenicol toxicity in the neonate is due to the free drug per se rather than due to its metabolic products. Anuric patients receiving chloramphenicol develop extremely high circulating levels of the glucuronic form of the drug with no untoward effects. Similarly, the glucuronic acid amide metabolite recovered from the urine of infants appears to have little demonstrable toxicity. The drug toxicity is a function of

1. the immaturity of the enzyme systems responsible for conjugation of the drug with glucuronic acid and
2. decreased renal clearance of the free form of the drug.

The quantity of hepatic glucuronyl transferase is diminished in the first three to four weeks of life. The quantitative inadequacy of this enzyme system is even greater in premature infants. In the newborn infant, glomerular filtration rates for insulin, mannitol, and creatinine are 30% to 50% of adult levels. This combination is responsible for increased circulating levels of free chloramphenicol and the resulting syndrome.

Erythromycin

Five reports have suggested maternal ingestion of erythromycin after the 32nd week of gestation may lead to early onset infantile hypertrophic pyloric stenosis. Theoretically, macrolide antibiotics may interact with gastric motilin receptors causing strong gastric and pyloric bulb contractions resulting in pylorus hypertrophy.

A retrospective cohort study utilizing Tennessee Medicaid prescription records linked to hospital discharge diagnosis and surgical procedure codes recorded on birth certificates. Of 260,799 mother/infant pairs studied, 13,146 had prescriptions for erythromycin and 621 received a nonerythromycin macrolide. No association of infantile hypertrophic pyloric stenosis with in utero exposure to erythromycin either in late pregnancy or at any stage of gestation. A weak association of infantile hypertrophic pyloric stenosis with nonerythromycin macrolide was apparent but causal inference was limited by the small number (three cases) of affected children.

Likewise, a surveillance study of 229,101 Michigan Medicaid recipients conducted between 1985 and 1992 reported that 6972 children had been subjected to erythromycin in the first trimester of pregnancy. In this study, 320 (4.6%) were found to have major birth defects compared with an expected number of 297 (4.3%). These data do not support an association of erythromycin and congenital malformations.

Philipson et al. (1973) studied erythromycin in pregnant women between the 10th and 18th weeks and reported peak serum levels ranged from 0.29 to 7.2 µg/mL and that peak concentrations were achieved at two hours in seven of nine patients and at four hours in the remaining two patients. Both erythromycin base and estolate were used in the study. Forty percent of their subjects were "low absorbers," defined by the authors as those whose peak serum levels were less than 20% of the arithmetic mean value for their group (Figs. 2 and 3).

Using an identical protocol, Larson and Glover (1998) studied the pharmacokinetics of erythromycin base in late pregnancy in 10 subjects, of which seven were in the third trimester. Eight subjects achieved peak serum levels within four hours, with individual concentrations ranging from 0 to 2.9 µg/mL. Two subjects had no detectable serum levels of erythromycin by four hours, of which one required hospital admission for rehydration and was found to have a serum level of 0.6 µg/mL three hours after the seventh dose. Serum levels reported by these investigators were lower than those of Philipson's study, with a mean serum level of 0.21 ± 0.19 µg/mL, compared with Philipson's mean level of 4.1 µg/mL. Although some patients have serum levels that reach the median minimal inhibitory concentration for such pathogens as *Neisseria gonorrhoeae* (0.1 µg/mL) and *Chlamydia trachomatis* (0.5 µg/mL), there remains a concern that patients who have no detectable levels, at least by four hours, are at risk for poor treatment outcomes. Additionally, such low maternal serum levels may limit fetal exposure to the drug.

Fluoroquinolones

Fluoroquinolones are synthetic, broad-spectrum anti-infective agents used to treat urinary tract and other systemic infections. They have activity against most *Enterobacteriaceae*, *Pseudomonas*, *Klebsiella*, and *Proteus* species as well as beta-lactamase–producing strains of *N. gonorrhoeae*. Data collected after introduction of these agents suggest an association of fluoroquinolones and cartilage defects in antibiotic-exposed infants may be a valid cause of concern. Although doses six times the usual daily human dose have not produced malformations in mice, rats, and rabbits, multiple doses of fluoroquinolones have been associated with lesions of cartilage in weight-bearing joints of laboratory animals.

Loebstein et al. conducted a multi-center prospective study of pregnancy outcomes following gestational exposure to fluoroquinolones. They concluded that the use of the fluoroquinolones during embryogenesis is not associated with increased risk of congenital malformations. Similarly, Wogelus P. et al. studied 87 women who received a fluoquinolone prescription at any time during pregnancy. The prevalence ratio of bone malformations was 2.2 (95% CL 0.7–6.7). What has been lacking to date is long term magnetic resonance imaging of fetuses that received fluoroquinolone therapy during osseous organogenesis and beyond to exclude subtle cartilage and bone damage.

Evaluation of the collective anomalies reported from eight reports fails to reveal a specific pattern of malformations in association with fluoroquinolone exposure. Until long-term follow-up using magnetic resonance imaging of the joints is done to exclude subtle cartilage and/or bone alterations, treatment with fluoroquinolones in pregnancy should be reserved for life-threatening infections that are unresponsive to other classes of antibiotic therapy. To date, there is no evidence that the fluoroquinolones are teratogenic.

Isoniazid

The use of isoniazid is not undertaken without some trepidation. Garibaldi et al. reported 21 cases of hepatitis, two fatal, among 2300 government employees receiving isoniazid prophylaxis. Isoniazid hepatitis is an entity observed primarily in elderly females. Because of the tendency for any hepatotoxic drug to be potentiated by pregnancy, the Centers for Disease Control (CDC) now recommend that pregnancy be considered a contraindication to the prophylactic use of isoniazid. A prodromal period marked by malaise, fatigue, and anorexia almost always precedes the appearance of jaundice. If isoniazid is stopped promptly, a serious outcome can be avoided. The decision to administer or not administer isoniazid to a gravida should be individualized. If therapy is given, the patient should be monitored clinically and biochemically.

Isoniazid administration during gestation has been incriminated in the development of mental retardation and (rarely) convulsions and myoclonia in the progeny, presumably due to the ability of its degradative products to interfere with the metabolism of pyridoxine. To counterbalance this possibility, when isoniazid is administered during pregnancy, it is advocated that vitamin B12, 50 µg daily, be given for possible fetal as well as maternal indications. Although it has been suggested that therapy with bacteriostatic drugs, including isoniazid, for tuberculosis in pregnant women may increase the risk of congenitally defective infants two- or threefold, this hypothesis is yet to be confirmed.

Streptomycin–Kanamycin–Amikacin

It has been shown that prolonged treatment with high doses of streptomycin during pregnancy may result in some degree

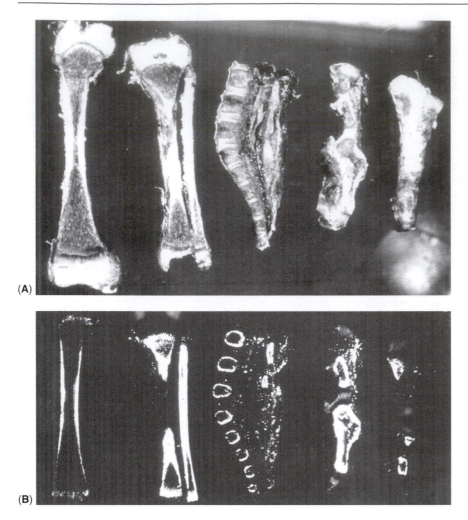

(A)

(B)

FIGURE 2 (**A**) Representative bones of a 28-week-old fetus whose mother had received 23 g tetracycline during gestation. (**B**) Sagittal section demonstrating the amount of autofluorescence due to deposition of tetracycline.

of irreversible bilateral sensorineural hearing loss and vestibular damage. These effects are less common when the fetus is exposed to the drug after the fifth month of pregnancy. Although the fetus is at risk, this appears to be a dose-related phenomenon. The existence of acceptable alternative forms of antituberculous therapy in pregnancy has relegated this form of drug toxicity to a phenomenon that reminds us that anti-biotics cross the placenta. Milliary tuberculosis, tuberculosis meningitis, and a strain of tubercle bacillus resistant to most other drugs constitute the only indications for the use of streptomycin in pregnancy. Despite causing less vestibular dysfunction, both kanamycin and amikacin are contraindicated in the treatment of pregnant women because of the risk of congenital hearing loss.

Sulfonamides

Sulfonamides administered during pregnancy equilibrate in maternal and fetal plasma within three hours. The plasma drug levels in the fetus are approximately 50% to 90% of those in the maternal plasma. This is dependent on the affinity of the sulfonamides for albumin, which differs considerably among the drugs in clinical use. Silverman and colleagues (1956), in a control study of two prophylactic antibacterial regimens in the therapeutic management of premature infants, noted an unexpected increase in mortality in the group receiving penicillin and sulfisoxazole. At necropsy, infants of this group had kernicterus 10 times

more frequently than those infants who received oxytetracycline. Most of the infants who died of kernicterus had shown bilirubin levels of less than 15 mg/100 mL.

It has subsequently been shown in vitro that sulfisoxazole successfully competes with bilirubin for binding sites on the serum albumin molecule. This competition of sulfonamides releases bilirubin from its protein-bound form and facilitates its diffusion into tissues and the development of kernicterus. The treatment of glucuronic transferase genetic-deficient rats with sulfonamides results in a marked increase in mortality despite low serum bilirubin concentrations. Just as the glucuronosyl transferase system is immature at birth, so is the acetylation mechanism that constitutes the alternative pathway for the detoxification of the sulfonamides.

The use of sulfonamides, especially the long-acting forms, should be restricted in the six weeks prior to parturition. Maternal treatment with sulfonamides at the time of parturition may necessitate exchange transfusion therapy for the newborn infant.

Trimethoprim

Trimethoprim is a diaminopyrimidine that competitively antagonizes folic and folinic acids. Trimethoprim is available as a single agent and is utilized effectively with sulfamethoxazole (Septra®, Bactrim®) in the treatment of urinary tract infections. The antimicrobial activity of this combination results from its action on two steps of the enzymatic pathway

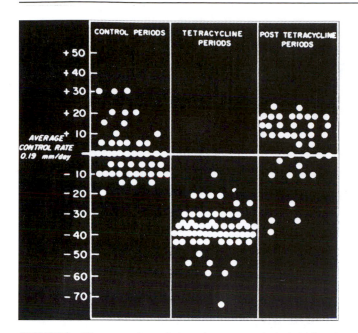

FIGURE 3 The control panel plots the percent deviation of each control fibula growth rate from the average control rate. Each white circle in the tetracycline and posttetracycline panels represents the percent deviation of each fibula growth rate as compared with the control rate.

for the synthesis of tetrahydrofolic acid. Recent reports suggest that use of trimethoprim in the first trimester may result in anatomic defects. A woman who was dieting in early pregnancy was treated for 10 days with a combination of trimethoprim–sulfamethoxazole for acute otitis media beginning in the third menstrual week. Dimenhydrinate was added as an antiemetic at the seventh week for hyperemesis. At 38 weeks, she delivered a 3225 g infant with lobar holoprosencephaly that included a median cleft lip and palate, a flat nose without nostrils, hypoplasia of the optic discs, a single ventricle, and fused thalami in the midline.

Richardson et al. (2000) have reported neural tube defects that occurred in the pregnancies of two HIV-infected women who received trimethoprim–sulfamethoxazole combination therapy for prophylaxis against *Pneumocystis carinii* concurrently with zidovudine and zalcitabine. Subsequently folic acid was added, but the date of initiation is in question. At term the woman delivered a female infant with an anomaly of the first lumbar vertebra and a protrusion of the second lumbar vertebra into the spinal cord. The other HIV-infected woman was taking trimethoprim–sulfamethoxazole at the booking visit (15 weeks), along with didanosine, stavudine, nevirapine, and a multivitamin that were prescribed prior to conception. Anatomic survey via ultrasonography at 19 weeks' gestation revealed spina bifida and ventriculomegaly. The pregnancy was terminated and at necropsy the fetus was found to have Arnold-Chiari malformation, ventriculomegaly, sacral spina bifida, and a lumbosacral meningomyelocele.

In a report from a multicenter case–control surveillance survey conducted in 80 maternity or tertiary care hospitals in the United States and Canada, the effects of exposure to folic acid antagonists on embryo and fetal development were evaluated. Folic acid antagonists were classified as follows: Group 1, dihydrofolate reductase inhibitors (methotrexate, aminopterin, sulfasalazine, pyrime-thamine, triamterene, and trimethoprim), and Group 2, drugs that affect other enzymes in folate metabolism, increase the metabolism of folate (phenobarbital, phenytoin, primidone, carbamazepine), and interfere with the absorption of folate. None of the controls took folic acid antagonists. Exclusions included infants with defects associated with a syndrome and those with neural tube defects. Analysis for trimethoprim exposure resulted in a relative risk of 4.2. These data appear to confirm that trimethoprim is a low level teratogen.

Miscellaneous Drugs

Ethionamide, pyrimethamine, and rifampin are in the category of drugs for which teratogenicity has been postulated or demonstrated in animal model systems.

Ethionamide, a drug used in the treatment of persistent tuberculosis, is potentially teratogenic and its use is contraindicated in pregnancy. In a 2000 report of 23 ethionamide-exposed infants, seven were found to have anomalies, including two with 21 trisomy syndrome.

Pyrimethamine is a diaminopyrimidine, which competitively antagonizes folic and folinic acids. Pyrimethamine (Daraprim®), in combination with a sulfonamide, has been used in the treatment of toxoplasmosis and some sensitive and multiresistant strains of *Plasmodium falciparum*. The mechanism of action is similar to that observed with trimethoprim and sulfamethoxazole in combination, namely, a sequential block resulting in an additive synergistic effect. This drug is a potential teratogen in experimental animals and must be used with great caution in pregnant patients.

Rifampin is a valuable second-line antituberculous drug used in the treatment of drug-resistant strains of *Mycobacterium tuberculosis* and atypical mycobacterial infection. Although no teratogenicity has been documented, its ability to inhibit DNA-dependent RNA polymerase questions its use during pregnancy.

Cycloserine crosses the placenta. There are limited data on safety in pregnancy. Its use in pregnancy should be only when there are no suitable alternatives.

Bioterrorism

In response to the presumed inhalation exposure to aerosol anthrax, the guidelines of CDC advocated the long-term administration of ciprofloxacin or doxycycline with or without anthrax vaccine administration.

With respect to pregnancy, the CDC 2001 guidelines state that in asymptomatic pregnant women, doxycycline should be used with caution and only when contraindications are indicated to use other appropriate antimicrobial drugs.

Any recommendation for drug administration in pregnancy needs to be analyzed under the "principle of dual effect" in which the combined benefits derived by mother and fetus/neonate are assessed against the maximum harm imposed upon either. To date, the theorized fetal adverse effects of 60 days of maternal doxycycline administration have been deemed acceptable within the context of a positive maternal/fetal risk–benefit ratio. That contention is open to serious challenge.

Potential Adverse Effects of Doxycycline

Characterization of tetracyclines' embryopathy is derived from observations and experiments involving the older tetracyclines. Formulation and dosage requirement of doxycyclines is sufficiently different to challenge whether old-generation tetracycline data have validity for doxycycline.

Animal experimental data strongly indicate that doxycycline retains tetracycline's ability to exert an adverse embryopathic effect on the developing fetus. Doxycycline reduces type X collagen epitope in avian explant cultures as well as decreases colagenase and gelatinase activities. It disrupts chondrocyte dif-ferentiation. Owing to its ability to inhibit matrix metalloproteinase as well as chelat divalent cations, doxycycline blocks angiogenesis in the chicken chorioallantoic membrane. Fetuses of albino pregnant rats fed the drug exhibit delayed primary ossification centers to their long bones. If doxycycline is fed during the second trimester, inbred mice exhibit impaired fetal development proportional to the dose administered.

The principal modifiers of a drug's embryopathic effect are (i) when in gestation, maternal drug therapy is initiated with respect to organogenesis and (ii) its duration of administration. The inhibition of protein synthesis by doxycycline will affect 100% of the fetuses to varying degrees. Data about maternal capacity for drug-binding over 60 days before back spillage in the form of free drug occurs are not currently available.

The absence of pharmacokinetic data as to drug accumulation at the end of 60 days focuses on the potential lethal induction of drug-induced hepatotoxicity. Dose-related hepatotoxicity was observed in pregnant women with the older-generation tetracyclines when they were administered in large doses or when the principal mode of drug elimination was compromised. A syndrome of fulminating hepatic decompensation has been described in pregnant women receiving tetracycline therapy, particularly when the renal portal of elimination is compromised. Direct renal effects include a diminished ability to concentrate urine and a rising serum blood urea nitrogen and creatinine content. The degradation of doxycycline differs from that of the other tetracyclines in that renal clearance is less important, thus providing some measure of safety when renal drug excretion is compromised.

Prophylactic administration of doxycycline for anthrax aerosol exposure by pregnant women requires a careful balancing of risks and benefits. Once antibiotic sensitivities of the attack strain are known, drug therapy should be changed from doxycycline to preferably an FDA Category B antibiotic.

SELECTED READING

Antibiotics in Pregnancy

Adamson K Jr, Joelsson I. The effects of pharmacologic agents upon the fetus and newborn. Am J Obstet Gynecol 1966; 96:437.

Audus KL, Soares MJ, Hunt JS. Characteristics of the fetal/maternal interface with potential usefulness in the development of future immunological and pharmacological strategies. J Pharmacol Exp Ther 2002; 301:402.

Briggs GG, Freeman RK, Yaffe SJ, eds. Drugs in Pregnancy and Lactation. 6th ed. Baltimore: Lippincott Williams & Wilken, 2002.

Charles D. Placental transmission of antibiotics. Br J Obstet Gynaecol 1954; 61:750.

Charles D. Dynamics of antibiotic transfer from mother to fetus. Semin Perinat 1977; 1:89.

Dash JS, Gilstrap LC 3rd. Antibiotics use in pregnancy. Obstet Gynecol Clin North Am 1997; 24:617.

Dunigan NM, Andrews J, Williams JD. Pharmacologic studies with lincomycin in late pregnancy. Br Med J 1973; 3:75.

Filippi B. Antibiotics and congenital malformations: evaluation of the teratogenicity of antibiotics. Adv Teratol 1967; 2:239.

Gibbs RS, Dinsmoor MJ, Newton E.R. Ramamurthy R.S. A randomized trial of intra-partum versus immediate postpartum treatment of women with intra-amniotic fluid infection. Obstet. Gynecol 1988; 72:803.

Good RG, Johnson GH. The placental transfer of kanamycin during late pregnancy. Obstet Gynecol 1971; 38:60.

Larson B, Glover DD. Serum erythromycin levels in pregnancy. Clin Ther 1998; 20:5.

Lucey JF. Drugs and intrauterine patient. Symposium on the placenta. Birth Defects 1965; 1:46.

Mertz HL, Ernest JM. Antibiotics and preterm labor. Curr Womens Health Rep 2001; 1:20.

Niebyl JR. Use of antibiotics for ear, nose, and throat disorders in pregnancy and lactation. Am J Otolaryngol 1992; 13:187.

Pacifici GM, Nottoli R. Placental transfer of drugs administered to the mother. Clin Pharmacokinet 1995; 28:235.

Philipson A, Sabath ND, Charles D. Transplacental passage of erythromycin and clindamycin. N Engl J Med 1973; 288:1219.

Smithells RW. Drugs and human malformations. Adv Teratol 1966; 1:251.

Weinstein AJ, Gibbs RS, Gallagher M. Placental transfer of clindamycin and gentamicin in term pregnancy. Am J Obstet Gynecol 1976; 124:688.

Yoshioko H, Monma T, Matsuda S. Placental transfer of gentamicin. J Pediatr 1972; 80:121.

Tetracyclines: Fetal Considerations (Teratogenic Potential)

Carter MP, Wilson F. Tetracycline and congenital limb abnormalities. Br Med J 1962; 2:407.

Carter MP, Wilson F. Antibiotics and congenital malformations. Lancet 1963; 1:1267.

LeBlanc AL, Perry JE. Transfer of tetracycline across the human placenta. Tex Rep Biol Med 1967; 25:541.

Woollam D, Miller J. Experimental mammalian teratology and the effect of drugs on the embryo. Proc R Soc Med 1963; 56:597.

Dental and Osseous Embryopathy

Cohlan SO, Bevelander G, Tiomsic T. Growth inhibition of the developing skeleton due to tetracycline deposition in bone: clinical and laboratory investigation. Am J Dis Child 1962; 104:480.

Davies PA, Little K, Ahearne W. Tetracyclines and yellow teeth. Lancet 1962; 1:743.

Harcourt JK, Johnson NW, Storey E. In vivo incorporation of tetracycline in teeth of man. Arch Oral Biol 1962; 7:431.

Kline Allen H, Blattner RJ, Lunin M. Transplacental effect of tetracyclines on teeth. J Am Med Assoc 1964; 188:178.

Kutscher Austin H, Zegarelli EV, Tovell HMM, Hochberg B. Discoloration of teeth induced by tetracycline administered antepartum. J Am Med Assoc 1963; 184:586.

Macaulay JC, Leistyna JA. Preliminary observations on the prenatal administration of demethylchlortetracycline HCL. Pediatrics 1964; 34:423.

Rendle-Short TJ. Tetracycline in teeth and bone. Lancet 1962; 1:1188.

Stewart DJ. The effects of tetracyclines upon the dentition. Br J Dermatol 1964; 76:374.

Wallman IS, Hilton HB. Teeth pigmented by tetracyclines. Lancet 1962; 1:827.

Witkop CJ, Wolf RO. Hypoplasia and intrinsic staining of enamel following tetracycline therapy. J Am Med Assoc 1963; 185:1008.

Tetracyclines: Maternal Considerations (Hepatotoxicity)

Allen ES, Brown WE. Hepatic toxicity of tetracycline in pregnancy. Am J Obstet Gynecol 1966; 95:12.

Horwitz ST, Marymont JH Jr. Fetal liver disease during pregnancy associated with tetracycline therapy. Obstet Gynecol 1964; 23:826.

Kunelis CT, Peters JL, Anderson HA. Fatty liver of pregnancy and its relationship to tetracycline therapy. Am J Med 1965; 38:359.

Lepper MH, Wolf CK, Zimmerman HJ, et al. Effect of large doses of aureomycin on human liver. Arch Intern Med 1953; 88:271.

Miller SEP, MacSween RNM, Glen ACA, et al. Experimental studies on the hepatic effects of tetracycline. Br J Exp Pathol 1967; 48:51.

Peters RL, Edmondson HA, Mikkelsen WP, Tatter D. Tetracycline-induced fatty liver in nonpregnant patients—a report of six cases. Am J Surg 1965; 113:622.

Schultz JD, Adamson JS Jr, Workman WW, Norman TD. Fatal liver disease after intravenous administration of tetracycline in high dosage. N Engl J Med 1963; 269:999.

Sheehan HL. The pathology of acute yellow atrophy and delayed chloroform poisoning. J Obstet Gynecol Br Emp 1940; 47:49–62.

Whalley PJ, Adams RH, Combes B. Tetracycline toxicity in pregnancy. J Am Med Assoc 1964; 189:357.

Wruble LD, Ladman AJ, Britt LG, Cumins AT. Hepatotoxicity produced by tetracycline overdosage. J Am Med Assoc 1965; 192:92.

Chloramphenicol

Burns LE, Hodgeman JW, Cass AB. Fatal circulatory collapse in premature infants receiving chloramphenicol. N Engl J Med 1959; 261:1318.

Lamboin MA, Waddel WW Jr, Birdsong M. Chloramphenicol toxicity in the premature infant. Pediatrics 1960; 25:935.

Lischner H, Seligman SJ, Krammer A, Parmelee AH Jr. An outbreak of neonatal deaths among term infants associated with administration of chloramphenicol. J Pediatr 1961; 59:21.

Morton K. Chloramphenicol overdose in a six-week old infant. Am J Dis Child 1961; 102:430.

Pendleton ME, Jewett JF. Three unexpected neonatal deaths. N Engl J Med 1960; 263:515.

Ross S, Burke RG, Sites J, et al. Placental transmission of chloramphenicol (Chloromycetin). J Am Med Assoc 1950; 142:1361.

Scott WC, Warner RF. Placental transfer of chloramphenicol (Chloromycetin). J Am Med Assoc 1950; 142:1331.

Snyder MJ, Woodward TE. The clinical use of chloramphenicol. Med Clin North Am 1970; 54:1187.

Sutherland JM. Fatal cardiovascular collapse of infants receiving large amounts of chloramphenicol. Am J Dis Child 1959; 97:761.

Weiss CF, Glazko AJ, Weston JK. Chloramphenicol in the newborn infant: a physiological explanation of its toxicity when given in excessive doses. N Engl J Med 1960; 262:787.

Fluoroquinolones

Loebstein R, Addis A, Ho E, et al. Pregnancy outcome following gestational exposure to fluoroquinolones: a multi-center prospective controlled study. Antimicrob Agents Chemother 1998; 42:1336.

Wogelus P, Norgaard M, Gislum M, et al. Further analysis of the risk of adverse birth outcomes after maternal. Int J Antimicrob Agents 2005; 26:323.

Doxycycline

Cole AA, Chubinskaya S, Luchene LJ, et al. Doxycycline disrupts chondrocyte differentiation and inhibits cartilage matrix degradation. Arthritis Rheum 1994; 37:1727.

Davies SR, Cole AA, Schmid TM. Doxycycline inhibits type X collagen synthesis in avian hypertrophic chondrocyte cultures. J Biol Chem 1997; 63:11.

Moutier R, Tchang F, Caucheteux SM, et al. Placental anomalies and fetal loss in mice after administration of doxycycline in food for tet-system activation. Transgenic Res 2003; 12:369.

Richardson M, Wong D, Lacroix S, et al. Inhibition by doxycycline of angiogenesis in chicken chorioallantoic membrane. Cancer Chemother Pharmacol 2005; 5:1.

Siddiqui MA, Janjua MZ. The effects of prenatal doxycycline administration on skeletal differentiation in ling bones of Albino rats. J Pak Med Assoc 2002; 52:211.

Sulfonamides

Fichter EG, Curtis JA. Sulfonamide administration in newborn and premature infants. Am J Dis Child 1955; 90:596.

Harris RC, Lucey JF, MacLean JR. Kernicterus in premature infants associated with low concentrations of bilirubin in the plasma. Pediatrics 1958; 21:875.

Johnson L, Sarmiento F, Blanc WA, Day R. Kernicterus in rats with an inherited deficiency of glucuronyl transferase. Am J Dis Child 1959; 97:591.

Nyhan WL. Toxicity of drugs in the neonatal period. J Pediatr 1961; 59:1.

Odell GB. Studies in kernicterus. I. The protein binding to the bilirubin. J Clin Invest 1959; 38:823.

Odell GB. The dissociation of bilirubin from albumin and its clinical implications. J Pediatr 1959; 55:268.

Silverman WA, Andersen DH, Blane WA, Crozier DN. A difference in mortality rate and incidence of kernicterus among premature infants allotted to two prophylactic antibacterial regimens. Pediatrics 1956; 18:614.

Streptomycin

Boletti M, Croato L. Sulla sordita da passaggio transplacentara di stretomicina (con illustrazione di un caso). Acta Paediatr Latina 1958; 11:1.

Conway N, Birt BD. Streptomycin in pregnancy: effect on foetal ear. Br Med J 1965; 2:260.

Kern G. Zur Frage der intrauterinen Streptomycinschadigung. Schweiz Med Wochenschr 1962; 92:77.

Rebattu JP, Lesner G, Megard M. Streptomycine, barriere placentaire, troubles cochleovestibulaires. J Fr Otorhinolaryngol 1960; 9:411.

Robinson GC, Combon KG. Hearing loss in infants of tuberculous mothers treated with streptomycin during pregnancy. N Engl J Med 1964; 271:949.

Sakula A. Streptomycin and foetus. Br J Tuberc 1954; 48:69.

Swift P. Streptomycin in fetal blood. Br Med J 1950; 2:787.

Isoniazid

Centers for Disease Control. Isoniazid-associated hepatitis. Morb Mortal Wkly Rep 1974; 23:97.

Charles D, MacAulay M. Use of antibiotics in obstetrics practice. Clin Obstet Gynecol 1970; 13:255.

Garibaldi RA, Drusin RE, Ferebee SH, Gregg MB. Isoniazid-associated hepatitis; report of an outbreak. Am Rev Respir Dis 1972; 106:357.

Ludford J, Doster B, Woolpert SF. Effect of isoniazid on reproduction. Am Rev Resp Dis 1973; 108:1170.

Maddrey WC, Boitnoff JK. Isoniazid hepatitis. Ann Intern Med 1973; 79:300.

Monnet P, Kalb JC, Pujol M. Toxic influence of Isoniazid on fetus. Lyon Med 1967; 218:431.

Varpela E. On the effect exerted by first line tuberculosis medicines on the fetus. Acta Tuberc Scand 1964; 45:53.

Miscellaneous Drugs

Goodman LS, Gilman A. The Pharmacological Basis of Therapeutics. 5th ed. New York: Macmillan, 1975.

Potworowska M, Sianozecka E, Szufladowicz R. Ethionamide treatment and pregnancy. Polish Med J 1966; 4:1152.

Antibiotics in Breast Milk

Catz SC, Giacola GP. Drugs and breast milk. Pediatr Clin North Am 1972; 19:151.

Knowles JA. Excretion of drugs in milk—a review. J Pediatr 1960; 66:1068.

Lien EJ, Kuwahara J, Koda RT. Diffusion of drugs into prostatic fluid and milk. Drug Intell Clin Pharm 1974; 8:470.

O'Brien TE. Excretion of drugs in human milk. Am J Hosp Pharm 1974; 31:844.

Vorherr H. Drug excretion in breast milk. Postgrad Med 1974; 56:97.

Timing of Antibiotic Therapy

FEVER

Fever has been the traditional early warning system to the physician for indicating the development of infectious complications as well as primary disease.

WHAT CONSTITUTES AN ABNORMAL TEMPERATURE

Any temperature greater than or equal to 38°C is abnormal. Any range of temperature between 37.6 and 37.9°C is called the "gray zone." It is a mandate, not for action but for concern. Should an abnormal temperature develop from a set of temperatures that have been in the gray zone, the probability of infection is great.

When monitoring a patient at high risk for an infectious complication, early-morning temperatures before breakfast often are harbingers of the subsequent temperature patterns. If the early-morning temperature is elevated above the anticipated baseline, the patient's temperature will probably spike in the late afternoon. The best action that can be practiced is administering preventive medicine; the next best is early intervention.

A significant number of patients with endomyometritis following cesarean section will have very minimal localized findings. Most patients have a significant amount of inflammatory induration involving the vaginal cuff following vaginal hysterectomy. Temperature elevations are often a mandate to an aggressive fever work-up. In the absence of a demonstrable nongenital cause for the fever, a commitment to exclude operative site disease is implemented. The following criteria have been derived primarily from patients with endomyometritis following cesarean section; however, they have proven to be highly adaptive for the majority of postoperative infectious complications.

1. Any temperature greater than or equal to 38.6°C. Obtain an immediate second reading, and if it confirms the validity of the initial reading, institute an immediate fever work-up.
2. Any two temperatures equal to 38°C or greater taken four hours apart for which the second temperature is higher by 0.2° than the first.
3. Three temperatures equal to 38°C or greater in any 24-hour period. The significance of temperature is in the first 24 hours postoperatively.

The standard definition of the American College of Obstetricians and Gynecologists disregards the validity of relatively minor temperature elevation in the first 24 hours (less than 38.6°C). These elevations are frequently attributed to postoperative atelectasis, urinary tract infection, and, in postpartum patients, breast engorgement. Unless associated with aspiration, atelectasis is not a cause of fever. One can tie off a bronchus and not induce fever. The incidence of postoperative atelectasis in oncology patients undergoing radical surgery documented by serial blood gases approaches 100%. Up to 20% of patients will have some roentgenographic evidence of atelectasis, yet the incidence of fever in this group is remarkably low in the first 24 hours. Finding greater than 100,000 colonies/mL of a single bacterial species in a urine specimen documents the presence of asymptomatic bacteriuria. Unless costovertebral angle tenderness or severe suprapubic and/or back pain is present, urinary tract infections are not a cause of fever.

When seeking an etiology for the development of febrile morbidity following an operative procedure, homage should be paid to Willie Sutton's first law: "Go where the gold is." Make a working hypothesis of operative site infection and then try to prove it wrong.

ANTICIPATED THERAPEUTIC RESPONSE

When dealing with monoetiological disease due to *Neisseria gonorrhoeae* or *Streptococcus pneumoniae* pneumonia, the response is often dramatic. The precipitous drop in temperature in response to appropriate antibiotic therapy is termed a monoetiological response. If the organ system in which disease occurs is prone to compartmentalization with varying patterns of perfusion, i.e., the kidney, the probability of seeing a pure mono-etiological curve is diminished. Most postoperative infections in obstetrics and gynecology are due to polymicrobial infection. With appropriate therapy, the time interval for normalization tends to be prolonged owing to the superimposition of multiple kill curves. Irrespective of whether it is monoetiological or polymicrobial therapy, the anticipated therapeutic result is the same. The patient should be afebrile within 24 to 36 hours. As long as each succeeding temperature is lower than the preceding temperature, even though it is above 38.6°C, one can still maintain a valid commitment to the antibiotic regimen utilized. Similarly, if, after 12 hours of antibiotic therapy, the patient's temperature continues to rise, it is unlikely the patient will benefit from 12 more hours of the same therapy. If a patient does not respond within 48 hours, one should question the validity of either the initial diagnosis or the antibiotic therapy.

A patient whose temperature comes down slowly over four or five days is a patient who is "curing herself." The initial antibiotic has contributed to her recovery by eliminating part of the bacterial flora, which could potentiate the infectious morbidity. But unless disease involves a site where bioavailability of antibiotic is a problem, the continued administration of antibiotics beyond five days is more

TIMING OF ANTIBIOTIC THERAPY ■ 25

for the physician's well-being than the patient's. If the patient is not responding to antibiotic therapy after 48 hours, both the patient and the physician have a problem.

ANTIBIOTIC ADMINISTRATION

The maximum dosage that can be safely administered should be given in the first 24 hours for concentration antibiotics. For time-dependant antibiotics, initial aggressive dosing is advocated for the first 24 hours. Thereafter, dosage should be cut back or tapered to the minimum dose appropriate unless there is a problem of bioavailability of drug, i.e., meningitis, septic arthritis, abscess formation, or reticuloendothelial intracellular sites of bacterial replication.

In most instances, the battle is usually won or lost in the first 24 hours. If won, subsequent drug administration is more medicolegal than therapeutic. If lost, the patient needs appropriate therapy, not more of the same. If infectious complications develop following the preoperative administration of an antibiotic, the use of an antibiotic with the same spectrum of coverage is not recommended.

WHEN TO DISCONTINUE PARENTERAL ANTIBIOTICS

The initial commitment to parenteral administration of antibiotics for hospitalized patients is totally warranted. The basic question is how long do you sustain this commitment? The decision as to when to discontinue parenteral antibiotic for oral administration is one that requires a great deal of individualization. The primary consideration is the drug's bioavailability with oral administration. Ideally, the conversion antibiotic should have 90% or greater bioavailability with oral administration. Conversion from intravenous to oral mode of antibiotic administration can be done 24 hours after evidence of resolution of infectious complication unless contraindicated by ileus, intestinal hypermotility, etc. Most patients can be converted to oral antibiotics within 24 hours after resolution of all evidence of infectious morbidity.

Early conversion to oral antibiotics reduces intravenous catheter-induced or related morbidity. Parent-eral antibiotics cost seven to ten times what the equivalent dose of oral medication costs.

AMBULATORY PARENTERAL ANTIBIOTIC THERAPY

Within obstetrics and gynecology, a rare instance may arise in which extended antimicrobial therapy is required. Cost considerations have been the driving force in developing ambulatory parenteral antibiotic therapy. The potential clinical situations requiring prolonged antimicrobial therapies tend to necessitate administration of aminoglycosides, amphotericin B, or vancomycin. Both the aminoglycosides and amphotericin B are concentration-dependent antimicrobials. Drug concentration at the critical target sites influences efficacy. Vancomycin is a time-dependent antibiotic. Care must be given to assure that drug concentration be about two to four times above the minimal inhibitory concentration for killing to proceed at a zero order rate. With appropriate care to dosage of drug, all three antimicrobial agents can be parenterally administered once a day.

SELECTED READING

DeMaio J. Outpatient parenteral antibiotic therapy. Infect Med 2004; 21:496.

Antibiotic-Induced Diarrhea

INTRODUCTION

Pseudomembranous enterocolitis (PME) is the consequence of filterable, heat-labile enterotoxin and cytotoxin elaborated by selected strains of *Clostridium difficile*. In selected cases, the antibiotic in question eradicates that portion of the gastrointestinal tract flora that suppresses the growth of *C. difficile*. The loss of bacterial interference permits the resistant *C. difficile* to numerically partially fill the biologic void created and, in so doing, elaborate the toxins. A single dose of an antibiotic given for cesarean section prophylaxis is capable of inducing disease. Privitera et al. (1991) studied *C. difficile* intestinal colonization following a single 2 g intravenous dose of either cephalosporin or mezlocillin. *C. difficile* was detected in 23% of patients who had received cephalosporin, in 3.3% of patients given mezlocillin, and in none of the 15 controls who had been given no antibiotics.

The probability of PME appears to be partially influenced by the route of antibiotic administration. This is particularly true of clindamycin. The incidence of this complication is significantly more frequent with oral administration than with parenteral administration.

The clinical manifestations of antibiotic-induced diarrhea are quite variable, running a spectrum from mild, nuisance diarrhea, which resolves spontaneously, to severe infections characterized by pseudomembranous colitis, toxic megacolon, or colonic perforation. In approximately 30% of cases, symptoms develop as late as several weeks after discontinuation of antibiotics.

A large number of antibiotics have functioned as inciting drugs for PME (Table 1). Antibiotics with significant activity against anaerobic bacteria alter the gut microbial ecosystem and put the patient at a greater risk for antibiotic-induced diarrhea. The use of multiple antimicrobial agents as well as more prolonged course of therapy further increases the potential of *C. difficile* colitis.

Initial symptomatology is simply that of an increased number of bowel movements (diarrheal syndrome). Symptoms of PME include cramping, hypogastric pain, profuse watery diarrhea (often with occult blood), and fever, usually not exceeding 38.9° C, in addition to small-bowel diarrhea. Symptoms usually evolve within three to nine days after antibiotic therapy is started. Definitive diagnosis of pseudomembranous colitis is made by proctoscopy. Raised, plaque-like pseudomembranes associated with erythema and edema are diagnostic of disease, with the degree depending on the severity of involvement (Fig. 1). Patients with diarrhea without pseudomembranes will exhibit only minimal edema without much overt inflammation.

Regardless of which condition is present, antibiotic therapy should be immediately discontinued. If antibiotic therapy is continued in a patient with pseudomembranous colitis, the proctoscopic findings become worse; the plaques gradually enlarge and coalesce. In the diarrheal syndrome, there is prompt amelioration of symptoms with the cessation of drug therapy. Patients with pseudomembranous colitis may continue to have multiple bowel movements for two to three weeks following discontinuation of therapy. In general, the longer the drug is given to patients with pseudomembranous colitis, the more prolonged the diarrhea is and the longer the proctoscopic examination is abnormal. In the absence of aggressive therapy, PME may progress to toxic megacolon, perforation of the bowel wall, peritonitis, and endotoxic shock.

DIAGNOSIS

Any patient who develops three or more uniform stools per day for at least two days in the setting of exposure to antimicrobial or antineoplastic agents can be considered to have antibiotic-associated diarrhea. Except in critically ill patients, laboratory evaluation is the principal diagnostic approach. *C. difficile* produces three virulence factors: an enterotoxin (toxin A), a cytotoxin (toxin B), and a substance that inhibits intestinal motility. Enzyme immunoassay (EIA) detects the presence of toxin A or B in stool filtrates and is a rapid technique for diagnosing *C. difficile* infection. The EIA assay has sensitivity and specificity ranges of 50% to 90% and 70% to 95%, respectively. Because of its low sensitivity, a repeat testing is ordered when a high index of suspicion exists.

Polymerase chain reaction detects toxigenic *C. difficile* by amplification of the toxin A or B gene or both genes. The cytotoxin assay detects toxin B in stool filtrates by observing the characteristic cytotoxin changes that this toxin produces in standardized tissue culture cell lines. Diagnostically, *C. difficile* cell culture cytotoxin assay is the gold standard with sensitivity and specificity of 93% and 89%, respectively.

A correctly performed stool culture is extremely sensitive in detecting the presence of *C. difficile*. Recovery of the

TABLE 1 Drugs with potential for PME

Level I: antibiotics commonly associated with PME
- Penicillin, penicillin/beta-lactamase inhibitors, cephalosporins, and clindamycin

Level II: antibiotics and drugs associated with PME
- Antibiotics: chloramphenicol, erythromycin, lincomycin, imipenem-cilastatin, quinolones, rifampin, tetracycline, trimethoprim-sulfamethoxazole
- Antineoplastics: doxorubicin, cisplatin, cyclophosphamide, fluorouracil, methotrexate

Level III: antibiotics rarely associated with PME
- Aminoglycosides, metronidazole, vancomycin

Abbreviation: PME, pseudomembranous enterocolitis.

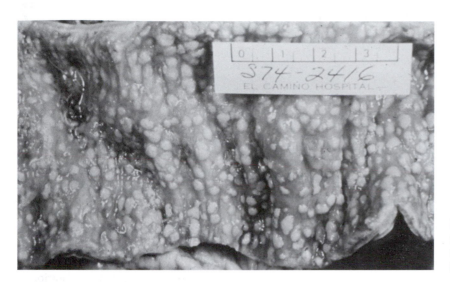

FIGURE 1 Raised, plaque-like pseudomembranes in the colon of a patient who died with clindamycin-induced enterocolitis. *Source:* Courtesy of S. Kabins, MD, Chicago, IL.

organism from stool culture does not document causability. About 25% to 60% of hospitalized patients, 10% to 25% of infants, and 3% of the general population in the United States are asymptomatic carriers of *C. difficile*. Not all strains of *C. difficile* are toxigenic. Definite diagnosis necessitates the identification of *C. difficile* toxin in the stool.

C. difficile is responsible for 10% to 15% of all cases of antibiotic-associated diarrhea and greater than 97% of all cases of antibiotic-associated pseudomembranous colitis. *Klebsiella oxytoca* has been implicated as the etiologic agent in antibiotic-associated hemorrhagic colitis. Patients who develop symptoms several days after completion of antibiotic therapy are at much higher risk of having antibiotic-associated diarrhea than nonspecific diarrhea. Individuals with a prior history of antibiotic-associated diarrhea who again develop diarrhea are likely to be infected with *C. difficile*. For those two categories of patients, empiric therapy with metronidazole or vancomycin should be considered while the cause of the diarrhea is being determined. In severe cases, flexible sigmoidoscopy can provide an immediate diagnosis.

Because of the progressive increase of *C. difficile* colonization in the community and, especially, in nursing homes, any woman admitted with severe diarrhea needs to be evaluated for *C. difficile* A and B toxins.

THERAPY

Whenever a patient is placed on antibiotic therapy, logging of a daily stool count is recommended. When the number of bowel movements increases to three per day for two days, antibiotic therapy should be discontinued.

If a patient develops diarrhea while on an antibiotic, the antibiotic should be discontinued immediately (Table 2). Electrolyte evaluations should be obtained and any electrolyte abnormalities corrected while carefully restoring the intravascular volume. If the diarrhea stops within 48 hours, there is no need for further evaluation. If diarrhea persists or other symptoms consistent with disease are present, the patient needs to be staged by proctoscopy.

Vancomycin has been the treatment of choice for severe antibiotic-associated diarrhea (Table 3). Metro-nidazole, bacitracin, teicoplanin, and fusidic acid are as effective as vancomycin for initial symptomatic resolution. Current evidence leads to uncertainty whether mild antibiotic-associated diarrhea needs to be treated. Patients with mild disease may resolve their symptoms as quickly without treatment. Metronidazole is the first drug of choice for antibiotic-associated diarrhea. Treatment with oral vancomycin is usually reserved for patients who have contraindications or intolerance to or who have failed to respond to metronidazole.

Vancomycin is given orally in doses of 125 mg four times daily for 10 days. This is directed against the etiologic agent. The drug must be given orally to provide high colonic levels. Once the drug is stopped, approximately 8% to 20% of patients treated will experience a relapse, with a recurrence of symptoms associated with reappearance of *C. difficile* toxin in the stool.

Metronidazole given a single 1.5 g per day dose for 10 days has achieved cure rates of 92% to 95%. However, in rare cases, this drug has been implicated as the precipitating agent of antibiotic-associated colitis.

Individuals experiencing relapse tend to be older and have had a higher frequency of recent surgery than those that did not relapse. Relapses are usually due to the persistence of antibiotic-resistant *C. difficile* spores rather than the development of antibiotic resistance by the vegetative

TABLE 2 Protocol for patients developing diarrhea while on antibiotics

1. (A) Discontinue antibiotics immediately. (B) Obtain electrolyte evaluations. (C) Correct any electrolyte abnormality while carefully restoring intravascular volume. (D) Pepto Bismol can be given, but avoid antiperistaltic drugs
2. If diarrhea stops within 24 hr, there is no need to institute further therapy
3. If diarrhea persists, examine patient with a proctosigmoidoscope. If raised yellowish-white plaques 2–5 mm in size superimposed on edematous colonic mucosa are identified, the patient has pseudomembranous enterocolitis—put the bowel to rest and obtain consultation from gastrointestinal medicine

TABLE 3 Therapy for pseudomembranous enterocolitis

Regimen of choice	Alternate regimen
Metronidazole: oral, 500 mg tid or 250 mg qid for 10 days	Vancomycin: oral 125–500 mg qid for 10 days or bacitracin[a]: oral, 25,000 units qid for 10 days

[a]Bacitracin therapy has a markedly inferior cure and relapse rate.

organism. In patients with relapses, re-treatment with the initial antibiotic achieves a greater than 90% cure rate. Recently, an experimental parenteral C. *difficile* vaccine containing toxoids A and B has been developed for potential therapeutic use in patients with multirecurrent C. *difficile*–associate diarrhea.

The emergence of vancomycin-resistant enterococci and/or staphylococci may influence drug therapy for antibiotic-associated diarrhea within a given institution.

NOSOCOMIAL COLONIZATION

Colonization, and subsequent disease, due to C. *difficile* is a potential nosocomial problem. When a nosocomial outbreak occurs, identification of asymptomatic carriers and their treatment have been effective in aborting the outbreak. However, for asymptomatic carriers, placebo administration can be as effective as vancomycin or metronidazole in eliminating C. *difficile*.

A heightened awareness of possible nosocomial transmission within intensive care units is necessary to prevent or arrest future clusters of cases. The diagnosis of one patient with this infection in a unit should prompt a review of all other patients within the unit. Implementation of a comprehensive hospital infection control policy has been effective in reducing the incidence of antibiotic-associated diarrhea.

Enteric infection control procedures including isolation of infected patients and frequent hand washing are additional important measures, which should be taken to minimize the development and spread of this nosocomial infection.

SELECTED READING

Alef K. *Clostridium difficile*-associated disease: implications for midwifery practice. J Nurse Midwifery 1999; 44:19.

Arsura EL, Fazio RA, Wickemesinghe PC. Pseudomembranous colitis following prophylactic antibiotic use in primary cesarean section. Am J Obstet Gynecol 1985; 151:87.

Bartlett JG. *Clostridium difficile*: clinical considerations. Rev Infect Dis 1990; 12(Suppl. 2):S243.

Bricker E, Garg R, Nelson R, et al. Antibiotic treatment of *Clostridium difficile*-associated diarrhea in adults. Cochrane Database Syst Rev 2005; CD004610.

Fekety R, Shah AB. Diagnosis and treatment of *Clostridium difficile* colitis. J Am Med Assoc 1993; 279:71.

Foulke GE, Silva J Jr. Clostridium difficile in the intensive care unit: management problems and prevention issues. Crit Care Med 1989; 17:822.

Gerding D, Johnson S, Peterson LR, et al. *Clostridium difficile*-associated diarrhea and colitis. Infect Control Hosp Epidemiol 1995; 16:459.

Guslandi M. Antibiotics for inflammatory bowel disease: do they work? Eur J Gastroenterol Hepatol 2005; 17:145.

Johnson S, Gerding DN. *Clostridium difficile*-associated diarrhea. Clin Infect Dis 1998; 26:1027.

Kelly CP, LaMont JT. *Clostridium difficile* infection. Annu Rev Med 1998; 49:375.

Kerr RB, McLaughlin DI, Sonnenberg LW. Control of *Clostridium difficile* colitis outbreak by treating asymptomatic carriers with metronidazole. Am J Infect Control 1990; 18:332.

McFarland LV, Mulligan ME, Kwok RYY, Stamm WE. Nosocomial acquisition of *Clostridium difficile* infection. N Engl J Med 1989; 320:205.

Mohan SC, McDermott BP, Parchuri S, Cunha BA. Lack of value of repeat stool testing for *Clostridium difficile* toxin. Am J Med 2006; 119:356.

Privitera G, Scarpellini P, Ortisi G, et al. Prospective study of *Clostridium difficile* intestinal colonization and disease following single-dose antibiotic prophylaxis in surgery. Antimicrob Agents Chemother 1991; 35:208.

Reinke CM, Messick CR. Update on *Clostridium difficile*-induced colitis, part 1. Am J Hosp Pharm 1994; 51:1771.

Satin AJ, Harrison CR, Hancock KC, Zahn CM. Relapsing *Clostridium difficile* toxin-associated colitis in ovarian cancer patients treated with chemotherapy. Obstet Gynecol 1989; 74:487.

Schroder O, Gerhard R, Stein J. Die antibiottika-assoziierte diarrho. Z Gastrointesterol 2006; 44:193.

Schroeder MS. *Clostridium difficile*-associated diarrhea. Am Fam Physician 2005; 71:921.

Sougioultzis S, Kyne L, Drudy D, et al. *Clostridium difficile* toxoid vaccine in recurrent C. *difficile*-associated diarrhea. Gastroenterology 2005; 128:764.

Surawicz CM, McFarland LV, Elmer G, Chinn J. Treatment of recurrent *Clostridium difficile* colitis with vancomycin and *Saccharomyces boulardii*. Am J Gastroenterol 1989; 84:1285.

Yarinsky S, Wheeler WE. Inappropriate antibiotic use and the development of *Clostridium difficile* colitis. W V Med J 1990; 86:239.

Waggoner SE, Barter J, Delgado G, Barnes W. Case–control analysis of *Clostridium difficile*-associated diarrhea on a gynecologic oncology service. Infect Dis Obstet Gynecol 1994; 2:154.

Prophylactic Antibiotics

INTRODUCTION

In women undergoing abdominal surgical procedures, the prophylactic administration of any antibiotic that is effective against the predominantly gram-positive spectrum will reduce in a statistically significant manner infectious morbidity in the postoperative period.

GROUND RULES FOR ANTIBIOTIC PROPHYLAXIS

Six guidelines governing the prophylactic use of antibiotics in obstetrical surgery were developed by Ledger:

1. Limit antibiotic use to a high-risk situation.
2. Establish tissue levels of the antibiotic before the incision.
3. Give a short course of therapy to minimize dose-related adverse drug reactions.
4. Use second- or third-line antibiotics.
5. Choose antibiotics that are effective against the anticipated pathogenic spectrum.
6. Be sure that benefits outweigh the possibility of an adverse drug reaction.

Limit Use to a High-Risk Situation

The purpose of prophylactic antibiotics is to avert the serious infections, which may intervene. Women with antedating problems (chronic cervicitis, repeated episodes of sexually transmitted disease with or without structural damage) and abnormal vaginal flora [bacterial vaginosis (BV) or bacterial excess syndrome (BES)] and individuals in whom hemostasis will be difficult to obtain for physiologic or anatomic reasons, or in whom surgery is anticipated to be difficult, are at augmented risk.

Establish Tissue Levels of the Antibiotic Before Incision

The theoretical basis for this guideline emanates from the experiments of Miles and Miles and their subsequent reduplication a decade later by Burke (1961). Both sets of investigators demonstrated in animal model systems that antibiotics administered before or simultaneously with local challenge with bacteria susceptible to the selected antibiotic were highly effective in aborting the infectious disease, whereas if the antibiotic was given as late as four hours after the microbes had been inoculated, it was essentially worthless. This preoperative interim has been called the "decisive period." Although this concept is probably valid in selected instances (e.g., for the orthopedic surgeon doing a total hip replacement who is concerned with coagulase-negative staphylococci), it is probably not as valid for vaginal hysterectomies. Postoperative infection, in these circumstances, is due to a polymicrobial infection. Consequently, antibiotic administration beyond the "decisive period" will be relatively effective. Rather than precluding initiation of the anaerobic progression, it would interrupt it prior to the induction of disease.

Minimize Dose-Related Adverse Reactions

The concept of minimizing the duration of therapy in order to minimize dose-related adverse reactions is endorsed in all situations in which antibiotics are administered prophylactically. It is probable that one can achieve a statistically comparable effect on the incidence of disease following cesarean section with a single bolus preoperative administration of an appropriate antibiotic as has been achieved with three-dose, three-day, and five-day regimens. There is no rationale for prolonged administration.

The antibiotic chosen for infection avoidance needs to be given in the immediate preoperative period. With more prolonged surgery, which is anticipated to exceed the antibiotic's half-life of efficacy, intraoperative administration of a second dose of the antibiotic has become standard procedure.

Use of a Second- or Third-Line Antibiotic

The goal in this instance is to minimize the emergence of strains that are resistant to the antibiotic in question. Cephalosporins, being second-line antibiotics and having little applicability in the practice of obstetrics and gynecology, fit this guideline ideally.

Antibiotics for the Anticipated Pathogens

What is achieved with the cephalosporins is the eradication of the minor constituents of the vaginal flora—corynebacteria, propionibacteria, lactobacilli, *Gardnerella vaginalis*, coagulase-negative staphylococci, viridans streptococci, some of the Enterobacteriaceae, etc.—leaving behind the enterococci, the cephalosporin-resistant Enterobacteriaceae, and the penicillin-resistant Bacteroidaceae. The cephalosporins do not effectively cover the anticipated pathogenic spectrum of polymicrobial infection, but can frequently disrupt the anaerobic progression.

Benefits Must Outweigh the Possibility of a Reaction

The potential for adverse drug reactions must be considerably less than the risk of postoperative infection when an antibiotic is given prophylactically. There must be a careful balancing of risks and benefits. The cephalosporins have been responsible for a number of surgical deaths due to anaphylaxis in cases in which the drugs were used prophylactically.

MECHANISM OF ACTION OF PROPHYLACTIC ANTIBIOTICS

Qualitative bacteriologic studies of women undergoing vaginal hysterectomy have shown that there are alterations of the bacteriologic flora as a consequence of the operative procedure, which occur independent of the selective influences of antibiotics. Only very rarely do preoperative antibiotics "sterilize" the posterior vaginal pool with any degree of regularity. Subsequent quantitative bacteriologic studies have shown that the reductions achieved in the total aerobic and anaerobic counts are transient. Postoperatively, the total aerobic and anaerobic counts approximate or exceed those obtained in the preoperative period. Prophylactic antibiotics eradicate selective constituents of the vaginal flora. The bacteria that have been eliminated are not usually considered to have pathogenic significance. After the prophylactic administration of a semisynthetic penicillin or a cephalosporin, the penicillin-resistant Bacteroidaceae including *Bacteroides fragilis*, *Prevotella* species, members of the Enterobacteriaceae, and the enterococci emerge as the dominant constituents of the vaginal flora. In short, we eradicate the nonpathogenic bacteria and leave behind the endogenous organisms, which have a recognized capacity to function as prime pathogens. Similarly, transient vaginal degerming with povidone–iodine has been shown to decrease the incidence of postcesarean endometritis, but had no demonstrable effect on the risk of wound infections.

The obvious question is "why then do prophylactic antibiotics work?" The answer appears to be that they interrupt the potential for the anaerobic progression. They eradicate the "facilitating flora," which may transform the microbiologic environment into one conducive for the replication of obligate anaerobes. Tangible evidence supporting this thesis has been gleaned by various investigators. Using meticulous surgical techniques and suction drainage, they were able to achieve results comparable to those observed with prophylactic antibiotics. The presumed reasons have to do with the understanding of the pathogenesis of anaerobic infection. Being gentle with tissue—practicing good hemostasis, using small clamps to minimize the amount of crush injury, and removing all foreign bodies—minimizes the probability of creating a microbiologic environment in which the oxidation–reduction potential is conducive to anaerobic infection. The use of T-tube drainage demonstrated that, after iatrogenically creating a microbiologic environment that will select for the anaerobic progression, mechanically removing it can circumvent the ensuing infectious morbidity. The studies on prophylactic antibiotics seem to corroborate this thesis. When Swartz attempted to use prophylactic antibiotics in conjunction with T-tube drainage, he was unable to alter his percentages in a statistically significant manner. This observation implies that both T-tube drainage and prophylactic antibiotics operate on the same mechanism, though presumably at different points.

PERIOPERATIVE ANTIBIOTICS TO PREVENT POSTPARTUM ENDOMETRITIS FOLLOWING CESAREAN SECTION

Prior to 1974, infections were the second leading cause of mortality in women undergoing cesarean section. The therapeutic efficacy of perioperative antibiotics in preventing postoperative infectious complications in patients undergoing vaginal hysterectomy prompted the clinical application of this concept to patients undergoing cesarean section. As in the case of patients undergoing vaginal hysterectomy, a statistically significant reduction in operative site infectious morbidity was demonstrated. Almost irrespective of the previous incidence of postcesarean endometritis, perioperative antibiotics will reduce the figure by at least 50%.

Not all women undergoing cesarean section are at equal risk for the development of postoperative endometritis. The risk of infection following cesarean section is markedly influenced by the socioeconomic status of the woman, duration of labor, rupture of the fetal membranes and/or labor, presence of an abnormal endogenous vaginal flora, presence of asymptomatic bacteriuria or known pathogen within the vaginal flora, presence of asymptomatic bacteriuria, and the operative skills of the surgeon.

Prior to the utilization of preoperative antibiotics, the incidence of endometritis following cesarean section varied between 35% and 60% in teaching hospitals as contrasted to private institutions in which the incidence of infection was usually below 20%.

Once a patient is designated as being at augmented risk for postoperative infection, the antibiotic for administration and the time of its administration should be selected so as to make it cost effective for the patient and to minimize potential effects on the bacterial flora of the newborn and neonatal intensive care nurseries.

The need to establish effective antibiotic concentration within tissues prior to making the initial incision is paramount to its effectiveness. Classen et al. (1992) observed a greater than sevenfold increase when prophylactic antibiotics were administered more than two hours before the operation when compared with cases in which drug administration occurred within the currently designated two-hour period. The use of perioperative antibiotics in women at the time of parturition differs from that in women undergoing vaginal or abdominal hysterectomy in that the physician treating a woman at the time of parturition is treating not one but rather two biologically unique individuals. All antibiotics, to one degree or another, traverse the placental barrier so that invariably a neonate whose mother was treated with antibiotics during parturition would be sent to the newborn nursery with a serum antibiotic level that in time could influence the composition of the bacterial flora of the newborn and neonatal intensive care nursery. The impact on the bacterial flora probably would be less significant if the antibiotic utilized had a limited spectrum of susceptibility that was restricted to the gram-positive bacteria; however, the second- and third-generation cephalosporins, because of their efficacy against selected members of the Enterobacteriaceae, theoretically could adversely influence the constituency of aerobic gram-negative bacterial flora. The first-generation cephalosporins do not penetrate the placental barrier well; consequently, suboptimal levels in newborn serum and amniotic fluid are achieved. Repetitive exposure to suboptimal concentrations of an antibiotic is a recognized mechanism for the in vitro induction of antibiotic resistance.

Clinical studies have demonstrated that the endogenous bacteria that cause postpartum endometritis can often be demonstrated in amniotic fluid at the time of cesarean section. Bacterial access to the endometrial cavity prior to parturition is a major factor that selects for disease. Those factors that enhance bacterial access prior to parturition are associated with an increased incidence of endometritis following cesarean section. The incidence of disease is significantly augmented for gravidae who are in active labor or who experience prolonged rupture of the fetal membranes in contradistinction to patients who undergo elective cesarean section.

The work of Burke (1961) was done in a closed animal system employing a single pathogen (*Staphylococcus aureus*). The postpartum endometrial cavity is an open system with physical continuity with the endocervical and vaginal bacterial flora. Disease is usually either the consequence of polymicrobial infection or due to a monoetiologic pathogen with enhanced virulence. The mechanism by which perioperative antibiotics aborted infection in the animal model system of Burke (2001) is eradication of the causative agent. The mechanism by which antibiotics most often decrease the incidence of postcesarean endometritis is by eradicating the so-called facilitating flora; more specifically, the bacteria within the vagina, which can accelerate alteration of the oxidation–reduction potential of the microbiologic environments to that point where no further lowering of the oxidation–reduction potential is required to ensure the replication of a single anaerobic genus of bacteria Postoperative administration of antibiotics achieves alteration of infectious morbidity by impacting on disease in evolution.

The drug advocated by the author to avert infectious morbidity following cesarean section is ampicillin. The reasons for its selection are its cost, spectrum of coverage, bioavailability in amniotic fluid, and ability to be integrated into the concept of triple therapy should infectious complications develop in the postpartum period. If endomyometritis does develop, it is not necessary to restart ampicillin. The existing gaps in the Gainesville Classification can be closed with clindamycin or metronidazole and an aminoglycoside, thus achieving the coverage of triple therapy. Ampicillin should be administered when the decision is made to commit to abdominal delivery and continued until parturition has been achieved plus one dose. Not waiting until the cord is clamped will favorably impact on the incidence of perinatal septicemia. Three decades of abuse of ampicillin in the neonatal intensive care units has not significantly altered its spectrum of efficacy.

If a cephalosporin is used for prophylaxis and maternal infectious complications ensue, the addition of clindamycin or metronidazole and an aminoglycoside will not achieve triple therapy equivalent. A gap will still exist for the enterococci (Category III).

PERIOPERATIVE ANTIBIOTICS TO PREVENT POSTOPERATIVE INFECTIONS FOLLOWING GYNECOLOGIC SURGERY

The ground rules governing antibiotic prophylaxis for gynecologic surgery were slower in evolution and modified by additional risk factors. While obstetrical surgery deals primarily with community-related bacteria in basically healthy individuals, gynecologic surgery has a greater tendency to involve a hospital-modified bacterial spectrum in an older, sicker population. Factors predisposing the risk of postoperative infection in gynecologic patients include

1. a hospital stay 72 hours prior to surgery,
2. preoperative exposure to antibiotics,
3. concomitant presence of disease, affecting small blood vessels, e.g., diabetes mellitus, irradiation, collagen vascular disease, and hypertension,
4. obesity, and
5. residency in a nursing facility.

Classically, antibiotic prophylaxis is advocated when the procedure is associated with a significant risk of postoperative infection. The antibiotic chosen is required to

1. impact on a significant portion of the bacteria that, through the anaerobic progression or individually, can cause disease and have been shown to be effective in clinical trials,
2. have an antibiotic half-life such that peak serum and tissue concentrations are functioning at the time of the operative procedure,
3. be not associated with significant adverse drug reactions, and
4. be relatively inexpensive.

The list of antibiotics that have been shown efficacious in prevention of infectious complications following gynecologic surgery has been engendered by commercial rather than scientific interests. Unlike antibiotic prophylaxis for obstetrical infection where there is no statistical significance between disease avoidance with the first-, second-, and third-generation cephalosporins, a closer probability of achieving statistical significance does occur with the broader spectrum antibiotic for gynecologic procedures. The problem with most studies of efficacy is their inability to control operative variables such as duration of procedure, operative skill, blood loss, meticulous tissue handling techniques, etc. The operations for which antibiotic prophylaxis is advocated are listed in Table 1.

For relatively simple gynecologic surgery, single- or two-dose cephalosporin prophylaxis is the usually accepted standard of care; however, when extensive surgery is contemplated, ampicillin/sulbactam combination has had the lowest incidence of postoperative wound infections.

Clinical studies have shown no value in continuing antimicrobial therapy beyond 24 hours in clean/contaminated

TABLE I Surgical procedures for which antibiotic prophylaxis is advocated

Therapeutic and nontherapeutic abortions
Uterine D&C where the potential for infection exists
Abdominal hysterectomies
Pregnancy termination[a]
Radical hysterectomy
Vaginal hysterectomy
Removal of infected intrauterine device or insertion in the presence of infection
Sterilization in the presence of potentially infected tissue
Cesarean section

[a]See Chapter 64.
Abbreviation: D&C, dilation and curettage.

surgery. Prolonged use of antibiotics on contaminated cases is considered therapeutic and not prophylactic administration.

Once an antibiotic has been given and an infectious operative site complication ensues, avoid restarting that or any close-related (in terms of spectrum of efficacy antibiotics) antibiotic.

FAILURE TO USE PROPHYLACTIC ANTIBIOTICS PROPERLY

Antibiotic prophylaxis requires proper case selection, use of an effective drug, proper dosage, proper route of administration, timing of administration, and intraoperative dosing for operations over two hours. The Health Care Quality Improvement Project of New York State reported that 27% to 54% of all patients did not receive antimicrobial prophylaxis in a proper or timely fashion. The principal misuse of prophylactic antibiotics involved duration of administration, timing of administration, and intraoperative dosing. Premature administration was most frequent for operations that occurred later in the day. With emergency surgery, administration of prophylactic antibiotics should be given in the operating room.

ANTIBIOTIC PROPHYLAXIS FOR INDUCED ABORTIONS

Periabortal antibiotic prophylaxis has been found to significantly reduce postabortal infections in women undergoing elective first trimester vacuum abortions. In a meta-analysis comprising over 5000 women, Sawaya et al. (1996) found an overall 42% decrease in interferon after analyzing results from 12 randomized trials. The American College of Obstetricians and Gynecologists and the Royal College of Obstetricians and Gynaecologists currently recommend the use of antibiotic prophylaxis at the time of induced abortions.

The duration of antibiotic prophylaxis is partially determined by the population being served. The overall protective effect of antibiotic prophylaxis is most significant in women who have the high-risk criteria for possible chlamydial infections. The duration of antibiotic administration should be considered so that it would minimally eradicate an underlying chlamydial infection. Penney et al. (1998) have reported that a strategy of universal prophylaxis is at least as

effective in preventing postabortal infection as a screen-and-treat strategy for *Chlamydia trachomatis* and *Neisseria gonorrhoeae*. Women with a single known partner or who have been recently tested for sexually transmitted disease can be prophylaxed with regimens as short as one day.

ANTIBIOTIC PROPHYLAXIS FOR PRETERM LABOR

Significant literature that deals with the use of prophylactic antibiotics in patients with preterm labor exists. In this clinical setting, antibiotic administration is hypothesized to delay or prevent preterm delivery. The underlying suppositions are that either women with preterm labor have an occult intrauterine infection or cervical/vaginal infection has initiated the prostaglandin cascade, which initiated labor. Studies in experimental animals have shown that early, but not delayed, antibiotic treatment prevents preterm delivery following experimental intra-amniotic infection.

Also in support of the former postulate is the ability of effective antibiotic therapy in cases of documented intrauterine *Listeria monocytogenes* infection to allow such a pregnancy to proceed to term. The ability of an abnormal cervico-vaginal bacterial flora to initiate labor has conceptual validity in theory, but has yet to be conclusively demonstrated.

A meta-analysis to evaluate the efficacy of antibiotic prophylaxis/therapy for preterm labor revealed a mixed outcome pattern, with only small improvements in pregnancy prolongation, estimated gestational weight, and birthweight. The data is considered insufficient to show a beneficial effect on neonatal morbidity or mortality. Key problems in evaluation of such data are the entry criteria for what constitutes preterm labor and, because of the rarity of morbidity and mortality, to the need to rely on surrogate outcomes. Among the antibiotics used in these studies, none demonstrated superiority to the others.

The majority of the studies reviewed excluded gravida with preterm labor associated with rupture of the fetal membranes. Ascending infection occurs in the setting of ruptured fetal membranes and to a lesser degree in gravida with marked cervical dilation but intact membranes. A few papers exist in which eradication of occult or overt chorioamnionitis resulted in pregnancy prolongation.

ENDOCARDITIS PROPHYLAXIS

The current recommendations for antibiotic prophylaxis are based not upon clinical trials, but rather on best-available evidence and consensus.

Historically, the aggressive use of antibiotic prophylaxis for women with known predisposing conditions for endocarditis in labor or undergoing an abortion has done a great deal in blunting the incidence of postpartum endocarditis (Tables 2 and 3).

The current recommendations of the American Heart Association classify cardiac conditions into high, moderate, and negligible risk. The third category is not felt to require prophylaxis.

TABLE 2 Recommendations of the American Heart Association categories of patients for prophylaxis (1997)

High risk
- All prosthetic heart valves (including bioprostheses and homografts)
- Previous bacterial endocarditis
- Complex cyanotic congenital heart disease and surgically constructed systemic pulmonary shunts

Moderate risk
- Congenital cardiac malformations (PDA, VSD, ostium primum, bicuspid aortic valve, and aortic coarctation)
- Acquired valvular heart disease (rheumatic heart disease, valvular stenosis, valvular regurgitation)
- Mitral valvular disease with regurgitation and/or myxomatous leaflets
- Hypertrophic cardiopathy

Abbreviations: PDA, patent ductus arteriosus VSD, ventricular septal defect.

The potential for acute endocarditis exists and should be kept in mind when women with postpartum or postaborted infectious complication exhibit an atypical clinical response to therapy or develop a murmur (Chapter 69). When patients are sensitive to penicillin or its degradative product, alternate regimens must be used.

Patients already taking antibiotics for another reason (particularly penicillin for rheumatic fever prophylaxis or current preoperative antibiotic prophylaxis) should be given an agent from a different class for endocarditis prophylaxis. Clindamycin 600 mg IV or cefazolin 1.0 g IM or IV given within 30 minutes before a procedure can be considered.

Mitral valve prolapse (MVP) occurs in approximately 6% to 10% of the population. The risk of endocarditis is projected to be five- to eightfold greater than that of individuals without MVP. Of 52 cases of failure of endocarditis prophylaxis, one-third occurred in individuals with MVP as their underlying cardiac lesion. The American Heart Association recommends prophylaxis specifically for MVP with evidence of regurgitation and/or myxomatous leaflets. Patients with MVP and only a systolic click represent a controversial subset and warrant prophylaxis or a vigilant search for evidence of intermittent regurgitation. The only patients with MVP who are not recommended for prophylaxis are those patients with isolated prolapse, normal

TABLE 3 Antibiotic prophylaxis recommendations for genitourinary tract procedures involving uninfected tissues

Ampicillin 2.0 g IV or IM plus gentamycin 1.5 mg/kg (up to 120 mg) within 30 min of starting procedure; followed by ampicillin 1.0 g IV or IM or amoxicillin 1 g orally 6 hr later

High risk
- Patients allergic to penicillin: vancomycin 1.0 g IV over 1–2 hr plus, gentamycin 1.5 mg/kg IV/IM (up to 120 mg) to be completed within 30 min of starting the procedure
Ampicillin 2.0 g orally 1 hr before the procedure or ampicillin 2.0 g IV/IM within 30 min of starting the procedure

Moderate risk
- Patients allergic to penicillin: vancomycin 1.0 g IV over 1–2 hr to be completed within 30 min of starting the procedure

Current recommendations do not include an erythromycin-based regimen for oral prophylaxis because of problems with pharmacokinetics and gastrointestinal tolerability.

appearing leaflets, no Doppler evidence of regurgitation, and no murmurs with maneuvers.

The American Heart Association recommends prophylaxis for vaginal delivery, despite the rarity of bacterial endocarditis after uncomplicated vaginal delivery. With vaginal delivery, if the membranes have been ruptured for any significant length of time or the patient has been in good labor and lost the mucous plug of pregnancy, the potential for uterine contamination exists.

GROUP B STREPTOCOCCAL DISEASE PROPHYLACTIC ANTIBIOTICS

In 1996, the Centers for Disease Control, American College of Obstetricians and Gynecologists, and the Academy of Pediatrics introduced two divergent approaches for the prevention of perinatal group B streptococcal disease (GBS). The first of these was predicated on prenatal maternal screening for GBS colonization at 35 to 37 weeks' gestation and offering intrapartum chemoprophylaxis. This approach was subsequently modified to include gravida with GBS bacteriuria and women who had previously given birth to a GBS-infected neonate. The second approach was contingent on the identification of one or more risk factors, which included preterm deliveries, preterm or prolonged rupture of the fetal membranes, intrapartum fever, prior-GBS neonatal disease, and GBS bacteriuria.

Both approaches had been successful in altering GBS neonatal and maternal morbidity and mortality. However, neither has completely eliminated the occurrence of GBS neonatal disease. The principal shortcoming of a risk-based approach was the fact that 20% of GBS neonatal disease occurred in women without demonstrable risk factors. With the bacteriologic screening approach for maternal GBS, the problems inherent in culturing on appropriate media, number of sites needed to exclude GBS, and the ultimate site/technique for obtaining the screening culture ensured less than 85% GBS detection.

Schrag et al. did a multistate retrospective cohort study involving 5144 births in which they compared the efficacy of the two officially recommended approaches. In the screened group, 18% of all gravida with GBS did not present with an identifiable maternal risk factor. These investigators found that the risk of early-onset GBS disease was significantly lower among infants of screened women than among the infants in the risk-based group by approximately 50%. The Centers for Disease Control and Prevention currently advocate only prepartum screening.

Prior to 1996, it had been demonstrated that the universal administration of penicillin to all neonates would profoundly alter, but not totally eliminate, the incidence of ensuing neonatal GBS. The switch from a pediatric-directed approach for GBS early-onset disease to an obstetrical-directed approach was justified argumentatively by the significant maternal morbidity caused by GBS at parturition. In terms of risk–benefit analysis, the justification is less clear. Both penicillin and ampicillin carry with their administration the risk of anaphylaxis. To date, anaphylaxis has not been described in a newborn.

If society's mandated goal on zero cases of early-onset GBS is to be met, it may require a combination of obstetrical approach based on culture surveillance and pediatric approach based on universal neonatal penicillin administration.

SELECTED READING

Operative Prophylaxis

Apuzzio JJ, Reyelt C, Pelosi M, et al. Prophylactic antibiotics for cesarean section: comparison of high- and low-risk patients for endomyometritis. Obstet Gynecol 1982; 59:693.

Ayangade O. Long- versus short-course antibiotic prophylaxis in cesarean section: a comparative study. J Natl Med Assoc 1979; 71:71.

Berkeley AS, Hirsh JC, Freedman KS, Ledger WJ. Cefotaxime for cesarean section prophylaxis in labor: intravenous administration vs lavage. J Reprod Med 1990; 35:214.

Burke JP. The effective period of preventive antibiotic action in experimental incisions and dermal lesions. Surgery 1961; 50:161.

Burke JP. Maximizing appropriate antibiotic prophylaxis for surgical patients: an update from LDS Hospital, Salt Lake City. Clin Infect Dis 2001; 33(Suppl 2):s78.

Carlson C, Duff P. Antibiotic prophylaxis for cesarean delivery: is an extended-spectrum agent necessary? Obstet Gynecol 1990; 76:343.

Classen DC, Evans RS, Pestonik SL, et al. The timing of prophylactic administration of antibiotics and the risk of surgical-wound infections. N Engl J Med 1992; 326:281.

Cooperman NR, Kasim M, Rajashekaraiah KR. Clinical significance of amniotic fluid, amniotic membrane, and endometrial biopsy cultures at the time of cesarean section. Am J Obstet Gynecol 1980; 137:536.

Dajani A, Taubert K, Wilson W, et al. Prevention of bacterial endocarditis: recommendations by the American Heart Association. J Am Med Assoc 1997; 277:1794.

Ehrenkranz NJ, Blackwelder WC, Pfaff SJ, et al. Infections complicating low-risk cesarean sections in community hospitals: efficacy of antimicrobial prophylaxis. Am J Obstet Gynecol 1990; 162:337.

Faro S, Phillips LE, Martens MG. Perspectives on the bacteriology of postoperative obstetric and gynecologic infections. Am J Obstet Gynecol 1988; 158:694.

Galask RP. The challenge of prophylaxis in cesarean section in the 1990s. J Reprod Med 1990; 35:1078.

Gilstrap LC, Cunningham FG. The bacterial pathogenesis of infection following cesarean section. Obstet Gynecol 1979; 53:545.

Gjonnaess H. Antimicrobial prophylaxis in gynecological and obstetric surgery. Scan J Infect Dis 1990; 70:52.

Goldenberg RI, Hauth JC, Andrews WW. Intrauterine infection and preterm delivery. N Engl J Med 2000; 342:1500.

Gordon JR, Phillips D, Blanchard K. Prophylactic cesarean section antibiotics: maternal and neonatal morbidity before or after cord clamping. Obstet Gynecol 1979; 53:151.

Grimes DA, Schulz KF, Cates WJ. Prophylactic antibiotics for curettage abortion. Am J Obstet Gynecol 1984; 150:689.

Hemsell DL, Heard MC, Hemsell PG, et al. Alterations in lower reproductive tract flora after single dose piperacillin and triple dose cefoxitin at vaginal and abdominal hysterectomy. Obstet Gynecol 1988; 72:875.

Hemsell DL. Prophylactic antibiotics in gynecologic and obstetric surgery. Rev Infect Dis 1991; 13:S821.

Henriques CU, Wilken JC, Thorsen, P, et al. A randomized controlled trial of prophylaxis of post-abortal infection: ceftriaxone versus placebo. Br J Obstet Gynaecol 1994; 101:610.

Houang ET. Antibiotic prophylaxis in hysterectomy and induced abortion: a review of the evidence. Drugs 1991; 41:19.

Kristensen GB, Beiter EC, Mather O. Single-dose cefuroxime prophylaxis in non-elective cesarean section. Acta Obstet Gynecol Scand 1990; 69:497.

Ledger WJ, Gee C, Lewis WP. Guidelines for antibiotic prophylaxis in gynecology. Am J Obstet Gynecol. 1975; 121:1038.

Matuschka PR, Cheadle WG, Burke JP. A new standard of care: administration of preoperative antibiotics in the operating room. Am Surg 1997; 63:500.

Osborne NG, Wright RC. Effect of preoperative scrub on the bacterial flora of the endocervix and vagina. Obstet Gynecol 1977; 50:148.

Probst JR, Benrubi GI, Sanchez-Ramos L, Todd M. Comparison of one dose cefazolin versus one dose cefotetan for cesarean section prophylaxis. J Fla Med Assoc 1989; 76:1027.

Ramsdale DR, Elliot TSJ, Wright P, et al. Guidelines for the prophylaxis of infective endocarditis in adults. http://www.bcs.com 2004:1.

Silver A, Eichorn A, Kral J, et al. Timeliness and use of antibiotic prophylaxis in selected inpatient surgical procedures: The antibiotic prophylaxis study group. Am J Surg 1996; 171:548.

Simmons NA. Recommendations for endocarditis prophylaxis. the endocarditis working party for antimicrobial chemotherapy. J Antimicrob Chemother 1993; 31:427.

Spruill FG, Minette LF, Sturner WO. Two surgical deaths associated with cephalothin. J Am Med Assoc 1974; 229:440.

Starr RV, Zurawski J, Ismail M. Preoperative vaginal preparation with povidone-iodine and the risk of postcesarean endometritis. Obstet Gynecol 2005; 105:1024.

Swartz WH, Grolle K. The use of prophylactic antibiotics in cesarean section, a review of the literature. J Reprod Med 1981; 26:595.

Swart WH, Tanaree P. T-tube suction drainage and/or prophylactic antibiotics. Obstet Gynecol 1976; 47:665.

Induced Abortion Prophylaxis

American College of Obstetricians and Gynecologists. Antibiotic prophylaxis for gynecologic procedures. ACOG Practice Bulletin Number 23, January 2001. In: 2002 Compendium of Selected Publications. Washington, DC: ACOG, 2002:268.

Darj E, Stralin E-B, Nilsson S. The prophylactic effect of doxycycline on postoperative infection after first-trimester abortion. Obstet Gynecol 1987; 70:755.

Lichtenberg ES, Grimes DA, Paul M. Abortion complications: prevention and management. In: Paul M, Lichtenberg ES, Borgatta L, Grimes DA, Stubblefield PG, eds. A Clinician's Guide to Medical and Surgical Abortion. New York, NY: Churchill Livingstone, 1999:197–216.

Lichtenberg ES, Paul M, Jones H. First trimester surgical abortion practices: a survey of National Abortion Federation members. Contraception 2001; 64:345.

Penney GC, Thomson M, Norman J, et al. A randomized comparison of strategies for reducing infective complications of induced abortion. Br J Obstet Gynaecol 1998; 105: 599.

Royal College of Obstetricians and Gynaecologists. The care of women requesting induced abortion. Evidence-Based Guideline Number 7. London, 2000.

Sawaya GF, Grady D, Kerlikowske K, Grimes DA. Antibiotics at the time of induced abortion: the case for universal prophylaxis based on a meta-analysis. Obstet Gynecol 1996; 87:884.

Sclar DA, Tartaglione TA, Fine MJ. Overview of issues related to medical compliance with implications for the outpatient management of infectious diseases. Infectious Agents Dis 1994; 3:266.

Endocarditis Prophylaxis

Baddour LM, Phillips TN, Bisno AL. Coagulase-negative staphylococcal endocarditis: occurrence in patients with mitral valve prolapse. Arch Intern Med 1986; 146:119.

Bor DH, Himmelstein DU. Endocarditis prophylaxis for patients with mitral valve prolapse: a quantitative analysis. Am J Med 1984; 76:711.

Durack DT, Kaplan EL, Bisno AL. Apparent failures of endocarditis prophylaxis: analysis of 52 cases submitted to a national registry. J Am Med Assoc 1983; 250:2318.

Fleming HA. Antibiotic prophylaxis against infective endocarditis after delivery. Lancet 1977; 1:144.

Henderson CE, Terribile S, Keefe D, Merkatz IR. Cardiac screening for pregnant intravenous drug abusers. Am J Perinatol 1989; 6:397.

Hickey AJ, MacMahon SW, Wilcken DEL. Mitral valve prolapse and bacterial endocarditis: when is antibiotic prophylaxis necessary? Am Heart J 1985; 109:431.

Kaye D. Prophylaxis for infective endocarditis: an update. Ann Intern Med 1986; 104:419.

Sugrue D, Blake S, Troy P, MacDonald D. Antibiotic prophylaxis against infective endocarditis after normal delivery—is it necessary? Br Heart J 1980; 44:499.

GBS Prophylaxis

Committee on Infectious Diseases and Committee on Fetus and Newborn. Guidelines for prevention of group B streptococcal (GBS) infection by chemoprophylaxis. Pediatrics 1992; 90:776.

Gigante J, Hickson GB, Entman SS, Oquist NL. Universal screening for group B streptococcus: recommendations and obstetricians' practice decisions. Obstet Gynecol 1995; 85:440.

Katz VL, Moos MK, Cefalo RC, et al. Group B streptococci: results of a protocol of antepartum screening and intrapartum treatment. Am J Obstet Gynecol 1994; 170:521.

Minkoff H, Mead P. An obstetric approach to the prevention of early-onset group B beta-hemolytic streptococcal sepsis. Am J Obstet Gynecol 1986; 154:973.

Ohlsson A, Myhr TL. Intrapartum chemoprophylaxis of perinatal group B streptococcal infections: a critical review of randomized controlled trials. Am J Obstet Gynecol 1994; 170:910.

Pylipow M, Gaddis M, Kinney JS. Selective intrapartum prophylaxis for group B streptococcus colonization: management and outcome of newborns. Pediatrics 1994; 93:631.

Rouse DJ, Goldenberg RL, Cliver SP, et al. Strategies for the prevention of early-onset group B streptococcal sepsis: a decision analysis. Obstet Gynecol 1994; 83:483.

Schrag SJ, Zell ER, Lynfield R, et al.: A population-based comparison of strategies to prevent early-onset group B streptococcal disease in neonates. N Engl J Med 2002; 347:233.

Schuchat A, Whitney C, Zangwill K. Prevention of perinatal group B streptococcal disease: a public health perspective. Morb Mortal Wkly Rep 1996; 45:1.

Congenital Viral Infections

Prior to the advent of virologic and immunologic techniques, congenital viral infection was defined as a disease present at birth or developing before the shortest known incubation period for the virus in the immediate neonatal period. Although still a valid documentation of congenital infection, it results in the recognition of only a limited spectrum of transplacental viral transmission and excludes those cases of congenital infection whose incubation period is one standard deviation removed or whose viral challenge is insufficient to produce clinical disease.

Congenital infection does not require either overt clinical disease or the presence of histologic lesions. As has been pointed out by René Dubos, "the determinants of the disease are not the same as the determinants of infection." In its most rigid form, the definition of congenital infection is the exposure in utero of the developing embryo or fetus to the antigenic determinants of presumably infectious virus particles and the subsequent elaboration of specific immunoglobulin M (IgM) antibodies of fetal origin.

Antigenic stimulation of the fetus in utero may result in the quantity of IgM immunoglobulins detectable in cord or neonatal serum being elevated above the anticipated values. Approximately 25% of infants with congenital rubella syndrome have appreciable elevations of their IgM level. In general, there is a positive correlation between elevated serum IgM and the severity of the clinical involvement.

When maternal viral infection occurs in gestation at any time other than the immediate perinatal period, the demonstration of persisting antibodies beyond three months of age constitutes highly suggestive evidence of congenital viral infection. Complete documentation of congenital infection is contingent on the recovery of the virus at parturition from presumptive sites of recovery, e.g., placenta, products of conception, fetal or newborn organs, urine, or cerebrospinal fluid. When dealing with abortion material or very early embryos, virus isolation and the use of organism-specific DNA products are the principal means of specifically documenting congenital viral infection.

Cytomegaloviruses

INTRODUCTION

Phylogenetically, the cytomegaloviruses (CMVs) are among the oldest viruses known. Their differentiation parallels that of individual species so that it is not unusual to have relative or absolute species specificity. As a result of years of adaptive evolution, the bulk of human infection is predominantly subclinical. CMVs establish a latent infection after the acute phase of the infection has resolved.

Taxonomically, the CMVs belong to the herpesvirus group, which includes herpes simplex viruses types 1 and 2 (HSV-1 and HSV-2), varicella-zoster virus, the Epstein-Barr virus, and herpes viruses 6, 7, and 8 (HSV-6, HSV-7, and HSV-8). A CMV particle measures approximately 1800 to 2000 Å in diameter and is made up of a single molecule of double-stranded DNA and sequential layers composed of an icosahedral protein coat and a lipid envelope. The site of viral DNA synthesis is within the host cell nucleus (Fig. 1). Consequently, histologic evidence of virus replication can be observed in the form of an intranuclear inclusion body, which is characterized by both cytoplasmic and nuclear gigantism. The mature "owl-eye" lesion of the CMV is distinct from the intranuclear inclusion bodies of herpes simplex and varicella-zoster viruses. The magnitude of diametric increase of the cell is two to three times that observed with other members of the herpesvirus group. The intranuclear inclusion retains a circular to ovoid configuration, stains basophilic with hematoxylin and eosin, and is Feulgen positive. The intranuclear inclusion body of the HSV is irregular in contour, stains eosinophilic with hematoxylin and eosin, and is negative in a Feulgen reaction.

Infection with the CMV results in the establishment of latent infection. Unlike the case with either the HSV-1, HSV-2, or the varicella-zoster virus, clinically overt manifestations of virus replication are seldom seen. Except in the immunologically compromised individual and in the developing human fetus, the CMVs rarely exhibit virulence for humans.

The CMVs spread by intimate contact with biologic fluids containing infectious material, specifically tears, saliva, urine, endocervical mucus, colostrum, and transfused blood. The demonstration of CMV in semen makes venereal transmission of the infection a distinct possibility.

EPIDEMIOLOGY AND TRANSMISSION

CMV causes a primary infection that can subsequently reactivate during pregnancy. Congenital in utero infection is primarily the consequence of the hematogenous dissemination as a consequence of the viremia of initial infection. Approximately 50% of women of childbearing in the United States lack antibodies to CMV. Of these serosusceptible women, 1% to 8% will ultimately acquire primary CMV infection during pregnancy. Approximately 28% of the infected fetus will have clinically overt disease at birth or in the neonatal period. The risk of infection is highest during the first trimester. After that time, infection poses a diminishing risk to the fetus in terms of morbidity.

If a woman is seropositive prior to her pregnancy, the risk of congenital infection is 1% or less. The vast majority of these neonates born to gravidae whose CMV antedated pregnancy will be asymptomatic.

Virus dissemination is by intimate contact with biologic fluids containing infectious material, specifically, tears, salvia, urine, mucus, colostrums, and transfused blood. The demonstration of CMV in semen and cervical secretions makes sexual transmission of CMV probable. CMV is recoverable from endocervical secretions in 1% to 2% of

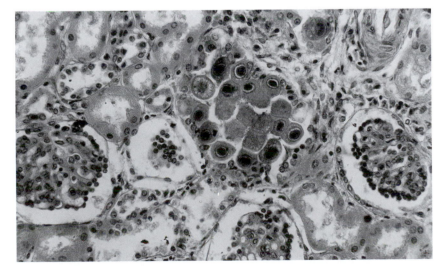

FIGURE I Classical intranuclear inclusion bodies in the renal tubular cells of an infant with congenital cytomegalovirus infection (H&E, ×420).

women undergoing routine examination in a private practice setting.

Seropositive women frequently reactivate and shed CMV during lactation. Newborns can acquire CMV owing to consumption of virus-containing breast milk. For healthy neonates at term, acquisition of CMV infection appears to be of little significance; however, for premature, medically compromised neonates, the added acquisition of CMV infection translates into increased morbidity and mortality.

Prior immunity to CMV may not protect the fetus from clinical disease in a subsequent pregnancy. Reinfection with a different CMV strain during pregnancy can lead to congenital infection.

CLINICAL INFECTION

Infectious Mononucleosis-Like Syndrome

Being so well adapted to the human host, the CMVs rarely produce clinically overt disease. The principal clinical syndrome that may alert a physician to possible primary maternal CMV infection is that of an infectious mononucleosis-like syndrome. This pattern of disease is characterized by febrile illness with high, irregular fevers lasting as long as three weeks. Clinically, the patient demonstrates lethargy, malaise, and hematologic alterations indistinguishable from those of infectious mononucleosis. The most important physical findings are the absence of the tonsillitis or pharyngitis and the cervical lymphadenopathy, which are characteristic of infectious mononucleosis. These two negative findings strongly reinforce the possibility of CMV infection.

Clinically, both relative and absolute lymphocytosis are present, with abundant atypical lymphocytes (12–55%). Levels of serum aspartate lactotransferase, serum aspartate aminotransferase, and alkaline phosphatase may or may not be abnormally elevated at this time. Although biochemical evidence of hepatitis may exist, the hepatic tenderness associated with either infectious mononucleosis or hepatitis type A or B viruses is characteristically absent. In rare instances, evidence of myocarditis or a rubella-like rash may be present. Specific tests for hepatitis-associated antigen and for the presence of specific antibodies to *Toxoplasma gondii* and the heterophil (Paul-Bunnell) reaction, if negative, aid in substantiating the diagnosis.

Significance of Prior Maternal Infection

Both primary and recurrent maternal CMV infections are important in the pathogenesis of congenital infection. The overall prevalence for a given population is governed in part by the prevalence of prior CMV infection. Women from middle to upper socioeconomic populations are less likely to have prior infection. Serosusceptibility in this population runs at 40% to 50% in contradistinction to 15% among those of low socioeconomic backgrounds. Although women from middle–upper class socioeconomic backgrounds are more susceptible, they are also less likely to acquire primary infection during gestation. Primary maternal infection during gestation accounts for approximately 63% of cases of congenital infection in this group as opposed to 25% of congenital infections in the progeny of women from lower socioeconomic groups. The age distribution of the population similarly influences both prevalence and mode of fetal acquisition of infection. Women from low socioeconomic backgrounds acquire disease early in life. In this group, congenital CMV is most often seen in the first born infant of teenage and young females. As a rule of thumb, the probability of vertical transmission associated with primary maternal infection is around 50%, whereas that associated with maternal CMV, which antedates a pregnancy reaction, is in the order of 1% to 3%.

While pregnancy per se does not alter the incidence of primary disease, viral shedding becomes a progressively more common phenomenon with time. On average, the prevalence of viral cervical and urinary tract shedding increases from 2.0% in the first trimester to 7.0% near term.

Age may also influence recurrent CMV shedding in the genital and urinary tracts of women. In low socioeconomic populations, the prevalence of CMV excretion in the genital tract is inversely related to age after puberty. The presence of CMV endocervical colonization is not a reliable marker for probable vertical transmission to the fetus. One cannot distinguish between viral excretion associated with primary disease and that of recurrent disease. Similarly, CMV viruria per se does not distinguish between primary infection and reactivation. Only when a high titer of urinary virus is present or demonstrable is there a markedly increased probability of delivery of a congenitally infected infant.

The overall incidence of congenital CMV among the progeny of seropositive women is approximately 1.8%. The overall incidence of congenital CMV infection in a general population is influenced by the composition of that population. It may range from 25 per 1000 live births for single black women under the age of 20 to 1.6 per 1000 live births for married white women over the age of 25. Although maternal immunity cannot completely eliminate transplacental transmission, it appears to reduce the morbidity and deleterious consequences for the fetus/neonate. Prospective studies now indicate that recurrent maternal CMV is responsible for more cases of congenital infection than primary infection. This is particularly true for low socioeconomic populations.

Congenital Cytomegalovirus Infection

Congenital CMV infection has a prevalence ranging between 0.5% and 2.0% of all live births. Approximately 40,000 neonates are born in the United States each year with congenital disease. Anywhere from 5% to 10% of these infants are clinically symptomatic at birth. Ninety percent of those who are symptomatic at birth develop major sequelae. Another 5% to 17% of neonates born with occult congenital infection will go on to develop varying degrees of complications during their preschool years. Anywhere from 2700 to 7600 babies are born each year who may develop developmental abnormalities caused by congenitally acquired infection.

Unlike congenital rubella, congenital infection with the CMV may occur despite the presence of strain-specific humoral immunity. Being latent viruses of man, the CMV may undergo reactivation as well as prolonged shedding in biologic fluid. Individuals with CMV infection tend to persistently or intermittently excrete virus in urine, breast milk, saliva, semen, cervical secretions, stools, and tears. Viral shedding after primary infection normally persists for months or even years. With reactivation of latent infection, the duration of shedding is significantly diminished. As a consequence of this type of reactivation of latent infection, there is a direct relationship between the incidence of congenital CMV and the rate of maternal seropositivity. Congenital infection resulting from recurrent CMV infection can and does occur in highly immune populations as well as in immunologically compromised individuals. There are at least three reports describing cases of congenital CMV infections in consecutive pregnancies.

Primary CMV infection occurs in 1.0% to 8.0% of pregnancies. With primary infection, fetal involvement occurs in 50% of the cases. Gestational age does not influence the rate of intrauterine infection following primary maternal infection. Stagno et al. prospectively followed 35 infants who were congenitally infected as a result of primary maternal infection. Only five neonates had clinical evidence of intrauterine infection at birth. The risk of primary maternal CMV infection leading to long-term sequelae is under 5%. The principal factor modulating this figure is that, when in gestation, primary maternal infection occurred. Lipitz et al. (1997) evaluated 63 pregnant women with primary CMV disease for congenital transmission. In this study, 22 (35%) of the pregnancies had virologic or immunologic evidence of vertical transmission. In nine (41%) of the 22 pregnancies with evidence of vertical transmission, abnormal ultrasonographic findings were recorded. The only pregnancy with prenatal ultrasonographic abnormalities that went to term resulted in an infant with neurologic sequelae. In the 37 pregnancies with no evidence of congenital infection that continued to term, only one of the ensuing pregnancies developed mild motor disability during a median of 23 months of follow-up.

Although based on limited observation, it appears that the CMVs are capable of infecting the products of conception irrespective of their gestational age and that the clinical manifestations of congenital CMV infection appear to be primarily a reflection of the duration of infection in utero.

Analogous to maternal infection with rubella virus in the first trimester, two patterns of involvement of infection of the products of conception exist: one in which infection is limited solely to the placenta and another in which both placental and panorgan fetal involvements occur.

First Trimester Infection

Early maternal disease does not invariably select for clinically overt disease; but when heightened neonatal morbidity occurs, it is most likely to do so in the progeny of women who acquired infection in the first trimester. The infants are usually premature or of a low birthweight for their term dates. The gross clinical presentation is often indistinguishable from the overt cases of congenital rubella, congenital toxoplasmosis, congenital herpes simplex virus infection, and congenital syphilis. The infant tends to be microcephalic (Fig. 2). Roentgenograms of the head demonstrate extensive calcification of the lateral ventricles and portions of the olfactory tract. These have their anatomic correlation in extensive dystrophic calcification within necrotic subependymal areas of the lateral ventricles (Fig. 3). Chorioretinitis is a frequent finding in those microcephalic infants with intracranial calcification. Hepatosplenomegaly due to extramedullary hemato poiesis, with or without superimposed hepatitis, is usually prominent. The infants may have evidence of disseminated intravascular coagulopathy. Petechiae due to thrombocytopenia may be present at birth.

Infants with symptomatic congenital CMV have a very high likelihood of developing long-term sequelae. The follow-up studies of symptomatic infants by Boppana et al. (1997) have revealed a 41% rate of developmental delays, 53% to 61% rate of mental retardation, and a 100% need for special education.

In contrast, permanent sequelae occurred in approximately 10% of asymptomatic congenital CMV infants. Ivarsson et al. (1997) reported that if infected infants were normal at one year of age, these children compared well in terms of neurologic development and intellectual status to their peers.

Necropsy material has demonstrated panorgan viral involvement. The characteristic nuclear inclusion bodies have been identified in, or the virus has been isolated from, every organ system. Primarily involved is the epithelial cell, within which both cytoplasmic and nuclear enlargement are evident. In the mature lesions, nuclear inclusion bodies show peripheralization of the chromatin and central Feulgen-positive DNA mass, which electron microscopy reveals to be composed of complete and incomplete virions.

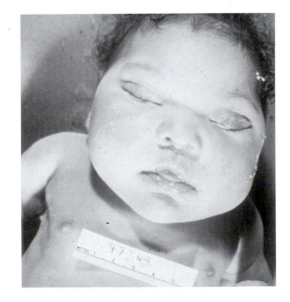

FIGURE 2 Marked microcephaly observed in fully developed congenital cytomegalovirus infection.

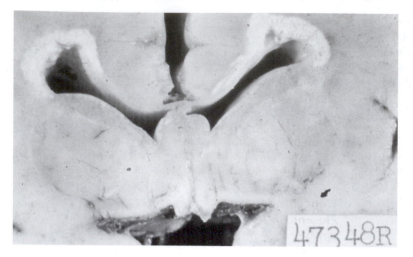

FIGURE 3 Extensive dystrophic calcification involving the lateral ventricles in an infant with congenital cytomegalovirus infection. *Source*: From Monif (1969).

The CMVs have been incriminated as a significant cause of fetal wastage. Griffiths and Baboonian (1984) have shown that fetal loss occurs in approximately 15% of gravida who contract CMV infection early in gestation as opposed to noninfected individuals (2.2%). Characteristic intranuclear inclusion bodies have been identified within alveolar macrophages of macerated small fetuses. The CMVs have been isolated from aborted material. Studies on abortion material reveal an incidence of virus recovery ranging from 0.5% to 10%. These figures may be inflated. A certain percentage of this merely represents contamination of the products of conception as they pass by virus present within the endocervix and birth canal and does not reflect true congenital involvement.

Second Trimester Infection

When second trimester congenital infection results in clinically overt symptoms and postnatal morbidity, the clinical manifestations are much more protean than those observed following first trimester involvement. Microcephaly occurs but is not associated with a predominantly subependymal pattern of CNS dystrophic calcification.

Chorioretinitis is much less frequently observed. Some infants are born with hepatosplenomegaly (Fig. 4) or hepatomegaly, with or without evidence of disseminated intravascular coagulopathy or jaundice. Other infants may have only elevated immunoglobulin M (IgM) levels as a consequence of congenital infection.

Third Trimester Infection

Third trimester involvement seems to be associated with a neonate who exhibits no early impairment of somatic growth or mental development. The infant tends to be normal by every parameter of gross measurement. Whereas specific IgM antibodies can be identified in cord serum, the IgM levels are only rarely elevated.

Late Developmental Sequelae

A primary question has been whether or not clinically inapparent disease might adversely affect the infant at a later date. What are the delayed morbid effects of occult neonatal infection? A longitudinal study of 16 infants with inapparent congenital CMV infection and elevated umbilical cord IgM levels revealed some degree of sensorineural hearing loss in 9 of the 16. An auditory handicap was either proven or considered likely in four infants. Evidence of congenital CMV infection can be detected in 12% of children with sensorineural hearing loss. This type of hearing loss is progressive.

A trend toward subnormal intelligence was observed in infected children. Hanshaw has postulated that clinically important mental and auditory impairment may occur in one out of every 1000 live births as a result of congenital CMV infection. Asymptomatic fetal CMV infection has been

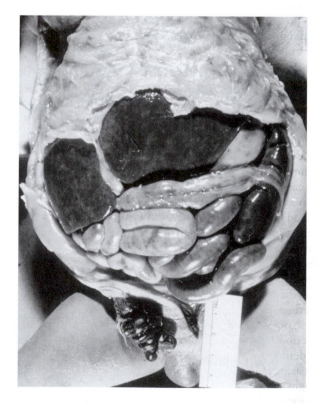

FIGURE 4 Hepatosplenomegaly, a finding characteristic of more severe chronic cases of intrauterine viral infection. *Source*: From Monif (1969).

shown to produce long-term damage in 10% to 15% of these infants. The long-term damage, which includes developmental problems, hearing loss, mental retardation, and motor deficiencies, usually manifests within the first two years of life. Congenital CMV infection is responsible for a substantial proportion of sensorineural hearing loss in children.

Postnatal Dissemination

Gestational age has a significant influence on the rate of maternal CMV excretion. On average, the prevalence of excretion increased from 2.6% in the first trimester to 7.6% near term. With parturition, breast milk becomes an additional vehicle for the transmission of virus from mother to progeny.

Although there is a poor correlation between cervical and urinary CMV excretion during pregnancy and fetal involvement, there is a positive correlation between maternal viral shedding and postnatal acquisition of infection. According to the data of Stagno et al., the two most efficient sources of transmission are infected breast milk, which resulted in a 63% rate of postnatal infection, and the infected genital tract, particularly in late gestation. The age of the mother influences the frequency of viral excretion into the genital tract and breast milk. Younger seropositive women from lower socioeconomic groups who breast-feed are at the greatest risk for transmitting virus to their progeny.

The incubation period of CMV infection acquired during the perinatal period ranges between 4 and 12 weeks (average 8 weeks). CMV infection acquired in the neonatal period occasionally results in clinical illness. The majority of infants with postnatally acquired CMV infection are asymptomatic. Postnatally acquired infection does not appear to adversely affect neurologic or psychomotor functions.

DIAGNOSIS

Maternal Infection

Virus can be isolated from a number of biologic fluids. Diagnostic specificity is usually established with polymerase chain reaction (PCR) techniques.

The serologic diagnosis of a primary maternal CMV infection can be confirmed by the appearance of specific antibodies in acute and convalescent sera (seroconversion). These antibodies, which can be detected by immunofluorescence, indirect hemagglutination, and enzyme-linked immunosorbent assay (ELISA), appear within two weeks after primary infection. Antibodies measured by complement fixation and neutralization tests follow with one- to two-week and four-week delays, respectively.

Serum-specific IgM antibodies can be demonstrated during the acute phase of primary CMV infection. Recent maternal infection can be inferred from a single serum specimen by the demonstration of IgM-specific antibody. IgM antibodies appear early in the course of the disease and persist for four to eight months depending on which test is used. Unless IgM-specific antibodies are present, a rise in antibody titer or a single high titer (>1:108) correlates poorly with vertical transmission. Of all the tests available for this purpose, ELISA appears to be the most reliable because in normal hosts,

including pregnant women, positive results occur only during the acute phase of primary infections and not with reactivations. With this test, specific IgM antibodies are detected in nearly 90% of women with a primary CMV infection, and the antibody response persists for up to four months. False-positive IgM tests can occur. The clinician needs to take care that a reliable laboratory is performing the test.

The development of the CMV IgG avidity test provides an additional test by which the probability of recent infection can be assessed. With low avidity, acute infection is inferred; with high avidity, past infection is more probable.

Congenital Infection
Placental Pathology

Gross and microscopic inspection may provide inferential evidence of the possibility of congenital CMV infection. The placenta tends to be large, pale, and edematous. Intranuclear inclusion bodies are difficult to find. Their identification is often contingent on a meticulous search. The villi and villous trunks frequently appear edematous. Focal collections of plasma cells intermixed with lymphocytes may be present (Fig. 5). Characteristically, there is persistence of Hofbauer cells. Focal hemosiderin pigment is often identified free and in macrophages in areas of apparent endothelial damage and fibrosis. Only 25% of CMV placenta have the demonstrable histologic criteria necessary for a definitive diagnosis. Immunohistochemistry can increase diagnostic sensitivity to 83%. PCR can detect 58% but if supplemented with Southern blot analysis after PCR, the combined sensitivity approaches 100%.

Cytology

Transformed renal cells shed into the neonate's urine can be diagnosed. Shedding of this type of cell is an intermittent phenomenon. The best urine sample for cytologic analysis is an early morning urinary specimen with a high specific gravity.

Serologic Diagnosis

Maternally derived specific IgG antibody undergoes degradative elimination in the neonate; consequently, irrespective of whether or not intrauterine infection has occurred, the complement fixation titer falls to nondetectable levels. The reappearance of specific complement fixation activity four to six months after birth is consistent with either congenital or postnatally acquired infection.

Evidence of possible intrauterine infection may be inferred by the presence of elevated IgM levels in cord serum or blood samples obtained by funipuncture. Techniques for identifying IgM-specific antibodies in cord blood are associated with a significant false-positive rate. Currently, the use of PCR testing on amniotic fluid for CMV is the best means of documenting in utero infection, short of viral recovery.

The immunoglobulins in the serum of the neonate, in the absence of congenital infection, reflect maternal experience with these agents and are predominantly of the IgG type. Since maternal IgM antibodies do not traverse the placenta and appear in the newborn serum, the finding of specific IgM or IgA antibodies is considered diagnostic of intrauterine

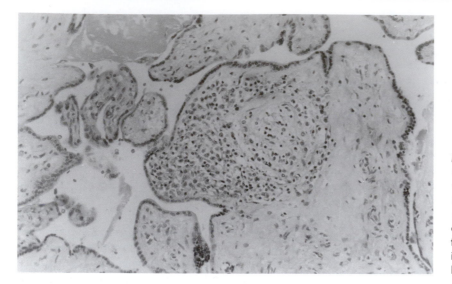

FIGURE 5 Cytomegalovirus placentitis: focal collection of plasma cells and lymphocytes within a chorionic villus. The presence of the characteristic intranuclear inclusion bodies is rare. The persistence of Hofbauer cells and the edematous, relatively avascular villi with focal fibrosis should suggest the possibility of congenital cytomegalovirus infection. *Source*: From Monif and Dische (1972a).

infection. Diagnosis of congenital infection can also be made by demonstrating virus-specific antigens using PCR or ligase chain reaction technology. Only 50% to 60% of CMV congenitally infected infants have IgM-specific antibodies at birth.

Virus Isolation

Amniocentesis can provide material for virus isolation or PCR testing. Amniotic fluid analysis for CMV viral isolation and CMV PCR testing are the most sensitive ways of diagnosing congenital infection. Both Davis et al. (1971) and French et al. (1977) used amniocentesis to document congenital infection in women who had an infectious mononucleosis-like syndrome in the first three months of gestation. Stagno et al. have reported failure to recover CMV infection from amniotic fluid in three cases of primary maternal CMV infection (two of whom had isolation of virus from fetal and/or placental tissue).

Failure to isolate CMV from amniotic fluid does not necessarily rule out fetal infection. The recovery of virus strongly infers that vertical transmission has occurred. Virus isolation techniques are applicable for the isolation and identification of the CMV from tissue sources or amniotic fluid. The CMV can replicate successfully in fibroblastic tissue culture lines of human origin; the one most commonly utilized for isolation is WI-38. Specimens for viral culture need to be processed as rapidly as possible. Holding a specimen at 4°C for 24 and 48 hours results in 14% and 32% false-negative rates, respectively. PCR and CMV shell vial assay to demonstrate the presence of virus-specific antigens has partially displaced viral isolation techniques.

PRENATAL COUNSELING OF THE GRAVIDA WITH EVIDENCE OF PRIMARY CMV INFECTION

Prenatal counseling of a gravida with primary CMV infection is difficult. Negative amniocentesis fluid analyzed by both viral culture and PCR testing confers a reasonably high probability that the fetus is not infected at that time;

however, vertical transmission is possible at a later date in gestation.

In the series reported by Lipitz et al. (1997), the use of a combination of prenatal tests resulted in an accurate diagnosis of all infected fetuses. Of the two procedures performed, amniocentesis provided the ability to identify all infected fetuses, using either amniotic culture or PCR analysis. The information yielded by funipuncture did not add to the ability of accurately diagnosing vertical transmission and, furthermore, had a sensitivity of only 77% in identifying infected fetuses. Regarding the two tests performed on amniotic fluid samples, the CMV culture identified all infected fetuses (among 13 tested), whereas the PCR identified 16 of 17 tested.

Although ultrasound has limited sensitivity in the detection of fetal infection, pregnancies with evidence of vertical transmission and definite ultrasonographic findings indicating suspected fetal damage (such as hydrocephaly, microcephaly, ventricular abnormalities characteristic of ventriculitis, or brain or liver calcifications) are at a significant risk of abnormal sequelae. Demonstration of fetal hypoechogenic bowel on ultrasonographic evaluation warrants obtaining a sample of amniotic fluid for viral isolation.

Therapy

Currently in the United States, four medications have been approved by the Food and Drug Administration to treat CMV infections. Cidofovir and ISIS 2922 are approved for CMV retinitis. Ganciclovir, valganciciclovir, and foscarnet are approved to treat visceral and disseminated CMV infections. Recently, therapy using CMV hyperimmune globulin has been described for congenitally infected fetuses. The documentation of maternal primary CMV infection during gestation and PCR confirmation of fetal involvement can be grounds for therapeutic abortion.

Ganciclovir, a homolog of acyclovir, has shown efficacy against CMV. It is the current drug of choice for life-threatening or visceral CMV in immunocompromised individuals. Use of this drug is restricted to congenitally infected neonates with severe disease manifestations.

Ganciclovir administration is associated with the induction of pan cellular bone marrow depression and requires skilled monitoring. Because of its teratogenicity and embryotoxicity in experimental animals, ganciclovir use is contraindicated in pregnancy. Attempts to use antiviral compounds in the treatment of severe congenital infection have met with mixed success.

There are no current recommendations for antiviral therapy in asymptomatic CMV neonates or infants. Neonates with congenital CMV infection treated with ganciclovir have been shown to have a significant decrease in hearing loss as compared to controls.

Prevention

The treatment of breast milk for premature infants born to seropositive mothers may need to be reviewed in light of its potential for containing CMV. Although pasteurization appears to be efficient in eliminating CMV infectivity in human milk, freeze-thawing of milk does not totally eliminate the risk of viral transmission.

SELECTED READING

Adler SP. Cytomegalovirus and pregnancy. Curr Opin Obstet Gynecol 1992; 4:670.

Adler SP. Congenital cytomegalovirus screening. Pediatr Infect Dis J 2005; 24:1105.

Ahlfors K, Ivarsson SA, Harris S, et al. Congenital cytomegalovirus infection and disease in Sweden and the relative importance of primary and secondary maternal infections. Preliminary findings from a prospective study. Scand J Infect Dis 1984; 16:129.

Alford CA, Stagno S, Britt WJ. Congenital and perinatal cytomegalovirus infections. Rev Infect Dis 1990; 12:5745.

Biron KK. Antiviral drugs for cytomegalovirus diseases. Antiviral Res 2006; 71:154.

Boppana SB, Fowler KB, Vaid Y, et al. Neuroradiographic findings in newborn period and longterm outcome in children with symptomatic congenital cytomegalovirus infection. Pediatrics 1997; 99:409.

Britt WJ, Vugler LG. Antiviral antibody responses in mothers and their newborn infants with clinical and subclinical congenital cytomegalovirus infections. J Infect Dis 1990; 161:214.

Daniel Y, Gulll, Peyser R, Lessing JB. Congenital cytomegalovirus infection. Eur J Obstet Gynecol Reprod Biol 1995; 63:7.

Davis LE, Tweed GV, Chin TDY, Miller GL. Intrauterine diagnosis of cytomegalovirus infection: viral recovery from amniocentesis fluid. Am J Obstet Gynecol 1971; 109:1217.

Demmler GJ. Summary of a workshop on surveillance for congenital cytomegalovirus disease. Rev Infect Dis 1991; 13:315.

Doerr HW. Cytomegalovirus infection in pregnancy. J Virol Methods 1987; 17:127.

Elliott GB, Elliott KA. Observations on cerebral cytomegalic inclusion disease of the foetus and neonate. Arch Dis Child 1962; 37:34.

Embil JA, Ozere RL, Haldane EV. Congenital cytomegalovirus infection in two siblings from consecutive pregnancies. J Pediatr 1970; 77:417.

Forsgren M. Cytomegalovirus in breast milk; reassessment of pasteurization and freeze-thawing. Pediatr Res 2004; 56:526.

Fowler KB, Stagno S, Pass RF. The outcome of congenital cytomegalovirus infection in relation to maternal antibody status. N Engl J Med 1992; 326:663.

French MLV, Thompson JF, White A. Cytomegalovirus viremia with transmission from mother to fetus. Ann Intern Med 1977; 86:748.

Grant S, Edmond E, Syme J. A prospective study of cytomegalovirus infection in pregnancy. I. Laboratory evidence of congenital infection following maternal primary and reactivated infection. J Infect Dis 1984; 3:24.

Griffiths PD, Baboonian C. Intrauterine transmission of cytomegalovirus in women known to be immune before conception. J Hyg 1984; 92:89.

Griffiths PD, Campbell-Benzie A. A prospective study of cytomegalovirus infection in pregnant women. Br J Obstet Gynaecol 1980; 87:308.

Griffiths PD, Baboonian C, Rutter D, Peckham C. Congenital and maternal cytomegalovirus infections in a London population. Br J Obstet Gynaecol 1991; 98:135.

Hagay ZJ, Birzan G, Ornoy A. Congenital cytomegalovirus infection: a long-standing problem seeking a solution. Am J Obstet Gynecol 1996; 174:241.

Hanshaw JB. Cytomegalovirus complement-fixing antibody in microcephaly. N Engl J Med 1966; 275:476.

Hanshaw JB. Congenital cytomegalovirus infection: a fifteen year perspective. J Infect Dis 1971; 123:555.

Hanshaw JB, Sheiner AP, Mosely AW, et al. School failure and deafness after "silent" congenital cytomegalovirus infection. N Engl J Med 1976; 195:468.

Hayes K, Danks DM, Givas H, Ian J. Cytomegalovirus in human milk. N Engl J Med 1972; 187:177.

Haymaker W, Girdany BR, Stephens J, et al. Cerebral involvement with advanced periventricular calcification in generalized cytomegalic inclusion disease in the newborn. J Neuropathol Exp Neurol 1954; 13:562.

Haywood LB, Abernathy MP. Cytomegalovirus infection. Semin Perinatol 1998; 22:260.

Hildebrandt RJ, Monif GRG. Congenital cytomegalovirus infection. Am J Obstet Gynecol 1969; 105:349.

Ivarsson SA, Lernmark B, Svanberg L. Ten-year clinical and developmental and intellectual follow-up of children without neurologic symptoms at 1 year of age. Pediatrics 1997; 99:800.

Kishikawa T, Kawarabayashi T, Hayasegawa J, et al. Intrauterine cytomegalovirus infection associated with fetal ascites and oligohydramnios. Asia Oceania J Obstet Gynaecol 1987; 13:297.

Krech U, Konjajev Z, Jung M. Congenital cytomegalovirus infection in siblings from consecutive pregnancies. Helv Paediatr Acta 1971; 26:355.

Kriel RL, Gates AG, Wulff H, et al. Cytomegalovirus isolates associated with pregnancy wastage. Am J Obstet Gynecol 1970; 106:885.

Kumar ML, Gold E, Jacobs IB, et al. Primary cytomegalovirus infection in adolescent pregnancy. Pediatrics 1984; 74:493.

Kumar ML, Nankervis GA, Gold E. Inapparent congenital cytomegalovirus infection: a follow-up study. N Engl J Med 1973; 288:1370.

Kumar ML, Nankervis GA, Cooper AR, Gold E. Postnatally-acquired cytomegalovirus infections in infants of CMV-excreting mothers. J Pediatr 1984; 154:674–679.

Kumar ML, Nankervis GA, Jacobs IB, et al. Congenital and postnatally acquired cytomegalovirus infections: long-term follow-up. J Pediatr 1984; 104:674.

Lang DJ, Kummer JR. Demonstration of cytomegalovirus in semen. N Engl J Med 1972; 287:756.

Leung AK, Loong EP, Chan RC, et al. Prevalence of cytomegalovirus cervical excretion in pregnant women in Hong Kong. Asia Oceania J Obstet Gynaecol 1989; 15:7708.

Monif GRG. Viral Infections of the Human Fetus. New York: Macmillan, 1969.

Monif GRG, Dische RM. Viral placentitis in congenital cytomegalovirus infection. Am J Clin Pathol 1972a; 58:445.

Monif GRG, Dische RM. Viral placentitis in congenital cytomegalovirus infection during varying stages in gestation with neonatal involvement. J Pediatr 1972b; 80:17.

Monif GRG, Daicoff GI, Flory LI. Blood as a potential vehicle for the cytomegalovirus. Am J Obstet Gynecol 1976; 126:45.

Nankervis GA, Kumar ML, Cox FE, Gold E. A prospective study of maternal cytomegalovirus infection and its effect on the fetus. Am J Obstet Gynecol 1984; 149:435.

Nankervis A, Kumar ML, Gold E. Primary infection with cytomegalovirus during pregnancy. Pediatr Res 1974; 8:487.

Pass RF. Congenital cytomegalovirus infection and hearing loss. Herpes 2005; 12:50.

Pass RF, Stango S, Myers GJ, Alford CA. Outcome of symptomatic congenital cytomegalovirus infection: results of long-term longitudinal follow-up. Pediatrics 1980; 66:758.

Peckham CS, Stark O, Dudgeon JA, et al. Congenital cytomegalovirus infection: a cause of sensorineural hearing loss. Arch Dis Child 1987; 62:1233.

Piper JM, Wen TS. Perinatal cytomegalovirus and toxoplasmosis: challenges of antepartum therapy. Clin Obstet Gynecol 1999; 42:81.

Preece PM, Pearl KN, Peckham CS. Congenital cytomegalovirus infection. Arch Dis Child 1984; 59:1120.

Preece PM, Tookey P, Ades A, Peckham CS. Congenital cytomegalovirus infection: predisposing maternal factors. J Epidemiol Community Health 1986; 40:205.

Reigstad H, Bjerknes R, Markestad T, Myrmel H. Ganciclovir therapy for congenital cytomegalovirus infection. Acta Pediatr 1992; 81:707.

Reynolds DW, Stagno S, Stubbs KG, et al. Inapparent congenital cytomegalovirus infection with elevated cord IgM levels: causal relation with auditory and mental deficiency. N Engl J Med 1974; 190:291.

Rosenstein DL, Navarrete-Reyna A. Cytomegalic inclusion disease: observation of the characteristic inclusion bodies in the placenta. Am J Obstet Gynecol 1964; 89:220.

Schleiss MR. Role of breast milk in acquisition of cytomegalovirus infection; recent advances. Curr Opin Pediatr 2006; 18:48.

Schopfer K, Laube E, Kreck U. Congenital cytomegalovirus infection in newborn infants of mothers infected before pregnancy. Arch Dis Child 1978; 53:536.

Sequin J, Cho CT. Congenital cytomegalovirus infection in one monozygotic twin. J Am Med Assoc 1988; 260:3277.

Stagno S, Pass RF, Cloud G, et al. Primary cytomegalovirus infection in pregnancy. Incidence, transmission to fetus, and clinical outcome. J Am Med Assoc 1986; 256:1904.

Stagno S, Reynolds DW, Huang E-S, et al. Congenital cytomegalovirus infection: occurrence in an immune population. N Engl J Med 1977; 296:1254.

Stagno S, Reynolds DW, Lakeman A, et al. Congenital cytomegalovirus infections: consecutive occurrence due to viruses with similar antigenic compositions. Pediatrics 1973; 52:788.

Stagno S, Reynolds DW, Pass RF, Alford CA. Breast milk and the risk of cytomegalovirus infection. N Engl J Med 1980; 302:1073.

Stagno S, Reynolds DW, Tsiantos A, et al. Cervical cytomegalovirus excretion in pregnant and non-pregnant women: suppression in early gestation. J Infect Dis 1975; 131:522.

Stern H, Tucker SM. Prospective study of cytomegalovirus infection in pregnancy. Br Med J 1973; 2:268.

Yow M, Williamson D, Leeds L, et al. Epidemiologic characteristics of cytomegalovirus infection in mothers and their infants. Am J Obstet Gynecol 1988; 158:1189.

Prenatal Diagnosis

Donner CL, Liesnard C, Brancraft F, Rodesch F. Accuracy of amniotic fluid testing before 21 weeks of gestation in the prenatal diagnosis of congenital cytomegalovirus infection. Prenat Diagn 1994; 14:1055.

Donner C, Liesnard C, Content J, et al. Prenatal diagnosis of 52 pregnancies at risk for congenital cytomegalovirus infection. Obstet Gynecol 1993; 82:481.

Grose C, Meehan T, Weiner C. Prenatal diagnosis of congenital cytomegalovirus infection by virus isolation after amniocentesis. Pediatr Infect Dis J 1992; 11:605.

Hohlfield P, Vial Y, Maillard-Brignon C, et al. Cytomegalovirus fetal infection: prenatal diagnosis. Obstet Gynecol 1991; 78:615.

Koga Y, Mizumoto M, Matsumoto Y, et al. Prenatal diagnosis of fetal intracranial calcifications. Am J Obstet Gynecol 1990; 163:1543.

Landry M, Ferguson D, Cohen S, et al. Effect of delay specimen processing on cytomegalovirus antigenemia test results. J Clin Microbiol 1995; 33:257.

Lipitz S, Vagel S, Shaler E, et al. Prenatal diagnosis of fetal primary cytomegalovirus infection. Obstet Gynecol 1997; 89:763.

Lynch L, Daffos F, Emanuel D, et al. Prenatal diagnosis of fetal cytomegalovirus infection. Am J Obstet Gynecol 1991; 165:714.

Newton ER. Diagnosis of perinatal torch infections. Clin Obstet Gynecol 1999; 42:59.

Ozono K, Mushiake S, Takeshma T, et al. Diagnosis of congenital cytomegalovirus infection by examination of placenta: application of polymerase chain reaction and in situ hybridization. Pediatr Pathol Lab Med 1997; 17:249.

Revello M, Baldanti F, Furione M, et al. Polymerase chain reaction for prenatal diagnosis of congenital human cytomegalovirus infection. J Med Virol 1995; 47:462.

Shulman LM, Rudich C, Sayer Y, et al. Detection of CMV-DNA in cells from peritoneal fluid of IPD/CAPD patients by polymerase chain reaction. Adv Perit Dial 1992; 8:258.

Stagno S, Reynolds DW, Tsiantos A, et al. Comparative serial virologic and serologic studies of symptomatic and subclinical congenitally and natally acquired cytomegalovirus infections. J Infect Dis 1975; 132:568.

Steimann F, Hayde M. A method to derive the time of onset of infection from serological findings. Meth Inform Med 1997; 36:51.

Weiner CP, Grose CF, Naides SJ. Diagnosis of fetal infection in the patient with an ultrasonographically detected abnormality but a negative clinical history. Am J Obstet Gynecol 1993; 168:6.

Enteroviruses

11

INTRODUCTION

The enteroviruses are small, spherical, nonenveloped (naked) viruses that have icosahedral symmetry and a diameter of 27 to 30 nm. The virion is composed of a core of single-stranded RNA of about 7500 bases, with a molecular weight of 2.6×10^6 daltons. The viruses have a protein shell containing four polypeptide chains, which are elements of 60 identical, four-segmented viral capsid protein subunits called protomers.

In terms of classification, the human enteroviruses are members of the picornaviruses. They are divided into four major groups. The enteroviruses are transmitted by both fecal-to-oral and oral-to-oral means. The ability to isolate enteroviruses in any age group is inversely proportional to age.

Enterovirus infections are common during pregnancy. Their prevalence in a given community is governed primarily by

1. the time of the year and
2. the presence or absence of prior immunity to antigenically related enterovirus serotypes.

In northern latitudes, enterovirus infections tend to occur during the summer and the fall. This seasonal periodicity is less pronounced in more tropical climates.

The majority of enterovirus infections result in asymptomatic or limited nonspecific febrile illness associated with primarily upper respiratory symptoms. Some patients will experience a brief but severe illness in which both fever and lower abdominal pain dominate. The abdominal pain tends to be midline and periumbilical in location and cramping in character. Experimental data suggest that a higher incidence of clinical infections occurs with pregnancy.

The sequelae of these clinical manifestations are potentially translatable into perinatal mortality. Although the bulk of maternal disease is subclinical or presents as nonspecific upper respiratory or gastrointestinal viral illness, maternal morbidity and mortality may develop as a consequence of meningoencephalitis, myocarditis, or poliomyelitis.

MATERNAL ENTEROVIRUS INFECTION/DISEASE

The enteroviruses are quite prevalent in the environment. Their mode of transmission involves hand-to-mouth or more commonly water-borne dissemination. The gastrointestinal tract is the primary portal of infection. As a consequence, the prevalence of disease in the community tends to take on an epidemic pattern and can be significantly influenced by socioeconomic factors.

Most enteroviruses are relatively well adapted to man. Prior to the development of the polio vaccines, for every case of paralytic poliomyelitis, there would be tens of thousands of asymptomatic infections. The incubation period for infection shows significant variability, primarily due to inoculum dose effect and individual host factors. Maternal illness manifests as gastrointestinal illness, "flu-like" symptomology, or aseptic meningitis.

Although maternal infection is a common event, transplacental transmission of the virus is rare. However, when it does occur, and when that event is early in gestation, the consequences for the fetus are significant.

Transplacental transmission of the enteroviruses is primarily governed by magnitude and duration of the maternal viremia and the availability of complementary fetal viral receptor sites. The potential morbid consequences are primarily a function of gestational age and strain virulence. Viral membrane receptors change qualitatively and quantitatively with gestational age.

MANAGEMENT OF ENTEROVIRUS INFECTION IN PREGNANCY

If acute maternal virus infection or disease is documented late in pregnancy, the fact that in rare instances, fetal disease may occur needs to be presented, but in proper context. With the exception of the coxsackie viruses, overt congenital disease is rare. The prognosis for the pregnancy outcome should be relatively optimistic. Management of maternal enterovirus infection is initially that of control of symptomatology. Marked elevations of maternal temperature need to be aggressively controlled.

CONGENITAL AND NEONATAL INFECTION/DISEASE CAUSED BY THE COXSACKIE GROUP A AND B VIRUSES

The coxsackie viruses currently account for 70% of all cases of serious neonatal disease due to the enteroviruses. The dominant virulent coxsackie B serotypes are B2, B3, B4, and B5.

In contrast to neonatal disease, overt congenital coxsackie virus infection is a rare entity. The majority of coxsackie outbreaks in intensive care units for the newborns have their genesis in premature birth or low birthweight of infant who had contracted disease in utero.

Extensive disease in utero probably results in abortion, stillbirths, or neonatal deaths. When fetal interstitial myocarditis is identified at necropsy, approximately half of these cases exhibit specific immunofluorescent staining for the coxsackie group A or B virus in the myocardium. The demonstration of significant fetal wastage caused by congenital coxsackie viruses, coupled with the existence of occult congenital disease, indicates that a parameter other than clinical illness at birth is necessary to assess the true incidence of involvement. The long-term consequences of occult congenital infection are not known.

Both congenital and neonatal infections with coxsackie group viruses have been responsible for fulminating disease in newborns characterized by meningoencephalitis, myocarditis, and hepatitis (Figs. 1 and 2).

The clinical manifestations are partially a function of the organ system that bears the brunt of the infection. One organ system usually dominates the clinical picture. If sought, multiorgan involvement usually can be clinically demonstrated.

The onset of overt disease may be sudden or preceded by a period in which the neonate refuses feedings and exhibits mottling and cyanosis of the skin. Clinical evidence of myocarditis may include bradycardia, tachycardia out of proportion to the temperature, gallop rhythm, or a poor first heart sound. Electrocardiographic changes consist for the main part of alterations in the T wave, either flattening or inversion, depressed ST segments, low voltage QRS, disturbances of rhythm and conduction, or, in some cases, an injury pattern compatible with anomalous origin of the left coronary artery. In other cases, central nervous system involvement may overshadow the myocardial or hepatic manifestations of disease. These neonates are often irritable and present with bulging fontanels and cerebrospinal fluid pleocytosis. Death usually follows vasomotor collapse.

A number of studies have suggested that congenital infection resulting in selective cytopathic effect within the beta cell of the pancreas could lead to childhood-onset diabetes mellitus. Dahlquist et al. (1995a,b) traced serum samples collected at the time of birth from 55 mothers whose children later developed insulin-dependent diabetes mellitus (IDDM) and matched them pairwise to control subjects who gave birth at the same hospital during the same month. The sera were analyzed for immunoglobulin M (IgM) antibodies to coxsackie B virus serotypes 2, 3, and 4 (CBV-2, -3, and -4) using a type-specific mu-antibody-capture radioimmunoassay. Despite a decreased power due

to the close matching by time of birth, they found a significantly higher frequency of CBV-3 IgM at delivery in mothers whose children later became diabetic compared with their matched control subjects.

Hyoty et al. (1995) initiated a prospective study designed to assess the role of coxsackie B and other enterovirus infections in the induction and acceleration of this process. Three separate series were studied:

1. An intrauterine exposure series comprising 96 pregnant mothers whose children subsequently manifested IDDM and 96 control mothers whose children remained nondiabetic
2. A cohort of 22 initially unaffected siblings of diabetic children who were followed until they developed clinical IDDM (mean observation time, 29 months) and 110 control siblings who remained nondiabetic
3. A case–control series comprising 90 children with newly diagnosed IDDM and 90 control subjects

Enterovirus infections were identified on the basis of significant increases in serum IgG, IgM, or IgA class antibodies against a panel of enterovirus antigens (capture radioimmunoassay). Enterovirus antibodies were significantly elevated in pregnant mothers whose children subsequently manifested IDDM, particularly in cases in which IDDM appeared at a very young age, before the age of three years ($p < 0.005$). Serologically verified enterovirus infections were almost two times more frequent in siblings who developed clinical IDDM than in siblings who remained nondiabetic (mean, 1.0 vs. 0.6 infections/follow-up year; $p < 0.001$). This difference was seen both close to the diagnosis of IDDM and several years before diagnosis.

Using the nationwide child-onset diabetes register in Sweden, Dahlquist et al. (1995a,b) traced children who contracted diabetes before the age of 15 years and who were born at a specific hospital in Sweden where maternal sera from delivery had been stored during the years 1969 to 1989. Sera obtained at delivery from 57 mothers of diabetic children were compared with sera from control subjects who

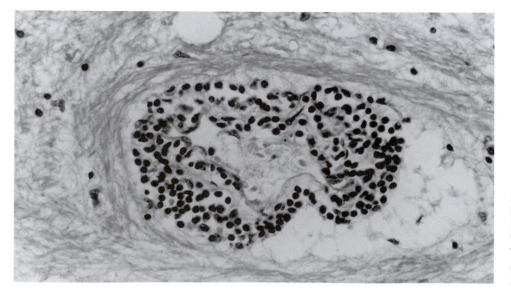

FIGURE I Photo of a neonatal brain infected with Coxsackie group B virus demonstrating perivascular "cuffing" with infiltration of the Virchow-Robin space by numerous mononuclear cells (H&E, ×280). *Source:* Monif (1969).

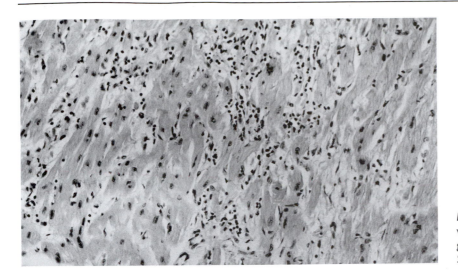

FIGURE 2 Interstitial myocarditis associated with myocardial necrosis in an infant with congenital coxsackie group B infection (H&E, ×280). *Source:* Monif (1969).

were delivered at the same hospital during the same time period. The sera were analyzed blindly using a group-specific enzyme-linked immunosorbent assay for specific IgM antibodies before and after urea wash as an avidity test. The mean absorbance values of enteroviral IgG antibodies against enteroviral antigens (echo-30, coxsackie B5, and echo-9) were significantly higher among mothers whose children later developed diabetes ($p = 0.002$, $p = 0.02$, and $p = 0.04$, respectively). When IgM activity and/or a significant decrease in avidity index, an indication of recent enterovirus infection, was used as a risk exposure, the odds ratio standardized for year of birth (95% confidence interval) was 3.19 (1.39–7.30).

These types of studies are part of a growing body of circumstantial evidence that may indicate that a fetal infection with the coxsackie viruses similar to rubella virus may initiate autoimmunity or cause persistent infection that may lead to progressive beta-cell destruction.

Diagnosis

Congenital infection with the coxsackie group B viruses is distinguished from its neonatal counterpart by the presence of the disease process at birth or its development in the first 48 hours of life. The diagnosis may be inferred prospectively or retrospectively on clinical or histologic grounds because of characteristic target organ involvement. However, involvement of brain, heart, and liver is not a constant occurrence. Formes frustes of the disease are more likely to predominate. The diagnosis of subclinical disease is contingent upon the recovery of the virus from the products of conception and/or the neonate or the demonstration of specific IgM-neutralizing antibody in the cord blood.

The enteroviral subgroups were originally differentiated from each other by their different effects in tissue cultures and in animals.

Even though many human tissue culture systems are capable of functioning as adequate indicator systems, virus recovery is best achieved in a biologic indicator system, such as less than 24-hour-old suckling mice. The identification of enteroviral types by neutralization in suckling mice or tissue cultures with antiserum pools is well defined.

Serologically, there are some minor cross-reactions between several enteroviral types, but there are no common group structural protein antigens of diagnostic importance.

Congenital and neonatal infections have been linked with many enteroviruses, and representatives of all four major enterovirus groups have been associated with disease in the neonate. The serologic diagnosis of enterovirus infection is impractical because there are no common group antigens, making identification by each specific virus very time consuming and costly.

Polymerase chain reaction (PCR) testing of cerebrospinal fluid, blood, urine, and tissue specimens is the principal method used to detect enterovirus DNA in cerebrospinal and amniotic fluids as well as in tissue specimens.

CONGENITAL ECHOVIRUS INFECTION

Transplacental dissemination of echoviruses occurs; infection in the fetus or neonate is usually subclinical. To date, no recognized embryopathy or teratogenic sequelae have been identified. Johansson et al. (1992) report a case of intrauterine fetal death in the 29th week of gestation. Echovirus 11 was isolated from the umbilical cord of the fetus. The mother had only serologic evidence of current echovirus 11 infection. Enterovirus PCR performed on paraffin-embedded specimens of various tissues (myocardium, lung, liver, and placenta) from the fetus yielded positive results in all cases. These findings together with supporting serologic and epidemiologic findings—e.g., proven echovirus 11 infection three weeks before in the 18-month-old son of a woman—constituted evidence that echovirus 11 infection was responsible for the fetal death.

POLIOVIRUS

A high incidence of abortion does occur among gravidas who contract clinically overt poliomyelitis during the acute phase of their disease. Among the progeny born to mothers who contracted their disease early in gestation, there is a definite increase in the incidence of prematurity and low-birthweight neonates. Some of these infants exhibited impaired somatic development.

Poliomyelitis early in pregnancy may result in abortion or stillbirth. Whereas some cases are presumably related to the attending toxemia and hypermetabolic state, others may be the direct consequence of transplacental infection. Viral infection of the fetus later in gestation may result in premature deliveries or overt clinical disease at parturition.

CONGENITAL POLIOVIRUS INFECTION/DISEASE

Rare cases of overt poliomyelitis in newborn infants at parturition or within the first four days of life have been identified. The application of virologic techniques to the products of conception or the progeny of mothers whose gestation had been complicated by the development of poliomyelitis has demonstrated a significant occurrence of asymptomatic congenital infection. The clinical expression of poliovirus injection is contingent on their neurotropism rather than viscerotropism. Although potentially of etiologic significance with respect to the heightened incidence of miscarriage and abortion observed during maternal infection with the polioviruses during gestation, congenital infection with visceral involvement is probably insufficient in most instances for the production of clinically overt neonatal disease. It is only when the virus has the additional ability to traverse the "blood–brain barrier" that in utero infection is manifested at birth or in the immediate neonatal period.

Overt congenital poliomyelitis, like its extrauterine counterpart, is a rare phenomenon with respect to the true incidence of infection. The meaning of visceral involvement in terms of somatic development and subsequent related morbidity has never been adequately evaluated because of lack of prospective virologic studies during the neonatal period and beyond.

The existence of both maternal and congenital subclinical diseases invalidates many of the statistics concerning the probability of transplacental transfer. With the advent of the live vaccines, this entity has been basically reduced to a theoretical academic issue.

NEONATAL POLIOMYELITIS

Neonatal poliomyelitis is acquired due to either ascending infection associated with prolonged rupture of the fetal membrane or contact infection in association with parturition. Infants born to mothers whose disease manifested itself in the postpartum period exhibit a higher probability of ensuing neonatal neurologic disease. This reflected the more prolonged and intimate exposure to the virus.

Congenital and neonatal poliomyelitis are clinically and pathologically indistinguishable. Characteristically, infants are lethargic and exhibit marked focal flaccidity. Cyanosis is a variable phenomenon predominantly related to the spinal cord involvement, affecting the muscles of respiration and/or the presence of interstitial pneumonia.

At necropsy, the dominant lesions involve the anterior horns of the spinal cord and the motor nuclei of the cranial nerves. The process is irregular in distribution and usually asymmetrical. As in "adult" poliomyelitis, interstitial myocarditis may occur. A focal interstitial pneumonitis may be present.

Diagnosis

The distinction between congenital and neonatal infections with the polioviruses is the presence of the disease process at birth or its development before the shortest documented incubation period for the polioviruses (five days). Both subclinical and overt congenital infections can be identified on the basis of virus isolation from placenta and neonate. Epithelial and fibroblastic tissue culture lines of human and primate origin afford adequate indicator systems for the recovery of the polioviruses. In dealing with necropsy material, primary monkey kidney tissue culture, in conjunction with agar overlay, constitutes the most sensitive indicator system for the isolation and tentative identification of any of the enteroviruses.

The diagnosis of congenital infection can be made on serologic grounds. This requires the demonstration of specific IgM antibody in cord serum or in the serum obtained in the immediate neonatal period.

Prophylaxis

One of the unresolved questions concerning therapy is whether a given patient with bulbar poliomyelitis should be allowed to go to term and, if so, the mode of delivery. Fragmentary reports suggest that certain patients benefit from the effect of terminating the pregnancy; however, it is stressed that the viability of the infant, progression of disease, and maternal vital capacity are the prime factors governing the mode of delivery.

The postpartum development of maternal poliomyelitis warrants immediate isolation of the infant. Once infection is initiated, gamma globulin is probably ineffective in aborting the disease or modifying the clinical severity of the disease.

A killed poliovirus vaccine can be administered during pregnancy when the clinical and epidemiologic indications warrant its administration. Live attenuated vaccine strains of the polioviruses in rare instances spread among susceptible family contacts and have produced clinical disease in vaccine recipients and family contacts.

LIVE VIRUS AND INACTIVATED VIRUS VACCINES

In 1998, the World Health Assembly resolved to eradicate polio worldwide. The global incidence decreased from 350,000 cases in 1988 to fewer than 2000 cases in 2005. Only Afghanistan, India, Nigeria, and Pakistan continue to have endemic outbreaks due to the wild strain of the polioviruses.

The risk of poliomyelitis is very small in the United States; however, epidemics could occur if the high immunity level of the general population is not maintained by vaccinating children routinely or if wild poliovirus is introduced into susceptible populations in communities with low immunization levels.

Two types of poliovirus vaccines are currently licensed in the United States: OPV (live virus) and eIPV (inactive). A primary vaccination series with either vaccine produces immunity to all three types of poliovirus in >95% of recipients. The primary series of OPV consists of three doses: two doses given six to eight weeks apart and a third dose given at least six weeks and customarily twelve months after the second. The primary series for eIPV consists of three doses: two doses each given four to eight weeks apart and a third dose given six to twelve months after the second. A primary vaccine series need not be given to adults living in the United States who have not had a primary series as children. However, for adults who have not had a primary series and who are at greater risk of exposure than the general population to wild polioviruses because of foreign travel or occupation, eIPV is preferred because the risk of OPV-associated paralysis is slightly higher among adults than among children. Poliovirus vaccine is not routinely recommended for persons older than 18 years. A small portion of immunodeficient individuals exposed to OPV have excreted vaccine-derived poliovirus over prolonged periods.

A new problem is arising: polio outbreaks due to vaccine-derived polioviruses, particularly in individuals with primary immunodeficiencies. Children of women with HIV should not receive live poliovirus vaccines.

Vaccine Adverse Reactions
Inactivated Poliovirus Vaccine
No serious side effects of currently available eIPV have been documented. Because eIPV contains trace amounts of streptomycin and neomycin, hypersensitivity reactions are possible among persons sensitive to these antibiotics. Persons with signs and symptoms of an anaphylactic reaction (e.g., hives, swelling of mouth and throat, difficulty in breathing, hypotension, or shock) after receipt of streptomycin or neomycin should not receive eIPV. Persons with reactions that are not anaphylactic are not at increased risk and may be vaccinated.

Oral Poliovirus Vaccine
In rare instances, administration of OPV has been associated with paralysis among healthy recipients and their contacts. The risk of vaccine-associated paralytic poliomyelitis is extremely small for immunologically normal vaccinees (approximately one case per 1.4 million first doses distributed and one case per 41.5 million subsequent doses) and for their susceptible immunologically normal household contacts (approximately one case per 1.9 million first doses distributed and one case per 13.8 million subsequent doses). However, vaccinees should be informed of this risk.

Vaccine Precautions and Contraindications
Inactivated Poliovirus Vaccine
No convincing evidence of adverse effects of eIPV for the pregnant woman or developing fetus exists; however, theoretically vaccination of pregnant women should be avoided. However, if immediate protection against poliomyelitis is needed, OPV, not eIPV, is recommended.

Oral Poliovirus Vaccine
Unlike other live virus vaccines that are administered parenterally, OPV is administered orally. Immunoglobulin and other antibody-containing blood products do not appear to interfere with the immune response to OPV.

OPV should not be administered to persons (i) who are or may be immunocompromised as a result of immune deficiency diseases, HIV infection, leukemia, lymphoma, or generalized malignancy and (ii) who are or may be immunosuppressed as a result of therapy with corticosteroids, alkylating drugs, antimetabolites, or radiation.

SELECTED READING

Coxsackie Viruses

Batcup G, Holt P, Hambling MH, et al. Placental and fetal pathology in Coxsackie virus A-9 infection: a case report. Histopathology 1985; 9:1227.

Bates HR. Coxsackie virus B-3 calcific pancarditis and hydrops fetalis. Am J Obstet Gynecol 1970; 106:629.

Benirschke K, Kibrick S, Craig JM. The pathology of fatal Coxsackie infection of the newborn. Am J Pathol 1958; 34:587.

Benirschke K, Pendleton ME. Coxsackie virus infection. An important complication of pregnancy. Obstet Gynecol 1958; 12:305.

Brightman VJ, Scott TFM, Westphal M, Boggs TR. An outbreak of Coxsackie B-5 virus infection in a newborn nursery. J Pediatr 1966; 69:179.

Burch GE, Sun SC, Colcolough HL, et al. Coxsackie B viral myocarditis and valvulitis identified in routine autopsy specimens by immunofluorescent techniques. Am Heart J 1967; 74:13.

Butler N, Skelton MO, Hodges GM, et al. Fatal Coxsackie B-3 myocarditis in a newborn infant. Br Med J 1962; 1:1251.

Dahlquist G, Frisk G, Ivarsson SA, et al. Indications that maternal Coxsackie B virus infection during pregnancy is a risk factor for childhood-onset IDDM. Diabetologia 1995a; 38:1371.

Dahlquist GG, Ivarsson S, Lindberg B, Forsgren M. Maternal enteroviral infection during pregnancy as a risk factor for childhood IDDM. A population-based case control study. Diabetes 1995b; 44:408.

Delaney TB, Fukunga FH. Myocarditis in a newborn infant with encephalomeningitis due to Coxsackie virus group B, type 5. New Engl J Med 1958; 259:234.

Fechner RE, Smith MG, Middlekamp JN. Coxsackie B virus infection of the newborn. Am J Pathol 1963; 42:493.

Helin I, Widell A, Borulf S, et al. Outbreak of Coxsackievirus A-14 meningitis among newborns in a maternity hospital ward. Acta Paediatr Scand 1987; 76:234.

Hosier DM, Newton WA Jr. Serious Coxsackie infection in infants and children. Am J Dis Child 1958; 96:251.

Hyoty H, Hiltunen M, Knip M, et al. A prospective study of the role of coxsackie B and other enterovirus infections in the pathogenesis of IDDM. Childhood Diabetes in Finland (DiMe) Study Group. Diabetes 1995; 44:652.

Jack I, Townley RRW. Acute myocarditis of newborn infants, due to Coxsackie viruses. Med J Aust 1961; 2:265.

Jahn CL, Cherry JD. Mild neonatal illness associated with heavy enterovirus infection. N Engl J Med 1966; 274:394.

Javett SN, Hymann S, Mundel B, et al. Myocarditis in the newborn infant: a study of an outbreak associated with Coxsackie group B virus infection in a maternity home in Johannesburg. J Pediatr 1956; 48:1.

Jenning RC. Coxsackie group B fatal neonatal myocarditis associated with cardiomegaly. J Clin Pathol 1966; 19:325.

Kibrick S, Benirschke K. Acute aseptic myocarditis and meningoencephalitis in the newborn child infected with Coxsackie virus group B type 3. New Engl J Med 1956; 255:883.

Kibrick S, Benirschke K. Severe generalized disease occurring in the newborn period and due to infection with Coxsackie virus, group B. Pediatrics 1958; 22:857.

Makower HK, Skurska A, Halazinska L. On transplacental infection with Coxsackie virus. Texas Rep Biol Med 1958; 16:346.

McLean DM, Donahue WL, Snelling CE, Wyllie JC. Neonatal encephalitis and myocarditis. Can Med Assoc J 1961; 85:1046.

Monif GRG. Viral Infection of the Human Fetus. New York: Macmillan, 1969.

Moossy J, Geer JC. Encephalomyelitis, myocarditis and adrenal cortical necrosis in Coxsackie B-3 virus infection. Arch Pathol 1960; 70:614.

O'Shaughnessey WJ, Buechner HA. Hepatitis associated with Coxsackie B-5 virus late in pregnancy. J Am Med Assoc 1962; 179:71.

Plager H, Beebe R, Miller JK. Coxsackie B-5 pericarditis in pregnancy. Arch Intern Med 1962; 110:735.

Rantakallio P, Saukkonen AL, Krause U, et al. Follow-up study of 17 cases of neonatal Coxsackie B5 meningitis and one with suspected myocarditis. Scand J Infect Dis 1970; 2:25.

Rapmund G, Gauld JR, Rogers NB, Holmes GB. Neonatal myocarditis and meningoencephalitis due to Coxsackie virus Group B type 4: virology study of a fatal case with simultaneous aseptic meningitis in the mother. New Engl J Med 1959; 260:819.

Robino G, Perlman A, Togo Y, Reback J. Fatal neonatal infection due to Coxsackie B-2 virus. J Pediatr 1962; 61:911.

Schurmann W, Statz A, Mertens T, et al. Two cases of Coxsackie B-2 infection in neonates: clinical, virological, and epidemiological aspects. Eur J Pediatr 1983; 140:59.

Simenhoff ML, Uys CJ. Coxsackie virus myocarditis of newborn: a pathological survey of four cases. Med Proc 1958; 4:389.

Strong BS, Young SA. Intrauterine Coxsackie virus, group B type 1, infection: viral cultivation from amniotic fluid in the third trimester. Am J Perinatol 1995; 12:78.

Susman ML, Strauss L, Hodes HL. Fatal Coxsackie group B virus infection in the newborn: report of a case with necropsy findings and brief review of the literature. Am J Dis Child 1959; 97:483.

Talsma M, Vegting M, Hess J. Generalized Coxsackie A-9 infection in a neonate presenting with pericarditis. Br Heart J 1984; 52:683.

Van Crevelds S, de Jager H. Myocarditis in newborns, caused by Coxsackie virus. Ann Paediatr 1956; 187:100.

Verlinde JD, van Tongeren HAE, Kret A. Myocarditis in newborns due to Group B Coxsackie virus: virus studies. Ann Paediatr 1956; 187:113.

Wright HT Jr, Okuyama K, McAllister RM. An infant fatality associated with Coxsackie B1 virus. J Pediatr 1963; 63:428.

Echoviruses

Berkovich S, Smithwick EM. Transplacental infection due to echo virus type 22. J Pediatr 1968; 72:94.

Bowen GS, Fisher MC, Deforest A, et al. Epidemic of meningitis and febrile illness in neonates caused by echo type II virus in Philadelphia. Pediatr Infect Dis 1983; 2:359.

Cheeseman SH, Hirsch MS, Keller EW, et al. Fatal neonatal pneumonia caused by echovirus type 9. Am J Dis Child 1977; 131:1169.

Cherry JD, Soriano F, Jahn CL. Search for perinatal viral infection: a prospective clinical virological and serological study. Am J Dis Child 1968; 116:245.

Cho CT, Janelle JG, Behbehani A. Severe neonatal illness associated with echo 9 virus infection. Clin Pediatr 1973; 12:304.

Georgieff MK, Johnson DE, Thompson TR, et al. Fulminant hepatic necrosis in an infant with perinatally acquired echovirus 21 infection. Pediatr Infect Dis 1987; 6:71.

Johansson ME, Holmstrom S, Abebe A, et al. Intrauterine fetal death due to echovirus 11. Scand J Infect Dis 1992; 24:381.

Jones MJ, Kolb M, Votava HA, et al. Intrauterine echovirus type II infection. Mayo Clin Proc 1980; 55:509.

Kibrick S. Viral infections of the fetus and newborn. In: Pollard M, ed. Perspective in Virology. Vol. 2. Minneapolis: Burgess Publishing Co, 1961:141.

Mostoufizadeh M, Lack EE, Gang DL, et al. Postmortem manifestations of echovirus 11 sepsis in five newborn infants. Hum Pathol 1983; 14:818.

Piraino FF, Sedmak G, Raab K. Echovirus 11 infections of newborns with mortality during the 1979 enterovirus season in Milwaukee. Wisc Public Health Rep 1982; 97:346.

Reyes MP, Ostrea EM Jr, Roskamp J, et al. Disseminated neonatal echovirus 11 disease following antenatal maternal infection with a virus-positive cervix and virus negative gastrointestinal tract. J Med Virol 1983; 12:155.

Rowan DF, McGraw MF, Eward RD. Virus infections during pregnancy. Obstet Gynecol 1968; 32:56.

Steinmann J, Albrecht K. Echovirus 11 epidemic among premature newborns in a neonatal intensive care unit. Zentralbl Bakteriol Mikrobiol Hyg 1985; 259:284.

Wreghitt TG, Gandy GM, King A, et al. Fatal neonatal echo 7 virus infection. Lancet 1984; 2:465.

Polioviruses

Abramson J, Greenberg MM, Maggee MC. Poliomyelitis in the newborn infant. J Pediatr 1953; 43:167.

Aycock WL. Personal communication cited by Shelokov A and Weinstein L. Poliomyelitis in the early neonatal period. J Pediatr 1951; 38:80.

Baker ME, Baker IG. Acute poliomyelitis in pregnancy. Minn Med 1947; 30:729.

Barsky P, Beale AJ. Transplacental transmission of poliomyelitis. J Pediatr 1957; 51:207.

Baskin JL, Soule EH, Mills SD. Poliomyelitis of the newborn: pathologic changes in two cases. Am J Dis Child 1950; 80:10.

Bates T. Poliomyelitis in pregnancy, fetus and newborn. Am J Dis Child 1955; 90:189.

Bergeisen GH, Bauman RJ, Gilmore RL. Neonatal paralytic poliomyelitis: a case report. Arch Neurol 1986; 43:192.

Biermann AH, Piszczdk EA. A case of poliomyelitis in a newborn infant. J Am Med Assoc 1944; 124:296.

Bowers VM Jr, Danforth DN. The significance of poliomyelitis during pregnancy: an analysis of 24 cases. Am J Obstet Gynecol 1953; 65:34.

Carter HM. Congenital poliomyelitis. Obstet Gynecol 1956; 8:373.

Cherry JD, Soriano F, Jahn CL. Search for perinatal viral infection: a prospective, clinical, virologic and serologic study. Am J Dis Child 1968; 116:245.

Elliott GB, McAllister JE. Fetal poliomyelitis. Am J Obstet Gynecol 1956; 72:896.

Harmon PH, Hoyne A. Poliomyelitis and pregnancy with special reference to the failure of fetal infection. J Am Med Assoc 1943; 123:185.

Horn P. Poliomyelitis in pregnancy. Obstet Gynecol 1955; 6:121.

Johnson JF, Stimson PM. Clinical poliomyelitis in the early neonatal period: report of a case. J Pediatr 1952; 40:733.

Schaeffer M, Fox MJ, Li CP. Intrauterine poliomyelitis infection. J Am Med Assoc 1954; 155:248.

Shelokov A, Weinstein L. Poliomyelitis in the early neonatal period: report of a case of possible intrauterine infection. J Pediatr 1951; 38:80.

Shelokov A, Havel K. Subclinical poliomyelitis in a newborn infant due to intrauterine infection. J Am Med Assoc 1956; 160:465.

Siegel M, Greenberg M. Polio in pregnancy: effect on the fetus and the newborn infant. J Pediatr 1956; 49:280.

Swarts CL, Kercher EF. A fatal case of poliomyelitis in a newborn infant delivered by cesarean section following maternal death due to poliomyelitis. Pediatrics 1954; 14:235.

12

The Hepatitis Viruses

INTRODUCTION

At least four distinct viruses causing human hepatitis have been distinguished to date on the basis of their biologic, physiochemical, and antigenic characteristics (Table 1).

HEPATITIS A VIRUS

Hepatitis A virus (HAV) belongs to the picornavirus group. The virus is approximately 27 nm in diameter and appears to have cubic symmetry. Degradative analysis has revealed four capsid polypeptides as well as the presence of a genome of linear single-stranded RNA. The polypeptides have molecular weights similar to three of the four polypeptides of enteroviruses. HAV is stable in the presence of ether at acid pH. Compared with the other picornaviruses, HAV is more resistant to heat. HAV exposed to temperatures of 60° C for up to 12 hours does not completely inactivate the virus. Survival of the virus in marine sediment, soil, water, and especially in seafood such as shellfish for weeks has been reported. In 1969, researchers succeeded in transmitting HAV to marmoset monkeys. The subsequent detection of hepatitis A antigen (HAAg) in the serum and liver of infected marmoset monkeys paved the way for the development of the current tests for hepatitis A antibody (anti-HAV).

Close personal contact by the fecal-oral route is the primary means of HAV transmission in the United States. The prime portal of infection in hepatitis A is the gastrointestinal tract. Disease follows an incubation period of 30 to 80 days. HAAg can be demonstrated in the stool for up to three weeks before the onset of illness and 8 days after the onset of jaundice. Shedding of antigen is maximal before onset of illness, but HAAg is still found in low amounts in about 50% of the serologically confirmed cases of hepatitis A during the first week of illness and in about 25% during the second week. This prolonged excretion of virus from the gastrointestinal tract is subclinical and designates humans as the prime reservoir of the virus. In infants and children, shedding from the stool may continue for extended periods of time. The disease has been reproduced in human volunteers following the oral ingestion of virus-containing material.

The virus resists heat inactivation at 56° C as well as freezing for one-half to one hour. It can maintain its infectiousness for prolonged periods. Because of the high probability of encountering virus-containing material, susceptible subjects are probably infected at an early age (Fig. 1). As might be anticipated, there is a seasonal nosologic distribution for HAV, with a low incidence in midsummer and a peak in late winter and early spring. The incidence of overt HAV infection is highest for individuals under 20 years of age. The peak incidence of disease in this age group can be interpreted as 2reflecting the prevalence of HAV and secondarily its contagiousness for susceptible contacts. Secondary cases are not uncommon. In these cases, hand-to-mouth dissemination appears to be the mode of transmission. Nevertheless, the majority of cases of both clinical and subclinical forms of hepatitis A are the result of water-borne viral spread (Figs. 2–5). Epidemics have been shown to occur under conditions of poor sanitation as water-borne epidemics or in association with the ingestion of raw oysters or hardshell clams bred in polluted water. The relative incidence of icteric versus nonicteric cases of hepatitis A is not known. The ratio between the two may be analogous to that of the poliovirus, where poliomyelitis is like the tip of an iceberg in contrast to the bulk of subclinical infection. Although rare, cases of intrauterine infected with HAV have been reported.

HEPATITIS B VIRUS

Hepatitis B virus (HBV) is grouped with the Hepadnaviridae. The virus gives rise to the appearance of various types of antigenic particles in the serum of affected individuals. The structure representing the causative virus is a double-shelled particle about 42 nm in diameter. It contains an inner core of distinct antigenicity, hepatitis B core antigen (HBcAg), which shows cubic symmetry and contains a molecule of circular double-stranded DNA of 1.6×10^6 daltons. The core particle is surrounded by a shell, hepatitis B surface antigen (HBsAg), and composed of carbohydrate, lipid, and protein. HBsAg carries a common determinant and a number of major subdeterminants (designated d, u, w, and r), which are coded by the viral genome. HBsAg may also occur in the form of 22 nm spherical particles and as filaments of similar diameter but of variable length. The 42 nm HBV particle contains a DNA-dependent DNA polymerase that uses the circular double-stranded DNA of the core as a primary template.

No cross-immunity between HAV and HBV has been demonstrated in vitro and in vivo. Individuals previously exposed to HAV are immune to rechallenge with HAV. The prime portal of entry for HBV was thought to be the parenteral injection of blood or blood products derived from a healthy carrier of serum hepatitis, but this need not be the case. The ingestion of infectious material can induce either infection or disease in presumably susceptible individuals. HBsAg has been detected in many human biologic fluids, including saliva, semen, cervical secretions, and leukocytes during acute infection. Person-to-person spread of hepatitis B has been documented among mentally retarded individuals in institutions and among intimate contacts, including sexual consorts of patients with hepatitis B or with persistent HBs antigenemia. Because HBV has a limited accessibility to a susceptible population, there is no peak incidence of disease,

TABLE I   Hepatitis nomenclature

	Abbreviation	Term	Definition/comments
Hepatitis A	HAV	Hepatitis A virus	Etiologic agent of "infectious" hepatitis; a picornavirus; single serotype
	Anti-HAV	Antibody to HAV	Detectable at onset of symptoms; lifetime persistence
	IgM anti-HAV	IgM class antibody to	Indicates recent infection with hepatitis A; detectable for 4–6 mo after infection
Hepatitis B	HBV	Hepatitis B virus	Etiologic agent of "serum" hepatitis; also known as Dane particle
	HBsAg	Hepatitis B surface antigen	Surface antigen(s) of HBV detectable in large quantity in serum; several subtypes identified
	HBeAg	Hepatitis Be antigen	Soluble antigen; correlates with HBV replication, high titer of HBV in serum, and infectivity of serum
	HBcAg	Hepatitis B core antigen	No commercial test available
	Anti-HBs	Antibody to HBsAg	Indicates past infection with and immunity to HBV, passive antibody from HBIG, or immune response from HB vaccine
	Anti-HBe	Antibody to HBeAg	Presence in serum of HBsAg carrier indicates lower titer of HBV
	Anti-HBc	Antibody to HBcAg	Indicates prior infection with HBV at some undefined time
	IgM anti-HBc	IgM class antibody to	Indicates recent infection with HBV; detectable for 4–6 mo after infection
Hepatitis C	PT-NANB	Parenterally transmitted	Diagnosis by exclusion; at least two candidate viruses, one of which has been proposed as hepatitis C virus; shares epidemiologic features with hepatitis B
	ET-NANB	Enterically transmitted	Diagnosis by exclusion; causes epidemics in Asia, Africa, and Mexico; fecal–oral or water borne
Delta hepatitis	HDV	Delta virus	Etiologic agent of delta hepatitis; can cause infection only in the presence of HBV
	HDAg and anti-HDV	Delta antigen and antibody to delta antigen	Detectable in early acute delta infection; indicates present or past infection with delta virus

Abbreviations: IgM, immunoglobulin M.
Source: From Monif (1993).

in contrast to the case with hepatitis A. Several valuable markers of hepatitis B were discovered during the 1970s. These include the following:

1. HBsAg and its respective antibody (anti-HBs or HBsAb)
2. HBcAg and its respective antibody (anti-HBc or HBcAb)
3. Hepatitis Be antigen (HBeAg) and its respective antibody (anti-HBe)

Both HBsAg and HBeAg are usually found in the serum of hepatitis B patients during late incubation and early clinical phases of the illness. Both antigens are detectable prior to the onset of jaundice or enzymatic abnormalities. HBsAg appears about one to three weeks after exposure and disappears after a period of three weeks to three months, while anti-HBs appears for several weeks to a month following the clearing of HBsAg from the serum. Once present, anti-HBs will persist for years. The case fatality rate is approximately 1.4%.

HBcAg is not detectable in serum; however, anti-HBc is usually demonstrable at the time of onset of jaundice and abnormal enzyme chemistries. Anti-HBc, like anti-HBs, tends to persist once it is present.

HBeAg is demonstrable by solid-phase radioimmuno-assay for a relatively short period of time and usually disappears before HBsAg has been cleared from the serum. The persistence of HBeAg tends to correlate with a prolonged course of illness and appears to have prognostic value late in the course of the disease.

Anti-HBe appears following the disappearance of HBeAg. Disease follows an incubation period of 41 to 108

days. The host may influence the clinical expression of the disease. Millman has noted that patients with Down's syndrome, leukemia, lepromatous leprosy, or chronic renal failure and those undergoing renal dialysis tend to develop a chronic anicteric form of hepatitis associated with the persistence of HBs antigen, in contrast to normal individuals, in whom the disease is clinically overt but of a shorter duration. In a small epidemic of hepatitis B among the patients and staff of a renal dialysis unit, infection occurred among nine patients and six staff members within one year. The disease among the staff members was characterized by acute overt clinical disease with elevated bilirubin levels and serum aspartate aminotransferase (AST) levels over 1000 units. The AST elevations were less than 10 weeks in duration. The patients undergoing dialysis exhibited SGPT levels under 1000 units, but these elevations persisted for 20 weeks or more.

Chronic Hepatitis B Infection

The serum of a small percentage of individuals with hepatitis B will exhibit a persistence of HBs antigenemia. Three patterns are evident among the chronic HBsAg carriers. Chronic infection may be characterized by the following:

1. A prolonged period of abnormal serum transaminase activity and by persistence of HBsAg, HBeAg, and anti-HBc
2. Persistence of HBsAg and anti-HBc associated with normal serum transaminase activity, the disappearance of HBeAg without the development of HBe-Ab

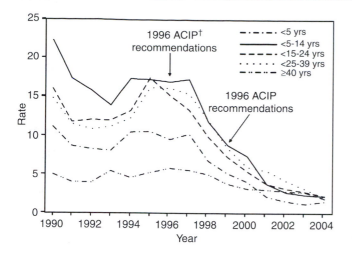

FIGURE 1 Rate of reported hepatitis A by age group and year, per 100,000 population (United States, 1990–2004). *Abbreviation*: ACIP, Advisory Committee on Immunization Practices. *Source*: From National Notable Diseases Surveillance System.

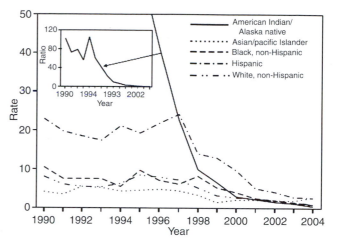

FIGURE 2 Rate of reported hepatitis A by race and ethnicity, per 100,000 population (United States, 1990–2004). *Source*: From National Notable Diseases Surveillance System.

3. Persistence of HBsAg and anti-HBc associated with normal serum transaminase activity, the disappearance of HBeAg, and the subsequent appearance and persistence of HBe-Ab

These forms of chronic hepatitis B pose unique problems for the offspring of mothers with HBs antigenemia. The rate of hepatitis B infection in infants born to mothers with the active type of chronic infection depends on their HBeAg and HBeAb status as follows if the newborns are not properly treated with immune globulin and HBV vaccine:

- HBsAg positive and HBeAg positive: 90%
- HBsAg positive and HBeAg positive: 25%
- HBsAg positive and HBeAg positive: 10%

HEPATITIS C

According to the National Health and Nutrition Examination Survey (1988–1994) and other population-based surveys, estimates of the incidence and prevalence of hepatitis C virus (HCV) infection have been made. Nearly four million Americans are infected with hepatitis C. The

infection is more common in minority populations (3.2% of African Americans and 2.1% of Mexican Americans) than in non-Hispanic whites (1.5%). The incidence of hepatitis C infection appears to be declining since its peak in 1989. Currently, approximately 30,000 acute new infections are estimated to occur each year, about 25% to 30% of which are diagnosed. Hepatitis C accounts for 20% of all cases of acute hepatitis. Currently, hepatitis C is responsible for an estimated 8000 to 10,000 deaths annually, and without effective intervention, that number is postulated to triple in the next 10 to 20 years. Hepatitis C is now the leading reason for liver transplantation in the United States.

Parenterally transmitted NANBH accounts for 20% to 40% of acute viral hepatitis in the United States. Although it has traditionally been considered a transfusion-associated disease, studies of community-acquired NANBH and data from the Centers for Disease Control (CDC) National Surveillance System have shown that 23% to 42% of NANBH cases are associated with IV drug use. In addition, 8% to 11% are attributed to blood transfusion and 4% to 8% to healthcare occupational exposure. However, for as many as 57%, no source of infection can be identified.

High rates of HCV infection in commercial sex workers and in persons with multiple sexual partners suggest a sexual

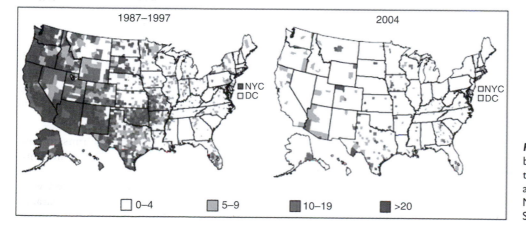

FIGURE 3 Rate of hepatitis A by county, per 100,000 population (United States, 1987–1997 and 2004). *Source*: From National Notable Diseases Surveillance System.

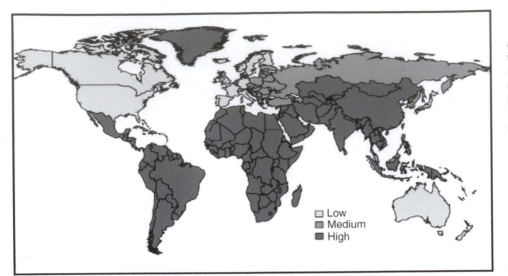

FIGURE 4 Geographic distribution of hepatitis A endemicity (2005). For multiple countries, estimates of prevalence of antibody to hepatitis A virus (anti-HAV), a marker of previous HAV infection, are based on limited data and might not reflect current prevalence. In addition, anti-HAV prevalence might vary within countries by subpopulation and locality. As used on this map, the terms "high," "medium," and "low" endemicity reflect available evidence of how widespread infection is within each country rather than precise quantitative assessments.

mode of transmission for HCV. However, this has not been proven to date. HCV RNA has been detected in semen and saliva. In cases where there has only been sexual exposure for a route of transmission for an explanation for infection, this provides additional evidence. At present, the exact risk of transmission by the sexual route is unknown, but is low. However, healthcare providers need to discuss this risk and encourage the use of barrier precautions.

The HCV is an RNA virus of the Flaviviridae family. Individual isolates consist of closely related yet heterogeneous populations of viral genomes (quasi-species). Probably as a consequence of this genetic diversity, HCV has the ability to escape the host's immune surveillance, leading to a high rate of chronic infection. Comparing the genomic nucleotide sequences from various HCV isolates enables classification of viruses into several genotypes and many more subtypes.

Based on genomic sequencing, there are at least six distinct genotypes. Some of these genotypes appear to be sufficiently divergent from each other to suggest the prob-

ability that they represent different serotypes biologically due to significant differences in their critical antigens.

HCV is a virus composed of a single strand of RNA containing approximately 10,000 nucleotides (Table 2). The virus is a spherical, lipid-enveloped virus with a mean diameter of 35 to 50 nm. Various strains of HCV demonstrate a remarkable degree of nucleotide sequence diversity.

Hepatitis C antigen is primarily a disease that is able to spread by transfusion or the use of drug paraphernalia. HCV antibodies are detected in approximately 0.6% of blood donors in the United States. Its overall prevalence worldwide is comparable. However, there are within these populations high-risk groups defined as multiply transfused hemophiliacs and intravenous drug addicts, in whom the prevalence of HCV antibodies may reach 60% to 70%. The distribution of HCV antibodies in different populations is listed in Table 3.

Primary Infection

After initial exposure, HCV RNA can be detected in blood in one to three weeks. Viremia is maximum at the onset of either clinical or subclinical disease. Within an average of 50 days (range: 15–150 days), virtually all patients develop liver

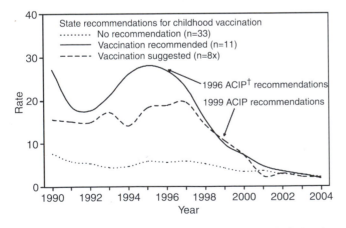

FIGURE 5 Rate of hepatitis A by region, recommendation for childhood vaccination and year (1990–2004), per 100,000 population. *Abbreviation*: ACIP, Advisory Committee on Immunization Practices. *Source*: From National Notable Diseases Surveillance System.

TABLE 2 Hepatitis C virus

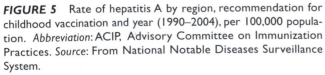

RNA virus: single strand
Configuration: Similar to flavivirus, which includes dengue yellow fever, Japanese encephalitis virus. Spherical, lipid-enveloped viruses with a mean diameter of 35–50 nm. Different strains of HCV demonstrate a remarkable degree of nucleotide sequence diversity. Based on genomic sequencing, there are at least six distinct genotypes. Some HCV genotypes appear to be sufficiently divergent from each other to suggest the probability that they represent different serotypes, biologically due to significant differences in critical antigens
Mode of transmission: Transfusion, intravenous drug user, occupation hazard; 75% anicteric. Extrahepatic manifestations not recognized
Serologic response: HCV antibodies appear 6–12 mo after the onset of infection/disease

Abbreviation: HCV, hepatitis C virus.

TABLE 3 Distribution of HCV antibodies by presumed mode of transmission

Parental transmission	2.1%
Blood transfusion	4.8%
Parental drug abusers	0.5%
Hemodialysis patients	1.8%
Nonparental transmission (sexual exposure)	7.1%

cell injury, as shown by elevation of serum alanine amino-transferase (ALT). The majority of patients are asymptomatic and anicteric. Only 25% to 35% develop malaise, weakness, or anorexia, and some become icteric. Clinically overt hepatitis in the course of primary disease is rare unless the Japanese serotype is involved, in which case it may be as high as 20% to 30%. Fulminant liver failure following HCV infection has been reported, but is a rare occurrence. Antibodies to HCV (anti-HCV) almost invariably become detectable during the course of illness. Anti-HCV can be detected in 50% to 70% of patients at the onset of symptoms and in approximately 90% of patients three months after the onset of infection. HCV infection is self-limited in only 15% of cases. Recovery is characterized by disappearance of HCV RNA from blood and return of liver enzymes to normal. There are no associated extrahepatic manifestations with acute, as opposed to chronic, hepatitis C infection.

Chronic Infection

About 85% of HCV-infected individuals fail to clear the virus by six months and develop chronic hepatitis with persistent, although sometimes intermittent, viremia. Multiple episodes due to this virus grouping can occur. This capacity to produce chronic hepatitis is one of the most striking features of HCV infection. The majority of patients with chronic infection have abnormalities in ALT levels that can fluctuate widely. About one-third of patients have persistently normal serum ALT levels. Antibodies to HCV or circulating viral RNA can be demonstrated in virtually all patients.

Chronic hepatitis C is typically an insidious process, progressing, if at all, at a slow rate without symptoms or physical signs in majority of patients during the first two decades after infection. A small proportion of patients with chronic hepatitis C, perhaps fewer than 20%, develop nonspecific symptoms, including mild intermittent fatigue and malaise. Symptoms first appear in many patients with chronic hepatitis C at the time of development of advanced liver disease.

The rate of progression is highly variable. Long-term studies suggest that most patients with progressive liver disease who develop cirrhosis have detectable ALT elevations; these can, however, be intermittent. The relationship is inconsistent between ALT levels and disease severity as judged histologically. Although patients with HCV infection and normal ALT levels have been referred to as "healthy" HCV carriers, liver biopsies can show histologic evidence of chronic hepatitis in many of these patients.

One of the major problems with chronic hepatitis, which progresses to cirrhosis, is that three quarters of the affected people would have no overt clinical signs or symptoms of disease. Extrahepatic manifestations of chronic hepatitis C do occur. Because of the immunologic responses, some of these patients will develop cryoglobulinemia with circulating polyclonal immunoglobulin G (IgG) and immunoglobulin M (IgM). Cryoglobulins may be detected in the serum of about one-third of patients with HCV, but the clinical features of essential mixed cryoglobulinemia develop in only about 1% to 2% of patients. These circulating immune complexes result in thyroid antibodies and, ultimately, Hashimoto's thyroiditis, vasculitis, or membranous proliferative glomerulonephritis. Chronic hepatitis C may be a major underlying cause of porphyria cutanea tarda.

Cirrhosis of the Liver

Chronic hepatitis C infection leads to cirrhosis in at least 20% of patients within two decades of the onset of infection. Cirrhosis and end-stage liver disease may occasionally develop rapidly, especially among patients with concomitant alcohol use. Alcohol appears to be a very important cofactor in the ultimate development of HCV-related cirrhosis.

Hepatocellular Carcinoma

Hepatocellular carcinoma (HCC) is a late complication of chronic HCV. The prevailing concept is that HCC occurs against a background of inflammation and regeneration associated with chronic hepatitis over the course of approximately three or more decades. Most cases of HCV-related HCC occur in the presence of cirrhosis.

The risk that a person with chronic hepatitis C will develop HCC appears to be 1% to 5% after 20 years, with striking variations in rates in various geographic areas of the world. Once cirrhosis is established, the rate of development of HCC increases to 1% to 4% per year. Among patients with cirrhosis due to hepatitis C, HCC develops more commonly in men than in women and in older than in younger patients.

DELTA VIRUS

Delta virus is a unique hepatotropic virus. It is composed of a single strand of RNA, of low molecular weight and an internal protein core. The delta virus is 35 to 37 nm in size and is coded with the HBsAg. Its uniqueness comes from the fact that in itself, it is incapable of attaching and hence infecting hepatocytes. Infection of the liver requires concomitant presence of the hepatitis B virus. The delta virus must borrow hepatitis B surface proteins, which permit attachment and subsequent infection of liver parenchymal cells. Without this critical step of attachment, there can be no infection.

The antibody response to delta virus infection is of both IgM and IgG character. The IgM anti-delta antibody appears early during acute delta virus infection and may persist for years owing to the presence of chronic infection. The IgG anti-delta antibody occurs later in the course of acute infection. Chronic delta hepatitis is usually associated with persisting high-titer IgG anti-delta. Delta virus infection is a complicating factor in the course of acute hepatitis due to the HBV. It occurs either as a coinfection in the form of a more fulminant type of hepatitis or as a superimposed infection in a patient who is an antecedent chronic HBV carrier. Coinfection with hepatitis B/delta virus usually causes an acute hepatitis. This infection is often clinically indistinguishable from that caused by the HBV alone. However, in selected instances, disease may exhibit a biphasic course. The second set of enzyme elevations represent in this instance superimposed delta virus infection. Coinfection appears to be associated with a higher rate of fulminant hepatitis; however, it does not increase the subsequent risk of becoming a chronic HBV carrier. The incubation period of hepatitis B/delta coinfection ranges from 4 to 20 weeks. Clinical manifestations of superinfection of an HBV carrier range from asymptomatic liver enzyme elevations to fulminant hepatitis. Superinfection frequently results in the establishment of persistent delta virus infection and constitutes the major reservoir of this virus. Chronic coinfection with HBV and delta virus is associated with the development of chronic active hepatitis and cirrhosis. The diagnosis of delta virus infection is made on the basis of detection of the delta virus in serum during early infection, immunofluorescent staining of delta antigen in liver, or the appearance of delta antibodies during or after infection. Testing for delta virus is currently indicated in fulminant HBV infection or, in the case of acute non-A hepatitis, infection occurring in a known HBV carrier.

Evidence of delta virus infection has been found in up to 30% to 50% of people with fulminant hepatitis B. Coinfection has been associated with fulminant hepatitis, particularly in drug abusers. Delta infection is often related to occult blood contact, suggesting sexual or inapparent percutaneous modes of dissemination similar to the HBV.

CLINICAL MANIFESTATIONS OF HEPATITIS VIRUS INFECTION

For most of the hepatitis viruses, overt disease tends to be more severe in adults than in children. During the prodromal phase of the disease, anorexia, lassitude, myalgia, arthralgia, headaches, and gastrointestinal symptoms are often manifested. In a significant number of cases of hepatitis B, a polyarthritis-like syndrome or arthralgias may occur several weeks before the onset of jaundice. The arthralgias tend to involve the smaller joints and are particularly evident at night. A small percentage of individuals, primarily women, may develop a maculopapular rash not unlike that of rubella or certain enterovirus exanthems. Fever, often accompanied by pseudochills, tends to occur shortly before the onset of clinically overt jaundice.

The earliest derangements of hepatic dysfunction are the appearance of bile in the urine. Darkening of the urine can be detected well in advance of clinical evidence of jaundice (this is usually indicative of a serum bilirubin level greater than 3 mg/100 mL). The urinary bilirubin test is useful in the detection of anicteric and preicteric hepatitis. Paralleling the rise in serum bilirubin is the increase in alkaline phosphatase. The ALT and AST exhibit maximum titers just prior to the onset of jaundice. Early in the course of hepatitis A, the cephalin flocculation and thymol turbidity tests become positive. An ALT/AST ratio of less than 1 is reputedly characteristic of viral hepatitis due to either type A or type B virus.

With the onset of jaundice, the liver tends to enlarge and becomes tender. Histologically, it exhibits focal hepatocytic necrosis associated with a predominantly mononuclear cell infiltration both in areas of cell death and within the portal triad, as well as bile plugs and early bile duct proliferation. Individual hepatocytes may exhibit a rounding up and hyalinization similar to the Councilman body described in yellow fever. With electron microscopy, it can be seen that the most uniform change is disruption of the rough endoplasmic reticulum (ER). This alteration of the rough ER seems to correlate best with decreased hepatocellular protein secretion. Hepatocellular death is indicated by the almost complete loss of glycogen and ER or by the occurrence of Councilman bodies, which are mummified whole cells. In these acidophilic bodies, the ER and even glycogen are preserved. A resultant increase in hepatic mass occurs because of the swelling of hepatocytes and the inflammatory infiltrate. They cause stretching of Glisson capsule, which is responsible for the right upper quadrant tenderness and the positive "hepatic punch," which is evocable at this time. Splenomegaly is not an uncommon finding and is said to be present in 25% of cases if carefully sought. If hyperbilirubinemia is prolonged, pruritus may be experienced.

The severity and persistence of hepatocellular destruction determine much of the subsequent clinical course. When hepatocellular necrosis is extensive, nausea, vomiting, and derangement of the higher cortical functions ultimately develop. This type of fulminating extensive hepatocellular destruction is more commonly due to HBV. It is to be noted that patients in coma may exhibit liver function tests indicative of a predominantly obstructive phenomenon. The ALT and AST levels may be only moderately elevated, in contrast to the marked elevations of bilirubin and alkaline phosphatase; nevertheless, the AST tends to be more elevated than the ALT. Coma is a reflection of a metabolic encephalopathy, which in turn is a consequence of too little functional hepatocellular tissue.

As a rule, the peak ALT and AST elevations occur within one or two days before or after the onset of jaundice. With massive necrosis, there is a collapse of the supporting reticulum for the destroyed hepatocytes. At this time, the liver is no longer palpable, and death is imminent if aggressive supportive therapy is not instituted promptly.

The differential diagnosis of hepatocellular necrosis during pregnancy is limited: the hepatitis may be due to HAV, HBV, HCV viruses, the cytomegaloviruses, Epstein-Barr (infectious mononucleosis) virus, idiopathic acute fatty metamorphosis of pregnancy, intravenous tetracycline therapy, alcoholic fatty metamorphosis, or chemical or drug hepatotoxicity. A careful history coupled with appropriate laboratory tests will provide the working diagnosis in most instances. For those cases in which a specific etiology cannot be inferred with a high degree of probability, a liver biopsy is indicated.

In general, the clinical course in adults lasts three to four weeks. Amelioration of symptoms with the return of appetite and loss of lassitude accompanies the return of normal hepatic function. A significant diuresis usually occurs at this time. Late sequelae, such as subacute hepatitis or cirrhosis, are rare following acute hepatitis. There is no predictable association between the severity of clinical manifestations of illness and the probability of these complications; however, it is worth noting that subacute hepatitis has a predilection for postmenopausal women over the age of 40.

CONGENITAL HEPATITIS

No question by an expectant mother is more poignant to an obstetrician than "will it affect my baby?" With respect to the hepatitides, the answer has been obscured by the previous inability to segregate cases of type B and type C from type A hepatitis.

In a number of retrospective cases, neonatal hepatitis was found to have developed in children born to mothers whose pregnancy had been complicated by hepatitis. These cases tended to lend weight to the possibility that a form of viral hepatitis in the mother could be transmitted in utero to her progeny. Additional data along these lines were derived from infants dying of neonatal hepatitis in the immediate postpartum period. At autopsy, they were found to have lesions ranging from diffuse hepatic cell necrosis to advanced cirrhosis. The maturity of the latter lesion and the short interim between birth and demise made it certain that the disease had developed in utero. A tendency for the lesions to be more pronounced in the left lobe of the liver reinforced the concept of hematogenous maternofetal dissemination. Because affected newborn infants exhibited the late sequelae of viral hepatitis, namely posthepatic cirrhosis, it must be presumed that other cases had undergone complete remission of infection in utero.

The first body of data consistent with the hypothesis of transplacental viral infection was the work of Stokes et al. (1951). In 1951, they were able to reproduce clinical and laboratory evidence of hepatitis in human volunteers, with serum from a newborn baby with neonatal hepatitis and from its mother, who had hepatitis during pregnancy. The failure to reproduce these findings obscured the issue until the recognition of HBsAg.

HAV Vertical Transmission

The ability of type A hepatitis to infect the fetus in utero has only recently been documented. Leiking et al. (1996) reported a case of maternal hepatitis at 20 weeks' gestation. At 27 weeks, ultrasound revealed polyhydramnios and fetal ascites. Through maternal testing, detailed fetal ultrasound, echocardiography, and funipuncture, the diagnosis was made by demonstrating abnormal liver tests, nonspecific findings of recent viral infection, and HAV IgM antibodies at the time of funipuncture. Maternal history and serologic testing also confirmed the diagnosis of hepatitis A in the mother four weeks before the appearance of fetal ascites.

Fetal meconium peritonitis has been reported after maternal HAV infection in pregnancy. Fetal in utero infection with HAV is low, but there are case reports, and mothers need to be informed of this possible transmission.

HBV Vertical Transmission

HBsAg can cross the placenta and has been demonstrated in cord serum. In a prospective study of maternofetal transmission of HBV in 125 healthy mothers who were carriers of HBsAg, Lee et al. (1978) showed that the most important determinant in such transmission was the presence of HBeAg in the mother. HBsAg was detectable by solid-phase radioimmunoassay in 33% of the amniotic fluid samples, 50% of cord blood samples, 71% of breast milk samples, and 95.3% of samples of gastric contents from newborns. The absence of a tight correlation between HBsAg in the amniotic fluid and cord blood and the subsequent development of antigenemia in the babies suggested that intrauterine infection is not a primary mode of maternofetal transmission. Intrauterine infection accounted for those babies who had HBsAg-positive cord blood and who had HBs antigenemia from one month after delivery onward. However, these babies constituted only a small percentage of the series. Shen et al. were conclusively able to demonstrate the presence of HBV DNA in the serum of 13 neonates and in leukocytes of two neonates born to 16 HBeAg-positive gravida.

Unlike most other viral infections capable of transplacental transmission and infection, congenital type B hepatitis in one child may not confer immunity to subsequent offspring. Multiple instances of disease in successive pregnancies or alternate pregnancies have been documented. Typical is a case of Gruber's in which a gravida developed anicteric hepatitis, presumably caused by HBV, in the sixth month of pregnancy. She gave birth to a child who died shortly after birth with giant-cell hepatitis (Fig. 6). A year later, another child died 48 hours after birth; at necropsy, the infant exhibited multinucleated giant cells and periportal fibrosis. A biopsy of the mother's liver at this time showed changes consistent with chronic hepatitis.

Acute HBV infection in the third trimester can give direct inoculation of the virus to the fetus in utero. The primary mode of transmission is inoculation during delivery. In addition, postnatal infection can occur via breast-feeding.

One point worthy of comment is that transplacental transmission can be a two-way phenomenon. Maternal and neonatal hepatitis have been observed following intrauterine transfusion, but it is probable that the mechanism by which this occurs is markedly different from that of congenital infection.

HCV Vertical Transmission

In one series, a vertical transmission has been documented in 10 of 31 babies born to women positive for serum HCV RNA. The statistics obtained by Ohto et al. (1994) are very similar to those previously published by Thaler et al. (1993). The Ohto study presented evidence that the strongest correlation for risk of transmission was the titer of serum HCV in the mother. HCV transmission to the

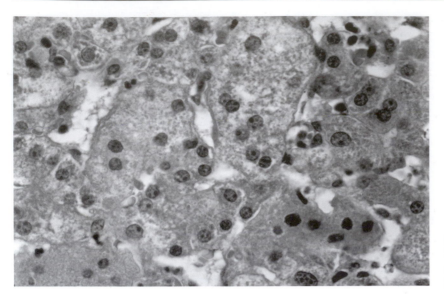

FIGURE 6 Giant-cell transformation characterized by ballooning of hepatocytes and dissolution of cell membranes in a case of neonatal hepatitis (H&E, ×480). *Source:* From Monif (1969).

newborn appears to occur prior to birth. This in utero transmission of HCV occurs in up to 50% of cases and is greater in mother coinfected with HIV and infected with HCV genotype 1. In these studies, it is not clear to what extent one is dealing with congenital transmission and to what extent one is dealing with transmission owing to breast-feeding. However, breast-feeding has been shown to have little effect on the rate of transmission of HCV virus.

NEONATAL HEPATITIS

Whereas congenital hepatitis is a relatively rare phenomenon, unfortunately neonatal hepatitis is not. Mothers with transient or persistent antigenemia at term can infect their offspring via body fluids. In the United States, an estimated 16,000 births occur to HBsAg-positive women each year. Approximately 4300 of these women are HBeAg positive. These pregnancies result in 3500 neonates becoming chronic HBV carriers. Vertical transmission of HBsAg from mother to fetus may occur transplacentally or during the birth process. If the mother has acute disease in the immediate periparturitional period or exhibits HBe antigenemia, the probability of subsequent neonatal antigenemia at some time during the first year of life is of the order of 70% to 90%. Once infected, the infant tends to remain HBsAg positive indefinitely, and the persistent HBs antigenemia is more likely to be associated with evidence of chronic hepatitis than if it were to occur in an adult. Up to 85% to 90% of infected infants will become chronic HBV carriers. It has been estimated that more than 25% of these carriers will die from primary HCC or cirrhosis of the liver. In Schweitzer's (1975) series of 20 infants whose mothers had hepatitis and who became HBs positive, two developed acute mild hepatitis at three months of age, promptly recovered, lost their antigenemia, and developed significant antibody titers at six months. The remaining 18, who did not develop overt hepatitis, have now been monitored up to five years of age and all have remained persistently HBsAg positive. Seven of these children have been monitored for at

least four years. Clinically, the children have had variable transaminase elevations. Liver biopsies, performed on 10 of the 18 children between 3 and 27 months of age, have demonstrated the presence of a chronic viral hepatitis.

MANAGEMENT OF HEPATITIS IN PREGNANCY

Maternal Considerations
Clinically Overt Maternal Disease
Jaundice in pregnancy is most commonly due to infection, namely viral hepatitis. It is commonly stated that during pregnancy, particularly during the second and third trimesters, the liver may be more susceptible to noxious stimuli than at other periods. Although this point is still moot, those workers who perform autopsies on pregnant women are impressed by the frequency with which fulminating hepatic disease is the cause of maternal mortality. This observation is the rationale for clinical management. Any pregnant woman with a rapidly rising AST and ALT should be hospitalized and observed until such time as it can be demonstrated that the transaminase values have passed their maximum and are clearly falling toward physiologic levels.

There is no evidence that prolonged bed rest or a high-protein diet alters the course of the more common form of the disease. A policy of gradual ambulation and a diet on demand suffices in the majority of cases. For hepatitis, appropriate isolation procedures should be instituted during hospitalization.

The determination of the type of hepatitis may predicate whether or not hepatitis immune serum globulin (ISG) should be administered to household contacts.

HBV Asymptomatic Infection
The CDC estimates that there are approximately 0.7 to 1.0 million chronic carriers of HBV in the United States and that this pool of carriers grows by 2% to 3% (8000 to 16,000 individuals) annually. Chronic carriers represent the largest human reservoir of HBV. More and more hospitals are instituting a prospective screening of all admissions

for the presence of HBsAg. The identification of a pregnant woman about to deliver presents two problems:

1. The possibility that she will function as an effective vehicle for the dissemination of hepatitis B within the immediate medical environment
2. The possibility that she will function as a potential horizontal and/or vertical vector for her progeny

HBV Nosocomial Impact

Nosocomial transmission of HBV to staff and patients can be minimized by appropriate practices and environmental measures. All patients who are known at the time of admission to be HBsAg positive should be placed on blood and discharge precautions. A mother may be HBsAg positive, either because she has acute hepatitis B during pregnancy or because she is a chronic carrier of the virus. The chronic carrier state is defined as HBs positivity at two points in time at least six months apart. The potential perinatal or nosocomial transmission is more dependent on the presence or absence of HBeAg than on whether the patient has acute or chronic hepatitis. HBeAg-positive individuals are also potential vectors for individuals in their immediate hospital environment. Susceptible medical personnel who receive a needle-stick puncture from an HBe antigen–positive gravida have a 20% chance of developing infection. In contrast, HBsAg-positive mothers who are HBe antigen negative seldom infect the neonates and these infants usually do not develop the chronic carrier state. Needle-stick injuries from HBe antigen–negative patients are much less likely to infect susceptible medical personnel. Nevertheless, the guidelines that have been developed by the CDC are recommended for all HBsAg-positive births regardless of the maternal HBe antigen status.

HCV Antibody–Positive Gravida

Management of an individual with anti-HCV antibodies requires the following:

1. *Challenging the validity of the initial enzyme immunoassay (EIA) observation.* Use a qualitative HCV polymerase chain reaction (PCR) assay. If the HCV PCR is negative or there is a questionable history of exposure or risk of HCV infection, the use of the recombinant immunoblot assay (RIBA) can be useful to determine a false-positive HCV EIA.
2. *Monitoring maternal serum ALT.* Patients with serologic evidence of HCV infection who demonstrate elevated HCV levels of their serum aminotransferase over 6 to 12 months should be deemed as having HCV infection and biopsy at some future date unrelated to pregnancy may be indicated.

The standard care of treatment for chronic HCV disease is combination therapy with peginterferone-alfa and ribavirin. HCV genotype determines the response to therapy. The best response is with patients infected with genotype 2 or 3. Therapy during pregnancy is lacking. When possible, general anesthesia should be avoided in gravida with anti-HCV antibodies and abnormal liver function tests.

PRENATAL SCREENING FOR HEPATITIS B AND C VIRUSES

All pregnant women should be tested routinely for HBsAg during an early prenatal visit (e.g., first trimester) in each pregnancy, even if they have been previously vaccinated or tested. Women who were not screened prenatally, those who engage in behaviors that put them at high risk for infection [e.g., injection-drug use, having had more than one sex partner in the previous six months or an HBsAg-positive sex partner, evaluation or treatment for a sexually transmitted disease (STD), or recent or current injection-drug use], and those with clinical hepatitis should be tested at the time of admission to the hospital for delivery.

The commercially available HBsAg tests have an extremely high sensitivity and specificity if positive tests are repeated and confirmed by neutralization as recommended by the manufacturers of the reagent kits. Testing for other markers of HBV infection, such as HBeAg, is not necessary for maternal screening. Mothers who are positive for both HBsAg and HBeAg have the highest likelihood of transmitting HBV to their newborns. However, infants of mothers who are HBsAg positive but HBeAg negative may become infected and develop severe, even fatal, fulminant hepatitis B during infancy. For this reason, hepatitis B immune serum globulin (HBIG) and HB vaccine treatment of all babies born to HBsAg-positive women is recommended. HBsAg-positive mothers identified during screening may have HBV-related acute or chronic liver disease and should be evaluated by a physician. Identification of women who are HBV carriers through prenatal screening presents an opportunity to vaccinate susceptible household members and sexual partners of HBV carriers.

Although HCV is not an official part of prenatal screening, it is only a question of time before it becomes one of the cornerstones of prenatal preventive care.

PERINATAL INFECTION

Most perinatal infection seems to occur at the time of delivery, not transplacentally or at the time of conception. Although maternal HBsAg has often been found in cord blood samples, its presence has not correlated closely with neonatal infection. Either external contamination of samples or maternal blood entering the placenta after fetoplacental circulation has ceased may account for this poor correlation.

The probability of developing the carrier state in infected neonates can be greatly reduced by using HBIG, provided it is used soon enough. A large clinical trial of HBIG, reported from Taiwan, showed that administering HBIG to infants within seven days of birth was unsuccessful, but using HBIG within 48 hours of birth (usually in the delivery room) proved highly successful in preventing the development of the carrier state in infants of mothers who were both HBsAg and HBeAg positive. Delay in administration of HBIG to infants of carrier mothers will decrease the efficacy of therapy. In the studies that demonstrated the highest efficacy (85–95%) of combined HBIG and HB vaccine prophylaxis, HBIG was administered within 2 to 12 hours after birth.

In one study in which only HBIG was used for prophylaxis, no efficacy was found if HBIG was given more than seven days after birth, and a significant decrease in efficacy was observed if it was given more than 48 hours after birth. If the prenatal population can be prospectively screened, HBIG administration can be done in the delivery room. Infants born to these women should receive HBIG. The initial dose is 0.5 mL intramuscularly in the delivery room, if possible, and certainly within 48 hours of birth. The injection site should be thoroughly cleaned before HBIG administration. The infant is born covered with maternal blood and other secretions containing the HBV, and these enter the eyes, mucous membranes, gastrointestinal tract, and sometimes the circulatory system. Cesarean section delivery does not prevent HBV infection. These infectious secretions constitute a risk not only to the neonate but also to those attending the delivery. "Blood precautions" should be taken to protect staff and prevent environmental contamination that could lead to infection of others. Care should be taken with maternal blood and secretions before, during, and after delivery. Attendants at delivery should wear gloves, face mask, and glasses to keep infective material from splashing onto eyes or mucous membranes, and should be careful to avoid punctures from sharp instruments. The delivery room and instruments should be carefully cleaned and sterilized. Dressings soiled with lochia or wound exudates should be carefully handled. Sitz baths should be thoroughly cleaned and then wiped with a suitable high-level disinfectant. A 1/2 cup per gallon solution of 5.25% sodium hypochlorite is recommended. Infants whose mothers are chronic carriers will be continuously exposed to HBV throughout their childhood; therefore, these infants should receive HB vaccine in conjunction with HBIG administration. The presence of passively acquired antibody from the mother or that which results in HBIG administration does not appear to affect active immunization. Vaccination of individuals who possess antibodies against HBV from a previous infection or by passive acquisition will not cause an adverse effect. Such individuals will have a postvaccination increase in their anti-HBs levels.

Even if the neonate is infected at birth, active viral replication will not occur for several weeks. After thoroughly washing off external contamination, the infant need not be separated from his mother or placed in special isolation. Washing and rinsing should be thorough and done carefully by a gloved attendant using soap or detergent and water. Vitamin K injections can wait until after the bath.

Lamivudine (a cytosine analog) can treat HBV during pregnancy. It can also reduce transmission of HBV to the fetus and newborn. Studies performed in China and Holland showed the effectiveness of this therapy in pregnancy as well as its safety.

CDC RECOMMENDATIONS FOR BREAST-FEEDING FOR HBsAg-POSITIVE WOMEN

The question of breast-feeding usually arises in discussions of perinatal transmission. Although HBsAg has been detected in some samples of breast milk, some investigators required special concentration techniques to do so. Significant exposure to HBV via breast milk appears to be unlikely, especially after the relatively massive exposure occurring during the birth process. Studies from Taiwan have shown that breast-fed infants of carrier mothers are no more likely to be infected at one year than are infants for whom breast-feeding was withheld. Cracked nipples, abscesses, or other breast lesions, however, could mix breast milk with highly infectious serous exudates, and feeding should be temporarily suspended from that breast until the lesion is healed.

The CDC states there is no evidence that breast-feeding spreads HCV. HCV-positive mothers should consider abstaining from breast-feeding if their nipples are cracked or bleeding. The American Academy of Pediatrics states that breast-feeding is not contraindicated for infants born to mothers who are HBsAg positive and mothers who are infected with HCV (HCV antibody or HVC RNA–positive blood).

DIAGNOSIS

Hepatitis A

Documentation of hepatitis A is predicated upon the serologic demonstration of a significant increase in anti-HAV titer during the acute stage of the disease. Anti-HAV is present at the onset of jaundice, and the absence of antibody at this stage of the disease excludes HAV as the etiologic agent of the illness. The titer of antibody increases rapidly during the first two weeks of illness. After infection, anti-HAV is usually present in the serum for life. If titers are obtained late in the course of the disease, a high titer of anti-HAV will be present. The ability to document a four-fold rise in titer may not be possible. In this situation, the diagnosis of acute infection can be confirmed by the demonstration of anti-HAV antibody of the IgM class. Specific IgM antibodies are synthesized during the first two to three months of hepatitis A.

Hepatitis B

Detection of markers of hepatitis B, namely HBsAg, anti-HBs, anti-HBc, HBeAg, or anti-HBe, by the EIA has been adapted. Although the presence of HBsAg documents the diagnosis of hepatitis B infection, it does not address the issue of infectivity.

The presence or absence of IgM antibody to the core antigen of HBV (IgM anti-HBc) provides a means of distinguishing between acute infection and chronic disease. Almost all patients with acute hepatitis B have high titers of IgM anti-HBc at the time of initial examination, whereas chronic carriers of the virus have only low titers or no detectable IgM anti-HBc at all, but will have high titers of IgG anti-HBc. The presence of high-titer IgM anti-HBc generally indicates the patient has acute hepatitis B (hepatitis delta coinfection is not excluded), whereas a negative test in an HBsAg-positive patient with hepatitis should prompt the consideration of other possibilities, especially hepatitis delta superinfection or HCV hepatitis. With respect to the diagnosis of acute hepatitis B, IgM anti-HBc is arguably the best serologic marker.

Hepatitis C

A variety of tests are available for hepatitis C diagnosis. Tests that can detect antibody against the virus include the EIAs, which contain HCV antigens from the core and nonstructural genes, and the RIBAs, which contain the same HCV antigens as EIA in an immunoblot format. In addition, several PCR-based assays for HCV RNA have been developed to detect the RNA virus directly.

Only about 70% of patients with acute hepatitis C develop detectable antibodies to HCV antigen within six weeks of the onset of signs or symptoms. The diagnosis of acute HCV infection may require follow-up testing at 12 weeks.

Although serum ALT and other enzymes indicative of hepatocellular destruction are reasonable indicators of the presence of disease, they are poor indicators of activity. Over half of all viremic patients will have normal ALT levels. ALT levels are often normal or near normal even in patients with biopsy-proven advanced liver disease. As a consequence, normal ALT levels do not preclude the presence of chronic HCV infection.

Serologic testing for HCV is currently the only way of documenting infection or disease. The newer immunoassays for HCV, composed of multiple HCV-specific antigens, have both sensitivities and specificity in the range of 95%. False-negatives occur due to the heterogeneity of the virus. Current EIAs are based on the predominant genotype of HCV found in U.S. patients. False-positive results occur in patients with hypergammaglobulinemia and connective tissue disorders.

RIBA, which uses recombinant proteins derived from HCV, is used to confirm EIA results. This test contains four HCV-specific antigens blotted as separate bonds on a nitrocellulose strip. A confirmatory RBA test result demonstrates reactivity to two or more of these antigens. As with the EIA test, false-negative tests do occur. Patients infected with less common HCV genotypes are less likely to satisfy the diagnostic criteria required.

Direct detection of HCV viral genomic RNA can be done using PCR. This test is available as primarily a research tool. The presence of anti-HCV antibodies in human serum or plasma does not necessarily indicate ongoing NANBH, but may be a remnant of a past infection with the HCV. Levels of antibody are usually undetectable in early stages of an infection.

Anti-HCV antibodies appear as early as four weeks and as late as one year after infection. The mean delay between onset of hepatitis symptoms and seropositivity is 15 weeks. In acute posttransfusion hepatitis, the mean delay between transfusion (infection) and appearance of anti-HCV is 22 weeks. Once the antibodies develop, they persist for years. Unlike hepatitis B, the "window period" is variable. When the diagnosis of hepatitis C is strongly suspected, sequential repeat testing for anti-HCV is recommended. The major usefulness of the test is to screen out blood donors who

could transmit HCV. A positive test for the presence of anti-HCV will assist in the diagnosis of individuals with recent or prior signs, symptoms, and/or biochemical evidence of hepatitis. A negative test is of limited value.

False-positive reactions with the EIA for hepatitis C have been seen in some patients with hypergammaglobulinemia and in patients whose serum has been stored improperly or for a prolonged period. False-negative antibody studies in acute HCV disease are related mainly to the slow development of antibodies during convalescence.

To establish a diagnosis of perinatal/neonatal hepatitis C, virologic testing requires the use of branched chain DNA (bDNA) amplification assay or PCR. These tests are required because passively transferred maternal antibodies against HCV can interfere with EIA tests. Infants born to HCV-infected mothers should be tested before breast-feeding is initiated or within 12 months of birth. If positive, the bDNA assay or PCR should be repeated between 12 and 15 months of age. After 15 months of age, the infant can be monitored serologically using anti-HCV assay for indigenous antibody production indicative of HCV infection.

PASSIVE IMMUNOTHERAPY

Diagnostic Evaluation for Hepatitis C

A negative EIA test is sufficient to rule out infection. However, low-risk individuals with positive EIA tests should undergo a supplementary RIBA testing. If the RIBA is negative, the anti-HCV EIA result is likely to have been a false positive, and the patient is unlikely to have hepatitis C. If the RIBA is positive, the patient can be assumed to have or to have had hepatitis C. These patients can benefit by testing for HCV RNA by PCR, the result of which will indicate whether the patient has ongoing viremia. A single positive assay for HCV RNA by PCR confirms HCV infection; unfortunately, a single negative assay does not prove that the patient is not viremic or has recovered from hepatitis C. Follow-up testing for ALT levels and perhaps repeating the HCV RNA in the future may be needed.

Individuals with even mildly elevated ALT levels, with or without risk factors for hepatitis C, should be tested for anti-HCV by EIA, and, if positive, the results should be confirmed by either supplemental RIBA or qualitative HCV RNA by PCR. Obviously anti-HCV testing is very helpful in all patients with clinical liver disease.

In patients presenting with biochemical or clinical evidence of liver disease (e.g., repeatedly elevated ALT levels), a positive EIA test is sufficient to diagnose hepatitis C infection, especially if risk factors are present. A qualitative HCV RNA test can be used for confirmation. If a patient is being considered for anti-viral therapy, liver biopsy is of value to assess disease severity.

Testing for HCV RNA by PCR can be very helpful in initial diagnosis, but repeat testing over time is generally not helpful in the management of untreated patients; almost all remain viremic, and a negative result may merely reflect a transient fall of viral titer below the level of detection rather than permanent clearance. On the other hand, repeat testing for HCV RNA during antiviral therapy can be helpful because loss of HCV RNA with treatment is a strong predictor of a sustained beneficial response.

Liver biopsy is considered the gold standard for assessment of patients with chronic hepatitis. When combined with serial determinations of ALT levels, liver biopsy is very helpful in judging the severity or activity of the liver disease and the stage or degree of fibrosis. Liver biopsy is recommended before treatment to assess the grade and stage of disease and to exclude other forms of liver disease or complications (such as concurrent alcoholic liver disease, medication-induced liver injury, and iron overload). However, liver biopsy is expensive and is associated with some morbidity. Therefore, serial ALT and qualitative HCV RNA testing are recommended for monitoring patients under treatment.

Contraindications to treatment with interferon that must be carefully considered are history of major depressive illness, cytopenias, hyperthyroidism, renal transplant, and convincing evidence of autoimmune disease. Data suggest a benefit from interferon treatment with higher clearance of HCV RNA in patients with acute hepatitis C. In light of these findings, interferon treatment of patients with acute hepatitis C could be recommended.

The adjunctive drug with the most promise, at present, is ribavirin, an oral antiviral agent that, when used alone, reduces serum ALT levels in approximately 50% of patients. However, ribavirin by itself does not lower serum HCV RNA levels, and relapses occur in virtually all patients when therapy is stopped. Of greater promise are recent reports that the combination of interferon alfa and ribavirin leads to sustained virologic response rates (40–50%) higher than for interferon alfa alone in six-month clinical trials. Ribavirin has not been licensed or approved for use in hepatitis C by the Food and Drug Administration (FDA).

For pregnant patients with chronic active hepatitis due to HCV, general anesthesia is best avoided when cesarean section is indicated. Some neonatologists empirically administer immune globulin to the progeny of such gravida with high titer of HCV antibodies. Currently there is little scientific data to support or negate this approach. In utero transmission is an unexplored possibility.

Hepatitis A

The efficacy of ISG for the prevention or modification of hepatitis A depends on the following:

1. The degree and type of exposure
2. The dose of ISG and its antibody content
3. The time interval between exposure and the administration of ISG

Optimal passive immunization following presumed exposure requires the use of high-titered, HBsAg-negative ISG, administered in the shortest possible time after exposure. Different lots of ISG may vary as much as 16-fold in anti-HAV content. It will be imperative in the future for licensed lots of ISG to be marked as to anti-HAV titer.

Administration of ISG early in the incubation period of type A hepatitis is capable of modifying or arresting the infection. A dose of 0.02 mL/kg body weight affords effective protection for short-term exposure.

Pregnancy per se does not alter the recommendations for ISG prophylaxis. The administration of ISG is indicated following known exposure to HAV or in anticipation of entering an area where disease is endemic and intermittent exposure probable. Under most circumstances, protection is afforded by giving 0.01 mL ISG/lb of body weight (approximately 0.02 mL/kg). Larger doses provide longer-lasting, but not necessarily more, protection and are indicated when an individual plans to reside in a high-risk area for a prolonged period. A dosage as high as 0.05 mL/lb every five to six months has been advocated.

Although HAV does not traverse the placenta, maternal infection immediately prior to delivery, unless appropriate isolation procedures are instituted and ISG is administered, raises the possibility of neonatal dissemination of disease from mother to infant in the postpartum period.

Hepatitis B

The ability to answer the question as to the efficacy of standard ISG as prophylaxis against hepatitis B has been largely negated by the significant variation in anti-HBs from lot to lot. Most lots of standard ISG have contained low or undetectable levels of anti-HBs. The development of an HBIG preparation with an anti-HBs titer about 25,000 to 50,000 times higher than that of standard ISG has demonstrated that partial efficacy may be achieved through passive immunization.

HBIG should be given immediately, at a dose of 0.06 mL/kg body weight, to individuals who are exposed by a contaminated needle or by contact with infective blood splashed onto a mucous membrane or a skin cut, or to those who have had intimate physical contact with a person who has hepatitis B infection. This dose should be repeated in 28 days. An individual given a blood transfusion that, in retrospect, is discovered to be infected with HBsAg may be given large doses of HBIG (0.5 mL/kg). Large doses of HBIG or high-titered plasma are of no value in the treatment of ongoing infection.

In infants whose mothers had hepatitis B during pregnancy or have persistent antigenemia, the probability of ensuing postnatal hepatitis tends to be influenced by the presence or absence of other viral markers in the mother. The attack rate of hepatitis B in infants born to mothers with a persistence of HBsAg, HBeAg, and anti-HBc usually exceeds 90%. Large doses of HBIG are recommended for these infants. The probability of hepatitis B in infants born to mothers with a persistence of HBsAg and anti-HBe is usually less than 10%. The accumulated evidence to date indicates that HBsAg-positive and HBeAg-positive blood is highly infectious, whereas HBsAg-positive and HBeAB-positive blood is minimally infectious. The many known ways to limit dissemination or acquisition of infection must not be neglected. With effective surveillance of patients and personnel exposed to hepatitis B, proper washing of hands, and stringent aseptic technique for eliminating HBs-positive blood products, the potential for spread of HBV disease is reduced.

ACTIVE IMMUNIZATION

Hepatitis A Virus

Only vaccines made from inactivated HAV have been evaluated for efficacy in controlled clinical trials (Tables 4–7). The vaccines containing HAV antigen that are currently licensed in the United States are HAVRIX® (manufactured by GlaxoSmithKline, Rixensart, Belgium) and VAQTA® (manufactured by Merck & Co., Inc., Whitehouse Station, New Jersey) and the combination vaccine TWINRIX® (containing both HAV and HBV antigens; manufactured by GlaxoSmithKline). The vaccines are administered intramuscularly into the deltoid muscle.

Hepatitis B Virus
RECOMBIVAX HB®: Hepatitis B Vaccine and ENGERIX-B®

RECOMBIVAX HB® [hepatitis B vaccine (recombinant)] and ENGERIX-B® are noninfectious subunit viral vaccines derived from HBsAg produced in yeast cells. A portion of the HBV gene coding for HBsAg is cloned into yeast and the vaccine for hepatitis B is produced from cultures of this recombinant yeast strain. The vaccine against hepatitis B, prepared from recombinant yeast cultures, is free of association with human blood or blood products.

Infants born to HBsAg-positive mothers are at high risk of becoming chronic carriers of HBV and of developing the chronic sequelae of HBV infection. Well-controlled studies have shown that administration of three 0.5 mL doses of HBIG starting at birth is 75% effective in preventing establishment of the chronic carrier state in these infants during the first year of life. Protection can be transient, whereupon the effectiveness of the HBIG would decline thereafter. Results from clinical studies indicate that administration of one 0.5 mL dose of HBIG at birth and three 20 mg (1.0 mL) doses of hepatitis B vaccine, the first dose given within one week after birth, was 85% to 93% effective in preventing establishment of the chronic carrier state in infants born to HBsAg- and HBeAg-positive mothers.

The immunization regimen consists of three doses of vaccine:

- First dose, with HBIG
- Second dose, one month later
- Third dose, six months after the first dose

The protective efficacy of hepatitis B vaccine has been demonstrated in neonates born of mothers positive for both

TABLE 4 Recommended doses of IG for hepatitis A preexposure and postexposure prophylaxis

Setting	Duration of coverage	Dose(mL/kg)[a]
Preexposure	Short-term (1–2 mos)	0.02
	Long-term (3–5 mos)	0.06[b]
Postexposure		0.02

[a]IG should be administered by intramuscular injection int either the deltoid or gluteal muscle. For children aged <24 months, IG can be administered in the anterolateral thigh muscle.
[b]Repeat every 5 months if continued exposure to hepatitis A virus occurs.
Abbreviation: IG, Immune globulin.

TABLE 5 Licensed dosages of VAQTA®[a]

Vaccine recipient's age	Dose (U)[b]	Vol. (mL)	No. of doses	Schedule (mos)[c]
12 mos–18 yrs	25	0.5	2	0, 6–18
≥19 yrs	50	1.0	2	0, 6–18

[a]Hepatitis A vaccine, inactivated, Merck & Co., Inc. (Whitehouse Station, New Jersey).
[b]Units.
[c]0 months represents timing of initial dose; subsequent numbers represent months after the initial dose.

HBsAg and HBeAg. In a clinical study of infants who received one dose of HBIG at birth followed by the recommended three-dose regimen of hepatitis B vaccine, efficacy in prevention of chronic hepatitis B infection was 94% in 93 infants at six months and 93% in 57 infants at nine months as compared with the infection rate in untreated historical controls. Significantly fewer neonates became chronically infected when given one dose of HBIG at birth followed by the recommended three-dose regimen of hepatitis B vaccine when compared with historical controls who received only a single dose of HBIG. Testing for HBsAg and anti-HBs is recommended at 12 to 15 months of age. If HBsAg is not detectable, and anti-HBs is present, the child has been protected. The recommended treatment regimen for infants born of HBsAg-positive mothers is shown in Table 8.

THERAPY

Chronic Hepatitis B

Updated guidelines for the treatment of chronic HBV infected patients were reported by the American Association for the Study of Liver Diseases in 2003. Medications included in these guidelines are interferon-alpha, lamivudine, and adefovir dipivoxil.

Chronic Hepatitis C

A multicenter, randomized, controlled trial recently demonstrated that treatment with three million units of recombinant alpha interferon three times weekly for six months is associated with normalization or near-normalization of hepatic enzyme levels in 46% of patients, compared with 28% of patients receiving lower doses of interferon and 8% of those receiving no interferon.

Although several different forms of interferon have been evaluated in the treatment of patients with chronic hepatitis C, the bulk of available evidence pertains to the alpha interferons (interferon alfa). The efficacy of interferon alfa therapy currently is defined biochemically as normalization of serum

TABLE 6 Licensed dosages of HAVRIX®[a]

Vaccine recipient's age	Dose (EL.U.)[b]	Vol. (mL)	No. of doses	Schedule (mos)[c]
12 mos–18 yrs	720	0.5	2	0, 6–12
≥19 yrs	1,440	1.0	2	0, 6–12

[a]Hepatitis A vaccine, inactivated, GlaxoSmithKline (Rixensart, Belgium).
[b]Enzyme-linked immunosorbent assay units.
[c]0 months represents timing at initial dose; subsequent numbers represent months after the initial dose.

TABLE 7 Licensed dosages of TWINRIX®[a]

Vaccine recipient's age	Dose (hepatitis A/ hepatitis B)	Vol. (mL)	No. of doses	Schedule (mos)[b]
≥18 yrs	720 EL.U.[c]/20 μg	1.0	3	0, 1,6

[a]Combined hepatitis A and hepatitis B vaccine, GlaxoSmithKline (Rixensart, Belgium).
[b]0 months represents timing of initial dose; subsequent numbers represent months after the initial dose.
[c]Enzyme-linked immunosorbent assay units.

ALT and virologically as loss of serum HCV RNA. Therefore, serial ALT testing is recommended for monitoring patients during treatment to document biochemical responses, and testing for HCV RNA by qualitative PCR is recommended at selected time points to document virologic responses.

Many therapeuticians obtain a liver biopsy before initiating therapy with interferon. Laboratory tests that should be obtained before starting therapy include liver chemistries (serum ALT, bilirubin, albumin, prothrombin time), complete blood count (CBC) with differential and platelet count, antinuclear antibodies, thyroid stimulating hormone, serum HCV RNA, and glucose. Monitoring during therapy should be done at two- to four-week intervals with serum ALT and CBC. Both serum ALT and serum HCV RNA testing should be done after three months to assess whether the patient is responding to therapy. This should be repeated at the end of therapy to document end-of-treatment response. Follow-up testing with serum ALT and serum HCV RNA should be done six months after therapy is stopped to determine whether there has been a sustained response.

TABLE 8 Recommended schedule of hepatitis B immunoprophylaxis to prevent perinatal transmission of hepatitis B virus infection

Infant born to mother known to be HBsAg positive	
Vaccine dose[a]	Age of infant
First	Birth (within 12 hr)
HBIG[b]	Birth (within 12 hr)
Second	1 mo
Third	6 mos[c]
Infant born to mother not screened for HBsAg	
Vaccine dose[d]	Age of infant
First	Birth (within 12 hr)
HBIG[b]	If mother is found to be HBsAg positive, administer dose to infant as soon as possible, not later than 1 wk after birth
Second	1–2 mos[e]
Third	6 mos[c]

[a]Use appropriate dose.
[b]HBIG—0.5 mL administered intramuscularly at a site different from that used for vaccine.
[c]If four-dose schedule (Engerix-B) is used, the third dose is administered at 2 mos of age and the fourth dose at 12–18 mos.
[d]First dose is for infant of HBsAg-positive mother. If mother is found to be HBsAg positive, continue that dose; if mother is found to be HBsAg negative, use an appropriate dose for that situation.
[e]Infants of women who are HBsAg negative can be vaccinated at 2 mos.
Abbreviations: HBsAg, hepatitis B surface antigen; HBIG, hepatitis B immune globin.
Source: From CDC (1991).

Three months after beginning an initial course of therapy, patients who are unlikely to respond to that dosage and frequency can be identified by persistent elevation of serum ALT levels and presence of HCV RNA in the serum. In this situation, therapy should be discontinued because the likelihood of future response is extremely low. If either HCV RNA is negative or ALT levels are normal (or both), therapy should be continued for 12 months.

The important factors associated with a favorable response to treatment include HCV genotype 2 or 3, low serum HCV RNA level (less than 1,000,000 copies/mL), and absence of cirrhosis.

Flu-like symptoms (fever, chills, malaise, headache, arthralgia, myalgia, tachycardia) occur early in the majority of patients who receive interferon but generally diminish with continued therapy. Later side effects include fatigue, alopecia, bone marrow suppression, and neuropsychiatric effects such as apathy, cognitive changes, irritability, and depression. Relapse of drug and/or alcohol abuse may occur. Nocturnal administration of interferon reduces the frequency of side effects, and the flu-like syndrome is ameliorated by pretreatment with acetaminophen. A reduction in interferon dosage is required in 10% to 40% of patients because of side effects, and treatment must be discontinued in 5% to 10%. Higher dosages tend to be associated with higher rates of side effects.

Chronic Hepatitis C

Combination therapy with pegylated interferon and ribavirin is the treatment of choice for chronic infection HBV resulting in sustained response rates of 40% to 80% [up to 50% for patients infected with the most common genotype found in the United States (genotype 1) and up to 80% for patients infected with genotype 2 or 3]. Interferon monotherapy is generally reserved for patients in whom ribavirin is contraindicated. Ribavirin, when used alone, does not work. Combination therapy using interferon and ribavirin is now approved by the FDA for the use in children aged 3 to 17 years.

For pregnant patients with chronic active hepatitis due to HCV, general anesthesia is best avoided when cesarean section is indicated.

Patients most likely to respond to therapy are those

1. without cirrhosis,
2. with evidenced chronic hepatitis/periportal inflammation on biopsy,
3. with low HCV RNA levels,
4. with low serum ferritin,
5. with low gamma-glutamyl transpeptidase, and/or
6. with HCV genotype 2.

SELECTED READING

Alter HJ, Seeff LB, Kaplan PM, et al. Type B hepatitis: the infectivity of blood positive for e antigen and DNA polymerase after accidental needlestick exposure. N Engl J Med 1979; 295:909.
Bayer MD, Blumberg BS, Werner B. Particles associated with Australia antigen in the sera of patients with leukemia, Down's syndrome and hepatitis. Nature 1968; 218:1057.

Beasley RP, Stevens CE, Shiao IS, Meng HC. Evidence against breast-feeding as a mechanism for vertical transmission of hepatitis B. Lancet 1975; 2:740.

CDC. Morb Mortal Wkly Rep 1991; 40:1.

Dienstag JL, Purcell RH, Alter HJ, et al. Non-A, non-B post-transfusion hepatitis. Lancet 1977; 1:560.

Editorial. Vaccination against hepatitis B. Lancet 1976; 1:1391.

Feinman SV, Berris B, Sinclair JC, et al. e antigen and anti-e in HBsAg carriers. Lancet 1975; 2:1173.

Fox RA, Niazi SP, Sherlock S. Hepatitis-associated antigen in chronic liver disease. Lancet 1969; 2:609.

Guntupalli SR, Steingrub J. Hepatic disease and pregnancy: an overview of diagnosis and management. Crit Care Med 2005; 33:S332–S339.

Heathcote J, Cameron CH, Dane DS. Hepatitis B antigen in saliva and semen. Lancet 1974; 1:71.

Hindman SH, Gravelle CR, Murphy BL, et al. 'e' antigen, Dane particles, and serum DNA polymerase activity in HBsAg carriers. Ann Intern Med 1976; 85:458.

Hoofnagle HJ, Gerety RJ, Smallwood MS, et al. Subtyping of hepatitis B surface antigen and antibody by radioimmunoassay. Gastroenterology 1977; 72:290.

Kaplan PM, Greenman RL, Gerin JL. DNA polymerase associated with human hepatitis B antigen. J Virol 1973; 12:995.

Koff RS, Isselbacher KJ. Changing concepts in the epidemiology of viral hepatitis. N Engl J Med 1968; 278:1371.

Krugman S, Giles JP, Hammond J. Infectious hepatitis: evidence for two distinctive clinical epidemiological and immunological types of infection. J Am Med Assoc 1967; 300:365.

Linneman CC Jr, Goldberg S. HBAg in breast milk. Lancet 1974; 2:155.

Monif GRG. Viral Infection of the Human Fetus. New York: Macmillan, 1969.

Monif GRG. Viral hepatitis. In: Charles D, ed. Obstetrics and Perinatal Infections. Mosby Year Book Inc, 1993.

Nishioka K, Levin AG, Simons MJ. Hepatitis B antigen, antigen subtypes, and hepatitis B antibody in normal subjects and patients with liver disease. Bull WHO 1975; 52:293.

Ogra P. Immunologic aspects of hepatitis-associated antigen and antibody in human body fluids. J Immunol 1973; 110:1197.

Okada K, Kamiyama I, Inomata M, et al. e antigen and anti-e in the serum of asymptomatic carrier mothers as indicators of positive and negative transmission of hepatitis B virus to their infants. N Engl J Med 1976; 294:746.

Prince AM, Hargrove RI, Szmuness W, et al. Immunologic distinction between infectious and serum hepatitis. N Engl J Med 1970; 282:987.

Policy Statement. Breastfeeding and the use of human milk. Pediatrics 2005; 115:496–506.

Shih JW-K, Tan PL, Gerin JL. Antigenicity of the major polypeptides of hepatitis B surface antigen (HBsAg). J Immunol 1978; 120:520.

Shikata T, Karasawa T, Abe K, et al. Hepatitis B e antigens and infectivity of hepatitis B virus. J Infect Dis 1977; 136:571.

Wright RA. Hepatitis B and the HBsAg carrier. An outbreak related to sexual contact. J Am Med Assoc 1975; 232:717.

Viral Hepatitis in Pregnancy

Adams RH, Combes B. Viral hepatitis during pregnancy. J Am Med Assoc 1965; 192:195.

Cahill KM. Hepatitis in pregnancy. Surg Gynecol Obstet 1962; 114:545.

Frucht HL, Metcalfe J. Mortality and late results of infectious hepatitis in pregnant women. N Engl J Med 1954; 251:1094.

Hammouda AA. Acute virus hepatitis and pregnancy. Br J Obstet Gynaecol 1962; 69:680.

Lyons KP, Guzb LB. Australia antigen-associated hepatitis: radioimmunoassay in mother and infant. J Am Med Assoc 1971; 215:981.

Martin R, Ferguson FC Jr. Infectious hepatitis associated with pregnancy. N Engl J Med 1947; 237:114.

Mickel A. Infectious hepatitis in pregnancy. Am J Obstet Gynecol 1951; 62:409.

Naidu SS, Visvanathan R. Infectious hepatitis in pregnancy during Delhi epidemic. Indian J Med Res 1957; 45:71.

Peretz A, Paldi D, Brandstaedter S, Barzilai D. Infectious hepatitis in pregnancy. Obstet Gynecol 1959; 14:435.

Rose G. Acute yellow atrophy of the liver of viral etiology in pregnancy. Med J Aust 1962; 49:284.

Siegler AM, Keyser J. Acute hepatitis in pregnancy: a report of ten cases and review of the literature. Am J Obstet Gynecol 1963; 86:1068.

Smithwick FM, Go SC. Hepatitis-associated antigen in cord and maternal sera. Lancet 1970; 2:1080.

Stevens CE, Beasley RP, Tsui J, Lee WC. Vertical transmission of hepatitis B antigen in Taiwan. N Engl J Med 1975; 292:771.

Stokes J Jr, Berk JE, Malamut LL, et al. Carrier state in viral hepatitis. J Am Med Assoc 1954; 154:1059.

Stokes J Jr, Wolman JJ, Blanchard MC, Farquhar JD. Viral hepatitis in the newborn: clinical features, epidemiology and pathology. Am J Dis Child 1951; 82:213.

Tolentino P, Braito A, Tassara A. HAA and congenital biliary atresia. Lancet 1971; 1:398.

Tong MJ, Thursby M, Rakela J, et al. Studies of the maternal-infant transmission of the viruses which cause acute hepatitis. Gastroenterology 1981; 80:999.

Zondek B, Bromberg YM. Infectious hepatitis in pregnancy. J Med Mount Sinai NY 1947; 14:222.

Congenital or Neonatal Hepatitis

Adams H, Anderson RC, Richdorf LF. Four siblings with hepatic disease leading to cirrhosis. Am J Dis Child 1952; 84:168.

Aterman K. Neonatal hepatitis and its relation to viral hepatitis of mother. Am J Dis Child 1963; 105:395.

Aziz MA, Khan G, Khanum T, et al. Transplacental and postnatal transmission of the hepatitis-associated antigen. J Infect Dis 1973; 127:110.

Beasley RP, Stevens CE, Shiao I-S, et al. Evidence against breast-feeding as a mechanism of vertical transmission of hepatitis B. Lancet 1975; 2:740.

Beasley RP, Trepo C, Stevens CE, et al. The E antigen and vertical transmission of hepatitis B surface antigen. Am J Epidemiol 1977; 105:94.

Collins DL. Neonatal hepatitis including a case associated with hepatitis during pregnancy. Can Med Assoc J 1956; 75:828.

Derso A, Boxall EH, Tarlow MJ, et al. Transmission of HBsAg from mother to infant in four ethnic groups. Br Med J 1978; 1:949.

Dible JH, Hunt WE, Pugh YW, et al. Foetal and neonatal hepatitis and its sequelae. J Pathol Bact 1954; 67:195.

Ehrlich JC, Ratner JM. Congenital cirrhosis of liver with kernicterus: report of two cases in siblings with discussion of relationship to so-called neonatal hepatitis and to iso-immunization disease. Am J Pathol 1955; 31:1013.

Gillespie A, Dorman D, Walker-Smith JA, Yu JS. Neonatal hepatitis and Australia antigen. Lancet 1970; 2:108.

Hutchinson DL, Iskandar GB, Faggney PC. Maternal and neonatal jaundice and hepatitis associated with intrauterine fetal transmission. J Am Med Assoc 1965; 194:199.

Keys TF, Hobel CJ, Oh W, et al. Maternal and neonatal Australia antigen. Clin Res 1971; 19:184.

Kohler PF. Hepatitis B virus infection in pregnancy, neonate. Perinatal Care 1978; 2:7.

Krainin P, Lapan B. Neonatal hepatitis in siblings. J Am Med Assoc 1956; 160:937.

Krugman S. Vertical transmission of hepatitis B and breast-feeding. Lancet 1975; 2:916.

Krugman S. Hepatitis B infection and pregnancy. Infect Dis Letters Obstet Gynecol 1980; 2:26.

Lee AKY, Pi HMH, Wong VCW. Mechanisms of maternal-fetal transmission of hepatitis B virus. J Infect Dis 1978; 138:668.

Leiking E, Lysikiewicz A, Garry D, Tejani N. Intrauterine transmission of hepatitis A virus. Obstet Gynecol 1996; 88:690.

Merrill DA, Dubois RS, Kohler PF. Neonatal onset of the hepatitis associated antigen carrier state. N Engl J Med 1972; 287:1280.

Okada K, Kamiyama I, Inomata M, et al. e antigen and anti-e in the serum of asymptomatic carrier mothers as indicators of positive and negative transmission of hepatitis B virus to their infants. N Engl J Med 1976; 294:746.

Okada K, Yamada T, Miyakawa Y, Mayumi M. Hepatitis B surface antigen in the serum of infants after delivery from asymptomatic carrier mothers. J Pediatr 1975; 87:360.

Papaevangelou G, Hoofnagle J, Kremastinou J. Transplacental transmission of hepatitis-B virus by symptom-free chronic carrier mothers. Lancet 1974; 2:746.

Peace R. Fatal hepatitis and cirrhosis in infancy: a critical analysis of 32 cases studied at necropsy. Arch Pathol 1956; 61:107.

Ruebner B. The pathology of neonatal hepatitis. Am J Pathol 1960; 36:151.

Schweitzer IL. Vertical transmission of the hepatitis B surface antigen. Am J Med Sci 1975; 270:287.

Schweitzer IL, Dunn AE, Peters RL, Spears RL. Viral hepatitis B in neonates and infants. Am J Med 1973; 55:762.

Schweitzer IL, Mosley JW, Ashcavai M, et al. Factors influencing neonatal infection by hepatitis B virus. Gastroenterology 1973; 65:277.

Schweitzer IL, Wing A, McPeak C, Spears RL. Hepatitis and hepatitis associated antigen in 56 mother-infant pairs. J Am Med Assoc 1972; 220:1092.

Shapiro VS. Primary hepatitis in children associated with infectious hepatitis of the mother during pregnancy. Sov Med 1958; 23:42.

Shen HD. Hepatitis B virus infection of cord blood leukocytes. J Med Virol 1987; 22:211.

Skinhoj P, Sardemann H, Cohn J, et al. Hepatitis associated antigen (HAA) in pregnant women and their newborn infants. Am J Dis Child 1972; 123:380.

Stevens CE, Neurath RA, Beasley RP, Szmuness W. HBeAg and anti-HBe detection by radioimmunoassay: correlation with vertical transmission of hepatitis B virus in Taiwan. J Med Virol 1979; 3:237.

Stevens CE, Toy PT, Tong MJ, et al. Perinatal hepatitis B virus transmission in the United States. J Am Med Assoc 1985; 253:1740.

Hepatitis A Virus

Bell BP, Shapiro CN, Alter MJ, et al. The diverse pattern of hepatitis A epidemiology in the United States: implications for vaccination strategies. J Infect Dis 1998; 178:1579–1584.

Centers for Disease Control. Prevention of hepatitis A through active or passive immunization. Morb Mortal Wkly Rep 2006; 55(RR07):1–23.

Innis BL, Snithbham R, Kunasol P, et al. Protection against hepatitis A by an inactivated vaccine. J Am Med Assoc 1994; 271:1328–1334.

McDuffie RS Jr, Bader T. Fetal meconium peritonitis after maternal hepatitis A. Am J Obstet Gynecol 1999; 180:1031–1032.

Nissen E, Konig P, Feinstone SM, et al. Inactivation of hepatitis A and other enteroviruses during heat treatment (pasteurization). Biologicals 1996; 24:339–341.

Hepatitis B Virus

Center for Disease Control. A comprehensive immunization strategy to eliminate transmission of hepatitis B virus infection in the United States. Morb Mortal Wkly Rep 2005; 54(RR16):1–23.

Guan-Guanv S, Kong-Han P, Nian-Feng Z, et al. Efficacy and safety of lamivudine treatment for chronic hepatitis B in pregnancy. World J Gastroenterol 2004; 15:910–912.

Lok AS, McMahon BJ. Chronic hepatitis B: update of recommendations. Hepatology 2004; 34:1–5.

Hepatitis C Virus

Alter MJ, Hadler SC, Judson FN, et al. Risk factors for acute non-A, non-B hepatitis in the United States and association with hepatitis C virus infection. J Am Med Assoc 1990; 264:2231.

Alter MJ, Kruszon-Moran D, Nainan OV, et al. The prevalence of hepatitis C virus infection in the United States, 1988 through 1994. N Engl J Med 1999; 341:556–562.

Center for Disease Control. Recommendations for prevention and control of hepatitis C virus (HCV) infection and HCV-related chronic disease. Morb Mortal Wkly Rep 1998; 47(RR19):1–39.

Chemello L, Alberti A, Rose K, Sirnonds P. Hepatitis C serotype and response to interferon therapy. N Engl J Med 1994; 330:1.

Dusheiko G, Schmilovitz-Weiss H, Brown D, et al. Hepatitis C virus genotypes: an investigation of type specific differences in geographic origin and disease. Hepatology 1994; 19:13.

Esteban LL, Gonzalez A, Hernandez JM, et al. Evaluation of antibodies to hepatitis C virus in a study of transfusion-associated hepatitis. N Engl J Med 1990; 323:1107.

Eyster ME, Alter HJ, Aledort LM, et al. Heterosexual cotransmission of hepatitis C virus (HCV) and human immunodeficiency virus (HIV). Ann Intern Med 1991; 15:764–768.

Gerolami V, Halfon P, Bourliere M, et al. Hepatitis C virus genotypes in chronic hepatitis and response to interferon-alpha therapy. J Infect Dis 1993; 168:1328.

Gross JB Jr., Pershing DH. Hepatitis C: advances in diagnosis. Mayo Clin Proc 1995; 70:2962.

NIH Consensus Development Conference Statement. Management: management of hepatitis C:2002-June10-12,2002. Hepatology 2002; 36:S3–S20.

Seef LB, Buskell-Bales Z, Wright EC, et al. Long-term mortality after transfusion-associated non-A, non-B opiates. N Engl J Med 1992; 327:1906.

Mok J, Pembrey L, Tovo PA, Newell ML. When does mother to child transmission of hepatitis C virus occur? Arch Dis Child Fetal Neonatal Ed 2005; 90:F156–160.

Weinstock HS, Bolan G, Reingold AL, Polish LB. Hepatitis C virus infection among patients attending clinic for sexually transmitted diseases. J Am Med Assoc 1993; 269:392.

Hepatocellular Carcinoma

Tanaka K, Hrohata T, Koga S, et al. Hepatitis C and hepatitis B in the etiology of hepatocellular carcinoma in the Japanese population. Cancer Res 1991; 151:2842.

Tsukuma H, Hlyama T, Tanaka S, et al. Risk factors for hepatocellular carcinoma among patients with chronic liver disease. N Engl J Med 1993; 1328:1797.

Yu MC, Tong MJ, Coursaget P, et al. Prevalence of hepatitis B and C viral markers in black and white parents with hepatocellular carcinoma in the United States. J Natl Cancer Inst 1990; 82:1038.

Vertical Transmission

Inoue Y, Miysmura T, Unayama T, et al. Maternal transfer of HCV. Nature 1991; 353:6G9.

Ohto H, Terazawa S, Sasaki N. Transmission of hepatitis C virus from mothers to infants. N Engl J Med 1994; 330:744.

Riesiro S, Suarez A, Rodrlgo L. Transmission of hepatitis C. Ann Intern Med 1990; 113:411.

Thaler MM, Park C-K, Landus, et al. Vertical transmission of hepatitis C. Lancet 1993; 338:17.

Delta Virus

Alessandro ZR, Elisabetta T, Pierino F, Enrico M. Vertical transmission of the HBV associated delta agent. Prog Clin Biol Res 1983; 143:172.

Redeker A. Delta virus and hepatitis B. Ann Intern Med 1983; 98:542.

Rizzetto J. The delta agent. Hepatology 1983; 3:729.

Shen HD. Hepatitis B virus infection of cord blood leukocytes. J Med Virol 1987; 22:211.

Zanetti AR, Ferroni P, Magliano EM, et al. Perinatal transmission of the hepatitis B virus and of the HBV-associated delta agent from mothers to offspring in northern Italy. J Med Virol 1982; 9:139.

Passive Immunotherapy

Beasley RP, Hwang L, Lee GC, et al. Prevention of perinatally transmitted hepatitis B virus infections with hepatitis B immune globulin and hepatitis B vaccine. Lancet 1983; ii:1099.

Beasley RP, Hwang L, Stevens CE, et al. Efficacy of hepatitis B immune globulin for prevention of perinatal transmission of the hepatitis B virus carrier state: final report of a randomized double-blind, placebo-controlled trial. Hepatology 1983; 3:135.

Desforges JF, Matt RA, Smith AL, Hollenberg MK. Use of high-titer immune serum globulin for hepatitis A prophylaxis. N Engl J Med 1977; 296:1477.

Dosik H, Jhaveri R. Prevention of neonatal hepatitis B infection by high-dose hepatitis B immune globulin. N Engl J Med 1978; 298:602.

Grady GF, Lee VA. Hepatitis B immune globulin: prevention of hepatitis from accidental exposures among medical personnel: a preliminary report of a cooperative multi-center trial. N Engl J Med 1975; 293:1067.

Grady GF, Lee VA, Prince AM, et al. Hepatitis B immune globulin for accidental exposures among medical personnel: final report of a multicenter controlled trial. J Infect Dis 1978; 138:625.

Knodell RG, Conrad ME, Ginsberg AL, Bell CJ. Efficacy of prophylactic gammaglobulin in preventing non-A, non-B post-transfusion hepatitis. Lancet 1976; 1:557.

Krugman S. The prevention of viral hepatitis. Ann Clin Res 1976; 8:216.

Mayumi M, Miyakawa Y. Prevention of neonatal hepatitis B infection. N Engl J Med 1978; 299:46.

Prince AM, Szmuness W, Mann MK, et al. Hepatitis B immune globulin: final report of a controlled multicenter trial of efficacy in prevention of dialysis-associated hepatitis. J Infect Dis 1978; 137:131.

Redeker AG, Mosley JW, Gocke DJ, et al. Hepatitis B immune globulin as a prophylactic measure for spouses exposed to acute type B hepatitis. N Engl J Med 1975; 293:1055.

Reesink HW, Reerink-Brongers EE, Lafeber-Schut BJT, et al. Prevention of chronic HBsAg carrier state in infants of HBsAg-positive mothers by hepatitis B immunoglobulin. Lancet 1979; 2:436.

Seeff LB, Wright EC, Zimmerman HJ, et al. Type B hepatitis after needlestick exposure: prevention with hepatitis B immune globulin: final report of Veterans Administration Cooperative Study. Ann Intern Med 1978; 88:285.

Seeff LB, Zimmerman HJ, Wright EC, et al. Efficacy of hepatitis B immune serum globulin after accidental exposure: preliminary report of the Veterans Administration Cooperative Study. Lancet 1975; 2:939.

Active Immunotherapy

Beasley RP, Hwang L-Y, Lee CG-Y, et al. Prevention of perinatally transmitted hepatitis B virus infections with hepatitis B immune globulin and hepatitis B vaccine. Lancet 1983; 2:1099.

Brook MG, Lever AM, Kelly D, et al. Antenatal screening for hepatitis B is medically and economically effective in the prevention of vertical transmission: three years experience in a London hospital. Q J Med 1989; 71:313.

CDC. Inactivated hepatitis B virus vaccine. Morb Mortal Wkly Rep 1982; 31:317.

CDC. Hepatitis surveillance 1981; Report 47:1.

CDC. Hepatitis B virus vaccine safety. Morb Mortal Wkly Rep 1982; 31:465.

CDC. Suboptimal response to hepatitis B vaccine given by injection into the buttock. Morb Mortal Wkly Rep 1985; 34:105.

CDC. Recommendations for protection against viral hepatitis. Morb Mortal Wkly Rep 1985; 34:313.

Krugman S. Viral hepatitis type B: prospective for active immunization. Am J Med Sci 1975; 270:391.

Maupas P, Corsaget P, Goudeau A, Drucker J. Immunization against hepatitis B in man. Lancet 1976; 1:1367.

Okun NB, Larke RP, Waters JR, Joffres MR. Success of a program of routine prenatal screening for hepatitis B surface antigen: the first 2 years. Can Med Assoc J 1990; 143:1317.

Recombinant Hepatitis B Vaccine

Beasley RP, Hwang L, Stevens CE, et al. Efficacy of hepatitis B immune globulin for prevention of perinatal transmission of the hepatitis B virus carrier state: final report of a randomized double-blind, placebo-controlled trial. Hepatology 1983; 3:135.

CDC. Suboptimal response to hepatitis B vaccine given by injection into the buttock. Morb Mortal Wkly Rep 1985; 34:105.

Recommendation of the Immunization Practices Advisory Committee (ACIP). Recommendations for protection against viral hepatitis. Morb Mortal Wkly Rep 1985; 34:313.

Robinson WS. Hepatitis B virus and the delta virus. In: Mandell GL, Douglas RG, Bennett JE, eds. Principles and Practice of Infectious Diseases. Vol. 2. New York: John Wiley & Sons, 1985:1002–1029.

Stevens CE, Toy PT, Tong MJ, et al. Perinatal hepatitis B virus transmission in the United States. J Am Med Assoc 1985; 253:1740.

Herpes Simplex Viruses, Types 1 and 2

13

David A. Baker and Gilles R. G. Monif

INTRODUCTION

The herpesviruses are composed of a single molecule core of double-stranded DNA, an icosahedral structure with 162 capsomers, a granular zone, and a lipid envelope, which contains predominantly viral-specific glucoproteins. As a characteristic of the herpesvirus group, virus replication occurs in the cell nucleus. Six to eight hours after infection, synthesis and assembly of virus particles can be observed with an electron microscope. A basophilic Feulgen-positive mass centrally displaces the nuclear chromatin. Electron microscopy reveals this viral DNA core to be surrounded by a protein coat. There is a subsequent movement of the virus particle from the nucleus to the cytoplasm. This is paralleled by morphologic changes in the intranuclear inclusion body. The central ovoid intranuclear inclusion body loses both its basophilia and its affinity for DNA stains. The lesion is characterized by an eosinophilic, irregular central intranuclear inclusion body rimmed by peripheral fragments of chromatin at the margins of the nuclear membrane (Fig. 1). The virion obtains its final envelope from the nuclear membrane.

The DNA viruses of the herpesvirus group do not undergo immune elimination. Despite the presence of specific antibody, they persist as latent viruses. Recrudescence of herpes simplex virus (HSV) replication may be triggered by a variety of exogenous factors (e.g., cold, fever, intense sunlight, emotional stress, menstruation). Recurrent infection occurs in the presence of complement-fixing and neutralizing antibodies and is rarely associated with serologic evidence of a booster-type effect. In contrast to primary infection, it is unassociated with systemic symptoms and most often occurs at the site of initial infection.

Two types of herpesvirus can be identified on the basis of divergent biologic properties and are designated types 1 and 2 (HSV-1 and HSV-2; Table 1). They can also be differentiated by minor differences in antigenic composition and biochemical characteristics. Although they are distinct, the degree of sharing of antigenic determinants between the type 1 and 2 viruses results in cross-reacting antibodies capable of extensively neutralizing the heterologous virus type.

Initial contact with HSVs usually occurs early in childhood and involves HSV-1. Less than 10% of primary infections with HSV-1 are clinically overt.

HSV-1 is the causative agent for most nongenital herpetic lesions: herpes labialis, gingivostomatitis, and keratoconjunctivitis. Infection of the female genital tract by HSV-1 may occur at this time; however, the virus can often be simultaneously cultured from nongenital sites, suggesting that genital involvement is most often a secondary phenomenon.

FEMALE GENITAL TRACT INVOLVEMENT

Approximately 30% of the female population in the United States is infected with HSV-2 as determined by using sensitive HSV type-specific antibody studies performed on collected and stored sera. HSV of the genital

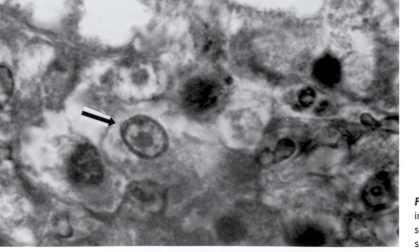

FIGURE I Characteristic mature intranuclear inclusion body (arrow) due to HSV-2 within tissue (H&E, ×1000). *Abbreviation*: HSV-2, herpes simplex virus type 2.

TABLE I Major distinguishing biologic and epidemiologic characteristics of type 1 and type 2 herpes simplex viruses

Characteristic	Type I	Type 2
Pock size on chorioallantoic membrane	Small	Large embryonated eggs
Plaques in chick embryo tissue cultures	None	+++
Neurovirulence for mice	++++	+
Sensitivity to idoxuridine (5-iodo-2′-deoxyuridine)	+++	+
Principal sites of viral replication	Nongenital	Genital
Group in which genital involvement occurs	Prepuberty, adolescence	Postpuberty, sexually active years
Principal mode of dissemination	Hand-to-mouth	Venereal

tract is one of the most common viral sexually transmitted diseases (STDs) with an estimated 40 million men and women infected with genital herpes. Approximately 1.6 million new cases of genital herpes occur annually. Most cases of HSV infection are occult or misdiagnosed. The genital tract of the female patient can be infected with HSV type 1 or type 2 virus. In the United States, the majority of genital infections is from HSV-2 virus. Up to 30% of first episode cases of genital herpes are caused by HSV-1. The vast majority of primary genital infections are caused by HSV-2.

Primary infection of the genital tract can produce clinical disease with symptoms or can be subclinical. Five percent of reproductive age women will give a history of genital herpes virus infection. Genital infection with HSV is associated with the age of the patient, years of sexual activity, race, one or more episodes of other genital infections, lower annual family income, and multiple sex partners. After clinically apparent primary genital herpes infection with HSV-2, almost all patients will experience recurrences; however, recurrences with HSV-2 tend to be much less frequent.

Type 2 antibodies usually appear first about the time of puberty and exhibit a significant increase during the prime reproductive years. The greatest incidence of overt type 2 infection occurs in women in their late teens and early twenties.

HSV-2 is recovered predominantly from the female genital tract. Epidemiologic data strongly support the thesis that dissemination of the type 2 strain is primarily but not exclusively contingent on venereal transmission. The incidence of specific antibody approaches 100% among prostitutes. Following exposure to males with active herpetic lesions of the genitalia, 50% to 90% of susceptible sexual partners develop infection.

Primary Infection

Primary genital infection due to HSV-2 may be asymptomatic or may be associated with severe symptoms. In primary vulvovaginitis, the genital lesions occur on the vulva, vagina, cervix, or all three between 2 and 14 days following exposure to infectious virus (Fig. 2). Like those in primary herpes labialis, the lesions are multiple and larger than those observed in recurrent disease or in those who have had prior

infection with HSV-1. At this time, patients usually experience vaginal discharge, discomfort, and pain. The mucocutaneous lesions are prone to trauma. The initial vesicles rupture and may become secondarily infected (Fig. 3). They subsequently appear as shallow, eroded, painful ulcers covered by a shaggy white membrane. Regional lymphadenopathy is readily demonstrated as the consequence of virus replication in the sites of lymphatic drainage as well as nodal stimulation by secondary bacterial infection.

Whereas local symptoms of dysuria, soreness of the vulva and vagina, dyspareunia, and a sudden increase of discharge are common in both primary and recurrent infections, systemic symptoms (malaise, myalgia, and fever) are virtually restricted to primary herpetic infection (Table 2). These symptoms reflect the viremia engendered during primary infection. The lesions tend to persist for one to three weeks without therapy. However, when secondary bacteria or mycotic infection is not treated, the lesions may persist for two to six weeks (Fig. 4).

Primary herpetic infection may occur on the cervix. The appearance of extensive cervical involvement may mimic that observed with squamous cell carcinoma of the cervix. Significant symptomatic and subclinical shedding can be found from the lower genital tract of the women. During the first six months after healing of primary genital HSV-2 lesions, subclinical cervical and vulvar shedding was more frequent. Asymptomatic shedding occurs around the time of symptomatic recurrences.

Recurrent Infection

Confinement of the ulcers to one area of the vulva, vagina, or cervix is more common in recurrent forms of the disease. The ulcers tend to be limited in size and number. Cervical involvement may occur as a diffuse cervicitis or as a single large ulcer. Local symptoms predominate over systemic symptoms, with increased vaginal discharge or pain being the usual presenting complaint. In certain women, it can be demonstrated that once it is involved, the genital tract is the site of intermittent virus replication. Virus shedding without a lesion (asymptomatic shedding) can occur from the vulva and cervix intermittently in subsequent years after primary infection. The titer of virus is significantly reduced compared with the level of recoverable virus when clinically overt lesions are present.

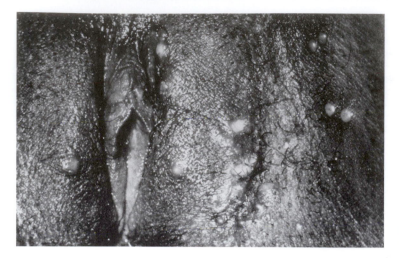

FIGURE 2 Vesicular and vesiculopustular lesions characteristic of genital herpes.

Asymptomatic shedding of virus lasts an average of 1.5 days and the quantity of virus is lower; however, a susceptible partner can acquire this virus during times of asymptomatic shedding. Shedding of virus without any symptoms or signs of clinical lesions (asymptomatic shedding) makes this viral STD difficult to control and prevent. Patients will experience recurrent disease after clinical or asymptomatic primary HSV genital infection. Recurrences of genital HSV infection can be symptomatic or asymptomatic and there is significant variation from patient to patient in the frequency, severity, and duration of symptoms and viral shedding. Young adult women tend to acquire the first episode of genital herpes between the ages of 20 and 24 years. Direct contact with an individual who is infected is required for the transmission of this viral infection. This may be genital to genital contact or contact of the genital tract from an area that is infected with HSV such as oral to genital contact. Direct sexual contact is the most common source of genital HSV transmission to women.

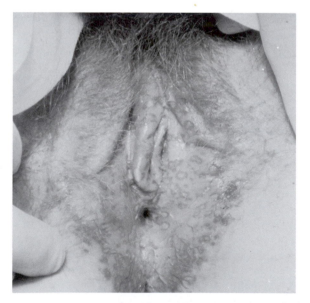

FIGURE 3 Classical primary herpetic vulvovaginitis. Note the multiplicity of the ulcers and the fact that the majority of them have become secondarily infected.

Symptomatic herpetic recurrence on the buttocks has been shown, depending on the dermatomes involved, to correlate with genital isolation of HSV. Kerkering et al. reviewed the records of 151 women with herpetic buttock recurrences. In the absence of genital lesions, HSV was isolated from the genital area on 7% of days during a buttock recurrence.

Diagnosis

Maternal herpes infection may be documented in several ways. Being DNA viruses, the HSV produce histologic stigmata indicative of virus replication. Papanicolaou smears of a given lesion may demonstrate large multinucleated cells containing eosinophilic intranuclear inclusion bodies (Fig. 5). Cytological tests have a maximum sensitivity of 60% to 70% when dealing with overt clinical disease. Both the Papanicolaou and Zanck smears are poor screening procedures. The presence of multinucleated giant cells is predominantly a phenomenon of herpetic involvement at free surfaces, as opposed to the single intranuclear inclusion body observed within organ tissues. Biopsy in conjunction with cytologic analysis of a cell preparation from the lesion very often leads to a diagnosis, even in the absence of virus isolation studies.

Isolation of virus by cell culture remains the standard and the most sensitive test for the detection of infectious herpes virus from clinical specimens. Numerous factors in sampling and transport of the specimen determine the sensitivity of this technique. False-negative cultures are not uncommon in patients with recurrent infection or healing lesions.

Newer techniques such as polymerase chain reaction (PCR) are three to four times more sensitive than culture techniques. As in cultures, false-negative results may occur. Because of cost and availability, PCR testing has not yet completely replaced virus isolation techniques.

Early first episode ulcers yield virus in 80% of patients, whereas ulcers from recurrent infections are less likely to be culture-positive and only 25% of crusted lesions contain recoverable virus. In culturing for HSV, overt lesions that are not in the ulcerated state should be unroofed and the fluid sampled. Virus isolation can be readily achieved in many primary or continuous human tissue culture cell lines.

TABLE 2 Clinical differences between primary and recurrent vulvovaginitis due to herpes simplex virus type 2

Signs or symptoms	Primary	Recurrent
Number of lesions	Multiple	Scattered 1 to 3
Location of lesions	Tend to involve both labia and vagina; cervix may be concomitantly involved	Limited involvement of vulva, vagina, or cervix
Size of lesions	Variable; tends to be larger than those observed in recurrent disease	Tends to be smaller
Inguinal adenopathy	Present	Usually absent
Viremia	Occurs	Absent
Systemic symptoms (malaise, myalgia, fever)	Present[a]	Absent
Local symptoms (dysuria, itching, dyspareunia)	Present	Present
Specific antibody titer	Greater than fourfold rise observed between postconvalescent sera	Usually no significant change between pre- and

[a]Only in the absence of preexisting antibodies to herpes simplex type 1.

The newly available serologic type-specific glycoprotein G (gG)–based assays can distinguish infection between HSV type 1 and 2 antibodies. These new immunoglobulin G (IgG) tests have excellent sensitivity (80–98%) and specificity (>96%) in comparison with Western blot assay; however, early in the course of infection, false-negative tests may occur. The older nonspecific antibody tests are of limited value owing to the frequency of cross-reacting antibodies to heterologous virus. IgM antibody test for HSV-1 and HSV-2 should not be used to diagnose acute infection.

HSV-2 is considered to reside primarily in the genital tract. A demonstration of HSV-2 type-specific antibodies by a gG-based assay is deemed evidence of genital tract infection.

The newer gG-based test requires three weeks to turn positive and should not be repeated for at least 8 to 12 weeks to test for serological conversion. One-third of the patients with recurrent herpes mount an IgM response. IgM testing for HSV cannot definitively differentiate new from recurrent infection.

Therapy

Numerous treatment options are available to the clinician to treat patients with genital herpes. These compounds are nucleoside analogs, and they selectively inhibit viral replication and produce little or minimal effects on the cell. Acyclovir was the first drug developed in this classification. This drug possessed a high safety profile along with being selective against herpesvirus-infected cells. Further advances with antiviral therapy have focused on greater bioavailability and therefore better absorption and higher plasma levels of compound with fewer daily doses of medication.

Acyclovir

Acyclovir was the first purine nucleoside analog with a new and selective activity against virus infected with HSV-1 and HSV-2. The drug stops HSV viral DNA replication and acts selectively against a viral-coded protein, thymidine kinase. The drug has been shown to be very safe, with few side effects. However, it has poor oral absorption. Only

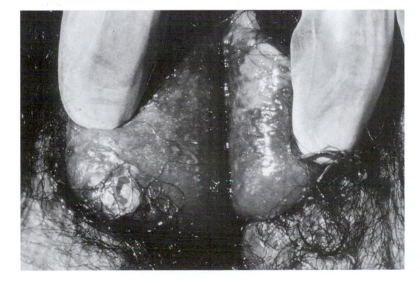

FIGURE 4 Painful herpetic ulcers with a shaggy white membrane and marked bilateral labial edema as a consequence of secondary bacterial infection. *Source:* Courtesy of MS Amstey, MD, Rochester, NY.

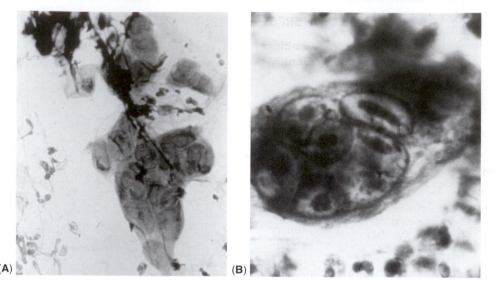

FIGURE 5 Multinucleated giant cells exhibiting intranuclear inclusion bodies, due to herpes simplex type 2 virus found in a cytological smear of a herpetic ulcer. **(A)** A more active lesion. The classical irregular eosinophilic intranuclear inclusion body is not present. The nuclei exhibit gigantism with a ground-glass background in which is scattered chromatin fragments (Papanicolaou stain, ×610). **(B)** A mature multinuclear giant cell. Each nucleus has a discrete central intranuclear inclusion body surrounded by a halo (Papanicolaou stain, ×1200).

approximately 20% of an oral dose is absorbed. The Food and Drug Administration (FDA) has approved acyclovir for the treatment of primary genital herpes, treatment of episodes of recurrent disease, and daily treatment for suppression of outbreaks of recurrent genital herpes.

Approximately 3% of isolates obtained from healthy patients demonstrate in vitro resistance to acyclovir. The frequency of in vitro resistance has not changed from that prior to its introduction. The demonstration of in vitro resistance has only rarely been associated with clinical failure in immunocompetent individuals. Foscarnet, a phosphonate viral DNA inhibitor, or cidofovir, an acyclic nucleoside phosphonate, has been used in infected AIDS patients with acyclovir-resistant isolates of herpes virus.

Valacyclovir

This newer antiviral is acyclovir with a valine ester. This drug is only for oral administration and, because there is an enzyme in the gut that cleaves the valine, the bioavailability is three to five times greater than oral acyclovir. The safety profile is that of acyclovir with a less frequent dosing schedule. The FDA has approved valacyclovir for the treatment of primary genital herpes, treatment of episodes of recurrent disease, daily treatment for suppression of outbreaks of recurrent genital herpes, and reduction of transmission of genital herpes to a susceptible sexual partner.

Famciclovir

Famciclovir is a prodrug of penciclovir. Bioavailability is good, but its clinical long-term use is less than that of acyclovir. Famciclovir requires less frequent dosing than acyclovir, but more frequent dosing than valacyclovir.

All cases of primary genital herpes should be treated with antiviral medication (Table 3). Currently, the FDA has approved acyclovir, valacyclovir, and famciclovir for the treatment of primary genital herpes, recurrent episodes of genital herpes (episodic therapy), and daily suppressive therapy of this disease. The bioavailability of the newer agents, valacyclovir and famciclovir, is greater; so they may require a less frequent dosing schedule to get as good

therapeutic benefit as from acyclovir. Acyclovir treatment of primary genital herpes infections reduces viral shedding, reduces pain, and heals lesions statistically significantly faster than placebo. Antiviral therapy should be administered as early in the course of the disease as possible for the greatest therapeutic benefit. With all these antiviral medications, therapy for the primary infection does not alter the natural history of genital herpes or the frequency of recurrent disease. Newer information concerning symptomatic and asymptomatic shedding within the first three to six months after primary infection may direct the clinician that in selective patients continued therapy after the first 10 days may be indicated. Therapy for the initial months after primary infection appears to significantly suppress symptomatic and asymptomatic shedding.

The clinician can select patient-initiated episodic or daily suppressive therapy to control this disease in immunocompetent patients. All three medications have been studied and have received approval for these forms of therapy. Patient-initiated episodic therapy can be effective in limiting each episode of recurrent disease, but this mode of therapy does not prevent recurrences. Famciclovir has been shown to be effective in treating genital herpes with episodic therapy as compared to placebo. Valacyclovir compared to the standard dose of acyclovir has been tested in more than 2500 patients with self-initiated episodic treatment for recurrent genital herpes. Valacyclovir is as effective as acyclovir in treating genital herpes episodically. In 50% of patients that have taken valacyclovir early in the prodromal phase, it appears to prevent lesion development.

With the high frequency of recurrent disease in patients who acquire genital herpes, daily suppressive therapy is a management mode that may benefit many patients. Antiviral therapy would be justified in patients after initial therapy for primary infection to reduce the increased symptomatic and asymptomatic shedding. A long-term safety and efficacy study has recently been concluded in which more than 1140 immunocompetent patients with frequent recurrences of genital herpes (more than 12 episodes per year) were treated with acyclovir for the first 10 years of the study

TABLE 3 Uses of antiviral therapy

For the treatment of initial genital herpes infections in nongravida, the recommended adult dosage of oral acyclovir is 200 mg every 4 hr while awake (5 times daily) for 7–10 days or until clinical resolution occurs (initiated within 6 days of onset of lesions), or acyclovir 400 mg orally 3 times a day for 7–10 days or valacyclovir 1 g orally twice a day for 7–10 days, or famciclovir 250 mg orally 3 times a day for 7–10 days

For the intermittent treatment of recurrent episodes, the recommended adult dosage of acyclovir is 200 mg every 4 hr while awake (5 times daily) for 5 days or, alternatively, 800 mg twice daily for 5 days (initiated within 2 days of onset of lesions); of fanciclovir is 125 mg twice a day; of valacyclovir is 500 mg twice a day for 5 days

For chronic prophylaxis of recurrent episodes, the recommended adult dosage of acyclovir is 200 mg 2–5 times daily or 400 mg twice daily; of famciclovir is 125 mg twice daily; and valacyclovir 500 mg once a day for patients with 9 or fewer recurrences a year, 250 mg twice a day or 1000 mg once for women who experience more than 9 episodes a year

and then valacyclovir in the 11th year. Goldberg et al. (1993) summarize the first five-year data from that study. There is a statistically significant reduction in recurrent disease when acyclovir is used at 400 mg twice a day. There was a 75% to 90% reduction in recurrent disease in each three-month quarter over the five-year period. This long-term study provides major insights and information concerning suppressive therapy. Adverse reactions to the medication were minimal, and, after the first year, less than 2% of patients reported any one side effect. Nausea, diarrhea, headache, and rash were seen during the study. Fife et al. (1994) showed that six years of continuous daily acyclovir suppressive therapy did not produce the emergence of acyclovir-resistant isolates in immunocompetent patients. Approximately 3% of patients required a higher dose to control symptoms than the standard dose of 400 mg acyclovir twice a day. This study has continued for 11 years, and the data were recently reported at a national clinical meeting.

Suppressive Therapy

Suppressive therapy can reduce the frequency of genital recurrences by 70% to 80% among individuals with frequent recurrences (six or more per year).

Daily oral acyclovir therapy not only significantly reduces symptomatic recurrences but also suppresses subclinical viral shedding. Valacyclovir therapy of 500 to 1000 mg orally once day, famciclovir 250 mg orally twice a day is effective in suppressing recurrent genital herpes. Patients on long-term suppressive therapy with oral acyclovir 400 mg twice a day can be changed to valacyclovir 500 mg once a day and maintain the safety and effectiveness of this therapy. Valacyclovir 500 mg once a day may be less effective than its higher dose or acyclovir dosing regimens in women who experience 10 or more outbreaks in a year.

Recently, daily valacyclovir (500 mg) suppressed overt acquisition of HSV-2 in susceptible sexual partners. Overall acquisition, symptomatic and asymptomatic, was reduced by 48% in the valacyclovir group compared with the placebo group.

HERPES IN PREGNANCY

Problems in Distinguishing Primary and Recurrent Genital Herpes

In the absence of systemic symptomology, the distinction between primary and secondary herpetic infections appears to be more difficult than previously assumed. Henseleigh et al. evaluated serologically and virologicaly 23 women with severe first clinical outbreak of genital herpes in the second and third trimesters of pregnancy. They were classified as having true primary (no HSV type 1 or type 2 antibodies), nonprimary (heterologous HSV antibodies present), and recurrent (homologous antibodies present) infections. Only one of the 23 women with clinical illnesses consistent with primary genital HSV infections had serologically verified primary infection. This primary infection was caused by HSV type 1. Three women had nonprimary type 2 infections, and 19 women had recurrent infections.

This report demonstrates the need for careful serological evaluation of all cases of presumed first episode of genital herpes in pregnant women. In the absence of homologous and heterologous antibodies, the risk of congenital infection exists. Recurrent herpes may not be associated with vertical transmission unless a uterine site of reactivation is involved.

Disseminated Maternal Herpetic Infection and Pregnancy

Disseminated herpetic infection in an adult is distinct from herpetic encephalitis, although the latter may occur as part of the widespread organ system involvement. Disseminated disease in adults is thought to represent primary infection in a partially immunocompromised host, whereas herpetic encephalitis functions independent of systemic humoral or cellular immunity. Severe disseminated HSV may occur in normal immunocompetent pregnant women.

There are several patient populations in whom disseminated disease may occur: neonates, immunocompromised adults, particularly individuals with thymic dysplasias, and pregnant women. Disseminated herpetic infection in pregnancy is an extremely rare event. The manifestations of systemic dissemination in pregnancies tend to be viscerotropic rather than neurotropic. Its principal presentation is that of a fulminating hepatitis. Herpetic hepatitis is extremely rare, with a maternal mortality rate of 43%. Classically, disease occurs in the third trimester. Often there is viral-like prodromal illness in association with vulvar or oropharyngeal vesicular or vesiculopustular lesions. Despite elevated liver enzymes, most of the cases are anicteric. In some cases, no clinically overt site of primary herpetic infection can be identified. Chatelan et al. (1994) identified 14 cases in the literature. Of the 14 patients reported, six died. Four patients treated with parenteral acyclovir survived and two patients treated with the antiviral agent vidarabine also survived; however, five of seven patients who did not receive antiviral therapy died.

Herpetic hepatitis should be included in the differential diagnosis of hepatic dysfunction in the third trimester. Any pregnant patient with primary infection in the third trimester should be closely watched for any evidence of disseminated disease. In the absence of herpetic lesions elsewhere, a diagnosis can be inferred by the demonstration of characteristic intranuclear inclusion bodies within a liver biopsy specimen. Once the diagnosis is made, acyclovir should be initiated to reduce maternal mortality.

In every case, dissemination has occurred in the late-second and third trimester at a time when maternal T-cell function is partially compromised. Both type 1 and 2 HSV viruses have been isolated from gravidas with disseminated disease in pregnancy.

Fetal Considerations: Infection and Fetal Wastage

Preliminary data indicate a threefold increase in the rate of abortion following primary maternal genital infection with HSV early in pregnancy. The probability of abortion appears to be directly related if the maternal infection is primary. It is yet to be determined whether this increased fetal wastage is related to infection of the conceptus or is secondary to the maternal response to disease.

Congenital Infection

During gestation, primary herpetic infection, in the absence of cross-protecting antibodies, theoretically may result in hematogenous dissemination of the virus to the conceptus.

Congenital herpetic infection can affect organogenesis or may produce visceral disease. In utero infection in the first 12 to 14 weeks of gestation may produce a cluster of anomalies clinically indistinguishable from those caused by the cytomegaloviruses. Chalhub et al. (1977) reported a case of a premature neonate with microcephaly and periventricular calcifications, bilateral lenticular opacities, and extensive hepatomegaly with secondary dystrophic calcification, who did not develop overt evidence of characteristic herpetic infection until the fifth day. The fetal membranes ruptured 30 minutes before parturition. At necropsy the infant had characteristic lesions involving the brain, liver, and adrenals. Eosinophilic Cowdry type A intranuclear inclusion bodies were present in hepatocytes adjacent to areas of bland necrosis and dystrophic calcification. Predicated on the clustering of ocular lesions, microcephaly with dystrophic periventricular calcification and hepatosplenomegaly, this case could have been attributed to the cytomegalovirus. Similarly, an increased rate of premature births had been found in infants whose mothers had genital infection after the 20th week of pregnancy. This was particularly true with primary maternal herpetic vulvovaginitis.

The limited perception of the ability of HSV to cause disease in utero has been a partial function of the criteria used to define congenital infections. The rigid adherence to documented herpetic infection present at birth and/or within 24 hours of rupture of the fetal membranes (ROM) had effectively excluded a significant number of cases. In the absence of well-established placental or fetal pathology that clearly antedated potential access of the virus to the products of conception by means of ascending infection, the cases of congenital herpes reported by Von Herzen and Benirschke (1977), Altshuler (1984), and Witzleben and Driscoll (1965) could have been challenged. Gagnon (1968) reported a case

of what typically would have been considered a case of neonatal disease developing on the fifth day of life. Had umbilical cord blood and placenta not been cultured for virus at the time of delivery, parturitional acquisition of disease would have been inferred. Similarly, Pettay (1979) described a case of overt acute neonatal disease, which developed on the sixth day of life; however, HSV-2 had been recovered from an amniotic fluid specimen one week prior to parturition and at a time when the fetal membranes were intact.

The mucus plug of pregnancy and the presence of intact fetal membranes are a formidable barrier to ascending viral infection; however, once dissolution of the membranes occurs, the herpes viruses can obtain direct access to amniotic fluid and/or the fetus without ensuing vaginal delivery. For the term congenital herpetic infection to imply vertical hematogenous dissemination from the mother to the fetus, disease must develop within the shortest known incubation period required to induce overt disease in experimental animals from ROM, or a virally induced effect on organogenesis must be identified in fetuses or neonates with documented herpetic infection. The criteria that can be used to make the diagnosis of congenital infection due to the HSVs include

1. documented herpetic infection present at birth and/or within 24 hours of ROM (Fig. 6),
2. effects of herpetic infection on organogenesis, which antedate dissolution of the fetal membrane, and
3. evidence of herpetic and/or viral placentitis, the induction of which antedates ROM, which is associated with documented disseminated herpetic infection of the newborn.

Without virological confirmation, the baby described by Schaffer and Avery (1971) would have been attributed to the cytomegalovirus. South et al. (1969) reported a case of a premature neonate with microcephaly, intracranial calcifications, micro-ophthalmus, and retinal dysplasia, who had vesicular skin lesions from which HSV-2 was recovered. Fagnant and Monif (1989) identified 15 cases of congenital transplacental HSV using three criteria:

1. herpetic infection and altered organogenesis of inflammatory etiology that antedates dissolution of the fetal membranes,
2. documented herpetic infection present at birth and within 24 hours of ROM, and
3. evidence of viral herpetic placentitis, the induction of which antedates rupture of the membranes.

In this series, disease manifesting after the shortest recognized incubation period for the induction of the disease in experimental animals did not necessarily preclude transplacental acquisition.

The Centers for Disease Control (CDC) conducted an 18-month hospital-based surveillance study in which 184 cases of neonatal HSV infection were analyzed. Only 22% of mothers had a history of genital HSV infection and only 9% had genital lesions at the time of delivery. Cesarean delivery initiated prior to membrane rupture failed to prevent infection in 15 cases. Their data confirm previous

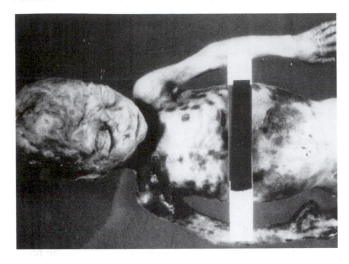

FIGURE 6 Fetus aborted at 28 weeks who demonstrated multiple ulcerative lesions from which herpes simplex virus type 2 was isolated. *Source*: Monif et al. (1985).

observations that most mothers of infected neonates have no history of genital HSV and are asymptomatic at delivery. They concluded that intrauterine infection was an important route of transmission, which underscores the limitations of our current prevention strategy.

Neonatal Infection

Neonatal herpes affects as many as 1 per 3200 live births. Neonatal infection is the consequence of delivery of a neonate through an infected birth canal. Neonatal involvement characteristically appears between the fourth and the tenth days. The length of the incubation period is a partial function of the inoculating dose of virus.

The infants may eat poorly and become listless and irritable. Cutaneous herpetic vesicles may or may not develop. In the next few days, depending on the organs involved and the extent of infection, the neonates may exhibit fever or subnormal temperature, cough, increased respiratory distress, cyanosis, tachycardia, jaundice, vomiting, diarrhea, irritability, and convulsions. A hemorrhagic diathesis associated with thrombocytopenia or gastrointestinal bleeding from herpetic gastric ulcers or esophagitis may occur. The clinical course may terminate in irreversible vasomotor collapse or respiratory arrest.

At necropsy, affected infants exhibit miliary focal necrosis involving primarily the liver, lungs, and adrenal glands (Fig. 7). Microscopically, these lesions demonstrate focal, coagulative necrosis (Fig. 8). At the margin of these areas of necrosis, the characteristic intranuclear inclusion bodies can be identified.

Fifty percent of infected progeny will develop disease, which results in the death of 50% to 60% of cases with disseminated disease and neurological damage in up to 70% of survivors with central nervous system involvement, even with antiviral therapy. Of the 326 cases of neonatal herpes summarized by Nahmias et al. (2006), 59% died. An additional 20% who survived had permanent ocular or central nervous system sequelae.

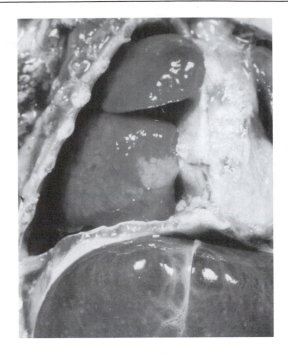

FIGURE 7 Miliary focal necrosis. Miliary involvement of liver and segmented involvement of the lungs of a term neonate who died of disseminated disease acquired at the time of parturition.

Probability of Neonatal Involvement

The simple presence of virus within the birth canal is not the sole determinant of disease. In the absence of any demonstrable lesion, sensitive virological techniques can demonstrate the presence of HSV in endocervical tissue of 1% to 2% of all gravid females. The incidence of isolation appears to increase in the third trimester. Asymptomatic occult shedding of HSV-2 can be demonstrated in 0.65% to 3.03% of cultures from pregnant women with a history of recurrent genital herpes. When serial specimens for culture are obtained, at least one episode of asymptomatic reactivation is detected in 2.3% to 14% of pregnant women with a history of genital herpes. As the number of antepartum culture specimens increases, so does the incidence of culture-proven asymptomatic excretion. Among women with recurrent genital herpes antedating pregnancy, the mean number of recurrences per trimester increased from 0.01 to 1.26 to 1.63 in the first trimester through third trimester. In a very real sense, one infant in 50 to 100 live births has been delivered through a birth canal harboring infectious virus, yet the incidence of disseminated herpetic infection of the newborn is extremely low, i.e., 1:20,000. The difference between these patients and gravida with overt herpetic vulvovaginitis is that in the former case, the quantity of virus present is limited to a few plaque-forming units, whereas in the latter the quantity of virus present is in the order of several logs of virus. While the quantity of virus present is a major factor in determining the probability of ensuing neonatal disease, almost equally important may be the duration of exposure to a given minimum quantum of virus, the genetic constitution of the infant, and the presence of specific homologous neutralizing antibodies. The risk of infection for an infant born to a mother

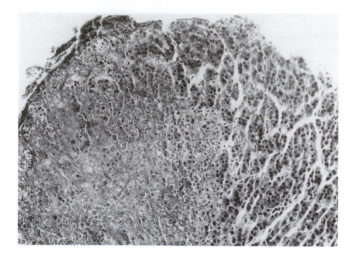

FIGURE 8 Photomicrograph of an adrenal gland exhibiting coagulative necrosis due to herpes simplex type 2 virus (H&E, ×120).

with primary herpetic vulvovaginitis is 30% to 45%. With active recurrent herpetic disease at the time of parturition, the risk of infection is estimated to be between 5% and 8%.

The significant ability of careful patient selection and antiviral prophylaxis to decrease the incidence of neonatal disseminated herpetic infection from the neonatal nursery has focused on the question of resultant maternal morbidity. Once a disease is eradicated, the cost of its eradication is re-evaluated. Cesarean section carries with it significant maternal morbidity and, in rare instances, mortality.

The rarity of neonatal disease has fostered the concept that cesarean section is unwarranted for recurrent herpetic vulvovaginitis. How completely maternal antibody will protect a neonate from infection during a recurrence is not well established. There have been several case reports describing neonatal herpetic disease in progeny born to mothers with high serum IgG antibody titers to HSV-2. Preexisting homologous and probably heterologous antibodies appear to afford relative protection against congenital but not neonatal disease.

Local neonatal infection may result from the use of fetal scalp electrode monitoring in which the portal of infection was the site of attachment of the scalp electrode used in internal fetal monitoring. If vesicular or vesiculopustular lesions develop at this site, it is imperative that immediate cytologic evaluation be carried out. If multinucleated giant cells with intranuclear inclusion bodies are identified, systemic chemotherapy should be instituted immediately.

Nosocomial Neonatal Herpetic Infection

The major emphasis has been placed on preventing acquisition of neonatal infection by avoiding delivery through an infected or potentially infected birth canal. The success of preventing "baby and virus from ever meeting" has overshadowed the fact that neonatal infection may be acquired independently of the events involved with parturition. Transmission of virus to the neonate may be mediated by individuals other than the mother and from sites other than the genital tract. The neonate, and particularly the

premature neonate, is uniquely susceptible to the HSV. Postnatally, nosocomially acquired disease can be as lethal as that acquired by virtue of delivery through an infected birth canal. Oropharyngeal or cutaneous lesions can be an effective source of virus as primary herpetic vulvovaginitis. Most strains of HSV responsible for nosocomial neonatal disease are type 1 rather than type 2. One of the big problems in devising a management sequence is our current inability to document immunological competence on the part of the neonate. Should the infant contract herpetic infection after 15 to 20 days, the baby may become sick; however, permanent sequelae or mortality rarely ensues. Only when we can document T-cell competence for HSV in a given neonate, can the recommendations concerning the duration of relative isolation have validity. Given a woman with one or more active lesions at term, the policy is to institute appropriate isolation procedures (routine gown and glove isolation). Masks are added to the isolation regimen only if an oropharyngeal lesion is identified. Although isolation precautions need to be implemented, bonding should be permitted. Although separation of mother from her neonate up to one week of age can be implemented, concern must be given to the potential adverse effect on the establishment of a satisfactory mother–child relationship later in life. The mode of dissemination of the herpes virus is basically that of direct contact (hand-to-mouth type of dissemination). Care is taken to screen the father and other family contacts for the presence of oral lesions. The neonate born to a mother with prior primary infection during gestation will be isolated from other infants only if that child is at risk for congenital involvement. These children will be handled as potentially infected children and removed from the normal newborn nursery to a semi-isolated situation.

Nosocomial Dissemination via Breast Milk

The question of breast-feeding in the immediate postpartum period has been complicated by the demonstration of neonatal HSV-1 infection. Serological studies demonstrated postnatal acquisition of infection for which breast milk was the vehicle of dissemination. The mother was found to have HSV-1 in her breast milk. She had no history of genital lesions. Viral cultures of cervix, vagina, and throat were negative for HSV-1. Previously, Quinn and Lofberg reported the death of an eight-day-old breast-fed neonate with disseminated HSV-2. The mother was subsequently found to have bilateral herpetic nipple lesions; however, concomitant cultures of the vulva and cervix also grew HSV-2. The presence of HSV in breast milk is not surprising. The cytomegalovirus, which is also a herpesvirus, is not an uncommon isolate from breast milk. The major question that needs to be resolved is whether the concomitant presence of specific secretary IgA antibody can adequately function to render an infant relatively immune to infection. It is the opinion of the Committees on Fetus and Newborn and on Infectious Diseases of the American Academy of Pediatrics (1980) that breast-feeding can be attempted; however, careful attention to hygienic measures must be implemented to adequately protect the infant. The nipple should be examined to exclude the presence of herpetic lesions. In view of the occult transmission of the HSVs in breast milk, it may be wise to individualize each case.

Management of Active Herpetic Vulvovaginitis in Pregnancy

When a pregnant patient presents with genital herpes, the physician must determine whether he is dealing with primary or recurrent herpetic infection. In most instances, the solution does not require sophisticated laboratory backup, but can be made on clinical grounds: the number of lesions, their size, their distribution, the presence or absence of systemic symptomatology, etc. In primary herpetic infection, the immediate focus of management (beyond that of maternal pain and discomfort) is to determine whether or not an effective maternal viremia has occurred. Most people with primary infection to HSV-2 have preexisting cross-reacting antibodies to HSV-1, which will effectively abort type 2 viremia. A history of cold sores or the absence of systemic symptomatology argues against an effective viremia having been engendered. The critical focus of attention becomes the immediate antepartum period and the exclusion of recurrent infection. If the gravida gives a history of fever, pseudochills, myalgia, or arthralgia, these should be interpreted as indicative of an effective maternal viremia, and the possibility of congenital herpetic infection is raised. It was previously advocated that, approximately four to six weeks after primary infection, an amniocentesis should be performed and the amniotic fluid cultured for the virus. Based on observation derived from cases of congenital cytomegalovirus and rubella, it was postulated that recovery of herpes virus from amniotic fluid would be presumptive evidence of in utero infection, and consequently, should overt disease be detected at the time of parturition, no advantage would accrue from cesarean section. This postulate may not be invariably correct for the HSV. To date, there has been a poor correlation between effective viremia as documented by systemic symptomatology and/or the absence of cross-reacting antibodies to the heterologous strain of HSV and congenital infection. Out of several hundred patients studied by amniocentesis, only three isolates have been achieved from amniotic fluid. In one instance, the neonate was free of any stigmata of disease at the time of parturition. In the other two cases, the infants were infected in utero. This observation, coupled with the rarity with which HSV functions teratogenically for the human fetus, has led to questioning the wisdom of resorting to such a procedure except within academic settings. Currently, culture of amniotic fluid for virus or analysis of amniotic fluid for viral antigens is not recommended unless the fluid is to be obtained for another diagnostic purpose or a high index of suspicion exists that in utero infection has occurred.

Given a patient with recurrent herpetic vulvovaginitis during pregnancy, no maternal viremia is engendered and, consequently, there is no potential for fetal involvement. Here management focuses on whether or not disease is present at the time of parturition. Given one or more maternal lesions at the time of parturition, the probability of neonatal disseminated infection is in the order of 5% to 8%. The two most important variables that determine the probability of neonatal infection are

1. the amount of virus present and
2. the duration of labor.

Both variables must function in concert to achieve neonatal involvement with any degree of regularity.

In the presence of one or more lesions, it is our recommendation that cesarean section be performed. The cardinal point of therapy is that delivery must not occur through the birth canal harboring virus. In the absence of congenital involvement, cesarean section prior to the ROM is effective in circumventing neonatal infection. Once the fetal membranes have been ruptured, both HSV-1 and HSV-2 have the ability to ascend and infect the fetus in utero. With the advent of antiviral therapy of the newborn, the duration of rupture of membranes is not the important clinical factor, but the estimated time of delivery once the mother presents in labor.

Scott et al. (1996) have reported a small, randomized, double-blind clinical trial in which women with clinically first-episode genital herpes during pregnancy received daily acyclovir treatment initiated in week 36 of gestation. They were able to demonstrate a reduced need for cesarean section. The ability of acyclovir, famciclovir, and valacyclovir to diminish viral shedding has brought into question the use of antiviral therapy for gravida with lesions in close proximity to parturition, but not fulfilling guidelines for cesarean section. Sheffield et al. (2006) evaluated the efficacy of valacyclovir suppression late in pregnancy. In this study, 170 women were treated with valacyclovir and 168 were treated with placebo. At delivery, 13% of gravidas in the placebo group required cesarean section delivery as opposed to 4% in the valacyclovir group. Despite an overrepresentation of women with recurrent genital herpes, with only 6% of study participants having primary genital herpes, the investigators interpreted the data as showing valacyclovir suppression significantly reduced HSV shedding that required cesarean delivery.

The CDC and Glaxo-Welcome have maintained a voluntary registry of women who have received acyclovir or valacyclovir during pregnancy. Women who received acyclovir in the first trimester and whose birth outcomes were known had a 2.3% prevalence of birth defects as compared to a background rate of 3%. A theoretical concern is the development of obstructive uropathy in newborns, secondary to acyclovir crystals.

Virological Monitoring During Pregnancy

Whatever management scheme that is to be developed for the prevention of neonatal herpetic disease will be predicated on less than optimal scientific data. The future schema will probably be built around two basic tenets:

1. the probability of fetal–neonatal involvement increases following primary herpetic vulvovaginitis in pregnancy and
2. the probability of neonatal disease is greater when one or more active lesions are present at the time of parturition.

Influence of Primary Herpetic Vulvovaginitis on Neonatal Outcome

Brown et al. (1986) prospectively followed 29 patients who had acquired genital herpes during pregnancy. While 15 patients had a primary episode of genital HSV-2, 14 had a nonprimary first episode. Six of the 15 gravida with primary genital herpes, but none of the 14 with nonprimary first episode infection, had infants with serious perinatal morbidity. Four of the five infants whose mothers acquired primary HSV in the third trimester had perinatal morbidity, which included prematurity, intrauterine growth retardation, and neonatal infection with HSV-2. Perinatal complications occurred in one of the five infants whose mothers acquired primary HSV-2 during the first trimester as well as one of the five infants who had primary HSV-2 during the second trimester. Asymptomatic cervical shedding of HSV-2 was detected at 10.6% of weekly visits made after a primary first episode as compared to 0.5% of visits made after a nonprimary first episode.

One of the factors selected for the increased prevalence for neonatal involvement following primary herpes appears to be the occurrence of in utero hematogenous involvement. Fagnant and Monif (1989) have identified 15 well-documented cases of congenital involvement in which disease or its impact on organogenesis clearly antedated the ROM. When well-documented cases of congenital involvement as well as those of probable congenital acquisition were combined, they constituted approximately 5% of all the cases that had been reviewed.

Significance of Subclinical Viral Shedding

A second factor that influences the probability of an adverse fetal outcome is the greater incidence of clinically overt recurrent infection as well as asymptomatic shedding in gravida whose primary disease occurs during gestation. Brown et al. (1986), in another study, documented that asymptomatic secretion from the genital tract was more common in women whose first episode of genital herpes was acquired during pregnancy (33%) than in women whose disease antedated pregnancy (12.9%; $p < 0.05$). Following primary infection there may be continued viral shedding in the absence of clinically discernible disease.

A third factor selecting for a higher probability of disease induction is the amount of virus present. In most cases of asymptomatic shedding, the amount of virus present is low (less than one log). When one or more lesions are present, the quantity of virus recovered from such lesions is in the order of four or five logs of virus.

About 50% to 70% of neonates with HSV infection are born to mothers who do not have a history of peripartum genital herpes infection. HIV-positive women have an increased tendency for genital shedding of virus; herpetic lesions persist longer and may become chronic ulcerations.

Who and When to Culture

Virological monitoring has proven to be both costly and noneffective. The correlation between asymptomatic viral shedding and ensuing neonatally acquired disease is poor.

Unless a portal of infection is incidentally established, i.e., scalp electrode site, and in the absence of lesions in the periparturitional period, the probability of ensuing neonatal disease appears to be exceedingly low. Prior disease that antedates this gestation is not a sensitive predictor of ensuing fetal disease. Negative cultures probably do not preclude the possibility of subsequent neonatal involvement. Current policy is not to institute virological monitoring in gravida whose onset of disease antedated pregnancy or whose sexual consorts have had herpetic lesions. Similarly, current information does not support the value of culturing asymptomatic patients with a history of recurrent disease.

There is no justification for cesarean delivery in women with merely a history of HSV infection but no active disease during the last weeks of pregnancy. In the absence of herpetic lesions in the periparturitional period, the probability of ensuing neonatal disease appears to be exceedingly low. A critical determinant of whether or not to do a cesarean section for a gravida with a genital lesion is whether or not the lesion present is due to HSV. In a longitudinal study from 1989 to 1999, Gardella et al. demonstrated a poor correlation between the clinical diagnosis of genital herpes at the time of labor and HSV detection from genital sites or lesions by culture or PCR. Although the presence of virus at parturition in a gravida whose disease antedates this gestation is not a sensitive predictor of ensuing fetal disease, the current guidelines for neonatal HSV prevention recommend cesarean delivery for women with genital lesion or prodromal symptomology at the time of labor.

Negative cultures probably do not preclude the possibility of subsequent neonatal involvement. The reason for this is that type 1 disease, which occurs in the neonate, may be acquired from family contact and nursing personnel and may not be the consequence of delivery through an infected birth canal. Identifying the 1% to 2% of gravida whose herpetic infection antedates gestation and who are excreting virus at the time of parturition requires that 200 to 500 cultures be obtained. If these women with low titers of virus are then allowed to deliver vaginally, estimated probability of neonatal involvement is significantly less than 1%.

Just as current monitoring policies have failed to totally preclude neonatal involvement, it must be understood that the new policies will fail to preclude sporadic occurrence of disease in the neonate. The difference between previous and currently advocated positions is that the latter are more rational and more cost effective. Failure of the current policies will occur because of

1. asymptomatic primary herpetic infection during gestation and subsequent hematogenous dissemination to the fetus may occur,
2. ROM introducing distinct potential for ascending infection,
3. direct mechanical inoculation associated with the use of a scalp electrode in an asymptomatic shedder, and
4. distinguishing nosocomially acquired disease from parturitionally acquired disease may be difficult.

Primary Infection During Pregnancy

These individuals constitute a higher risk group than do gravida whose disease antedates gestation. The absence of episodes of symptomatic genital HSV infection throughout pregnancy does not eliminate the risk of asymptomatic shedding at delivery. There are limited data concerning prevention of disease in the fetus with maternal antiviral therapy. Acyclovir, famciclovir, and valacyclovir can reduce viral shedding and shorten the duration of lesions. In theory, the reduction of the magnitude of the viremia and its duration should lessen the risk of transplacental viral dissemination in a nonimmune gravida.

If the fetus develops an abnormal biophysical profile, an amniotic fluid sample can be obtained for either culture or testing for virus-specific antigens using PCR technology.

Maternal Herpetic Genital Tract Disease Antedating Gestation or History of Genital Tract Disease in Sexual Consort

If there are no recurrences during pregnancy and no lesions are present at the time of parturition, vaginal delivery has been advocated.

Presence of Clinically Overt Disease at Parturition

The presence of one or more lesions at parturition is a contraindication to vaginal delivery. Clearly when primary disease is present, there will be near unanimity on this point. With limited recurrent disease, even though the estimated risk may also be less than 5%, the ability to lower it to less than 1% mandates implementation of current protocol, which uses cesarean section.

There is a continued need to identify gravida who have any risk factor that antedates gestation. Gravida with prior herpetic genital tract infection, those with herpes infection in consort, and women who are on immunosuppressant therapy should be prospectively identified to the neonatologists.

A unique situation arises when maternal genital HSV infection manifests in an immature, nonviable gestation in conjunction with documented ROM. What we would do after an informed consent is obtained is to put the patient on parenteral antiviral therapy and manage the patient as one would any other gravida with ROM and a previable fetus whose gestational age precluded reasonable lung maturity. The use of corticosteroids to accelerate pulmonary maturity needs to be carefully evaluated. Parenteral antiviral therapy is continued until termination of viral synthesis is documented. Thereafter, conversion to oral drug is implemented and therapy is continued until parturition. This approach is totally experimental.

Therapy in Pregnancy

Approximately 1500 to 2000 newborns in the United States contact neonatal herpes each year. Infections occur in the perinatal period from contact with infected maternal secretions in the majority of cases. Mothers who do not know they are infected with genital herpes and shed the virus without lesions or symptoms give rise to most infected newborns. Alternative management of these women to prevent the transmission of this virus is being studied. The current management that relies on cesarean delivery has many disadvantages.

A viable alternative is antiviral therapy of the mother to prevent maternal symptomatic and subclinical viral shedding during the intrapartum period.

Other examples of prophylactic antiviral therapy have been shown to be safe and effective in reducing the spread of HIV from mother to newborn. In cases of disseminated HSV, herpes pneumonitis, herpes hepatitis, and herpes encephalitis, antiviral therapy using acyclovir has been life saving to mother and fetus. The use of antiviral medication in the last few weeks of pregnancy to suppress recurrent disease is being studied. Acyclovir, valacyclovir, and famciclovir are class B medication as categorized by the FDA. When acyclovir or valacyclovir is given by the oral or intravenous route to the mother, the drug crosses the placenta, is concentrated in amniotic fluid and breast milk, and reaches therapeutic levels in the fetus. Starting in 1984, an acyclovir pregnancy registry has been compiled. The CDC published data in 1993 showing there was no increase in fetal problems in women who received acyclovir in the first trimester of their pregnancy. The registry continues to accumulate this information.

The newer recommendations to reduce the number of newborns infected with HSV will combine serological testing of all pregnant women for antibodies to HSV-1 and HSV-2 using a type-specific glycoprotein gG-based test and the use of antiviral therapy starting at 36 weeks in selected cases. Intervention is aimed primarily at preventing primary infection in those women at risk for HSV.

Prevention of Sexual Transmission

Abstinence is advised when prodromal symptoms develop or one or more lesions are identified. Antiviral therapy, by suppressing viral replication, may result in decreased transmission of infection to sexual partners in discordant couples. In theory, the use at the time of intercourse of nonoxynol-9 and a condom may afford another layer of protection; however, given the wide distribution of herpes during reactivation, these measures may not suffice.

In stable, established relationships, serological type-specific testing is advised. Often transmission of infection has occurred.

Information and its sharing are the keys to prevention. An HSV-infected woman needs to know about the risk that HSV can be sexually transmitted, how to detect the earliest symptoms of disease, the availability of suppressive therapy, the ability to obtain type-specific testing of sexual partners, and the potential dangers to the newborn when disease is present at parturition.

Pregnant women who are not infected with HSV-2 should be advised to avoid intercourse during the third trimester with men who have had genital herpes. Pregnant women who are not infected with HSV-1 should be counseled to avoid cunnilingus with any partner with prior oral herpes and genital intercourse with a partner with genital HSV-1 infection.

SELECTED READING

Herpes and Pregnancy

Amstey MS, Monif GRG. Genital herpes virus infection in pregnancy. Obstet Gynecol 1974; 44:394.

Amstey MS, Monif GRG, Nahmias AJ, Josey WE. Cesarean section and genital herpes virus infection. Obstet Gynecol 1979; 53:641.

Ashley RL. Sorting out the new HSV type specific antibody tests. Sex Trans Infect 2001; 77:232.

Arvin AM, Hensleigh PA, Prober CG, et al. Failure of antepartum maternal cultures to predict the infant's risk of exposure to herpes simplex virus at delivery. N Engl J Med 1986; 315:796.

Baker D, Brown Z, Hollier LM, et al. Cost-effectiveness of herpes simplex virus type 2 serologic testing and antiviral therapy in pregnancy. Am J Obstet Gynecol 2005; 192:483.

Benedetti J, Corey L, Ashley R. Recurrence rate in genital herpes after symptomatic first-episode infection. Ann Intern Med 1994; 121:847.

Brown ZA, Berry S, Vontver LA. Genital herpes simplex virus infections complicating pregnancy: natural history and peripartum management. J Reprod Med 1986; 31(5 suppl):420.

Brown ZA, Gardella C, Wald A, et al. Genital herpes complicating pregnancy. Obstet Gynecol; 106:845.

Bryson Y, Dillon K, Bernstein DI, et al. Risk of acquisition of genital herpes simplex virus type 2 in sex partners of persons with genital herpes: a prospective couple study. J Infect Dis 1993; 167:942.

Catalano PM, Merritt AO, Mead PB. Incidence of genital herpes simplex virus at the time of delivery in women with known risk factors. Am J Obstet Gynecol 1991; 164:1303.

Cook CR, Gall SA. Herpes in pregnancy. Infect Dis Obstet Gynecol 1994; 1:298.

Growdon WA, Apodaca L, Cragun J, et al. Neonatal herpes simplex virus infection occurring in second twin of an asymptomatic mother: failure of a modern protocol. J Am Med Assoc 1987; 257:508.

Hensleigh PA, Andrews WW, Brown Z, et al. Genital herpes during pregnancy: inability to distinguish primary and recurrent infections clinically. Obstet Gynecol 1997; 89:891.

Johnson RE, Nahmias AJ, Magder LS, et al. A seroepidemiologic survey of the prevalence of herpes simplex virus type 2 infection in the United States. N Engl J Med 1989; 321:7.

Kerlering K, Gardella C, Selka S, Krantz E, Corey L, Wald A. Isolation of herpes simplex virus from the genital tract during symtomatic recurrence on the buttock. Obstet Gynecol 2006; 108:947.

Koelle DM, Benedetti J, Langenberg A, Corey L. Asymptomatic reactivation of herpes simplex virus in women after the first episode of genital herpes. Ann Intern Med 1992; 116:433.

Kulhanjian JA, Soroush V, Au DS, et al. Identification of women at unsuspected risk of primary infection with herpes simplex virus type 2 during pregnancy. N Engl J Med 1992; 326:916.

Major C, Towers C, Lewis D, Asrat T. Expectant management of patients with both preterm premature rupture of membranes and genital herpes. Am J Obstet Gynecol 1991; 164:248.

Prober C, Hensleigh P, Boucher F, et al. Use of routine viral cultures at delivery to identify neonates exposed to herpes simplex virus. N Engl J Med 1988; 318:887.

Prober CG, Sullender WM, Yasukawa LL, et al. Low risk of herpes simplex virus infections in neonates exposed to the virus at the time of vaginal delivery to mothers with recurrent genital herpes simplex virus infections. N Engl J Med 1987; 316:240.

Scott LL, Sanchez PJ, Jackson GJ, et al. Acyclovir suppression to prevent cesarean delivery after first-episode genital herpes. Obstet Gynecol 1996; 87:69.

Wald A, Zeh J, Selke S, Ashley RL, Corey L. Virologic characteristics of subclinical and symptomatic genital herpes infections. N Engl J Med 1995; 333:771.

Wittek AE, Yaeger AS, Au DS, Hensleigh PA. Asymptomatic shedding of herpes simplex virus from cervix and lesion site during pregnancy. Am J Dis Child 1984; 138:439.

Woods GL. Update on laboratory diagnosis of sexually transmitted diseases. Clin Labs Med 1995; 15:665.

Disseminated Maternal Herpetic Infection and Pregnancy

Anderson JM, Nicholls NWN. Herpes encephalitis in pregnancy. Br Med J 1972; 1:632.

Chatelan S, Neumann DE, Alexander SM. Fatal herpetic hepatitis in pregnancy. Obstet Gynecol 1994; 1:236.

Fiewett TH, Parker RGB, Philip WM. Acute hepatitis due to herpes simplex virus in an adult. J Clin Pathol 1969; 22:60.

Frederick DM, Bland D, Gollin Y. Fatal disseminated herpes simplex virus infection in a previously healthy pregnant woman: a case report. J Reprod Med 2002; 47:5911.

Gozette RE, Donowho EM, Hieper LR, Plunrett GD. Fulminant herpes virus hominis hepatitis during pregnancy. Obstet Gynecol 1974; 43:191.

Goyert GL, Bottoms SF, Sokol FJ. Anicteric presentation of fatal herpetic hepatitis in pregnancy. Obstet Gynecol 1985; 65:585.

Grover L, Kane J, Kravitz J, et al. Systemic acyclovir in pregnancy: a case report. Obstet Gynecol 1985; 65:284.

Hensleigh PA, Glover DB, Cannon M. Systemic herpes virus hominis in pregnancy. J Reprod Med 1979; 22:171.

Hillard P, Seeds J, Cefalo R. Disseminated herpes simplex in pregnancy: two cases and a review. Obstet Gynecol Surv 1982; 37:449.

Jewett JF. Committee on maternal welfare: herpes simplex encephalitis. N Engl J Med 1975; 292:531.

Klein NA, Mabie WC, Shaver DC, Latham PS, et al. Herpes simplex virus hepatitis. Gastroenterology 1991; 100:239.

Kobberman T, Clark L, Griffin WT. Maternal death secondary to disseminated herpesvirus hominis. Am J Obstet Gynecol 1980; 137:742.

Lagrew DC, Furlow TG, Hager D, et al. Disseminated herpes simplex virus infection in pregnancy: successful treatment with acyclovir. J Am Med Assoc 1984; 252:2058.

Peacock JE, Sarubbi FA. Disseminated herpes simplex virus infection during pregnancy. Obstet Gynecol 1983; 61(suppl 3):13s.

Wertheim RA, Brooks BJ, Rodriguez FH, et al. Fatal herpetic hepatitis in pregnancy. Obstet Gynecol 1983; 62(suppl 3):38s.

Young EJ, Allen PK, Grune JF. Disseminated herpesvirus infection-association with primary genital herpes in pregnancy. J Am Med Assoc 1976; 235:2731.

Congenital Herpesvirus

Altshuler G. Pathogenesis of congenital herpesvirus infection: case report including a description of the placenta. Dis Child 1984; 127:427.

Chalhub EG, Baenziger J, Feigen RD, et al. Congenital herpes simplex type II infection with extensive hepatic calcification, bone lesions and cataracts: complete postmortem. Develop Med Child Neurol 1977; 19:527.

Fagnant RJ, Monif GRG. How rare is congenital herpes simplex: a literature review. J Reprod Med 1989; 34; 6:417.

Florman AL, Gershon AA, Blackett PR. Intrauterine infection with herpes simplex virus: resultant congenital malformations. J Am Med Assoc 1973; 275:129.

Gagnon RA. Transplacental inoculation of fatal herpes simplex in the newborn: report of two cases. Obstet Gynecol 1968; 31:682.

Hain J, Doshi N, Harger JH. Ascending transcervical herpes simplex infection with intact fetal membranes. Obstet Gynecol 1980; 56:106.

Hutchison DS, Smith RE, Haughton PB. Congenital herpetic keratitis. Arch Ophthalmol 1975; 93:70.

Monif GR, Kellner KR, Donnelly WH Jr. Congenital infection due to herpes simplex type II virus. Am J Obstet Gynecol 1985; 152:1000.

Nahmias AJ, Alford CA, Korones SB. Infection of the newborn with Herpesvirus hominis. Adv Pediatr 1970; 17:185.

Pettay O. Intrauterine and perinatal viral infections: a review of experiences and remaining problems. Ann Clin Res 1979; 11:258.

Schaffer AJ, Avery ME. Diseases for the Newborn. 3rd ed. Philadelphia: WB Saunders Co, 1971:656.

Sieber OE Jr, Fulginiti VA, Brazie J, et al. In utero infection of the fetus by herpes simplex virus. Pediatrics 1966; 69:30.

South MA, Tompkins WAF, Morris CR, et al. Congenital malformation of the central nervous system associated with genital type (type 2) herpesvirus. J Pediatr 1969; 75:13.

Strawn EY, Scrimenti RJ. Intrauterine herpes simplex infection. Obstet Gynecol 1971; 5:581.

Von Herzen JL, Benirschke K. Unexpected disseminated herpes simplex infection in a newborn. Obstet Gynecol 1977; 50:728.

Witzleben CL, Driscoll SG. Possible transplacental transmission of herpes simplex infection. Pediatrics 1965; 36:192.

Neonatal Herpetic Infection

Amann St, Fagnart RJ, Chartrand SA, Monif GRG. Herpes simplex infection with short-term use of a fetal scalp electrode. J Reprod Med 1992; 37:372.

Monif GRG. Viral Infections of the Human Fetus. New York: Macmillan, 1969.

Nahmias AJ, Josep WE, Naib ZM, Freeman MG, et al. Perinatal risk associated with maternal genital herpes simplex infection. Am J Obstet Gynecol 1971; 110:825.

Nahmias AJ, Keyserling HH, Kerrick G. Herpes simplex. In: Remington JS, Klein JO, eds. Infectious Diseases of the Fetus and Newborn Infant. 2nd ed. Philadelphia: WB Saunders, 1983:156.

Sieber OF Jr, Fulginiti VA, Brazie J, Umlauf HJ Jr. In utero infection of the fetus by herpes simplex virus. J Pediatr 1966; 69:30.

Stone K, Brooks C, Guinana M, Alexander E. National surveillance for neonatal herpes simplex virus infections. Sex Transm Dis 1989; 16:152.

Whitley RJ, Hutto C. Neonatal herpes simplex virus infections. Pediatr Rev 1985; 7:119.

Whitley RJ, Nahmias AJ. Therapeutic challenges of neonatal herpes simplex infection. Scand J Infect Dis 1985; (suppl)47:97.

Whitley R, Arvin A, Prober C, et al. Predictors of morbidity and mortality in neonates with herpes simplex infection. N Engl J Med 1991; 324:450.

Whitley R, Corey L, Arvin A, et al. Changing presentation of herpes simplex virus infection in neonates. J Infect Dis 1988; 158:109.

Nosocomial Herpes

Adams G, Purohit DM, Bada HS, Andrews BR. Neonatal infection by herpes virus hominus type 2: a complication of intra-partum fetal monitoring. Pediatr Res 1975; 9:337.

Augenbraun M, Feldman J, Chirgwin K, et al. Increased genital shedding of herpes simplex type 2 in HIV-seropostive women. Ann Intern Med 1995; 123:845.

Douglas JM, Schmidt O, Corey L. Acquisition of neonatal HSV-1 infection from a paternal source contact. J Pediatr 1983; 103:908.

Dunkle LM, Schmidt RR, O'Connor DM. Neonatal herpes simplex infection possibly acquired via maternal breast milk. Pediatrics 1979; 63:250.

Francis DP, Hermann KL, MacMahon JR, et al. Nosocomial and maternally acquired herpesvirus hominis infections: a report of four cases of neonates. Am J Dis Child 1975; 129:889.

Gardella C, Browm ZA, Wald A, Morrow RA, Selke S, Krantz E, Corey L. Poor correlation between genital lesions and detection of herpes simplex virus in women in labor. Obstet Gynecol 2005; 106:869.

Golden SM, Merenstein GB, Todd WA, Hill JM. Disseminated herpes simplex neonatorum: a complication of fetal monitoring. Am J Obstet Gynecol 1977; 129:917.

Goldkrand JW. Intrapartum inoculation of herpes simplex virus by fetal scalp electrode. Obstet Gynecol 1982; 59:163.

Hammerberg O, Watts J, Chernesky M, et al. An outbreak of herpes simplex virus type 1 in an intensive care nursery. Pediatr Infect Dis 1983; 2:290.

Kilbrick S. Herpes simplex virus in breast milk. Pediatrics 1979; 64:290.

Light IJ. Postnatal acquisition of herpes simplex virus by the newborn infant: a review of the literature. Pediatrics 1979; 63:480.

Pannuti CS, Finck MCDS, Grimbaum RS, et al. Asymptomatic perinatal shedding of herpes simplex virus type 2 in patients with acquired immunodeficiency syndrome. Arch Dermatol 1977; 133:180.

Quinn PT, Lofberg JV. Maternal herpetic breast infection: another hazard of neonatal herpes simplex. Med J Aust 1978; 21:411.

Therapy

Baker DA. Valacyclovir in the treatment of genital herpes and herpes zoster. Expert Opin Pharmacother 2002; 3:51.

Baker DA, Blythe JG, Miller JM. Once daily valacyclovir for suppression of recurrent genital herpes. Obstet Gynecol 1999; 94:103.

Centers for Disease Control. Pregnancy outcomes following systemic acyclovir exposure. June 1, 1984–June 30, 1993. Morb Mortal Wkly Rep 1993; 42:806.

Dracker JL, Miller JM, and The International Valacyclovir Study Group. Once-daily valacyclovir sustains the suppressive efficacy and safety record of acyclovir in recurrent genital herpes. Proceedings of the First European Congress of Chemotherapy (Abstract). Glasgow, UK. 1996.

Fife KH, Crumpacker CS, Mertz GJ, et al. and the Acyclovir Study Group. Recurrence and resistance patterns of herpes simplex virus following cessation of >6 years of chronic suppression with acyclovir. J Infect Dis 1994; 169:1338.

Goldberg LK, Kaufinan R, Kurtz TO, et al. Long-term suppression of recurrent genital herpes with acyclovir. Arch Dermatol 1993; 129:582.

Lavoie SL, Kaplowitz LG. Management of genital herpes infections. Sem Dermatol 1994; 13:248–255.

Patel R, Crooks JR, Bell AR, and the International Valacyclovir Study Group. Once-daily valacyclovir for the suppression of recurrent genital herpes—the first placebo controlled clinical trial. Presented at the First European Congress of Chemotherapy. Glasow, UK. 1996.

Sarag P, Chastong C, Bertin L, et al. Efficacy and safety equivalence of 1000 mg once-daily and 500 mg twice daily valaciclovir in recurrent genital herpes. Proceedings of the 36th ICAAC, New Orleans. ASM. 1996; Abstract HI 13.

Scott LL, Sanchez PJ, Jackson GL, et al. Acyclovir suppression to prevent cesarean delivery after first episode genital herpes. Obstet Gynecol 1996; 87:69.

Sheffield JS, Fish DN, Hollier LM, et al. Acxyclovir concentration in human breast milk after valvacyclovir administration. Am J Obstet Gynecol 2002; 186:100.

Sheffield JS, Hill JB, Hollier LM, et al. Valacyclovir prophylaxis to prevent recurrent herpes at delivery. Obstet Gynecol 2006; 108:141.

Tyring SK, Baker D, Snowden W. Valacyclovir for herpes virus infection: long term safety and sustained efficacy after 20 years' experience with acyclovir. J Infect Dis 2002; 186 (suppl. 1):40s.

Wald A. New therapies and prevention strategies for genital herpes. Clin Infect Dis 1999; 28 (suppl 1):4.

Wald A, Zeh J, Barnum G, et al. Suppression of subclinical shedding of herpes simplex virus type 2 with acyclovir. Ann Intern Med 1996; 124(1, pt 1):8–15.

Human Immunodeficiency Virus

David J. Garry

14

INTRODUCTION

The acquired immune deficiency syndrome (AIDS) epidemic was discovered in 1981, when the U.S. Centers for Disease Control and Prevention (CDC) reported a cluster of *Pneumocystis carinii* pneumonia in five homosexual men in Los Angeles. In 1983, scientists led by Luc Montagnier at the Pasteur Institute in France first discovered the virus that causes AIDS and named it "lymphadenopathy-associated virus" (LAV). Gallo and colleagues in the United States confirmed the virus and renamed it "human T lymphotropic virus type-III" (HTLV-III). In 1986, the new term "human immunodeficiency virus" (HIV) was adopted. HIV is classified in the genus *Lentivirus*, part of the family of Retroviridae. Lentiviruses are transmitted as single-stranded, positive-sense, enveloped RNA viruses. They enter the target cell, and the viral RNA genome is converted to double-stranded DNA by a virally encoded reverse transcriptase. Then the viral DNA is integrated into the cellular DNA by a virally encoded integrase so that the genome can be transcribed. Once the virus has infected the cell, there are two possible pathways: either the virus becomes latent with the infected cell continuing to function, or the virus is activated and replicates.

Two species of HIV can infect humans: HIV-1 and HIV-2. HIV-1 probably originated in southern Cameroon after jumping from wild chimpanzees (*Pan troglodytes troglodytes*) to humans during the 20th century. HIV-2 most probably originated from the Sooty Mangabey (*Cercocebus atys*), an Old World monkey of Guinea-Bissau, Gabon, and Cameroon. HIV-1 is the most virulent, is the easiest transmitted, and is the cause of the majority of HIV infections globally. The earliest known instance of HIV-1 infection in humans is a plasma sample taken in 1959 from an adult male living in what is now the Democratic Republic of Congo. HIV-2 is less transmittable and is largely confined to West Africa. Although a variety of theories exist elucidating the transfer of HIV to humans, no single hypothesis is accepted and the topic remains controversial.

TRANSMISSION

The methods of transmission of HIV can be summarized into the following three methods: (*i*) sexual, (*ii*) blood and blood products, and (*iii*) maternal-to-child transmission (MTCT). Although HIV virus can be detected in minimal amounts in saliva, tears, urine, and other bodily fluids, the risks of transmission are negligible. Although per-act transmission risk from unprotected exposure to a partner known to be HIV positive is relatively low for various types of

exposure, different nonoccupational exposures are associated with distinctive levels of risk (Table 1).

The CDC estimates that 70% of the 11,442 AIDS cases diagnosed among female adults and adolescents in 2004 were attributed to high-risk heterosexual contact: 12% of these cases are from heterosexual contact with an injection-drug user and 58% from sexual contact with high-risk partners such as bisexual men or HIV-infected men with unidentified risk factors. Of the cases in female adults and adolescents, 28% were attributed to injection-drug use and 2% to other or unidentified risk factors. The virus appears to concentrate in the seminal fluid, particularly in situations where there are increased numbers of lymphocytes and monocytes in the fluid, as in genital inflammatory conditions such as urethritis or epididymitis. The virus has also been demonstrated in cervical smears and vaginal fluid. There is a strong association of transmission of HIV with receptive anal intercourse, probably due to a thin, fragile rectal mucosal membrane and microtrauma associated with anal intercourse. Sexual practices that overtly traumatize the rectal mucosa will increase the likelihood of infection. Although the vaginal mucosa is several layers thicker than the rectal mucosa and less likely to be traumatized during intercourse, it is clear that the virus can be transmitted to either partner

TABLE I Estimated at risk for acquiring HIV by exposure without condom usage

Exposure route	Risk per 10,000 exposures	Reference
Blood transfusion	9000	Donegan et al. (1990)
Maternal–child transmission	2500	Coovadia (2004)
Needle-sharing/ IV drug use	67	Kaplan and Heimer (1995)
Receptive anal intercourse	50	European Study Group (1992) and Varghese et al. (2002)
Insertive anal intercourse	6.5	European Study Group (1992) and Varghese et al. (2002)
Receptive vaginal intercourse	10	European Study Group (1992), Varghese et al. (2002), and Leynaert et al. (1998)
Insertive vaginal intercourse	5	European Study Group (1992) and Varghese et al. (2002)
Receptive oral sex	1	Varghese et al. (2002)
Insertive oral sex	0.5	Varghese et al. (2002)
Percutaneous needle stick	30	Bell (1997)

Source: Adapted from Smith et al. (2005).

through vaginal intercourse. In women with genital ulcers, secondary to sexually transmitted diseases (STDs), and menstruating women having unprotected intercourse, there is an increase in transmission of the virus. Gonorrhea, *Chlamydia*, and trichomoniasis have been identified as risk factors for the enhancement of HIV transmission in women.

An estimated 700,000 healthcare workers are stuck with needles or other sharp instruments in the United States annually, and there is a small occupational risk of HIV transmission to healthcare workers and laboratory personnel. Large studies have shown that the risk of HIV transmission following skin puncture from a needle or a sharp object that was contaminated with blood from a documented HIV-positive person is approximately 0.3%, and after a mucous membrane exposure, it is 0.09%. Transmission of HIV through intact skin has not been documented. The risks for HIV infection following percutaneous exposures to HIV-infected blood are inversely associated with the amount/quantity of blood involved. A large quantity of blood, as in an appliance visibly contaminated with the patient's blood, a procedure that involves a needle placed directly in a vein or artery, or a deep penetrating injury, is more likely to result in transmission of the virus. In addition, the risk increases for exposures to blood from patients with advanced-stage disease, probably owing to the higher viral load of HIV in the blood and the presence of a more virulent strain of virus. The use of antiretroviral drugs such as postexposure prophylaxis (PEP) decreases the risk of infection compared to historic controls in occupationally exposed healthcare workers (Fig. 1).

Three modes of MTCT are possible: (*i*) in utero, (*ii*) intrapartum, during labor and delivery, and (*iii*) postpartum, primarily due to breast-feeding. Prior to antiretroviral therapy, the MTCT rates were 14% to 25% in industrialized areas and 25% to 40% in developing countries. These differences may be related to the adequacy of prenatal care, severity of HIV disease, or to the general health of the mother. The factor most closely associated with higher rates of transmission is the presence of high maternal viral load. Other potential factors associated with higher MTCT are low maternal CD4+ T-cell lymphocyte counts, prolonged interval between membrane rupture and delivery, presence of chorioamnionitis at delivery, STDs during pregnancy, drug use during pregnancy, preterm delivery, and certain obstetric procedures (amniocentesis, amnioscopy, and fetal scalp electrodes). In one report of 552 singleton gestations in the United States, the rate of MTCT was 0% among women with <1000/mL copies of HIV RNA, 16.6% among women with 1000 to 10,000/mL, 21.3% among women with 10,001 to 50,000/mL, 30.9% among women with 50,001 to 100,000/mL, and 40.6% among women with >100,000/mL.

Breast-feeding is an important mode of transmission of HIV infection in resource-poor countries. The risk factors for MTCT of HIV via breast-feeding are not completely understood, and the factors that increase the likelihood of transmission include detectable levels of HIV in breast milk, mastitis, a low maternal CD4+ count, and maternal vitamin A deficiency. The risk of MTCT through breast-feeding is highest in the early months, and interestingly, exclusive breast-feeding has been reported to have a lower risk of HIV transmission than mixed feeding. In developed countries, where formula is readily available, breast-feeding should be avoided. In countries where breast milk is the only source of nutrition or culture dictates breast-feeding, there have been several approaches using antiretroviral therapies to reduce transmission. Intermittent administration of nevirapine, which has a relatively long half-life, to uninfected babies breast-feeding from infected mothers has been shown to decrease the incidence of MTCT.

DIAGNOSIS

The standard screening test for HIV infection is an enzyme-linked immunosorbent assay (ELISA) or an enzyme immunoassay (EIA). This screening test has a sensitivity of >99.5% in detecting antigens from both HIV-1 and HIV-2. These EIAs are extremely sensitive but not optimal with regard to specificity. In low-risk individuals, only 10% of EIA-positives are subsequently confirmed to have HIV infection. Factors associated with the false-positive EIA tests are antibodies to class II antigens, autoantibodies, hepatic disease, recent influenza vaccination, and acute viral infections. Thus, anyone having a positive or inconclusive EIA result must have the result confirmed with a more specific assay, the confirmatory western blot test. The western blot utilizes multiple HIV antigens of different, well-characterized molecular weights that can be separated and detected as discrete bands. A negative western blot is one in which no bands are present at molecular weights corresponding to HIV gene products. A western blot demonstrating antibodies to the major gene products of HIV (*gag*, *pol*, and *env*) is conclusive evidence of HIV infection. Western blot patterns that do not fall into the positive or negative categories are considered "indeterminate." There are two possible explanations for an indeterminate western blot result. The most likely explanation is that the patient being tested has antibodies that cross-react with one of the proteins of HIV. The most common cross-reactivity patterns are antibodies that react with p24 or p55. Another, less likely explanation is that the patient is infected with HIV and is early in the process of mounting a classic antibody response. Any "indeterminate" western blot should be repeated in four to six weeks. Although the western blot is an excellent confirmatory test for HIV infection, it is an inadequate screening test.

When screening for HIV infection, the appropriate initial test is the EIA. If the initial result is negative, unless there is strong reason to suspect early HIV infection, the diagnosis is ruled out and retesting should be performed only as indicated. If the EIA is indeterminate or positive, the test should be repeated. If the repeat test is negative on two occasions, then that initial positive reading was most likely secondary to a technical error and the patient is HIV negative. If the repeat is indeterminate or positive, then proceed to the western blot testing.

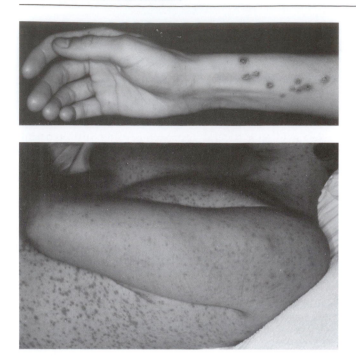

FIGURE I Kaposi's sarcoma with extensive involvement of extremities and trunk.

SCREENING

The CDC currently recommends diagnostic HIV testing with opt-out HIV screening as a part of routine clinical care in all healthcare settings while preserving the patient's option to decline HIV testing. Opt-out testing for HIV is explaining to the patient that an HIV test will be included in the standard battery of tests (e.g., prenatal tests performed on all pregnant women), and that she may refuse the HIV test or "opt-out." The CDC recommendations are intended for providers in all healthcare settings, including hospital emergency departments, inpatient services, urgent-care clinics, outpatient STD clinics, tuberculosis (TB) clinics, substance-abuse treatment clinics, community clinics, correctional healthcare facilities, and primary care settings. The guidelines do not modify the existing guidelines concerning HIV counseling, testing, and referral for persons at high risk for HIV who seek or receive HIV testing in nonclinical settings (e.g., community-based organizations, outreach settings, or mobile vans).

2006 CDC RECOMMENDATIONS: SCREENING FOR HIV INFECTION

Universal

- Screening HIV infection should be performed routinely in all healthcare settings in patients aged 13 to 64 years.
- Healthcare providers should initiate screening unless prevalence of undiagnosed HIV infection in their patients has been documented to be <0.1%. In the absence of existing data for HIV prevalence, healthcare providers should initiate voluntary HIV screening until they establish that the diagnostic yield is <1/1000

patients screened, at which point such screening is no longer warranted.

- All patients initiating treatment for TB should be screened routinely for HIV infection.
- All patients seeking treatment for STDs should be screened routinely for HIV during each visit for a new complaint, regardless of whether the patient is known or suspected to have specific behavior risks for HIV infection.
- Healthcare providers should subsequently test all persons likely to be at high risk for HIV at least annually. Persons likely to be at high risk include injection-drug users and their sex partners, persons who exchange sex for money or drugs, sex partners of HIV-infected persons, and men who have sex with men or heterosexual persons who themselves or whose sex partners have had more than one sex partner since their most recent HIV test.
- Healthcare providers should encourage patients and their prospective sex partners to be tested before initiating a new sexual relationship.
- Repeat screening of persons not likely high risk for HIV should be performed on the basis of clinical judgment.
- Unless recent HIV test results are immediately available, any person whose blood or body fluid is the source of an occupational exposure for a healthcare provider should be informed of the incident and tested for HIV infection at the time the exposure occurs.

Consent and Pretest Information

- Screening should be voluntary and undertaken only with the patient's knowledge and understanding that HIV testing is planned.
- Patients should be informed orally or in writing that HIV testing will be performed unless they decline (opt-out screening). Oral or written information should include an explanation of HIV infection and the meanings of positive and negative test results, and the patient should be offered an opportunity to ask questions and to decline testing. With such notification, consent for HIV screening should be incorporated into the patient's general informed consent for medical care on the same basis as are other screening or diagnostic tests; a separate consent form for HIV testing is not recommended.
- Easily understood informational materials should be made available in the languages of the commonly encountered populations within the service area. The competence of interpreters and bilingual staff to provide language assistance to patients with limited English proficiency must be ensured.
- If a patient declines an HIV test, this decision should be documented in the medical record.

Diagnostic Testing for HIV Infection

- All patients with signs or symptoms consistent with HIV infection or an opportunistic illness characteristic of AIDS should be tested for HIV.
- Clinicians should maintain a high level of suspicion for acute HIV infection in all patients with a compatible

clinical syndrome and who report recent high-risk behavior. When acute retroviral syndrome is a possibility, a plasma RNA test should be used in conjunction with an HIV antibody test to diagnose acute HIV infection.

- Patients or persons responsible for the patient's care should be notified orally that testing is planned, advised of the indication for testing and the implications of positive and negative test results, and offered an opportunity to ask questions and to decline testing. With such notification, the patient's general consent for medical care is considered sufficient for diagnostic HIV testing.

Pregnant Women

- HIV screening should be included in the routine panel of prenatal screening tests for all pregnant women.
- HIV screening is recommended after the patient is notified that testing will be performed unless the patient declines (opt-out screening).
- Separate written consent for HIV testing should not be required; general consent for medical care should be considered sufficient for HIV testing.
- Repeat screening in the third trimester is recommended in jurisdictions with elevated rates of HIV infection among pregnant women (with at least one diagnosed HIV case per 1000 pregnant women per year).

THE INCUBATION PERIOD

Seroconversion for antibodies to HIV usually occurs within three to six weeks following infection. In isolated instances, the appearance of a specific antibody does not appear until months later. The viral subtypes appear to be one of the variables influencing the time interval prior to antibody production. The onset of symptoms following infection with the HIV-1 virus (and presumably HIV-2) is thought to range from six months to ten or more years.

SYMPTOMS

Many manifestations of HIV infection are similar in both men and women. Infection with HIV may have nonspecific symptoms even early in disease, including low-grade fevers, night sweats, fatigue, and weight loss. Other conditions, however, occur in different frequencies in men and women. HIV-infected men are at an eightfold increased risk than HIV-infected women to develop Kaposi's sarcoma. In some studies, women had higher rates of herpes simplex infections than men. Data from several studies conducted by the Community Programs for Clinical Research on AIDS (CPCRA) have described HIV-infected women to be more likely than HIV-infected men to develop bacterial pneumonia.

Women also experience HIV-associated gynecologic problems, many of which occur in uninfected women but with less frequency or severity. Vaginal candidiasis, common and easily treated in most women, is often persistent and difficult to treat in HIV-infected women. Other

vaginal infections may occur more frequently and with greater severity in HIV-infected women, including bacterial vaginosis, gonorrhea, chlamydia, and trichomoniasis. Severe herpes simplex virus (HSV) ulcerations, which are sometimes unresponsive to therapy, can severely compromise a woman's quality of life. Idiopathic genital ulcers, with no evidence of an infectious organism or cancerous cells in the lesion, are a unique manifestation of HIV infection. These ulcers, for which there is no proven treatment, are sometimes confused with those caused by HSV. Human papillomavirus infection, the etiology of cervical dysplasia and cervical cancer, occurs more frequently in HIV-infected women. Pelvic inflammatory disease (PID) appears to be more common and more aggressive in HIV-infected women compared to uninfected women. Menstrual irregularities have been described as similar when comparing HIV-infected women and at-risk HIV negative women; however, women with CD4+ T-cell counts <50/mm^3 of blood were more likely to report amenorrhea than uninfected women or HIV-infected women with higher CD4+ T-cell counts.

The CDC categorization of HIV is based on the lowest documented CD4 cell count and on previously diagnosed HIV-related conditions (Table 2). The CDC divides HIV infection into clinical categories that are defined as follows:

Category A consists of one or more of the conditions described below in an adolescent or adult (≥13 years) with documented HIV infection. The conditions listed in Categories B and C must not have occurred.

- Asymptomatic HIV infection
- Persistent generalized lymphadenopathy
- Acute (primary) HIV infection with accompanying illness or history of acute HIV infection

Category B consists of symptomatic conditions in an HIV-infected adolescent or adult that are not included among conditions listed in clinical Category C and that meet at least one of the following: (i) the conditions are attributed to HIV infection or are indicative of a defect in cell-mediated immunity; (ii) the conditions are considered by physicians to have a clinical course or to require management that is complicated by HIV infection. Some examples of conditions

TABLE 2 CDC classification system for HIV-infected adults and adolescents

CD4 cell categories	Clinical categories		
	A: (asymptomatic, acute HIV, or PGL)	B: (symptomatic conditions)	C: (AIDS indicator conditions)
1 (≥500 cells/µL)	A1	B1	C1
2 (200–499 cells/µL)	A2	B2	C2
3 (<200 cells/µL)	A3	B3	C3

Abbreviations: CDC, Centers for Disease Control and Prevention; PGL, persistent generalized lymphadenopathy.
Source: Adapted from CDC (1992).

in clinical Category B include, but are not limited to, the following:

- Bacillary angiomatosis
- Candidiasis, oropharyngeal (thrush)
- Candidiasis, vulvovaginal; persistent, frequent, or poorly responsive to therapy
- Cervical dysplasia (moderate or severe)/cervical carcinoma in situ
- Constitutional symptoms, such as fever (38.5°C) or diarrhea lasting greater than one month
- Hairy leukoplakia, oral
- Herpes zoster (shingles), involving two or more distinct episodes or more than one dermatome
- Idiopathic thrombocytopenic purpura
- Listeriosis
- PID, particularly if complicated by tubo-ovarian abscess
- Peripheral neuropathy

Category C includes the clinical conditions listed in the AIDS surveillance case definition. In this classification, once a Category C condition has occurred, the person will remain in Category C:

- Candidiasis of bronchi, trachea, esophagus or lungs
- Cervical cancer (invasive)
- Coccidioidomycosis, disseminated or extrapulmonary
- Cryptococcosis, extrapulmonary
- Cryptosporidiosis, chronic intestinal (greater than one month's duration)
- Cytomegalovirus disease (other than liver, spleen, or nodes)
- Cytomegalovirus retinitis (with loss of vision)
- Encephalopathy, HIV related
- Herpes simplex: chronic ulcer(s) (more than one month's duration); or bronchitis, pneumonitis, or esophagitis
- Histoplasmosis, disseminated or extrapulmonary
- Isosporiasis, chronic intestinal (more than one month's duration)
- Kaposi's sarcoma
- Lymphoma, Burkitt's (or equivalent term)
- Lymphoma, immunoblastic (or equivalent term)
- Lymphoma, primary, of brain
- Mycobacterium avium complex or *M. kansasii*, disseminated or extrapulmonary
- *Mycobacterium tuberculosis*, any site (pulmonary or extrapulmonary)
- *Mycobacterium*, other species, disseminated or extrapulmonary
- *P. carinii* pneumonia
- Pneumonia, recurrent
- Progressive multifocal leukoencephalopathy
- Salmonella septicemia, recurrent
- Toxoplasmosis of brain
- Wasting syndrome due to HIV

If a patient had a condition that once met the criteria for Category B but now is asymptomatic, the patient would remain in Category B. Additionally, categorization is based on specific conditions, as indicated in Table 2. Patients who met the definition of categories A3, B3, and C1 through C3 are considered to have AIDS.

DISEASE PROGRESSION

The immunologic hallmark of progressive HIV disease is the decline in the CD4+ lymphocyte count. Clinical manifestations are closely related to the CD4+ T-lymphocyte count which in otherwise healthy individuals declines at a rate of approximately $75/\mu L$ per year. In general, HIV-infected individuals do not manifest immune deficiency complications when the CD4+ lymphocyte count is $500/\mu L$ or above and rarely when the counts are above $350/\mu L$. As counts decline below $350/\mu L$, symptoms such as oral or recurrent vaginal candidiasis, weight loss, herpes zoster, diarrhea, unexplained prolonged fevers, seborrhea dermatitis, and the risk for other opportunistic infections increases. Bacterial infections such as pneumonia and listeriosis occur both early and late in the progression of induced immune deficiency. *Streptococcus pneumoniae* and *Hemophilus influenzae* are the most commonly identified pathogens. The risk of full blown disease and death occurs at CD4+ T-cell counts of 100 to $150/\mu L$.

Prior to 1996, HIV-infected individuals would develop AIDS within 10 years after becoming infected. This time varied greatly from person to person and depended on many factors, including a person's health status and health-related behaviors. Since 1996, the introduction of improved antiretroviral therapies has dramatically expanded the time between HIV infection and the development of AIDS. In addition to retroviral therapies, alterations in sexual behavior practices, complementary alternative medication usage, media attention, and many other changes have occurred that have changed HIV infection into a chronic disease state.

A vaccine, either for treatment or for prevention of transmission, is the ideal way to contain and even eradicate the HIV epidemic. However, it is not possible to use a "live" attenuated retroviral vaccine in humans due to safety reasons. In preliminary, experimental vaccine data, the results are disappointing, and there are potential hazards with "killed" whole virus used in the vaccine. An effective vaccine needs to stimulate both systemic and mucosal immunity and there are many difficulties in performing a Phase III trial using volunteers. Due to the HIV virus' capacity to integrate its genetic information into the DNA of target cells quickly, a vaccine response must be quick and effective in preventing HIV entry (by inducing production of neutralizing antibodies) and potent in finding and killing infected cells (by inducing activation of killer T-cells). First attempts at developing a vaccine from 1984 to 1990 used unmodified forms of the HIV protein envelope gp120 with the goal of introducing neutralizing antibodies that could block virus entry, thereby possibly achieving complete protection from infection. This approach failed in animal model (monkey) tests because the neutralizing antibodies are short lived and unable to block infection by a broad range of HIV strains. The emphasis then switched to inducing T-cell–mediated immunity, involving production of killer T-cells. Trials in infected monkeys did not produce complete protection but kept virus at low levels for more than one year. There are two arguments in favor of this approach. First, successful vaccines do not necessarily have to achieve complete protection; for example, in vaccinated individuals exposed to poliovirus, the virus replicates in the gut before the recall immune response targets the virus. Second, some argue that with HIV, there is no other choice because we cannot achieve broadly reactive, enduring neutralizing antibodies. In addition, there have been some reports of broadly reactive neutralizing antibodies raised against primary isolates of HIV and of new candidate vaccines that achieve this goal. Therapeutic vaccines would be designed and tested in HIV-infected persons as therapeutic supplements after initial antiretroviral therapy. The outcome of the vaccine therapeutically would be a lack of viral rebound after interruption of drug therapy. Also, on another front of therapeutic modalities, there have been encouraging data with candidate microbicidal agents such as the cyclodextrins, which block infection when delivered at portals of entry.

RESISTANCE AND RESISTANCE TESTING

The reported prevalence of antiretroviral drug resistance varies depending on several factors, including characteristics of the population studied, prior and current exposure to antiretroviral drugs and type of regimen (highly active vs. non-highly active antiretroviral therapy), geographic area, and type of resistance assay used (genotypic vs. phenotypic). Genotypic resistance investigations from the United States and Europe of newly infected, naïve persons demonstrate rates of primary resistance mutations to be as high as 23% and increasing over time. The presence of high-level phenotypic resistance has increased from 3.4% in 1995–1998 to 12.4% in 1999–2000 in a retrospective analysis from 10 U.S. cities. These phenotypic resistance changes have been associated with longer time to viral suppression and shorter time to virologic failure.

In newly diagnosed HIV infection (drug-naïve persons) of unknown duration, antiretroviral drug resistance has been reported to range from 8.3% to 10.8%. The highest rates of antiretroviral drug resistance are in antiretroviral treatment-experienced individuals, with resistance rates as high as 88% reported in viremic individuals currently receiving therapy and 30% in individuals with a past history of treatment.

Resistance testing, genotype and phenotype, is recommended for all antiretroviral-naïve pregnant women before initiating treatment or prophylaxis if prior resistance testing has not been performed. Testing should be considered at a preconception visit to allow for optimum selection of an antiretroviral drug regimen to be used during pregnancy. The prevalence of resistance in antiretroviral-naïve patients is increasing and that baseline resistance may be associated with adverse virologic outcomes. For these reasons, baseline HIV resistance testing is now recommended for all patients with established infection, including pregnant women, prior to initiating treatment. Resistance testing is recommended before initiation of therapy or

prophylaxis in pregnant women who received prophylaxis in a previous pregnancy. The identification of baseline resistance mutations may allow selection of more effective and durable antiretroviral regimens; however, there is no evidence that baseline resistance testing in pregnancy is associated with a reduction in MTCT. In women presenting late in the third trimester (>34 weeks), resistance testing can be performed; however, test results may not be back in time to allow effective reduction of viral load before delivery.

There are limited data about the prevalence of antiretroviral drug resistance in pregnant women; however, data suggest that rates of resistance are similar in pregnant women and nonpregnant individuals, with antiretroviral drug resistance being more frequent among antiretroviral-experienced women. There are several features unique to pregnancy that potentially increase the possibility of developing resistant strains of virus. One scenario includes the following: (*i*) antiretrovirals used during pregnancy solely for prophylaxis of MTCT and then discontinued after delivery in women who do not meet requirements for therapy outside of pregnancy; (*ii*) regimens used for prophylaxis include drugs with significant differences in half-life, such as nevirapine combined with two-nucleoside analog drugs; discontinuation of all regimen components simultaneously postpartum may result in functional monotherapy and increase the risk of development of nevirapine resistance; (*iii*) problems such as nausea and vomiting in early pregnancy that may compromise adherence and increase the risk of resistance in women receiving antiretroviral treatment; (*iv*) patient noncompliance with antiretroviral therapy secondary to fears of "harming the baby," which can increase risks of resistance.

In women who have documented zidovudine (ZDV) resistance and whose antepartum regimen does not include ZDV, intravenous ZDV during labor should still be administered. If the woman's antepartum regimen includes stavudine, the stavudine should be stopped during the intrapartum period and restarted after delivery secondary to the antagonistic properties to ZDV. For an infant born to a woman with known a ZDV-resistant virus, most clinicians choose to provide additional antiretroviral agents to the infant in combination with ZDV. Such a decision must be accompanied by a discussion with the woman of the potential risks and benefits. The optimal prophylactic regimen for newborns of women with antiretroviral drug-resistant virus is unknown. The rationale for including ZDV intrapartum and to the infant when a woman is known to have ZDV-resistant virus has been based on several factors. In woman with mixed populations of wild-type virus and virus with low-level ZDV resistance, only wild-type virus has been transmitted to the infant. Efficacy of the pediatric AIDS clinical trial group (PACTG) 076 ZDV regimen appears to be based not only on reduction of HIV levels, but also on pre- and PEP in the infant. ZDV crosses the placenta readily and has one of the highest maternal-to-cord blood ratios among the nucleoside analog agents. Additionally, ZDV has been shown to be metabolized to the active triphosphate within the placenta and may provide additional protection against transmission. ZDV reduces genital HIV-1 RNA levels, and genital viral levels have been correlated with MTCT rates. ZDV also has better penetration into the central nervous system compared to most other nucleoside analogs. Thus intrapartum and neonatal ZDV for reduction of MTCT, even in the presence of known ZDV resistance, should be utilized due to the unique characteristics of ZDV and the evidence in reducing perinatal transmission.

CHEMOPROPHYLAXIS

The following recommendations for use of antiretroviral chemoprophylaxis to reduce the risk for MTCT are based on situations that may be commonly encountered in clinical practice (Table 3). The current standard ZDV dosing regimen for adults is 200 mg thrice daily or 300 mg twice daily. Because the mechanism by which ZDV reduces MTCT is not known, these dosing regimens may not have equivalent efficacy to that observed in PACTG 076. However, a regimen of two to three times daily is expected to increase adherence to the regimen. The recommended ZDV dosage for infants was derived from pharmacokinetic studies performed among full-term infants. ZDV is primarily cleared through hepatic glucuronidation to an inactive metabolite. The glucuronidation metabolic enzyme system is immature in neonates, leading to prolonged ZDV half-life and clearance compared with older infants (ZDV half-life: 3.1 hours vs. 1.9 hours; clearance: 10.9 vs. 19.0 mL/min/kg body weight, respectively).

When initiating treatment, a woman's adherence to therapy is crucial, and secondly, the choice of a first-line therapy should include a consideration of the possible failure of that regimen. Intermittent compliance with antiretroviral therapy can potentially lead to development of resistant virus. Even very brief drug holidays have been associated with the replacement of wild-strain virus with mutant strains that are resistant to therapeutic agents. Therefore, it is critical that healthcare providers educate patients about the need to start treatment and needed adherence to complex therapies. With regard to factoring the possible need for future therapy due to failure of initial therapy, it is useful to choose a regimen that "spares" one class of antiretroviral agent. Thus, a regimen should spare protease inhibitors or nonnucleoside reverse-transcriptase inhibitors or both. In fact, there are therapies that use three nucleoside reverse-transcriptase inhibitors alone. When those therapies are used, the patient is assured that if resistance develops, there are classes of drugs.

Current recommendations for care of HIV-infected pregnant individuals include highly active antiretroviral therapies (HAART), which include a protease inhibitor or protease inhibitors (indinavir, nelfinavir, ritonavir + saquinavir, ritonavir + indinavir, ritonavir + lopinavir) or a nonnucleoside reverse-transcriptase inhibitor (efavirenz in the nonpregnant patient) in combination with one of several two-nucleoside reverse-transcriptase inhibitor combinations. Because the genotypic barrier to resistance is greatest with protease

inhibitors, a protease inhibitor with two-nucleoside reverse-transcriptase inhibitors should be the preferred initial therapy. Abacavir (ABC) with two-nucleoside reverse-transcriptase inhibitors, a triple-nucleoside reverse-transcriptase inhibitors therapy, has been used with success but may have short-lived efficacy when the baseline viral load is >100,000 copies/mL. Certain individuals may have a genetic predisposition to a rash associated with ABC, a rash that can be a harbinger of a fatal reaction. In all circumstances, a rash signals the need to immediately discontinue therapy. Dual therapy with nucleoside reverse-transcriptase inhibitors is less likely to persistently suppress viral loads below detectable levels than HAART's and should be used only if more potent therapies are not possible. Use of antiretroviral agents as monotherapy is contraindicated, except when there are no other options, or, as noted above, in pregnant women with very low viral loads when it is being used solely to reduce MTCT.

Healthcare providers who are treating HIV-1–infected pregnant women and their newborns are advised to report instances of prenatal exposure to antiretroviral drugs (either alone or in combination) to the Antiretroviral Pregnancy Registry. This registry is an epidemiologic project to collect observational, nonexperimental data regarding antiretroviral exposure during pregnancy for the purpose of assessing the potential teratogenicity of these drugs. Registry data have been used to supplement animal toxicology studies and assist clinicians in weighing the potential risks and benefits of treatment for individual patients. Table 4 describes the antiretroviral medications, their categories, and the neonatal-to-maternal concentrations of the medications. Long-term study data regarding carcinogenic possibilities of antiretroviral therapies and potential harm based on animal teratogen studies are presented in Table 4. The Antiretroviral Pregnancy Registry[a] is a collaborative project of pharmaceutical manufacturers with an advisory committee of obstetric and pediatric practitioners. The registry does not use patient names and obtains birth outcomes with follow-up information from the reporting physician.

SPECIFIC ANTIRETROVIRAL-RELATED COMPLICATIONS

Nevirapine

There have been reported increases in hepatic transaminase levels [alanine aminotransferase (ALT) and aspartate aminotransferase (AST)] associated with rash or systemic symptoms, which has been observed during the first 18 weeks of treatment with nevirapine. These toxicities have been reported in patients on chronic therapy, and have not been reported in women or infants receiving single- or two-dose nevirapine for prevention of MTCT. Signs and symptoms of systemic toxicity may be nonspecific, and can include fatigue, malaise, anorexia, nausea, jaundice, liver tenderness, or hepatomegaly, with or without initially abnormal hepatic transaminases. The development of severe nevirapine-associated skin rash has been reported to be five to seven times

TABLE 3 Clinical scenarios and recommendations regarding mode of delivery to reduce MTCT of HIV-1

Clinical scenario	Recommendations
Scenario A HIV-1–infected women presenting in late pregnancy (≥36 wk of gestation), known to be HIV-1 infected but not receiving antiretroviral therapy, and who have HIV-1 RNA level and lymphocyte subsets pending but unlikely to be available before delivery	Therapy options should be discussed in detail. The woman should be started on antiretroviral therapy including at least the PACTG 076 ZDV regimen. The woman should be counseled that scheduled C/S is likely to reduce the risk of transmission to her infant. She should also be informed of the increased risks to her of C/S, including increased rates of postoperative infection, anesthesia risks, and other surgical risks. If C/S is chosen, the procedure should be scheduled at 38 wk of gestation based on the best available clinical information. When scheduled C/S is performed, the woman should receive continuous intravenous ZDV infusion beginning 3 hr before surgery and her infant should receive 6 wk of ZDV therapy after birth. Options for continuing or initiating combination antiretroviral therapy after delivery should be discussed with the woman as soon as her viral load and lymphocyte subset results are available
Scenario B HIV-1–infected women who initiated prenatal care early in the third trimester, are receiving highly active combination antiretroviral therapy, and have an initial virologic response, but have HIV-1 RNA levels that remain substantially over 1000 copies/mL at 36 wk of gestation	The current combination antiretroviral regimen should be continued as the HIV-1 RNA level is dropping appropriately. The woman should be counseled that although she is responding to the antiretroviral therapy, it is unlikely that her HIV-1 RNA level will fall below 1000 copies/mL before delivery. Therefore, scheduled C/S may provide additional benefit in preventing intrapartum transmission of HIV-1. She should also be informed of the increased risks to her of C/S, including increased rates of postoperative infection, anesthesia risks, and surgical risks. If she chooses scheduled C/S, it should be performed at 38 wk of gestation according to the best available dating parameters, and intravenous ZDV should be begun at least 3 hr before surgery. Other antiretroviral medications should be continued on schedule as much as possible before and after surgery. The infant should receive oral ZDV for 6 wk after birth. The importance of adhering to therapy after delivery for her own health should be emphasized
Scenario C HIV-1–infected women on highly active combination antiretroviral therapy with an undetectable HIV-1 RNA level at 36 wk of gestation	The woman should be counseled that her risk of MTCT of HIV-1 with a persistently undetectable HIV-1 RNA level is low, probably 2% or less, even with vaginal delivery. There is currently no information to evaluate whether performing a scheduled C/S will lower her risk further. C/S has an increased risk of complication for the woman compared to vaginal delivery, and these risks must be balanced against the uncertain benefit of C/S in this case
Scenario D HIV-1–infected women who have elected scheduled C/S but present in early labor or shortly after rupture of membranes	Intravenous ZDV should be started immediately since the woman is in labor or has ruptured membranes. If labor is progressing rapidly, the woman should be allowed to deliver vaginally. If cervical dilatation is minimal and a long period of labor is anticipated, some clinicians may choose to administer the loading dose of intravenous ZDV and proceed with C/S to minimize the duration of membrane rupture and avoid vaginal delivery. Others might begin oxytocin augmentation to enhance contractions and potentially expedite delivery. If the woman is allowed to labor, scalp electrodes and other invasive monitoring and operative delivery should be avoided if possible. The infant should be treated with 6 wk of ZDV therapy after birth

Abbreviations: C/S, cesarean section; MTCT, maternal-to-child-transmission; PACTG, pediatric AIDS clinical trial group; ZDV, zidovudine.
Source: Adapted from AIDSinfo (2006).

more common in women than men, and has been reported in pregnant women. Other studies have found that hepatic adverse events with systemic symptoms (predominantly rash) were threefold more common in women than men. The risk for hepatic toxicity varies with CD4+ cell count. In a summary analysis of data from 17 clinical trials of nevirapine therapy, women with CD4+ counts >250 cells/mm^3 were 9.8 times more likely than women with lower CD4+ counts to experience symptomatic, rash-associated, nevirapine-related hepatotoxicity. Higher CD4+ cell counts have also been associated with increased risk of severe nevirapine-associated skin rash. Severe or life-threatening rash occurs in approximately 2% of patients receiving nevirapine. Women initiating nevirapine with CD4+ counts >250 cells/mm^3, including pregnant women receiving antiretroviral drugs solely for the prevention of MTCT, have an increased risk of developing symptomatic, often rash-associated, nevirapine-related hepatotoxicity, which can be severe, life threatening, and in some cases fatal. Nevirapine should therefore be used as a component of a combination regimen in this setting only if the benefit clearly outweighs the risk. Regardless of maternal CD4+ cell count, if nevirapine is used, healthcare providers should be aware of this potential complication and carefully monitor clinical symptoms and hepatic transaminases (ALT and AST), particularly during the first 18 weeks of therapy. Patients who develop possible clinical symptoms with elevations in serum transaminase levels (ALT and/or AST), or who have asymptomatic but severe transaminase elevations, should stop nevirapine and not receive nevirapine therapy in the future.

Protease Inhibitors

Hyperglycemia, new-onset diabetes mellitus, exacerbation of existing diabetes mellitus, and diabetic ketoacidosis have been reported with usage of protease-inhibitor antiretroviral drugs. Pregnancy, a diabetogenic state, in combination with protease inhibitors, may increase the risk for gestational diabetes. Healthcare providers caring for HIV-1–infected pregnant women who are receiving protease-inhibitor therapy should be aware of the risk and may screen for gestational diabetes in the second (early screening) and third (traditional) trimesters.

Antiretroviral Medications and Methergine Usage

Women having postpartum hemorrhage secondary to uterine atony are often managed with methergine as a first-line agent. However, methergine should not be coadministered with drugs that are potent CYP3A4 enzyme inhibitors, including protease inhibitors and the nonnucleoside reverse-transcriptase inhibitors efavirenz and delavirdine. The concomitant use of ergotamines and protease inhibitors has been associated with exaggerated vasoconstrictive responses. When uterine atony results in excessive postpartum bleeding in women receiving protease inhibitors or efavirenz or delavirdine as a component of an antiretroviral regimen, methergine should only be used if alternative treatments (prostaglandin F2-alpha, misoprostol, or oxytocin) are not available.

Mitochondrial Toxicity and Nucleoside Analog Medications

Nucleoside analog drugs induce mitochondrial dysfunction due to the drugs having an affinity for mitochondrial gamma DNA polymerase. This affinity interferes with mitochondrial replication, resulting in mitochondrial DNA depletion and dysfunction. The relative potency of the nucleosides in inhibiting mitochondrial gamma DNA polymerase in vitro is highest for zalcitabine (ddC), followed by didanosine (ddI), stavudine (d4T), ZDV, 3TC, ABC, and tenofovir. Toxicity related to the mitochondrial dysfunction generally resolves with discontinuation of the drugs; a possible genetic polymorphism allows susceptibility for toxicities. These toxicities may be of particular concern for pregnant women and infants with in utero exposure to nucleoside analog drugs.

The clinical picture of mitochondrial toxicity includes neuropathy, myopathy, cardiomyopathy, pancreatitis, hepatic steatosis, and lactic acidosis. Symptomatic lactic acidosis and hepatic steatosis may have a female predominance, and these syndromes have similarities to complications that occur during pregnancy, especially during the third trimester: acute fatty liver, or preeclampsia with hemolysis, elevated liver enzymes, and low platelets (HELLP syndrome).

These pregnancy-related complications may be associated with a recessively inherited mitochondrial abnormality in the fetus/infant that results in an inability to oxidize fatty acids. With a maternal heterozygotic carrier state of the gene mutation, the risk for liver toxicity is increased during pregnancy since the mother is unable to properly oxidize either maternal or fetal accumulating fatty acids properly. Thus this inability to oxidize fatty acids during the third trimester may play a role in the development of acute fatty liver of pregnancy or in development of HELLP syndrome. The development of lactic acidosis with hepatic steatosis is a toxicity related to nucleoside analog drugs that is related to mitochondrial toxicity; it has been reported to occur in infected persons treated with nucleoside analog therapies for periods of more than six months. The typical initial symptoms included one to six weeks of nausea, vomiting, abdominal pain, dyspnea, and weakness. Metabolic acidosis with elevated serum lactate and elevated hepatic enzymes occurs mostly in overweight females. The syndrome incidence is increasing as there is increased use of combination nucleoside analog therapy and increased recognition of the complication. The frequency of this syndrome in pregnant HIV-1–infected women receiving nucleoside analog treatment is unknown, and the reported incidence of symptomatic hyperlactatemia ranges from 0.8% for all patients to 1.2% for patients receiving a regimen including d4T. Italian investigators reported a case of severe lactic acidosis in an HIV-positive pregnant woman who was receiving d4T-3TC from conception and throughout pregnancy: she experienced symptoms and fetal death at 38 weeks of gestation. The pharmaceutical company Bristol-Myers Squibb reported three maternal deaths due to lactic acidosis among women who were either pregnant or postpartum and had antepartum therapy including d4T and ddI with other antiretroviral agents. All women were receiving treatment with these agents at the time of conception and continued throughout pregnancy, and the women presented late in gestation with symptomatic disease, which progressed to death in the postpartum period. Nonfatal cases of lactic acidosis in pregnant women receiving combination d4T-ddI have also been reported. Pregnancy can mimic some of the early symptoms of the lactic acidosis/hepatic steatosis syndrome

[a]Antiretroviral Pregnancy Registry: Research Park, 1011 Ashes Drive, Wilmington, NC 28405, U.S.A. Phone: 1–800–258–4263; fax: 1–800–800–1052; website: www.APRegistry.com.

TABLE 4 Clinical data relevant to the use of antiretrovirals in pregnancy

Antiretroviral drug	FDA category	Placental passage (N:M ratio)	Long-term animal carcinogenicity studies	Animal teratogen studies
Nucleoside and nucleotide analog reverse-transcriptase inhibitors				
Abacavir (Ziagen, ABC)	C	Y	Positive (malignant and nonmalignant tumors of liver, thyroid in female rats)	Positive [rodent anasarca and skeletal malformations at 1000 mg/kg (35×human exposure) during organogenesis; not in rabbits]
Didanosine (Videx, ddI)	B	Y (0.5)	Negative	Negative
Emtricitabine (Emtriva, FTC)	B	U	Not completed	Negative
Lamivudine (Epivir, 3TC)	C	Y (1.0)	Negative	Negative
Stavudine (Zerit, d4T)	C	Y (0.76)	Positive (mice and rats, at very high dose exposure, liver and bladder tumors)	Negative (but sternal bone calcium decreases in rodents)
Tenofovir DF (Viread)	B	Y	Positive (hepatic adenomas in female mice at high doses)	Negative (osteomalacia in juvenile animals at high doses)
Zalcitabine (HIVID, ddC)	C	Y (0.40)	Positive (rodent, thymic lymphomas)	Positive (rodent—hydrocephalus at high dose)
Zidovudine (Retrovir, AZT, ZDV)	C	Y (0.85)	Positive (rodent, noninvasive vaginal epithelial tumors)	Positive (rodent—near lethal dose)
Nonnucleoside reverse-transcriptase inhibitors				
Delavirdine (Rescriptor)	C	U	Positive (hepatocellular adenomas and carcinomas in male and female mice but not rats, bladder tumors in male mice)	Positive (rodent—ventricular septal defect)
Efavirenz (Sustiva)	D	Y (1.0)	Positive (hepato-cellular adenomas and carcinomas and pulmonary alveolar/bronchiolar adenomas in female mice)	Positive (cynomolgus monkey—anencephaly, anophthalmia, microphthalmia)
Nevirapine (Viramune)	C	Y (1.0)	Positive (hepato-cellular adenomas and carcinomas in mice and rats)	Negative
Protease inhibitors				
Amprenavir (Agenerase)	C	U	Positive (hepato-cellular adenomas and carcinomas in male mice and rats)	Negative (but deficient ossification and thymic elongation in rats and rabbits)
Atazanavir	B	U	Positive (hepato-cellular adenomas in female mice)	Negative
Darunavir (Prezista)	B	U	Not completed	Negative
Fosamprenavir (Lexiva)	C	U	Positive (benign and malignant liver tumors in male rodents)	Negative (deficient ossification with amprenavir but not fosamprenavir)
Indinavir (Crixivan)	C	Y (min)	Positive (thyroid adenomas in male rats at highest dose)	Negative (but extra ribs in rodents)
Lopinavir/ritonavir (Kaletra)	C	U	Positive (hepato-cellular adenomas and carcinomas in mice and rats)	Negative (but delayed skeletal ossification and increase in skeletal variations in rats at maternally toxic doses)
Nelfinavir (Viracept)	B	Y (min)	Positive (thyroid follicular adenomas and carcinomas in rats)	Negative
Ritonavir (Norvir)	B	Y (min)	Positive (liver adenomas and carcinomas in male mice)	Negative (but cryptorchidism in rodents)
Saquinavir (Fortovase)	B	Y (min)	Negative	Negative
Tipranavir (Aptivus)	C	U	In progress	Negative (decreased ossification and pup weights in rats at maternally toxic doses)
Fusion inhibitors				
Enfuvirtide (Fuzeon)	B	U	Not done	Negative

Abbreviation: FDA, Food and Drug Administration.
Source: Adapted from AIDSinfo (2006).

or be associated with other disorders of liver metabolism; these reports emphasize the need for physicians caring for HIV-1–infected pregnant women receiving nucleoside analog drugs to be attentive for signs of this syndrome. Pregnant women receiving nucleoside analog drugs should have hepatic enzymes and electrolytes assessed more frequently during the third trimester of pregnancy, with any suggestive symptoms evaluated. Healthcare providers should prescribe this antiretroviral combination during pregnancy with caution following these reports of maternal mortality secondary to lactic acidosis after prolonged use of the combination of d4T and ddI.

Conflicting data have been reported regarding whether mitochondrial dysfunction is associated with antenatal/perinatal antiretroviral exposure. If there is an association, the development of severe or fatal mitochondrial disease seems to be extremely rare. There is clear benefit of antiretroviral prophylaxis in reducing MTCT of infection by 70% or more. Mitochondrial dysfunction should be considered in uninfected children with perinatal antiretroviral exposure who present with severe clinical findings of unknown etiology, particularly neurologic findings.

Efavirenz and Neural Tube Defects

Efavirenz may be teratogenic when used during the first trimester of pregnancy. No adequate and well-controlled studies have been performed in pregnant women. In prospective reports, birth defects have occurred in 5 of 188 live births after first-trimester maternal exposure; none were neural tube defects. Four retrospective reports identified findings consistent with neural tube defects, including meningomyelocele, in mothers exposed to efavirenz during the first trimester. Although a causal relationship has not been established, similar defects have been observed in preclinical studies of efavirenz.

Two methods of birth control, with a barrier method in combination with a nonbarrier method, should be used to avoid pregnancy in women taking efavirenz. Before initiating therapy with efavirenz, women of childbearing potential should undergo pregnancy testing. It is recommended that efavirenz not be given to pregnant women except in situations in which there are no therapeutic alternatives. It is not known if efavirenz is secreted into breast milk in humans; however, efavirenz is distributed into the milk of laboratory animals. Breast-feeding is not recommended with efavirenz therapy.

MOTHER-TO-CHILD TRANSMISSION

Management of HIV during pregnancy should include antiretroviral therapy to suppress plasma HIV-1 RNA to undetectable levels. Labor and delivery management of HIV-1–infected pregnant women should focus on minimizing the risks of MTCT of HIV-1 and the potential for maternal and neonatal complications. Several publications performed prior to routine viral load testing showed that cesarean delivery before labor and rupture of membranes (scheduled) was associated with a significant decrease from 80% to 55% in MTCT of HIV-1 compared with other delivery modes. Table 5 summarizes the relationship of antiretroviral treatment to vertical transmission rates.

A meta-analysis comprised of 15 prospective cohort studies with >7800 mother–child pairs analyzed the rate of MTCT of HIV-1 among women undergoing elective cesarean delivery and found a significantly lower MTCT compared to women having either nonelective cesarean or vaginal delivery, regardless of zidovudine administration. In an international randomized trial of mode of delivery, transmission was 1.8% among women randomized to elective cesarean delivery. Additionally, in both studies, nonelective cesarean delivery (performed after onset of labor or rupture of membranes) was not associated with a significant decrease in transmission compared with vaginal delivery. The American College of Obstetricians and Gynecologists' (ACOG) Committee on Obstetric Practice has issued a Committee Opinion concerning route of delivery, recommending consideration of scheduled cesarean delivery for HIV-1–infected pregnant women with HIV-1 RNA levels >1000 copies/mL near the time of delivery. More recently, pregnant women have been receiving HAART with MTCT rates of 1.2% to 1.5% reported. Given the low transmission rates among women on HAART, the benefit of elective cesarean delivery is difficult to evaluate. Until further data are available, elective cesarean delivery should continue to be recommended for women on HAART who have HIV RNA levels >1000 copies/mL near delivery. Elective cesarean delivery should not be routinely provided for women on therapy who have HIV RNA <1000 copies/mL, unless the woman chooses this procedure after counseling regarding uncertain benefits and known risks.

In a report of transmission of women with HIV RNA <1000 copies/mL at delivery, among the subset receiving therapy (primarily ZDV), transmission occurred among none of 270 women who delivered by scheduled or urgent cesarean; transmission occurred among 1.8% (7/396) of women who delivered vaginally ($p = 0.05$). More recent data have demonstrated the benefit of HAART for reduction in MTCT of HIV. Data from PACTG 316 demonstrated an overall transmission rate of 1.5% among women on antiretroviral therapy during pregnancy; 23% of the women were on ZDV, 36% on nucleoside analog combination regimens, and 41% on combinations including protease inhibitors. Data from PACTG 367, a chart review study of 2756 women, found a transmission rate of 34 (1.3%) of 2539 women on multiagent antiretroviral therapy. In a recent report from the European Collaborative Study that included data from 4525 women, the overall transmission rate among the subset of women on HAART was 11 (1.2%) of 918. Data from PACTG 367 do not suggest benefit from elective cesarean delivery among women with HIV RNA levels <1000 copies/mL. Women with HIV RNA levels <1000 copies/mL on multiagent therapy had MTCT rates of 0.8% with elective cesarean delivery and 0.5% with all other delivery modes. Among the subset of 560 women from the European Collaborative Study, with undetectable HIV RNA levels (200–500 copies/mL, depending on site), elective

TABLE 5 Relationship of antiretroviral treatment to vertical transmission

Antiretroviral treatment regimen	Percentage of vertical transmission
Nothing	33%
Nothing + breast-feeding	50%
PACTG 076 study AZT	8.3%
C/S + AZT	2%
HAART	Less than 1%
Bangkok oral AZT	9.4%
Uganda Nevirapine	13.3%

Abbreviations: AZT, azidothymidine (zidovudine); C/S, cesarean section; HAART, highly active antiretroviral treatment; PACTG, pediatric AIDS clinical trial group.

cesarean delivery was associated with a significant reduction in MTCT on univariate analysis [odds ratio (OR) 0.07, 95% confidence interval (CI) 0.02–0.31, $p = 0.0004$]. However, after adjustment for antiretroviral therapy (none vs. any), the effect was no longer significant (adjusted OR 0.52, 95% CI 0.14–2.03, $p = 0.359$). These data do not confirm or rule out benefit from elective cesarean delivery among women with HIV RNA <1000 copies/mL who are receiving antiretroviral therapy. Pregnant women on antiretroviral therapy with HIV RNA levels <1000 copies/mL should be counseled regarding the low baseline rate of transmission, the uncertain benefits, and the known risks of elective cesarean delivery. Women on HAART with HIV RNA >1000 copies/mL near delivery should be counseled regarding the potential benefits of scheduled cesarean delivery and the known risks of cesarean delivery versus vaginal delivery. Until further data are available, elective cesarean delivery should continue to be recommended for women on HAART with HIV RNA levels >1000 copies/mL near delivery.

POSTPARTUM FOLLOW-UP OF WOMEN

The care of the HIV-positive woman in the postpartum period should include both medical services and support services. Components of care include (*i*) primary obstetric and pediatric care; (*ii*) HIV specialty care; (*iii*) family planning services; and if needed (*iv*) mental health/substance-abuse treatment. Maternal medical services during the postpartum period should be coordinated between obstetric healthcare providers and HIV specialists. Continuity of antiretroviral therapies if treatment is required for the woman's HIV infection is especially important. Adherence to antiretroviral therapies during the postpartum period can become difficult with the physical and hormonal changes coupled with the stresses and demands of caring for a new baby. Poor adherence has been shown to be associated with virologic failure, development of resistance, and decreased long-term effectiveness of antiretroviral therapy. Efforts to maintain good adherence during the postpartum period might prolong the effectiveness of therapy.

Data from PACTG 076 and 288 have not demonstrated adverse effects through 4+ years postpartum among women who received ZDV during pregnancy. Women who have received only ZDV chemoprophylaxis during pregnancy should receive appropriate evaluation to determine the need for antiretroviral therapy during the postpartum period. Continuation of antiretroviral therapy during the postpartum period and thereafter should follow CDC guidelines (Table 6).

Postpartum or in any woman of reproductive age, antiretroviral therapy selection should account for the possibility of pregnancy. Sexual activity, reproductive plans, and use of effective contraception should be discussed with the woman. As part of the evaluation for initiating therapy, women should be counseled about the potential teratogenic risks of the various antiretroviral therapies discussed previously and in Table 4. Known therapies that are teratogenic should be avoided in women who are trying to conceive or are not using reliable contraception. Various protease inhibitors and nonnucleoside reverse-transcriptase inhibitors are known to interact with oral contraceptives, resulting in possible decreases in ethinyl estradiol or increases in estradiol or norethindrone levels (Table 7). These changes may decrease the effectiveness of the oral contraceptives or increase risk of estrogen/progestin-related side effects. Healthcare providers should be aware of these drug interactions and an alternative/additional contraceptive method should be considered. Amprenavir (and probably fosamprenavir) increases blood levels of both estrogen and progestin components, and oral contraceptives decrease amprenavir levels as well; therefore, these drugs should not be coadministered. Only minimal information about drug interactions and the newer hormonal contraceptive methods (i.e., patch, vaginal ring, progesterone insert) is currently available. Women who express a desire to become pregnant should be referred for preconception counseling, including discussion of special considerations with antiretroviral therapy during pregnancy.

PRECONCEPTION COUNSELING IN HIV-POSITIVE WOMEN

The CDC and ACOG recommend offering all women of childbearing age the opportunity to receive preconception counseling and care as a component of routine primary medical care. The purpose of preconception care is to optimize

TABLE 6 Guidelines for antiretroviral therapy in HIV-positive adults and adolescents

Antiretroviral therapy is recommended for all patients with history of an AIDS-defining illness or severe symptoms of HIV infection regardless of CD4+ T-cell count
Antiretroviral therapy is recommended for asymptomatic patients with <200 CD4+ T-cells/mm³
Asymptomatic patients with CD4+ T-cell counts of 201–350 cells/mm³ should be offered treatment
For asymptomatic patients with CD4+ T-cell of >350 cells/mm³ and plasma HIV RNA >100,000 copies/mL, most experienced clinicians defer therapy but some clinicians may consider initiating treatment
Therapy should be deferred for patients with CD4 1 T-cell counts of >350 cells/mm3 and plasma HIV RNA ,100,000 copies/mL

Source: Adapted from AIDSinfo (2006).

TABLE 7 Interactions with protease inhibitors or nonnucleoside reverse-transcriptase inhibitors with oral contraceptives

Antiretroviral agent	Effect with oral contraceptive	Change in management
Atazanavir (ATV)	Ethinyl estradiol AUC increased 48%, norethindrone AUC increased 110%	Use lowest effective dose or alternative methods
Fosamprenavir (fAPV)	An increase in ethinyl estradiol and norethindrone levels occurred with APV, and APV levels decrease 20%	Do not coadminister; alternative methods of contraception are recommended
Darunavir with ritonavir (DRV/RTV)	Potential for decreased ethinyl estradiol from RTV	Use alternative or additional method with DRV/RTV
Indinavir (IDV)	Norethindrone increased 26%. Ethinyl estradiol increased 24%	No dose adjustment
Lopinavir with ritonavir (LPV/r)	Ethinyl estradiol decreased 42%	Use alternative or additional method
Nelfinavir (NFV)	Norethindrone deceased 18%. Ethinyl estradiol decreased 47%	Use alternative or additional method
Ritonavir (RTV)	Ethinyl estradiol decreased 40%	Use alternative or additional method
Saquinavir (SQV)	No data	No data
Tipranavir with ritonavir (TPV/RTV)	Ethinyl estradiol AUC decreased 50%	Use alternative or additional method. Women on estrogen may have increased risk of nonserious rash
Delavirdine (DLV)	Ethinyl estradiol may increase	Clinical significance is unknown
Efavirenz (EFV)	Ethinyl estradiol increased 37%. No data on progesterone	Use alternative or additional methods
Nevirapine (NVP)	Ethinyl estradiol decreased 20%	Use alternative or additional methods

Abbreviation: AUC, area under the plasma concentration–time curve.
Source: Adapted from AIDSinfo (2006).

health prior to conception by identifying risk factors for adverse maternal and/or fetal outcome, providing education and counseling aimed at the patient's individual needs, and treating identified medical conditions for improved outcome. Most pregnancies are unplanned and, therefore, HIV health-care providers who routinely see women of reproductive age have an important role in promoting preconception health. The fundamental principles of preconception counseling and care have been outlined by the CDC Preconception Care Work Group in their publication "Recommendations to Improve Preconception Health and Health Care." The following CDC recommendations should be considered in pre-conception care in HIV-infected women:

- Select effective and appropriate contraceptive methods to reduce the likelihood of unintended pregnancy. Providers should be aware of potential interactions of antiretroviral drugs with hormonal contraceptives that could lower contraceptive efficacy.
- Counsel on safe sexual practices that prevent HIV transmission to sexual partners and protect women from acquiring STDs and the potential to acquire more virulent or resistant HIV strains.
- Counsel on eliminating alcohol, illicit drug use, and cigarette smoking.
- Educate and counsel women about risk factors for MTCT of HIV, strategies to reduce those risks, and potential effects of HIV or treatment on pregnancy course and outcomes.
- When prescribing antiretroviral treatment to women of childbearing potential, considerations should include regimen effectiveness for treatment of HIV disease and the drug's potential for teratogenicity should pregnancy occur. Women who are planning to get pregnant should strongly consider using antiretroviral regimens

that do not contain efavirenz or other drugs with teratogenic potential.

- Attain a stable, maximally suppressed maternal viral load prior to conception in women who are on antiretroviral therapy and wish to become pregnant.
- Evaluate and control for therapy-associated side effects that may adversely impact maternal–fetal health outcomes (e.g., hyperglycemia, anemia, hepatic toxicity).
- Evaluate for appropriate prophylaxis for opportunistic infections and administration of medical immunizations (e.g., influenza, pneumococcal, or hepatitis B vaccines) as indicated.
- Encourage sexual partners to receive HIV testing and counseling and appropriate HIV care if infected.
- Counsel regarding available reproductive options, such as intrauterine or intravaginal insemination, that prevent HIV exposure to an uninfected partner.
- Breast-feeding by HIV-infected women is not recommended in the United States secondary to risk of HIV transmission and availability of alternative food sources.

SUMMARY OF RECOMMENDATIONS DURING PREGNANCY

- All pregnant women should have prenatal HIV screening test on initial exam. In populations at "high risk," repeat HIV screening in the third trimester should be considered.
- If no prior HIV screening has been performed during pregnancy, then testing should be performed in the intrapartum (in the labor and delivery area) and/or neonatal period.
- All HIV-infected women should be monitored with
  1. viral loads monthly until the virus is undetectable and then every two to three months,

2. CD4 counts (absolute number or percent) each trimester, and
3. resistance testing on initial exam and/or if they have failed therapy.

- Pregnant women should have access to all of the same therapies as nonpregnant women with the following exceptions:
  1. efavirenz,
  2. hydroxyurea,
  3. stavudine/didanosine in combination (should be used only if other regimens are not available).

- Undetectable viral loads is the goal during pregnancy.
- All pregnant women should receive antiretroviral therapy. A highly active regimen that includes zidovudine should be part of the therapy. If a woman has a low viral load that would not require therapy if she were not pregnant (<1000 copies), then use of monotherapy can be considered, with the understanding that there may be a small risk of the development of resistance.
- An HIV-infected women in labor and the neonate should be treated with one of the following:
  1. Zidovudine in labor and six weeks to the neonate
  2. Nevirapine, a single dose to the mother in labor and a single dose to the neonate
  3. Zidovudine–lamivudine in labor and to the neonate for one week
  4. Both nevirapine as above and the zidovudine regimen as above.
- Cesarean delivery should be recommended to all women with a viral load >1000 copies.

SUGGESTED READING

American College of Obstetricians and Gynecologists. ACOG practice bulletin number 47, October 2003: prophylactic antibiotics in labor and delivery. Obstet Gynecol 2003; 102:875–882.

American College of Obstetricians and Gynecologists. The importance of preconception care in the continuum of women's health care. ACOG Committee Opinion No. 313. American College of Obstetricians and Gynecologists. Obstet Gynecol 2005; 106:665–666.

AIDSinfo Website: http://AIDSinfo.nih.gov "Recommendations for use of antiretroviral drugs in pregnant HIV-1-infected women for maternal health and interventions to reduce perinatal HIV-1 transmission in the United States." Published October 12, 2006. Accessed November 2006.

Barré-Sinoussi F, Chermann JC, Rey F, et al. Isolation of a T-lymphotropic retrovirus from a patient at risk for acquired immune deficiency syndrome (AIDS). Science 1983; 220:868–871.

Barret B, Tardieu M, Rustin P, et al. Persistent mitochondrial dysfunction in HIV-1-exposed but uninfected infants: clinical screening in a large prospective cohort. AIDS 2003; 17:1769–1785.

Baylor MS, Johann-Liang R. Hepatotoxicity associated with nevirapine use. J Acquir Immune Defic Syndr 2004; 35:538–539.

Bell DM. Occupational risk of human immunodeficiency virus infection in healthcare workers: an overview. Am J Med 1997; 102: 9–15.

Bersoff-Matcha SJ, Miller WC, Aberg JA, et al. Sex differences in nevirapine rash. Clin Infect Dis 2001; 32:124–129.

Birkus G, Hitchcock MJ, Cihlar T. Assessment of mitochondrial toxicity in human cells treated with tenofovir: comparison with other nucleoside reverse transcriptase inhibitors. Antimicrob Agents Chemother 2002; 46:716–723.

Blanche S, Tardieu M, Rustin P, et al. Persistent mitochondrial dysfunction and perinatal exposure to antiretroviral nucleoside analogues. Lancet 1999; 354:1084–1089.

Boucher FD, Modlin JF, Weller S, et al. Phase I evaluation of zidovudine administered to infants exposed at birth to the human immunodeficiency virus. J Pediatr 1993; 122:137–144.

Branson BM, Handsfield HH, Lampe MA, et al. Centers for Disease Control and Prevention (CDC). Revised recommendations for HIV testing of adults, adolescents, and pregnant women in healthcare settings. MMWR Recomm Rep 2006; 55:1–17.

Brinkman K, Ter Hofstede HJM, Burger DM, et al. Adverse effects of reverse transcriptase inhibitors: mitochondrial toxicity as common pathway. AIDS 1998; 12:1735–1744.

Bristol-Myers Squibb Company. Healthcare Provider Important Drug Warning Letter. January 5, 2001.

CDC. 1993 revised classification system for HIV infection and expanded surveillance case definition for AIDS among adolescents and adults. MMWR Recomm Rep 1992; 41:1–19.

CDC. Revised guidelines for HIV counseling, testing, and referral. MMWR 2001; 50:1–62.

Chuachoowong R, Shaffer N, Siriwasin W, et al. Short-course antenatal zidovudine reduces both cervicovaginal human immunodeficiency virus type 1 RNA levels and risk of perinatal transmission. J Infect Dis 2000; 181:99–106.

Coovadia H. Antiretroviral agents—how best to protect infants from HIV and save their mothers from AIDS. NEJM 2004; 351:289–292.

Donegan E, Stuart M, Niland JC, et al. Infection with human immunodeficiency virus type 1 (HIV-1) among recipients of antibody-positive blood donations. Ann Intern Med 1990; 113:733–739.

Dorenbaum A, Cunningham CK, Gelber RD, et al. Two-dose intrapartum/newborn nevirapine and standard antiretroviral therapy to reduce perinatal HIV-1 transmission: a randomized trial. JAMA 2002; 288:189–198.

Dube MP, Sattler FR. Metabolic complications of antiretroviral therapies. AIDS Clinical Care 1998; 10:41–44.

European Study Group on Heterosexual Transmission of HIV. Comparison of female to male and male to female transmission of HIV in 563 stable couples. BMJ 1992; 304:809–813.

Eastone JA, Decker CF. New-onset diabetes mellitus associated with use of protease inhibitor [letter]. Ann Intern Med 1997; 127:948.

European Collaborative Study. Mother-to-child transmission of HIV infection in the era of highly active antiretroviral therapy. Clin Infect Dis 2005; 40:458–465.

Fortgang IS, Belitsos PC, Chaisson RE, et al. Hepatomegaly and steatosis in HIV-infected patients receiving nucleoside analogue antiretroviral therapy. Am J Gastroenterol 1995; 90:1433–1436.

Gallo RC, Sarin P. S, Gelmann EP, Robert-Guroff M, et al. Isolation of human T-cell leukemia virus in acquired immune deficiency syndrome (AIDS). Science add to p.117 1983; 220(4599):865–867.

Gao F, Bailes E, Robertson DL, et al. Origin of HIV-1 in the Chimpanzee Pan troglodytes troglodytes. Nature 1999; 397:436–441.

Gerard Y, Maulin L, Yazdanpanah Y, et al. Symptomatic hyperlactatemia: an emerging complication of antiretroviral therapy. AIDS 2000; 14:2723–2730.

Giaquinto C, De Romeo A, Giacomet V, et al. Lactic acid levels in children perinatally treated with antiretroviral agents to prevent HIV transmission. AIDS 2001; 15:1074–1075.

Grimbert S, Fisch C, Deschamps D, et al. Effects of female sex hormones on mitochondria: possible role in acute fatty liver of pregnancy. Am J Physiol 1995; 268:G107–G115.

Guay LA, Musoke P, Fleming T, et al. Intrapartum and neonatal single-dose nevirapine compared with zidovudine for prevention of mother-to-child transmission of HIV-1 in Kampala, Uganda: HIVNET 012 randomised trial. Lancet 1999; 354:795–802.

Hitti J, Frenkel LM, Steck AM, et al. (for the PACTG 1022 Study Team). Maternal toxicity with continuous nevirapine in pregnancy: results from PACTG 1022. J Acquir Immune Defic Syndr 2004; 36:772–776.

Ibdah JA, Yang Z, Bennett MJ. Liver disease in pregnancy and fetal fatty acid oxidation defects. Mol Genet Metab 2000; 71:182–189.

Ibdah JA, Bennett MJ, Rinaldo P, et al. A fetal fatty-acid oxidation disorder as a cause of liver disease in pregnant women. NEJM 1999; 340:1723–1731.

Ickovics JR, Wilson TE, Royce RA, et al. Prenatal and postnatal zidovudine adherence among pregnant women with HIV. J Acquir Immune Defic Syndr 2002; 30:311–315.

Ioannidis JPA, Abrams EJ, Ammann A, et al. Perinatal transmission of human immunodeficiency virus type 1 by pregnant women with RNA virus loads <1000 copies/mL. J Infect Dis 2001; 183:539–545.

Johnson K, Posner SF, Biermann J, et al. (CDC/ATSDR Preconception Care Work Group; Select Panel on Preconception Care). Recommendations to improve preconception health and health care—United States. A report of the CDC/ATSDR Preconception Care Work Group and the Select Panel on Preconception Care. MMWR Recomm Rep 2006; 21; 55:1–23.

Kaplan EH, Heimer R. HIV incidence among New Haven needle exchange participants: updated estimates from syringe tracking and testing data. J Acquir Immune Defic Syndr Hum Retrovirol 1995; 10:175–176.

Keele BF, van Heuverswyn F, Li YY, et al. Chimpanzee reservoirs of pandemic and nonpandemic HIV-1. Science 2006; 313:523–526.

Kendell RE, Chalmers JC, Platz C. Epidemiology of puerperal psychoses. Br J Psychiatry 1987; 150:662–673.

Knudtson E, Para M, Boswell H, Fan-Havard P. Drug rash with eosinophilia and systemic symptoms syndrome and renal toxicity with a nevirapine-containing regimen in a pregnant patient with human immunodeficiency virus. Obstet Gynecol 2003; 101:1094–1097.

Lallemant M, Jourdain G, Le Coeur S, et al. Single dose perinatal nevirapine plus standard zidovudine to prevent mother-to-child transmission of HIV-1 in Thailand. NEJM 2004; 351:217–228.

Landreau-Mascaro A, Barret B, Mayaux MJ, et al. Risk of early febrile seizure with perinatal exposure to nucleoside analogues. Lancet 2002; 359:583–584.

Leynaert B, Downs AM, de Vincenzi I. Heterosexual transmission of human immunodeficiency virus: variability of infectivity throughout the course of infection. European Study Group on Heterosexual Transmission of HIV. Am J Epidemiol 1998; 148:88–96.

Luzzati R, Del Bravo P, Di Perri G, et al. Riboflavine and severe lactic acidosis. Lancet 1999; 353:901–902.

Mallal S, Nolan D, Witt C, et al. Association between presence of HLA-B*5701, HLA-DR7, and HLA-DQ3 and hypersensitivity to HIV-1 reverse-transcriptase inhibitor abacavir. Lancet 2002; 359:727–732.

Mandelbrot L, Kermarrec N, Marcollet A, et al. Case report: nucleoside analogue-induced lactic acidosis in the third trimester of pregnancy. AIDS 2003; 17:272–273.

Mazhude C, Jones S, Murad S, et al. Female sex but not ethnicity is a strong predictor of non-nucleoside reverse transcriptase inhibitor-induced rash. AIDS 2002; 16:1566–1568.

Melbourne KM, Geletko SM, Brown SL, et al. Medication adherence in patients with HIV infection: a comparison of two measurement methods. The AIDS Reader 1999; 9:329–338.

Melvin AJ, Burchett SK, Watts DH, et al. Effect of pregnancy and zidovudine therapy on viral load in HIV-1-infected women. J Acquir Immune Defic Syndr Hum Retrovirol 1997; 14:232–236.

Miller LG, Liu H, Hays RD, et al. How well do clinicians estimate patients' adherence to combination antiretroviral therapy? J Gen Intern Med 2002; 17:1–11.

Murri R, Ammassari A, Gallicano K, et al. Patient reported nonadherence to HAART is related to protease inhibitor levels. J Acquir Immune Defic Syndr 2000; 24:123–128.

Popovic M, Sarngadharan MG, Read E, Gallo RC. Detection, isolation, and continuous production of cytopathic retroviruses (HTLV-III) from patients with AIDS and pre-AIDS. Science 1984; 224:497–500.

Poirier MC, Divi RL, Al-Harthi L, et al. Long-term mitochondrial toxicity in HIV-uninfected infants born to HIV-infected mothers. J Acquir Immune Defic Syndr 2003; 33:175–183.

Qian M, Bui T, Ho RJY, Unadkat JD. Metabolism of 3'-azido-3'-deoxythymidine (AZT) in human placental trophoblasts and hofbauer cells. Biochem Pharmacol 1994; 48:383–389.

Reeves JD, Doms RW. Human immunodeficiency virus type 2. J Gen Virol 2002; 83:1253–1265.

Sandberg JA, Binienda Z, Lipe G, et al. Placental transfer and fetal disposition of 2',3'-dideoxycytidine and 2',3'-dideoxyinosine in the rhesus monkey. Drug Metab Dispos 1995; 23:881–884.

Sarner L, Fakoya A. Acute onset lactic acidosis and pancreatitis in the third trimester of pregnancy in HIV-1 positive women taking antiretroviral medication. Sex Transm Infect 2002; 78:58–59.

Shapiro D, Tuomala R, Pollack H, et al. Mother-to-child HIV transmission risk according to antiretroviral therapy, mode of delivery, and viral load in 2895 U.S. women (PACTG 367). Oral presentation at the 11th Conference on Retroviruses and Opportunistic Infections; February, 2004; San Francisco, CA. Abstract 99.

Sims HF, Brackett JC, Powell CK, et al. The molecular basis of pediatric long-chain 3-hydroxyacyl Co-A dehydrogenase deficiency associated with maternal acute fatty liver of pregnancy. Proc Natl Acad Sci USA 1995; 92:841–845.

Smith DK, Grohskopf LA, Black RJ, et al. Antiretroviral postexposure prophylaxis after sexual, injection-drug use, or other nonoccupational exposure to HIV in the United States (http://www.cdc.gov/mmwr/preview/mmwrhtml/rr5402a1.htm). MMWR 2005; 54:1–20.

Sperling RS, Shapiro DE, Coombs RW, et al. Maternal viral load, zidovudine treatment, and the risk of transmission of human immunodeficiency virus type 1 from mother to infant. Pediatric AIDS Clinical Trials Group Protocol 076 Study Group. NEJM 1996; 335:1621–1629.

Sperling RS, Shapiro DE, McSherry GD, et al. Safety of the maternal-infant zidovudine regimen utilized in the Pediatric AIDS Clinical Trials Group 076 Study. AIDS 1998; 12:1805–1813.

Stern JO, Robinson PA, Love J, et al. A comprehensive hepatic safety analysis of nevirapine in different populations of HIV infected patients. J Acquir Immune Defic Syndr 2003; 34:S2133.

Strauss AW, Bennett MJ, Rinaldo P, et al. Inherited long-chain 3-hydroxyacyl-CoA dehydrogenase deficiency and a fetal-maternal interaction cause maternal liver disease and other pregnancy complications. Semin Perinatol 1999; 23:100–112.

The European Mode of Delivery Collaboration. Elective cesarean-section versus vaginal delivery in prevention of vertical HIV-1 transmission: a randomized clinical trial. Lancet 1999; 353:1035–1039.

The International Perinatal HIV Group. The mode of delivery and the risk of vertical transmission of human immunodeficiency virus type 1—a meta-analysis of 15 prospective cohort studies. NEJM 1999; 340:977–987.

The Perinatal Safety Review Working Group. Nucleoside exposure in the children of HIV-infected women receiving antiretroviral drugs: absence of clear evidence for mitochondrial disease in children who died before 5 years of age in five United States cohorts. J Acquir Immune Defic Syndr Hum Retrovirol 2000; 25:261–268.

Varghese B, Maher JE, Peterman TA, Branson BM, Steketee RW. Reducing the risk of sexual HIV transmission: quantifying the per-act risk for HIV on the basis of choice of partner, sex act, and condom use. Sex Transm Dis 2002; 29:38–43.

Wade NA, Birkhead GS, Warren BL, et al. Abbreviated regimens of zidovudine prophylaxis and perinatal transmission of the human immunodeficiency virus. NEJM 1998; 339:1409–1414.

Zhu T, Korber BT, Nahmias AJ, Hooper E, Sharp PM, Ho DD. An African HIV-1 sequence from 1959 and implications for the origin of the epidemic. Nature 1998; 391:594–559.

Human Papilloma Viruses

15

Stanley Gall / *Revised by* David A. Baker

INTRODUCTION

The spectrum of clinical disease that has been identified necessitates the use of the term "human papillomavirus" (HPV) infection rather than genital warts or condyloma acuminata. This spectrum has been extended to include entities such as subclinical HPV infection of the cervix, vagina, vulva, penis, and scrotum, a relationship of HPV to intraepithelial neoplasia of the vulva, vagina, and cervix, Bowen's disease, and juvenile laryngeal papillomatosis. Because of the relationship to malignant disease and because HPV infection is among the most widespread of the STDs and difficult to treat, it has become a disease of potentially great concern.

There are four morphological types of genital warts: (*i*) condyloma acuminata, which have the appearance of small cauliflowers; (*ii*) smooth papular warts, which are dome-shaped, flesh-covered, 1 to 4 mm papules; (*iii*) keratotitic genital warts, which resemble a common wart or a seborrheic keratosis (thick horny layer); and (*iv*) flat warts, which are flat to slightly raised, flat-topped papules (Fig. 1).

VIROLOGY

Genital warts are caused by specific types of HPV. HPV is classified with the papovavirus family (standing for papilloma, polyoma, simian kidney cell vacuolating virus). It is composed of double-stranded DNA with an average molecular weight of 5×10^5 daltons. The viral DNA is present as a supercoiled covalently closed circle with an icosahedral capsid composed of one major structural protein. Papillomaviruses are highly host and site specific and possess the ability to transform epithelial cells. HPV has not been convincingly cultured in tissue systems, probably because productive viral infection requires a degree of keratinocyte differentiation that has not yet been achieved.

HPV DNA has been molecularly cloned, and more than 70 HPV types have been identified by DNA homologies. HPV types are correlated with anatomic sites and biologic behavior (Table 1). Genital warts are associated with HPV types 6, 11, 16, 18, 31, 33, 35, 39, 42, 43, 44, 45, 51, 52, 56, 58, 66, and 68 (Table 1). HPV types 6 and 11 are the most prevalent viral types in exophytic warts while HPV types 16, 18, 31, 33, 35, 45, and 56 are the types most associated with genital neoplasia (Fig. 2).

The genomes of HPV as well as other papillomaviruses have been sequenced. The HPV genome does not need to be integrated into the host genome to induce transformation.

Integration of HPV into the host genome has been associated with malignancy (Table 2). HPV DNA sequences can be found in basal layer keratinocytes, but complete viral particles are found only in terminally differentiated cells in the superficial layers of the dermis.

The DNA regions with protein-coding potential are termed open reading frames (ORFs), which are divided into early and late capsid ORFs. The remainder of the circular viral DNA (15%) is a noncoding segment termed the upstream regulatory region located between the end of the "late" region and the beginning of the "early" region. The products of ORFs E6 and E7 are the primary inducers of oncogenic transformation and logically receive considerable investigative attention. E6 and E7 interfere with the functions of cellular proteins RB and p53, which are the critical elements in the control of the cellular "clock." ORF E1 specifies proteins required for regulated episomal (nonintegrated) DNA replication. ORF E2 encodes proteins that regulate viral transcription. ORFs L1 and L2 encode the major and minor capsid proteins, respectively.

With benign and precancerous HPV-related lesions, the viral DNA tends to be episomal (i.e., a free, self-replicating, extrachromosomal, circular nuclear plasmid). In invasive cancerous lesions, it is integrated (i.e., spliced into the host chromosomes by covalent bonds). This phenomenon occurs in particular with HPV 16– and HPV 18– containing tumors. Altered unregulated expression of E6 and E7 ORFs is hypothesized to be a consequence of viral integration into the host genome.

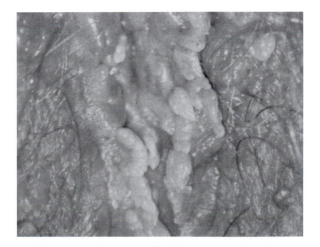

FIGURE 1 Vestibular condyloma presenting as pink, whitish or pigmented sessile projections with a lobulated surface.

TABLE 1 Human papilloma viruses: type of disease and anatomic location and malignant potential

Type	Disease and/or anatomic site	Malignant potential
1	Plantar and palmar warts	Benign
2	Common skin warts, occasionally associated with anogenital condylomata	Benign
3, 10, 28	Juvenile flat warts may be associated with epidermodysplasia verruciformis, genital infection and common warts	Rarely malignant
4	Plantar and common skin warts	Benign
5, 8	Epidermodysplasia verruciformis associated with congenital or reduced cell-mediated immune deficiency	30% malignancy
6, 11	Anogenital condylomata acuminata flat condylomas, CIN 1, 2, juvenile and laryngeal papillomas	Usually benign
7	Common warts of meat and animal handlers	Benign
9, 12, 14, 15, 17, 19–25, 36, 40	Epidermodysplasia verruciformis	Several progress to malignancy
12, 17, 20, 16, 18, 31 33, 35, 39, 45 51, 52, 56, 58	CIN 2, 3, carcinoma in situ of genital tract, Bowenoid papulosis, Bowen's disease, laryngeal, esophageal and some bronchial carcinomas	Frequent progression to malignancy
13, 32	Oral focal epithelial hyperplasia	Possible progression to malignancy
26, 29	Cutaneous warts, immunodeficient patients	Unknown
30, 40	Laryngeal carcinoma	Malignant
34	Nongenital Bowen's disease	CIS
37	Keratoacanthoma	Benign
38	Epidermodysplasia verruciformis	Malignant
41	Condylomas, cutaneous flat warts	Benign
42, 43, 44	Genital warts	Benign

Abbreviations: CIN, cervical intraepithelial neoplasia CIS, carcinoma in situ.

EPIDEMIOLOGY

HPV infections of the genital tract are one of the most common sexually transmitted viral infections. Both the incidence and prevalence of genital HPV infection are increasing. A survey of private office-based physicians showed that consultations for genital warts increased 580% in a decade. With an increasing awareness that many HPV infections are subclinical, most reports seriously underestimate the frequency of HPV infection. Current epidemiology data show that the probability of infection with at least one of the genital HPV types approaches 80% or more over a woman's lifetime. Fortunately, the vast majority of these infections are cleared by the host immune response without detection or treatment. This suggests that a vaccine approach should be feasible.

Cervical cytology and histology have been used to estimate the prevalence of genital HPV infection. These studies have shown cytologic evidence of HPV infection in 1.85% to 3% of unselected Papanicolaou (Pap) smears.

Routine cervical cytologic examination alone is inadequate for diagnosing all cervical HPV infections. HPV DNA sequences have been detected in greater than 50% of women attending an STD clinic who had normal Pap smears and normal colposcopic examination. In Seattle, cervical HPV infection diagnosed by Pap smear, immunoperoxidase stains, or DNA hybridization was detected in 18% of nonselected women attending an STD clinic.

In an important study from the University of California health service, women presenting for nongynecologic complaints had a cervical and vulvar scrape for detection of HPV. Polymerase chain reaction (PCR) analysis showed that 32% of scrapes from the cervix and 42% of scrapes from the vulva were positive for HPV.

An effort to identify asymptomatic HPV infection in males has been initiated but has not been well accepted by patients or the medical community. Diagnostic methods include koilocytosis of exfoliated uroepithelial cells, tissue biopsies, and acetowhitening of penile skin viewed through a colposcope (Table 3). In one study of male partners of women with condyloma acuminatum, of the 88% who had

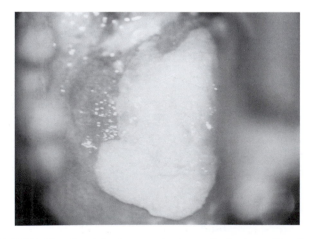

FIGURE 2 Condyloma acuminatum of the cervix after application of acetic acid.

TABLE 2 Association of HPV types and cervical malignancies

Risk	HPV types
High-risk HPV	16, 18, 31, 33, 35, 39, 45, 51, 52, 56, 58, 59, 66, 68
Low-risk HPV	6, 11, 40, 42, 43, 44

Abbreviation: HPV, human papillomavirus.

histologic evidence of penile condyloma, 16% had visible lesions and 72% had asymptomatic infection detected colposcopically after application of 5% acetic acid.

The male:female ratio of genital HPV infection varied from 1:1.7 to 2:1, with the peak age at 20 to 24 years.

Sexual transmission of HPV is the commonly accepted mode of transmission. Transmission rates vary from 59% to 95%. Infectivity of genital warts may decrease with time; so warts present for greater than one year may be less likely to be transmitted than warts present less than one year. Genital warts in children have been associated with child abuse but are not necessarily confirmatory for sexual contact.

HUMAN PAPILLOMA VIRUS AND MALIGNANCY

The association between HPV infection and genital malignancy has been investigated most intensively for cervical neoplasia, HPV infection of the vulvar, vaginal, anal, and penile can cause dysplasia and cancer. The concern today is that HPV is a carcinogen and/or cocarcinogen throughout the genital tract and other parts of the body and that simple HPV infections should be taken seriously by the patient and clinician. (Table 4)

The potential role of HPV in the etiology of neoplasia was originally suspected following observations of malignant

TABLE 3 Colposcopic index[a]

sign	0 points	1 point	2 points
Margin	Condylomatous or micropapillary contour. Indistinct acetowhitening. Flocculated or feathered margins. Angular or jagged margins. Satellite lesions and acetowhitening beyond transformation zone	Regular lesions with smooth, straight outlines	Rolled, packing edges. Interval of demarcation appearances
Color	Shiny snow-white color. Indistinct acetowhitening	Intermediate shade (shiny gray)	Dull oyster-white
Vessels	Fine-caliber vessels. Poorly formed patterns. Condylomatous micropapillary lesions	Absent vessels. Punctuation or mosaic	Definite

[a]Colposcopic score: 1–2 = SPI or CIN 1; 3–5 = CIN 1, 2; 6–8 = CIN 2, 3 "aneuploid lesions."
Abbreviations: CIN, cervical intraepithelial neoplasia; SPI, subclinical papillomavirus infection.
Source: From Reid and Scalzi (1985).

TABLE 4 Cancers associated with HPV and percentage attributable to oncogenic HPV (United States, 2003)

Cancer	Cases[a]	% Attributable to oncogenic HPV[b]
Cervix[c]	11,820	100
Anus[d]	4,187	90
Vulva[d]	3,507	40
Vagina[d]	1,070	40
Penis[d]	1,059	40
Oral cavity and pharynx[d]	29,627	≤12

[a] U.S. Cancer Statistics Working Group. United States cancer statistics: 2003. Incidence and mortality. Atlanta, GA: US Department of Health and Human Services, CDC, and the National Cancer Institute: 2006.
[b] Parkin M. The global health burden of infection-associated cancers in the years 2000. Int J Cancer 2006: 118:3030–44.
[c] A total of 70% attributed are HPV types 16 or 18.
[d] Majority of these cancers attributable to HPV type 16.

conversion of HPV-induced skin and mucosal tumors. HPV DNA was first detected in squamous cancers arising in epidermodysplasia verruciformis (a disease of multiple flat warts of nongenital skin in persons with congenital impairment of cellular immunity). The HPV DNA found in these cancers were types 5 and 8 in more than 90% of patients. An average of 20 years elapsed between the onset of verrucosis and cancer, and the preferential location of carcinomas on sunlight-exposed skin implied that malignant conversion depended on the activity of other cocarcinogens.

The association of HPV infection and cervical neoplasia was first reported with the finding that koilocytes, a possible marker for HPV infection, were present in 70% of cytologic and biopsy specimens showing cervical intraepithelial neoplasia (CIN) (Fig. 3). It has also been recognized that as the grade of CIN increases, the detection of koilocytes decreases, and they are absent in frank carcinoma. Similarly, the detection of HPV antigens shows a similar decrease in higher grades of CIN. It is believed that permissive factors for productive viral infection are absent in higher grades of dysplasia and carcinoma. However, HPV DNA has been found in all grades of CIN as well as invasive cancer. The association with cervical neoplasia is strong, with as much as 91% of CIN lesions containing HPV DNA compared to 10% of controls.

HPV DNA types are not equally present in neoplastic lesions. Types 16 and 18 are present in 70% of cancers, and types 10, 11, 31, 33, 35, 46, 51, and 56 are present in small percentages. However, types 16 and 18 are found in only a small percentage of genital warts, while type 6, the most common type found in genital warts, is found much less often in genital cancer. This has led to the concept of "high-risk" HPV types. The finding of HPV types 16 and 18 in genital lesions anywhere in the genital tract implies a greater tendency toward advanced grade neoplasia (as high as 85% in one study). The corollary is that the finding of HPV DNA type 6/11 indicates the lesion will usually not progress but will regress.

There seems to be an anatomic site selection for various HPV types. Types 16 and 18 seem to be detected in cervical neoplasia while HPV types 6 and 11 are more frequently found in the lower vaginal and vulvar lesions as well as in subclinical infection.

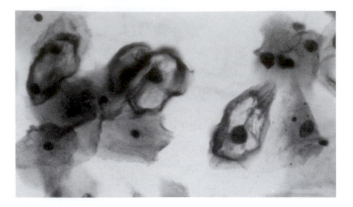

FIGURE 3 Koilocytotic changes demonstrable on cytologic smears (Papanicolaou's stain, ×490).

It has now been determined that about 100% of invasive cervical squamous carcinomas contain HPV DNA. The viral DNA has been detected both in primary and in metastatic cancers, with HPV 16 being the most prevalent type. Equally interesting is the finding of HPV DNA in histologically normal genital tissue in women with invasive carcinoma. This helps to confirm the concept that HPV infection is a generalized lower-genital-tract epithelial infection and is not localized to the area of the genital wart or the CIN lesion and the therapy must be commensurate with the extent of the lesion.

CLINICAL MANIFESTATIONS

Clinical versus Subclinical

The extent and spectrum of genital HPV infection has not been fully appreciated by patients or by most clinicians. The spectrum of the disease has become much broader than previously recognized because of newer diagnostic tools such as HPV DNA typing and the application of the colposcope for the detection of subclinical disease. Many clinicians still regard the presence of a vulvar condyloma as a nuisance local problem and do not consider its potential presence throughout the genital tract. HPV infection must be considered an infectious disease that in many cases will be present throughout the genital tract. Acceptance of this concept will significantly improve the chances for diagnosis and application of appropriate therapy techniques.

Vulva

The incidence of vulvar condylomata has increased 460% in the United States in the last 15 years. Age incidence is similar to other STDs, with peaks at 16 to 25 years. Vulvar condylomas appear as pink, whitish, or pigmented sessile tumors, with the surface of lobulated or pointed finger-like projections. The most common sites are the posterior introitus, perineal skin, labia minora, labia majora, and urethral orifice. Less common sites are the anus, clitoris, mons pubis, and crural folds. Small sessile warts or flat condyloma-like lesions, which are minimally elevated, pink papules, and plaques with a smooth surface may be missed during routine examination.

Generally, the majority of women with type 6 or 11 infection will not experience local complications. There is a direct association with HPV infection in the vagina and cervix, and, therefore, colposcopic examination is indicated as well as careful cytological surveillance.

Subclinical vulvar HPV infection may be detected by colposcopic examination of the vulva after application of 5% acetic acid. The acetic acid removes the surface mucus and causes the individual cells to swell, giving a white color to warty or neoplastic epithelium. Colposcopic patterns involve three distinct types of subclinical papillomavirus infection (SPI). These are the presence of vestibular papillae, fused papillae, and acetowhite epithelium.

The vestibular papillae are small, multiple villous projections largely confined to mucous membranes. Each villous projection resembles the individual aspirates of an exophytic condyloma. Histology will show a central capillary surrounded by koilocytotic dyskeratotic epithelium.

Fused papillae refer to individual papillae that have grown together, giving the vulvar skin a granular rather than villous appearance. These areas will show whitening with acetic acid and are associated with burning vulvar discomfort that is erroneously attributed to chronic *Candida albicans* infection.

Acetowhite epithelium is a flat, normal-appearing epithelium that turns white with application of 5% acetic acid. This may be found in vulvar areas and may act as a reservoir for high-risk HPV types. Acetowhite epithelium is usually multifocal.

Vagina

Vaginal HPV infection has been given less attention than vulvar or cervical because the lesions

1. seem to be asymptomatic,
2. seem to have less malignant potential,
3. may be more difficult to diagnose, and
4. are more difficult to treat satisfactorily.

Vaginal condylomas can be detected in as many as one-third of patients who have vulvar condylomas.

The condylomas are usually present in the upper and lower one-third, with "high-risk" DNA types more frequently found in the upper one-third and "low-risk" DNA types found in the lower one-third. Condylomas in the vagina are usually multiple. The lesions are small, raised, dense, white elevations with small aspirates. Although vaginal condylomas may be asymptomatic, vaginal discharge and pruritus frequently accompany the infection. In patients with recurrent episodes of bacterial vaginosis or monilial vaginitis, the presence of HPV infection should be investigated.

Subclinical vaginal HPV infection is more common than overt condyloma. Most changes can be seen with the colposcope after application of 5% acetic acid. In addition, staining the vaginal walls with Lugol's solution will aid in making the diagnosis.

A common lesion consists of elongated vaginal papillae, made up of clustered epithelial projections with a central capillary. These lesions are analogous to the fronds seen in classic condyloma. Histologic features include koilocytotic atypia and dyskeratosis. Capsid antigen is present in 30%, indicating infectivity.

A second colposcopically detectable lesion is acetowhite epithelium following 5% acetic acid application. Sharply demarcated areas of flat white epithelium are detected. Vascular patterns may be present and the small capillary loops are of uniform caliber. This lesion is more common in the upper one-third of the vagina. Punctuation and mosaicism are quite common in the upper vagina.

A third and most common colposcopically detectable lesion is that of "reverse punctuation." This is defined as a diffuse pattern of minimally elevated white dots against the pink background of the vaginal mucosa. The appearance is made more prominent by staining with quarter-strength Lugol's solution. The parakeratotic "dots" will turn yellow. Histologic findings include minimal basal hyperplasia, mild koilocytosis, variable dyskeratosis, and prominent intraepithelial capillaries.

Cervix

Condyloma acuminatum of the cervix which are clinically apparent lesions can now be seen in 20% of HPV-infected women. These lesions are recognized by papillary projections often with irregular vascular loops beneath the epithelium. HPV infection is usually detected within the transformation zone but can involve the original squamous epithelium of the portico.

Subclinical cervical HPV infection is generally accepted as being most common and becoming visible with application of acetic acid. Cervical HPV infection is one of the most common STDs. The cytopathic effects of HPV include koilocytotic atypia, dyskeratosis, and multinucleation.

Colposcopic differentiation of SPI and significant grades of CIN can be difficult. A colposcopic index devised by Reid and Scalzi aids in the process by using four colposcopic signs (lesion margin, color, vascular patterns, and iodine staining) as a means to direct biopsies to the most severe areas (Table 3). SPI represents the earliest stage in the CIN continuum that leads to invasive cancer. The evidence is strong that women with koilocytotic atypia on Pap smear will show CIN and that approximately 25% will progress to CIN 3 within two years. The spontaneous regression rate is low (11%). The transit time to CIN 3 today for these groups of women is shorter than that described 20 years ago and probably reflects the impact of HPV on the process.

Anus

Clinical vulvar condylomas extend into the anal canal and perianal region in about 18% of women. Lesions can be found above the dentate line in the lower rectum. Growth in the perianal region tends to be luxuriant, painful, and difficult to treat.

Subclinical infection is common and 5% acetic acid should be applied prior to colposcopic evaluation. Histology shows characteristic HPV infection.

DIAGNOSIS OF HPV INFECTION

The diagnosis of HPV infection may be easy or very difficult. Diagnostic techniques include physical examination, colposcopy, cytologic studies, histologic studies, HPV antigen detection, ploidy studies of HPV DNA molecular hybridization, PCR assay, hybrid capture, and Southern and dot blots.

Southern blot and dot blot use radioactive probes and are labor intensive. They require a significant sample size. DNA hybridization involves nonradioactively labeled DNA probes. It can be performed on formalin-fixed, paraffin-embedded tissues and requires little specialized equipment.

Physical examination of the genital tract is simple and noninvasive. However, this method alone fails to detect most cervical HPV infections and an unknown proportion of vaginal, vulvar, anal, and penile lesions.

If wart-like lesions are present on the vulva, visual diagnosis is 90% correct. It is appropriate to initiate therapy on the basis of visual diagnosis. However, should the patient fail to respond to therapy or the "warts" (*i*) appear atypical, (*ii*) are pigmented or change color, (*iii*) are fixed to underlying tissues, (*iv*) exceed 1 cm (possible Buschke-Lowenstein growths), an excisional biopsy should be seriously considered.

The differential diagnosis includes the following:
1. Normal anatomic structures
2. Vestibular papillae
3. Sebaceous glands
4. Molluscum contagiosum
5. Seborrheic keratoses
6. Lichen planus
7. Skin tags
8. Melanocytic nevi
9. Condyloma latum

Colposcopic examination after the application of acetic acid is time consuming but detects most of the SPI. The colposcope will help the clinician find the areas that need to be biopsied. The colposcopic examination must include the vulva, vagina, cervix, and anus. The entire area should be exposed to acetic acid for at least five minutes prior to examination.

Cytologic studies are a relatively inexpensive method of diagnosing HPV infection on epithelial surfaces from which exfoliated cells can be obtained (Fig. 3). The cytologic findings of koilocytosis, dyskaryosis, atypical parabasal cells, and multinucleation can be seen. Anal cytology has been demonstrated to be useful in screening for anal HPV infection, but urinary cytology was not useful as a screening procedure for HPV infection in male consorts of women with genital warts. It is not known whether penile or vulvar cytology is useful or practical.

The histologic findings of genital warts are basal cell hyperplasia, acanthosis, papillomatosis, koilocytosis, parakeratosis, and mild nuclear atypia (Figs. 4–6). Koilocytosis is probably the most specific marker for HPV infection; however, the specificity of koilocytosis is poor for lesions caused by HPV DNA types 16 and 18, especially in advanced grades of CIN.

HPV antigens can be detected in cytologic or histologic specimens by immunoperoxidase-staining techniques utilizing antisera made in rabbits immunized to BPV. The cells carrying the virus are well-differentiated keratinocytes and often koilocytes. As the dysplasia becomes progressive, it becomes increasingly difficult to detect HPV antigens. Similarly, lesions containing HPV 16 and 18 have poor sensitivity for detection of HPV antigens.

The diagnostic tests that give the clinician the most information are the detection and typing of HPV DNA in clinical specimens. This may be in conjunction with a Pap smear or "Thin Prep" cytological analysis. HPV DNA detection and typing allows a risk assessment on the presence of high-risk or low-risk virus, which can be used to monitor and manage treatment. Two types of tests are currently available. One, called "hybrid capture," indicates the presence of low-risk or high-risk virus without specific type information. The other indicates the presence of a series of the most prevalent high-risk and low-risk viruses in a type-specific manner. This is a fast-moving field that is likely to have a big impact on patient management.

THERAPY FOR HPV INFECTION

The classic standard therapy for genital warts has been based on the assumption that the grossly visible warty tissue needs to be destroyed and that the virus resides only where the warts exist. The recognition of subclinical disease in addition to overt disease and the association with genital neoplasia forces a reevaluation of the standard approach. HPV infection must be regarded as having the potential for infecting the entire genital tract, and only very early disease tends to be localized. Therapy is also complicated by the fact that HPV may be present in normal skin and in colposcopically, cytologically, and histologically normal epithelium. Wart recurrence after any therapy is common, and whether a virologic "cure" can be accomplished is unknown. Practically all clinical trials address only overt visible disease. Wart recurrence after therapy is difficult to assess. It is not known whether recurrence indicates failure of therapy, failure to treat all areas involved, resistant virus, or reinfection. Most recurrences are seen within three months of therapy. If disease is present for six months despite repetitive attempts at therapy, it is called resistant and persistent.

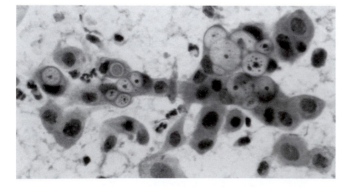

FIGURE 4 Koilocytotic changes involving glandular cells (Papanicolaou's stain, ×360).

Therapy uses agents that are keratolytic [podophyllin, tri- or bichloracetic acid, 5-fluorouracil (5-FU)], physical agents (electric cautery, laser therapy, cryotherapy), and immunotherapy (vaccine, interferon inducers). Since the classic standard approach must be modified to account for subclinical infection and the frequent presence of HPV throughout the genital tract, no single agent or combination of agents has emerged as standard treatment at this time.

Options

Currently available treatments for visible genital warts are patient-applied therapies: podofilox (Condylox®) and imiquimod (Aldara®); and provider-administered therapies: cryotherapy, podophyllin resin, trichloroacetic acid (TCA), bichloracetic acid, interferon (Intron, Alferon), and surgery. Most patients have one to ten genital warts, with a total wart area of 0.5 to 1.0 cm², which is amenable to most treatment modalities. Factors that may influence selection of treatment include wart size, wart count, anatomic site, wart morphology, patient preference, financial cost of treatment, and clinician's experience. It is important to have a treatment plan or protocol since many patients will require a course of therapy rather than a single treatment. The treatment should be no worse than the disease. In general, warts on moist surfaces and/or located in intertriginous areas respond better to topical treatment such as TCA, podophyllin, podofilox, and imiquimod than do warts on drier surfaces.

After the utilization of provider-administered treatments, if there has not been significant improvement after three treatment sessions, or complete clearance after six treatment sessions, the treatment modality should be changed. The risk–benefit ratio of treatment should be evaluated throughout the course of therapy in order to avoid overtreatment. Providers should be knowledgeable about, and have available to them, at least one patient-applied and one provider-administered modality.

When employed properly, complications of wart treatment are rare but can occur. Scarring in the form of persistent hypo- or hyperpigmentation may occur with ablative modalities. Depressed or hypertrophic scars are rare but can occur especially when the patient has not had sufficient time to heal between treatments. Overly aggressive treatment can result in disabling chronic pain syndrome such as vulvodynia or hypoesthesia of the treatment.

Patient Applied
Podofilox 0.5% Solution or Gel (Condylox®)

Podofilox, being an antimitotic, causes localized tissue necrosis. The 5% solution or gel does not contain the mutagenic flavanoid compounds found in the provider-applied analog podophyllin. Patients may apply podofilox solution with a cotton swab, or podofilox gel with a finger, to visible genital warts twice daily for three days, followed by four days of no therapy. This cycle may be repeated as necessary for a total of four cycles. Total wart area treated should not exceed 10 cm², and a total volume of podofilox should not exceed 0.5 mL per day. If possible, the healthcare provider

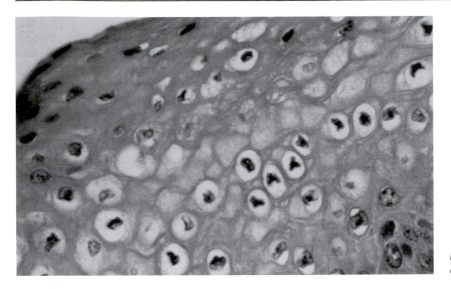

FIGURE 5 Histological demonstration of koilocytes with variable dyskeratosis (H&E stain, ×375).

should apply the initial treatment to demonstrate the proper application technique and identify which warts should be treated. The use of podofilox is contraindicated during pregnancy. Between 45% and 82% of patients treated for four to six weeks achieve total clearance of warts; however, 10% to 90% can be anticipated to experience recurrences.

Imiquimod 5% Cream (Aldara®)
Imiquimod is a topically active, nonnucleoside, heterocycline amine, immune-response enhancing agent. It is a potent inducer of interferon-alpha and other cytokines. Patients should apply imiquimod cream with a finger, at bedtime, three times per week, for up to 16 weeks. It is recommended that 6 to 10 hours following the application, the treatment area be washed with mild soap and water. Many patients may be clear by 8 to 10 weeks or sooner. The use of imiquimod is contraindicated in pregnancy.

This therapeutic approach is unique in that the host's cell-mediated immunity is used to destroy the warts. Imiquimod is used to sensitize the patient, and when this is accomplished, the imiquimod is placed in a cream which is placed on the wart. A delayed hypersensitivity reaction occurs that destroys the wart. The difficulties of therapy include an inability to sensitize the patient, varying sensitivity with potential for severe reaction, and the patient's resistance to a hypersensitivity reaction in the perineal area.

Between 37% and 85% of patients treated with 5% cream exhibit wart clearance after therapy. Between 13% to 19% of these patients can be expected to have recurrences.

Provider Administered Cryotherapy
Cryotherapy causes cryocytolysis, resulting in tissue sloughing. Cryotherapy of anogenital warts employs either single or repetitive one- to two-minute freeze–thaw cycles to destroy wart tissue. Cryotherapy may be performed by probe or liquid nitrogen. Most patients require three to six treatments to clear the warts. In comparative studies, cryotherapy is more effective than podophyllin and is as effective as electrical cautery and laser therapy. Between 60% and 97% will have

total clearing by three to six weeks. Wart recurrences may occur in 20% to 79% of patients so treated.

Keratolytic Agents
Podophyllin Resin 10% to 25%: This is a compound tincture of benzoin. Podophyllin is an extract from May apples, and there are four active ingredients which vary in concentration in different lots of podophyllin. It acts by poisoning the mitotic spindle and causing intense vasospasm. A small amount should be applied to each wart and allowed to air dry. To avoid the possibility of problems with systemic absorption and toxicity, some experts recommend that application be limited to ~0.5 mL or ~10 cm^2 of warts per session.

The patient is instructed to wash off the podophyllin in four to six hours. It is applied to warts weekly until the

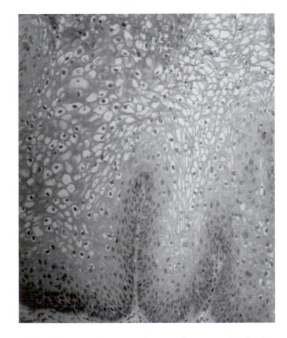

FIGURE 6 Elongated rete ridges with extensive koilocytotic change (H&E stain, ×220).

wart disappears. The side effects are unpredictable and include severe local reaction at initiation and ulceration and systemic toxicity from excessive absorption. Podophyllin is contraindicated in pregnancy because of teratogenesis and possible carcinogenesis.

Podophyllin's success is dependent on the size and number of lesions and is indicated in patients with minimal vulvar or anal disease. It is generally not used for vaginal or cervical HPV infection. Its use has diminished significantly.

TCA (Bichloracetic Acid) 80% to 90%: The mode of action of TCA is by precipitation of surface proteins and, therefore, it is less effective when applied to keratinized epithelium. It should be used at a strength of 85%. Application should be via small cotton-tipped applicator. It is not necessary to apply paraffin to adjacent skin as this is cumbersome and counterproductive. Powder with talc or sodium bicarbonate (baking soda) is used to remove unreacted acid if an excess amount is applied. TCA has been used on occasion on lesions of the cervix and seems to be well tolerated and effective. However, no randomized clinical trial of TCA therapy of cervical HPV disease has been published. Clearance rates between 50% and 100% have been reported. Between 6% and 50% of patients so treated may develop recurrences.

5-Fluorouracil: This agent is a pyrimidine antimetabolite that causes necrosis and sloughing of growing tissue. The 5% 5-FU cream is applied by several protocols:

1. *Vulvar or anal lesions*: 5-FU is applied directly to the lesion on a daily basis until erythema to vesiculation occurs. This will generally occur on about the 7th to 10th day of therapy. The course may be repeated to any remaining lesions following initial healing. A preferable alternative therapy is the administration of 5-FU on two consecutive days per week for 10 to 12 weeks. This seems to diminish the inflammatory reaction that results from 7 to 10 days of consecutive therapy.

3. *Vaginal lesions*: A vaginal tampon should be placed at the introitus to prevent the 5-FU from getting to the vulva.

A preferable alternative method is to use 5-FU once weekly for 10 to 12 weeks to diminish the vaginitis from the more intensive course of therapy. This has been found to be equally effective as the more intensive course. Randomized, placebo-controlled studies have demonstrated total wart clearance in 55% to 65% of patients. Between 30% and 45% of patients will have recurrences within three months after the completion of therapy.

5-FU is a mutagen and is contraindicated in pregnant and lactating women.

Surgical Removal
Tangential scissor excision, tangential shave excision, curettage, and electrosurgery have all been utilized with varying degrees of success.

Laser Therapy
Laser therapy is widespread and has the theoretical advantages of precise control of depth, margins, and hemostasis.

Laser ablation has the disadvantages of being under operator control as well as being able to treat only visible disease. Recurrences occur in 25% to 100% of cases. Some clinicians have extended their field of treatment to account for latent HPV at the margins, but more than one-half of these women have recurrences and the morbidity is excessive. The use of 5-FU immediately following laser therapy of the vagina has been proposed, in which 5-FU is placed intravaginally daily for five days. The success and morbidity rates need to be confirmed. The use of electrical cautery destruction of warts has been found to be very effective. It is particularly useful for office destruction of small lesions. It may be used for larger warts but the laser offers more precision.

Cytokine Immunotherapy
Interferons are a family of proteins with antiviral, antiproliferative, and immunomodulatory properties. Interferon has been shown to induce reversion of BPV-transformed mouse cells and elimination of extrachromosomal viral DNA.

Leukocyte interferon, alpha-recombinant interferon, beta interferon, and lymphoblastoid interferon have been used in the treatment of warts topically, intralesionally, and systemically. Generally speaking, the topical therapy is least effective; intralesional therapy is effective for a small wart number or volume; and systemic therapy is effective for large wart numbers and volumes and especially for intravaginal warts. Although the preparations of interferon doses and treatment regimens varied, the studies have reported positive results; however, only the responses of clinically overt lesions have been evaluated. The potential advantages of therapy with systemic interferon include therapy of all wart-affected areas at the same time, the potential of eliminating the HPV from the patient, and lower morbidity than other techniques. Interferon is administered parenterally either by intralesional or by subcutaneous routes. The intralesional route is recommended by the package inserts and has Food and Drug Administration approval. This route is very painful to the patient because wart tissue is very dense and distention with even small amounts of interferon is very uncomfortable. The usual scenario that occurs is that the clinician injects the wart intralesionally with the first injection; however, on the subsequent injections, the clinician places the interferon under the wart, i.e., subcutaneously, and therefore the injection is painless. We have found that a superior method without the loss of efficacy is the patient's self-administration of interferon subcutaneously in the anterior thigh. The administration is with a 29 gauge needle and TB syringe. The dosage of interferon should be 2.5 or 3.0 million units three times per week for eight weeks. The patient should have a complete blood count with platelets, and liver function tests determination prior to initiation of interferon. If the pulmonary tests are normal, no additional testing is necessary. This program will result in a clearing of the condyloma in 65% to 70% of the patients. Follow-up data from patients achieving a complete clearing of the condyloma showed a recurrence rate of <5% in two years.

Side effects are dose dependent and are minimal at 3 million units three times per week. Side effects will occur in less than 10% of patients at this dosing level. The most frequent side effects at this dose level are transient malaise, fatigue, and headache. Experience with interferon therapy has shown that if any external genital warts remain after eight weeks of therapy, interferon may be continued for another four weeks. An alternative therapy for condyloma at the conclusion of the primary interferon course is the use of CO_2 laser, cryotherapy, or surgical excision. The combination of laser ablation as primary therapy plus interferon 1.0 million units three times per week for 10 weeks may be successful for the patient who wants immediate wart removal.

Therapy of HPV in Pregnancy

The true incidence of genital HPV infection during pregnancy is unknown, but it is probably greater than in the general population. Existing lesions tend to enlarge during pregnancy, probably in response to diminished cell-mediated immunity (Fig. 7). These lesions may become large and friable, causing pain and hemorrhage. The fetal effects are those of the possibility of passage of HPV to the fetus during delivery. Congenital, infant, and childhood genital condylomas have been reported in children born to mothers known to have genital warts; however, it is not known how many pregnant women harbor HPV. The number of children with respiratory papillomatosis is low. Recent data from the Perinatal Collaborative Study reported no cases in a seven-year followup of 44,000 deliveries. Recurrent respiratory papillomatosis Is rare with a prevalence of 4 In 100,000 children.

Therapy with podophyllin is contraindicated in pregnancy because of toxicity and teratogenesis. Agents such as bleomycin and 5-FU are also contraindicated because of their antimitotic and cytotoxic action. TCA (85%) solution is useful and can be applied weekly either to skin or to mucous membranes. Cryotherapy and CO_2 laser have been found to be helpful in reducing the number and volume of

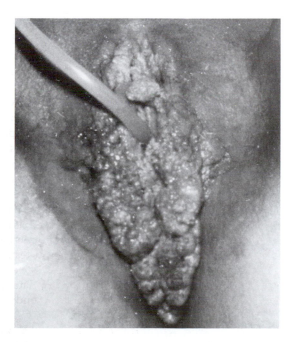

FIGURE 7   Extensive fused vulvar condyloma in pregnancy.

warts. Most of the time, the warts will diminish significantly after delivery.

A registry of Gardasil Inadvertent administration during the clinical vaccine trials in presented in Table 5.

Impact of HIV on HPV

The concomitant epidemic of HIV and HPV more than overlap each other. Findings from a number of clinical studies suggest that while HPV does not appear to alter the course or frequency of HIV infections, HIV-induced immunosuppression does increase the severity and duration of anogenital warts. Also, it is probable that it increases the period of infectiousness and decreases the probability of a good clinical response to conventional therapy. The impact of HIV on HPV pathogenesis appears to extend beyond increased clinical recognition of conventional lesions and severity of disease. If demographic studies are correct, preinvasive and ultimately invasive cervical neoplasia are becoming more common manifestations in patients with dual infections.

The magnitude of host immunosuppression influences the probability of premalignant and/or preinvasive histological changes. Spinillo et al. (1992) evaluated the prevalence of lower-genital neoplasia and HPV-related genital lesions in each cohort of 75 women infected with HIV 1 at different stages of the disease. The overall rate of CIN in the group studies was 29.3% (22/75). Eight out of ten high-grade CIN lesions contained "high-risk" HPV DNA 16/18 and/or 31/35/51 as demonstrated by in situ hybridization with biotinylated probes. Vulvar and/or perianal condylomata were histologically diagnosed in 14 patients (18.7%); nine of these biopsies contained detectable HPV DNA, which was always related to HPV 6/11.

The rate of high-grade CIN-symptomatic HIV-infected patients was 28% (7/25), compared to 6% (3/50) of the other cases ($p = 0.02$). CD4+ lymphocyte counts, white blood cell counts, the CD4+/CD8+ cell ratio, and the percentage of CD4+ lymphocytes were lower in patients with high-grade CIN than in patients with negative colposcopic and/or

TABLE 5   Pregnancy outcomes in the quadrivalent HPV vaccine phase III database

Outcome	Quadrivalent HPV vaccine		Placebo	
	No.	(%)	No.	(%)
Women with pregnancies	1115	(10.7)	1151	(12.6)
No. of pregnancies	1244		1272	
Infants/fetuses with known outcomes	996		1018	
Live births[a]	621	(62.3)	611	(60.0)
Spontaneous miscarriage[a]	249	(25.0)	(257)	(25.2)
Late fetal deaths[a]	11	(1.1)	8	(0.8)
Congenital anomalies[a]	15	(1.5)	16	(1.6)

[a]Percentage of those with known outcomes.
Source: Food and Drug Administration. Vaccines and Related Biological Products Advisory Committee, May 18, 2006: FDA GARDASIL briefing information. Rockville, MD: US Department of Health and Human Services, Food and Drug Administration: 2006.

cytological examinations. After adequate standard treatment (cryotherapy, electrocauterization, cold-knife conization), only one case of CIN 2 recurred during the two-year follow-up period. The prevalence of lower-genital neoplasia and HPV-related lesions among HIV-infected women is high (compared with 9% of 76 intravenous drug users who were HIV negative and 4% of 526 new high-risk women) and therefore seems to correlate with the severity of HIV disease.

Johnson et al. correlated HPV DNA testing with CD4 T-cell status in 32 HIV-infected women using colposcopy, Pap smears, and PCR. Women with a CD4 T-cell count below 200/mL were considered to be functionally immunosuppressed. The frequency of HPV positivity was fivefold higher among immunocompromised women (9 of 10) than in relatively immunocompetent HIV-infected women (4 of 22). Four immunosuppressed women, compared with no immunocompetent subjects, showed evidence of HPV DNA without signs of HPV-associated lesions by cytology or histology (i.e., latent HPV infection). Furthermore, four of the nine immunocompromised subjects, compared with four of the 21 immunocompetent subjects, had CIN. HPV 18 was detected in five of the ten women with CD4 T-cell counts below 200/mL and in only one of the 22 with CD4 T-cell counts above that level. These results suggest that impaired immune status, as reflected by the CD4 T-cell count, was an important factor in increasing the severity of HPV-induced cervical infection in their population.

HPV is not a true opportunistic infection; however, its apparent progression to cervical neoplasia can be viewed as an opportunistic complication of a concomitant infection/disease. Laga et al. (1992) followed 47 HIV-seropositive and 48 HIV-seronegative patients. Thirty-eight percent of the HIV-seropositive and eight percent of the seronegative women (odds ratio = 6.8; $p = 0.001$) had HPV DNA. This was found using

1. Vira Type (a dot-blot assay which detects specific genital HPV types) or
2. low-stringency Southern blot (a blot that detects all HPV types).

Eighty-two women (86%) had an interpretable Pap smear; 11 of 41 (27%) HIV-seropositive women and one of 41 (3%) seronegative women had CIN (odds ratio = 14.7; $p = 0.002$). HPV was detected in 8 of 11 (73%) seropositive women with CIN.

As many as 12% of all HIV-infected individuals develop malignant lymphoma, primarily of non-Hodgkin's B-cell phenotype. The etiology is unclear, but may be facilitated by long-term Ayidothymidine therapy. HIV may be associated with reactivation of a chronic hepatitis B virus (HBV) infection, and HBV itself may induce HIV replication in latently infected cells, through its X gene. When viewed in an abstract sense, the STD wars are a collective tribute to what can be achieved as a consequence of the diversity of the genetic pool. It should be a warning to those who would seek to limit genetic diversity.

Vaccines and Immunotherapy

HPV infection is a very common event. However, host immunity typically resolves most infections. Only a small fraction of acquired infections progress to detectable disease.

In the early 1990s, several groups showed that production of the HPV virus major coat protein L1 in an rDNA system resulted in the formation of virus-like particles (VLPs). VLPs are arrays of L1 proteins arranged in a manner similar to that of the outer surface of a papillomavirus. This vaccine design had previously been used for the rDNA hepatitis B vaccine licensed in the mid-1980s. Two HPV vaccines have been developed using this method. A quadrivalent vaccine with HPV 6/11/16/18 Gardasil ™ (Merck) and a bivalent HPV 16/18 Cervarix TM (GlaxoSmithKline(GSK), consisting of L1 coat proteins in the form of VLPs.

Protection provided by these vaccines appears to be by the production of IgG serum neutralizing antibody that Is type specific after IM administration of these vaccines. The current studies show that vaccine antibody titers are higher then those generated by natural Infection and persist for at least 5 years. Several Important features of these vaccines must be emphazied. these vaccines do not contain any HPV DNA and are non-Infectious. they are made up of the L! protein of the specific virus type plus and adjuvant. Side effects are listed In (Table 6 and 7).

Endpoints for the clinical studies were the precursor of Invasive cervical (vulvar, vaginal) cancer High-grade CIN

TABLE 6 Injection-site adverse events among female participants aged 9–23 years in the detailed safety data, days 1–5 after any vaccination with quadrivalent HPV vaccine

Adverse event	Quadrivalent HPV vaccine (% occurrence)	Aluminum-containing placebo (% occurrence)	Saline placebo (% occurrence)
Pain	83.9	75.4	48.6
Mild to moderate	81.1	74.1	48.0
Severe	2.8	1.3	0.6
Swelling[a]	25.4	15.8	7.3
Mild to moderate	23.3	15.2	7.3
Severe	2.0	0.6	0
Erythema[a]	24.7	18.4	12.1
Mild to moderate	23.7	18.0	12.1
Severe	0.9	0.4	0

[a]Intensity of swelling and erythema was measured by size (inches): mild, 0 to ≤1: moderate, >1 to ≤2: severe, >2.
Source: Food and Drug Administration. Product approval information—licensing action, package insert: GARDASIL (quadrivalent human papillomavirus types 6, 11,16, and 18), Merck & Co. Whitehouse Station, NJ: Food and Drug Administration: 2006.

TABLE 7 Systemic clinical adverse events among female participants aged 9–23 years in the population with detailed safety data, days 1–15 after vaccination with quadrivalent HPV vaccine

Adverse event (1–15 days postvaccination)	Quadrivalent HPV vaccine (N =5,088)	Placebo (N =3,790)
Pyrexia	13.0	11.2%
Nausea	6.7%	6.6%
Nasopharyngitis	6.4%	6.4%
Dizziness	4.0%	3.7%
Diarrhea	3.6%	3.5%
Vomiting	2.4%	1.9%
Myalgia	2.0%	2.0%
Cough	2.0%	1.5%
Toothache	1.5%	1.4%
Upper respiratory tract infection	1.5%	1.5%
Malaise	1.4%	1.2%
Arthralgia	1.2%	0.9%
Insomnia	1.2%	0.9%
Nasal congestion	1.1%	0.9%

Source: Food and Drug Administration. Product approval information—licensing action, package insert: GARDASIL (quadrivalent human papillomavirus types 6,11,16, and 18). Merck & Co. Whitehouse Station, NJ: FDA; 2006

(CIN 2/3). (Table 8). In placebo-controlled randomized clinical trials of women approximately 15 to 26 years of age, both vaccines showed close to 100% protection against CIN grades 2 or 3 caused by the types of HPV VLPs included in the vaccines. The vaccines have had no impact on preexisting infection or disease. The vaccines encompassing HPV 16 and 18 cover approximately 70% of the anticipated high-grade cervical lesions. The GSK vaccine contains HPV types 16 and 18. The Merck vaccine contains types 16 and 18 as well as types 6 and 11, which are the most common HPV that induce nonmalignant genital warts.

The quadrivalent Merck vaccine was licensed for use in the United States in june of 2006. The GSK vaccineis still under review by the FDA. In 2077, the ACIP published the recommended age for vaccination is 11–12 years; vaccine can be administered to females as young as age 9 years. At the beginning of a vaccination program, females aged >12 years will exist who did not have the opportunity to receive vaccine at age 11–12 years. Catch-up vaccination is recommended for females aged 13–26 years who have not yet been vaccinated. The vaccine is given intramuscularly in a three-dose regimen at zero, two, and six months for the Merck vaccine.

HPV vaccines provide the opportunity to prevent, rather than treat, a significant portion of cervical, vulva and vaginal cancer.

SELECTED READING

Barnes W, Delgado G, Kurman RJ, et al. Possible prognostic significance of human papillomavirus type in cervical cancer. Gynecol Oncol 1988; 29:267.

Beckman AM, Myerson D, Doling Jr, et al. Detection of human papillomavirus DNA in carcinomas by in-situ hybridization with biotinylated probes. J Med Virol 1985; 16:265.

Billingham RP, Lewis RG. Laser versus electrical cautery in the treatment of condylomata acuminata of the anus. Surg Gynecol Obstet 1982; 155:865.

TABLE 8 Summary of quadrivalent HPV vaccine efficacy studies in the per protocol populations[a]

Outcome and protocol	Quadrivalent vaccine		Placebo		% Efficacy	(95% CI)
	No[b]	Cases	No.	Cases		
HPV 16-or 18-related CIN 2/3 or AIS[a]						
Protocol 005[c]	755	0	750	12	100.0	(65. 1–100.0)
Protocol 007	231	0	230	1	100.0	(−3734.9–100.0)
Protocol 013	2,200	0	2,222	19	100.0	(78.5–100.0)
Protocol 015	5,301	0	5,258	21	100.0[b]	(80.9–100.0)
Combined protocols[e]	8,487	0	8,460	53	100.00[d]	(92.9–100.0)
HPV 6-, 11-, 16-, 18-related CIN (CIN 1, CIN 2/3) or AIS						
Protocol 007	235	0	233	3	100.0[d]	(−137.8–100.0)
Protocol 013	2,240	0	2,258	37	100.0[d]	(89. 5–100.0)
Protocol 015	5,383	4	5,370	43	90.7	(74.4–97.6)
Combined protocols[e]	7,868	4	7,861	83	95.2	(87.2–98.7)
HPV 6-, 11-, 16-, 18-related genital warts						
Protocol 007	235	0	233	3	100.0	(−139,5–100.0)
Protocol 013	2,261	0	2,279	29	100.0	(86.4–100.0)
Protocol 015	5,401	1	5,387	59	98.3	(90.2–100.0)
Combined protocols[e]	7,897	1	7,899	91	98.9	(93.7–100.0)

Note: Point estimates and confidence intervals are adjusted for person-time of follow-up.
[a]Populations consisted of persons who received all 3 vaccinations within 1 year of enrollment, did not have major deviations from the study protocol, and were naïve (polymerase chain reaction-negative and serogative) to the relevant HPV type(s), (types 6, 11, 16, and 18) before dose 1 and through 1 month post dose 3 (month 7). Median follow-up time for protocols 007, 013, and 015 was 1.9 years; median follow-up time for protocol 005 was 3.9 years.
[b]Number of persons with at least 1 follow-up visit after month 7. [c]Evaluated only the HPV 16 L1 VLP vaccine component of GARDASIL. [d]P values were computed for pre-specified primary hypothesis tests. All p-values were < 0.001. supporting the following conclusions: efficacy against HPV 16/18-related CIN 2/3 is >0 (protocol 015); efficacy against HPV 16/18-related CIN 2/3 in >25% (combined protocols): and efficacy against HPV 6/11/16/18-related CIN is >20% (protocol 013). [e]Analyses of the combined trials were prospectively planned and included the use of similar study entry criteria.
Abbreviations: CI, confidence interval; CIN, cervical intraepithelial neoplasia; CIS, carcinoma in situ.
Source: Adapted from Food and Drug Administration. Product approval information—action, package insert: GARDASIL (quadrivalent human papillomavirus types 6, 11, 16, and 18), Merck & Co. Whitehouse Station, NJ: FDA; 2006.

Cullen AP, Reid R, Camion MJ, Lorincz AT. Analysis of the physical state of different papilloma virus DNAs in intraepithelial and invasive cervical neoplasms. J Virol 1991; 65:606.

Eron LF, Judson F, Tucker S, et al. Interferon therapy for condylomata acuminata. N Engl J Med 1986; 315:1059.

Felix JC, Wright TC. Clarification of equivocal history: HPV testing by in-situ hybridization and polymerase chain reaction of lesions clinically considered to be condyloma. Arch Pathol Lab Med 1994; 118:39.

Ferenczy A, Mitao M, Nagai N, et al. Latent papillomavirus and recurring genital warts. N Engl J Med 1985; 313:784.

Fuchs PG, Girardi F, Pfister H. Human papillomavirus DNA in normal, metaplastic, preneoplastic and neoplastic epithelia of the cervix uteri. Int J Cancer 1988; 41:41.

Gall SA, Hughes CE, Trofatter KF. Interferon for the therapy of condyloma acuminatum. Am J Obstet Gynecol 1985; 153:157.

Harper DM, Franco EL, Wheeler Cm et al. Sustained efficacy up to 4.5 years of a bivalent L1 virus-like particle vaccine against human papilloma viurs type 16 and 18: follow-up from a randomized control trial. Lancet. 2006; 367:1247.

Helmrich G, Stubbs TM, Stoerkor J. Fetal maternal laryngeal papillomatosis in pregnancy. Am J Obstet Gynecol 1992; 166:524.

Johnson JC, Burnett AF Willet JD, et al. High frequency of latent and clinical human papilloma virus cervical infections in immunocompromised human immunodeficiency virus-infected women. Obstet Gynecol 1992; 79:321.

Krebs HB. Prophylactic topical 5-fluorouracil following treatment of human papillomavirus associated lesions of the vulva and vagina. Obstet Gynecol 1986; 68:837.

Lorinez AT, Reid R, Jensen AB, et al. Human papillomavirus infection of the cervix: relative risk associated actions of 115 common anogenital types. Obstet Gynecol 1992; 79:328.

Reid R, Scalzi P. Genital warts and cervical cancer VII: an improved colposcopic index for differentiating benign papillomavirus infections from high grade cervical intraepithelial neoplasia. Am J Obstet Gynecol 1985; 153:611.

Tidy JA, Mason WP, Farrell PJ. A new and sensitive method of screening for human papillomavirus infection. Obstet Gynecol 1989; 74:410.

Vermund SH, Kelley KF, Klein RS, et al. High risk of human papilloma virus infection and cervical squamous intraepithelial lesions among women with symptomatic human Immunodeficiencey virus infection. Am J Obstet Gynecol 1991; 165:392.

Villa LL, Costa RI, Petta CA et al. High sustained efficacy of a prophylactic quadrivalent human papilloma virus types 6/11/16/18 L1 virus-like particle vaccine through 5 years of follow-up. Br J Cancer, 2006; 95:1459.

Reviews

Center for Disease Control. Quadrivalent Human Papillomavirus Vaccine. MMWR, 2007; 56RR-2:1.

Kirby P, Corey L. Genital human papillomavirus infection. Infect Dis Clin North Am 1987; 1:123.

Lorinez A, Reid R. Human papilloma virus II. Obstet Gynecol Clin N Am 1996; 23.

Lorinez A, Reid R. Human papilloma virus I. Obstet Gynecol Clin N Am 1996; 23.

Reid R, ed. Human papilloma virus. Obstet Gynecol Clin North Am 1987; 14:2.

Stanley M. Prophylactic HPV vaccines. JClin Pathol. 2007; 60:961.

Tasca RA, Clarke RW. Recurrent respiratory papillomatosis. Archives Dis Childhoo. 2006; 91:689.

HIV/HPV

Braun L. Role of human immunodeficiency virus infection in the pathogenesis of human papillomavirus-associated cervical neoplasia. Am J Pathol 1994; 144:209–214.

Clottey C, Dallabetta G. Sexually transmitted diseases and human immunodeficiency virus. Sex Transm Dis 1993; 7:753.

Elfgren K, Jacobs M, Jan MM, et al. Rate of human papillomavirus clearance after treatment of cervical intraepithelial neoplasia. Obstet Gynecol 2002; 100:965.

Franco EL, Villa LL, Sobrinobo JP, et al. Epidemiology of acquisition and clearance of cervical human papillomavirus in women from a high-risk area for cervical cancer. J Infect Dis 1991; 180:1415.

Henry-Stanley MJ, Simpson M, Stanley MW. Cervical cytology findings in women infected with the human immunodeficiency virus. Diagn Cytopathol 1993; 9:508–509.

Icenogle JP, Laga M, Miller D, et al. Genotypes and sequence variants of human papillomavirus DNAs from human immunodeficiency virus type I-infected women with cervical Intraepithelial neoplasia. J Infect Dis 1992; 166:1210–1216.

Johnson JC, Burnett AF, Willet GD, et al. High frequency of latent and clinical human papilloma virus cervical infection in immunocompromised human immunodeficiency virus-infected women. Obstet Gynecol 1992; 79:321–327.

KiviatNB, Koutsky LA, Critchlow CW, et al. Prevalence and cytological manifestations of human papilloma virus (HPV) types 6, 11, 16, 18, 33, 35, 42, 43, 44, 45, 51, 52, and 56 among 500 consecutive women. Int J Gynecol Path 1992; 11:197.

Kohl PK. Epidemiology of sexually transmitted diseases. What does it tell us? Sex Transm Dis 1994; 21:S81–S83.

Kreiss JK, Kiviat NB, Plummer FA, et al. Human immunodeficiency virus, human papillomavirus, and cervical intraepithelial neoplasia in Nairobi prostitutes. Sex Transm Dis 1992; 19:54–59.

Laga M, Icenogle JP, Marsella R, et al. Genital papillomavirus infection and cervical dysplasia Ñ opportunistic complication of HIV infection. Int J Cancer 1992; 50:45.

MMWR. Sexually transmitted diseases treatment guidelines. 1993; 42:1–102.

Northfelt DW. Cervical and anal neoplasia and HPV infection in persons with HIV infection. Oncology 1994; 8:3340.

Northfelt DW, Palefsky JM. Human papillomavirus-associated anogenital neoplasia in persons with HIV infection. AIDS Clin Rev 1992:241–259.

Quinn TC. Recent advances in diagnosis of sexually transmitted diseases. Sex Transm Dis 1994; 21:S19–S27.

Quinn TC, Zenilman J, Rompalo A. Sexually transmitted diseases: advances in diagnosis and treatment. Adv Intern Med 1994; 39:149–196.

Spinillo A, Tenti P, Zappatore R, et al. Prevalence, diagnosis and treatment of lower genital neoplasia in women with human immunodeficiency virus infection. Eur J Obstet Gynecol Reprod Biol 1992; 43:3541.

Vernon SD, Icenogle JP, Johnson PR, Reeves WC. Human papillomavirus, human immunodeficiency virus, and cervical cancer: newly recognized associations? Infect Agents Dis 1992; 1:319–324.

Woodman CBJ, Collins S, Winters H, et al. Natural history of cervical human papilloma-virus infection in young women: a longitudinal cohort study. Lancet 2001; 357:1831.

Human B-19 Parvovirus

Newton G. Osborne

16

INTRODUCTION

Parvovirus B-19, one of the parvoviruses known to infect humans, belongs to the family Parvoviridae, which includes two general DNA vertebrate viruses: genus parvovirus (autonomously replicating parvoviruses) and genus dependovirus (parvoviruses that require a helper virus, such as adenovirus or herpesvirus, for replication), and one genus of invertebrate viruses. Parvovirus B-19, discovered by Yvonne Cassart in 1970, is in the genus parvovirus, which includes a number of animal parvoviruses such as the canine parvovirus and feline panleukopenia virus. The parvoviruses tend to be species specific; only adeno-associated parvoviruses (members of the dependovirus genus) and B-19 are known to infect humans. Animal parvoviruses are known to cause fetal infection, nonimmune hydrops fetalis, intrauterine death, and abortion. Cerebral hypoplasia in kittens and pseudo-Down syndrome in hamsters have been attributed to intrauterine parvovirus infection.

B-19 parvovirus, a nonenveloped, single-stranded DNA virus about 20 nm in diameter, is responsible for benign illness in children (fifth disease) and in adults (arthritis). Acute or chronic anemia may occur following the lysis of its target cell, the erythroid progenitor.

CLINICAL DISEASE

Erythema Infectiosum (Fifth Disease)

The most commonly recognized illness associated with B-19 infection is erythema infectiosum (EI). The incubation period is usually 4 to 14 days, but can be as long as 20 days. The individual is contagious prior to the development of a rash. Aerosol spread is the principal method of dissemination. Respiratory secretions contain the virus up to the time of onset of rash or arthralgia and rarely thereafter. EI is a mild exanthematous childhood illness which begins as a bright red facial rash ("slapped cheek" appearance), and spreads to the trunk and extremities. As it fades, it produces a reticulated or lace-like appearance. Reappearance of the rash may occur for several weeks following nonspecific stimuli such as change in temperature, sunlight, and emotional stress. Typically, the patient is otherwise well at rash onset but often gives a history of mild systemic symptoms one to four days before rash onset. In some outbreaks, pruritus has been a common clinical feature.

Maternal parvovirus B-19 infection is often atypical or asymptomatic. Asymptomatic disease occurs in approximately 20% of the cases. Rash or fever, which is common in children, may not develop in adults. Viremia precedes the rash.

In adults, infection often produces a symmetrical peripheral polyarthropathy. Joints in the hands are most frequently affected, followed by the knees and wrists. Symptoms are usually self-limited but may persist for several months. Joint symptoms, more common in adults, may occur as the sole manifestation of infection.

The highest rate of attack is in school-age children and household contacts. Although commonly observed in children aged 2 to 12 years, approximately 40% of the individuals over 12 years of age are serosusceptible.

In adult patients, particularly women, arthralgia or arthritis has been associated with up to 80% involvement. The process usually starts in the small joints of the hand and progresses to larger joints. The presence of a rash involving primarily the face, or B-19 infection in the community, should suggest the possibility of fifth disease; however, arthralgia, arthritis, or arthrophy may occur in the absence of a rash.

Transient Aplastic Crisis

Human parvoviruses have a special affinity for rapidly dividing cells and, in particular, marrow erythroid progenitor cells. The virus attacks immature erythroblasts, arresting red blood cell (RBC) production. Destruction of erythroid lineage cells may involve apoptosis induced by the nonstructural protein of the virus. Parvovirus B-19 infections have been implicated in the induction of aplastic crisis in patients with sickle cell diseases, hereditary spherocytosis, and other chronic hemolytic anemias.

Parvovirus B-19 is the primary etiologic agent causing transient aplastic crisis (TAC) in patients with chronic hemolytic anemias (e.g., sickle cell disease, hemoglobin SC disease, hereditary spherocytosis, beta-thalassemia, and autoimmune hemolytic anemia). It can also cause TAC in other conditions in which increased red cell production is necessary to maintain stable red cell indices, as may occur in anemia due to blood loss. Patients with TAC typically present with pallor, weakness, and lethargy and may report a nonspecific prodromal illness in the preceding one to seven days. Few patients with TAC report a rash. In the acute phase of the illness, patients usually have a moderate to severe anemia with absence of reticulocytes, and bone marrow examination shows a hypoplastic or an aplastic erythroid series with a normal myeloid series. Recovery is indicated by a return of reticulocytes in the peripheral smear approximately seven to ten days after their disappearance. TAC may require transfusion and hospitalization and can be fatal if not treated promptly. In immunocompromised individuals, B-19 parvovirus may cause pure red cell aplasia.

HUMAN PARVOVIRUS INFECTION AND PREGNANCY

Approximately 50% of pregnant women have serological evidence of prior parvovirus B-19 infection. Prior infection confers immunity. Maternal disease is usually self-limited, but the effects on the fetus can be devastating.

Human parvovirus B-19 is a recognized cause of nonimmune hydrops fetalis. Hydrops fetalis is more likely to occur when there is fetal infection between the 10th and 20th weeks of gestation. It is diagnosed by demonstrating the accumulation of fluid in two or more body cavities of the fetus. The presence of fetal ascites, edematous fetal skin, pleural effusion, placental enlargement, placental edema, pericardial effusion, hepatosplenomegaly, and cardiomegaly can be detected with ultrasonography (Figs. 1–8). Infection is accompanied by characteristic intranuclear inclusions in fixed and circulating RBC precursors. These inclusions have been shown to contain virus particles by electron microscopy and in situ hybridization. Recent work has shown that parvovirus B-19 can infect cells other than erythroid precursors, such as myocardial cells. Infected fetuses are not always hydropic. Bailão et al. and Bonilla-Musoles et al. (2005) have reported that infection of fetal myocardial cells in the first trimester may cause fetal congestive heart failure, which in turn causes increased nuchal translucency (Figs. 7–10).

Maternal infection results in increased abortion and stillbirth. Early infected fetuses are particularly vulnerable to premature demise owing to their high erythrocyte turnover rate and limited hematologic reserves. The overall risk of fetal loss following maternal exposure is much less than previously thought, and may be less than 3% in the first 20 weeks of gestation with maternal exposure, or approximately 10% if the mother is actually infected. Although parvoviruses are teratogenic in animals, there is no evidence that B-19 is a significant human teratogen.

Parvovirus B-19 infection appears to be a significant cause of second-trimester abortions. Nyman et al. (2002) assessed the frequency of first-trimester fetal loss associated with parvovirus B-19 infection during a nonepidemic period in Sweden. Using B-19 DNA-specific polymerase chain reaction (PCR) in placental tissue, only 1 of 36 placentae examined from first-trimester losses contained detectable parvovirus B-19 DNA. In second-trimester fetal losses, 8 of 64 samples were B-19 DNA positive.

Ananda et al. (1987) have reported six women with serological evidence of having contracted human parvovirus infection during pregnancy. Two of the women had mid–third-trimester abortions. Both abortuses were grossly hydropic with anemia. Histopathological analysis revealed a pronounced leukoerythroblastic reaction, hepatitis, excess iron pigment in liver, and degenerative changes in the hematopoietic cell nuclei. Dot hybridization with radiolabeled human parvovirus probes revealed viral DNA in several tissues of both fetuses. The remaining four women had uncomplicated pregnancies and delivered apparently healthy babies, none of whom had human parvovirus–specific immunoglobulin M (IgM) antibodies at delivery.

Maeda et al. (1988) reported two cases of nonimmunologic hydrops fetalis associated with intrauterine human parvovirus B-19 infection. In these cases, hydrops fetalis was diagnosed with ultrasound at 21 and 22 weeks of gestation after 10 or more days of maternal flu-like symptoms. The outcome was stillbirth in one case and neonatal death in the other. In both cases, intrauterine infection by human parvovirus B-19 was confirmed based on two findings: maternal serum positive for human parvovirus B-19 IgM antibody, and human parvovirus B-19 DNA detected in the fetal organs using Southern blotting and hybridization with a labeled probe. Laboratory tests on cord blood demonstrated an RBC count of 163×10^4 mL nucleated

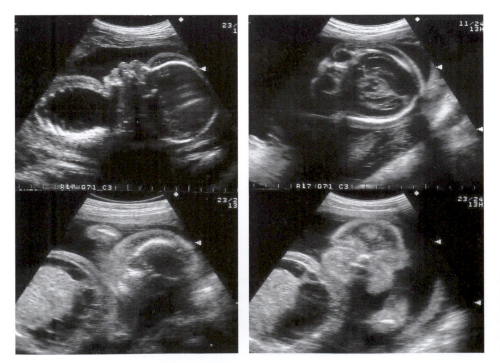

FIGURE I Two-dimensional (*upper frames*) and three-dimensional (*lower frames*) ultrasound images of second-trimester fetus with nonimmune hydrops fetalis. Observe the marked edema of the skin and ascites.

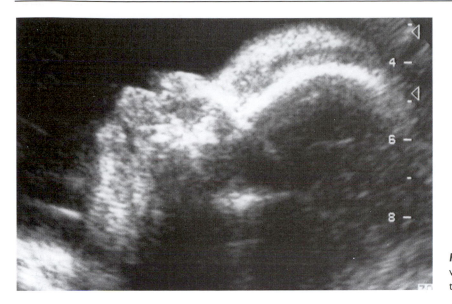

FIGURE 2 Sagittal two-dimensional ultrasound view of infected fetus with facial edema. Observe the skin separation from the fetal skull.

red cells, numbering 1267 per 50 white cells in the live-birth case. Histologic examinations of fetal tissues demonstrated leukoerythroblastic reaction in the liver and spleen, granular hemosiderin deposition in hepatocytes and Kupffer cells, and bilirubin deposition in the intercellular space in the liver. Hydropic changes may be induced by the sudden decrease in oxygen-carrying capacity of the blood due to severe anemia caused by the infection (Fig. 11).

Schwarz et al. (1990) serologically confirmed 80 acute cases of parvovirus B-19 infection in pregnancy using enzyme-linked immunosorbent assay (ELISA). Of the 80 pregnancies, four were terminated. Of the remaining 76 pregnancies, no fetal complications were observed in 36 (47.4%), hydrops fetalis occurred in 18 (23.7%), and no further information was available in 22 (28.9%). Of the 18 fetuses with hydrops, 15 died (83.3%). Intrauterine transfusion was performed in the remaining three fetuses and pregnancy continued without further complications.

Sheikh et al. (1992) reported two cases of fetal parvovirus B-19 infection with documented hydrops at 24 and 30 weeks of gestation. Serial sonograms demonstrated that the hydrops resolved spontaneously over three to five weeks after initial diagnosis. Both infants appeared normal at birth and developed normally through the first year of life.

Hager et al. (1998) studied 618 pregnant women exposed to parvovirus B-19. Of the 618 pregnant women, 307 (49.7%) were immune to B-19, 259 remained susceptible after exposure, and 52 (16.7% of all susceptibles) contracted B-19 infection. None of the 52 fetuses of infected women developed nonimmune hydrops, and there were no fetal deaths attributed to B-19 in this group. The risk of maternal B-19 infection in pregnancy was significantly higher when the source of exposure was her own child. Maternal symptoms of polyarthralgia (46%), fever (19%), and nonspecific rash (38%) were significantly more common ($p < 0.001$) in IgM-positive patients than in noninfected women

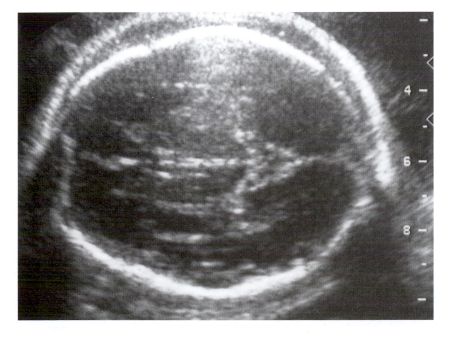

FIGURE 3 Transverse two-dimensional ultrasound view of the skull of the infected edematous fetus seen in Figure 2. Observe the skin separation from the skull due to fetal edema.

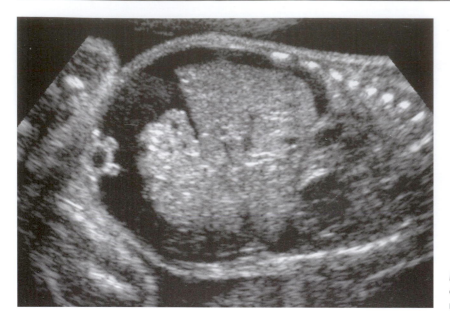

FIGURE 4 Two-dimensional ultrasound image of infected second-trimester hydropic fetus with marked fetal ascites.

1(4.1%, 2.8%, and 5.7% respectively). Only 17 (33%) of the IgM-positive women were entirely asymptomatic.

In the most comprehensive study done to date, Rodis et al. (1998) retrospectively surveyed the progeny of 113 immunoglobulin-positive women. The 113 pregnancies resulted in 103 term singletons, two sets of twins (of which one neonate died of complications of prematurity), one hydropic stillborn, four spontaneous abortions, and one ectopic pregnancy. The mean gestational age at time of exposure was 15.6 weeks. The median age of the liveborn infants in study and comparison groups was four years. Eight of the 108 (7.3%) surviving children, one set of twins (exposed at 27 weeks), and six singletons (exposed at 7, 8, 9, 20, 27, and 35 weeks) had developmental delays in speech, language, information processing, and attention. Their conclusion was that while there was no apparent increase in the frequency of developmental delays in children with exposure in utero to parvovirus, larger studies are needed. No increased incidence of congenital anomalies was identified.

Congenital Postnatal Infection

Adverse fetal/neonatal consequences are not limited to erythroid cells. The virus can infect and cause disease in myocardial and endothelial cells. Neonatal cases of myocarditis, hepatitis, and systemic necrotizing vasculitis have been described in infected infants.

In suspected cases of fetal infection, cordocentesis can be performed. If the technology is available, B-19–infected fetal erythroblasts can be detected by standard histological staining methods and in situ hybridization using a digoxigenin-labeled B-19 DNA probe and PCR.

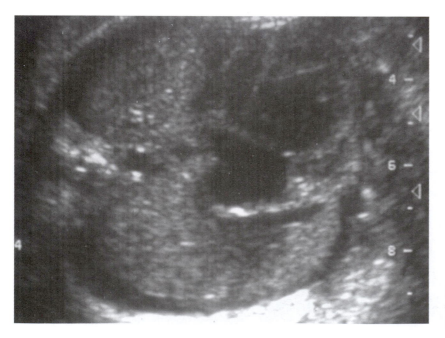

FIGURE 5 Two-dimensional ultrasound image of infected second-trimester hydropic fetus with pleural and pericardial effusions.

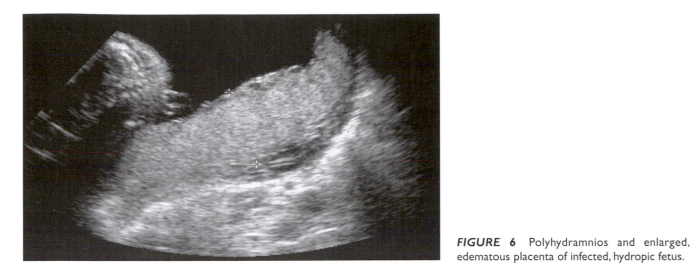

FIGURE 6 Polyhydramnios and enlarged, edematous placenta of infected, hydropic fetus.

Rather than being teratogenic, intrauterine human parvovirus infection appears to be embryocidal. No increase in the incidence of antiparvovirus antibodies occurs in malformed infants as compared with normal infants.

DIAGNOSIS

While a presumptive diagnosis can be inferred on clinical grounds, definite diagnosis requires serological confirmation. Immunoglobulin G (IgG) and IgM titers are available through the Centers for Disease Control (CDC) laboratories on a limited basis for women with clear-cut exposure to parvovirus B-19 infection during pregnancy. The most sensitive serological test to detect recent infection is the IgM antibody assay. Parvovirus B-19 IgM antibody can be detected by capture-antibody radioimmunoassay or enzyme immunoassay in approximately 90% of cases by the third day after symptoms of TAC or EI begin. The titer and the percentage of positives begin to decline 30 to 60 days after onset. Maternal IgM titers may drop to low or undetectable levels depending on the interval between maternal infection

and fetal signs of involvement. B-19 IgG antibody is usually present by the seventh day of illness and persists for years.

There are several methods to diagnose parvovirus infection. They rely on antibodies to the virus, PCR for detection of the virus, and histopathology.

An IgG antibody response occurs usually within a week of IgM antibody production. IgG antibody is protective and, if positive in the absence of IgM-specific antibodies, represents past exposure. The diagnosis by antibody testing is limited by the assay and reagents employed. Assays using serum-derived or recombinant antigens are significantly better than those using peptide antigens.

PCR assays for the detection of parvovirus DNA have been developed and applied to the clinical diagnosis of this disease. Amniotic fluid appears to be a good source to test for parvovirus DNA by PCR for the diagnosis of in utero infection.

Histological studies looking for inclusion-bearing cells (finding of characteristic intranuclear inclusions in nucleated erythroid cells in formalin-fixed placental or fetal tissues) can suggest the diagnosis of this infection.

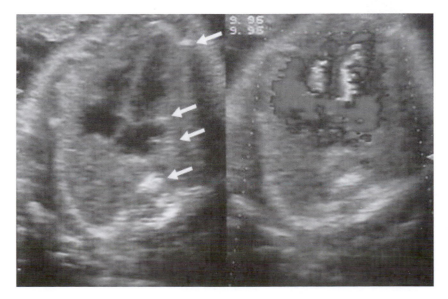

FIGURE 7 Myocardial infection in third-trimester fetus. Observe areas of cardiac calcification and pericardial effusion on the left frame. The right frame is a Doppler image that shows right ventricular enlargement secondary to congestive heart failure.

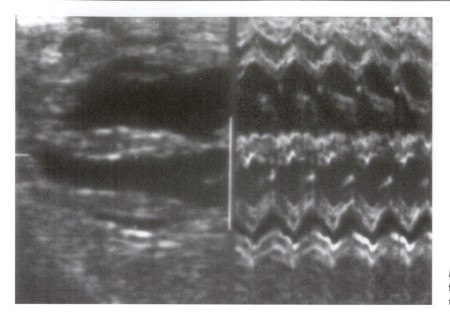

FIGURE 8 M mode image of heart of infected fetus with pericardial effusion and with right ventricular enlargement.

Fetal/neonatal serological response to infection can also exhibit variability. Only a minority of viral DNA confirmed cases of congenital infection will have a B-19 positive response. Infants exposed to the virus earlier in gestation are less likely to produce an IgM immune response; infants infected in the last trimester almost invariably do. The most definitive way to document infection is the demonstration of viral DNA in infected tissue samples.

For women with a documented infection, maternal serum alpha-fetoprotein levels and diagnostic ultrasound examina-

tions have been used to identify adversely affected fetuses. The sensitivity and specificity of these tests are 94.1% and 93.3% respectively. Fetal anemia caused by parvovirus infection can be detected noninvasively by Doppler ultrasonography on the basis of an increase in the peak velocity of systolic blood flow in the middle cerebral artery (Fig. 4).

The fetuses of gravidas with only IgG-specific antibodies are not at risk for the in utero development of nonimmune hydrops. If the mother has IgM-specific and no IgG-specific antibodies to human parvovirus B-19, the fetus is at risk. One-third of the progeny may develop an aplastic

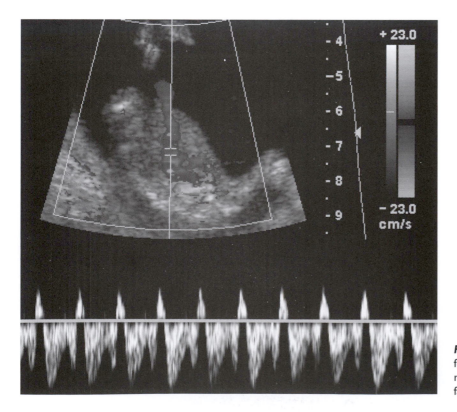

FIGURE 9 Doppler image of ductus venosus in fetus with myocardial infection. Observe the reverse flow resulting from fetal congestive heart failure.

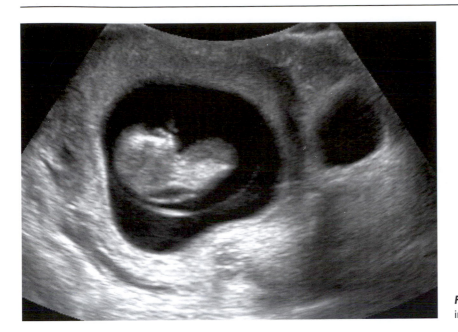

FIGURE 10 First-trimester infected fetus with increased nuchal translucency.

crisis resulting in fetal hydrops (Figs. 1 and 2). Current management dictates careful serological, clinical, and ultrasonographic evaluation of the fetus for evidence of hydrops fetalis (Table 1).

Nonimmune hydrops is the presence of excessive fetal body fluid accumulated in the tissues and serous cavities in the absence of RBC antibodies. Ultrasonic diagnosis includes subcutaneous edema (>5 mm), ascites, pleural effusion, pericardial effusion, excessive amniotic fluid, and placental edema (>6 cm) (Figs. 1–5). Hydrops fetalis can be diagnosed by ultrasonography as early as 10 to 14 days after maternal illness. The majority of fetuses that develop hydrops after maternal parvovirus infection do so within six to eight weeks of infection. Weekly ultrasound studies are recommended for eight weeks from the time of maternal infection or six weeks from the documented convalescent titer if the precise time of maternal infection is unknown.

When a fetus presents with hydrops, a diagnosis of parvovirus fetal infection can be made by detection of viral agents in amniotic fluid using PCR or ligase chain reaction tests.

THERAPY

The immune response to the virus is largely humoral and directed against limited numbers of epitopes. Persistent infection is due to failure to produce neutralizing antibodies. Because viral infection is prevalent in the population, therapeutic immune globulin preparations are a good source of anti–B-19 antibodies. IgG administration can lead to cure of anemia in the congenitally immunodeficient patient and to its amelioration in AIDS patients with persistent parvovirus infection. Treatment strategies may include supportive care, analgesic medications, transfusions with RBC, and administration of intravenous immunoglobulin, depending on the clinical circumstances.

Maternal therapy is largely symptomatic. Care should be given to limiting exposure to other gravidas.

TABLE I Management of material/fetal parvovirus infection

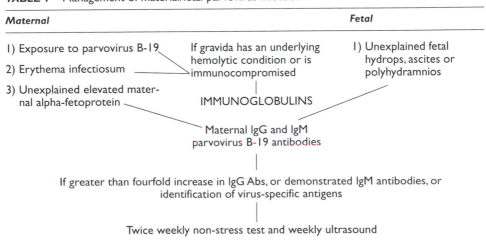

Maternal		*Fetal*
1) Exposure to parvovirus B-19	If gravida has an underlying hemolytic condition or is immunocompromised	1) Unexplained fetal hydrops, ascites or polyhydramnios
2) Erythema infectiosum		
3) Unexplained elevated maternal alpha-fetoprotein	IMMUNOGLOBULINS	

Maternal IgG and IgM parvovirus B-19 antibodies

If greater than fourfold increase in IgG Abs, or demonstrated IgM antibodies, or identification of virus-specific antigens

Twice weekly non-stress test and weekly ultrasound

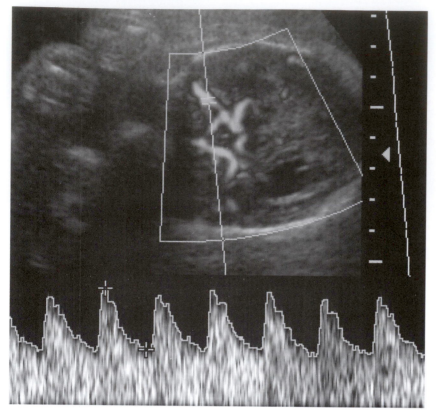

FIGURE 11 Doppler image of middle cerebral artery of infected fetus. Observe the increase in diastolic flow secondary to the reduced cerebral vascular impedance that results from chronic fetal hypoxia.

In the presence of hydrops at or beyond 20 weeks of gestation, diagnostic cordocentesis is recommended. The fetal blood should be tested for fetal hematocrit, reticulocyte count, platelet count, white blood cells, IgM antiparvovirus B-19 antibodies, and parvovirus B-19 DNA (using PCR).

While fetal hydrops may spontaneously regress, intrauterine transfusion is the cornerstone of management when the biophysical profile begins to change. Rodis (1999) recommends transfusing the fetus sufficiently to raise the fetal hematocrit to 45%. Because fetal aplasia is transient, being related to fetal viremia, a single transfusion usually suffices. Fetal anemia with a reticulocyte count of 10^5 to 10^9mL suggests that the fetus is in the recovery phase of the infection. These fetuses should be followed closely with fetal biophysical profiling and Doppler evaluation of the fetal circulation (Figs. 8, 9, 11).

At some future date, an attenuated live virus vaccine will be available. At such time, a prenatal strategy, not dissimilar to that employed for rubella, may be implemented. No studies have been conducted to determine whether preexposure or postexposure prophylaxis with commercially available immune globulin preparations would prevent infection or modify the course of illness during community outbreaks.

SELECTED READING

Ananda A, Gray ES, Brown T, et al. Human parvovirus infection in pregnancy and hydrops fetalis. N Engl J Med 1987; 316:183.

Anderson MJ, Khousam MN, Maxwell DJ, et al. Human parvovirus B-19 and hydrops fetalis. Lancet 1988; 1:535.

Bailão LA, Rizzi MCS, Bonilla-Musoles F, Osborne NG. Ultrasound markers of intrauterine infection. Ultrasound Quarterly 2000; 16(4):221–233.

Bailão LA, Osborne NG, Rizzi MCS, Bonilla-Musoles F, Duarte G, Bailão TCS. Ultrasound markers of fetal infection. Part I: viral infections. Ultrasound Quarterly 2005; 22(1):295–308.

Bonilla-Musoles F, Raga F, Blanes J, Osborne NG, Da Cunha-Branco J, Remohí J. Triple dimensión ecográfica en el estudio del embrión y del feto normales durante el primer trimestre del embarazo y el inicio del segundo. En: Carrera JM y Kurjak A. Medicina del Embrión. Colección de Medicina Materno-Fetal. Barcelona: Masson, 1997, 163–188.

Barton LL, LaxD, Shehab ZM, Keith JC. Congenital cardiomyopathy associated with human parvovirus infection and systemic necrotizing vasculitis. Am Heart J 1997; 133:131.

Berry PJ, Gray ES, Porter HJ, Burton PA. Parvovirus infection of the human fetus and newborn. Semin Diagn Pathol 1992; 9:4.

Boley TJ, Popek EJ. Parvovirus infection in pregnancy. Semin Perinatol 1993; 17:410.

Bond PR, Caul EO, Usher J, et al. Intrauterine infection with human parvovirus. Lancet 1986; 1:448.

Brown T, Ritchie LD. Infection with parvovirus during pregnancy. Br Med J 1985; 290:559.

Bruu AI, Nordbo SA. Evaluation of five commercial tests for detection of immunoglobulin M antibodies to human parvovirus B19. J Clin Microbiol 1995; 33:1363.

Cassinotti P, Weitz M, Siegel G. Human parvovirus B19 infections: routine diagnosis by a new nested PCR assay. J Med Virol 1993; 40:228.

Cohen BJ. Parvovirus B19: an expanding spectrum of disease. Br Med J 1995; 311:1549.

Cosmi E, Maxi G, Chiaie LD, et al. Noninvasive diagnosis by Doppler ultrasonography of fetal anemia resulting from parovirus infection. Am J Obstet Gynecol 2002; 187:1290.

de Krjger RR, van Elsacker-Niele AMW, Mulder-Stapel A, et al. Detection of parvovirus B19 infection in the first and second trimester fetal loss. Ped Pathol Lab Med 1998; 18:23.

Fairley CK, Smoleniec JS, Caul OE, Miller E. Observational study uuof effect of intrauterine transfusions on outcome of fetal hydrops after parvovirus B19 infection. Lancet 1995; 346:1335.

Finkel TH, Ferguson PJ, Durigon EL, et al. Chronic parvovirus infection and systemic necrotizing vasculitis: opportunistic infection or etiological agent. Lancet 1994; 343:1255.

Franciosi RA, Tattersall P. Fetal infection with human parvovirus B-19. Hum Pathol 1988; 19:489.

Fridell E, Cohen BJ, Wahren B. Evaluation of a synthetic peptide enzyme linked immunosorbent assay for immunoglobulin M to human parvovirus B19. J Clin Microbiol 1991; 29:1376.

Gloning KP, Schramm T, Brusis E, et al. Successful intrauterine treatment of fetal hydrops caused by parvovirus B-19 infection. Behring Inst Mitt 1990; 85:79.

Gray ES, Anand A, Brown T. Parvovirus infections in pregnancy. Lancet 1986; 1:208.

Hager JH, Adler SP, Koch WC, Hager GF. Prospective evaluation of 618 pregnant women exposed to parovirus B19: risks and symptoms. Obstet Gynecol 1998; 91:413.

Hedrick J. The effects of human parvovirus B19 and cytomegalovirus during pregnancy. J Perinat Neonatal Nurs 1996; 10:30.

Holzgreve W, Curry CJR, Golbus MS, et al. Investigation of nonimmune hydrops fetalis. Am J Obstet Gynecol 1984; 150:805.

Humphrey W, Magoon M, O'Shaughnessy R. Severe nonimmune hydrops fetalis secondary to parvovirus B19 infection: spontaneous reversal in utero and survival of a term infant. Obstet Gynecol 1991; 78:900.

Im SS, Rizos N, Joutsi P, et al. Nonimmunologic hydrops fetalis. Am J Obstet Gynecol 1984; 148:566.

Jordan EK, Sever JL. Fetal damage caused by parvoviral infections. Reprod Toxicol 1994; 8:161.

Katz VL, McCoy MC, Kuller JA, Hansen WF. An association between fetal parvovirus B19 infection and fetal anomalies: a report of 2 cases. Am J Perinatol 1996; 13:43.

Kinney JS, Anderson LJ, Farrar J, et al. Risk of adverse outcomes of pregnancy after human parvovirus B-19 infection. J Infect Dis 1988; 157:663.

Knott PD, Welply GAC, Anderson MJ. Serologically proved intrauterine infection with parvovirus. Br Med J 1984; 189:1660.

Koch WC, Harger JH, Barnstein B, Adler SP. Serologic and virologic evidence for frequent intrauterine transmission of human parovirus B19 with primary maternal infection during pregnancy. Pediatr Infect Dis 1988; 17:489.

Kovacs BW, Carlson DE, Shahbahrami B, Piatt LD. Prenatal diagnosis of human parvovirus B-19 in nonimmune hydrops fetalis by polymerase chain reaction. Am J Obstet Gynecol 1992; 167:461.

Lagrew DC. Management of nonimmune hydrops. Perinatal Coordinating Center News XIV, Number 3, March 1988.

Maeda H, Shimokawa H, Satoh S, et al. Nonimmunologic hydrops fetalis resulting from intrauterine human parvovirus B-19 infection: report of two cases. Obstet Gynecol 1988; 72:482.

Markenson GR, Yancey MK. Parvovirus B19 infection in pregnancy. Semin Perinatol 1998; 22:309.

Margolis G, Kilham L. Problems of human concern arising from animal models of intrauterine and neonatal infections due to viruses: a review. II. Pathological studies. Prog Med Virol 1975; 20:144.

Metzman R, Anand A, DeGiulio A, Knisely AS. Hepatic disease associated with intrauterine parvovirus B19 infection in a premature infant. J Pediatr Gastroenterol Nutr 1989; 9:112.

Mortimer PP, Cohen BJ, Buckley MM, et al. Human parvovirus and the fetus. Lancet 1985; 2:1012.

Nyman M, Tolfvenstam T, Petersson K, et al. Detection of human parvovirus B19 infection. Obstet Gynecol 2002; 99:795.

Odibo AO, Campbell WA, Feldman D, et al. Resolution of parvovirus B19-induced nonimmune hydrops after intrauterine transfusion. J Ultrasound Med 1998; 17:547.

Porter HJ, Khong TY, Evans MF, et al. Parvovirus as a cause of hydrops fetalis: detection by in situ DNA hybridization. J Clin Pathol 1988; 41:391.

Public Health Laboratory Service Working Party on Fifth Disease. Prospective study of human parvovirus B19 infection in pregnancy. Br Med J 1990; 300:1166.

Qari M, Qadri SM. Parvovirus B19 infection. Associated diseases, common and uncommon. Postgrad Med 1996; 100:246.

Rodis JF. Parvovirus infection. Clin Obstet Gynecol 1999; 42:107.

Rodis JF, Rodner C, Hasen AA. Long-term outcome of children following maternal human parvovirus B19 infection. Obstet Gynecol 1998; 91:125.

Samra JS, Obhrai MS, Constantine G. Parvovirus infection in pregnancy. Obstet Gynecol 1989; 73:832.

Schwarz TF, Nerlich A, Roggendorf M. Parvovirus B-19 infection in pregnancy. Behring Inst Mitt 1990; 85:69.

Sheikh AU, Ernest JM, O'Shea M. Long-term outcome in fetal hydrops from parvovirus B-19 infection. Am J Obstet Gynecol 1992; 167:337.

Torok TJ. Human parvovirus B-19 infections in pregnancy. Pediatr Infect Dis J 1990; 9:772.

Influenza Viruses

17

INTRODUCTION

Influenza virus infections occur every year in the United States but vary greatly in incidence and geographic distribution. Infections may be asymptomatic or they may produce a spectrum of manifestations ranging from mild upper respiratory infection to pneumonia and death.

Influenza epidemics are frequently associated with deaths in excess of the number normally expected. More than 200,000 excess deaths are estimated to have occurred in association with influenza epidemics in the United States during 1968 to 1982. Excess deaths in this period were attributable mainly to influenza A viruses, although influenza B epidemics were occasionally associated with excess deaths during 1979 to 1980.

INFLUENZA A AND B VIRUSES

Type A influenza viruses occur frequently in humans and domestic animals. These pathogens all have a core of RNA. This internal component is antigenically stable, but the two envelope proteins of the virus may vary. The World Health Organization nomenclature for influenza A viruses includes their strain designation and a description of hemagglutinin (H) and neuraminidase (N), the two surface antigens. The presence of these two proteins provides a basis for dividing influenza A viruses into subtypes. Three subtypes of hemagglutinin (H1, H2, and H3) and two subtypes of neuraminidase (N1 and N2) are recognized among influenza A viruses that have caused widespread human disease. Immunity to these antigens, especially hemagglutinin, reduces the likelihood of infection and the severity of disease if a person does become infected. However, there may be sufficient antigenic variation (antigenic drift) within the same subtype over time, so that infection or vaccination with one strain may not induce immunity to distantly related strains of the same subtype. Although influenza B viruses have shown much more antigenic stability than influenza A viruses, antigenic variation does occur. As a consequence, the antigenic characteristics of current strains provide a basis for selecting virus strains to be included in the vaccine. Human and animal influenza A viruses are interrelated, but not identical.

Between epidemics, there are minor degrees of antigenic drift because of the passage of human influenza A viruses in partially immune people. This process selects mutants that are responsible for the seasonal illnesses experienced every year or so. Major antigenic change probably results from recombination of animal and human influenza A viruses. Influenza A virus may cross the species line periodically and cause major alterations of one or both of the envelope proteins. Laver (at Canberra) and Webster (at Memphis) have

postulated that new human strains appear by recombination of viruses from animals and humans. They suggest that A2/Hong Kong/68 strain was a recombinant that gets its N2 moiety from an Asian H2N2 strain and its H3 from another unknown donor. The influenza B viruses have no known animal reservoirs.

INFLUENZA

Viral influenza can include any of these symptoms: fever, muscle aches, headache, lack of energy, dry cough, sore throat, and sometimes runny nose. The fever and body aches can last three to five days. Cough and lack of energy may last for two or more weeks. Diagnosis based upon purely clinical presentation is problematic. A number of other infectious agents including *Mycoplasmae pneumoniae*, adenovirus, respiratory syncytial virus, rhinovirus, parainfluenza viruses, and *Legionella* species can mimic the initial symptoms of influenza. Even when the diagnosis of influenza is documented by commercial rapid diagnostic tests, superimposed bacterial infection must be ruled out.

INFLUENZAL PNEUMONIA

Analysis of virologicaly confirmed fatal cases of influenza indicate three broad patterns of respiratory involvement: pure influenza virus pneumonia, postinfluenzal bacterial pneumonia, and pneumonia due to concomitant virus and bacterial infection. In terms of their therapeutic ramifications as well as their pathogenesis, the latter two categories can be considered as one, namely, influenza-associated bacterial pneumonia. The translation of infection into mortality or into disease sufficiently severe to force hospitalization has led to early recognition of the fact that influenza constitutes a special hazard to patients with cardiopulmonary disease and to gravidas. Pure influenza virus pneumonia functions as a lethal disease almost exclusively in these special circumstances. In the 1957–1958 epidemic, influenzal pneumonia was the leading cause of maternal mortality in Minnesota, but what was more significant was the observation that gravidas died from pure influenza virus pneumonia and not from superimposed bacterial infection.

Pure Influenza Virus Pneumonia

A wide spectrum of modes of onset of symptoms and signs is observable with influenza virus pneumonia. Nevertheless, sufficient common denominators are discernible to permit a generalized description of the typical fatal course. Usually there is a short antecedent illness of 6 to 12 hours characterized by malaise, myalgia, and chilly sensation, followed by the onset of fever, headaches, pain on ocular movement, nasal congestion, or mild sore throat. Between the second and third day, cough, dyspnea, hemoptysis, and occasionally pleuritic chest pain develop. These symptoms usually herald the onset of clinical deterioration. Analysis of the white blood cell (WBC) count at this time reveals that it is either within normal limits or slightly elevated. There is no marked shift to the left in terms of the WBC differential. The cough becomes productive of frothy blood-stained sputum. Frank hemoptysis is frequent. Marked cyanosis secondary to pulmonary decompensation and shock due to cardiovascular collapse precede death. Almost invariably, fetal death occurs before maternal death. If maternal demise occurs, it does so most commonly about the fourth day following the prodromal illness, and within 24 to 48 hours after the onset of the clinical features of pneumonia.

Physical examination during the clinical course reveals diffuse bilateral crepitant basilar inspiratory rales. The chest roentgenograms correlate closely with the physical findings. Characteristically, there are diffuse, fluffy bilateral infiltrates radiating from the hilum to the peripheral portion of the lung fields. These infiltrates are not uncommonly sparse. Gram-stained sputum smears are noteworthy in that they fail to demonstrate significant numbers of pathogenic bacteria. At necropsy, the lungs are heavy, bulky, and plum colored. Numerous subpleural hemorrhages are discernible. These changes are most pronounced in the lower lobes. The cut surface of the lung reveals blood-stained frothy fluid as well as hemorrhage both in bronchi and in the lung parenchyma. The microscopic features are characteristic, with widespread necrosis of the tracheobronchial epithelium as low as the respiratory bronchioles and alveolar ducts. Similar cytopathologic effects are observable within alveolar macrophages. Scattered foci of interstitial mononuclear cell infiltrate can be identified. Intra-alveolar hemorrhage secondary to capillary disruption is characteristic. Rare capillary thrombi and hyaline membranes lining the intra-alveolar surface are also present.

Influenza-Associated Bacterial Pneumonia

Purulent sputum, shaking chills, or pleuritic chest pain frequently indicate superimposed bacterial infection. Although the symptoms of pure viral pneumonia may blend directly with and be indistinguishable from those of secondary bacterial pneumonia, in certain instances, a short period of improvement intervenes. In the absence of bacteremia, the recognition of secondary bacterial pneumonia depends on the identification of bacterial pathogens in gram-stained sputum. Roentgenographic findings in these two entities may mimic each other exactly; however, pleural effusion, lobar consolidation, or cavitation within the involved lung segments strongly suggests superimposed bacterial pneumonia.

DIAGNOSIS

The diagnosis of influenza pneumonia is usually presumptive and is based on a characteristic pattern of disease or roentgenograms occurring at a time when influenza infection is prevalent in the community. Diagnostic tests available for influenza include viral culture, rapid antigen processing, polymerase chain reaction, and immunofluorescence assays. Among respiratory specimens for viral isolation or rapid detection, nasopharyngeal specimens are more effective than throat specimens. Among the respiratory specimens for viral isolation or rapid detection, nasopharyngeal specimens are more effective than throat specimens. Rapid diagnostic tests can detect influenza viruses in approximately 30 minutes. The various rapid diagnostic tests commercially available differ in the type of influenza viruses they detect and in their ability to distinguish between influenza types. Different tests can detect (i) only influenza A; (ii) both influenza A and B viruses, but not distinguish between the two types; (iii) both influenza A and B viruses and distinguish between the two types. The rapid tests have lower sensitivity than viral cultures. When interpreting results of a rapid influenza test, physicians should consider the possibility of false-negative rapid tests results. Most of the rapid tests are approximately 70% sensitive for detecting influenza and approximately greater than 90% specific.

None of the rapid diagnostic tests provide information as to the subtype present. For this reason, submission of clinical specimens to a state laboratory for viral culture is an important public health commitment.

Infection can be retrospectively documented. A greater than eightfold rise in serum influenza-specific antibodies between acute and convalescent serums is deemed diagnostic of infection. Routine serological testing for influenza does not provide results to help with clinical decision-making.

MANAGEMENT

The frequent inability to distinguish between the two entities dictates a common therapeutic approach. Once the diagnosis of severe influenza pneumonia is made, the patient should be hospitalized, with appropriate precautions made to isolate the patient from potential antibiotic-resistant strains of bacterial pathogens indigenous to the hospital environment. Chemoprophylaxis with amantadine, rimantadine, or the neuraminidase inhibitors, zanamivir or oseltamivir, is recommended for exposed family member and those who will be providing care who have not been recently vaccinated.

Baseline blood gas values should be obtained. Clinical amelioration or deterioration can be monitored by serial determinations of blood pH, PCO_2, and O_2 saturation.

Contraction of the intravascular space should be anticipated and intravenous therapy should be directed at restoring the intravascular volume, replacing the insensible water loss due to hyperventilation and hyperthermia, and maintaining electrolyte balance. Aggressive intravenous therapy necessitates careful monitoring of the intravascular compartment by a central venous catheter. Should vascular overload occur, rapid but cautious digitalization is indicated. Marked hypoxia increases the probability of an adverse drug reaction as a consequence of digitalization. The development of shock may require large intravenous doses of corticosteroids.

Vigorous pulmonary therapy includes administration of oxygen and intermittent positive pressure breathing. Progressive deterioration as indicated by blood gas studies may necessitate intubation. Therapy at this point should be performed by specialists.

Operative intervention with evacuation of the uterus, rather than contributing to clinical amelioration, appears to be associated with significantly increased maternal mortality. Because many of the medications used for inducing analgesia or anesthesia may have adverse effects on pulmonary function, it is imperative to involve the anesthesiologist early in the disease. In general, the pregnancy becomes of secondary consideration, and the patient is treated for acute pulmonary decompensation.

Staphylococcal pneumonia is now recognized as the prime bacterial complication in fatal cases of influenza pneumonia. However, a high incidence of disease due to *Streptococcus pneumoniae* is to be anticipated. *Escherichia coli* is the next most frequent pathogen observed. The spectrum of antibiotic therapy instituted for presumptive bacterial superinfection (nafcillin and gentamicin) should encompass these three major pathogens. The possibility of intrahospital epidemics has focused on the desirability of restricting hospital visits by relatives and friends.

MATERNAL RISK DUE TO PREGNANCY

Without a massive epidemiologic study, it is not established how much added risk influenza imposes on pregnancy. Fragmentary data and anecdotal experience suggest that pregnant women may be at greater risk.

In the 1918 and 1957–1958 epidemics, many pregnant women were among those who developed severe and rapidly fatal pneumonia. In analyzing maternal mortality in these situations, investigators found that most pregnant women died of influenza pneumonia rather than of secondary bacterial infection. In the 1957–1958 epidemic, influenza pneumonia was the leading cause of maternal death in Minnesota. Again, the women died of viral pneumonia and not of a superimposed bacterial infection. After describing a case of fatal maternal influenza in the third trimester, one author stated: "Pregnant women are at increased risk when infected with influenza virus ... Perhaps prior vaccination would have averted the disaster."

Only two deaths were reported as a direct consequence of the 1979 swine flu outbreak: one, a military recruit who reputedly left sick bay and ran to catch up to his unit; the other, a pregnant 17-year-old with no underlying disease. Figures on morbidity and pregnancy are elusive, but assessment of mortality is not difficult. What is notable about pregnant women is that they die of pure viral pneumonia rather than bacterial superinfection. The only other groups who consistently die of pure viral pneumonia are those with mitral stenosis and chronic bronchopulmonary disease.

POSSIBLE FETAL CONSEQUENCES

Stanwell-Smith et al. (1994) studied the possible association of influenza infection with fetal or perinatal mortality.

They conducted an epidemiological investigation that focused on a small cluster of early and late fetal deaths in early 1986. Women whose pregnancies were affected (cases) were compared with women whose pregnancies had a normal outcome (controls). Case pregnancies were distinguished by a significant excess of recent flu-like illness ($p = 0.006$), and were significantly more likely than controls to have serological evidence of influenza A infection ($p = 0.00067$), predominantly the influenza A H3N2, Christchurch/4/85-like strain. The cluster was recognized because most cases were patients of one health center. Larger epidemiological studies will be needed to confirm an association between influenza A and fetal death, but this cluster suggests that influenza A may have an adverse influence on fetal survival.

In a limited number of animal model systems, influenza A virus may have some teratogenic abilities. Weak circumstantial evidence has been advanced that purports a linkage between maternal infection in pregnancy and a number of late-manifesting neurological defects or childhood leukemia.

All know viral teratogens function either by direct cytopathic effect or by indirect inhibition of DNA replication. Except for a case reported by Yawn et al. (1971), there is no added data that document the ability of the influenza viruses to traverse the placental barrier.

VACCINATION IN PREGNANCY

The Centers for Disease Control (CDC) have designated women who are in the second or third trimester of pregnancy during the influenza season as individuals at increased risk for complication and hence a vaccine-target population (Table 1). Should a pregnant woman have a chronic metabolic disease such as diabetes mellitus, significant renal dysfunction, hemoglobinopathies, or chronic disorders of the pulmonary or cardiovascular system, or be immunosuppressed, including drug-induced immunosuppression or human immunodeficiency infection/disease, these conditions constitute additive risk factors.

In addition, women who are healthcare workers and other individuals in close contact with persons at high risk should be vaccinated to decrease the risk for transmitting infection to persons at risk.

Inactivated Influenza Vaccine

Inactivated influenza vaccine should not be administered to persons known to have anaphylactic hypersensitivity to eggs or other vaccine components. Influenza vaccines contain three strains, two type A and one type B, representing the influenza viruses likely to be circulating in the United States during the winter. Different manufacturers may use additional compounds as a preservative such as thimerosal, a mercury-containing compound, or they may use an antibiotic to prevent bacterial contamination. Before administering a vaccine, the package insert should be consulted and the vaccine recipient questioned as to known allergies. Currently, no scientifically conclusive evidence exists documenting harm from thimerosal preservative-containing

TABLE I CDC recommendations for influenza vaccination

Annual vaccination is strongly suggested
(1) For women who will be in the second or third trimester of pregnancy during the influenza season
(2) For women over the age of 64 years

Conditions predisposing to such increased risk include
(1) Acquired or congenital heart disease with actual or potential alterations in circulatory dynamics (e.g., mitral stenosis, congestive heart failure, or pulmonary vascular overload)
(2) Any chronic disorder or condition that compromises pulmonary function (e.g., chronic obstructive pulmonary disease, bronchiectasis, heavy smoking, tuberculosis, severe asthma, cystic fibrosis, neuromuscular and orthopedic disorders with impaired ventilation, bronchopulmonary dysplasia following neonatal respiratory distress syndrome)
(3) Chronic renal disease with azotemia or nephrotic syndrome
(4) Diabetes mellitus or other metabolic diseases
(5) Severe chronic anemia, such as sickle cell disease
(6) Conditions that compromise the immune mechanism, including certain malignancies and immunosuppressive therapy

influenza vaccine; nevertheless, consideration should be given to using thimerosal-reduced or thimerosal-free influenza vaccine to pregnant women.

The effectiveness of an influenza vaccine is a function primarily of the recipient's age, immunocompetence, and the degree of similarity between viruses in the vaccine and those in circulation. When the vaccine and circulating viruses are antigenically similar, influenza vaccine is 70% to 90% effective. Immunity declines in the year following vaccination.

A 0.5 mL dose of either the whole- or the split-virus vaccine administered intramuscularly is recommended for women. Immunogenicity and side effects of whole and split-virus vaccines are similar among adults when administered at the recommended dosages. Little or no improvement in antibody response is observed when a second dose of the vaccine is administered in the same season.

Both local and systemic side effects occur. Soreness at the site of vaccination is common and may last for up to two days. Fever, malaise, and myalgia tend to occur in individuals with little prior exposure to the viral antigens in the vaccine. Immediate allergic reactions are rare.

Live, Attenuated Influenza Vaccine

Live, attenuated influenza vaccine (LAIV) is a live, trivalent, intranasally administered vaccine that has been attenuated so as to produce minimal signs or symptoms of disease. The live influenza strains are temperature sensitive. This property restricts viral replication at temperatures found within the tracheobronchial confines. In experimental animals, LAIV viruses replicate in the mucosa of the nasopharynx, inducing local protective immunity, but are inefficient in replicating in the tracheobronchial tree and lungs. LAIV is marketed under the name FluMist.

Adults vaccinated with LAIV can shed vaccine virus for approximately two to three days postvaccination. The amount of virus produced is lower than that associated with wild-type influenza viruses. In isolated cases, shed vaccine virus can be transmitted from vaccinees to nonvaccinated individuals. In clinical trials, viruses shed by vaccine recipients have been phenotypically stable. The potential advantages of LAIV include induction of both mucosal and systemic immunity, ease of administration, and acceptability of intranasal over intramuscular route of administration. Currently, pregnant women should not be vaccinated with LAIV. The CDC recommends that they receive inactivated influenza vaccine.

CHEMOPROPHYLAXIS

Antiviral drugs for influenza are an adjunct to the vaccine. Four influenza antiviral drugs have been licensed for use in the United States: amantadine, rimantadine, zanamivir, and oseltamivir.

Amantadine and rimantadine are chemically related antiviral drugs with activity against influenza A, but not influenza B. They interfere with the influenza virus lifecycle. Both are approved for the treatment and prophylaxis of influenza A virus infection. When administered prophylactically to healthy adults before and throughout the epidemic period, they are 70% to 90% effective in preventing illness caused by naturally occurring strains of type A influenza viruses.

Zanamivir and oseltamivir are neuraminidase inhibitors with activity against both influenza A and B viruses. Both are approved for the treatment of uncomplicated influenza infections. Only oseltamivir is approved for prophylaxis, but both drugs appear to afford similar effectiveness in preventing febrile illness in community-based studies.

Antiviral agents taken prophylactically can prevent illness but not subclinical infection. Individuals taking these drugs, if infected, will develop immune responses that may protect them when they are exposed to antigenically related viruses in later years. The recommended daily dosages of influenza medications for treatment and prophylaxis are listed in Table 2.

Although annual vaccination is the primary strategy for prevention of influenza virus infection, antiviral medication with activity against influenza viruses can be effective for chemoprophylaxis and treatment of influenza. Chemoprophylaxis can be considered for persons with immune deficiency in whom a less than optimal response to vaccination is anticipated. Such patients should be closely monitored for adverse drug reactions if chemoprophylaxis is administered.

Chemoprophylaxis should not be used in lieu of vaccinations. Antiviral therapy is indicated for nonvaccinated individuals after an outbreak of influenza A has begun in the community. Individuals in this situation should still be vaccinated.

The development of antibodies takes 8 to 14 days; hence the rationale for concomitant chemoprophylaxis during an influenza outbreak for high-risk women. Amantadine and rimantadine do not interfere with antibody response to the vaccine. When inactivated influenza A virus vaccine is unavailable or contraindicated, amantadine may be administered for up to 90 days in cases of epidemic exposure. Amantadine must be taken each day for the duration of

TABLE 2 Recommended daily dosage of antiviral medications for treatments and prophylaxis

Antiviral agent	13–64 yr	≥65 yr
Amandadine[a]		
Treatment	100 mg twice daily	≤100 mg/day
Prophylaxis	100 mg twice daily	≤100 mg/day
Rimantadine[b]		
Treatment[c]	100 mg twice daily	100 or 200 mg/day[d]
Prophylaxis	100 mg twice daily	100 or 200 mg/day[d]
Zanamivir[e,f]		
Treatment	10 mg twice daily	10 mg twice daily
Oseltamivir		
Treatment[g]	75 mg twice daily	75 mg twice daily
Prophylaxis	75 mg/day	75 mg/day

[a]The drug package insert should be consulted for dosage recommendations for administering amantadine to persons with creatinine clearance ≤50 mL/min/1.73 m².
[b]A reduction in dosage to 100 mg/day of rimantadine is recommended for persons who have severe hepatic dysfunction or those with creatinine clearance ≤10 mL/min. Other persons with less severe hepatic or renal dysfunction taking 100 mg/day of rimantadine should be observed closely, and the dosage should be reduced or the drug discontinued, if necessary.
[c]Only approved treatment among adults.
[d]Elderly residents of nursing homes should be administered only 100 mg/day of rimantadine. A reduction in dosage to 100 mg/day should be considered for all persons aged ≥65 years of age if they experience side effects when taking 200 mg/day.
[e]Zanamivir is administered via inhalation by using a plastic device included in the package with the medication. Patients will benefit from instruction and demonstration of correct use of the device.
[f]Zanamivir is not approved for prophylaxis.
[g]A reduction in the dose of oseltamivir is recommended for persons with creatinine clearance <30 mL/min.
Source: Adapted from Centers for Disease Control (2001).

the epidemic or until active immunity has an opportunity to develop after vaccination.

No clinical studies have been conducted regarding the safety or efficacy of amantadine, rimantadine, zanamivir, or oseltamivir for pregnant women. Both amantadine and rimantadine have been demonstrated to be teratogenic and embryotoxic in animal studies when administered in very high doses. Because of the unknown effects of these drugs on the developing fetus, all anti-influenza virus drugs should be used during pregnancy only when benefits justify the potential risk to the embryo or fetus. These drugs are secreted into breast milk.

Side effects associated with amantadine and rimantadine are usually mild and cease soon after discontinuing the drug. Side effects can diminish or disappear after the first week despite continued drug ingestion.

In nonpregnant, otherwise healthy adults, when administered within two days of illness onset, amantadine and rimantadine can reduce the duration of uncomplicated influenza A illness. Similarly, zanamivir and oseltamivir can reduce the duration of uncomplicated influenza A and B illness by approximately one day. Data concerning the effectiveness of the four antiviral agents in preventing serious influenza-related complications are limited.

Influenza A virus resistance to amantadine and rimantadine can emerge rapidly during treatment. To reduce the emergence of antiviral drug-resistant influenza viruses, chemoprophylaxis should be discontinued once the threat of the epidemic has subsided.

SELECTED READING

Influenza Viruses and Pregnancy
Barker WH, Mullooly JP. Influenza vaccination of elderly persons. Reduction in pneumonia and influenza hospitalizations and deaths. J Am Med Assoc 1980; 244:2547.
Barker WH, Mullooly JP. Impact of epidemic type A influenza in a defined adult population. AM J Epidemiol 1980; 112:798.
Centers for Disease Control. Prevention and control of influenza: recommendation of the advisory committee on immunization practices (ACIP). MMWR 1996; 45:1–24.
Centers for Disease Control. Neuraminidinase inhibitors for treatment of influenza A and B infections. MMWR 1999; 48/No. RR-14:1.
Centers for Disease Control. Prevention and control of influenza: recommendations of the Advisory Committee on Immunization Practices. MMWR 2001; 50/No. RR-4:1.
Centers for disease Control. Prevention and control of influenza: recommendations of the Advisory Committee on Immunization Practices. MMWR 2005; 54/No. RR-8:1.
Dowdle WR, Coleman MT, Gregg MB. Natural history of influenza type A in the United States, 1957–1972. Prog Med Virol 1974; 17:91.
Editorial. Influenza zoo. Lancet 1979; 2:197.
Freeman DW, Barno A. Deaths from Asian influenza associated with pregnancy. Am J Obstet Gynecol 1959; 78:1172.
Gall SA. Influenza and current guidelines for its control. Infect Dis Obstet Gynecol 2001; 9:193.
Greenberg M, Jacobziner H, Parker J, Weisl BAG. Maternal mortality in the epidemic of Asian influenza, New York City, 1957. Am J Obstet Gynecol 1958; 76:897.
Hamburger V, Habel K. Teratogens and lethal effects of influenza A and mumps virus on early chick embryos. Proc Soc Exp Biol 1947; 66:608.
Hardy JB. Viral infection in pregnancy. A review. Am J Obstet Gynecol 1965; 93:1052.
Hardy JB, Azarowica EN, Mannini A, et al. The effect of Asian influenza on the outcome of pregnancy. Baltimore, 1955–1958. Am J Public Health 1961; 51:1182.
Harris JW. Influenza occurring in pregnant women. J Am Med Assoc 1919; 72:975.
Ingelfinger FJ. Thou shalt be vaccinated. N Engl J Med 1976; 294:1060.
Jewett JG. Committee on maternal welfare: influenzal pneumonia at term. N Engl J Med 1974; 291:256.
MacKenzie S, Houghton M. Influenza infections during pregnancy: association with congenital malformations and with subsequent neoplasms in children and potential hazards of live virus vaccines. Bacteriol Rev 1974; 38:356.
Monif GRG, Sowards DL, Eitzman DV. Serologic and immunologic evaluation of neonates following maternal influenza infection during the second and third trimesters of gestation. Am J Obstet Gynecol 1972; 114:239.
Neuzil KM, ReedGM, Mitchell EF, et al. Impact of influenza on acute cardiopulmonary hospitalizations in pregnant women. Am J Epidemiol 1998; 148:1094.
Nolan TF Jr, Goodman RA, Hinman AR, et al. Morbidity and mortality associated with influenza B in the United States, 1979–1980. A report from the Centers for Disease Control. J Infect Dis 1980; 142:360.
Stanwell-Smith R, Parker AM, Chakraverty P, et al. Possible association of influenza A with fetal loss: investigation of a cluster of spontaneous abortions and stillbirths. Commun Dis Rep Rev 1994; 4:R28.
Weinstein L. Influenza-1918, a revisit? N Engl J Med 1976; 294:1058.
Yawn DH, Pyeatte JC, Joseph JM, et al. Transplacental transfer of influenza virus. J Am Med Assoc 1971; 216:1022.

Influenzal Pneumonia in Pregnancy
Freeman DW, Barno A. Deaths from influenza associated with pregnancy. Am J Obstet Gynecol 1959; 78:1172.
Harris JW. Influenza occurring in pregnant women. J Am Med Assoc 1919; 72:975.

Hers JF, Masurel N, Mulder J. Bacteriology and histopathology of the respiratory tract and lungs in fatal sign influenza. Lancet 1958; 2:1141.

Hopwood HG Jr. Pneumonia in pregnancy. Obstet Gynecol 1965; 25:875.

Louria DB, Blumenfeld HL, Ellis JT, et al. Studies of influenza in the pandemic of 1957–1958. II: pulmonary complications of influenza. J Clin Invest 1959; 38:213.

Martin CM, Kunin CM, Gottlieb LS, et al. Asian Influenza A in Boston, 1957–1958. Arch Intern Med 1959; 103:515.

Masterson J. Respiratory complications of epidemic influenza. J Ir Med Assoc 1969; 62:37.

Petersdorf RG, Fusca JJ, Harter DH, Albrink WS. Pulmonary infections complicating Asian influenza. Arch Intern Med 1959; 103:262.

Robertson L, Caley JP, Moore J. Importance of Staphylococcus aureus in pneumonia in the 1957 epidemic of influenza A. Lancet 1958; 2:233.

Influenza Virus Vaccine

Barker WH, Mullooly JP. Pneumonia and influenza deaths during epidemics: implications for prevention. Arch Intern Med 1982; 142:85.

Hammond GW, Cheang M. Absenteeism among hospital staff during an influenza epidemic: implications for immunoprophylaxis. Can Med Assoc J 1984; 131:449.

Kaplan JF, Katona P, Hurwitz ES, Schonberger LB. Guillain-Barré syndrome in the United States, 1979–1980 and 1980–1981: lack of an association with influenza vaccination. J Am Med Assoc 1982; 248:698.

Kilborne ED. Influenza. New York. Plenum Publishing Corp, 1987.

LaMontagne JR, Noble GR, Quinnan GV, et al. Summary of clinical trials of inactivated influenza vaccine—1978. Rev Infect Dis 1983; 5:723.

Meinick JL. Viral vaccines. New problems and prospectives. Hosp Prac 1978; 13:104.

MMWR. Prevention and control of Influenza, 1983–1984. 1987; 36(24):73.

National Institute of Allergy and Infectious Diseases. Amantadine: does it have a role in the prevention and treatment of influenza? A National Institutes of Health Consensus Development Conference. Ann Intern Med 1980; 92:256.

Schonberger LB, Hurwitz ES, Katona P, et al. Guillain-Barré syndrome: its epidemiology and associations with influenza vaccination. Ann Neurol 1981; 9(suppl):31.

18

Measles

INTRODUCTION

Measles virus is a paramyxovirus. Its virions have a diameter of 100 to 250 nm and consist of a helical ribonucleoprotein core surrounded by a lipid envelope. The virions replicate predominantly in the cytoplasm and are released from the cell surface by budding. The envelope of the virion is composed of at least two glycoproteins: F, which causes membrane fusion and is crucial for infectivity; and H, which is the hemagglutinin. Antibodies to F glycoprotein inhibit viral infectivity.

Measles is an extremely infectious disease entity. The virus is disseminated predominantly by droplet transmission from an infected individual to a susceptible subject in close proximity. Transmission by articles soiled by respiratory secretions may occur. Although any mucosal surface potentially provides a portal of entry, the principal portal of infection is the upper respiratory tract.

The usual incubation period between initiation of infection and onset of the first symptoms (prodrome) is approximately 10 days. Approximately 10 to 14 day intervals between exposure and exanthema occur in 80% of individuals, 15 to 19 days in 14%, and less than 10 days in 6%.

Measles is most communicable during the prodrome and catarrhal stage of infection rather than during the period of the exanthema. Individuals with measles should be considered infectious from the onset of the prodrome (about four days before the appearance of the exanthema) until three days after the onset of the exanthema. The risk of contagion abruptly diminishes 48 hours after the rash appears. Measles virus is readily recovered from respiratory secretions from two days before until one or two days after the onset of the rash.

Before licensing of live measles vaccines, the incidence of measles in pregnancy ranged from 0.4 to 0.6 cases of measles per 10,000 pregnancies. The decline in the incidence of measles can be attributed to the widespread use of the measles–mumps–rubella (MMR) vaccine. Liberman et al. demonstrated that 8.2% of women seronegative to rubella were also seronegative to rubeola, compared to 0.8% if the woman was rubella seropositive. Over half of the adult cases of measles that now occur are believed to result from primary vaccine failure or nonadministration of vaccine. At present, there is no evidence that immunity induced by wild-strain measles wanes with time.

CLINICAL MANIFESTATIONS

The prodrome typically begins 10 to 11 days after exposure, with fever and malaise, followed within 24 hours by coryza, sneezing, conjunctivitis, and cough. During the next two to three days, this catarrhal phase is accentuated with markedly infected conjunctivae and photophobia. Toward the end of the prodrome, Koplik's spots appear. These are tiny (no larger than a pinhead), granular, slightly raised, white lesions surrounded by a halo of erythema.

The rash, which appears 12 to 14 days after exposure, begins on the head and neck, especially behind the ears and on the forehead. At first, the lesions are red macules 1 to 2 mm in diameter, but during a period of two or three days, they enlarge, becoming maculopapules of 1 cm or greater. By the second day, the exanthema spreads to the trunk and upper extremities. The lower extremities are involved by the third day. The lesions are most prominent in those regions where the exanthema appears first, namely, the face and upper trunk. By the third or fourth day, the exanthema begins to fade in the order of its appearance. A brown staining of the lesions often persists for 7 to 10 days and is followed by fine desquamation.

The clinical course of measles can be altered by administration of immune globulin (IG) during the incubation period. In modified measles, the catarrhal phase may be completely suppressed and the exanthema limited to a few macules on the trunk.

The principal complications associated with measles are pneumonia, encephalitis, and myocarditis. Encephalitis occurs in one per 10,000 cases of measles. Measles encephalitis has a mortality rate approaching 10%. Liver enzyme elevations may occur in 50% to 75% of young adults. It is not uncommon for adults with arrested tuberculosis to have an acute flare-up following measles.

MEASLES IN PREGNANCY

The incidence of death and other complications from measles during pregnancy may be higher than expected for age-comparable, nonpregnant women (Table 1). Pneumonia, which is a relatively rare complication in the general population, is increased in pregnancy.

Eberhart-Phillips et al. (1993) identified 58 gravidae with measles. Of these, 35 (60%) were hospitalized for measles, 15 (26%) were diagnosed with pneumonia, and 2 (3%) died of measles complications.

In Packer's series of cases, 6 of 18 pregnant women with measles were said to suffer from "severe" disease. Christensen et al. (1953) describe an epidemic of measles in Greenland. Pregnant women were nearly three times as likely to die from their infections as nonpregnant women with measles aged 15 to 54 years. In a hospital-based study of women in Houston, seven gravidae with measles had pneumonia. One died.

PERINATAL WASTAGE

Measles in pregnancy may lead to high rates of fetal loss and prematurity, especially within the first two weeks after onset of the rash. In Eberhart-Phillips' series, excluding three induced abortions, 18 pregnancies (31%) ended prematurely; five were spontaneous abortions; and 13 were preterm deliveries. All but 2 of the 18 pregnancies that terminated early did so within 14 days after onset of the rash. Two term infants were born with minor congenital anomalies, but their mothers had measles late in their third trimester.

CONGENITAL MEASLES

Because the usual incubation period from infection to the first appearance of the exanthema is 13 to 14 days, measles exanthemas acquired in the first 10 days of life are considered transplacental in origin, whereas those appearing at 14 days or later are probably postnatally acquired.

By and large, the outcome of gestational measles on the fetus is relatively benign. The spectrum of disease in congenital measles varies from a mild illness in which a rash and Koplik's spots may or may not be present to fulminating fetal disease in which pneumonia is the leading complication. Mortality, if it occurs, tends to do so in a premature infant. The case fatality ratio is not well established and is probably significantly influenced by the gestational age and maternal/fetal immune response. Administration of IG at birth may decrease the mortality. The dose usually administered has been 0.25 mg/kg.

Overt neonatal disease usually is seen when maternal disease occurs in the periparturitional period. Disease in the newborn is not associated with enhanced virulence or an expanded pattern of disease. There is no evidence to incriminate the measles virus as a teratogen for the human fetus.

Neonatal disease is usually but not invariably at the same stage of development as that of the mother. Most of the progeny of pregnancies that have been complicated by maternal measles during gestation exhibit apparent immunity when subsequently exposed to rubeola virus.

Most women of childbearing age in urban areas are immune to measles because of previous natural infection or vaccination. Haas et al. (2005) identified 16.5% of women presenting for prenatal care as being serosusceptible to rubeola. Infants born to immune mothers are usually protected in the neonatal period by transplacentally acquired antibodies. Consequently measles outbreaks in newborn nurseries are rare events.

DIAGNOSIS

Maternal
A definitive diagnosis of maternal measles can be inferred on purely clinical grounds when there is history of recent exposure and the typical catarrhal phase is followed by

TABLE I Adverse fetal consequences of maternal rubeola (measles) in pregnancy

Abortion[a]
Fetal death in utero[a]
Congenital infection

[a]Fetal wastage is probably as contingent upon the severity of maternal disease as on the gestational age of the fetus.

Koplik's spots and a maculopapular exanthema in the characteristic distribution. Koplik's spots are deemed to be pathognomonic.

More characteristically, the clinical impression is confirmed by serological testing. For routine determinations of antibodies in paired human sera, the hemagglutination inhibition test is faster, less cumbersome, and less expensive than the neutralization or enzyme-linked immunosorbent assay (ELISA) test. For detecting antibodies after infection in the remote past or for predicting immunity, the neutralization test is somewhat more sensitive. Recent maternal infection can be inferred by the demonstration of immunoglobulin M (IgM) antimeasles antibodies in the ELISA test system. Serum antibodies appear shortly after the appearance of the rash and peak in three to four weeks. A definitive diagnosis of rubeola is contingent on the demonstration of IgM-specific antibodies, a fourfold or greater rise in paired sera run in the same test or isolation of the virus.

The measles virus is best isolated using primary cultures of human embryonic kidney or rhesus monkey kidney. Presumptive isolates of measles virus are identified by typing with known antiserum in hemadsorption inhibition or plaque-reduction tests or by polymerase chain reaction (PCR) technology.

Congenital
The diagnosis of congenital measles is contingent upon the disease process being present at birth or developing in the first 12 days of life and either recovery of virus and PCR confirmation or the demonstration of specific IgM or IgA virus antibodies in neonatal blood.

THERAPY AND PREVENTION

Management of maternal myxovirus infection is largely supportive in terms of symptomatology. If hyperthermia develops, fever must be aggressively controlled. Antibiotics are indicated if pulmonary secondary bacterial superinfection occurs.

MANAGEMENT OF THE EXPOSED GRAVIDA

Mothers with an unequivocal history of either previous natural measles or vaccination with live-attenuated measles virus are assumed not to be at risk when exposed to measles in the neonatal period. If a mother without a history of previous measles or measles vaccination is exposed 6 to 15 days antepartum, she may be in the incubation period and capable of transmitting measles infection during the postpartum period. In the absence of a previous maternal history of measles, the neonate should remain in the newborn nursery.

Both mother and the neonate should receive IG, 0.25 mg/kg intramuscularly, to prevent or modify subsequent measles infection that might have been incubating at the time of delivery. If exposed less than six days antepartum, she would not be capable of transmitting measles by the respiratory route until at least 72 hours postpartum.

PROPHYLAXIS

The identification of serosusceptibility to rubella virus argues for postpartum vaccination with a combined MMR live virus vaccine rather than rubella alone.

For the serosusceptible gravida with intimate exposure to rubeola, the administration of gamma globulin during the virus' incubation period should be seriously considered.

IG prophylaxis given to a pregnant woman within 72 hours of exposure appears to prevent infection in the majority of instances. Efficacy diminishes linearly with time after 72 hours. The recommended dose of IG is 0.25 mL/kg IM (not to exceed 15 mL).

Nonpregnant adults who are exposed to measles and who have no or uncertain documentation of live measles vaccination on or after their first birthday, no record of physician-diagnosed measles, and no laboratory evidence of immunity should be vaccinated within 72 hours after exposure. If the exposure did not result in infection, the vaccine will more likely than not induce protection against subsequent measles infection.

All infants born to mothers with active measles in the six days before delivery should receive IG.

POSTPARTUM VACCINATION

Measles combination, live-attenuated virus vaccines produce a mild or inapparent noncommunicable infection. Virus-specific antibodies can be demonstrated in 90% to 95% of susceptible individuals.

Vaccine Adverse Reactions

A temperature may develop among approximately 5% to 15% of vaccinees, usually beginning between the fifth and twelfth days after vaccination; fever usually lasts one to two days and, rarely, up to five days.

Rashes have been reported among approximately 5% of vaccinees. Encephalitis after measles vaccination is extremely rare, and its incidence cannot be discerned from the background incidence of encephalitis of an unknown etiology.

Vaccine Precautions

Vaccination should not be postponed because of a minor illness such as a mild upper respiratory infection. However, vaccination of persons with severe febrile illnesses should be postponed until recovery. Vaccine should be given 14 days before—or deferred for at least six weeks and preferably three months after—a person has received IG, whole blood, or other blood products containing antibody.

Persons with a history of any sign or symptom of a prior anaphylactic reaction should be given measles vaccine only after detailed analysis of the circumstances surrounding the event and then with extreme caution.

Persons with reactions that are not anaphylactic are not at increased risk and can be vaccinated. Because of a theoretical risk to the developing fetus, measles vaccine should not be given to pregnant women.

The vaccine also should not be given to persons who are immunocompromised as a result of immune deficiency diseases, leukemia, lymphoma, or generalized malignancy or who are immunosuppressed as a result of therapy with corticosteroids, alkylating drugs, antimetabolites, or radiation.

SELECTED READING

Atmar RL, Englund JA, Hammill H. Complications of measles during pregnancy. Clin Infect Dis 1992; 14:217.

Cerf L. Rougeole, Épidémiologie, Immunologie, Prophylaxie. Paris: Masson et Cie, 1926.

Christensen PE, Schmidt H, Bang HO, et al. An epidemic of measles in Southern Greenland, 1951: measles in virgin soil. II. The epidemic proper. Acta Med Scand 1953; 144:430.

Connelly JP, Reynolds S, Crawford JD, Talbot NB. Viral and drug hazards in pregnancy. Clin Pediatr 1964; 3:587.

Dyer I. Measles complicating pregnancy. Report of 24 cases with three instances of congenital measles. Southern Med J 1940; 33:601.

Eberhart-Phillips JE, Frederick PD, Baron RC, et al. Measles in pregnancy: a descriptive study of 58 cases. Obstet Gynecol 1993; 82:797.

Gazala E, Karplus M, Liberman JR, Sarov I. The effect of maternal measles on the fetus. Pediatr Infect Dis J 1985; 4:203.

Gershon AA. Chickenpox, measles, and mumps. In: Remington JS, Klein JO, eds. Infectious Diseases of the Fetus and Newborn Infant. Philadelphia: WB Saunders, 1990:395.

Haas DM, Flowers CA, Congdon CL. Rubella, rubeola and mumps in pregnancy; susceptibilities and strategies for testing and vaccinating. Obstet Gynecol 2005; 106:295.

Khon J. Measles in newborn infants (maternal infection). J Pediatr 1933; 3:176.

Kincaid DP. Measles in a child contracted in utero. Memphis Med Monthly 1917; 38:86.

Kugel RB. Measles in a newborn premature infant. Am J Dis Child 1957; 93:306.

Liberman MD, Behr MA, Martel N, Ward BJ. Rubella susceptibility precedes measles susceptibility: implication for postpartum immunization. Clinic Infect Dis 2000; 31:1501.

Manson MM, Logan WPD, Loy RM. Rubella and other virus infections during pregnancy. Ministry of Health Report on Public Health and Medical Subjects, No. 101, London, Her Majesty's Stationery Office, 1960.

Mariani JA. La rougeole congénital et la rougeole des premiers mois de la vie. Thesis No. 45, Paris, 1925.

Musser JH. Six cases (in an epidemic) of measles in the newborn. Med Clin North Am 1927; 2:619.

Packer AD. Influence of maternal measles on the unborn child. Med J Aust 1950; 1:835.

Plimpton CC. Measles contracted in utero. Homeop J Obstet 1891; 13:131.

Richardson DL. Measles contracted in utero. Rhode Island Med J 1920; 3:13.

Rosa C. Rubella and rubeola. Semin Perinatol 1998; 22:318.

Smith I. Delivery: the mother suffering from prodomata of measles; the disease developing in both mother and child on the succeeding day. Am J Med Sci 1870; 59:282.

Swan C, Tostevin AL, Moore B, et al. Congenital defects in infants following infectious diseases during pregnancy, with special reference to relationship between German measles and cataract, deaf mutism, heart disease and microcephaly, and to period in pregnancy in which occurrence of rubella was followed by congenital abnormalities. Med J Aust 1943; 2:201.

van Reuss A. Die Krankheiten des Neugeborenen. J Springer, 1914:435.

Mumps

19

INTRODUCTION

The mumps virus, like the measles virus, is also a member of the paramyxovirus family. The mumps virus contains a hemagglutinin neuraminidase glycoprotein or viral (V) antigen associated with the envelope, a hemolysis cell fusion (F) glycoprotein antigen also associated with the envelope, and a soluble (S) antigen associated with the ribonucleoprotein core.

The mumps virus is transmitted primarily by droplet, saliva, and fomites. The initial site of virus replication is the upper respiratory tract from which a viremia is engendered, which results in metastatic, glandular, and central nervous system (CNS) involvement.

Haas et al. (2005) found that 16.3% of women seeking prenatal care were serosusceptible to mumps virus.

Mumps is an acute, generalized, communicable disease whose most distinctive feature is swelling of one or both parotid glands. Involvement of other salivary glands, the meninges, the pancreas, and the testes of postpubertal males occurs with some frequency.

The usual incubation period, between exposure to infection and onset of parotitis is 14 to 18 days. Extremes between 7 and 23 days have been identified.

The prodrome consists of fever, malaise, and myalgia. Parotitis, if it is to develop, does so in the next 24 hours. Parotid gland involvement progresses for two to three days and then gradually regresses.

MUMPS IN PREGNANCY

When mumps is superimposed on pregnancy, the resultant disease is not appreciably more severe than it is in non-pregnant women. In general, the clinical course of mumps in pregnancy is relatively benign. Mumps virus has been isolated from breast milk.

PERINATAL WASTAGE

Like measles, mumps infection when superimposed upon pregnancy may adversely affect its outcome. Small studies have demonstrated a greater than twofold increase in perinatal wastage. Mumps differs from measles in the sense that some studies have identified an increased incidence in congenital defects as well as abortions; however, in the largest series involving 501 cases, no significant difference in terms of fetal complications could be demonstrated between gravida whose pregnancy had been complicated by mumps and the control group, irrespective of the stage of pregnancy at which infection occurred. Unlike fetal deaths or abortions associated with measles, those associated with mumps are closely related temporally to the maternal infection.

CONGENITAL INFECTION

In extremely rare incidences, maternal mumps has produced congenital disease. The infants present with parotitis at birth or develop it in the ensuing 10 days of life. In general, the disease tends to pursue an uneventful course. Occasionally severe systemic involvement is noted. Lacour et al. (1993) reported a case in which the mother developed bilateral parotitis beginning the day of the delivery. The child was subsequently severely ill and suffered from fever, splenomegaly, and thrombocytopenia, however, without parotitis or pancreatic involvement. Both mother and child recovered with symptomatic treatment. When maternal disease occurs in the immediate periparturitional periods, the neonate may develop parotitis or aseptic meningitis.

MUMPS EMBRYOPATHY

The prime controversy concerning maternal mumps during gestation centers around the question of whether there is a mumps embryopathy. Retrospective studies have noted a higher incidence of delayed hypersensitivity to mumps in infants with endocardial fibroelastosis than in the control groups. This observation has not been universally substantiated. Despite the ability of the mumps virus to induce congenital malformations in experimental animals, there is no definite evidence of teratogenicity for the mumps virus in humans.

There is a question as to whether maternal disease in gestation is causally related to childhood-onset diabetes mellitus. Fine et al. (1985) conducted a long-term follow-up study of 3076 subjects who were exposed to viral infection in utero and who at the time of analysis were up to 40 years of age. Mortality and morbidity were compared with those in a control population matched for sex, date of birth, and area of birth. There was evidence of an increased risk of diabetes among those exposed to mumps during the first trimester (four cases among 128 subjects against none of 148 controls).

DIAGNOSIS

The diagnosis of mumps is not problematical on clinical grounds when bilateral, painful parotitis develops, especially when a history of recent exposure is available. The virus can be recovered from saliva or urine by cultivation on a variety of cell tissue culture lines. Definite diagnosis requires either serological confirmation, virus isolation, or specific documentation using polymerase chain reaction.

Serologically, the diagnosis of mumps is established by demonstrating a rising antibody titer in paired acute and convalescent sera. Complement fixation, hemagglutination inhibition, and neutralization tests can demonstrate sero-conversion to mumps V antigen. These test systems have largely been replaced by the introduction of highly sensitive enzyme-linked immunosorbent assay (ELISA) tests, which are capable of identifying both immunoglobulin G (IgG) and immunoglobulin M (IgM) antimumps antibodies. IgM mumps antibodies can also be measured using a variation of the ELISA known as antibody capture.

THERAPY

Treatment is largely symptomatic. Application of cold packs to the parotid glands in conjunction with the liberal use of analgesics may be beneficial. If mastitis develops, cold packs can be applied. Mumps vaccine may be used to immunize serosusceptible individuals in the home or hospital environment. Mumps vaccine is not recommended for pregnant women. Immunoglobulin is of little value in aborting mumps or its complications.

MUMPS VACCINE

Live mumps virus is currently administered in a combined live-virus vaccine that contains measles, rubella viruses (MMR) or measles, mumps, and varicella viruses (Pro-Quad 0). Vaccine administered subcutaneously provides protective and long-lasting levels of antibody. Clinical vaccine efficacy reports range between 75% and 95%.

VACCINE INDICATIONS

Mumps vaccine is indicated for all adults believed to be susceptible. Persons should be considered susceptible to mumps unless they have documentation of physician-diagnosed mumps, adequate immunization with MMR vaccine on or after their first birthday, or laboratory evidence of immunity. Most adults born before 1957 are likely to have been infected naturally and can be considered immune, even if they did not have clinically recognizable mumps disease.

VACCINE ADVERSE REACTIONS

Parotitis and fever after vaccination have been reported rarely. Allergic reactions including rash, pruritus, and purpura have been associated temporally with mumps vaccination but are uncommon, usually mild, and of brief duration. The frequency of reported CNS dysfunction after mumps vaccination is not greater than the observed background incidence rate in the general population.

VACCINE PRECAUTIONS

Because of the theoretical risk of fetal harm after administration of a live-virus vaccine to a pregnant woman, avoiding administering mumps vaccine to pregnant women is prudent.

Mumps vaccine should not be given to persons who are immunocompromised as a result of immune deficiency diseases, leukemia, lymphoma, or generalized malignancy or to persons who are immunosuppressed as a result of therapy with corticosteroids, alkylating drugs, antimetabolites, or radiation.

SELECTED READING

Aase JM, Noren GR, Reddy DV, et al. Mumps-virus infection in pregnant women and the immunologic response of their offspring. N Engl J Med 1972; 286:1379.

Baumann B, Danon L, Weitz R, et al. Unilateral hydrocephalus due to obstruction of the foramen of Monro: another complication of intrauterine mumps infection? Eur J Pediatr 1982; 139:158.

Bertoye P, Monnet P, Bret J, Touraine R. Congenital cardiopathy in dizygotic twins due to embryopathy (maternal mumps). Case J Méd Lyon 1952; 33:391.

Boriskin Y, Booth JC, Yamada A. Rapid detection of the mumps virus by the polymerase chain reaction. J Virol Methods 1993; 42:23.

Bowers D. Mumps during pregnancy. West J Surg Obstet Gynecol 1953; 61:72.

Brid NS, Kulkarni Ag. Double viral infection during pregnancy. J Assoc Physician India 1995; 43:288.

Chen S-C, Thompson MW, Rose V. Endocardial fibroelastosis: family studies with special reference to counseling. J Pediatr 1971; 79:385.

Chiba Y, Ogra PA, Nakao T. Transplacental mumps infection. Am J Obstet Gynecol 1975; 122:904.

Dutta PC. A fatal case of pregnancy complicated with mumps. J Obstet Gynecol Br Emp 1935; 42:869.

Editorial. Mumps and the endocardium. N Engl J Med 1966; 275:393.

Fine PE, Adelstein AM, Snowman J, et al. Long term effects of exposure to viral infection in utero. Br Med J Clin Res Ed 1985; 290:509.

Garcia A, Pereira J, Vidigal N, et al. Intrauterine infection with mumps virus. Obstet Gynecol 1980; 56:756.

Gersony WM, Katz SL, Nadas AS. Endocardial fibroelastosis and the mumps virus. Pediatrics 1966; 37:430.

Gold E. Almost extinct diseases: measles, mumps, rubella, and pertussis. Pediatr Rev 1966; 17:207.

Greenberg MW, Beilly JS. Congenital defects in the infant following mumps during pregnancy. Am J Obstet Gynecol 1966; 38:309.

Grönvall H, Selander P. Some virus diseases during pregnancy and their effect on the fetus. Nord Med 1948; 37:409.

Guneroth WG. Endocardial fibroelastosis and mumps. Pediatrics 1966; 38:309.

Hardy JB. Viral infection in pregnancy. A review. Am J Obstet Gynecol 1965; 93:1052.

Hodes D, Brunell PA. Mumps antibody: placental transfer and disappearance during the first year of life. Pediatrics 1970; 45:99.

Holowach J, Thurston DL, Becker B. Congenital defects in infants following mumps during pregnancy. A review of the literature and a report of chorio-retinitis due to fetal infection. J Pediatr 1957; 50:689.

Hyatt H. Relationship of maternal mumps to congenital defects and fetal deaths, and to maternal morbidity and mortality. Am Pract Dig Treat 1961; 12:359.

Jones JF, Ray G, Fulginiti VA. Perinatal mumps infection. J Pediatr 1980; 96:912.

Katz M. Is there mumps embryopathy? An unanswered question. Clin Pediatr 1967; 6:321.

Kilham L. Mumps virus in human milk and in milk of infected monkey. J Am Med Assoc 1951; 146:1231.

Kleiman M. Mumps virus infections. In Lennette EH, ed. Laboratory Diagnosis of Viral Infections. New York: Marcel Dekker, 1985; 369–384.

Korones SB. Uncommon virus infections of the mother, fetus, and newborn: influenza, mumps and measles. Clin Perinatol 1988; 15:259.

Kurtz J, Tomlinson A, Pearson J. Mumps virus isolated from a fetus. Br Med J 1982; 284:471.

Haas DM, Flowers CA, Congdon CL. Rubella, rubeola, and mumps in pregnant women: susceptibilities and strategies for testing and vaccinating. Obstet Gynecol 2005:106:295.

Lacour M, Maherzi M, Vienny H, Suter S. Thrombocytopenia in a case of neonatal mumps infection: evidence for further clinical presentations. Eur J Pediatr 1993; 152:39.

Monif GR. Maternal mumps infection during gestation: observations on the progeny. Am J Obstet Gynecol 1974; 119:549.

Moore JH. Epidemic parotitis complicating late pregnancy: report of a case. J Am Med Assoc 1931; 97:1625.

Nahmias AJ, Armstrong G. Mumps virus and endocardial fibroelastosis. N Engl J Med 1966; 275:1449.

Reman O, Freymuth F, Laloum D, et al. Neonatal respiratory distress due to mumps. Arch Dis Child 1986; 61:80.

Robertson GG, Williamson AP, Blattner RJ. Origin and development of lens cataracts in mumps-infected chick embryos. Am J Anat 1964; 115:473.

Schwartz HA. Mumps in pregnancy. Am J Obstet Gynecol 1950; 60:875.

Shone JD, Muañoz Armas S, Manning JA, et al. The mumps antigen skin test in endocardial fibroelastosis. Pediatrics 1966; 37:423.

Shouldice D, Mintz S. Mumps in utero. Can Nurse 1955; 51:454.

Siddall RS. Epidemic parotitis in late pregnancy. Am J Obstet Gynecol 1937; 33:524.

St Geme JW Jr, Davis CWC, Peralta HJ, et al. The biologic perturbations of persistent embryonic mumps virus infection. Pediatr Res 1973; 7:541.

St Geme JW Jr, Peralta H, Farias E, et al. Experimental gestational mumps virus infection and endocardial fibroelastosis. Pediatrics 1971; 48:821.

Sterner G, Grandien M. Mumps in pregnancy at term. Scan J Infect Dis 1990; Suppl 71:36.

Swan C. Congenital malformations associated with rubella and other virus infections. In Banks HS, ed. Modern Practice in Infectious Fevers, Vol. 2. New York: PB Hoeber, 1951; 528–552.

Vosburgh JB, Diehl AM, Liu C, et al. Relationship of mumps to endocardial fibroelastosis. Am J Dis Child 1965; 109:69.

Ylinen O, Järvinen PA. Parotitis during pregnancy. Acta Obstet Gynecol Scand 1953; 32:121.

Mumps Vaccine

Cochi SL, Preblud SR, Orenstein WA. Perspectives on the relative resurgence of mumps in the United States. Am J Dis Child 1998; 142:499.

Fahlgren K. Two doses of MMR vaccine—sufficient to eradicate measles, mumps and rubella? Scand J Soc Med 1988; 16:129.

Hersh BS, Fine PEM, Kent WK, et al. Mumps outbreak in a highly vaccinated population. J Pediatr 1994; 119:187.

Rubella 20

INTRODUCTION

Clinical rubella was first described in Germany by De Bergen in 1752 and Orlow in 1758. Considered sort of a "bastard measles," it was given several names, the principal ones being rotheln, rubeola, and German measles. The latter name was engendered by the early interest of these German investigators.

In 1886, Veale formally proposed the name "rubella" for the disease:

> The name of a disease is always a matter of importance. It should be short for the sake of convenience in writing, and euphonious for ease in pronunciation. It should not be a question-begging appellative. Rotheln is harsh and foreign to our ears, rubeola notha and Rosalia idiopathica are too long for general use, and are certainly expressive of conclusions which have yet to be proved. I therefore venture to propose Rubella as a substitute for Rotheln.

During the early 1970s, most cases of rubella occurred in children and young adolescents. By 1999, adults accounted for 86% of cases. Seventy-three percent of individuals with rubella were Hispanic. Most of these persons were foreign born. Recent outbreaks of rubella occurred in individuals from Mexico and Central America.

The rash characteristic of rubella virus is a maculopapular eruption. It usually begins on the upper thorax or face and spreads in a wavelike pattern to involve first the thorax, then the abdomen, and finally the extremities over approximately a three-day period. It is not uncommon for the rash to be fully developed on the lower extremities at the same time that there is early fading of the rash around the face and neck. Characteristically, the rash lasts for three days; hence its popular name "the three-day measles," as contrasted to that of rubeola, the "seven-day measles."

Arthralgia (and occasional instances of arthritis) is not an uncommon complication in adults, particularly young women. Depending on the strain virulence of the virus, the incidence of clinically significant arthralgia may approach 20%.

Not all viral infections associated with an exanthema of three-days duration are rubella. Exanthemas comparable to that observed with rubella infection have been described with echovirus and coxsackie virus infections and type A hepatitis. The diagnosis of rubella can be inferred on clinical grounds by the additional finding of postauricular adenopathy. The postauricular adenopathy may be detectable six to seven days prior to the onset of rash and persists for one to two weeks after its disappearance.

CONGENITAL RUBELLA FOLLOWING MATERNAL INFECTION

The aggressive use of childhood and strategic vaccination programs have dramatically reduced the incidence of congenital rubella cases. In 2004, a panel convened by the Centers for Disease Control and Prevention concluded that rubella was no longer endemic in the United States. Nine cases of rubella occurred in 2004. Between 2001 and 2004, only four cases of congenital rubella were identified. Both maternal rubella and congenital rubella cases now occur in foreign-born mothers.

The probability of involvement of the developing fetus by rubella virus is in part a function of when in gestation maternal infection occurs. An inverse relationship exists between clinical manifestations of the teratogenic potential of rubella virus and the age of the embryo at the time of maternal infection within the first 90 days of pregnancy. The earlier in development maternal infection occurs, the greater the probability of significant fetal involvement. In light of the augmented knowledge concerning congenital rubella, it is apparent that there are no adequate statistics that can translate the true incidence of infection in utero into a problematic figure. Nevertheless, certain principles are evident:

1. The further advanced the pregnancy is from the tenth week, the less the probability of overt fetal involvement. If congenital involvement occurs, fetal involvement is more likely to result further in an incomplete form or *forme fruste* of the syndrome rather than the full-blown congenital rubella syndrome (CRS).
2. Even within the period of maximum susceptibility to the teratogenic effect of the virus, although the incidence of involvement of the fetus per se is markedly increased, it is nonetheless a random phenomenon. Gestational age is just one of the many variables for fetal involvement.

Based on epidemiologic data, the chances of having an infant with CRS as a consequence of maternal infection in the first trimester are estimated to be between 18% and 20% (Table 1). Although statistics are an adequate reflection of the teratogenicity of rubella virus, they fail to delineate the total morbidity resulting from congenital infection. *Formes frustes* of rubella embryopathy due to continuous virus–cell interaction ("the expanded CRS") have gone unrecognized. Once it was recognized that infection of the fetus could still result in normal-appearing neonates, it

TABLE I Probability of fetal involvement following maternal infection in gestation

Month of maternal infection	Probability of overt congenital rubella	Probability of congenital rubella
First	50%	The inability to quote a precise probability of involvement is due to a number of factors.
Second	25%	(i) The "normal"-appearing infants, who harbor rubella virus in their biological fluids, are readily missed when only clinical parameters are used to calculate the incidence of involvement.
Third	10%	(ii) Many of the symptoms are not detectable early in life, i.e., in two separate studies, only 50% of the malformations presented signs or symptoms at birth. In another study, while deafness was detected in 6% of the infants at 2 yr of age, it was found in 13% of the same group at 3 yr of age.
Fourth	1–2%	(iii) The mother can contract subclinical rubella.

became apparent that the incidence of transplacental infection could not be monitored from clinically overt disease alone. Involvement of the fetus and the persistence of viral infection into the first year of life meant that delayed morbidity was to be anticipated because of continued virus–cell interaction during somatic growth. Previous statistical assessments of the possibility of fetal involvement as opposed to teratogenicity were invalid, owing to their failure to include congenital rubella infants without overt rubella syndrome or *formes frustes*.

Only fragmentary data exist that might shed some light on the probability of congenital infection as well as its translation into morbidity and mortality. The effect of the 1964 epidemic in Baltimore on the outcome of pregnancy was studied prospectively in 1086 women enrolled in a prenatal program at Johns Hopkins Medical Center. When maternal infection occurred in the first trimester, four of the seven live-born infants had defects compatible with rubella syndrome; six of the seven were small for their age. The seventh was normal in all clinical aspects tested; however, rubella virus was recovered from the throat washings on two occasions.

Morbidity from congenital rubella is not restricted to maternal infection in the first 90 days. Hardy et al. described variants of rubella embryopathy in the progeny of mothers who contracted infection in the early part of the second trimester. They reported on 24 women with clinical and laboratory evidence of rubella between the 14th and 31st weeks of pregnancy. In the two cases of fetal loss, the rubella virus was recovered from the products of conception. Although the 22 live-born infants were incompletely sampled, the virus was isolated from three of them. Of the 22 infants, seven were clinically normal and had no detectable antibody at six months of age. Of the remaining 15 infants suspected to be abnormal, six had elevated immunoglobulin M (IgM) levels and 10 had detectable levels of antibodies after six months of age. Although morbidity may occur as a consequence of second-trimester fetal involvement, the incidence of congenital malformations by the fifth month approaches its background norm.

PATHOGENESIS

Following maternal infection in the first trimester, rubella virus is recoverable from the products of conception in up to 64% of cases. If maternal rubella is prospectively confirmed, either by viral isolation or by serologic conversion, the incidence of recovery approaches 100%. Involvement of the conceptus is almost invariably the result of hematogenous dissemination associated with maternal viremia. Involvement of the conceptus takes either of the two principal forms:

1. Recovery of virus is limited to the placenta
2. Concomitant widespread organ involvement

It is this latter pattern of viral infection that correlates with congenital rubella. Once infection of a given organ system is achieved, virus replication may continue throughout gestation and well into the first year of life.

Despite widespread organ involvement, the teratogenic manifestations of rubella virus are primarily limited to those organ systems with a limited capacity to regenerate (Table 2). Certain facets of rubella embryopathy require not only the establishment of infection within that organ system, but also its involvement at a critical phase of organogenesis. As with drug-induced embryopathy, vulnerability of the developing fetus is partly a function of time, wherein minimal insult, either direct, in the form of virus–cell interaction resulting in necrobiosis, or indirect, in the form of inhibition of mitosis, can have an exaggerated effect. Both of these possibilities are functional postulates in the pathogenesis of congenital rubella (Fig. 1).

An inverse relationship exists between manifestations of the teratogenic potential of rubella virus and gestational age within the first 90 days of life. This may be a partial function of alterations in placental structure during early growth and development or the loss of the complementary viral receptor sites on cell surfaces.

Even when fetal infection has occurred within the first 90 days of gestation, in rare instances, the infants, although possessing virus in all their biologic fluids except blood, have been deemed normal by every clinical parameter. In these instances, the effects of rubella virus have been either negligible or offset by the limited regenerative capacity of those tissues that are compromised in the classic rubella syndrome.

Virus persistence and continued virus–cell interaction during in utero existence is responsible for a wide spectrum of clinical disease in the neonatal period. Thrombocytopenia, hemolytic anemia with extramedullary hematopoiesis, hepatitis, interstitial pneumonitis, myocarditis, myocardiopathy,

TABLE 2 Clinical findings in symptomatic neonates with the "expanded" congenital rubella syndrome

Organ system	Clinical findings
Bone	Micrognathia
	Bony radiolucencies
Cardiovascular system	Pulmonary arterial hypoplasia
	Patent ductus arteriosus
	Coarctation of aortic isthmus
	Interventricular septal defect
	Interauricular septal defect
	Myocardial necrosis
	Myocarditis
Central nervous system	Encephalitis
	Microcephaly
	Dystrophic calcification
	Bulging fontanel
	Neurologic deficits
	Progressive panencephalitis
Ear	Hearing defects
	Peripheral
	Central
Eye	Retinopathy
	Cataracts
	Cloudy cornea
	Glaucoma
	Microphthalmos
Genitourinary system	Hypospadias
	Unilateral agenesis
	Renal artery stenosis with hypertension
Hematopoietic system	Anemia
	Dermal erythropoiesis (blueberry muffin syndrome)
	Immunologic dyscrasias
	Leukopenia
	Thrombocytopenia with/without purpura
Liver	Hepatitis
	Hepatosplenomegaly
	Jaundice (regurgitative)
Lungs	Interstitial pneumonitis (acute, subacute, chronic)
Pancreas (growth and development)	Diabetes mellitus
	Growth retardation
	Intrauterine
	Extrauterine
	Prematurity
	Psychomotor retardation: intellectual, behavioral, autistic, educational difficulties

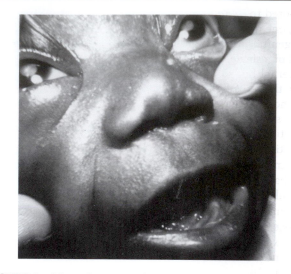

FIGURE 1 Bilateral congenital cataracts which, with cardiovascular, central nervous system, and inner ear abnormalities, constitute the so-called classic stigmata of congenital rubella.

has been isolated from the brain biopsy of one such patient.

POSTNATAL PERSISTENCE

The postnatal persistence of rubella virus is one of the major enigmas in our understanding of the pathogenesis of rubella embryopathy. Acquisition of rubella infection in the neonatal period or later results in a limited period of virus replication within internal organ systems and at free epithelial surfaces. Thirty days after the onset of rash, there is no evidence of continued virus replication, a finding that is in sharp contrast to the condition as it exists in an infant with congenital rubella. Once the fetus is infected in utero, virus replication persists throughout gestation. Approximately 90% of all neonates with CRS have virus in most of their extravascular biologic fluids, such as CSF, urine, tears, and swabbings of the conjunctiva or posterior part of the oropharynx.

The earliest postulate advanced to account for viral persistence was immune paralysis, namely, that the fetus exposed to an antigen in appropriate quantity in utero would be rendered incapable of synthesizing specific antibodies to the antigen. Congenital rubella furnished an exciting model system in which infection could antedate implantation.

Analysis of the serum of infants with congenital rubella shows it to contain a composite of specific IgG and IgM antibodies. Because IgM of maternal origin is excluded from the fetal circulation, this finding constituted presumptive evidence of congenital infection. At the age of 34 months, infants with congenital rubella do not exhibit significant absence of neutralizing or hemagglutination-inhibition antibodies, as would be anticipated if the titers were totally contingent on transplacentally acquired maternal immunoglobulins.

That the IgM antibodies are functional is suggested by the infrequency of recovery of rubella virus from the serum of neonates in the neonatal and postnatal periods, as

interstitial nephritis, encephalitis, interstitial pancreatitis, and osteomyelitis have all been observed in infants with congenital rubella (Table 2). These manifestations of cellular dysfunction and necrobiosis have prompted the use of the term "the expanded CRS."

Infants with congenital rubella develop a neurologic syndrome, progressive rubella panencephalitis, during the second decade of life. The progressive neurologic deterioration observed is characterized by motor spasticity, ataxia, intellectual deterioration, and seizures. Examination of the cerebrospinal fluid (CSF) reveals elevated protein and gamma-globulin levels, in conjunction with a high rubella antibody titer in both the serum and the CSF. Rubella virus opposed to its recovery from multiple organs. Having said this, one must focus on what perhaps is the critical issue in congenital infection. The response of host to virus is not that of a single, but of a dual, biologic system in which the maternal host is capable of a more accelerated response than the fetus. The fetus at the time of immunologic competence is involved in antigenic processing and initial antibody synthesis. The maternal host has already responded to infection and is now flooding the fetal compartment with a high titer of specific antibody. What is the influence of specific maternal IgG antibody on the immune response?

It has been clearly demonstrated, either in vivo or in vitro, in multiple animal systems, and in humans, that exogenous administration of specific antibody may suppress in vivo endogenous production of antibody to that immunogen. The best example of this is probably the use of Rho(D) human immune globulin to prevent sensitization of an Rh-negative woman. The function of a specific antibody is postulated to result in the destruction of immunologically committed lymphocytes. The possibility that this phenomenon functions in fetuses has been suggested by three sets of observations:

1. There is a prolonged phase of IgM antibody synthesis in congenital rubella as opposed to that in neonatally acquired infection. In the latter, the conversion from the IgM to the IgG antibody response occurs 6 to 20 weeks prior to that observed in congenital rubella.
2. Some 10% of infants with congenital rubella exhibit dysgammaglobulinemia or hypogammaglobulinemia. The characteristic pattern is an elevated IgM level with a low IgG level and absence of IgA. Eventually, there is a reemergence of the IgG and IgA classes of immunoglobulins.
3. Some infants with documented congenital rubella fail to produce specific antibodies to rubella virus in the first two years of life.

Having touched on the conversion from specific IgM to IgG, we can now see the ramifications. A total of 80% of IgM is maintained within the intravascular space as contrasted to 20% at the interstitial sites of virus replication. With the conversion, the interstitial distribution of immunoglobulins is markedly altered, so that a threefold increase in specific antibody is achieved at the interstitial site of replication (60% of IgG is extravascular). Marked similarity exists between the curves of apparent immune elimination of the virus and the emergence of specific IgG. The correlation is not absolute for a given case. Although the shift in the type of immunoglobulin synthesis is probably of great importance in the ultimate nonrecovery of virus, other factors function concomitantly. Otherwise, a tighter correlation between the two phenomena would be anticipated.

Many investigators have explored the possibility that chronic rubella viral infection may be the result of defective cellular immunity. Although decreased delayed hypersensitivity can be demonstrated in infants with congenital rubella, it is not unlike that observed in normal individuals during acute viral infection and following administration of viral vaccines. While delayed hypersensitivity plays a prominent role

in certain facets of the histopathology of congenital rubella, it is yet to be demonstrated that chronic viral infection is primarily the result of defective cellular immunity.

Clinical Significance of Persistence

Approximately 50% of infants with congenital rubella will have recoverable virus in their biologic fluids at six months of age. Rubella virus has been recovered from lens fragments as long as three years following birth.

The persistence of rubella virus has very pragmatic ramifications. Infants with congenital rubella are a source of infection among nurses and are responsible for the "second generation" congenitally malformed infants in pregnant females caring for these children. Consequently, prophylactic measures need to be instituted to guard the immediate paramedical and medical personnel within the delivery suite and on the obstetric ward.

The inability to supply prospective identification of all potentially infected infants, owing to occult maternal illness or the lack of maternal participation in a prenatal program, should prompt the screening of all potential vectors within the nursing and medical community. It is not enough to merely determine the antibody status of the women who are currently pregnant or may soon become so. A susceptible nurse may become infected and may serve as a vector in disseminating infection among a young childbearing population. Although the diagnosis of congenital rubella may be made after parturition, it is often recognized within the incubation period of rubella virus. Thus, prospective knowledge of the susceptibility of the nursing staff permits both the following:

1. Assessment of the probability of the subsequent development of infection among personnel exposed to the infant, the amniotic fluid, or the placenta
2. Initiation of proper quarantine

DIAGNOSIS

Congenital

Laboratory diagnosis of congenital rubella infection only requires any one of the following:

1. Demonstration of a rubella-specific IgM antibody or infant IgG rubella antibody level that persists at a higher level and for a longer time than expected from passive transfer of maternal antibody (i.e., rubella titer that does not drop at the expected rate of a twofold dilution per month). Approximately 20% of infected infants tested for rubella IgM might have detectable titers before the age of one month. Infant with symptoms consistent with congenital rubella who tested negative soon after birth should be retested at the age of one month.
2. Isolation of rubella can be obtained from nasal, blood, throat, urine, or CSF specimens. The best results are from throat swabs. An infant with CRS should be considered infectious until two cultures of clinical specimens obtained one month apart are negative for rubella virus.
3. Detection of virus by reverse transcription and polymerase chain reaction methodology (RT-PCR). This

process can be used to detect the presence of rubella virus after growth in tissue culture or directly in clinical specimens.

RT-PCR has been used to document rubella placentitis; however, demonstration of rubella virus in the placenta correlates poorly with secondary dissemination to the fetus.

Maternal

A clinical case of adult rubella is defined as an illness characterized by (*i*) acute onset of a generalized maculopapular rash; (*ii*) temperature greater than 37.2° C (99.0° F); and (*iii*) arthralgia/arthritis, lymphadenopathy (usually suboccipital, postauricular, and cervical), or conjunctivitis.

Maternal rubella is most commonly documented serologically with the demonstration of a greater than eightfold rise in the specific antibody titer obtained from specimens drawn on or before the rash and 7 to 10 days following its clinical appearance.

Not infrequently, the obstetrician or gynecologist is confronted with a gravida who had a rash three or four days earlier. Paired serologic specimens obtained within the first five days following may still demonstrate possible serologic conversion (rubella infection). When more than five days have elapsed since the onset of a rash, the presence of postauricular adenopathy in conjunction with a high rubella titer containing specific IgM antibodies can substantiate the diagnosis of recent infection. Rubella IgM antibodies appear one week after the onset of infection and persist for approximately one month. To document recent maternal infection with rubella virus, the IgM enzyme-linked immunosorbent assay test should be utilized.

EXPOSURE TO RUBELLA DURING GESTATION

One of the most common problems of clinical management is that of a gravida with known exposure to rubella virus. At the time of the initial visit, it is imperative to obtain a sample of serum for testing. Since antibodies first appear at the time of the rash, any significant titer of specific antibody prior to the presumed onset of rash or possible subclinical illness (days 11–17) is indicative of prior infection. A gravida with preexisting antibody can be reassured about the safety of her fetus in terms of the potentially deleterious effects of rubella virus. Absence of specific antibody indicates susceptibility. The patient is given an appointment to return in 18 to 20 days or at the time of clinical symptoms (fever, malaise, arthralgia, and rash), whichever comes first. At the time of this follow-up visit, the patient is carefully reevaluated for postauricular adenopathy (Fig. 2). Approximately 25% to 30% of maternal infections can be expected to be subclinical. Although rash may not develop, postauricular adenopathy not infrequently does. Postauricular adenopathy, even in the absence of rash, should arouse a high index of suspicion of infection with rubella virus. Definitive diagnosis is contingent on the demonstration of an eightfold increase in specific antibody titer. An eightfold increase in the convalescent specimen drawn 21 to 24 days after exposure, or 7 to 10 days after the onset of the rash,

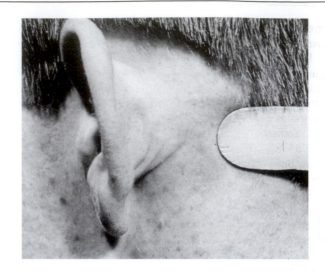

FIGURE 2 Postauricular adenopathy associated with rubella virus infection.

serologically confirms the diagnosis. Serologic evaluation at the time of the rash is still valid, since the peak antibody titers will not be reached for another 7 to 10 days.

There is no place for gamma-globulin in the clinical management. Administration of specific antirubella antibodies can only suppress the clinical manifestation of rubella and the appearance of endogenous specific antibody. If gamma-globulin has been given to susceptible individuals following intimate exposure to rubella virus, serologic surveillance must be extended for at least another 30 days. In the experimental model systems, the concomitant administration of exogenous specific antibody with an immunogen results in partial suppression or ablation of the immune response.

Once a case of rubella is confirmed, the appropriate health agencies must be immediately notified. Even one documented case needs to be treated as a potential outbreak. Since 30% to 50% cases of rubella infections are subclinical, investigation of an apparently isolated case may reveal the occurrence of additional cases.

VACCINATION OF WOMEN OF CHILDBEARING AGE

The advent of rubella vaccines has markedly altered the natural history of both rubella and congenital rubella and delineated new responsibilities for the discipline of obstetrics and gynecology, namely, vaccination of women of childbearing age. Estimates of susceptibility to rubella among reproductive-aged women in the United States ranges between 10% and 18%. In other countries, susceptibility to rubella virus may reach 40%.

The major impediment to the vaccination of women of childbearing age is the recognition that vaccine strains of rubella virus can, in very rare instances, reach the products of conception. That intrauterine rubella infection may follow immunization of the gravida underscores the need for careful selection and monitoring of the populations to be vaccinated. Prior to vaccination, the criteria that must be met include documented susceptibility, absence of pregnancy, and demonstration of a reliable form of contraception.

Prior to vaccination, the patient should undergo a pregnancy test and should use an effective modus of contraception, which should be continued for three menstrual cycles after vaccination. Noteworthy is the immediate postpartum period as a time for vaccination; also attractive as a situation for vaccination is the family planning clinic.

No CRS defects have been noted when pregnant women have been vaccinated with RA 27/3 vaccine. Rubella vaccine viruses, including the RA 27/3 strain, can cross the placenta and infect the fetus. Approximately 1% to 2% of infants born to susceptible gravidae vaccinated in pregnancy had serologic evidence of subclinical infection, regardless of vaccine strain. The risk of placental or fetal infection from RA 27/3 vaccine appears to be minimal. In view of the data collected through 1985, the Advisory Committee on Immunization Practices (ACIP) continues to state that

1. pregnancy remains a contraindication to rubella vaccination because of the theoretical albeit very small risk of CRS,
2. reasonable precautions should be taken to preclude vaccination of pregnant women, including asking women if they are pregnant, excluding those who say they are, and explaining the theoretical risks to the others, and
3. if vaccination does occur within three months before or after conception, the risk of CRS is so small as to be negligible; thus, rubella vaccination of a pregnant woman should not ordinarily be a reason to consider interruption of pregnancy. The patient and her physician, however, should make the final decision.

The success of childhood vaccination against rubella coupled with postpartum vaccination of serosusceptible women has, in part, masked a new mandate in women's healthcare, the extension of broad immunization protection to nonpregnant women who recently immigrated from countries without rubella control programs. They need to be evaluated from possible serosusceptibility to measles and mumps as well as rubella.

Identification of serosusceptibility to rubella virus may indicate a broader susceptibility to other viruses. Serosusceptibility to rubella virus frequently marks for serosusceptibility to measles and/or mumps. Haas et al. (2005) identified that twice the number of serosusceptible women to either measles or mumps viruses existed for each woman seronegative to rubella virus. Consideration should be given to the use of combination rubella, measles, and mumps (MMR) vaccine when vaccinating serosusceptible women in the postpartum period.

SELECTED READING

Maternal Rubella
Alysworth AA, Monif GRG. Delayed serological evidence of infection with rubella virus after the administration of gamma globulin. Obstet Gynecol 1971; 38:752.

Centers for Disease Control. Prevention of rubella: evaluation and management of suspected outbreaks, rubella in pregnant women, and surveillance for congenital rubella. MMWR 2001; 50/No. RR-12:1.

Centers for Disease Control. Achievements in public health: elimination of rubella and congenital rubella syndrome—United States, 1969–2004. MMWR 2005; 54:1.

Cradock, Watson JE. Laboratory diagnosis of rubella: past, present and future. Epidemiol Infect 1991; 107:1–15.

Hardy J, Monif GRG, Medearis D, Sever JL. Postnatal transmission of rubella virus to nurses. J Am Med Assoc 1965; 191:1034.

Herrmann KL. Rubella in the United States: toward a strategy for disease control and elimination. Epidemiol Infect 1991; 107:55.

Parkman PD, Buescher EL, Artenstein NS. Recovery of rubella virus from army recruits. Proc Soc Exp Biol Med 1962; 111:225.

Sever JL, Brody JA, Schiff GM, McAlister R, Culting R. Rubella epidemic on St. Paul Island in the Pribilofs, 1963. II: Clinical and laboratory findings for intensive study population. J Am Med Assoc 1965; 191:624.

Sever JL, Heubner RI, Fabiyi A, et al. Antibody response in acute and chronic rubella. Proc Soc Exp Biol Med 1966; 122:513.

Weller TH, Neva FA. Propagation in tissue culture of cytopathic agents from patients with rubella-like illness. Proc Soc Exp Biol Med 1962; 111:215.

Congenital Rubella
Alford CA, Neva FA, Weller TH. Virologic and serologic studies on human products of conception after maternal rubella. N Engl J Med 1964; 271:1275.

Avery GB, Monif GRG, Sever JL, Leikin SL. Rubella syndrome after apparent maternal illness. Am J Dis Child 1965; 110:444.

Brody JA, Sever JL, McAlister R, et al. Rubella epidemic on St. Paul Island in Pribilofs, 1963. I: epidemiologic, clinical and serological findings. J Am Med Assoc 1965; 191:619.

Cooper LZ, Krugman A. Diagnosis and management: congenital rubella. Pediatrics 1966; 37:335.

Centers for Disease Control. Import case of congenital rubella—New Hampshire, 2005. MMWR 2005; 54:1160.

Hardy JB, McCracken GH Jr, Gilkeson MR, Sever JI. Adverse fetal outcome following maternal rubella after the first trimester of pregnancy. J Am Med Assoc 1969; 207:2414.

Hardy JB, Monif GRG, Sever JL. Studies in congenital rubella, Baltimore 1964–65. Part II: clinical and virologic. Johns Hopkins Med J 1966; 118:97.

Korones SB, Ainger LE, Monif GRG, et al. Congenital rubella syndrome: new clinical aspects with recovery of virus from affected infants. J Pediatr 1965; 67:166.

Kunakorn M, Petchclai B, Liemsuwan C. Laboratory diagnosis of congenital and maternal rubella infection: a review. J Med Assoc Thai 1992; 75:1:282.

McCracken GH, Hardy JB, Gilkeson MR, Sever JL. Serum gamma M levels as a screening test in congenital rubella. The Society for Pediatric Research, 38th Annual Meeting, Atlantic City, 1968:151.

Monif GRG. Viral Infection of the Human Fetus. New York: Macmillan, 1969.

Monif GRG, Jordan PA. Rubella virus and rubella vaccine. Semin Perinatol 1977; 1:41.

Monif GRG, Avery GB, Korones SB, Sever JL. Isolation of the rubella virus from the organs of three children with rubella syndrome defects. Lancet 1965; 1:723.

Monif GRG, Hardy J, Sever JL. Studies in congenital rubella, Baltimore 1964–65. Part I: epidemiologic and virologic. Johns Hopkins Med J 1966; 118:85.

Monif GRG, Sever JL, Schiff GM, Traub RG. Isolation of rubella virus from products of conception. Am J Obstet Gynecol 1965; 91:1143.

Phillips CA, Melnick JL, Yow MD, et al. Persistence of virus in infants with congenital rubella and in normal infants with a history of maternal rubella. J Am Med Assoc 1965; 193:1027.

Plotkin SA, Oski FA, Hartnett EM, et al. Congenital syndrome. Some recently recognized manifestations of the rubella syndrome. J Pediatr 1965; 64:182.

Robinson J, Lemay M, Vaudry WL. Congenital rubella after anticipated maternal immunity: two cases and a review of the literature. Pediatr Infect Dis J 1994; 13:812.

Rosa C. Rubella and rubeola. Perinatol Semin 1988; 22:318.

Rudolph AJ, Yow MD, Phillips CA, et al. Transplacental rubella infection in newly born infants. J Am Med Assoc 1965; 191:843.

Tanemura M, Suzumori K, Yagami Y, et al. Diagnosis of fetal rubella infection with reverse transcription and nested polymerase chain reaction: a study of 34 cases diagnosed in fetuses. Am J Obstet Gynecol 1996; 174:578.

Tondury G, Smith DW. Fetal rubella pathology. J Pediatr 1966; 68:867.

Townsend N, Baringer JR, Wolinsky JS, et al. Progressive rubella panencephalitis: late onset after congenital rubella. N Engl J Med 1975; 292:990.

Weil ML, Itabeshi HH, Cremer NE, et al. Chronic progressive panencephalitis due to rubella virus stimulating SSPE. N Engl J Med 1975; 292:994.

Rubella Vaccine

Best JM. Rubella vaccines: past, present and future. Epidemiol Infect 1991; 107:17.

Centers for Disease Control. Rubella vaccination during pregnancy—United States, 1971–1981. MMWR 1982; 31:477.

Centers for Disease Control. Rubella in hospitals—California. MMWR 1983; 32:37.

Chin L, Werner SB, Kusumoto HH, Lennette EH. Complications of rubella immunization in children. Calif Med 1971; 114:7.

Crawford GE, Gremilion DH. Epidemic measles and rubella in Air Force recruits: impact of immunization. J Infect Dis 1981; 144:403.

Hinman AR, Orenstein WA, Bart KJ, Preblud SR. Rational strategy for rubella vaccination. Lancet 1983; 1:39.

Kilroy AW, Schaffner W, Fleet WF Jr, et al. Two syndromes following rubella immunization: clinical observations and epidemiological studies. J Am Med Assoc 1970; 214:2287.

Monif GRG, Jortan PA. Rubella virus and rubella vaccine. Semin Perinatol 1977; 1:41.

Noble IS, Wand M. Catcher's crouch and rubella immunization. J Am Med Assoc 1971; 217:212.

Preblud SR, Gross F, Halsey NA Jr, et al. Assessment of susceptibility to measles and rubella. J Am Med Assoc 1982; 247:1134.

Preblud SR, Serdula MK, Frank NA Jr, et al. Rubella vaccination in the United States: a ten-year review. Epidemiol Rev 1980; 2:171.

Rubella Vaccination in Pregnancy

ACIP. Rubella prevention. MMWR 1984; 33:301–310, 315–318.

American Academy of Pediatrics, American College of Obstetricians and Gynecologists. Guidelines for prenatal care. Fifth ed. Elk Groove Village (IL); Washington, DC: ACOG, 2002.

Balfour HH Jr, Groth KE, Edelman CK, et al. Rubella viraemia and antibody responses after rubella vaccination and reimmunization. Lancet 1981; 1:1078.

Banatvala JE, O'Shea S, Best JM, et al. Transmission of RA 27/3 rubella vaccine strain to products of conception (Letter). Lancet 1981; 1:392.

Barts SW, Stetler HC, Preblud SR, et al. Fetal risk associated with rubella vaccine: an update. Rev Infect Dis 1985; 7(suppl 1):595.

Bernstein DI, Ogra PL. Fetomaternal aspects of immunization with RA 27/3 live attenuated rubella virus vaccine during pregnancy. J Pediatr 1980; 97:467.

Centers for Disease Control. Rubella vaccination during pregnancy—United States, 1971–1981. MMWR 1982; 31:477.

Centers for Disease Control. Rubella vaccination during pregnancy—United States, 1971–1982. MMWR 1983; 32:429–432, 437.

Centers for Disease Control. Rubella and congenital rubella—United States, 1983. MMWR 1984; 33:237.

Centers for Disease Control. Rubella vaccination during pregnancy—United States, 1971–1985. MMWR 1986; 35:275.

Desmond MM, Montgomery JR, Melnick JL, et al. Congenital rubella encephalitis: effects on growth and early development. Am J Dis Child 1969; 118:30.

Enders G. Rubella antibody titers in vaccinated and nonvaccinated women and results of vaccination during pregnancy. Rev Infect Dis 1985; 7(suppl 1):S103.

Gall SA, Reef S. Rubella prenatal testing and postpartum vaccination. ACOG Clin Rev 2002; 7:1.

Haas DM, Flowers CA, Congdon CL. Rubella, rubeola and mumps in pregnant women; susceptibilities and strategies for testing and vaccinating. Obstet Gynecol 2005; 106:295.

Libman MD, Behr MA, Martel N, Ward BJ. Rubella susceptibility predicts measles susceptibility: implications for postpartum vaccination. Clin Infect Dis 2000; 31:1501.

O'Shea S, Parsons G, Best JM, et al. How well do low levels of rubella antibody protect? Lancet 1981; 2:1284.

Preblud SR, Stetler HC, Frank JA Jr, et al. Fetal risk associated with rubella vaccine. J Am Med Assoc 1981; 246:1413.

INTRODUCTION

Varicella-zoster virus (VZV) is a member of the herpesvirus family. The mature particle is approximately 1800 Å in diameter and consists of a linear double-stranded DNA molecule center core surrounded by an icosahedral capsid and a lipid envelope. The capsid is composed of 162 elongated hexagonal prisms, called capsomeres.

The outer envelope is derived from the inner nuclear membrane of the host cell. Having a significant phospholipid component, it is sensitive to both ether and chloroform degradation. The site of biosynthesis of viral DNA is the nucleus of the whole cell. Even though the site of assembly of viral particles is cytoplasmic as well as nuclear, virus replication within a cell produces an eosinophilic intranuclear inclusion body.

VARICELLA (CHICKENPOX)

The average incubation period is 11 days; the range is from 10 to 21 days. With direct parenteral inoculation, disease may develop in as few as nine days. Fever is usually the first sign of illness. Within a day, a maculopapular rash appears on the skin and mucous membranes. The lesions rapidly undergo vesiculation and appear as superficial thin-walled vesicles that appear in crops and are intensely pruritic. All stages from maculopapular to encrusted lesions can be observed simultaneously. This pattern distinguishes varicella from variola (smallpox), in which all the lesions are synchronous. The patient's temperature is in the range 101° F to 103° F. VZV usually can be obtained from vesicular fluid but rarely from other sites. Individuals with varicella should be considered to be infectious from 24 to 48 hours before to five days following the appearance of the first vesicles when the scabs have become dried. The infectivity period of herpes zoster is about the same as for varicella. Varicella is spread primarily by the respiratory route and is extremely contagious. Late winter and early spring are the times varicella becomes epidemic. Transmission of varicella is by close intimate contact. In the United States, varicella is a disease of childhood. Ninety percent of cases occur in children younger than 13 years of age. The estimated population in the United States over the age of one year is estimated to be 10%. Mortality for adults contracting disease is 15 times greater than that observed in immunocompetent normal children.

HERPES ZOSTER

Herpes zoster represents the reactivation of latent chickenpox. After the patient recovers from varicella, the virus persists in a latent form within the peripheral nervous system. The triggering mechanism for reactivation of viral synthesis is poorly understood, but may be related to diminishing specific immunity with age. Its clinical manifestation is shingles, in which the cutaneous lesions, rather than being generalized, are restricted to one to three dermatomes. Because of the sensorineural ganglion involvement, intense pain is characteristic of this manifestation of the VZV. Pain precedes lesion formation by two to three days and may confuse the initial diagnosis until lesions develop. The vesicular rash develops over three to five days, with the total duration of herpes zoster lasting up to 15 days. The trunk is the major area of disease involvement. Less frequently involved are the head, limbs, and genital area. Patients older than 50 years have as great as 50% risk of developing postherpetic neuralgia.

Varicella is uncommon in the first three months of life. The transplacental transfer of maternal antibody appears to be able to modify clinical expression of postnatally acquired varicella-zoster infection such that the infant develops zoster rather than chickenpox. The factors responsible for preventing the activation of latent VZV are unknown. Although it is postulated that serum antibody is the critical determinant, evidence is accumulating that cell-mediated immunity may be a more important factor. The risk of developing herpes zoster appears to be augmented in immunosuppressed patients and patients with Hodgkin's disease who have lost their cell-mediated responses. Varicella occurs more frequently during the late winter and early spring. Since herpes zoster is not caused by exogenous reinfection, it occurs with equal frequency throughout the year. The incidence of herpes zoster increases with age, whereas most cases of varicella occur in children. Herpes zoster afflicts about 10% to 20% of the population. Patients aged 60 years or older have the highest incidence of zoster. A second episode of zoster occurs in only 4% of afflicted individuals.

VARICELLA AND PREGNANCY

Varicella superimposed upon pregnancy causes three distinct sets of problems:

1. Enhanced maternal morbidity and mortality
2. Adverse impact in utero on organogenesis and growth
3. Potentially lethal parturitional disease in the neonate

Maternal Morbidity and Mortality

Greater than 90% of children have serological evidence of varicella-zoster before they reach adolescence or adulthood. The incidence of chickenpox among women of childbearing age is under 5%. The attack rate in pregnancy is between one and two cases per 10,000 pregnancies. These figures are probably conservative estimates owing to the underreporting of mild cases.

Varicella, when it occurs in an adult, tends to be more severe than in preadolescence. While the incidence of chickenpox is no higher in pregnant than in nonpregnant women, in pregnant women in advanced stages of gestation, infection is more likely to run a complicated course, with possible development of pneumonia, encephalitis, hepatitis, pancreatitis, and/or nephritis.

MATERNAL EXPOSURE TO VARICELLA

Inquiry should be made as to prior history of varicella or zoster. Barring gross alterations of the patient's immune state, prior disease confers life-long immunity. If the patient is uncertain about prior diseases and one or more family members cannot confirm its occurrence, a serological test to determine immune status should be performed. Maternal virus-specific immunoglobulin G (IgG) antibody levels as determined by enzyme-linked immunosorbent assay (ELISA) or the fluorescent antibody test for membrane antigen can be done. If exposure was beyond the standard incubation period for varicella-zoster by more than five days, and if maternal IgG antibody is detected, the serum specimen should be retested to determine whether IgM-specific antibodies are concomitantly present. If IgM antibodies are demonstrated, a second serum sample should be tested five to seven days later. The presence of IgM antibodies are indicative of recent infection. The presence of IgM-specific antibodies and a greater than fourfold rise in titer of a pair of specimens in parallel is diagnostic of acute infection.

If acute maternal infection or seronegativity (with the risk of continued intimate exposure) is documented, the patient can be offered varicella-zoster immune globulin (VZIG). The usual dose of VZIG is 125 units per 10 kg body weight, administered intramuscularly, up to a maximum of 625 units (five vials). The cost of VZIG varies between US$100 and US$600. While reasonably effective in preventing or attenuating varicella if given within four days of exposure, the value of VZIG in the presence of acute disease is not well established. Currently, the availability of VZIG is a problem and may not be produced at a future date.

VARICELLA-ZOSTER (CHICKENPOX) PNEUMONIA IN PREGNANCY

Much speculation exists as to whether varicella in pregnancy is complicated by an increased incidence of pneumonitis. The incidence of pneumonia in adults is probably about 16%. In a review of 173 cases of varicella complicated by pneumonia, Harris and Rhoades (1965) found 30 deaths, or a mortality rate of 17%. Of the 17 cases of varicella pneumonia complicating pregnancy, seven terminated in maternal deaths, giving a mortality rate of 41%.

Most cases of varicella pneumonia in pregnancy have occurred in the third trimester at a time when it has been demonstrated that maternal cell-mediated immunity is depressed.

Respiratory symptoms usually develop when the cutaneous lesions have been present for two to five days (Fig. 1). The initial sign is a dry, nonproductive cough. In many instances, this may be the sole manifestation of pulmonary involvement, and no symptomatic progression beyond this stage may be noted. In those patients with more severe disease, the cough, after 36 to 48 hours, becomes productive of a mucoid sputum, which may become blood-streaked; frank hemoptysis can occur. Dyspnea, tachypnea, and cyanosis may subsequently develop. Chest pain indicates parenchymal disease extending to the pleural surface. Symptoms may progress with frightening rapidity. Physical examination usually reveals minimal abnormal findings despite extensive roentgenographic evidence of pulmonary parenchymal involvement. The X-ray films characteristically reveal a widespread bilateral acinonodular infiltrate. The nodular densities seem to be superimposed on markedly increased bronchovascular markings. The infiltrates are most accentuated in the hilar regions, and while apices may be relatively spared, no areas are completely free of disease. In moderately severe cases, the respiratory symptoms may persist for 7 to 10 days.

The sudden increase in tachypnea and tachycardia may be signs of impending cardiovascular collapse. Clinicians must be aware of the insidious nature of the disease and of the gross disparity between initial relatively mild symptoms and potentially fulminating lethal disease.

Varicella pneumonia is but the clinical manifestation of disseminating disease. If sought for, evidence can be occasionally demonstrated for multiple organ involvement (pericarditis, myocarditis, hepatitis, pancreatitis, encephalitis).

The pathologic process is primarily an extensive mononuclear cell infiltration of the interstitium, with focal areas of coagulative necrosis associated with alveolitis. Septal cells may become cuboidal and form multinucleated giant cells. Within septal cells or macrophages, the characteristic intranuclear inclusion body of the VZV may be identified.

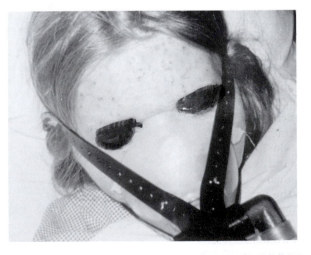

FIGURE 1   Varicella pneumonia complicating gestation in the third trimester. Oxygen saturation measurements on room air were as low as 57%. Following her recovery, the patient delivered at term a normal healthy infant.

The National Institutes of Health Study Group has recently identified two maternal risk factors. Women who are smokers and women with extensive cutaneous lesions (100 or more lesions) who contract varicella during pregnancy are at greater risk for developing the pneumonic complications.

Diagnosis

The differential diagnosis is usually not in doubt in view of the characteristic cutaneous and pulmonary findings, and the frequent history of chickenpox in progeny or household contacts. Laboratory analyses are not particularly helpful. The white blood cell count tends to be normal or slightly elevated, with a shift to the left, and the Gram smear of the sputum is unremarkable. The definite diagnosis of varicella-zoster infection resides in either serologic confirmation or virus isolation.

Therapy

Supportive therapy is comparable to that utilized in influenzal pneumonia. Salient features of management include the following:

1. Administration of oxygen, primarily via a positive pressure apparatus. This is often helpful in relieving the dyspnea.
2. Intravenous maintenance of fluids and electrolyte balance. As a rule, patients with varicella-zoster pneumonia tend to have intravascular hypovolemia.
3. If central venous pressure rises, digitalization of the patient before acute pulmonary edema occurs.
4. Transfusion therapy with concomitant digitalization, in case of significant hemoptysis, especially in a patient with preexisting anemia.
5. Obtaining serial sputum smears and cultures, and antibiotics, if secondary bacterial infection is suspected.

If a pregnant woman develops VZV, antiviral therapy is indicated to prevent severe and life-threatening complications. In the United States, acyclovir has been approved for the treatment of acute VZV.

Acyclovir has been used in gravidae with varicella pneumonia in the late second and third trimester. Most case reports involve the use of intravenous acyclovir 5 to 18 mg/kg every eight hours for 5 to 10 days. Pulmonary function improved in most women with therapy, but one patient died after increasing pulmonary dysfunction.

Smego et al. (1991) retrospectively evaluated the use of acyclovir in 21 women with varicella pneumonia in their second or third trimester of pregnancy. Sixteen of the women were previously reported in the literature and five of the women were newly reported by the investigator. Those women received a short course of oral acyclovir 600 to 800 mg four to five times daily for five days following intravenous therapy. Due to pneumonia, ventilatory assistance was required in five of twelve women in their second trimester and in seven of nine women in their third trimester. Deaths associated with uncontrolled infection or complications occurred in 2 of 21 (14%) women. Among

the women who died, two of the three infants born also died. One infant was stillborn and one infant was born prematurely. Women at highest risk for fatality were those in their third trimester of pregnancy who required mechanical ventilation. Preliminary evidence suggests that acyclovir is safe and the drug is safe for the developing fetus when given during the last trimester.

The antiviral drugs acyclovir, valacyclovir, and famciclovir have been approved for treating herpes zoster.

Some physicians have used oral valacyclovir, 1 g three times a day for 7 to 10 days in the therapy of acute VZV in pregnancy.

Huang et al. (2001) have shown that the combination of intravenous immunoglobulin (IVIG) and acyclovir intravenously administered seven days after the onset of maternal rash can effectively prevent perinatal varicella.

IVIG should be offered to pregnant, varicella-seronegative women with significant exposure to VZV.

The patient who develops varicella pneumonia near term may require hospitalization. To counteract possible nosocomial spread, respiratory isolation with dressing precautions should be instituted. This means a private room with the door closed at all times; use of masks, gloves, and gowns; restricting equipment to use only in that room (an article possibly contaminated by direct contact or secretions must be handled as infectious and disposed of properly); handwashing upon leaving the room; and restricting personnel who care for the patient to those with a history of prior varicella or those over the age of 30 years and not pregnant.

Fetal Wastage

Postpartum goals are focused clearly on the neonate and on maximizing its well-being. The possibility of congenital involvement, that is, the occurrence of disease at birth or before the tenth day of life, must be assessed. In those cases in which maternal disease occurs immediately prior to the delivery, strict isolation must be instituted.

In general, maternal infection with VZV during the first trimester does not result in a detectable increase in fetal wastage, unless it is associated with severe maternal illness.

Abortion may ensue in those instances complicated by varicella pneumonia. Early abortion or prematurity is thought to be secondary to maternal hypoxia and febrile response. The degree of maternal hypoxia can be marked. The interstitial pneumonitis creates an alveolar–capillary block upon which is imposed intra-alveolar hemorrhage.

In Utero Varicella

Although the bulk of fetal wastage associated with varicella is the consequence of the severity of the maternal disease, congenital varicella may occur as a result of both clinical and subclinical maternal infection. Congenital varicella is defined as disease occurring in the neonate before the tenth day of life. Maternal and neonatal disease most often are nonsynchronous. This discrepancy in the stage of development of lesions between mother and neonate strongly suggests the possibility that transplacental infection depends on the second viremia from placental sites. Although most cases of congenital infection in the world literature are varicella, congenital herpes zoster does occur.

Up to 25% of progeny born to gravidae whose pregnancies were complicated by varicella will have serological evidence of congenital infection; however, the incidence of overt congenital anomalities ranges from 0% to 9%. The best test for predicting morbidity as opposed to infection is ultrasonography. Ultrasound findings suggestive of congenital varicella include ventriculomegaly, microcephaly, limb abnormalities, intrauterine growth retardation, and dysmorphic calcification in multiple organs, especially the liver.

There is little evidence to suggest that subclinical infection modifies the ability of the virus to establish infection in utero. Varicella rarely has an incubation period shorter than 10 days. Congenital varicella is defined as (*i*) a disease occurring before the tenth day of life; (*ii*) the characteristic syndrome of developmental anomalies associated with maternal chickenpox in the first 15 days of life; or (*iii*) presence of IgM- or IgA-specific antibodies at birth.

Transplacental transmission of VZV is not limited by gestational age nor by the severity of maternal disease. VZV is not recoverable in the neonates whose mothers had chickenpox in the first trimester, despite morphological and serological evidence of in utero infection or disease. The most probable consequence of second-trimester and early third-trimester congenital varicella-zoster is complete resolution in utero. In an unpublished prospective study by Ann Arvins of 43 pregnant women whose gestations were complicated by maternal varicella, 8 of the 43 resultant progeny demonstrated immunologic evidence of in vitro infection. Only one of these eight neonates had viral-induced anomalies. This baby was one of 11 neonates born

to mothers who contracted their disease in the first trimester.

VARICELLA-ZOSTER EMBRYOPATHY

The time in gestation that varicella occurs markedly influences the pattern of ensuing disease. Chickenpox, which occurs early in gestation, may be associated with multiple developmental abnormalities (Table 1). La Foret and Lynch, in 1947, were the first to describe a syndrome characterized by low birth weight, areas of critical skin scarring (Fig. 2), hypotrophic limbs (Fig. 3), eye abnormalities, and neonatal growth retardation. The ophthalmologic lesions include microphthalmia, cataracts, optic atrophy, and chorioretinitis. The demonstrable neurologic defects include motor and sensory deficits, overt paralysis, and/or dysphagia. Postnatally, such infants may exhibit a failure to thrive. Psychomotor retardation and seizures are not uncommon. Necropsy analysis supports the thesis that the observed embryopathy is the result of viral cytopathic effects that are magnified by incomplete organogenesis.

Sauerbrei et al. (1960) using polymerase chain reaction demonstrated VZV DNA in formalin-food samples of lung, spleen, adrenal glands, bulbus oculi, and placenta from a 34-week-old stillborn with hypophthamos, hypoplasia of the extremities, and skin lesions.

The full-blown La Foret–Lynch syndrome occurs in neonates whose mothers contracted chickenpox during the first 15 weeks of gestation. The syndrome is not constant. Some neonates exhibit the complete spectrum of pathology whereas others have only one or two organ systems involved.

Congenital VZV infection can occur in the absence of overt maternal illness. Mustonen et al. (2001), in their study of 201 neonates, identified four babies with neurological

TABLE I Clinical and laboratory findings in five infants born following maternal varicella in early pregnancy

Findings	Individual cases						
	1	2		3		4	5
Gestational varicella	8 wk	13–14 wk		11 wk		9 wk	13–15 wk
Low birth weight for gestational age							
Skin lesions							
Hypotrophic limb	Right lower	Right lower		Right upper		Left upper	Left lower
Seizures							
Cortical atrophy						NR	
Ophthalmologic observations	Bilateral optical atrophy	Chorioretinitis		Chorioretinitis		Left Horner syndrome	Microphthalmia, cataracts, chorioretinitis
Virus isolation	NR	Negative		NR		NR	Negative
Varicella-zoster antibody titer (complement-fixing)	NR	Day 13	Day 63	5 mo	8 mo	6 wk	Day 2	5 mo
Infant		1:16	1:32	1:32	1:8	1:40	1:256	1:128
Mother		1:64	1:8	NR	1:320	1:128	1:64

Abbrevation: NR, not reported.
Source: Modified from Srabstein et al. (1974).

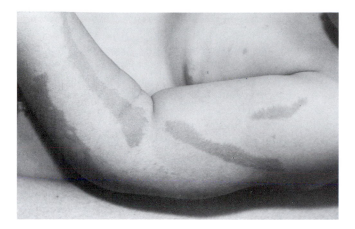

FIGURE 2 Cutaneous scars in a child suspected of having had congenital varicella. Source: Courtesy of WE Bell, MD, Iowa City, IA.

varicella-induced sequelae whose mothers had asymptomatic infection during pregnancy.

PERIPARTURITIONAL VARICELLA

When gravidae develop varicella late in the third trimester, within 17 days of delivery, 24% of the ensuing progeny will develop overt disease. The incubation period from onset of maternal rash to the onset of rash in the newborn is 11 days (range 9–15 days). This discrepancy between maternal and neonatal lesions suggests that transplacental infection is dependent on a second viremia from fetal endothelial sites within the placenta and that only occasionally is the congenital form of the disease a consequence of the primary viremia in the maternal host. In rare cases, the primary maternal viremia induces simultaneous disease in both mother and fetus. One study reported the presence of congenital varicella at birth in fraternal twins whose mother developed the disease on the day prior to delivery. Similarly, Harris (1967) reported two cases of congenital varicella in which maternal and neonatal lesions were in a comparable stage of development. With the exception of these four cases, varicella in the mother and in the newborn are nonsynchronous.

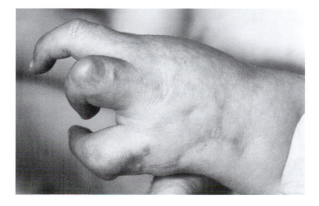

FIGURE 3 Digital anomalies in the same child as in Figure 2. *Source:* Courtesy of WE Bell, MD, Iowa City, IA.

Timing of maternal disease is a critical factor for neonatal outcome. When maternal disease has occurred within five days prior to delivery, at 5 to 10 days of life, the ensuing progeny are prone to develop a severe form of varicella characterized by disseminated intravascular coagulopathy superimposed upon viral pneumonitis and hepatitis. Thirty percent of these neonates die. If the onset of maternal rash is more than five days postpartum and the neonate develops a disease in the first four days of life, the morbidity and mortality are significantly modified by the presence of specific maternally derived antibodies.

The order of appearance and the distribution of the eruptions in the newborn are similar to the pattern seen in adults. The initial lesions appear on the torso and then spread centrifugally. Successive crops of lesions develop in such a manner that later in the disease, an infant may exhibit macules, vesicles, and pustules simultaneously. Respiratory difficulty may develop between the second and third day after the initial cutaneous lesions. This time interval between the onset of cutaneous lesions and respiratory distress is comparable to that of varicella pneumonia in the adult. The development of respiratory distress carries with it an ominous prognosis.

The placenta exhibits both gross and microscopic foci of miliary coagulative necrosis. The adjacent intervillous spaces are filled with necrotic material, leukocytes, and nuclear fragments. Some of the villi may exhibit granulomatous lesions in the stroma consisting of areas of necrosis surrounded by epithelioid cells, a few foreign-body giant cells, and mononuclear elements. Some of the decidual cells contain intranuclear inclusion bodies consisting of an eosinophilic central mass surrounded by a clear halo and rimmed by fragments of chromatin along the nuclear membrane.

Fatal cases of congenital and neonatal varicella are indistinguishable on anatomic and histologic grounds. Postmortem examinations have revealed widespread systemic involvement, with characteristic areas of focal necrosis associated with intranuclear inclusion bodies and secondary hemorrhage. The most important lesions involve the lungs. The pulmonary parenchyma exhibits areas of focal necrosis. In some cases, an interstitial pneumonitis may be present. Miliary areas of coagulative necrosis may be identified, involving liver, pancreas, esophagus, stomach, adrenal cortices, thymus, spleen, and bone marrow. At the margins of these lesions, eosinophilic intranuclear inclusion bodies are present in adjacent epithelial cells.

NOSOCOMIAL VARICELLA IN THE NEWBORN NURSERY

Nosocomial spread of varicella is an uncommon event owing to the underlying presence in most neonates of transplacentally acquired specific maternal antibodies. Even when chickenpox occurs (after the ninth day of life) as a result of postnatal nursery exposure, it is usually attenuated. Infants born of mothers who contracted varicella within two weeks prior to delivery should be regarded as potentially incubating the virus. Such infants are best isolated to minimize the possibility of horizontal transmission of infection to other neonates, postpartum mothers, or hospital personnel. If the baby does not develop the disease and lacks specific antibodies, it is best to isolate the baby from the mother if she still has evidence of the disease.

NEONATAL HERPES ZOSTER

The fetus may develop an infection with varicella-zoster in utero that resolves before birth. Such infants harbor the virus, which later in life reactivates to cause zoster. This association of maternal chickenpox during gestation and early onset of zoster in the child has been reasonably well documented. Brunell et al. (1981) reported a series of cases of zoster in children ranging from three and a half months to two years of age. In each case, the mother had experienced clinically overt varicella during pregnancy. None of these infants had any stigmata of intrauterine varicella-zoster infection at birth. Infants who acquire varicella in utero appear to have difficulty in maintaining virus in its latent state. Ordinarily, zoster is a disease of the elderly.

DIAGNOSIS

Maternal

A presumptive diagnosis of varicella or herpes zoster is made primarily on the basis of a characteristic pattern of disease. Definitive documentation requires serologic confirmation or virus isolation or demonstration.

Rapid diagnosis of varicella or zoster infection can be done using a fluorescein-conjugated VZV monoclonal antibody test. Cell scrapings obtained from the base of one or more vesicles are smeared onto a glass slide and air-dried. The cells are then probed with the conjugated VZV-specific monoclonal antibody. Vesicular fluid collected with a sterile tuberculin syringe is appropriate material for virus isolation in cell cultures.

Complement-fixing antibodies to the virus are demonstrable four to five days after the onset of the disease, and the titer continues to rise for about two weeks. Viral neutralization and immunofluorescent and ELISA identification can be used. The availability of such methods for serologic identification, as well as viral isolation, tends to be variable. Demonstration of VZV-specific antibodies during the course of disease similarly documents etiology.

Immunofluorescent tests and ELISA are reliable tests for documenting prior infection with VZV.

Congenital Disease

Congenital varicella is usually defined as varicella occurring in a neonate before the tenth day of life. This definition is based on the shortest incubation period accepted for varicella. A study using human volunteers suggests that eight rather than nine days may represent the shortest incubation period for varicella. In those cases in which maternal disease occurred prior to delivery and congenital varicella ensued in the immediate postpartum period, an eight-day interim between the two events was not uncommon.

Although the gross and microscopic pathologies of varicella embryopathy are sufficiently characteristic to warrant a high index of suspicion as to the probable etiologic agent, the specific incrimination of VZV resides in the occurrence of classic maternal disease, serologic confirmation of prior specific infection, and/or virus isolation.

Immunofluorescent tests have been adapted to detect VZV-specific IgM antibodies.

PROPHYLAXIS AND THERAPY

Maternal Disease

The pruritus can be controlled with local applications of calamine lotion. Systemic antipruritics are rarely required, and until their effects in the fetus are established, it would be wise to avoid their use in pregnant women. The skin should be kept clean by daily bathing to prevent secondary infection. Complications such as pneumonia, encephalitis, myocarditis, hemorrhagic disorders, or nephritis are managed with therapeutic agents directed at the specific problems.

There are no specific guidelines for the management of a pregnant woman who is exposed to or develops varicella early in gestation. Pregnant women with a history of previous chickenpox or prior chickenpox in their immediate progeny are probably not at risk. VZIG is the only apparent potentially therapeutic modality.

Some experts have recommended VZIG administration for pregnant women with negative or uncertain prior histories of varicella who are exposed in the first or second trimester to prevent congenital varicella syndrome or in the third trimester to prevent neonatal varicella. However, there is no evidence that administration of VZIG to a susceptible, pregnant woman will prevent viremia, fetal infection, or congenital varicella syndrome. In the absence of evidence that VZIG can prevent congenital varicella syndrome or neonatal varicella, the primary indication for VZIG in pregnant women would be to prevent complications of varicella in a susceptible adult patient rather than to prevent intrauterine infection. VZIG is supplied in vials containing 125 units per vial (volume is approximately 1.25 mL). The recommended dose is 125 units per 10 kg (22 lbs) body weight, up to a maximum of 625 units (i.e., five vials). Fractional doses are not recommended. VZIG has not been evaluated as a prophylactic measure for prevention or attenuation of varicella in normal adults.

VZIG is mandatory, 1.25 mL (one vial) IM, for all progeny of mothers with onset of rash less than five days.

If VZIG is not available, 1.0 to 1.5 mL/kg of immune globulin will not prevent but may attenuate disease.

In 1995, the Food and Drug Administration (FDA) approved a live-attenuated VZV vaccine for children. The vaccine is recommended for all nonpregnant susceptible women of childbearing age. Pregnancy should be avoided for three months after vaccination. The vaccination regimen requires two doses one month apart. Protection has been reported to be >94% of immunized persons; vaccine use in pregnancy is contraindicated.

Neonatal Disease

If a neonate is delivered during the incubation period of the mother but before viremia, the risk of neonatal chickenpox is minimal, unless the infant is exposed to the virus. The period of greatest risk for severe and potentially lethal disease occurs when the infant is born within one day before or four days after the onset of maternal varicella.

The progeny of mothers with onset of rash less than five days prior to parturition should receive VZIG as soon as possible. Zaia et al. (1983) reported no deaths in 133 neonates who received VZIG in the first 24 hours. Slightly over 50% of the VZIG recipients developed mild disease. The recommended dose of VZIG for the neonate is 1.25 mL (one vial) IM. If VZIG cannot be obtained, high doses of immune serum globulin (1.0–1.5 mL/kg) should be used, although it will probably not prevent infection. The use of intravenous acyclovir, prophylactically and therapeutically, has not been assessed in clinical studies.

Since its licensure on February 1, 1981, VZIG has been produced and distributed in Massachusetts by the Massachusetts Public Health Biologic Laboratories (MPHBL) and distributed elsewhere by the American Red Cross Services—Northeast Region through regional blood centers.

PREVENTION

In 1995, the FDA approved a live attenuated varicella vaccine. Children 12 to 18 months of age now receive the vaccine as well as any susceptible older children and adults. In rare instances, transmission of vaccine virus to susceptible individuals in the immediate environment has been reported. The number of cases of zoster in vaccinated individuals is comparable to baseline values. The immunity induced by vaccination appears to be long lasting.

Live virus vaccines have been used to increase immunity against subsequent development of zoster in older individuals. In a large placebo-controlled study of 38,000 individuals 60 years of age or older, vaccine administration reduced the incidence of zoster by 50%.

In October 2006, the FDA approved PROQUAD, a live virus vaccine that includes measles, mumps, rubella, and varicella viruses.

SELECTED READING

Varicella-Zoster Infection in Pregnancy
Balducci J, Rodis JF, Rosengren S, et al. Pregnancy outcome following first-trimester varicella infection. Obstet Gynecol 1992; 79:5.
Brunnel PA. Varicella in pregnancy, the fetus, and the newborn: problems in management. J Infect Dis 1992; 166(suppl 1): S412.
Chodos WS. Varicella in pregnancy: report of case and review of the literature. J Am Osteopath Assoc 1982; 81:644.
Drips RC. Varicella in a term pregnancy complicated by postpartum varicella pneumonia and varicella in the newborn infant. Obstet Gynecol 1963; 22:771.

Enders G. Varicella-Zoster virus infection in pregnancy. Prog Med Virol 1984; 29:166.
Fish SA. Maternal death due to disseminated varicella. J Am Med Assoc 1960; 173:978.
Gilbert-Gwendolyn L. Infections in pregnant women. Med J Aust 2002; 176:229.
Heuchan AM, Issacs D. The management of varicella-zoster virus exposure and infection in pregnancy and the newborn period. Australasian Subgroup in Paediatric Infectious Diseases of Australasian Society for Infectious Diseases. Med J Aust 2001; 174:288.
McCarter-Spaulding DE. Varicella in pregnancy. J Obstet Gynecol Neonatal Nurs 2001; 30:667.
Mendelow DA, Lewis GC Jr. Varicella pneumonia during pregnancy. Obstet Gynecol 1969; 33:98.
Paryani SG, Arvin AM. Intrauterine infection with varicella-zoster virus after maternal varicella. N Engl J Med 1986; 314:1542–1546.
Purtilo DT, Bhawan J, Liao S, et al. Fatal varicella in a pregnant woman and a baby. Am J Obstet Gynecol 1977; 127:208.
Sauerbrei A, Muller D, Eichorn U, Wutzler P. Detection of varicella-zoster virus in congenital varicella syndrome. Obstet Gynecol 1960; 88:687.
Stagno S, Whitley RJ. Herpesvirus infections of pregnancy. Part II: Herpes simplex virus and varicella-zoster virus infections. N Engl J Med 1985; 313:1327.
Trlifajova J, Benda R, Benes C. Effect of maternal varicella-zoster virus infection on the outcome of pregnancy and the analysis of transplacental virus transmission. Acta Virol (Praha) 1986; 30:249.

Varicella Pneumdonia
Boeles JS, Ehrenkranz NJ, Marks A. Abnormalities of respiratory function in varicella pneumonia. Ann Intern Med 1964; 60:183.
Fritz RH, Meiklejohn G. Varicella pneumonia in adults. J Med Sci 1956; 232:489.
Harge JH, Errnest JM, Thurnau GR, et al. Risk factors and outcome of varicella-zoster virus pneumonia in pregnant women. J Infect Dis 2002; 185:422.
Harris RE, Rhoades ER. Varicella pneumonia complicating pregnancy: report of a case and review of literature. Obstet Gynecol 1965; 25:734.
Hockberger RS, Rothstein RJ. Varicella pneumonia in adults: a spectrum of disease. Ann Emerg Med 1986; 15:931.
Smego RA Jr, Asperilla MO. Use of acyclovir for varicella pneumonia during pregnancy. Obstet Gynecol 1991; 78:1112.
Weber DM, Pellecchia JA. Varicella pneumonia. J Am Med Assoc 1965; 192:572.

Congenital/Neonatal Varicella
Alber C. Neonatal varicella. Am J Dis Child 1964; 197:492.
Brunell PA. Placental transfer of varicella-zoster antibody. Pediatrics 1966; 38:1034.
Brunell PA. Fetal and neonatal varicella-zoster infections. Semin Perinatol 1983; 7:47.
Cosgrove AK, Samuel J. A case of congenital chickenpox. Malayan Med J 1934; 9:68.
Ehrlich RM, Turner JAP, Clark M. Neonatal varicella. J Pediatr 1958; 53:139.
Essex-Cater A, Heggarty H. Fatal congenital varicella syndrome. J Infect 1983; 7:77.
Freud P. Congenital varicella. Am J Dis Child 1958; 96:730.
Garcia AGP. Fetal infection in chickenpox and alastrim with histopathological study of the placenta. Pediatrics 1963; 32:895.
Harris LE. Spread of varicella in nurseries. Am J Dis Child 1967; 105:315.
Henderson WV. Chickenpox in an eight-day-old infant. J Pediatr 1934; 4:668.
Huang YC, Lin TY, Lin YJ, et al. Prophylaxis of intravenous immunoglobulin and acyclovir in perinatal varicella. Eur J Pediatr 2001; 160:91.

Jodar EO. Neonatal chickenpox. Henry Ford Hospital Med Bull 1957; 5:296.

La Russa P. Perinatal herpesvirus infections. Pediatr Ann 1984; 659:668.

Mustonen K, Mustakangas P, Valanne L, et al. Congenital varicella-zoster virus infection after maternal subclinical infection: clinical and neuropathological findings. J Perinatol 2001; 21:141.

Petignat P, Vial Y, Laurini R, Hohlfeld P. Fetal varicella-herpes zoster syndrome in early pregnancy: ultrasonographic and morphological correlation. Prenat Diagn 2001; 21:121.

Sauerbrei A, Wutzler P. Neonatal varicella. J Perinatol 2001; 21:545.

Congenital Zoster

Bennet R, Forsgren M, Herin P. Herpes zoster in a two-week-old premature infant with possible congenital varicella encephalitis. Acta Paediatr Scand 1985; 74:979.

Bokay J von. Uber den atiologischen Zusammenhand der Varizellen mit gewissen Fallen von Herpes zoster. Wien Klin Wochenschr 1909; 22:1323.

Brunell PA, Kotchmar GS Jr. Zoster in infancy: failure to maintain virus latency following intrauterine infection. J Pediatr 1981; 98:71.

Duehr PA. Herpes zoster as a cause of congenital cataract. Am J Ophthalmol 1955; 39:157.

Feldman GV. Herpes zoster neonatorum. Arch Dis Child 1952; 83:421.

Helander I, Arstila P, Terho P. Herpes zoster in a 6-month-old infant. Acta Derm Venereol 1983; 63:180.

Varicella Embryopathy

Dessemond M, Laurent JL, Chappard D, Robberts JM. Is varicella virus teratogenic? Lancet 1977; 1:362.

Dodison-Framson J, DeKegel D, Thiry L. Congenital varicella-zoster infection related to maternal disease in early pregnancy. Scand J Infect Dis 1973; 5:149.

Harger JH, Ernest JM, Thurau GR, et al. Frequency of congenital varicella syndrome in a prospective cohort of 347 pregnant women. Obstet Gynecol 2002; 100:260.

La Foret EG, Lynch CL. Multiple congenital defects following maternal varicella. Report of a case. N Engl J Med 1947; 236:534.

McKendry JBJ, Bailey JD. Congenital varicella associated with multiple defects. Can Med Assoc J 1973; 108:66.

Petignat P, Vial Y, Laurini R, Hohlfeld P. Fetal varicella-herpes zoster syndrome in early pregnancy: ultrasonographic and morphological correlation. Prenat Diagn 2001; 21:121.

Rinvik R. Congenital varicella encephalomyelitis in surviving newborn. Am J Dis Child 1969; 114:231.

Savage MO, Moosa A, Gordon RR. Maternal varicella infection as a cause of fetal malformations. Lancet 1973; 1:352.

Srabstein MD, Morris N, Larke RPB, et al. Is there a congenital varicella syndrome? J Pediatr 1974; 84:239.

Williamson AP. The varicella-zoster virus in the etiology of severe congenital defects: a survey of eleven reported instances. Clin Pediatr 1975; 14:553.

Neonatal Varicella

Mossner E (cited by Alber C). Neonatal varicella. Am J Dis Child 1964; 107:492.

Multach D, Kaufman H. Varicella in the newborn. J Fla Med Assoc 1963; 50:448.

Murphy K, O'Brien N, Hillary I. Congenital varicella. Ir J Med Sci 1985; 154:316.

Neustadt A. Congenital varicella. Am J Dis Child 1963; 106:96.

Newmann CGH. Perinatal varicella. Lancet 1965; 2:1159.

Odessky L, Newman B, Wein GB. Congenital varicella. NY J Med 1954; 54:2849.

O'Neil RR. Congenital varicella. Am J Dis Child 1962; 104:491.

Oppenheimer EH. Congenital chickenpox with disseminated visceral lesions. Johns Hopkins Med J 1944; 74:240.

Paryani SG, Arvin AM. Intrauterine infection with varicella-zoster virus after maternal varicella. N Engl J Med 1986; 314:1542.

Pearson HE. Parturition varicella-zoster. Obstet Gynecol 1963; 23:21.

Raine DN. Varicella infection contracted in utero: sex, incidence and incubation period. Am J Obstet Gynecol 1966; 94:1144.

Readett MD, McGibbon C. Neonatal varicella. Lancet 1961; 1:644.

Rinvik R. Congenital varicella encephalitis in surviving newborn. Am J Dis Child 1969; 117:231.

Shuman HH. Varicella in the newborn. Am J Dis Child 1939; 48:564.

Steen J, Pedersen RV. Varicella in a newborn girl. J Oslo City Hosp 1959; 9:36.

Waddington HK. Congenital chickenpox: report of a case of twins. Obstet Gynecol 1956; 7:319.

Zaia JA, Levin MJ, Preblud SC, et al. Evaluation of varicella-zoster immune globulin: protection of immunosuppressed children after household exposure to varicella. J Infect Dis 1983; 147: 737–743.

Varicella-Zoster Immune Globulin and Vaccines

Brunell PA. Varicella-zoster virus. In Monif GRG, ed. Infectious Diseases in Obstetrics and Gynecology. Hagerstown: Harper & Row, 1974.

Brunell PA, Roxx A, Miller L, Kuo B. Prevention of varicella by zoster immune globulin. N Engl J Med 1969; 280:1191.

Duff P. Varicella in pregnancy: five priorities for clinicians. Infect Dis Obstet Gynecol 1996; 1:163.

Hanngren K, Grandien M, Granstrom G. Effect of zoster immunoglobulin for varicella prophylaxis in the newborn. Scand J Infect Dis 1985; 17:343.

Oxman MN, Levin MJ, Johnson GR. A vaccine to prevent zoster and postherpetic neuralgia in older adults. N Engl J Med 2005; 352:2271.

Ross AH. Modification of chickenpox in family contacts by administration of gamma globulin. N Engl J Med 1962; 267:369.

Seward JF, Watson BM, Peterson CL, et al. Varicella disease after introduction of varicella vaccine in the United States, 1995–2000. JAMA 2002; 287:505.

Trimble GX. Attenuation of chickenpox with gamma globulin. Can Med Assoc J 1975; 77:697.

Varicella-Zoster immune globulin for the prevention of chickenpox. Recommendations of the Immunization Practices Advisory Committee, Centers for Disease Control. Ann Intern Med 1984; 100:859.

Vazquez M, La Russa PS, Gershon AA, et al. Effectiveness over time of varicella vaccine. JAMA 2004; 291:851.

Acyclovir and Pregnancy

Boyd K, Walker E. Use of acyclovir to treat chickenpox in pregnancy. Br Med J 1988; 296:393.

Eder S, Apuzzio JJ, Weiss G. Varicella pneumonia during pregnancy: treatment of two cases with acyclovir. Am J Perinatol 1988; 5:16.

Glaser J. Varicella infection in pregnancy. N Engl J Med 1986; 315:1416.

Hankins GD, Gilstrap LC 3rd, Patterson AR. Acyclovir treatment of varicella pneumonia in pregnancy. Crit Care Med 1987; 15:336.

Hockberger RS, Rothstein RJ. Varicella pneumonia in adults: a spectrum of disease. Ann Emerg Med 1986; 15:931.

Landsberger EJ, Hager WD, Grossman JH 3rd. Successful management of varicella pneumonia complicating pregnancy: a report of three cases. J Reprod Med 1986; 31:311.

Smego R. Use of acyclovir for varicella infection during pregnancy. Obstet Gynecol 1991; 78:1112.

Klebsiella granulomatis (Calymmatobacterium granulomatis)

INTRODUCTION

Granuloma inguinale was first recognized in 1882 by McLeod, who named it serpiginous ulcerations of the groin. In 1905, Colonel Donovan described the intracellular, rod-shaped bodies known since as Donovan bodies.

The ultrastructure of *Klebsiella granulomatis* in human tissue is typical of gram-negative bacteria. A distinguishing feature is the large capsule around the bacterium within mononuclear cells. The demonstration of phage material within *K. granulomatis* has suggested the possibility that *K. granulomatis* is a phage-modified bacterium. Phage modification may be the necessary prerequisite to translate fecal bacterial contamination into the disease state.

The determinants of disease and the factors responsible for the pathogenic expression of this organism are poorly understood. Although disease can be produced with some regularity with infected human material, as a rule, organisms grown on appropriate culture media fail to produce infection when inoculated into human volunteers.

It has been postulated that *K. granulomatis* is primarily a constituent of the gastrointestinal tract that is autoinoculated from the rectum into sites of both sexual and nonsexual trauma. Poor personal hygiene is thought to be a contributing factor. Disease is usually endemic in areas with both high temperatures and humidity. In the United States, disease occurs primarily in port cities in the southern part of the United States.

The disease is apparently not very contagious. While a significant mode of transmission involves sexual contact, the disease does not invariably affect conjugal partners despite repeated contact.

NATURAL HISTORY OF THE DISEASE

Donovanosis is a chronic, progressive ulcerative disease involving primarily the genital region. The predilection of lesions for the genital areas and the occasional occurrence of disease in sexual partners of infected individuals constitute the prime evidence to support the concept of granuloma inguinale as a venereal disease.

The prevalence of the disease among pederasts and the predominant anal and perianal predilection of the lesions strongly suggest that rectal coitus is the prime means of transmission of infection, either by contamination of the skin directly through anal intercourse (whether it be heterosexual or homosexual) or indirectly by faulty hygiene. Further evidence supporting the inferred thesis of venereal disease transfer, secondary to rectal coitus, can be drawn from the observations that the disease process is infrequent among prostitutes. In the preantibiotic era, individuals in the florid stage of the disease only occasionally transmitted infection to their sexual partners. From clinical studies, an incubation period of 17.4 days has been calculated; however, experimental infection of human volunteers has produced disease in 50 days.

The disease is only mildly contagious. In most cases, lesions cannot be demonstrated in sexual consorts. Evidence of infection as opposed to disease is detected in 12% to 52% of marital or steady sexual partners.

The common sites for lesions, in women, are the labia minora, fourchette, and labia majora. The perianal region also can be affected. Bedi (1980) has reported an unusual case of nonvenereal transmission of perianal granuloma inguinale in a child. Another site that may occasionally be affected by this disease is the oral cavity.

Clinically, the disease presents as painless, progressive ulcerative lesions without regional lymphadenopathy. The initial lesion usually begins as a reddish-brown, flat-topped papule that often spreads and then ulcerates in the center. Not infrequently, other papules appear at about the same time. When they ulcerate, the lesions eventually coalesce.

The ulcer may show variation in its morphology:

1. The ulcerative or ulcerogranulomatous form—the fleshy, exuberant lesion—presents as a beefy-red granulomatous ulcer, usually single, which is nontender, nonindurated, and bleeds profusely on touch (owing to its high vascularity).
2. The hypertrophic or verrucous form consists of an ulcer or growth with a raised, irregular edge or surface, drier than the ulcerative variety, with an elevated, granulomatous base.
3. The necrotic type gives rise to extensive destruction of genitalia with profuse, foul-smelling exudate.
4. The sclerotic or cicatricial variety presents as a band-like scar in and around the genitalia.

As a rule, the ulcer tends to have a clean base composed of fresh granulation tissue and to have well-defined borders. The advancing edge of the lesion exhibits a scrolled appearance owing to epithelial hyperplasia and acanthosis of the squamous epithelium (Fig. 1). The degree of hyperplasia (and not infrequently dysplasia) in response to infection may cause an erroneous diagnosis of low-grade squamous cell carcinoma. The lesion or lesions may develop secondary bacterial infection or may be coinfected with another sexually transmitted pathogen.

Spread of the disease may be by contiguous contact, autoinoculation, or lymphatic extension. The histologic

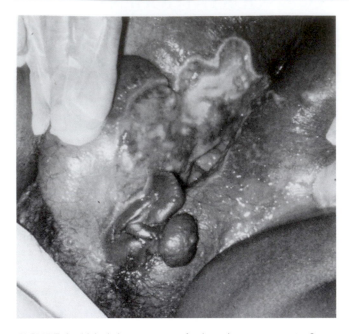

FIGURE I Vulval donovanosis of relatively recent origin. Some of the lesions are separate, others confluent. The margin of the lesion is raised and scrolled, and the base is granular and covered imperfectly by a thin gray slough.

demonstration of lymph node involvement and the development of pseudobubo in males stress the role of lymphatic dissemination from the superficial genital lesion (Table 1). In females, the regional lymph nodes enlarge somewhat and are occasionally tender, but they do not suppurate unless gross secondary infection of the initial lesion is present.

Biopsy of the initial lesion reveals, in addition to the secondary epithelial change, a granulomatous proliferative response and a secondary connective tissue attempt at repair. The histopathologic feature of the ulcer of donovanosis is a dense granulomatous tissue reaction consisting mainly of small lymphocytes, with a scattering of the typically large mononuclear cells, which may contain the pathognomonic Donovan bodies. Small collections of polymorphonuclear neutrophils (microabscesses) secondary to superimposed bacterial infection are typical. In the absence of secondary infection, neutrophils are conspicuously absent. Within the granulation tissue, capillaries tend to be prominent, owing to reactive hyperplasia of their endothelial cells. Even in the

absence of Donovan bodies, the histopathology of infection due to *Calymmatobacterium granulomatis* is sufficiently characteristic to warrant a presumptive diagnosis.

The more advanced lesions represent a composite of the two processes of exuberant granulomatous proliferation and fibroblastic repair. With partial resolution of infection, isolated foci of plasma cells and lymphocytes appear, as well as occasional macrophages within the interstices of connective tissue. With arrest of the disease process, the granulation tissue is replaced by newly grown connective tissue.

One of the less commonly seen features of the disease is a gross local swelling of the affected area. It may develop before treatment or during the phase when the ulcers are healing. These hard, knobby swellings are due to obliteration of predominantly efferent lymphatics. Biopsy of such a lesion reveals grossly dilated lymphatics.

With secondary infection of the initial ulcers, the gross appearance of the lesions changes, owing to extension of the area of ulceration deep into the underlying dermis with excavation and undermining of the margins. With appropriate therapy, the fibroblastic component predominates, leaving scar formation as the end-stage lesion of genital involvement. In 6% of the cases, extragenital lesions are observed. Metastatic hematogenous infection as well as involvement of the oral cavity has been described. The infection, particularly after delivery or abortion, infrequently extends from the cervix and may involve the uterus, fallopian tubes, and ovaries.

With extensive disease and secondary infection, systemic signs such as fever, anemia, weight loss, malaise, and leukocytosis may occur. Although the diagnosis may be inferred because of the clinical presentation and the exclusion of other disease processes, a definitive diagnosis is still contingent upon the demonstration of Donovan bodies.

DONOVANOSIS AND CARCINOMA

Infection with *K. granulomatis* is thought to influence the high incidence of carcinoma of the vulva in very young patients in Jamaica. Occasionally, concomitant active donovanosis and carcinoma have been identified in the same patient. Carcinoma of the vulva occurring only a year or two after apparent cure of granuloma inguinale is one of the urgent reasons for thorough treatment and careful follow-up.

TABLE I Differential diagnosis of inguinal adenopathy associated with a presumed venereal disease

Disease	Genital lesion	Nodal involvement	Cutaneous lesions
Granuloma inguinale	Extensive in males, less evident in females	Involvement of lymph nodes; draining cutaneous sinuses late in the course of the disease, nodes become tender	Primary skin infection with superficial ulceration
Lymphogranuloma venereum	Occurs, but is extremely transient In nature	Bilateral node involvement idetermined by site of primary lesion	Multiple sinus tracts draining a thick, creamy exudate
Chancroid	Usually present	Primarily unilateral with limited involvement of lymph nodes	Acute, with craterlike slough
Genital tuberculosis	None	With extensive involvement of female genital tract, bilateral inguinal adenopathy	Pleomorphic, often with sinus tract draining scanty thick exudate
Syphilis	Usually present	Bilateral; firm, rubbery nodes	Protean in its clinical manifestations

DIAGNOSIS

Many clinicians examining their first case of donovanosis think it is carcinoma, regardless of whether the lesion is of the vulva or of the cervix. Adequate biopsies must be taken and carefully studied. Pathologists can also be misled. The hyperplasia and dysplasia of squamous epithelium at the edge of an ulcer can easily be mistaken for low-grade squamous cell carcinoma. Occasionally, however, the diagnosis is carcinoma.

The clinical diagnosis is suggested by the clinical appearance of the lesion or lesions. Owing to the degree of vascularization, the lesions appear beefy-red. Confirmation can be obtained on the basis of histologic examination of punch biopsy material taken from the edge of active lesions, on scrapings taken from the edge of lesions, or on a crush preparation made from granulation tissue obtained with a thin scalpel. In all cases, active lesions should be cleansed with physiological saline prior to sampling. Smear preparations should be stained with either Giemsa or Wright stain. Fixed embedded tissue specimens require the long Giemsa or silver stains. An indirect immunofluorescence test is available. This test is both sensitive and specific. Its utilization is limited by the paucity of positive control material.

A definitive diagnosis of granuloma inguinale is almost invariably based on the identification of classic Donovan bodies in biopsy material. Donovan bodies appear as clusters of blue or black staining with an organism's "safety pin" appearance (from bipolar chromatin) in the cytoplasm of large mononuclear cells. Biopsies should be taken radially through the edge of the ulcer and include some of its base. The affinity of the intracysts of *C. granulomatis* for silver salts facilitates the recognition of the Donovan bodies. Because Donovan bodies are very hard to find, they may be more readily demonstrated in tissue spreads stained with Giemsa stain than in histologic sections stained with either hematoxylin and eosin or silver stains. In either case, success in their identification depends on the sharp eyes and persistence of the pathologist, who often has to search many slides in order to establish the diagnosis of donovanosis.

No Food and Drug Administration-cleared polymerase chain reaction tests for the detection of *K. granulomatis* DNA currently exist; however, such a test may be available at a future date.

THERAPY

K. granulomatis is susceptible to a wide number of antibiotic preparations that interfere with protein synthesis. Doxycycline 100 mg orally twice a day is the recommended initial therapy. An alternative regimen includes ciprofloxacin 750 mg po two times a day for at least three weeks and until the lesions completely heal, erythromycin 500 mg orally four times a day for 21 days and until the lesions completely heal, azithromycin 1 g orally per week for three weeks, or trimethoprim–sulfamethoxazole two 800 mg/160 mg tablets every 12 hours for at least three weeks and until the lesions completely heal. For any of these regimens, addition of an aminoglycoside (such as gentamicin 1 mg/kg IV every eight hours) should be considered if lesions do not respond within the first few days of therapy. Doxycycline, trimethoprim–sulfamethoxazole, and ciprofloxacin are contraindicated in pregnancy.

Both ampicillin and erythromycin have been found to be somewhat erratic in efficiency; the combination of ampicillin and erythromycin or azithromycin has been found to be satisfactory in the treatment of pregnant patients. Published data for treating granuloma inguinale during pregnancy are lacking.

When possible, strong consideration should be given to the addition of a parenteral aminoglycoside if improvement is not evident within the first three to four days of therapy. Treatment should be continued until the lesions have healed completely, which usually takes three weeks. Prolonged duration of therapy is often required to permit granulation and reepithelialzation of the ulcers. Longstanding lesions may be so mutilating that adjunctive surgical care may be necessary. The elimination of secondary infection by topical cleansing and antimicrobial therapy accelerates healing.

Relapses may occur within 6 to 18 months later despite effective initial therapy; some cases require prolonged courses of antibiotic therapy. It is wise to treat infection vigorously and to insist on compulsive follow-up even after apparent cure.

The local areas of "elephantiasis" remaining after effective treatment of active infection are often uncomfortable and cause cosmetic embarrassment. Once infection is cured, local excision of such focal swelling can be carried out.

MANAGEMENT OF SEX PARTNERS

Persons who have had sexual contact with a patient who has granuloma inguinale within the 60 days before onset of the patient's symptoms should be examined and treated if clinical signs and symptoms are present. The value of empiric therapy in the absence of lesions has not been established.

SELECTED READING

Davis CM. Granuloma inguinale. J Am Med Assoc 1970; 211:632.

Davis CM, Collins C. Granuloma inguinale: an ultrastructural study of Calymmatobacterium granulomatis. J Invest Dermatol 1969; 53:315.

Hart G. Granuloma inguinale. In: Mandell GL, Douglas RG, Bennet JE, eds. Principles and Practice of Infectious Diseases. Wiley Medical School Publication, 1979:1902–1904.

Kuberski T. Granuloma inguinale (donovanosis). Sex Transm Dis 1980; 7:29.

Kuberski T, Papdimitron JM, Phillips P. Ultrastructure of Calymmatobacterium granulomatis in lesions of granuloma inguinale. J Infect Dis 1980; 147:744.

Marmell M, Santora E. Donovanosis: granuloma inguinale incidence, nomenclature, diagnosis. Am J Syph 1950; 34:83.

Natural History of Disease

Bhagwandeen SB, Mottiar YA. Granuloma venereum. J Clin Pathol 1972; 25:812.

Dienst RB, Reinstein Cr, Kupperman HS, Greenblatt RB. Studies on the causal agent of granuloma inguinale. Am J Syph Gono Vener Dis 1947; 31:614.

Goldberg J. Studies on granuloma inguinale. IV. Growth requirements of D. granulomatis and its relationship to the natural habitat of the organism. Br J Vener Dis 1959; 32:266.

Goldberg J. Studies on granuloma inguinale. V. Isolation of a bacterium resembling D. granulomatis from feces of a patient with granuloma inguinale. Br J Vener Dis 1962; 38:99.

Goldberg J. Studies on granuloma inguinale. VII. Some epidemiological considerations of the disease. Br J Vener Dis 1964; 40:140.

Las S, Nicholas C. Epidemiological and clinical features in 165 cases of granuloma inguinale. Br J Vener Dis 1970; 46:461.

Nayer M, Chandra M, Saxena HMK, et al. Donovanosis: a histopathological study. Ind J Pathol Microbiol 1981; 24:71.

Sehgal VN, Prasad ALS. A clinical profile of donovanosis in a non-endemic area. Dermatology 1984; 168:273.

Sehgal VN, Shyam-Prasad ALS. Donovanosis: current concepts. Int J Dermatol 1986; 25:8.

Sehgal VN, Prasad ALS, Beohar PC. The histopathology of donovanosis. Br J Vener Dis 1984; 60:45.

Female Genital Tract Involvement

Bedi TR. Perianal granuloma inguinale in a child (nonvenereal transmission). Ind J Dermatol Venereol Leprol 1980; 46:45.

Lawson JB, Steward DB. Obstetrics and Gynecology in the Tropics. London: Arnold, 1966.

Leiman G, Markowitz S, Margolius KA. Cytologic detection of cervical granuloma inguinale. Diagn Cytophal 1986; 2:138.

MMWR. Sexually Transmitted Diseases Treatment Guidelines, 2006, Vol. 55 No. RR-11.

Murugan S, Venkatram K, Renganathan PS. Vaginal bleeding in granuloma inguinale. Br RR-11. J Vener Dis 1982; 58:200.

Pund ER, Gotcher VA. Granuloma venereum (granuloma inguinale) of uterus, tubes and ovaries. Surgery 1948; 3:34.

Sehgal VN, Prasad AL. Donovanosis: current concepts. Int J Dermatol 1986; 25:8.

Sehgal VN, Sharma NL, Bhargava NC, et al. Primary extragenital disseminated cutaneous donovanosis. Br J Dermatol 1979; 101:353.

Stewart DB. The gynecological lesions of lymphogranuloma venereum and granuloma inguinale. Med Clin North Am 1964; 48:773.

INTRODUCTION

Chancroid is a superficial infection of the external genital tract caused by *Haemophilus ducreyi*. The bacteria are small gram-negative rods measuring 0.5 mm by 1.5 to 2.0 mm, and are often seen in short chains or parallel arrays ("school-of-fish" or "fingerprint" patterns). They may be cultivated with considerable difficulty, are nonmotile, and are not acid fast. Bipolar staining is often demonstrable.

H. ducreyi has a worldwide distribution but is found more frequently in tropical and subtropical countries. Within the United States, there is geographic variation in disease prevalence and recognition.

CHANCROID

Chancroid has had a cyclic history in the United States. Reported cases of chancroid peaked in 1947 and then declined until 1978, when the numbers of reported cases began to rise. This increase continued through 1987, and only recently has the number of reported cases begun to decline. Considered a relatively uncommon sexually transmitted disease, chancroid has become a matter for greater concern as studies have indicated that genital ulcer is a risk factor in the transmission of HIV. The infection is disseminated venereally. Genital lesions appear 3 to 14 days after sexual contact and may be single or multiple. The initial lesion is usually one or more small erythematous macules that rapidly become vesicular pustules. The lesion ruptures, leaving behind a small circumscribed ulcer with an erythematous base (Table 1). The ulcer is painful and tender to palpation and is characterized by a nonindurated base, painful overhanging edges, and ragged margins. The lesion frequently has an erythematous halo. The base of the ulcer is covered with a dirty-looking, necrotic, grayish exudate. Lymphadenitis occurs in approximately 30% of the cases. The lymphadenopathy is regional and is often unilateral (generally on the same side as the lesion). Without adequate therapy, there may be extension of the process from the lymph nodes to the overlying skin, resulting in draining sinuses.

Superinfection of the ulcer or ulcers, especially by fusospirochetes, may lead to extensive destruction of the external genitalia (phagedenic chancroid).

TABLE I   Clinical characteristics of chancroid ulcer

Number:	Usually multiple but may occur as an isolated lesion
Shape:	Irregular
Depth:	Deep
Purulence:	Present
Tenderness:	Present

DIAGNOSIS

Diagnosis is inferred by the demonstration of small gram-negative rods with the so-called "school-of-fish" appearance (Fig. 1), occurring in strands on smears stained with Gram or Wright stain, and an ulcer characterized by noninduration of the base and painful, ragged, overhanging margins. Specific fluorescent antibody staining of bacteria in smears from suspected lesions provides a means for substantiation of the diagnosis; unfortunately, the availability of this diagnostic procedure is limited. Biopsy of the lesion is useful since it eliminates granuloma inguinale, syphilitic chancre, and herpetic ulcer from diagnostic consideration.

A definitive diagnosis is established with the isolation of the organism. Gonococcal agar supplemented with bovine hemoglobin and fetal calf serum or Mueller-Hinton agar supplemented with chocolatized horse blood are required to maximize recovery on primary isolation.

H. ducreyi grows best at 35°C in an atmosphere of 5% CO_2 in a moist environment. Single colonies are not visible until after 48 to 96 hours of incubation. Colonies are typically raised, opaque, compact, granular, tan or yellowish, and difficult to pick up with a loop, as colonies characteristically slide over the agar surface intact. It is the sole human *Haemophilus* species with a requirement only for X factor as determined by the porphyrin test.

H. ducreyi, being a fastidious organism that is not easily isolated and having few biochemically distinguishing features that can be used to identify it, causes concern about the sensitivity of culture identification. Many reports have suggested that the sensitivity of culture, using clinical diagnosis as the gold standard, is between 35% and 80%, and these estimates appear to depend strongly on the laboratory setting; laboratories that deal with populations with a high prevalence of chancroid tend to be better able to both culture *H. ducreyi* and diagnose chancroid. Even with specialized culture media, the sensitivity of culture identification is less than 80%. Unfortunately, a definitive diagnosis by culture is not widely available from commercial sources.

A number of molecular diagnostic methods exist. These include DNA probes for the direct detection of *H. ducreyi*, monoclonal antibodies for detecting *H. ducreyi* in smears, and polymerase chain reaction (PCR) assays. The former two methods lack either the specificity or the sensitivity desirable in a nonculture approach for detection and identification of *H. ducreyi*. PCR, which uses specific primers to amplify the intervening DNA sequences, offers a sensitive and specific alternative approach for the diagnosis of chancroid.

No Food and Drug Administration–cleared PCR test for *H. ducreyi* is available in the United States, but various

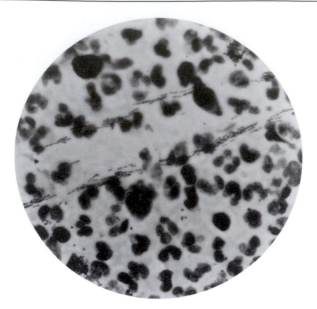

FIGURE 1 Chancroid. Gram-stained smear revealing the classic "school-of-fish" pattern. *Source:* From Parker (1964).

clinical laboratories do PCR testing using their own PCR test. PCR is a useful method for the detection of *H. ducreyi* in genital lesions, particularly those in female patients where normal flora may complicate culture, and in bubo aspirates that yield positive cultures less readily than ulcers. PCR can be especially valuable for epidemiologic studies where poor culture sensitivity is a major problem, especially in studies conducted with high-risk patients who are likely to have ulcers that contain multiple etiologic agents where culture sensitivity may be poorer.

Because of the possibility of concomitant syphilitic infection, dark-field analysis of all lesions should be performed. Serologic tests for syphilis should be obtained during therapy. If the antimicrobial agent utilized will not eradicate incubating syphilis, the serological test should be repeated six to eight weeks after its termination.

A probable diagnosis for both clinical and surveillance purposes may be made if the person has one or more painful genital ulcers; and (*i*) no evidence of *Treponema pallidum* infection is found by dark-field examination of ulcer exudate or by a serologic test for syphilis performed at least seven days after onset of ulcers; (*ii*) the appearance of the genital ulcers and regional lymphadenopathy, if present, are typical for chancroid; and (*iii*) a test for herpes simplex virus is negative. The combination of a painful ulcer with tender inguinal adenopathy (which occurs among one-third of patients) is suggestive of chancroid and, when accompanied by suppurative inguinal adenopathy, is almost pathognomonic.

HIV and Chancroid

Women with HIV infection do not respond as well to treatment as do HIV-negative women. Patients should be tested for HIV infection at the time chancroid is diagnosed and retested three months later if the initial test results were negative.

THERAPY

The emergence of *H. ducreyi* that is resistant to multiple antibiotics has limited the effectiveness of many antimicrobials for therapy of chancroid. Trimethoprim sulfamethoxazole (160/800 mg twice a day for seven days) had been a drug of choice. Resistance to sulfonamides is mediated by a nonconjugative 4.9 mega Dalton plasmid. Because of an increasing number of treatment failures, tetracycline is no longer used for the treatment of chancroid. Worldwide, occasional isolates with intermediate resistance to ciprofloxacin or erythromycin have been reported.

Recommendations for antibiotic therapy include azithromycin (1 g orally in a single dose), erythromycin (500 mg three times a day orally for seven days), ceftriaxone (250 mg IM in a single dose), or ciprofloxacin 500 mg orally twice a day for three days (Table 2).

Although it is highly effective in the treatment of chancroid, erythromycin can cause significant gastrointestinal discomfort, leading to suboptimal compliance.

Azithromycin and ceftriaxone offer the advantage of single-dose therapy. Ciprofloxacin is contraindicated in pregnant and lactating women. Worldwide, several isolates with intermediate resistance to either ciprofloxacin or erythromycin have been reported.

Ulcers in HIV-positive women do not appear to heal as readily as would be anticipated. Such patients may benefit from more intensive therapy. Irrespective of culture data, women with persisting ulcer following therapy should be considered still infected.

With effective therapy, a clinical response, first subjective and then objective, should be apparent within several days of instituting therapy. A subjective response (diminished tenderness and pain) occurs within 48 hours of institution of antimicrobials. An objective response generally occurs within 72 hours and almost always within seven days. Healing takes 10 to 11 days after institution of therapy. Large ulcers may require relatively longer time periods to heal. Patients should be seen seven days after beginning therapy, when objective signs of ulcer healing will be present in virtually all successfully treated patients, and adenopathy should be less painful and usually smaller. Some nodes may progress to fluctuation despite adequate therapy and require needle aspiration through normal skin to prevent spontaneous drainage. Ernst et al. (1995) have advocated incision and drainage, with subsequent irrigation and packing of the bubo cavity. The use of a more extensive surgical procedure appears potentially applicable to large, confluent, fluctuant nodes. Incisional drainage may be preferred as it will reduce the need for subsequent drainage procedures.

TABLE 2 Centers for Disease Control 2006 recommended regimens

Azithromycin	1 g orally in a single dose
Ceftriaxone	250 mg IM in a single dose
Ciprofloxacin	500 mg orally bid for 3 days
Erythromycin base	500 mg orally tid for 7 days (alternative regimen)

While ulcers in successfully treated patients respond to therapy quickly, adenopathy may not, and progression to fluctuation is not necessarily a sign of treatment failure.

If by day seven, a clinical response has occurred and therapy has been taken as directed, therapy need not be continued. If a clinical response is not apparent, the clinician should reconsider the clinical diagnosis of chancroid or, if it has been confirmed by a culture, consider a mixed infection, e.g., herpes and chancroid, HIV and chancroid.

Sexual contacts of patients with chancroid should be examined and treated with an effective antimicrobial regimen, whether lesions are present or not, if they have had sexual contact with the patient during the 10 days preceding the patient's onset of symptoms. Asymptomatic carriage of *H. ducreyi* appears to be uncommon, but colonization of the vagina, penis, and mouth in the absence of lesions has been described.

Initial treatment guidelines recommended that therapy be continued for at least 10 days and until clinical resolution of ulcer(s) and adenopathy. Subsequent studies have shown a high efficacy for one- to seven-day courses of therapy and indicate that antimicrobial courses of 10 days offer no therapeutic advantage over shorter courses, even though ulcers have not completely healed and adenopathy is persistent.

SELECTED READING

Albritton WL. Infections due to Haemophilus species other than Haemophilus influenzae. Ann Rev Microbiol 1982; 36:199.

Ballard RC, Ye H, Matta A, et al. Treatment of chancroid with azithromycin. Int J STD AIDS 1996; 7(suppl 1):9.

Blackmore CA, Limpakarnjanarat K, Rigau-Perez JG, et al. An outbreak of chancroid in Orange County, California: descriptive epidemiology and disease control measures. J Infect Dis 1985; 151:840.

Centers for Disease and Prevention. Sexually transmitted disease treatment guidelines. MMWR 2002; 51(RR-6):1.

Ernst AA, Marvez-Valis E, Martin DH. Incision and drainage of fluctuant buboes in the emergency department during an epidemic of chancroid. Sex Trans Dis 1995; 22:217.

Johnson SR, Martin D, Cammarata C, Morse SA. Development of a polymerase chain reaction assay for the detection of Haemophilus ducreyi. Sex Trans Dis 1994; 21:13.

Karim QN, Finn GY, Easmon CS, et al. Rapid detection of Haemophilus ducreyi in clinical and experimental infections using monoclonal antibody: a preliminary evaluation. Genitourin Med 1989; 65:361.

Latif AS, Van D, Crocchiolo PR, et al. Thiamphenicol in the treatment of chancroid in men. Sex Transm Dis 1984; 11:454.

Lykke-Elesen L, Larsen L, Pedersen TG, et al. Epidemic of chancroid in Greenland 1977–1978. Lancet 1979; 1:654.

MMWR. Sexually transmitted diseases treatment guidelines. 2006; 55(RR-11).

Morse SA. Chancroid and Haemophilus ducreyi. J Clin Microbiol 1989; 2:137.

Museyi KE, Van Dyck E, Vervoort T, et al. Use of an enzyme immunoassay to detect serum IgG antibodies to Haemophilus ducreyi. J Infect Dis 1988; 157:1039.

Nsanze H, Plummer FA, Maggwa ABN, et al. Comparison of media for the primary isolation of Haemophilus ducreyi. Sex Transm Dis 1984; 11:6.

Oberhofer TR, Back AE. Isolation and cultivation of Haemophilus ducreyi. J Clin Microbiol 1982; 15:625.

Odumeru JA, Wiseman GM, Ronald AR. Virulence factors of Haemophilus ducreyi. Infect Immunol 1984; 43:607.

Parker RT. In: Holly R, ed. Gynecology-Obstetrics Guide. Chicago: Commerce Clearing House, 1964.

Parsons LM, Shayegani M, Waring AL, Bopp LH. DNA probes for the identification of Haemophilus ducreyi. J Clin Microbiol 1989; 27:1441.

Plummer FA, Nsanze H, D'Costa LJ, et al. Single-dose therapy of chancroid with trimethoprim-sulfamethoxazole. N Engl J Med 1983; 309:67.

Ronald AR, Plummer FA. Chancroid and Haemophilus ducreyi. Ann Intern Med 1985; 102:705.

Rossau R, Duhamel M, Jannes G, et al. The development of specific rRNA-derived oligonucleotide probes for Haemophilus ducreyi, the causative agent of chancroid. J Gen Microbiol 1991; 137:277.

Sanson-Lepors MJ, Casin I, Ortenberg M, et al. In vitro susceptibility of 30 strains of Haemophilus ducreyi to several antibiotics including six cephalosporins. J Antimicrob Chemother 1983; 11:271.

Schmid GP. Treatment of chancroid, 1997. Clin Infect Dis 1999; 28(suppl 1):14.

Schmid GP, Sanders LL, Blount JH, et al. Chancroid in the United States: re-establishment of an old disease. J Am Med Assoc 1987; 258:3265.

Schulte JM, Martich FA, Schmid GP. Chancroid in the United States 1981–1990: evidence for underreporting of cases. MMWR 1992; 41:57.

Taylor DN, Pitarangsi C, Echeverria P, et al. Comparative study of ceftriaxone and trimethoprim-sulfamethoxazole for the treatment of chancroid in Thailand. J Infect Dis 1985; 152:1002.

Thomson JA, Bilgeri YR. Plasmid-coded ampicillin resistance in Haemophilus ducreyi. Antimicrob Agents Chemother 1982; 22:689.

INTRODUCTION

The bacterium *Haemophilus influenzae* was initially described by Pfeiffer who presumed it to be the causative agent for the 1889–1891 influenza pandemic. The organism is a gram-negative aerobic bacillus that requires both X factor (hemin) and V factor (nicotinamide adenine dinucleotide). X factor is released into the medium by red blood cells. Although V factor is also present in red blood cells, it is not released into the medium unless the cells are lysed. Consequently, *H. influenzae* will not grow on blood agar except as satellite colonies around other colonies that produce hemolysis.

H. influenzae is classifiable by virtue of its capsular polysaccharides into six typeable serotypes (a, b, c, d, e, and f) and into nontypeable strains. The type b and nontypeable strains are the principal causes of disease. Of the typeable strains, type b is the most virulent.

Based upon three biochemical reactions, the organism can be classified into six biotypes. Most *H. influenzae* type b are biotypes I and II, whereas most nontypeable strains are biotypes II through VI (Table 1). Nearly all genital isolates of *H. influenzae* from puerperal women with endometritis and hematogenous isolates from infected neonates are biotype IV (Table 2). In contrast, biotype I accounts for 80% of septicemic isolates in children. Respiratory isolates from well children and children whose illness was not caused by *H. influenzae* were rarely serotypeable (1%) or were biotype I (8%). The predominance of biotype I in invasive disease argues that these strains possess unique virulence determinants.

H. influenzae is a rare constituent of the vaginal flora. Khuri-Bulos and McIntosh (1975) failed to recover *H. influenzae* in 325 cervical cultures obtained from obstetric patients. Other studies have shown rates of isolation of less than 0.02%.

As a monoetiological pathogen, *H. influenzae* produces four disease entities that are specific for the female genital tract and/or products of conception: acute bacterial vulvovaginitis, hematogenous and ascending chorioamnionitis, endometritis, and perinatal septicemia.

In addition, the nontypeable strains can function as part of the anaerobic progression.

CLINICAL DISEASE

Acute Bacterial Vulvovaginitis

H. influenzae can be a cause of vulvovaginitis and should be treated as an exogenous pathogen in this clinical setting.

It produces a purulent vaginitis. The onset of the disease is sudden. Vaginal erythema and pressure tenderness are two characteristics. The recovery of this bacterial species from the female genital tract should have the same significance to a clinician as that of group A beta-hemolytic streptococci.

Chorioamnionitis/Perinatal Septicemia

In contrast to the group B streptococci with their high prevalence of genital tract colonization but low attack rate, *H. influenzae* appears to have a low prevalence, but a high attack rate in terms of maternal and neonatal infection. When present, the organism has the potential to cause both local and systemic disease. If rupture of the fetal membranes ensues, chorioamnionitis frequently ensues; however, the majority of affected infants are born to mothers for whom rupture of the fetal membranes did not constitute a significant antepartum obstetric complication, implying hematogenous dissemination. In the majority of cases of neonatal septicemia, maternal colonization or infection with *H. influenzae* can be demonstrated. In one series of 10 cases of neonatal septicemia due to *H. influenzae*, type b was responsible for disease in four of the neonates. The strains were not typeable in four and not typed in the remaining two cases.

Maternal infectious febrile morbidity occurred within 24 hours of fetal membrane dissolution in 6 of the 10 cases. Prolonged rupture of the fetal membranes in combination with endocervical colonization has a higher correlation with postpartum maternal infectious morbidity than with neonatal disease. Rusin et al. (1991) analyzed the records of all mothers and neonates infected with *H. influenzae* over a 10-year period. Of the 18 infected mothers, 13 had chorioamnionitis, endometritis, or both. Of the 23 infected neonates, 15 presented with early sepsis and/or pneumonia and nine had conjunctivitis. During the period of the study, only group B streptococci and *Escherichia coli* were more common as causes of early neonatal bacteremia. In this retrospective study, maternal infection predicted neonatal infection.

TABLE 1 Relationship of serotypes and biotypes of *Haemophilus influenzae*

Serotype	Biotype
Type b strains	Biotype I and biotype II (I and II)
Nontypeable strains	Biotypes II through VI

TABLE 2 Relationship of serotypes to specific disease entities due to *Haemophilus influenzae*

Type B strain	Nontypeable strains
Meningitis[a]	Acute sinusitis
Otitis media	Chronic bronchitis
Cellulitis[a]	Acute tracheobronchitis
Epiglottitis[a]	Pneumonia
Septic arthritis[a]	Chorioamnionitis (ascending)
Chorioamnionitis	
Endometritis (hematogenous)	
Perinatal septicemia	
Vulvovaginitis	

[a]Specific for type b strains.

Endometritis

In the female genital tract, nonencapsulated *H. influenzae* organisms appear to function as pathogens when there is preexisting disease. *H. influenzae* has been recovered from cases of chronic endometritis associated with the Lippes loop intrauterine contraceptive device (IUD) and from tubo-ovarian abscesses.

Salpingitis

Salpingitis due to *H. influenzae* has traditionally been associated with IUD usage. Recently Carmeci and Gregg (1997) have reported a case of *H. influenzae* acute salpingitis in a patient who had no predisposing conditions.

DIAGNOSIS

As previously indicated, *H. influenzae* will not grow on blood agar, except as tiny colonies around other bacterial colonies that produce hemolysis of the red blood cells. Recovery of the bacteria can be readily achieved on chocolate agar. Dependence on X and V factors is demonstrable with horse blood and brain heart infusion plates. Definitive confirmation is achieved by the Quellung reaction using type-specific antiserum.

When present, capsular antigens can be detected by latex agglutination, enzyme-linked immunosorbent assay (ELISA), or polymerase chain reaction (PCR).

H. influenzae may be responsible for false-negative blood cultures if routine "blind" subcultures of grossly negative cultures are not performed within 12 to 16 hours after blood collection. Subcultures should be inoculated onto quadrants of chocolate agar plates that are incubated in 10% CO_2 for 48 hours.

THERAPY

Ampicillin was once considered the drug of choice; however, the therapy of the disease is complicated by the progressive development of antibiotic resistance due to the production of b-lactamases (Table 3). Approximately 25% of *H. influenzae* type b strains are resistant to penicillin and its semisynthetic analogs. Selected "third-generation" cephalosporins (cefuroxime 0.75–1.5 g every eight hours, ceftriaxone 1.0–2.0 g every 24 hours, or cefotaxime 1.5–2.0 g every eight hours) currently constitute the most commonly used antibiotics. The concomitant utilization of an aminoglycoside is recommended, given the spectrum of potential pathogens.

SELECTED READING

Abdul-Rauf A, Schreiber JR. Neonatal Haemophilus influenzae type b sepsis. Pediatr Infect Dis J 1990; 9:918.

Albritton WL, Penner S, Staney L, Brunton J. Biochemical characteristics of Haemophilus influenzae in relationship to source of isolation and antibiotic resistance. J Clin Microbiol 1978; 7:519.

Berczy J, Fernlund K, Kamme C. Haemophilus influenzae in septic abortion. Lancet 1973; i:1197.

Carmeci C, Gregg D. Haemophilus influenzae salpingitis and septicemia in an adult. Obstet Gynecol 1997; 89:863.

Courtney SE, Hall RT. Haemophilus influenzae sepsis in a premature infant. Am J Dis Child 1978; 132:1039.

TABLE 3 Therapeutic considerations for *Haemophilus influenzae*

Antibiotic	Limiting factors
Ampicillin Third-generation ephalosporins, i.e., ceftizoxime and cefotamine	25% of *H. influenzae* type b show resistance to penicillin and semisynthetic analogs

Frieson CA, Cheng TC. Characteristic features of neonatal sepsis due to Haemophilus influenzae. Rev Infect Dis 1986; 8:777.

Gibson M, Williams PP. Haemophilus influenzae amnionitis associated with prematurity and premature membrane rupture. Obstet Gynecol 1978; 52:705.

Hurley R. Haemophilus endometritis in women fitted with Lippes loop. Br Med J 1970; 2:560.

Ingman M. Neonatal Haemophilus influenzae septicemia. Am J Dis Child 1970; 119:66.

Khuri-Bulos N, McIntosh K. Neonatal Haemophilus influenzae infection. Am J Dis Child 1975; 129:57.

Kragsbjerg P, Nilsson K, Persson L, et al. Deep obstetrical and gynecological infections caused by non-typeable Haemophilus influenzae. Scand J Infect Dis 1993; 25:341.

Kristensen K. Haemophilus influenzae type b infections in adults. Scand J Infect Dis 1989; 21:651.

Lieberman JR, Hagay ZJ, Dagan R. Intraamniotic Haemophilus influenzae infection. Arch Gynecol Obstet 1989; 244:183.

Llien LD, Yeh TF, Novak GM, et al. Early onset Haemophilus sepsis in newborn infants: clinical, roentgenographic and pathologic features. Pediatrics 1978; 62:229.

Long SS, Teter MJ, Yirubra PH. Biotype of Haemophilus influenzae: correlation with Yirubra and ampicillin resistance. J Infect Dis 1983; 147:800.

Musher DM. Haemophilus influenzae infections. Hosp Pract 1983; 47:158.

Nicholls J, Yuille TB, Mitchell RG. Perinatal infections caused by Haemophilus influenzae. Arch Dis Child 1975; 50:739.

Ogden E, Amstey M. Haemophilus influenzae septicemia and midtrimester abortion. J Reprod Med 1979; 22:106.

Pastorek J 2d, Bellow P, Faro S. Haemophilus influenzae implicated in puerperal infection. South Med J 1982; 75:734.

Pinon G, Quentin R, Bosca G, et al. Haemophilus influenzae infections in infants and mothers. Nouv Presse Med 1982; 11:999.

Quentin R, Musser JM, Mellouet M, et al. Typing of urogenital, maternal, and neonatal isolates of Haemophilus influenzae and Haemophilus parainfluenzae in correlation with clinical source of isolation and evidence for a genital specificity of H. influenzae biotype IV. J Clin Microbiol 1989; 27:2286.

Rusin P, Adam RD, Peterson EA, et al. Haemophilus influenzae: an important cause of maternal and neonatal infections. Obstet Gynecol 1991; 77:92.

Silverberg K, Boehm FH. Haemophilus influenzae amnionitis with intact membranes: a case report. Am J Perinatol 1990; 7:270.

Skirrow MB, Prakash A. Tubo-ovarian abscess caused by a non-capsulated strain of Haemophilus influenzae. Br Med J 1970; 1:32.

Speer M, Rosen RC, Rudolph AJ. Haemophilus influenzae infection in the neonate mimicking respiratory distress syndrome. J Pediatr 1978; 93:295.

Wallace RJ Jr, Baker CJ, Quiones FJ, et al. Nontypeable Haemophilus influenzae (biotype 4) as a neonatal, maternal, and genital pathogen. Rev Infect Dis 1983; 5:123.

Wallace RJ Jr, Musher DM, Septimus EJ, et al. Haemophilus influenzae infection in adults: characterization of strains by serotypes, biotypes, and beta-lactamase production. J Infect Dis 1981; 144:101.

Winn HN, Egley CC. Acute Haemophilus influenzae chorioamnionitis associated with intact amniotic membranes. Am J Obstet Gynecol 1987; 156:458.

Winn HN, Egley CC. Haemophilus influenzae chorioamnionitis. Am J Obstet Gynecol 1989; 161:1419.

Listeria monocytogenes

INTRODUCTION

Listeria monocytogenes is a member of the family Corynebacteriaceae, order Eubacteriales. It is a small, slightly curved gram-positive and catalase-positive bacillus with rounded ends. The organism can exist in both a rough form and the predominantly pathogenic smooth form that is characterized by a peritrichous arrangement of flagella. These flagella are responsible for the tumbling motility seen when the organism is grown in cultures at room temperature. Old cultures, particularly if incubated at 37°C, show imperceptible movement. The organism ferments several carbohydrate substances; however, the fermentative reactions are neither sufficiently characteristic nor consistent enough to be of much diagnostic significance. *L. monocytogenes* produces soluble hemolysins that may cause a very narrow band of beta-hemolysis on blood agar plates.

There are 11 serotypes of *L. monocytogenes*, 1a, 1b, 2, 3a, 3b, 4a, 4b, 4ab, 4c, 4d, and 4e, based on analyses of somatic and flagellar antigens. It is generally stated that type 1 serotypes tend to be predominantly isolated from rodents, whereas type 4 serotypes tend to be isolated from herbivores; however, there is no absolute species specificity. Dissemination is believed to be primarily food borne.

The majority of human infections that have been serotyped belong to the group 3 serotypes. As might be anticipated from its characteristic pathology, abscess formation, the organism is a facultative anaerobe. Certain facets of the pathogenesis of the morphologic lesion are thought to be the consequence of host response to a toxin, even though no toxin has yet been identified.

Much speculation exists as to whether or not there may be a filterable L form of *L. monocytogenes*. The presence of an L form has been postulated as one of the reasons for the difficulties in isolating the bacterium from infected tissue as opposed to biologic fluids such as cerebrospinal fluid (CSF), urine, and blood.

CLINICAL DISEASE

Depending upon the patient population infected, *L. monocytogenes* produces primarily two diverging patterns of disease. In immunologically compromised or age-vulnerable populations, infection results in invasive disease. Among patients with advanced human immunodeficiency syndrome, listeriosis is approximately 100 times more frequent than in the general population. The clinical presentation tends to be sepsis, meningitis, meningoencephalitis, cerebritis, or brain abscess. Disease selection reflects the importance of the T-helper cell mononuclear phagocyte arm of the immune defense system in organismal containment. Fetuses and neonates constitute an age-vulnerable population.

In nonimmunocompromised or disease-compromised populations, clinical presentation is primarily that of a gastrointestinal illness or infectious mononucleosis-like syndrome.

Maternal Listeriosis

Infection has a predilection for pregnant women. *L. monocytogenes* produces a spectrum of disease. Because of the *forme fruste* of disease and the ability to mimic other infections, the clinical diagnosis of *L. monocytogenes* is often difficult.

When clinically overt, *L. monocytogenes* may present as one of three syndromes:

1. Infectious mononucleosis-like syndrome
2. Influenza-like syndrome
3. Typhoidal-like syndrome
4. Febrile gastroenteritis

Approximately 20% of infants with neonatal listeriosis are born to asymptomatic gravidae. The infectious mononucleosis-like syndrome is characterized by malaise, chills, fever, pharyngitis, lymphadenopathy, splenomegaly, and monocytosis. The influenza-like pattern is characterized by fever, headaches, and upper respiratory symptoms. Some women experience a very transient macular salmon-colored rash. Careful questioning of these patients reveals the majority to have one or more documented episodes of rigors. The typhoid-like syndrome is characterized by high spiking temperatures that are often associated with back pain or flank pain. In many instances, the diagnosis of pyelonephritis is made even though there is no subsequent substantiation by urinalysis or urine cultures. *L. monocytogenes* can cause a febrile gastroenteritis characterized by fever, musculoskeletal symptoms, nausea, vomiting, and diarrhea. Foods incriminated as the vehicle source have included soft cheese, shrimps, foods sold from delicatessen counters, rice salad, pork tongue in jelly, and undercooked chicken.

The dose inoculum of bacteria influences the timing and probability of disease. Although most of the gastrointestinal symptomology develops within a few days following ingestion of the contaminated food, Riedo et al. (1994) reported incubation periods in two pregnant women of 19 and 23 days.

Individuals infected with HIV appear to be at greater risk of infection with *L. monocytogenes* than the general population. Ewert et al. (1995) quantified the risk of listeriosis in persons with AIDS and HIV infection in Los Angeles County. The incidence of listeriosis was 95.8 and 8.8 cases per 100,000 person-years among persons with AIDS and all HIV-infected persons, respectively, but only 1.0 case per 100,000 person-years in the total population. When disease occurs in an immunocompromised gravida, greater morbidity is likely to ensue.

In the majority of instances, the mother is not critically ill, the symptoms are of relatively short duration, and with or without therapy the fever, pain, and associated symptoms will subside. The impact on the fetus is usually delayed for several days or weeks. Fetal death in utero may occur. This is usually heralded by diminution and finally total cessation of fetal movements. Alternatively, parturition may ensue, with delivery of a stillborn or severely ill infant. Occasionally, fever occurs or recurs with the onset of labor, and the amniotic fluid and fetal surfaces of the placenta are often suggestive of chorioamnionitis. In rare instances, careful inspection of the placenta reveals small miliary areas of necrosis. In many instances, the amniotic fluid will have a murky, discolored appearance. In those instances in which the gravida is febrile and symptomatic prior to parturition, she often becomes asymptomatic postpartum, and her clinical course tends to be uneventful even in the absence of therapy. In rare instances, maternal infection may result in meningitis that cannot be distinguished from meningitis due to other bacteria. There is no characteristic body of laboratory data or clinical profile. In most instances, the organism is readily identified in the CSF. In retrospect, one is often able to elicit a history of a prodrome of either gastrointestinal upset with diarrhea or respiratory infection and then ensuing headaches, myalgia, fever, chills, nausea, vomiting, and stiff neck. In the absence of therapy, mortality exceeds 70%. The correct diagnosis is usually made as a consequence of recovery of the organisms from the blood or CSF.

Patients without significant symptomatology will have the diagnosis of listeriosis made retrospectively, only after the delivery of an infected or stillborn infant. A significant number of cases of perinatal septicemia occur in the progenies born to asymptomatic mothers who experience no obvious illness during pregnancy. Maternal septicemia may occur with both disease and infection. What does maternal septicemia mean in terms of potential fetal involvement? Data in the literature indicate a near one-to-one correlation between symptomatic maternal listeriosis and subsequent involvement of the products of conception. *L. monocytogenes* can be isolated from amniotic fluid in cases of congenital infection and from the neonates or products of conception in cases after documented maternal septicemia. In the absence of therapy, when *L. monocytogenes* is isolated from the intravascular compartment of gravidae, the fetus almost invariably becomes infected.

Genital Listeriosis

There has been much speculation as to whether or not *L. monocytogenes* may result in prolonged colonization of the female genital tract. Circumstantial evidence indicates that *L. monocytogenes* may be spread by venereal modes of transmission. The organism has been isolated from urethral exudates of individuals with gonorrhea who shared a common sexual partner, as well as from the semen of consorts of women who had genital listeriosis. None of the men with genital listeriosis exhibited urethral symptoms; however, analyses of their semen prior to therapy showed reductions in sperm count, motility, and viability as well as incomplete

mucolysis of seminal fluid in the ejaculate. With therapy, the impaired sperm indices returned to normal. In European countries, there is a high incidence of isolation of the organism from women with histories of repeated abortions. In one study, *L. monocytogenes* was recovered from 25 of 34 women with a history of repeated abortion. Diagnosis was contingent on the isolation of the organism from at least three cultures taken at one to five day intervals. Three of the patients were pregnant and in the second trimester. All three aborted shortly thereafter. In one instance, *L. monocytogenes* was isolated from the amniotic fluid. The remaining eight gravidae were in their first trimester. They received antibiotic therapy, and no ensuing fetal deaths were observed.

Chronic infection of the female genital tract is thought to be manifested by continuous excretion of the microorganisms from the uterine cervix over long periods, which may result in abortion or stillbirth in a supervening pregnancy. The observations cited are only suggestive, and much more of the natural history of infection must evolve before these fragmentary pieces of knowledge can be put into proper perspective.

Congenital and Neonatal Infection (Granulomatosis Infantiseptica)

There have been recent attempts to divide neonatal listeriosis into early-onset and late-onset disease. Early-onset disease becomes clinically apparent within the first five days of life; late-onset, after more than five days. Unfortunately, this classification, borrowed from group B streptococcal infections, amalgamates congenital infection with early neonatally acquired infection despite their markedly different pathogeneses.

In most instances, congenital listeriosis is the consequence of seeding of the fetal compartment by a low-grade maternal septicemia. Almost invariably, microscopic listerial placentitis can be demonstrated, with involvement of the maternal placental component and subsequent extension of the disease process to the fetal compartment. The majority of mothers exhibit clinical illness characterized by pyrexia. Not infrequently, the amniotic fluid is discolored in appearance, resembling "murky dish water." When in gestation maternal disease occurs partially dictates the neonatal consequences in the absence of therapy. First-trimester maternal infection can result in abortion. Fetal death in utero is a common occurrence when disease occurs in the second trimester. Third-trimester infection or disease produces premature termination of pregnancy. Of those infants born alive, many die within minutes after parturition. The bacteria recovered from the female genital tract are of the same serotype as those that infect the infant. No particular serotype predominates. Congenital listeriosis may account for up to 20% of perinatal septicemia. Up to 60% of cases of congenital listeriosis present as preterm labor.

L. monocytogenes is endemic in both wild and domestic animals. A small but significant number of humans may function as fetal carriers of the organism for limited periods of time. It is probable that birds and mammals constitute the major reservoir of listeriosis and, in certain instances, are directly responsible for human infection. Direct contamination of fruits and vegetables as well as unpasteurized milk have been the source of miniepidemics. Schwartz et al. (1988) analyzed over 50 cases of perinatal listeriosis. The only statistically significant demographic difference was a history of having eaten uncooked hot dogs or undercooked chicken.

According to Farber and Losos (1988), *L. monocytogenes* can be recovered from a variety of dairy products, leafy vegetables, fish, and meat products. It can be isolated from refrigerated foods and is more heat resistant than most vegetative bacteria. Epizootic listeriosis occurs in laboratory animals and cattle. Disease in humans is a sporadic event; however, when it does occur, not infrequently, a second or third case will be identified at the same institution within several months of each other. Although occurring in unrelated patients, these miniclusters of cases are usually due to a common serotype. Other than some rare cases of apparent neonatal cross-infection in nurseries, person-to-person transmission, with the exception of the venereal route, has not been recognized.

L. monocytogenes is one of the more important bacterial infections that involve both the gravida and her fetus. The true incidence of perinatal infection with *L. monocytogenes* is higher than the 1 in 30,000 births reported in England by the Communicable Disease Surveillance Centre. In the past decade, the incidence of disease has increased such that, in a number of institutions in the United States, *L. monocytogenes* is the third most common bacterial cause of perinatal septicemia (septicemia in the first 24 hours of life).

The unique importance of *L. monocytogenes* is that, if left untreated, it results in a high perinatal mortality. Disease in the mother usually spontaneously regresses. Sixty percent of neonates die due to the infection. Another 30% have permanent sequelae. However, if identified and properly treated, the disease can be totally eradicated in utero.

Live-born infants exhibit evidence of central nervous system involvement, manifested by fever, abnormal patterns of respiration, and the subsequent onset of vasomotor collapse. Occasionally, a rash associated with cutaneous bacterial involvement is observed. The majority of infants with congenital infection will have roentgenographic abnormalities. These range from interstitial pneumonitis to nodular infiltrates. While group B streptococci can emulate these findings, it is relatively rare for *L. monocytogenes* to mimic the roentgenographic picture of hyaline membrane disease. The neonates surviving parturition are often critically ill and not infrequently succumb during the first or second week of life from cardiovascular collapse and pulmonary involvement. Therapy requires vigorous ventilatory support and aggressive antibiotic therapy with ampicillin. If evidence of a left-to-right shunt or pulmonary hypertension is documented and the infant cannot be adequately ventilated, attempts should be undertaken to combat the associated pulmonary vasospasm that seems to aggravate the hypoxemia.

Although congenital infection secondary to hematogenous dissemination is the most characteristic mechanism for granulomatosis infantiseptica, it does not represent the sole mechanism by which the fetus or neonate may become infected. Transperineal spread of the ingested *L. monocytogenes* can result in vaginal–cervical colonization and a possibility of ascending infection.

The probability of sexual transmission has been inferred by the identification of the organism in semen of sexual consorts of women with recurrent abortions. Once effective labor has been established and/or dissolution of the fetal membranes has occurred, the potential for ascending infection occurs. The clinical picture here is that of chorioamnionitis. An alternative presentation for these patients is relatively asymptomatic disease in the gravida with the major symptoms being that of premature labor. Transabdominal amniocenteses have documented that, in rare instances, the onset of labor in the late second or early third trimester was due to *L. monocytogenes*.

Infected neonates can be the source for hospital-acquired meningitis and enterocolitis within intensive-care nurseries.

Neonatally acquired listeriosis is somewhat analogous to the problems observed with group B streptococci. Two patterns of disease exist: an early-onset septicemia and a late-onset meningitis. The early-onset septicemic form is observed in progeny of mothers with obstetric complications; it has a proclivity for premature infants and is associated with a high neonatal mortality rate.

Neonatal presentation is primarily a function of the portal of infection. When the organism has been inhaled, the principal manifestations of disease are respiratory distress, apnea, cyanosis, hypothermia, and bradycardia. The majority of infants have roentgenographic evidence of disease. In other instances, the conjunctiva or nasopharynx provides the portal of infection. These patients present with a septicemic/meningitis type of onset that has been termed as late-onset as opposed to early-onset respiratory distress. These children develop hepatosplenomegaly, conjunctivitis, cutaneous manifestations of disseminated and vascular coagulopathy, and sometime ascites.

The characteristic pattern of late-onset disease is that of meningitis. Disease occurs in normal neonates with no antecedent history of infectious complications. In contrast to the meningitis due to *Haemophilus influenzae*, *Neisseria meningitidis*, or *Streptococcus pneumoniae*, disease tends to occur in the fourth week. The most frequent presenting manifestations, in addition to fever, are irritability and anorexia. Less-frequent signs include respiratory distress, lethargy, cyanosis, jaundice, tense anterior fontanelle, and convulsions. Differential cell counts of white blood cells in the CSF demonstrate a polymorphonuclear neutrophilic leukocytosis. A relative or absolute monocytosis occurs in approximately 30% of the cases.

The organisms responsible for late-onset neonatal meningitis tend to be serotypes 1 and 4. The mortality figures are far more favorable than those observed with early-onset septicemic disease. Approximately 50% of the infants survive; however, late sequelae including hydrocephalus and mental retardation may occur.

At autopsy, one finds widespread miliary micro- and macroabscesses, primarily involving the liver, spleen, adrenal glands, lung, gastrointestinal tract, central nervous system, and skin. These foci of septic necrosis are manifested as grayish white, often slightly raised, pinhead lesions. The hepatic abscesses characteristically border on central veins. The organism can be readily demonstrated with appropriate bacterial stains, both lying free and phagocytized within polymorphonuclear neutrophils. As is obvious from this description, granulomatosis infantiseptica is a misnomer. The name originated because the gross lesions resembled those seen in miliary tuberculosis.

DIAGNOSIS

The diagnosis requires a high index of suspicion. The presence of gram-positive coccobacilli in meconium gastric aspirates or CSF may make the presumptive diagnosis of neonatal listeriosis. The diagnosis can be inferred by finding widespread miliary microabscesses involving the placenta which, when Gram-stained, reveal the presence of the characteristic coccobacillus, both lying free and within Polymorphonuclear neutrophils. When available, definitive confirmation can be achieved using a direct immunofluorescent technique. Unless the laboratory is appropriately alerted to possible isolation of *L. monocytogenes*, because of the morphological similarities between *L. monocytogenes* and other members of the genus *Corynebacterium*, positive cultures may be discarded as diphtheroid contaminants. A laboratory report of diphtheroids, especially in pure culture from certain types of infection (i.e., meningitis, neonatal septicemia, or chorioamnionitis) should raise the possibility of false identification and a suspicion of underlying listeriosis. *L. monocytogenes* can be grown from blood and CSF; however, its isolation from tissue sources may be difficult. Once growth is achieved on an artificial medium, the bacteria grow well on common, commercially available media. If recovery of the organism is to be attempted from tissue, it is best that the material be kept at 4°C for one to two days before inoculation into a bacteriological media. *L. monocytogenes* can be differentiated from diphtheroids by its motility at 20°C to 30°C. A clinician who challenges the diagnosis of the diphtheroids can ask for the intraperitoneal inoculation of the isolate into seronegative mice. If the isolate is *L. monocytogenes*, intraperitoneal inoculation of 0.1 to 0.2 mL of a 24-hour culture of diphtheroids will result in the demise of the mouse in one to three days. Autopsy will reveal miliary abscesses involving primarily the liver, spleen, and mesenteric lymph nodes. A Gram stain of these nodes reveals gram-positive rods. In the majority of instances, the diagnosis of listeriosis is derived by bacteriological identification from blood or CSF. Polymerase chain reaction tests can be used to identify *L. monocytogenes* in CSF and blood.

THERAPY

The keynote of maternal therapy is prompt institution of effective antibiotic therapy. The variation in resistance to antibiotics exhibited by different strains of *L. monocytogenes* poses a problem in empiric treatment. Patients with overt listeriosis should receive parenteral therapy. At present, the combination of ampicillin and aminoglycoside appears to afford the best therapy.

If the gravida is allergic to penicillin (immediate type of reaction or definite history of hypersensitivity), trimethoprim–sulfamethoxazole, 20 mg/kg/day of the trimethoprim component in four divided doses or erythromycin 60 mg/kg/day intravenously in four divided doses can be utilized. Erythromycin traverses the placental barrier poorly. The recommended duration of therapy in symptomatic patients is 14 days; however, shorter courses of drug administration, five to seven days, have been effective. Because of the uncertainty of the initial maternal diagnosis, combined antibiotic therapy with ampicillin and an aminoglycoside is often used effectively. What is of the utmost importance is that when infection with *L. monocytogenes* is suspected, cephalosporins should not be used. The cephalosporins are ineffective in the therapy of listeriosis.

A growing number of reports indicate that a good reproductive outcome can be achieved if transplacental infection can be arrested in utero. Therapeutic concentrations of ampicillin can be achieved in amniotic fluid. A number of cases of maternal listeriosis septicemia have been reported in which systemic antibiotics resulted in a favorable pregnancy outcome. The growing documentability of successful treatment of potentially lethal fetal disease due to *L. monocytogenes* places a premium on excluding this disease entity when a gravida presents with rigors and/or flu-like syndrome.

SELECTED READING

Epidemiology

Dalton CB, Austin CC, Sobel J, et al. An outbreak of gastroenteritis and fever due to Listeria monocytogenes in milk. N Engl J Med 1997; 336:100.

Foodborne listeriosis. Bull World Health Org 1988; 66:421.

Ewert DP, Lieb L, Hayes PS, Reeves MW, Mascola L. Listeria monocytogenes infection and serotype distribution among HIV-infected persons in Los Angeles County, 1985–1992. J Acquir Immune Defic Syndr Hum Retrovirol 1995; 8:461.

Farber JIVI, Losos JZ. Listeria monocytogenes: a foodborne pathogen. Can Med Assoc J 1988; 138:413.

Gellin G, Broome CV, Bibb WF, et al. The epidemiology of listeriosis in the United States—1986. Listeriosis Study Group. Am J Epidemiol 1991; 133:392.

Gray JW, Barrett JF, Pedler SJ, Lind T. Faecal carriage of Listeria during pregnancy. Br J Obstet Gynaecol 1993; 100:873.

Linnan MJ, Mascola L, Lou XD, et al. Epidemic listeriosis associated with Mexican-style cheese. N Engl J Med 1988; 319:823.

Lorber B. Listeriosis. Clin Infect Dis 1997; 24:1.

McLauchlin J. Human listeriosis in Britain, 1967–85, a summary of 722 cases. 1. Listeriosis during pregnancy and in the newborn. Epidemiol Infect 1990; 104:181.

Real FX, Gold JW, Krown SE, Armstrong D. Listeria monocytogenes bacteremia in acquired immunodeficiency syndrome. Ann Intern Med 1984; 101:883.

Riedo FX, Pinner RW, Tosca ML, et al. A point-source foodborne listeriosis outbreak: documented incubation period and possible mild illness. J Infect Dis 1994; 170:693.

Schlech WF, Lavigne PM, Bortulussi R. Epidemic listeriosis—evidence for transmisson by food. N Engl J Med 1983; 308:203.

Schwartz B, Chieielski CA, Broome CV, et al. Association of sporadic listeriosis with consumption of uncooked hot dogs and undercooked chicken. Lancet 1988; 2:779.

Maternal/Perinatal Listeriosis

Boucher M, Yonekura ML. Listeria meningitis during pregnancy. Am J Perinatol 1984; 1:312.

Boucher M, Yonekura ML, Wallace R, Phelan JP. Adult respiratory distress syndrome: a rare manifestation of Listeria monocytogenes infection in pregnancy. Am J Obstet Gynecol 1984; 149:686.

Buchdahl R, Hird M, Gamsu H, Tapp A, et al. Listeriosis revisited: the role of the obstetrician. Br J Obstet Gynaecol 1990; 97:163.

Desprez D, Blanc P, Larrey D, et al. Acute hepatitis caused by Listeria monocytogenes infection. Gastroenterol Clin Biol 1994; 18:516.

Kelly CS, Gibson JL. Listeriosis as a cause of fetal wastage. Obstet Gynecol 1972; 40:91.

Larsson S. Listeria monocytogenes causing hospital-acquired enterocolitis and meningitis in newborn infants. Br Med J 1978; 2:473.

Liner RI. Intrauterine listeria infection: prenatal diagnosis by biophysical assessment and amniocentesis. Am J Obstet Gynecol 1990; 163:1596.

MacGowan AP, Cartlidge PH, MacLeod F, McLaughlin J. Maternal listeriosis in pregnancy without fetal or neonatal infection. J Infect 1991; 22:53.

MacNaughton MC. Listeria monocytogenes in abortion. Lancet 1962; 2:484.

Petrilli ES, D'Abiaing G, Ledger WJ. Listeria monocytogenes chorioamnionitis diagnosis by transabdominal amniocentesis. Obstet Gynecol 1980; 55:55.

Pezeshkian R, Fernando N, Carne CA. Listeriosis in mother and fetus during the first trimester of pregnancy: case report. Br J Obstet Gynaecol 1994; 91:85.

Rappaport F, Rabinovitz, Toaft R, Krochik N. Genital listeriosis as a cause of repeated abortion. Lancet 1960; 1:1273.

Romero R, Winn HN, Wan M, Hobbins J. Listeria monocytogenes chorioamnionitis and preterm labor. Am J Perinatol 1988; 5:286.

Valkenburg MH, Essed GG, Potters HV. Perinatal listeriosis underdiagnosed as a cause of pre-term labour? Eur J Obstet Gynecol Reprod Biol 1988; 27:283.

Congenital and Neonatal Listeriosis

Ahlfors CE, Goetzman BW, Halsted CC, et al. Neonatal listeriosis. Am J Dis Child 1977; 131:405.

Albritton WL, Wiggins GL, Feeley JC. Neonatal listeriosis: distribution of serotypes in relation to age at onset of disease. J Pediatr 1976; 88:481.

Bortolussi R. Neonatal listeriosis. Semin Perinatol 1990; 14:44.

Dungal M. Listeriosis in four siblings. Lancet 1961; 2:513.

Enocksson E, Wretlind B, Sterner G, Anzen B. Listeriosis during pregnancy and in neonates. Scand J Infect Dis 1990; 71:89.

Schwarze R, Bauermeiser CD, Ortel S, Wichmann G. Perinatal listeriosis in Dresden 1981–1986: clinical and microbiological findings in 18 cases. Infection 1989; 17:131.

Spencer JA. Perinatal listeriosis. Br Med J 1987; 295:349.

Teberg AJ, Yonekura ML, Salminen C, Pavlova Z. Clinical manifestations of epidemic neonatal listeriosis. Pediatr Infect Dis J 1987; 6:817.

Teberg A, Yonekura ML, Salminen C, Pavlova Z. Clinical manifestations of epidemic neonatal listeriosis. Pediatr Infect Dis J 1987; 6:817.

Yamazaki K, Price JT, Altshuler G. A placental view of the diagnosis and pathogenesis of congenital listeriosis. Am J Obstet Gynecol 1977; 129:703.

Nosocomial Perinatal Listeriosis

Lennon D, Lewis B, Martell C, et al. Epidemic perinatal listeriosis. Pediatr Infect Dis 1984; 3:30.

Levy E, Nassau E. Experience with listeriosis in the newborn. An account of a small epidemic in a nursery ward. Ann Paediatr 1960; 194:321.

Sinha SK, Jones D, Audurier A, Taylor AG. Perinatal listeriosis and hospital cross-infection. Arch Dis Child 1983; 58:938.

Therapy

Cruikshank DP, Warenski JC. First-trimester maternal Listeria monocytogenes sepsis and chorioamnionitis with normal neonatal outcome. Obstet Gynecol 1989; 73:469.

Fleming AD, Ehrlich DW, Miller NA, Monif GRG. Successful treatment of maternal septicemia due to Listeria monocytogenes at 26 weeks gestation. Obstet Gynecol 1985; 66:52.

Gordon RC, Barrett FF, Yow MD. Ampicillin treatment of listeriosis. Pediatrics 1970; 77:1067.

Hume OS. Maternal Listeria monocytogenes septicemia with sparing of the fetus. Obstet Gynecol 1976; 48:335.

Kalstone C. Successful antepartum treatment of listeriosis. Am J Obstet Gynecol 1991; 164:47.

Katz VL, Weinstein L. Antepartum treatment of Listeria monocytogenes septicemia. South Med J 1988; 75:1354.

Marget W, Seeliger HP. Listeria monocytogenes infections—therapeutic possibilities and problems. Infection 1988; 16:175.

Quentin C, Thibaut MC, Horovitz J, Bebear C. Multiresistant strain of Listeria monocytogenes in septic abortion. Lancet 1990; 336:375.

INTRODUCTION

Neisseria gonorrhoeae is a gram-negative, kidney-bean–shaped diplococcus measuring 0.6 to 1 mm in diameter. It is a strict aerobe and requires humidity and CO_2 for growth. Optimal growth occurs at 34° C to 36° C and a pH range of 7.2 to 7.6. Prior therapy with penicillin or its synthetic analogs can significantly alter both the characteristic bacterial morphology and the stainability, thus on occasion obscuring diagnosis from Gram-stained smears. Inhibition of cell wall synthesis by the penicillins causes the organism to lose its characteristic kidney-bean shape as well as its ability to stain gram-negative.

The organism is a pathogen for columnar and transitional epithelium. Infectivity appears to be in part a function of the presence of hair-like structures, pili, which may be important for the initial attachment of the gonococci to epithelial J-cells. Five distinct colony forms have been identified: fresh isolates exhibit colony forms T1 and T2 characterized by the presence of pili and by virulence on experimental inoculation into the urethra of male chimpanzees. Repeated subculturing of these isolates produces the T3, T4, and T5 colony forms, which lack pili and are less virulent.

The determinants of disease are difficult to distinguish. Prior infection does not confer immunity either systemically or at the portal of infection. Although volunteers with circulating antibodies are more resistant to experimental infection than those without, humoral immunity per se is not the critical factor in determining the attack rate. Disease can recur in the presence of specific antibodies. The virulence of *N. gonorrhoeae* may vary. Some men do not acquire the disease and others do when exposed to the same asymptomatic female carrier.

Two factors that permit infection to become disease are

1. dissolution of the anatomic–physiologic barrier constituted by endocervical mucosa and
2. the marked alteration in pH induced by menstrual blood.

The timing of the onset of acute salpingitis due to *N. gonorrhoeae* is such that it frequently occurs at or immediately following menses. In the gravid female, the rarity with which the gonococcus establishes overt disease in the endometrium and fallopian tubes after the first eight weeks of pregnancy indicates the efficacy of the endocervical barrier to ascending infection.

FEMALE GENITAL TRACT INVOLVEMENT

Acute Salpingitis

Gonococcal disease involving the female genital tract is characterized by

1. penetration of the glandular mucosa and
2. submucosal lymphatic and contiguous surface spread.

Once infection is established within the endometrial cavity, the gonococcus takes the path of least resistance. Involvement of the female genital tract is one of sequential infection due to contiguous bacterial replication and dissemination along the epithelial surfaces and to submucosal lymphatic spread. This is in marked contrast to the infectious mechanism of bacteria such as the group A streptococci, which, once having penetrated the glandular epithelium, pursue a transorgan route so as to involve sequentially the endometrium, the myometrium, and then adjacent soft tissues or the peritoneal serosa.

Peritonitis secondary to *N. gonorrhoeae* is primarily the consequence of spillage of organism and inflammatory exudate from the fimbriated ends of the fallopian tube into the peritoneal cavity, and not of transmural infection. Although the capsular surface of the ovary may be superficially involved in acute gonococcal salpingitis, it is resistant to penetration of the organism. Once having attained access to the peritoneal cavity, the gonococcus may again spread along free surfaces and up the paravertebral gutters to produce a perihepatitis known as the Stajano–Curtis–Fitz-Hugh syndrome (see the section titled Gonococcal Perihepatitis).

Currently, gonorrhea is the second most prevalent reportable infection in the United States, with over one and a half million new cases annually. Moreover, it is estimated that over 60 million new cases develop annually in the world. The relative inability to eradicate the disease is in part due to the fact that asymptomatic women with gonorrhea provide a great reservoir of infection that perpetuates the organism within the population. It is becoming apparent that significant control of the disease can only occur if routine cervical and anorectal cultures become a standard part of comprehensive female health care.

Clinical Aspects

Generally, in men, the initial symptoms of infection with the gonococcus appear three to five days after sexual exposure. In women, the interim between colonization and disease is so variable as to preclude a meaningful estimate. The susceptible genital areas that have been exposed are the urethra, paraurethral glands, and cervix. When the first two areas are involved, the symptoms produced may be so minimal that the patient is unaware of them. They include increased urinary frequency and slight burning on urination. When the endocervix is infected, vaginal leukorrhea frequently develops. The discharge may not be any more profuse than one which already existed; however, its appearance may be altered. It is now likely to be green or yellow-green and may be irritating to the vulvar tissues, whereas the previous discharge was not. Examination is rarely performed at this time, as the symptoms are usually not severe enough to compel the patient to seek medical advice.

The infection may extend to involve Bartholin's glands and may advance to abscess formation. It is a mistake to think that all Bartholin abscesses are gonorrheal, since they can develop from other types of infection also. Local redness, swelling, and edema as well as pain are present. As the abscess enlarges, it approaches the surface and may undergo spontaneous rupture. The pain may be sufficiently severe to require incision and drainage. Spontaneous resolution may occur, with cyst formation or the development of a nodular swelling that remains deep at the site of the gland. The symptoms generally subside after several days or a week, even if untreated. The gonococcus, if present at the start of the disease, is often eliminated from the site of infection by obligatory anaerobic bacteria once abscess formation is well established.

Progress of Disease

The organisms in the endocervix are probably prevented from progressing upward to the endometrium by cervical mucus. With the onset of menses, the bacteria may gain entrance to the uterine cavity. Menstruation not only negates the effect of cervical mucus and destroys the barrier constituted by the intact endometrium, but renders vaginal pH more alkaline, thus favoring the growth of N. gonorrhoeae.

Gonorrheal endometritis is transitory and heals spontaneously without leaving its mark. The organisms spread quickly and bilaterally to the endosalpinx and then, by virtue of the pus that pours from the fimbriated end of the tube, the infection spreads to the ovaries, the cul-de-sac, and the pelvic peritoneum, producing pelvic peritonitis.

N. gonorrhoeae by virtue of its replication alters the local microbiologic environment. The lowered oxidation–reduction potential permits selected constituents of the vaginal flora to successfully compete in this biologic niche. Initially, the bacteria recruited are Class I anaerobes. By virtue of local consumption of molecular oxygen, pH changes, and lowering of the oxidation-reduction potential, the microbiologic environment becomes progressively more conducive for anaerobic bacteria until a point is reached at which the aerobic bacteria, such as N. gonorrhoeae, undergo autoelimination. It is currently postulated that the critical site of infection in acute salpingitis is interstitial rather than intraluminal. As in patients with pyelonephritis, the consequence of basement membrane destruction secondary to the interstitial inflammatory process is healing by fibrosis. The destructive changes that alter the normal fallopian tube structure are due not primarily to N. gonorrhoeae, but to anaerobic bacteria, which function at these interstitial sites.

Although the endosalpingitis is the predominant feature of the infection, infection may spread both into the muscle wall of the tube and into the broad ligament tissues. The tube is grossly swollen, containing purulent material within its lumen that exudes from its fimbriated end. In severe cases, the tube may be covered with a shaggy fibrinous exudate. The vessels are engorged. The pelvic peritoneum and

ovaries are inflamed; turbid fluid or pus may be present in the pelvis. Microscopically, this stage is characterized by hyperemia, marked edema of the tubal folds, and leukocytic infiltration.

Symptomatically, there may be fever (up to 40° C); nausea and vomiting are not uncommon; and pain, moderate or severe, is usually present and generally located in both quadrants of the lower abdomen. Although one side may manifest greater involvement than the other, rarely will only one side be involved.

On examination, there is tenderness and variable rigidity in both lower quadrants; there may also be some distention. On pelvic examination, evidence of infection of the external genitalia and cervix may be present; motion of the cervix causes pain and there is tenderness in the lateral fornices.

Without the treatment, the symptoms and the findings described begin to subside in about 7 to 10 days and are usually gone in about 21 days. Uncomplicated gonococcal salpingitis responds to appropriate antibiotic therapy in 24 to 48 hours.

Acute Salpingitis and the Intrauterine Device

When a gonococcal infection occurs in a woman with a contraceptive intrauterine device (IUD), she has a three- to fourfold greater chance of developing acute salpingitis than an asymptomatic carrier without an IUD. Changes induced by the presence of an IUD on the endocervical/vaginal bacterial flora or the prior induction of a chronic anaerobic infection within the uterus by the IUD accelerates the anaerobic progression and effectively shortens the therapeutic window in which effective antimicrobial therapy can avert fallopian tube damage.

Gonococcal Septicemia

Most loci of gonococcal infection are the consequence of contiguous spread by the organism. There are two syndromes, which may either occur independently or coexist in a patient, that are the consequence of hematogenous dissemination: gonococcemia and gonococcal arthritis.

Not infrequently, a patient may exhibit small, raised macular skin lesions, which preferentially involve the wrists and distal joints. The lesions may become pustules (Fig. 1). Gonococcemia is usually associated with migratory polyarthralgia or arthritis. Fever occurs in 85% of the cases. The differential diagnosis includes meningococcemia, rickettsial infection, and subacute bacterial endocarditis. Unlike meningococcemia, gonococcemia is relatively benign in its morbidity and mortality. Since the initial clinical presentation may be indistinguishable from meningococcemia or subacute bacterial endocarditis, the patient should initially receive 20 million units of penicillin G intravenously in the first 24 hours after a minimum of three sets of blood cultures have been obtained. Once the diagnosis of N. gonorrhoeae septicemia has been documented, the dosage of penicillin can be substantially reduced.

Prolonged disseminated gonococcal infection, like meningococcemia, may be due to an inherent absence of

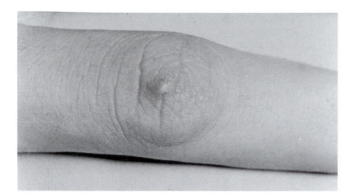

FIGURE I A vesiculopustular lesion on the middle finger of a young woman with disseminated gonococcal infection.

the fifth component of complement (C_5). The importance of C_5 in host susceptibility to invasive *Neisseria* infections has been inferred by epidemiological studies of females with this terminal complement component deficiency. Complement-mediated bacterial lysis appears to be important in human defense against bacteremic *Neisseria* infections. In families with the fifth component of complement deficiency recurrent invasive disease by either *Neisseria gonorrhoeae* or *Neisseria meningitis* may occur. Bacterial disease in the absence of C_5 due to *N. gonorrhoeae* usually occurs in adolescence and early childhood.

All patients with prolonged gonococcal bacteremia or gonococcemia should be analyzed for complement deficiency syndrome. Once identified, the entire family should be screened.

Although host considerations may be of prime importance in gonococcemia-like disease, the isolates from patient to patient with disseminated gonococcal infection (DGI) appear to be significantly different from other gonococcal isolates. The majority of the isolates are of an auxotype different from that of most other gonococci. They are not killed by sera from other patients with uncomplicated gonorrhea, even though these sera are bactericidal to other gonococci.

Gonococcal Arthritis

While acute gonococcal salpingitis in pregnancy is rare, gonococcal arthritis is not. The prompt and effective treatment of symptomatic primary gonorrhea has shifted the sex ratio of gonococcal arthritis. The majority of the current cases are in women, and, in particular, in gravidas. The absence of genitourinary signs often obscures early diagnosis and therapy. What is termed gonococcal arthritis is in most instances a tenosynovitis and not a true arthritis. Tenosynovitis, particularly of the wrist, is common in gonococcal arthritis, whereas it is rare in other types of pyogenic arthritis.

Gonococcal arthritis tends to take one of two forms: a septic form in which the patient gives a history of chills and fever, or a nonseptic form, in which there is no evidence of bacteremia or skin lesions comparable to those observed in meningococcemia. In approximately 85% of cases, the arthritis is polyarticular. Even in its septic mono- or oligoarthritis form, which involves large joints (knee, ankle, elbow), the clinician can usually elicit with careful questioning the history of an initial phase of migratory polyarthralgia. This monoarticular type of disease is a true arthritis. In most pyogenic arthritides, polyarthritis is rare. Once acute rheumatic fever has been excluded, the combination of polyarticular involvement, a lack of response to salicylates, fever, and joint swelling during pregnancy should be regarded as gonococcal arthritis.

In untreated septic monoarthritis due to *N. gonorrhoeae*, the clinician may find roentgenographic evidence of joint destruction. Before the introduction of antimicrobial agents, 23% of patients who recovered from gonococcal arthritis had residual joint damage. In rare instances of untreated gonococcal arthritis, osteomyelitis may develop in the contiguous bony structure. In general, with adequate therapy, resolution of either form is prompt and complete.

The diagnosis of gonococcal arthritis is often inferred rather than documented. A definitive diagnosis may be achieved by culturing joint fluid and blood on appropriate media. When joint fluid is available, *N. gonorrhoeae* can be demonstrated by direct immunofluorescence staining. Rarely, an exudative pharyngitis with subsequent recovery of *N. gonorrhoeae* may indicate the portal of infection. In most cases, the diagnosis is inferred from the recovery of the gonococcus from the endocervix or the anorectal area, and the dramatic clinical response to penicillin. Failure to achieve a dramatic response in 24 hours calls for a reevaluation of the working diagnosis. The strains of *N. gonorrhoeae* that cause disseminated infection are highly sensitive to penicillin. Prompt clinical amelioration has been achieved with both a low-dose regimen (procaine penicillin G, 600,000 units IM, given every 12 hours for up to 10 days) or a high-dose regimen of IV aqueous penicillin G, 10 million units daily for three days.

Gonococcal Endocarditis

In the preantibiotic era, 11% to 26% of all endocarditis was due to *N. gonorrhoeae*. The prevalence of gonococcal endocarditis has markedly declined in contrast to the increased incidence of the arthritis cutaneous variant of DGI. During the second and third trimesters of pregnancy, despite the relatively high incidence of DGI, there is not a concomitant increase in gonococcal endocarditis. Preliminary data have suggested that the more penicillin-sensitive strains of *N. gonorrhoeae* are more apt to produce clinical infections of the uterus and fallopian tubes or disseminated systemic disease than the more penicillin-resistant strains. In many instances, valvular involvement is aborted by relatively minimal therapy.

The majority of patients with gonococcal endocarditis experience a migratory polyarthritis, which usually precedes the signs of endocarditis. Weakness, high fever, chills, and rigors with diaphoresis are characteristic presenting complaints. Symptoms reputed to be unique to gonococcal endocarditis are the double-quotidian febrile spikes (two marked spikes in the same day) and concomitant jaundice secondary to hepatic involvement. These were not uncommonly seen in the preantibiotic era. Focal embolic manifestations involving the skin, conjunctiva, kidneys, lungs, and brain usually occur when one is dealing with well-established disease. The aortic, mitral, or pulmonary valve may be involved, in order of diminishing frequency. Right-sided valvular involvement is frequently silent until perforation occurs. The site of valvular involvement dictates whether systolic or diastolic murmurs are present. The most common electrocardiographic change is a bundle-branch block (usually right) or evidence of focal myocardial injury.

The diagnosis is readily established by the recovery of the organisms from the intravascular compartment. Liver biopsy during the investigation of a fever of unknown etiology may reveal leukocytes within the spaces of Disse with focal parenchymal necrosis. A presumptive diagnosis is based on the signs of progressive involvement of the cardiac valves in a patient with gonococcemia. Agglutinating antibodies to *N. gonorrhoeae* develop and titers may be of diagnostic significance. A definitive diagnosis can be established with echocardiography.

There are no set ground rules governing dosage or duration of therapy. Like *Streptococcus pneumoniae* and *Staphylococcus aureus*, *N. gonorrhoeae* produces an acute destructive process. Twenty million units of penicillin G per day by IV infusion followed by three weeks of oral ampicillin has been the regimen advocated. Current therapy is governed by the isolate's sensitivity profile to antibiotics.

In the preantibiotic era, the interim between initial manifestation and death was in the order of 10 weeks. Persistent heart failure or the presence of the murmurs of aortic insufficiency are strong indications for cardiac catheterization even in the absence of increasing left ventricular dilation and a wide pulse pressure. In our experience, successful treatment often necessitates valvular replacement. The failure of the temperature to normalize to its diurnal variation is often an antecedent to cardiac perforation.

Gonococcal Chorioamnionitis and Endometritis

Involvement of the fetal membranes and the subsequent clinical manifestation is the consequence of ascending gonococcal infection from glandular sites of bacterial replication. The status of the fetal membranes appears to be the major determinant of the pattern of ensuing maternal febrile morbidity. Dissolution of membrane integrity, in excess of 24 hours, may result in maternal pyrexia antenatally or in the immediate postpartum period. Examination of the placenta reveals morphologic evidence of an inflammatory process with varying degrees of vasculitis. The gonococcus is usually readily recoverable from the fetal or maternal surfaces of the placenta and from neonatal gastric aspirates. When the membranes have been ruptured for less than 24 hours, a more variable pattern in the timing of maternal disease is observed. Although pyrexia may still occur in the immediate postpartum period, the infectious morbidity frequently develops in the ensuing 24 hours. Not all patients with gonococcal endocervitis at parturition develop the postpartum endometritis.

In some patients, the clinical evidence of an endometritis does not develop until 4 to 20 days following delivery. This pattern tends to be more prevalent when the membranes are ruptured in the immediate antepartum period or at the time of parturition per se.

Gonococcal Ophthalmia Neonatorum

Before the introduction by Credé of silver nitrate, *N. gonorrhoeae* was reputed to be responsible for 12% of all blindness in the world. Gonococcal ophthalmia neonatorum is a consequence of the delivery of a neonate through an infected birth canal or its involvement in utero by *N. gonorrhoeae* following premature rupture of the membranes and ascending infection. Infection established before birth in this way is less likely to be aborted by silver nitrate than infection acquired during delivery.

Topical solutions of 1% silver nitrate, oxytetracycline, or erythromycin have been efficacious. An increase in the incidence of endocervical gonorrhea has engendered a proportionate increase in the number of cases of neonatal gonococcal ophthalmitis. Most of these cases occurred despite chemical or antibiotic prophylaxis. Periorbital edema and the tendency to resist manual opening of the eye on the part of the neonate contribute significantly to the problem of gonococcal ophthalmia neonatorum despite prophylaxis. The instillation of 1% silver nitrate may result in a chemical conjunctivitis requiring smear and cultures, but this is a small price to pay compared to acute gonococcal ophthalmitis. The silver nitrate should not be subsequently rinsed out with either saline or distilled water. A saline rinse following instillation of silver nitrate decreases the probability of efficacy. In addition to the diluent effect, the cation is precipitated by the use of the saline rinse, forming silver chloride. The chemical conjunctivitis from 1% silver nitrate is a self-limited entity. Any conjunctivitis present after 24 hours should be viewed with great suspicion. Gram-staining is important in early diagnosis. In addition to *N. gonorrhoeae*, *Haemophilus influenzae*, *Listeria monocytogenes*, and probably *S. pneumoniae* are all capable of producing a bacterial conjunctivitis. In the case of *L. monocytogenes* (a small gram-positive bacillus), one is dealing with a bacterial pathogen that is potentially lethal for the neonate.

The initial conjunctivitis of *N. gonorrhoeae* rapidly involves all of the contiguous portions of the eye. The resulting damage from healing by fibrosis may leave the neonate partially or completely blind. In the 1930s, isolated reports demonstrated the possible nosocomial spread of ocular gonococcal infection within newborn nurseries. This has not been a problem in the antibiotic era.

Any adequate prevention program must include not only silver nitrate prophylaxis but also early identification of infected women in the course of prenatal care and the eradication of maternal infection. It is imperative to treat sexual consorts to prevent reinfection. If gravidas are treated for bacteriologically documented gonorrhea during gestation but their consorts are not aggressively sought out and treated, approximately 30% will again harbor the organism at the time of parturition.

Prepubescent Gonococcal Vulvovaginitis

N. gonorrhoeae is one of the classic causes of vulvovaginitis in prepubescent girls. The anatomic–physiologic environment of the prepubescent vagina is ideal for the growth of the organism. The vaginal pH varies between 7 and 8 and is more conducive to gonococcal replication than the more acid adult vagina. Similarly, the absence of an estrogenic effect on the vaginal mucosa facilitates the establishment of infection.

Although gonorrhea is spread primarily by sexual congress, this is not the sole means of dissemination. Gonococcal vulvovaginitis occurs in epidemic forms, particularly in institutions with young girls. Some of these infections are probably transmitted by towels, common use of bathtubs, or the hands of infected individuals. Gonococcal vulvovaginitis readily responds to routine therapy.

Although gonococcal vulvovaginitis will occur given the opportunity, acute gonococcal salpingitis in prepubescent girls is rare. The failure of the disease to involve the endometrium and fallopian tubes appears to be primarily a function of the anatomic status of the cervix in children. The preadolescent cervix exhibits a cryptiform configuration and has been shown to be impermeable to high intravaginal fluid under pressure. The endocervical glands are at best rudimentary.

Gonococcal Pharyngitis

Changes in sexual behavior during pregnancy may include fellatio, with the result that the pharynx becomes a substantial reservoir of infection.

Gonococcal pharyngitis is seen primarily but not exclusively in patients who practice fellatio. Except following dental extraction, the gingiva, buccal mucosa, and tongue appear to be resistant to gonococcal infection. Gonococcal infection of the pharynx does not always produce clinical symptoms. When present, the most common clinical manifestation is an acute exudative pharyngitis; a less frequent presentation is chronic recurrent tonsillitis or pharyngitis. In approximately 15% of cases, asymptomatic pharyngeal infection has been the source of DGI.

Recovery of a gram-negative, catalase-positive diplococcus from the oropharynx is not sufficient to establish the diagnosis of gonorrhea. Because of the presence of other *Neisseria* species within the microbiologic flora of the oropharynx, confirmatory fermentation tests must be performed. When selecting sites for culture of *N. gonorrhoeae* in pregnant women, one should remember that the pharynx is a more common site of infection than the anorectal region. Pharyngeal gonococcal infection is more difficult to eradicate than infection of Skene's glands or the endocervical or anorectal glands. Tests of cure in women who practice fellatio should include follow-up cultures of the oropharynx.

Gonococcal Perihepatitis (Stajano–Curtis–Fitz-Hugh Syndrome)

Although originally described by Stajano in 1920, gonococcal perihepatitis was not perceived as a distinct entity until the early 1930s. In 1930, Curtis conceptually linked the association of "violin-string" or banded adhesions between the anterior surface of the liver and the parietal peritoneum with coexistent evidence of inflammatory disease of the pelvis. He believed that these adhesions were indicative of a previous gonococcal salpingitis and cites his discussions with other physicians who had observed flexure colitis, pleurisy, or gallbladder pain in female patients with gonorrhea. Fitz-Hugh characterized the acute clinical presentation of what Curtis had observed in end stage. He described three young women with pain in the right upper quadrant. One of them had been explored surgically for what was presumed to be cholecystitis. On the next day, recalling the article of Curtis, Fitz-Hugh reexamined the woman and was able to demonstrate, by Gram-staining, the presence of gram-negative intracellular diplococci in a smear of the wound drainage.

The syndrome is quite protean in its clinical manifestations. If not aware of its occurrence, the physician may be seduced into performing an exploratory laparotomy for what is a medical disease. Not infrequently, the presence of right upper quadrant pain may overshadow an antecedent history of bilateral lower quadrant pain. Failure to perform an adequate pelvic examination coupled with a lack of appreciation of the sequential pattern of pain precludes preoperative diagnosis of this entity.

There are two basic variants: the suprahepatic (phrenic) syndrome and the infrahepatic (subcostal) syndrome of Stajano. In the suprahepatic variant, gonococcal involvement may produce, in addition to fever and pain in the right upper quadrant, right supraclavicular pain, which is characteristic of rupture viscus. The infrahepatic form may produce symptoms and physical findings almost indistinguishable from those of acute cholecystitis, with a more or less localized point tenderness and pain referral along the 12th rib to the back. Roentgenograms may reveal elevation of the right hemidiaphragm. The patient experiences nausea without vomiting. The diagnosis is established by a positive smear or culture of *N. gonorrhoeae* from the cervix, prompt relief of symptoms with the appropriate antibiotic regimen, and a subsequent negative cholecystogram.

Care must be taken to distinguish this perihepatitis from the gonococcal hepatitis that can be seen in the course of DGI. In patients with DGI, an acute inflammatory infiltrate involving predominantly portal areas can be demonstrated by liver biopsies. Isolated neutrophils can be identified within the sinusoidal spaces. The pathogenesis of these two entities is sufficiently divergent to warrant a clear-cut distinction.

DIAGNOSIS

Specific diagnosis of infection with *N. gonorrhoeae* can be performed by testing endocervical, vaginal, or urine specimens. Culture, nucleic acid hybridization tests, and nucleic acid amplification tests (NAAT) are available for the detection of genitourinary infection with *N. gonorrhoeae*. Culture, nucleic acid hybridization, and NAAT identification require a female endocervical swab specimen. NAAT are cleared by the Food and Drug Administration (FDA)

164 ■ ORGANISMS ■ BACTERIA: EXOGENOUS PATHOGENS

for use with vaginal swabs and urine. Nonculture tests are not FDA cleared for use in the rectum and pharynx.

Gram Stain

The presence of intracellular gram-negative kidney-shaped diplococci within polymorphic neutrophils from an appropriate source is virtually pathognomonic of *N. gonorrhoeae*; nevertheless, the value of the Gram smear is limited compared to the cultural method of detecting *N. gonorrhoeae*. The Gram smear is used primarily as an important adjunct to cultural methods for the early diagnosis of gonorrhea in women.

Culture

A single culture from the endocervix plated on selective media and handled under near optimal conditions has a sensitivity of 84% to 89%.

The culture prerequisite for preheated culture plates, ambient CO_2, selective media, and marked organismal thermal liability has resulted in a gross underdiagnosing of subclinical infection. In many institutions, less than one-third of all subclinical carriers of gonorrhoeae are identified by bacterial cultures.

To obtain superior culture isolation results, certain ground rules need to be followed:

1. *Never culture a sample on a plate that is not at least at room temperature.* N. gonorrhoeae has an extremely limited thermal tolerance. Preferential growth occurs between 30° C and 36° C. Temperatures below room temperature will rarely sustain the replication of *N. gonorrhoeae* and often account for nonrecovery of the organism.
2. *Incubate cultures immediately.* N. gonorrhoeae does not tolerate drying. Again, the thermal liability of the organism is such that maintaining cultures at room temperature for more than one hour is destined to have a deleterious effect. One can almost establish a linear decay curve between recovery of organisms and prolonged exposure at suboptimal temperatures. If transport to a diagnostic laboratory is required, when possible, incubate the culture 6 to 10 hours before attempting transport.
3. *Be sure to provide a source of carbon dioxide.* In dealing with the Thayer-Martin plates, it is imperative that not only they be incubated, but that candle jars be utilized to provide the critical 5% CO_2 atmosphere required for the initiation of bacterial replication. Unless an extremely heavy inoculum of the bacteria is present, the likelihood of successfully culturing the organism is markedly reduced. This is probably the single greatest cause of failure.
4. *Roll the swab in a Z or W manner.* The swab when placed within the endocervical canal samples 360°; yet if one does not roll the swab, a maximum of 33% to 40% of the swab is sampled. One hundred percent sampling is exceedingly important when dealing with a situation where *N. gonorrhoeae* is present in quantities that are numerically reduced (e.g., the asymptomatic carrier or the patient with initial gonococcal salpingitis

who is now undergoing a facultative anaerobic superinfection at the endocervix).

Since roughly one-half of all women with gonorrhea have concomitant infection in the anorectal area, when cultures are indicated, samples for culturing should not be restricted to the endocervix. Obtaining an anorectal culture becomes even more imperative (*i*) when attempting to document causality in cases of presumed gonococcal arthritis and (*ii*) for documentation in cases of rape.

Because nonculture tests cannot provide antimicrobial susceptibility, in cases of persistent gonococcal infection after treatment, clinicians should perform both culture and antimicrobial susceptibility testing.

All patients suspected of gonorrhea should also be tested for other sexually transmitted diseases, including chlamydia, syphilis, and HIV.

DNA Probes

Due to the lower sensitivity of culture, primarily associated with delays in delivering specimens to the test laboratory, culture identification has been replaced by first DNA probes and then by NAAT.

DNA probes complementary to ribosomal RNA of *N. gonorrhoeae* allowed patient clinic facilities that relied on off-site laboratories to have specimens analyzed at a latter date as well as concomitant testing of *Chlamydia trachomatis*. DNA probes offer markedly superior sensitivity over suboptimally handled endocervical specimens.

The shortcoming of the probes as well as NAAT is that they cannot be used to identify the antibiotic-resistance pattern of a given gonococcal isolate.

Nucleic Acid Amplification Tests

Combination *N. gonorrhoeae*/*C. trachomatis* NAAT have largely displaced the DNA nonamplified probe assays. These tests not only have higher clinical sensitivity compared to conventional microbiological techniques, but also allow the assessment of noninvasive specimens. Comparable data have been demonstrated between specimens collected by the physician and those obtained by the patient.

ANTIMICROBIAL RESISTANCE

Antimicrobial resistance in the gonococcus can be plasmid mediated, chromosomally mediated, or both. In the United States, many variations have been identified. The three most important, from a public health standpoint, are plasmid-mediated resistance to penicillin (PPNG), chromosomally mediated resistance to penicillin (CMRNG), and plasmid-mediated, high-level tetracycline resistance (TRNG).

Plasmid-Mediated Resistance to Penicillin

PPNG are gonococcal strains that have acquired an extrachromosomal element or plasmid that encodes for beta-lactamase, an enzyme that destroys the beta-lactam ring of penicillin. Among the resistant strains, PPNG had the greatest impact on public health programs and resources in the mid-1980s.

Chromosomally Mediated Resistance to Penicillin

Unlike strains of plasmid-mediated resistance, strains with chromosomal resistance to penicillin do not produce beta-lactamase. Chromosomally mediated resistance is not limited to penicillin, but is a more general phenomenon that can include resistance to tetracycline, the cephalosporins, spectinomycin, and other aminoglycosides. In most instances to date, these strains have not been associated with treatment failure, either because the levels of resistance have been high or because the antibiotic in question was not used for therapy.

Plasmid-Mediated, High-Level Tetracycline Resistance

Gonococcal isolates with plasmid-mediated, high-level resistance to tetracycline (minimal inhibitory concentration >16 mg/mL) were first identified in 1985. Although many individual cases and clusters of TRNG have since been reported, investigation has shown that in most instances, Centers for Disease Control and Prevention (CDC) treatment guidelines were followed regarding dual therapy with penicillin and tetracycline, thus avoiding therapy failure. For nearly all patients with TRNG who have been treated with tetracycline alone, the therapy has not been effective.

Quinolone-Resistant N. gonorrhoeae

Cases of gonorrhea caused by *N. gonorrhoeae* resistant to fluoroquinolones is a growing problem.

Quinolone-resistant *N. gonorrhoeae* (QRNG) is widespread in parts of Europe, the Middle East, Asia, and the Pacific. In the United States, QRNG is becoming increasingly common. The fluoroquinolones should not be used in the treatment of infection that may have been acquired in Asia and the Pacific. The CDC has advised that quinolone not be used in California and Hawaii.

Gonococcal organisms with decreased in vitro susceptibilities to ciprofloxacin have deceased susceptibilities to all fluoroquinolones, including ofloxacin, enoxacin, iomefloxacin, levofloxacin, and norfloxacin. The dissemination of QRNG in the United States may increase to a point when fluoroquinolones can no longer be relied upon to eradicate gonococcal infections.

THERAPY

In terms of specific antibiotic therapy, the form of gonococcal disease dictates its therapy. The CDC 2006 guidelines for treatment of gonococcal infection in the United States take into account several observations: the high frequency of coexisting chlamydial and gonococcal infections, increased recognition of the serious complications of chlamydial and gonococcal infections, the difficulty in diagnosing chlamydial infection, the increasing incidence of infections due to both PPNG and CMRNG, and published reports of the emergence of tetracycline-resistant gonococci in some geographic areas (Table 1).

Women and men exposed to gonorrhea (e.g., within the past 60 days) should be examined, cultured, and treated prophylactically with a regimen that covers both gonococcal and chlamydial infections.

Meningitis and Endocarditis

Patients with gonococcal meningitis or endocarditis occurring in PPNG-endemic and hyperendemic areas should be treated with high-dose IV third-generation cephalosporins in consultation with an expert. Optimal therapy may be guided by results from in vitro susceptibility tests. Most authorities recommend treating patients with meningitis for 10 to 14 days and those with endocarditis for at least one month.

Ophthalmia

In PPNG-endemic and hyperendemic areas, adult patients with gonococcal ophthalmia should be treated with ceftriaxone, 1 g IM in a single dose. An ophthalmologist should evaluate the patient for ocular complications. Adjuvant topical antibiotics are not thought to offer any significant advantage. Irrigation of the eyes with saline or buffered ophthalmic solutions may be useful adjunctive therapy to eliminate discharge.

Gonococcal Ophthalmia in Neonates

Untreated gonococcal ophthalmia in neonates is highly contagious and may rapidly lead to blindness. All neonates with gonococcal ophthalmia in PPNG-endemic and hyperendemic areas should be treated with ceftriaxone, 25 to 50 mg/kg body weight/day, IV or IM. Topical antimicrobial preparations alone are not sufficient and are not required when appropriate systemic therapy is given. Irrigation of the eyes with saline or buffered ophthalmic solutions may be useful adjunctive therapy to eliminate discharge. Both the parents of newborns with gonococcal ophthalmia must be treated. Simultaneous ophthalmia infection with *C. trachomatis* has been reported and should be considered if a patient does not respond satisfactorily to recommended treatment.

Acute Salpingitis (Pelvic Inflammatory Disease)

Please refer to Chapter 75 on acute salpingitis.

MANAGEMENT OF SEX PARTNERS

Patients should be instructed to refer sex partners for evaluation and treatment. All sex partners of patients who have *N. gonorrhoeae* infection should be evaluated and treated for *N. gonorrhoeae* and *C. trachomatis* infections if their last sexual contact with the patient was within 60 days of onset of the patient's symptoms or diagnosis. If a patient's last sexual intercourse was more than 60 days before symptom onset or diagnosis, the patient's most recent sex partner should be treated. Patients should be instructed to avoid sexual intercourse until therapy is completed and patient and partner(s) are without symptoms.

NEONATAL PROPHYLAXIS AND PROPHYLACTIC TREATMENT

All newborns should receive ocular prophylaxis with either 1% silver nitrate solution, 1% tetracycline solution (or ointment), or 0.5% erythromycin ointment. Prophylaxis should

TABLE I Therapeutic recommendations for gonococcal infections

Uncomplicated gonococcal infections of the cervix, urethra, and rectum
■ *Recommended regimens*
  Cefixime 400 mg orally in a single dose or ceftriaxone 125 mg IM in a single dose or ofloxacin*
    400 mg orally in a single dose or ciprofloxacin* 500 mg orally in a single dose or levofloxacin*
    500 mg orally in a single dose
  Plus (if chlamydial infection is not ruled out)
  Doxycycline 100 mg orally twice a day for 7 days or azithromycin 1g orally in a single dose
■ *Alternate regimens*
  Spectinomycin 2 g in a single IM dose
  Single-dose cephalosporins (ceftizoxime 500 mg IM; ceftriaxone 500 mg IM)

Uncomplicated gonococcal infections of the pharynx
■ *Recommended regimens*
  Ceftriaxone 125 mg IM in a single dose or ciprofloxacin 500 mg IM in a single dose
■ *Plus (if chlamydial infection is not ruled out)*
  Azithromycin 1 g orally in a single dose or doxycycline 100 mg orally twice a day for 7 days or another regimen effective against
    C. trachomatis[a]

Disseminated gonococcal infection
■ *Recommended regimen*
  Ceftriaxone 1 g IM or IV every 24 hr
■ *Alternate regimens*
  Cefotaxime 1 g IV every 8 hr or ceftizoxime 1 g IV every 8 hr or for persons allergic to β-lactam drugs, spectinomycin 2 g IM every 12 hr.
    All regimens should be continued for 24–48 hr after improvement begins; then therapy may be switched to one of the following regimens
    to complete a full week of antimicrobial therapy: cefixime 400 mg orally twice a day or ciprofloxacin 500 mg orally twice times a day or
    ofloxacin 400 mg orally twice a day or levofloxacin 500 mg orally daily

Ophthalmia neonatorum caused by N. gonorrhoeae
■ *Recommended regimen*
  Ceftriaxone 25–50 mg/kg IV or IM in single dose, not to exceed 125 mg. Topical antibiotic therapy alone is inadequate and is unnecessary
    if systemic treatment is administered

Prophylactic treatment for infants whose mothers have gonococcal infection
■ Infants born to mothers who have untreated gonorrhea are at high risk for infection
■ Recommended regimen in the absence of signs of gonococcal infection
■ Ceftriaxone 25–50 mg/kg IV or IM, not to exceed 125 mg, in a single dose
■ Mother and infant should be tested for chlamydial infection
■ Azithromycin 2 g orally administered is effective against uncomplicated gonococcal infection but it is expensive and too often causes
  gastrointestinal distress to be used except in special situations

[a]Quinolones should not be used for infections acquired in Asia or the Pacific including California and Hawaii. The use of quinolones is probably inadvisable for the treatment of disease acquired in California and in other areas with increased prevalence of quinolone resistance. Pregnant women should not be treated with quinolones or tetracyclines. Gravidae infected with N. gonorrhoeae should be treated with a recommended or alternate cephalosporin. Women who can tolerate a cephalosporin should be administered a single dose of 2 g of spectinomycin IM.

be given within one hour after birth. No one regimen is completely effective. Tetracycline and erythromycin are also active against *C. trachomatis*. The prophylaxis failure rate of the antibiotic preparations for infections with resistant gonococcal strains is unknown. However, the intraocular antibiotic concentrations achieved with routine prophylaxis are high.

Neonates born to mothers with documented gonococcal infection peripartum should be treated with ceftriaxone 125 mg, IM, in one dose; low-birthweight infants should receive 25 to 50 mg/kg body weight.

TREATMENT FAILURES

If gonorrhea persists after treatment with one of the non-spectinomycin regimens, patients should be treated with spectinomycin 2.0 g IM. Recurrent gonococcal infections after treatment with the recommended schedules commonly are due to reinfection rather than treatment failure and indicate a need for improved sex-partner tracing and patient education. Since antimicrobial resistance is a cause of treatment failure, all posttreatment isolates should be tested for antimicrobial susceptibility.

RECOMMENDATIONS FOR THERAPY OF CONCOMITANT SYPHILIS

The concept that gonorrhea was a manifestation of syphilis resulted from John Hunter's experiment in 1767 of self-inoculation of pus from the urethra of an individual supposedly infected with gonorrhea. It was not until 1873 that Benjamin Bell clearly demonstrated that gonorrhea and syphilis were two separate disease entities. Nevertheless, this unfortunate experiment in self-inoculation serves to stress the fact that in approximately 1% to 2% of cases of gonorrhea, there is a concomitant infection with *Treponema pallidum*. Evidence of possible concomitant infection must be actively sought. The therapy for syphilis is inadequate for the treatment of gonorrhea, and vice versa.

Although long-acting forms of penicillin (such as benzathine penicillin G) are effective in the treatment of syphilis, they have no place in the treatment of gonorrhea. Penicillin preparations and cephalosporins not recommended for the treatment of gonorrhea include benzathine penicillin G, oral penicillin G, penicillin V, cloxacillin, dicloxacillin, cephradine, cephalothin, cephapirin, cefazolin, cephalexin, cefadroxil, and cefaclor.

SELECTED READING

Amstey MS, Steadman KT. Symptomatic gonorrhea and pregnancy. J Am Vener Dis Assoc 1976; 3:14.

Ashford WA, Adams JHU, Johnson SR, et al. Spectinomycin-resistant penicillinase-producing Neissera gonorrhoeae. Lancet 1981; 2:1035.

Bohnhoff M, Morello JA, Lerner SA. Auxotypes, penicillin susceptibility, and sero-groups of Neissera gonorrhoeae from disseminated and uncomplicated infections. J Infect Dis 1986; 154:225.

Bonin P, Tanino TT, Handsfield HH. Isolation of Neisseria gonorrhoeae on selective and non-selective media in a STD clinic. J Clin Microbiol 1984; 19:218.

Black JR, Sparling PF. Neisseria gonorrhoeae. In: Mandell GL, Douglas RG, Bennet JE, eds. Principles and Practice of Infectious Diseases. New York: John Wiley and Sons, 1985:1195.

Centers for Disease Control (CDC). Tetracycline-resistant Neisseria gonorrhoeae—Georgia, Pennsylvania, New Hampshire. MMWR 1985; 34:563.

Centers for Disease Control (CDC). Penicillinase-producing Neisseria gonorrhoeae—United States, Florida. MMWR 1986; 35:12.

Centers for Disease Control (CDC). Sexually Transmitted Diseases Treatment Guidelines 2002. MMWR 2002; 51:1.

Centers for Disease Control (CDC). Sexually Transmitted Diseases Recommended Guidelines 2006; 55:RR-11.

Crider SR, Colby SD, Miller LK, et al. Treatment of penicillin-resistant Neisseria gonorrhoeae with oral norfloxacin. N Engl J Med 1984; 311:137.

Faruki H, Sparling PF. Genetics of resistance in a non-beta-lactamase producing gonococcus with relatively high-level penicillin resistance. Antimicrob Agents Chemother 1986; 30:856.

Faruki H, Kohnescher, RN, McKinney WP, et al. A community-based outbreak of infection with penicillin-resistant Neisseria gonorrhoeae not producing penicillinase (chromosomally mediated resistance). N Engl J Med 1985; 313:607.

Heckels JE. Molecular studies on the pathogenesis of gonorrhoeae. J Med Microbiol 1984; 18:293.

Holmes KK, Johnson DW, Trostle HJ. An estimate of the risk of men acquiring gonorrhoeae by sexual contact with infected females. Am J Epidemiol 1970; 91:170.

Laga M, Plummer FA, Piot P, et al. Prophylaxis of gonococcal and chlamydia ophthalmia neonatorum: a comparison of silver nitrate and tetracycline. N Engl J Med 1988; 318:653.

Morse SA, Johnson SR, Biddle JW, et al. High-level tetracycline resistance in Neisseria gonorrhoeae is a result of acquisition of streptococcal tet M determinant. Antimicrob Agents Chemother 1986; 30:664.

Perine PL, Morton RS, Piot P, et al. Epidemiology and treatment of penicillinase-producing Neisseria gonorrhoeae. Sex Transm Dis 1979; 6:152.

Rice RJ, Thompson SE. Treatment of uncomplicated infections due to Neisseria gonorrhoeae. J Am Med Assoc 1986; 255:1739.

Rice RJ, Aral SO, Blount JH, Zaidi AA. Gonorrhea in the United States 1975–1984: is the giant only sleeping? Sex Transm Dis 1987; 14:83.

Rice RJ, Biddle JW, Jean Louis YA, et al. Chromosomally mediated resistance in Neisseria gonorrhoeae in the United States: results of surveillance and reporting 1983–1984. J Infect Dis 1986; 153:340.

Spence MR, Guzick DS, Kalla LR. The isolation of Neisseria gonorrhoeae: a comparison of three culture transport systems. Sex Transm Dis 1983; 10:138.

Wald ER. Gonorrhea: diagnosis by Gram stain in the female adolescent. Am J Dis Child 1977; 1131:1094.

Washington AE. Experience with various antibiotics for treatment of anorectal gonorrhea. Sex Transm Dis 1979; 6(suppl):148.

Whittington WL, Knapp JS. Trends in resistance of Neisseria gonorrhoeae to antimicrobial agents in the United States. Sex Transm Dis 1988; 15:202.

Wiesner PJ, Tronca E, Bonin P, et al. Clinical spectrum of pharyngeal gonococcal infections. N Engl J Med 1973; 288:181.

Gonococcol Arthritis

Davis CH. Gonorrheal arthritis complicating pregnancy treated with penicillin. Am J Obstet Gynecol 1945; 50:215.

Gantz NM, McCormack WM, Laughlin LW, et al. Gonococcal osteomyelitis: an unusual complication of gonococcal arthritis. J Am Med Assoc 1976; 236:2431.

Glaser S, Boxerbaum B, Kennel JH. Gonococcal arthritis in the newborn. Am J Dis Child 1966; 112:185.

Holmes KK, Counts GW, Beaty HN. Disseminated gonococcal infection. Ann Intern Med 1971; 74:979.

Holmes KK, Gutman LT, Belding ME, et al. Recovery of Neisseria gonorrhoeae from "sterile" synovial fluid. N Engl J Med 1971; 284:318.

Keiser H, Ruben FL, Wolinsky E, Kushner I. Clinical forms of gonococcal arthritis. N Engl J Med 1968; 279:234.

Kirsner AB, Hess EV. Gonococcal arthritis. Mod Treat 1969; 6:1130.

Metzger AL. Gonococcal arthritis complicating gonococcal pharyngitis. Ann Intern Med 1970; 73:267.

Nelson JD. Antibiotic concentration in septic joint effusions. N Engl J Med 1971; 284:349.

Niles JH, Lowe EW. Gonococcal arthritis in pregnancy. Med Ann DC 1966; 35:69.

Partain JO, Cathcart ES, Cohen AS. Arthritis associated with gonorrhea. Ann Rheum Dis 1968; 27:156.

Trentham DE, McCravey JW, Masi AT. Low-dose penicillin for gonococcal arthritis: a comparative therapy trial. J Am Med Assoc 1976; 236:2410.

Wheeler IK, Heffron WA, Williams RC Jr. Migratory arthralgias and cutaneous lesions as confusing initial manifestations of gonorrhea. Am J Med Sci 1970; 260:150.

Gonococcal Chorioamnionitis

Rothbard MJ, Gregory T, Slaerno LJ. Intrapartum gonococcal amnionitis. Am J Obstet Gynecol 1975; 121:565.

Thadepalli H, Rahmhatla K, Maldmen JE, et al. Gonococcal sepsis secondary to fetal monitoring. Am J Obstet Gynecol 1976; 126:510.

Disseminated Gonococcal Infections

Ackerman AB. Hemorrhagic bullae in gonococcemia. N Engl J Med 1970; 282:793.

Ackerman AB, Miller RC, Shapiro L. Gonococcemia and its cutaneous manifestations. Arch Dermatol 1965; 91:227.

Kahn G, Danielsson D. Septic gonococcal dermatitis. Arch Dermatol 1969; 99:421.

Knapp JS, Holmes KK. Disseminated gonococcal infection caused by Neisseria gonorrhoeae with unique nutritional requirements. J Infect Dis 1975; 132:204.

Masi AT, Eiskenstein BI. Disseminated gonococcal infection (DGI) and gonococcal arthritis (GCA). II: clinical manifestations, diagnosis, complications, treatment and prevention. Semin Arthr Rheum 1981; 10:173.

Mills J, Brooks GF. Disseminated gonococcal infections. In: Holmes KK, Mardh PA, Sparling PF, et al., eds. Sexually Transmitted Diseases. New York: McGraw-Hill, 1984:782.

Mitchell SR, Katz P. Disseminated neisserial infection in pregnancy: the empress may have a change of clothing. Obstet Gynecol Surv 1989; 44:780.

Schoolnick GK, Buchanan TM, Holmes KK. Gonococci causing disseminated gonococcal infections are resistant to the bacterial action of normal human sera. J Clin Invest 1976; 58:1163.

Strader KW, Wise CM, Wasilauskas BL, Salzer WL. Disseminated gonococcal infection caused by chromosomally mediated penicillin-resistant organisms. Ann Intern Med 1986; 104:365.

Gonococcal Endocarditis

Davis DS, Romansky MJ. Successful treatment of gonococcic endocarditis with erythromycin. Am J Med 1956; 21:473.

Gilson BJ, Trout ME, Alleman H. Gonococcic endocarditis. US Armed Forces Med J 1960; 11:1375.

Hancock EW, Shunway NE, Remington JS. Valve replacement in active bacterial endocarditis. J Infect Dis 1971; 123:106.

Holmes KK, Counts GW, Beaty HN. Disseminated gonococcal infection. Ann Intern Med 1971; 74:979.

John JF Jr, Nichols JT, Eisenhower EA, Farrar WE Jr. Gonococcal endocarditis. Sex Transm Dis 1977; 2:84.

Stone E. Gonococcal endocarditis. J Urol 1934; 31:869.

Tanowitz HB, Adler JJ, Chirito E. Gonococcal endocarditis. NY J Med 1972; 2:2782.

Thayer WS. On the cardiac complications of gonorrhea. Johns Hopkins Med J 1922; 33:361.

Trimble C. Gonococcal perihepatitis simulating acute cholecystitis. Surg Gynecol Obstet 1970; 130:54.

Thayer WS, Blumer G. Ulcerative endocarditis due to the gonococcus: gonorrheal septicemia. Johns Hopkins Med J 1896; 7:57.

Voight GC, Bender HW, Buckels LJ. Gonococcal endocarditis with severe aortic regurgitation: early valve replacement. Johns Hopkins Med J 1970; 126:305.

Williams RH. Gonococcal endocarditis. Arch Intern Med 1938; 61:26.

Williams C, Corey R. Neisseria gonorrhoeae endocarditis on a prosthetic valve. South Med J 1987; 80:1194.

Gonococcal Ophthalmia Neonatorum

Armstrong JH, Zacarias F, Rein MG. Ophthalmic neonatorum: a chart review. Pediatrics 1976; 57:884.

Csonk GW, Coufalik ED. Chlamydia, gonococcal and herpes virus infections in neonates. Post Med J 1977; 53:592.

Granstrom KO, Swanberg H, Wallmark G. Gonorrheal conjunctivitis of the newborn: report of eight cases. Opuse Med Stoch 1965; 10:8.

Hansen T, Burns RP, Allen A. Gonorrheal conjunctivitis: an old disease returned. J Am Med Assoc 1966; 195:1156.

Kober P. Gonorrhea neonatorum in spite of Crede's preventive method. Med Klin 1967; 64:424.

Pierog S, Nigam S, Marasigan DC, Dube SK. Gonococcal ophthalmia neonatorum: relationship of maternal factors and delivery room practices to effective control measures. Am J Obstet Gynecol 1975; 122:589.

Thompson TR, Swanson RE, Wiesner PJ. Gonococcal ophthalmia neonatorum. J Am Med Assoc 1974; 228:186.

Gonococcal Perihepatitis
(Stajano–Curtis–Fitz-Hugh Syndrome)

Curtis AH. A cause of adhesions in the right upper quadrant. J Am Med Assoc 1930; 94:1221.

Fitz-Hugh T. Acute gonococcal peritonitis of the right upper quadrant in women. J Am Med Assoc 1934; 102:2094.

Kimball MW, Knee S. Gonococcal perihepatitis in male, the Fitz-Hugh-Curtis syndrome. N Engl J Med 1970; 282:1082.

Lopez-Zeno JA, Keith LG, Berger GA. The Fitz-Hugh-Curtis syndrome revisited: changing perspectives after half a century. J Reprod Med 1985; 30:567.

Ris HW. Perihepatitis (Fitz-Hugh-Curtis syndrome): a review and case presentation. J Adolesc Health Care 1984; 5:272.

Trimble C. Gonococcal perihepatitis simulating acute cholecystitis. Surg Gynecol Obstet 1970; 130:54.

INTRODUCTION

The Salmonellae are short, plump rods that occur singly, in pairs, or in chains. The organisms stain gram-negative and are actively motile. All known *Salmonella* species are pathogenic for humans and domesticated animals. Isolates that fulfill the selected biochemical prerequisites of the genus fall into four groups: *typhi, cholerae, suis,* and *enteritidis.* Subclassification is achieved by serologic segregation based on the somatic (O) and flagella (H) antigens. More than 1400 serotypes have thus been identified; however, just 11 serotypes account for approximately 60% to 70% of human isolates. These include *S. enteritidis,* serotypes *typhimurium, enteritidis, copenhagen, newport, heidelberg, infantis, thompson, blockley, dergy,* and *S. typhi.*

PATHOGENESIS

The portal of infection is almost invariably the gastrointestinal tract. The ability to infect humans is primarily a quantum-related phenomenon. *S. typhi,* in small doses, may be rapidly eliminated, except when there has been an alteration of the acid barrier, as may occur in patients with partial gastrectomy, where as little as 10 organisms of *Shigella* may produce disease. An infective dose of 10^5 organisms or greater is required to produce salmonellosis.

The second important host defense mechanism is the bacterial flora of the gastrointestinal tract, which exerts a strong hemostatic influence. Many anaerobes produce short-chain fatty acids that are postulated to inhibit the growth of viral and bacterial enteric pathogens. Alteration of the enteric flora with antibiotic therapy increases the susceptibility of experimental animals and humans to enteric pathogens. Gastric acid buffering with antacids or compromising gastric function by disease or prior surgery may alter susceptibility. Patients with achlorhydria have been shown to have higher incidences of acute diarrheal disease.

A final factor potentially contributing to the induction of disease is the fact that selected strains of *S. typhi* possess a Vi surface antigen that may interfere with the bactericidal activity of serum and phagocytosis. *S. typhi* tends to elicit a predominantly mononuclear inflammatory response. Nontyphoid Salmonellae lead to a predominantly polymorphic response.

The Salmonellae characteristically invade the intestinal epithelium; however, extensive destruction of the intestinal mucosa does not occur. The lining epithelium is left relatively intact. A significant inflammatory exudative response is elicited in the lamina propria. Disease at this site has the potential to lead to septicemia.

With penetration of the bacteria through the intestinal mucosa, dissemination is initially by lymphatics to the regional nodes and ultimately by the intravascular compartment. *S. typhi* is one of the bacteria of humans that has a predilection for the reticuloendothelial system (RES). The initial bacteremia is rapidly cleared by the reticuloendothelial cells in the liver, spleen, and bone marrow. Although the liver, spleen, and mesenteric nodes are all enlarged as a consequence of hypertrophy of the RES, only splenic enlargement is commonly observed clinically. Bacterial replication occurs within these intracellular sites. The relative protection from host defense mechanisms afforded by the intracellular sites of replication accounts for bacterial persistence. Clinical disease becomes manifest when the bacteria reenter the vascular compartment from their intracellular sites of replication. The latent stage between ingestion and overt disease is usually of the order of 8 to 14 days, but it may range from 3 to 60 days. During this phase, the biliary tract becomes infected. The multiplication of typhoid bacilli in the bile leads to secondary seeding of the gastrointestinal tract and accounts for the increased number of *S. typhi* observed in the feces during the second and third weeks of clinical illness. Involvement of the lymphoid tissue in the intestinal tract, particularly the Peyer's patches in the terminal ileum, may be responsible for the subsequent diarrhea state, which is often associated with hemorrhage, and on rare occasions, may cause ileal perforation.

Immunity to *S. typhi* is not related to the presence of specific antibodies. There is no correlation between resistance to infection, recurrence, or relapse and the titer of antibodies to O, H, or Vi antigens of the typhoid bacillus. Resistance is presumably a function of cell-mediated immunity at the RES level.

All *Salmonella* serotypes are capable of producing a septicemia or typhoid-like picture. A transient bacteremia may be the rule rather than the exception in symptomatic *Salmonella* infections. The younger the patient, the greater is the probability of documented septicemia. Infants with *Salmonella* gastroenteritis under 90 days of age appear to be at greater risk for developing invasive disease. The frequency of nosocomial epidemics suggests that the infecting dose in newborns is considerably less than the 10^5 organisms usually needed to infect adults.

Mortality following *Salmonella* bacteremia is low compared with other Enterobacteriaceae. Of those with clinically overt bacteremia, less than 10% will develop severe, life-threatening sepsis or metastatic infections. If there is an underlying disease process, such as malnutrition, the ensuing mortality or the incidence of serious sequelae is significantly increased.

Metastatic infected foci may not be apparent at the time of initial clinical presentation, and osteomyelitis, for example, may manifest during or after initial therapy (Table 1).

Meningitis is almost exclusively a disease entity of children under one year of age. Even with optimum support, the results of therapy tend to be poor. The overall mortality is 60%. Morbidity, due to ventriculitis, subdural empyema, hydrocephalus, and chronic neurologic defects, is unfortunately common.

A sustained bacteremia in a gravid female introduces the possibility of transplacental infection and congenitally acquired disease.

FETAL INVOLVEMENT

Having fulfilled the major prerequisite, namely the ability to mount a sustained bacteremia, the Salmonellae have the potential to traverse the placental barrier and produce infection within the developing fetus. Involvement appears to be a two-step phenomenon in which the fetus is not affected until infection is established within the placenta and subsequent invasion of the fetal vascular compartment occurs. Pregnancy does not alter the maternal prognosis; however, the disease has a major effect on perinatal morbidity. An increased incidence of abortion or prematurity is observed when typhoid fever is superimposed on pregnancy. Much of the fetal mortality reported in the literature is secondary to the severity of maternal disease, rather than intrauterine involvement. When fetal exposure to maternal disease has been less than two or three weeks in duration, the typhoid bacillus has not been isolated at autopsy from the spleen, bone marrow, or liver of fetuses who have been aborted. This observation theoretically supports the contention that fetal involvement is a two-step phenomenon and the probability that early perinatal mortality and morbidity are due to the consequences of maternal disease; later in the course of the disease, fetal colonization and fetal infection may occur. In the majority of instances, even though the same strain of *S. typhi* is recovered from the alimentary tract of the newborn infant, the child is asymptomatic. The possibility that these isolates from the neonate were acquired during parturition as a consequence of delivery through an infected birth canal is unlikely. Fecal cultures are usually negative for *S. typhi* during the incubation period. Fetal involvement during the convalescent phase of the maternal disease carries with it a surprisingly good prognosis. Dildy et al. (1990) reported on a woman convalescing from typhoid fever who gave birth to a child with evidence of intrauterine dissemination. This child was isolated from the mother in the immediate postpartum period, yet *S. typhi* was repeatedly cultured from stools and a high titer of O and H typhoid agglutinins were demonstrable in the cord blood. A similar case was reported by Wing and Troppoli (1930). Again, the mother was convalescing from typhoid fever and gave birth to a child who had *S. typhi* in the feces and whose cord serum gave a positive Widal reaction. The Widal reaction is contingent on immunoglobulin M (IgM) antibodies. Since neither IgM nor IgA antibodies traverse the placental barrier, the presence of such agglutinins in cord blood indicates intrauterine exposure.

Awadalla et al. (1985) reported a case of a prima gravida who at 26 weeks of gestation developed a severe *S. typhi* gastroenteritis, sepsis, and disseminated intravascular coagulopathy. Shortly after the institution of antibiotic therapy, she spontaneously aborted a previable infant from whose intact gestational sac was recovered *S. typhi*. The amniotic fluid was grossly turbid.

Asymptomatic congenitally infected neonates as well as individuals with rectal carriage are the potential reservoir for nosocomial salmonellosis in newborn intensive-care nurseries.

In utero dissemination of maternal *salmonella* infection is not restricted to *S. typhi*. *S. enteritidis* can occasionally access the fetus in utero. Any *Salmonella* serotype producing a bacteremia lasting days to weeks can be responsible for induction of fetal infection/disease.

FEMALE GENITAL TRACT INVOLVEMENT

Hematogenous dissemination to the ovary has been reported. In a review of 8000 cases of salmonellosis, Cohen et al. (1987) identified nine cases of an ovarian abscess. The disease manifests as an acute abdomen with fever, abdominal pain, and a unilateral mass. Almost invariably, an abscess occurs in an ovary with some sort of preexisting lesion including simple cyst, dermoid, endometrioma, and cystadenoma. The corresponding fallopian tube is relatively free of disease.

DIAGNOSIS

Clinical Presentations

The nontyphoidal cases of salmonellosis usually present as acute-onset diarrhea in pregnancy. An unexplained splenomegaly in association with a relative lymphocytosis may be present.

In typhoidal-like disease (Table 2), once patients enter the septicemic stage, they commonly suffer from head pain, sore throat, chills, and persistent fever. The white blood cell count tends to be depressed and is often under $5000/mm^2$, with a marked shift to the right. What is impressive is the marked temperature–pulse dissociation. The patient tends to have a bradycardia that is disproportionate to the temperature. There are a number of cutaneous manifestations associated with the disease, varying from "rose spots" to transient erythematous maculopapular rashes. Once the organisms have reappeared in the stool, diarrhea, which may be bloody, is not uncommon. In rare instances, the patient may experience ileal perforation.

Salmonellosis is a disease of the small bowel. Careful history is helpful in distinguishing small-bowel versus large-bowel disease. The occurrence of large watery or bulky stools suggests a small-bowel origin. The presence of rectal pain and urgency to defecate is characteristic of large-bowel disease. The colicky pain of small-bowel

TABLE I Metastatic infectious complications of invasive *Salmonella septicemia*

Meningitis	Osteomyelitis
Pneumonia	Septic arthritis

TABLE 2 Common signs and symptoms of typhoid fever

Persistent fever
Abdominal pain
Diarrhea
Hypothermic response to antipyretics
Headache
Splenomegaly
Rose spots (small petechial hemorrhages)
Generalized malaise
Chills
Relative bradycardia
Relative leukopenia

disease tends to be periumbilical in distribution whereas terminal ileum and large-bowel pain occur in areas clearly below the umbilicus.

A second procedure that should be done in evaluating the significance of potentially infectious diarrhea in a gravid female is examination of stool for fecal leukocytes. The absence of fecal leukocytes depends on the integrity of the intestinal mucosa. Diseases that inflame or disrupt the intestinal mucosa frequently cause shedding of fecal leukocytes. Normal controls and diseases in which the intestinal mucosa remains relatively normal seldom cause excretion of fecal leukocytes. The demonstration of polymorphonuclear leukocytes in feces warrants the submission of feces for enteric pathogen culturing.

Procedure for Detection of Fecal Leukocytes
Examination for fecal leukocytes is easily performed by placing a small fleck of mucus (or stool if no mucus is present) on a clean microscope slide and mixing it thoroughly with two drops of Loeffler's methylene blue stain. A coverslip is then placed over the mixture, and after two to three minutes, the slide is examined microscopically. Leukocyte nuclei will appear blue with this technique. Specimens should be taken from the outside of stool specimens and not from the center or from the rectal swabs, which may give false-negative stains for leukocytes.

The absence of fecal leukocytes does not exclude an enteric pathogen etiology. Those agents that produce their diarrheic effect via enterotoxins usually are not associated with the presence of fecal leukocytes. The principal exceptions are the following:

1. *Shigella dysenteriae*
2. *Clostridium difficile*

The ultimate diagnosis rests on recovery of a pathogenic strain of *Salmonella* from stool or blood. The following procedure is recommended.

Stool Specimens for Microbiological Analysis
The stool sample should be fresh and warm and should be free of contamination from barium, bismuth, oils, antibiotics, antacids, or kaolin antidiarrheal agents.

The best specimen is a freshly passed stool obtained before the initiation of antimicrobial therapy. A rectal swab in a transport medium is a poor choice. Unless the specimen is taken immediately to the laboratory and properly handled there, a number of significant microorganisms will not survive the changes in pH that occur with a drop in temperature. This is especially true of most shigellae and an appreciable number of the Salmonellae.

Similarly, refrigeration markedly diminishes the probability of isolating enteric pathogens. While alternative methods do exist to diminish the changes in pH, the price is an increased incidence of false-negative bacteriological cultures. If sterile swabs are used in obtaining the specimen, they should be passed beyond the anal sphincter, carefully rotated, and withdrawn.

The definitive diagnosis of salmonellosis can be established by polymerase chain reaction tests.

THERAPY

Typhoidal and septicemic variants should be treated with antimicrobial drugs. The selection of initial antibiotic therapy is influenced by prior identification of resistant strains in the community.

Uncomplicated *Salmonella* gastroenteritis is usually not an indication for drug therapy per se unless the individual involved is at special risk (Table 3). Underlying conditions that would sanction antimicrobial therapy are the following:

1. Lymphoproliferative diseases
2. Vascular grafts
3. Aneurysms
4. Valvular heart disease
3. Sickle cell–related diseases

The current drugs of choice in nongravidas are the fluoroquinolones. Antibiotics commonly used in pregnancy are listed in Table 4.

When faced with life-threatening disease, maternal considerations should have priority over potential fetal adverse drug reactions.

TABLE 3 Therapeutic recommendations for nontyphoidal *Salmonella* infections

Uncomplicated enteritis in normal hosts	Antibiotics do not abbreviate period of symptoms or prolong asymptomatic excretion; however, relapse is more common when antibiotics are given; antibiotic therapy contraindicated
Enteritis with bacteremia	If toxicity persists and bacteremia more than transient event, give antibiotic therapy indicated
Colitis (characterized by fever, abdominal pain and tenesmus)	Antibiotic therapy indicated
Metastatic complications (meningitis, osteomyelitis, septic arthritis)	Antibiotic therapy indicated
Secretory diarrhea	Brief course of nonabsorbable antibiotic such as colistin sulfate or neomycin sulfate
Immunocompromised host	Individualization of each case

TABLE 4 Antimicrobial agents for potential use in the treatment of *Salmonella typhi* in pregnancy

Ampicillin, 8 g/day IV
Ceftriaxone, 75 mg/kg/day for 5 days
Amoxicillin, 4–6 g/day in four divided doses
Cefoperazone, 2 g b.i.d. IV to 4 g q.i.d.

SELECTED READING

Amster R, Lessing JB, Jaffa AJ, Peyser MR. Typhoid fever complicating pregnancy. Acta Obstet Gynecol Scand 1985; 64:685.

Ault KA, Kennedy M, Muhieddine A, et al. Maternal and neonatal infection with Salmonella heidelberg: A case report. Infect Dis Obstet Gynecol 1993; 1:46.

Awadalla SG, Mercer LJ, Brown LG. Pregnancy complicated by intraamniotic infection by Salmonella typhi. Obstet Gynecol 1985; 65:30s.

Balek AP, Fothergill R. Septic abortion due to invasive Salmonella agona. Postgrad Med J 1977; 53:155.

Buongiorno R, Schiraldi O. Treatment of typhoid fever in pregnancy. Chemioterapia 1984; 3:136.

Duff P, Engelsgjerd B. Typhoid fever on an obstetrics-gynecology service. Am J Obstet Gynecol 1983; 145:113.

Elliot DL, Tolle SW, Goldberg L, Miller JB. Pet-associated illness. N Engl J Med 1985; 313:985.

Gibb AP, Welsby PD. Infantile salmonella gastroenteritis in association with maternal mastitis. J Infect 1983; 6:193.

Gluck B, Ramim KD, Ramin SM. Salmonella typhi and pregnancy: a case report. Infect Dis Obstet Gynecol 1994; 2:186.

Lewis GJ. A rare cause of cholecystitis in pregnancy. Int J Gynaecol Obstet 1983; 21:175.

Nuttall ID, Wilson PD, Mandal BK. A suppurative ovarian cyst in pregnancy due to Salmonella typhi. Scand J Infect Dis 1980; 12:311.

Riggall F, Salkind G, Spellacy W. Typhoid fever complicating pregnancy. Obstet Gynecol 1974; 44:117.

Stamm AM. Salmonella bredeney mastitis during pregnancy. Obstet Gynecol 1982; 59:29.

Trettmar RE, Faithfull-Davies DN. Salmonella urinary tract infection in pregnancy. J Hosp Infect 1985; 6:227.

Fetal Involvement/Congenital Salmonellosis
Brown MA. Typhoid fever; pregnancy; miscarriage at seven and a half months; typhoid in the infant; death, autopsy. J Am Med Assoc 1901; 38:1135.

Dalaker K, Anderson BM, Lovslett K, et al. Septic abortion caused by Salmonella enteritidis. Acta Obstet Gynecol Scand 1988; 67:185.

Dildy GA III, Martens MG, Faro S, Lee W. Typhoid fever in pregnancy: a case report. J Reprod Med 1990; 35:273.

Freedman ML, Christopher P, Boughton CR, et al. Typhoid carriage in pregnancy with infection of neonate. Lancet 1970; 1:310.

Hicks TH, French H. Typhoid fever and pregnancy with special reference to fetal infection. Lancet 1905; 1:1491.

Lauderman TA, Hill OM. Salmonella enteritidis in the newborn: a maternal infant case study. W V Med J 1991; 87:249.

Lynch F. Fetal transmission of typhoid. J Am Med Assoc 1901; 36:1136.

Lyons RW, Samples CL, DeSilva HN, et al. An epidemic of resistant Salmonella in a nursery: animal-to-human spread. J Am Med Assoc 1980; 243:546.

Scialli AR, Rarick TL. Salmonella and second-trimester pregnancy loss. Obstet Gynecol 1992; 79:820.

Sengupta BS, Ramachander N, Zamah N. Salmonella septic abortion. Int Surg 1980; 65:183.

Seoud M, Saade G, Uwaydah M, Azoury R. Typhoid fever in pregnancy. Obstet Gynecol 1988; 71:711.

Wing ES, Troppoli DV. Intrauterine transmission of typhoid. J Am Med Assoc 1930; 95:405.

Zettel LA, Jelsema RD, Isada NB. First-trimester septic abortion due to Salmonella enteritidis oranienburg. Infect Dis Obstet Gynecol 1995; 2:239.

Extraintestinal Disease
Cohen JI, Bartlett JA, Corey RC. Extra-intestinal manifestations of salmonella infection. Medicine 1987; 66:349.

Lalitha MK, John R. Unusual manifestations of salmonellosis: a surgical problem. Q J Med 1994; 87:301.

INTRODUCTION

Streptococcus pneumoniae is a catalase-negative, gram-positive coccus that replicates in chains in liquid medium. Clinical isolates of *S. pneumoniae* contain an external capsule; only rarely have unencapsulated isolates been implicated as the cause of infection. Pneumococci produce a substance that breaks down hemoglobin, causing a green color; as a result, pneumococcal colonies are surrounded by a green zone during growth on blood agar plates. More than 80 serotypes of *S. pneumoniae* have been identified based on antigenic differences in their capsular polysaccharides.

S. pneumoniae is not a normal constituent of vaginal bacterial flora; however, given the opportunity, *S. pneumoniae* can be a significant pathogen for the female genital tract.

Classically, involvement with the female genital tract has occurred in conjunction with primary pulmonary disease, engenderment of bacteremia, and subsequent metastatic involvement.

S. PNEUMONIAE (PNEUMOCOCCAL) PNEUMONIA IN PREGNANCY

With the advent of antibiotics and in the absence of underlying chronic disease or acute alcoholism, death due to *S. pneumoniae* is a rarity. Yet, lobar pneumonia is still associated with a 2% to 3% maternal mortality when significant disease occurs in pregnancy. Fetal mortality approaches 30%. Both maternal and fetal mortality and morbidity are influenced by the extent of disease and the aggressiveness of therapy. Although a history suggestive of virus-like upper respiratory infection can be elicited not infrequently, the onset of disease often occurs with dramatic suddenness. The patient develops fever, cough, and malaise. The initial stage of pulmonary parenchymal involvement is characterized by marked vascular engorgement, serous exudate, and rapid bacterial proliferation. The thick, mucoid capsule of the bacterium impedes immediate phagocytosis and is responsible for the virulence of the organism. In contrast to the group A streptococci, the virulence of *S. pneumoniae* is primarily a function of the organism's ability to replicate and evoke an acute inflammatory reaction, rather than one of exo- or endotoxins or extracellular enzymes. The pneumococcus is a classic example of an organism that is highly pathogenic by virtue of its replicative ability. The pneumococci are numbered from 1 to 81 in the order in which they were identified.

The cough is sequentially productive first of turbid, watery sputum, which rapidly converts to purulent and grayish green, and then assumes the characteristic rust color. The changes in the sputum parallel those within the lung parenchyma. The initial serous exudate and vascular engorgement give way to a precipitous increase in neutrophils, extravasation of red blood cells, and precipitation of fibrin. The confluent exudative reaction tends to obscure the pulmonary architecture.

With the extension of the disease process to the pleural surfaces and the disruption of vascular elements, the patient experiences pleuritic chest pains, chills, and tremor. Shortness of breath, orthopnea, and cyanosis tend to reflect the extent to which the vital capacity of the lung parenchyma has been compromised. In pregnant women, the degree of oxygen unsaturation is often greater than anticipated. On physical examination, the patient exhibits a diminution of breath sounds associated with fine crepitant rales. With consolidation, increased tactile and vocal fremitus and bronchial breath sounds occur.

Prior to the advent of antibiotics, the disease usually persisted for seven to nine days. Extreme hypoxia and generalized vasomotor collapse usually led to death. In patients who ultimately recovered, a period of apparent clinical deterioration occurred about the eighth day, preceding recovery by crisis. Tachypnea and tachycardia increased, and the sensorium became obtunded. Then, precipitously, the breathing became less labored, the pulse rate dropped, and the fever lysed. Within hours, the seemingly moribund patient was transformed into a convalescent patient. Fortunately, in terms of morbidity and mortality, recovery is no longer a quantitative and possibly qualitative function of antibody synthesis.

METASTATIC FETAL INVOLVEMENT

The primary deleterious consequence of severe maternal pneumonia due to *S. pneumoniae* is fetal wastage. Beyond the question of possible maternal demise, a certain component of fetal wastage is difficult to avoid, owing to a failure to curtail aggressively maternal hyperthermia.

S. pneumoniae is capable of affecting the products of conception by other hematogenous involvement or ascending infection. Either mechanism results in chorioamnionitis and/or perinatal septicemia.

FEMALE GENITAL TRACT INVOLVEMENT

Vaginal carriage of *S. pneumoniae*, when present within the vaginal flora, is a rare occurrence. The microorganism may have a higher invasion-to-colonization ratio than the group B streptococci. At the time of parturition or rupture of the fetal membranes, bacteria have the ability to ascend and infect the amniotic sac and secondarily the fetus.

Involvement of the female genital tract as a metastatic process secondary to maternal septicemia due to *S. pneumoniae* was a relatively well-documented phenomenon in the preantibiotic era.

The occurrence of cases of chorioamnionitis and/or perinatal septicemia in the absence of pulmonary involvement indicated the possibility of contiguous spread from the vaginal/cervical reservoir and subsequent involvement of the female upper genital tract. Hughes et al. (2001) described a case of neonatal pneumococcal sepsis in the product of a 37-week uneventful gestation. The mother simultaneously developed bacteremia with the same serotype organism and died from septic shock. DNA fingerprinting confirmed the identicality of both isolates. Nallusamy (1998) reported two cases of invasive early-onset neonatal pneumococcal sepsis. One neonate was born with no maternal risk factors present and the other was preterm at 35 weeks. Evidence of infection was not present at parturition. Despite penicillin therapy, both neonates died. Kahke et al. (2000) described a case of pneumococcal peritonitis that occurred four weeks after the patient had given birth to a healthy boy. High vaginal, blood, and operative cultures were all positive for *S. pneumoniae*.

Genital tract disease due to *S. pneumoniae* has been reported in nonpregnant females. Isolated cases of spontaneous pneumococcal peritonitis have been described. Hadfield et al. (1990) reported a case of a 46-year-old woman with bilateral tubo-ovarian masses. Biopsy specimens from both tubes and from the wall of the abscesses demonstrated gram-positive, lancet-shaped diplococci that were documented to be *S. pneumoniae* by immunoperoxidase staining. Rahav et al. (1991) reported a case of postmenopausal pneumococcal tubo-ovarian abscess from which *S. pneumoniae* was recovered. The fallopian tubes in these two cases of spontaneous peritonitis due to *S. pneumoniae* were described as being swollen and hyperemic with pus emanating from the ends. What was described is not a specific disease entity (spontaneous peritonitis) but more probably a progressive consequence of salpingitis. Rare causes of acute salpingitis due to *S. pneumoniae* have been reported. *S. pneumoniae* appears to be able to function as a primary pathogen for the fallopian tubes. The entire pathogenic spectrum previously attributable to *Neisseria gonorrhoeae* can potentially be mimicked by *S. pneumoniae*.

DIAGNOSIS

A presumptive diagnosis is inferred from the presence of encapsulated, lancet-shaped diplococci in significant numbers on a Gram-stained smear of the sputum. Immunization of rabbits stimulates the appearance of antibodies that cause serotype-specific agglutination or microscopic demonstrability of the capsule (the Quellung reaction). This reaction is due to not only capsular swelling, often said to be responsible, but also the increased visibility of the capsule, because the interaction with antibody renders it retractile.

This reaction can be used for quick identification and typing of the organism. In adults, types I through VIII are responsible for about 80% of the cases of pneumococcal pneumonia and for more than one-half of the fatalities from pneumococcal bacteremia. Ultimate confirmation of the diagnosis rests with bacteriologic identification of the organism.

Pneumococci are identified in the routine microbiology laboratory by three reactions:

1. The so-called alpha-hemolysis of blood agar.
2. Catalase negativity.
3. Solubility in bile salts or susceptibility to ethyl hydrocupreine (optochin). In recent years a number of isolates have been found to be optochin resistant, which has led cautious microbiologists to rely more on the use of bile solubility for definitive identification.

While *S. pneumoniae* will grow on 5% to 7% sheep blood agar culture when incubated in a CO_2 environment, the recovery of alpha-hemolytic streptococci is usually not worked up any further and is often reported as "mixed vaginal flora." Recovery of alpha-hemolytic streptococci from patients with acute salpingitis needs to be microbiologically evaluated to exclude the possibility that these isolates are *S. pneumoniae*.

THERAPY

Penicillin has been, and still is, the drug of choice for susceptible or intermediately resistant strains of *S. pneumoniae*. *S. pneumoniae* with reduced susceptibility to penicillin has become common. About 20% to 30% of isolates exhibit reduced susceptibility to the beta-lactam antibiotics. The increase in antibiotic-resistant *S. pneumoniae* carriage and disease appears to be directly related to antibiotic use in the community.

Selection for antibiotics for pneumococcal disease is further complicated by the development of drug-resistant *S. pneumoniae* (DRSP). Penicillin resistance to the beta-lactam antibiotics can coexist with multidrug resistance to macrolides, sulfonamides, and third-generation cephalosporins, which limits therapeutic options. Seven serotypes (6A, 6B, 9V, 14, 19A, 19F, and 23F) account for most DRSP.

Most outpatient illnesses caused by *S. pneumoniae* end up being treated empirically, without identification of the organism. Ciprofloxin is not infrequently prescribe for patients with upper respiratory infections. The susceptibility to ciprofloxin has progressively decreased so as to be deemed marginal at best. When empirical therapy is given for potential pneumococcal disease, provision should be made for close follow-up.

In dealing with pneumococcal disease requiring hospitalization, community-specific antibiotic susceptibility data should be used in selecting initial therapy. In most cases, it is prudent to presume the existence of a resistant strain and treat accordingly with "best fit for spectrum." If a bacteriostatic antibiotic is to be used in conjunction with a bacteriocidal antibiotic, it is recommended that the bacteriocidal antibiotic be given at least half an hour before the bacteriostatic antibiotic. If the isolate is sensitive to penicillin, the "drug of choice" concept applies.

TABLE I Recommendations for pneumococcal vaccine use

Immunocompromised adults at increased risk for pneumococcal disease include those:
1. With chronic cardiovascular disease
2. With chronic pulmonary disease
3. With diabetes mellitus
4. With alcoholism/cirrhosis
5. Aged 65 yr or over

PREVENTION

Pneumococcal vaccination is an important part of pneumococcal disease prevention. In the past, uncertainty about local reactions and the duration of protection have limited the use of pneumococcal vaccination. Currently, the use of pneumococcal vaccine should be predicated on (*i*) the risk to the patient population; and (*ii*) whether a pneumococcal vaccination has been procured six years or more previously.

S. pneumoniae remains a major cause of morbidity and mortality in both developed and underdeveloped countries. To address the need for protection in infancy, maternal immunization with the newer pneumococcal vaccines has been aggressively advanced as a strategy to prevent disease during a period of increased vulnerability in infants.

The pneumococcal vaccine available before 1983 was a 14-valent pneumococcal vaccine. The currently licensed pneumococcal polysaccharide vaccine is composed of 23 capsular polysaccharides. Many of these antigens are of poor immunogenicity in infants under the age of five years, but not in adults.

Patients recommended for primary vaccination or revaccination are listed in Table 1. Immunocompromised individuals with splenic dysfunction, lymphoma, multiple myeloma, chronic renal failure, nephrotic syndrome, transplantation, or hepatitis C virus have an increased risk of pneumococcal disease.

SELECTED READING

Pneumonia
Austrian R, Gold J. Pneumococcal bacteremia with special reference to bacteremia pneumococcal pneumonia. Ann Intern Med 1964; 60:759.
Butler JC, Hofmann J, Cetron MS, et al. The continued emergence of drug-resistant Streptococcus pneumoniae in the United States: an update from the Centers for Disease Control and Prevention pneumococcal sentinel surveillance system. J Infect Dis 1996; 174:986.
Centers for Disease Control. Assessment of susceptibility testing practices for Streptococcus pneumoniae—United States, February 2000. MMWR 202; 51:392.
Greenhill JP. Obstetrics, 13th ed. Philadelphia: WB Saunders, 1965:170.
Nuckols HH, Hertig AT. Pneumococcus infection of the genital tract in women especially during pregnancy and the puerperium. Am J Obstet Gynecol 1938; 35:782.
Oxhorn H. The changing aspects of pneumonia complicating pregnancy. Am J Obstet Gynecol 1955; 70:1007.
Taylor ES. Back's Obstetrical Practice, 9th ed. Baltimore: Williams & Wilkins, 1971:353.

Genital Tract Involvement
Alzahawi MF, Stack TA, Shrestha TL. Pneumococcal neonatal colonization and sepsis in association with maternal genital pneumococcal colonization. Br J Obstet Gynaecol 1988; 95:1198.
Austrian R, Gold J. Pneumococcal bacteremia with special reference to bacteremia pneumococcal pneumonia. Ann Intern Med 1964; 60:759.
Carvalho BT, Carneito-Sampia MM, Sole D, et al. Transplacental transmission of serotype specific pneumococcal antibodies in a Brazilian population. Clin Diag Lab Immunol 1999; 6:50.
DiNello CH, Chaisilwattana R, Fagnant RJ, Monif GRC. Neonatal Streptococcus pneumoniae septicemia and meningitis. J Reprod Med 1990; 35:297.
Duff P, Gibbs RS. Acute intraamniotic infection due to Streptococcus pneumoniae. Obstet Gynecol 1993; 61:25.
Gomez RJ, Padilla B, Delgado IA, et al. Streptococcus pneumoniae peritonitis secondary to genital tract infection in a previously healthy woman. Clin Infect Dis 1992; 15:1060.
Hadfield TL, Neafie R, Lanoie LO. Tubo-ovarian abscess caused by Streptococcus pneumoniae. Hum Pathol 1990; 21:1288.
Hughes BR, Mercer JL, Gosbel LB. Neonatal pneumococcal sepsis in association with maternal pneumococcal sepsis. Aust NZ J Obstet Gynecol 2001; 41:457.
Jensen LS. Primary pneumococcal peritonitis. Ann Chir Gynaecol 1984; 73:95.
Kahke V, Fischer A, Schroder J. Streptococcus pneumoniae peritonitis postpartum. Infection 2000; 28:114.
Nallusamy R. Fatal early-onset neonatal sepsis due to Streptococcus pneumoniae. Med J Malaysia 1998; 53:442.
Nuckols HH, Hertig AT. Pneumococcus infection of the genital tract in women especially during pregnancy and the puerperium. Am J Obstet Gynecol 1938; 35:782.
Oxhorn H. The changing aspects of pneumonia complicating pregnancy. Am J Obstet Gynecol 1955; 70:1007.
Rahav G, Ben DL, Persitz E. Postmenopausal pneumococcal tubo-ovarian abscess. Rev Infect Dis 1991; 13:896.
Robinson EN Jr. Pneumococcal endometritis and neonatal sepsis. Rev Infect Dis 1990; 12:799.
Westh H, Skibsted L, Korner B. Streptococcus pneumoniae infections of the female genital tract and in the newborn child. Rev Infect Dis 1990; 12:416.

Group A Beta-Hemolytic *Streptococcus* (*Streptococcus pyogenes*)

INTRODUCTION

The group A beta-hemolytic streptococci are gram-positive cocci. Within actively spreading lesions, diplococcal forms predominate, whereas in purulent exudates, chain formation tends to occur.

The organisms have a capsule containing hyaluronic acid; the cell wall has three components:

1. A protein component containing M, T, and R antigens
2. The carbohydrate moiety that contains rhamnose *N*-acetylglucosamine, the group-specific carbohydrate for the group A streptococci
3. The peptidoglycan moiety

The M protein is closely associated with the virulence of group A streptococci. It interferes with the ingestion of the streptococci by phagocytic cells.

In terms of pathogenicity, the group A beta-hemolytic streptococci must be deemed to possess the most impressive enzymatic and cellular armamentarium of any human pathogen. They produce a minimum of 20 extracellular products, including streptokinase (fibrinolysin) and streptodornase (deoxyribonuclease), hyaluronidase, diphosphopyridine nucleotidase, and hemolysins (streptolysin O and S).

The fibrinolysin and deoxyribonuclease function to liquefy viscous inflammatory exudates and, in this way, facilitate dissemination of the organism. The fibrinolysin is effective in the breakdown of the fibrin barrier, which normally forms at the margins of inflammation, thus negating an additional host defense mechanism. Certain strains elaborate a diphosphopyridine nucleotidase that appears to possess the ability to kill leukocytes. Bacterial hyaluronidase can split hyaluronic acid, an important component of the ground substance of connective tissue, thus aiding in the spread of infection through connective tissue and fascial planes.

The streptolysin O is a protein that is hemolytically active in its reduced state. It is antigenic and forms the basis for the antistreptolysin titer; however, it is the streptolysin S (which is nonantigenic for humans) that is responsible for the beta-hemolysis on the surface of blood agar plates.

FEMALE GENITAL TRACT INVOLVEMENT

The syndromes attributable to group A beta-hemolytic streptococci and whose occurrence and clinical manifestation directly involve the disciplines of obstetrics and gynecology are puerperal sepsis, prepubertal vulvovaginitis, endometritis–salpingitis, and necrotizing fasciitis.

Puerperal Sepsis

Although group A beta-hemolytic streptococci are unique in terms of their potential pathogenicity, their mere presence within the bacterial flora of the female genital tract is not sufficient to produce disease. What is required is some breach of the mucosal barrier. Parturition is usually the event that provides the organism with an effective portal of infection. In rare instances, trauma associated with coitus late in gestation may precipitate infection.

Antepartum infection due to the group A beta-hemolytic streptococci utilizes a route of infection different from that observed in the postpartum period. Infection spreads from the cervix or endocervix through the tissue planes of the uterus. Clinically, the patient presents with very high fever. Physical examination reveals nothing more than significant uterine tenderness. When the organism attains either the vascular implantation site or the serosal surface, signs and symptoms of septicemia ensue. At no time is there evidence of an exudative process at the endocervix. Maternal pyrexia and septicemia occur before fetal involvement (Fig. 1). Even when the pregnancy is not at term, if the fetus is treated effectively with chemotherapy, an adverse fetal outcome may be totally averted.

In the pathogenesis of postpartum puerperal sepsis, two phases of disease can be discerned.

Phase of Lymphangitic Spread

Classically, the symptoms occur early—within 2 to 48 hours postpartum. Onset of the disease within the first 18 hours suggests that the group A beta-hemolytic streptococci resided within the patient's vaginal flora, whereas onset after 24 hours suggests possible acquisition of the organism from environmental sources.

Infection confined to the uterus and pelvis (parametrium) is clinically characterized by fever (38–40°C), leukocytosis (12,000–20,000 WBC/mL), tachycardia (110–120 heartbeats/min), and an edematous, soft uterus (uterine subinvolution). Exquisite pelvic tenderness involving both the adnexa and the cul-de-sac is usually demonstrable. The vaginal discharge tends to be serosanguineous and virtually free of odor. There is a pronounced diminution in the volume of lochia. Because of their invasiveness and virulence, the group A streptococci may produce fulminating infection with relatively unobtrusive localizing signs until peritonitis develops.

Peritonitis and Systemic Phases

With the extension of the infection beyond the pelvis and the resultant peritonitis, patients develop the classic signs

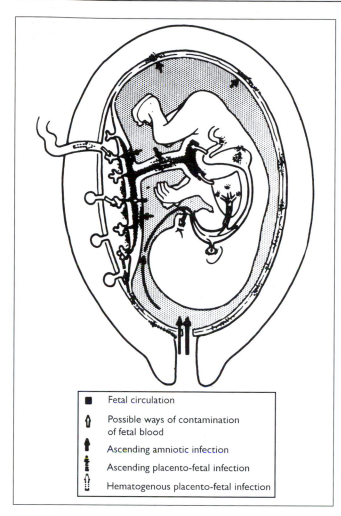

Fetal circulation

Possible ways of contamination of fetal blood

Ascending amniotic infection

Ascending placento-fetal infection

Hematogenous placento-fetal infection

FIGURE I Routes of fetal infection. *Source*: Blanc WAP. J Pediatr 1961; 59:473.

of puerperal sepsis, including shaking chills, flushed cheeks, glassy eyes, euphoria, distended tympanic abdomen, and absence of bowel sounds, in addition to those referable to infection limited to the pelvis. If the infection is not eradicated prior to this stage, bacteremia results, with possible secondary involvement of the lung parenchyma or heart valves and disseminated intravascular coagulopathy. These complications may be manifested as a friction rub, evidence of pulmonary consolidation, the development of a cardiac murmur, and petechiae or oozing from surgical wounds, respectively. Death is usually imminent.

In the Sloane Hospital epidemic of 1927 reported by Watson and by Meleney et al., there were 25 cases of puerperal sepsis, with nine deaths. All but one of the patients who died in this epidemic exhibited positive blood cultures. Careful bacteriologic investigation clearly indicated that the vagina was the portal of entry. With the recognition of the natural history of the disease and the institution of rigid antiseptic and aseptic precautions, childbed fever due to group A streptococci should have been relegated to the history of medicine. Yet every now and then, the organism circumvents precautionary measures and surveillance systems, and epidemic infection

among puerperal patients occurs. In an epidemic in Boston, prompt and massive administration of penicillin in the early stages of the disease was responsible for limiting septicemia and thus the hazard of death. Even when septicemia occurred, no maternal mortality was observed.

Group A streptococcal infection of the female genital tract is often a hospital-acquired infection rather than an infection from an organism endogenous to the vaginal flora. The recovery of this organism from a case of puerperal sepsis should alert the physician to the possibility not only of hospital acquisition but, even more importantly, of the potential for nosocomial spread. The individual responsible for bacteriologic surveillance in the institution should be notified immediately. If the infection is not an isolated occurrence, every attempt should be made to trace the pathway of bacterial dissemination and to institute rigid quarantine and isolation of known cases. The epidemiologic branch of the Centers for Disease Control may be of valuable assistance. In the Boston epidemic, penicillin was prophylactically administered to every new patient at admission and to the physicians intimately involved in therapy, in the hopes of eliminating organisms before they could either replicate to the point of clinical illness or become a source for additional dissemination.

Diagnosis

The clinical recognition of beta-hemolytic streptococci as being markedly more virulent than their nonhemolytic counterparts prompted a classification based on the type of hemolysis and carbohydrate reaction. It was not until Lancefield demonstrated by precipitation tests that the streptococci contained group-specific carbohydrate substances (see groups B, C, D and G streptococci) that the natural history of disease for the various subgroups was delineated. The hemolytic activity of the streptococci is the most misapplied feature of streptococcal classification and has engendered an inordinate amount of taxonomic confusion. Not all beta-hemolytic streptococci belong to the Lancefield group A. Beta-hemolysis does not necessarily imply pathogenicity; neither does an alpha- or gamma-hemolysis exclude it. The group A *Streptococcus pyogenes* are, in general, very susceptible to very low concentrations of bacitracin. The combination of these two characteristics, beta-hemolysis and bacitracin susceptibility, is presumptively diagnostic of *S. pyogenes*. Definitive identification is based on serologic testing for the group A polysaccharide antigen. This diagnosis has great potential consequences for the patient in view of the associated nonsuppurative sequelae (rheumatic carditis and glomerulonephritis), which are observed exclusively with the group A organisms.

Therapy

The key to therapy is antibacterial chemotherapy in the form of potassium penicillin G administered intravenously. Erythromycin may be administered when patients demonstrate hypersensitivity to penicillin. Every effort should be made to ensure that there are no retained products of conception in the uterus. If any are identified, antibiotic coverage should be broadened to include *Bacteroides fragilis*, *Peptococcus*, *Peptostreptococcus*, and *Prevotella*. The volume of the intravascular compartment should be restored. The patient should be isolated, and every attempt should be made to exclude an exogenous source of infection. Any hospital employee with a positive isolate from a nasopharyngeal, throat, skin, or rectal culture should receive 400,000 units of phenoxymethyl penicillin (penicillin V) orally four times a day for 10 days. Once the culture is negative, the individual may return to work.

Antenatal Streptococcal Infection

Group A streptococcal infection in a pregnant patient with intact membranes may produce a distinct syndrome in the antenatal period. The prerequisite necessary to transform vaginal colonization into disease is presumed to be a breach of the mucosal–epithelial barrier. The portal of infection determines the ensuing symptom complex. When the labia minora or introitus is the site of initial infection, the patient presents with fever that is in excess of 39.5°C and is extremely rapid in onset. Involvement of the external portion of the urethral meatus results in dysuria upon initiation of micturition. Physical examination reveals marked mucosal erythema and tenderness. When the cervix is traumatized by coitus late in gestation, the clinical presentation is virtually identical: sudden onset of significant fever. The pertinent physical findings are restricted to the uterus and peritoneum. Pelvic examination reveals diffuse uterine tenderness with or without parametrial tenderness. Rigors indicate involvement of the maternal implantation sites. The pathway of infection, with its ultimate involvement of the fetus, appears to be one of contiguous spread. Fetal infection occurs after maternal involvement. From the portal of infection, disease sequentially involves the endocervix, uterus, and products of conception. If maternal therapy is instituted early in the course of disease, the pregnancy is often unaffected.

Streptococcal Vulvovaginitis

The group A, B, C, and G beta-hemolytic streptococci can produce an acute vulvovaginitis in prepubertal children and adults. Heller et al. (1969) have demonstrated group A streptococci (*S. pyogenes*) to be the etiologic agent in 10% of children seen at the Baltimore City Hospital with vulvovaginitis.

Vulvovaginal disease is due to direct mechanical transport of the bacteria from the nasopharynx to the vulvovaginal area. The same serotype of group A streptococci can be frequently demonstrated in both the vulvar and the pharyngeal sites.

Clinically, the patients present with vulvar pain, pruritus, and frequently dysuria (at the beginning of micturition). The vaginal discharge varies significantly in character so as to be nondiagnostic. The presence of diffuse vulvovaginal pain associated with a markedly erythematous mucosa should alert the clinician to the possibility of group A streptococcal vulvovaginitis. A presumptive diagnosis can be made from the Gram stain, but a definitive diagnosis is based upon bacterial confirmation. Because of the inability to differentiate group A streptococcal vulvovaginitis from that due to *Neisseria gonorrhoeae*, appropriate tests need to be employed that encompass these organisms.

Streptococcal disease readily responds to an oral penicillin or semisynthetic penicillin. Erythromycin can be effectively used in the penicillin-allergic patient.

Group A Streptococcal Endometritis Salpingitis–Peritonitis

Disease due to group A beta-hemolytic streptococci in the nongravida female is not generally recognized. An acute endomyometritis may be triggered by the insertion of an intrauterine contraceptive device when group A beta-hemolytic streptococci are present in the vaginal flora. Characteristically, patients have the onset of a high, spiking fever within 24 hours following insertion. Physical examination reveals the virtual absence of any inflammatory exudate. The only pertinent physical finding is exquisite uterine tenderness. If the infection is allowed to progress untreated, death may ensue.

The advent of culdocentesis coupled with anaerobic technology has radically altered our conception of what was once thought to be a well-defined entity, acute salpingitis. Monif et al. (1977) demonstrated that *S. pyogenes* can be recovered as the sole isolate from the cul-de-sac. The recovery of the organism and the ability to exclude the concomitant presence of class III obligatory anaerobes have focused on the probability that the group A streptococci under selective conditions can be a rare cause of acute salpingitis in the nonpregnant woman.

A bacterium of unique virulence, the group A *streptococcus* requires a specific event such as a mechanical disruption of the cutaneous and mucosal barrier to initiate overt infection. The onset of menstruation appears to be an effective initiating event; consequently, the disease has a proximity to the onset of the menses, which is not dissimilar from that characteristic of *N. gonorrhoeae*. The clinical manifestations are indistinguishable from those associated with *N. gonorrhoeae*. The incidence of acute salpingitis due to the group A *streptococcus* is low. Monif et al. (1977) identified a single case in a study of 92 patients with acute salpingitis. Eschenbach et al. (1975), in their study of 241 cases of acute pelvic inflammatory disease, recovered *S. pyogenes* from the cul-de-sac in a single instance. In their case, as in that reported by Monif et al. (1977), a pure culture of group A streptococci was recovered from the cul-de-sac.

Therapy involves IV penicillin G. Because of occasional nonsusceptibility, clindamycin and the tetracyclines are not deemed first-line drugs for group A streptococci.

Necrotizing Fasciitis

As long ago as the Civil War, necrotizing fasciitis was recognized as a clinical entity. At that time it was known as "hospital gangrene." The condition was first formally described in 1924 by Meleney, who applied the name "hemolytic streptococcal gangrene." His description and therapy for this disease process are applicable even today.

The only significant alteration in therapy has been the introduction of antibiotics.

Clinical Course

The portal of infection is established by a prior surgical procedure. The clinical course is rapid, with the patient exhibiting fever (38–39°C) and tachycardia, which occasionally is out of proportion to the fever. With the onset of the disease, the patient usually experiences pain and swelling of the affected part. Chills and tremor are not uncommon. The initial pain is replaced by numbness, which, in conjunction with the toxic metabolic state, usually renders the patient indifferent to her illness. On the second to fourth day of illness, the pathognomic signs of streptococcal gangrene occur; to quote Meleney, "these are dusky hue of the skin, edema with blisters, from which can be expressed a dark serosanguinous fluid. The margins are red, and swelling is neither raised nor clearly demarcated."

On the fifth to eighth day, the discolored areas become frankly black or gray from gangrenous necrosis. Proportional to the severity of the disease, bacteremia is a common complication, with frequent metastatic involvement of the lung parenchyma. The disease process is one of extensive cellulitis complicated by abscess within fascial planes and widespread superficial fascial necrosis, resulting in separation and infarction of the overlying skin.

Streptococcal hyaluronidase is probably responsible for the destruction of connective tissue and the spread of infection along fascial planes. The fascia becomes liquefied and sloughs off. This disease entity is distinct from progressive synergistic bacterial gangrene, also described by Meleney, which is caused by microaerophilic streptococci in synergism with other organisms. It is interesting to note that Meleney's recorded mortality of 20% to 50% with the disease is the same as that indicated by present data. This high mortality and morbidity is partially the result of failure to recognize the pathognomic features of this disease and institute early treatment. The late stage of the disease is difficult to check.

Diagnosis

Although a presumptive diagnosis can be inferred from the Gram stain, definitive diagnosis is contingent on bacteriologic identification. The organisms are found only in the subcutaneous slough. The surrounding edema is sterile. The causative agent is the group A *Streptococcus*. Secondary or associated organisms, such as *Staphylococcus aureus*, *Pseudomonas*, and diphtheroids, may be present, necessitating a distinction of this condition from progressive bacterial synergistic gangrene.

Therapy

The wound must be widely opened and the necrotic material removed. Long incisions to the ends of the necrotic areas are necessary to expose the involved tissue adequately. They are generally made in a stellate fashion out from the wound. The viable overlying skin may be left intact. The whole area is irrigated and packed open. Large doses of penicillin, administered intravenously, are also necessary. Because of the nature of the destructive process and the debridement,

secondary closure is not possible and healing is by secondary intention. Grafting is sometimes necessary. Ventral hernias are frequent because of the loss of the abdominal wall fascia.

Streptococcal Toxic Shock Syndrome

The group A streptococci that cause a toxic shock-like syndrome belong to the M1 or M3 serotypes. They have been demonstrated to have the *S. pyogenes* exotoxin A gene, a superantigen, and can stimulate T-cells to proliferate nonspecifically and cause the release of massive amounts of lymphokines and monokines. The exotoxin produces rapid skin and soft-tissue necrosis with fever, septic shock, and multiple organ failure. Bacteremia due to streptococci belonging to just the M1 serotype increased from 18% in 1979 to 64% in 1989–1990.

The group A beta-hemolytic streptococci can produce a clinical syndrome not too dissimilar from that due to the toxigenic strains of *S. aureus*. Disease usually occurs in a previously healthy individual and is characterized by marked systemic toxicity, rapidly progressive multisystem organ failure, and a mortality of 30% to 60%.

Streptococcal pelvic infections are often associated with diffuse, nonlocalizing signs and symptoms. A prodroma of gastrointestinal symptoms such as vomiting and diarrhea and/or headache and myalgia may occur. Cervical exudate is usually sparse, with little or no odor. Regardless of the site of primary infection, the patient presents with acute onset of very high fever and pain in the affected area; however, occasionally, symptomatology referable to the primary site may not be conspicuous. Hypotension tends to develop in the first 24 hours. Mental status changes, oliguria, disseminated intravascular coagulopathy, biochemical evidence of hepatic dysfunction, and leukocytosis will manifest prior to respiratory and cardiovascular collapse; mortality exceeds 25%.

Streptococcal toxic shock has occurred with necrotizing fasciitis, endomyometritis, abortions, and postpartum endocarditis. When streptococcal toxic shock syndrome occurs in conjunction with necrotizing fasciitis, prompt and aggressive surgical removal of involved tissues is critical. Therapy entails aggressive use of beta-lactam antibiotics in conjunction with one or two doses (depending on renal status) of an aminoglycoside and, where indicated, surgical intervention in conjunction with use of a central venous line and intensive care support.

SELECTED READING

Holmes OW. The contagiousness of puerperal fever. N Engl J Med Surg 1843; 1:503.

Iffy L. Contribution of Semmelweiss to the problem of puerperal fever. Am J Obstet Gynecol 1968; 102:1180.

Jewett JF, Reid DE, Safon LE, Easterday CL. Childbed fever—a continuing entity. J Am Med Assoc 1968; 206:344.

Ledger WJ, Headington JT. Group A beta-hemolytic streptococcus. An important cause of serious infections in obstetrics and gynecology. Obstet Gynecol 1972; 39:474.

Marshall BR, Helper JK, Masaharu SJ. Fatal Streptococcus pyogenes septicemia associated with an intrauterine device. Obstet Gynecol 1973; 41:83.

Martens PR, Mullie A, Goessen L. A near-fatal case of puerperal sepsis. Anaesth Intensive Care 1991; 19:108.

McGregor J, Ott A, Villard M. An epidemic of "childbed fever." Am J Obstet Gynecol 1984; 150:385.

McIntyre DM. An epidemic of Streptococcus pyogenes. Puerperal and postoperative sepsis with an unusual carrier site—the anus. Am J Obstet Gynecol 1968; 101:308.

Meleney FL, et al. Epidemiologic and bacteriologic investigations of the Sloane Hospital epidemic of hemolytic streptococcus puerperal fever in 1927. Am J Obstet Gynecol 1928; 16:180.

Nathan L, Peters MT, Ahmed AM, Leveno KJ. The return of life threatening puerperal sepsis caused by group A streptococci. Am J Obstet Gynecol 1993; 169:571.

Ogden E, Amsty MS. Puerperal infection due to group A beta-hemolytic streptococcus. Obstet Gynecol 1978; 52:53.

Ooe K, Serikawa T, Sekine M, et al. A new type of fulminant group A streptococcal infection in obstetric patients: report of two cases. Hum Pathol 1997; 28:509.

Schwartz B, Fracklam RR, Breiman RF. Changing epidemiology of group A streptococcal infection in the USA. Lancet 1990; 336:1167.

Silver RM, Heddleston LN, McGregor JA, Gibbs R. Life-threatening puerperal infection due to group A streptococci. Obstet Gynecol 1992; 79:894.

Tancer ML, McManus JE, Bellotti G. Group A, type 33, hemolytic streptococcus outbreak on a maternity and newborn service. Am J Obstet Gynecol 1969; 103:1028.

Watson BP. An outbreak of puerperal sepsis in New York City. Am J Obstet Gynecol 1928; 16:157.

Watson BP. Practical measures in the prevention and treatment of puerperal sepsis. J Am Med Assoc 1934; 103:1745.

Webb LG, Silberstein N. Severe puerperal sepsis. Med J Aust 1985; 143:316.

Antenatal Fetal Infection

Monif GRG. Antenatal group A streptococcal infection. Am J Obstet Gynecol 1975; 123:213.

Neonatal Infection

Ginsberg H, Cohen I. Late onset group A streptococcal bacteremia in a neonate. J La State Med Soc 1987; 139:39.

Lehtonen OP, Kero P, Ruuskanen O, et al. A nursery outbreak of group A streptococcal infection. J Infect 1987; 14:263.

Shanks GD, Anderson RT, Lazoritz S, Hemming VG. Bilateral neonatal group A streptococcal hydrocele infection associated with maternal puerperal sepsis. Pediatr Infect Dis 1986; 5:107.

Streptococcal Vulvovaginitis

Boisvert PL, Walchen DN. Hemolytic streptococcal vaginitis in children. Pediatrics 1948; 2:24.

Emans SJ, Goldstein DO. The gynecologic examination of the prepubertal child with vulvovaginitis: use of the knee-chest position. Pediatrics 1980; 65:758.

Heller RH, Joseph JM, David HJ. Vulvovaginitis in the premenarchal child. J Pediatr 1969; 74:370.

Group A Endometritis/Salpingitis/Peritonitis

Eschenbach DA, Buchanan TM, Pollock HM, et al. Polymicrobial etiology of acute pelvic inflammatory disease. N Engl J Med 1975; 293:166.

Marshall BR, Hepler JK, Jinguji MD. Fatal Streptococcus pyogenes septicemia associated with an intrauterine device. Obstet Gynecol 1973; 41:83.

Monif GRG, Williams BT, Dase DF. Group A streptococcus as a cause of endometritis/salpingitis/peritonitis. Obstet Gynecol 1977; 50:509.

Necrotizing Fasciitis

Beathard GA, Guckion JC. Necrotizing fasciitis due to group A beta-hemolytic streptococcus. Arch Intern Med 1967; 120:63.

Buchanon CS. Necrotizing fasciitis to group A beta-hemolytic streptococci. Arch Dermatol 1970; 101:664.

Collins RN, Nadel MS. Gangrene due to the hemolytic streptococcus—a rare but treatable disease. N Engl J Med 1965; 272:578.

Crosthwait RW Jr, Crosthwait RW, Jordan GL. Necrotizing fasciitis. J Trauma 1964; 4:149.

Gryska PF, O'Dea AE. Postoperative streptococcal wound infection: the anatomy of an epidemic. J Am Med Assoc 1970; 213:1189.

Mastro T, Farley TA, Elliot JA, et al. An outbreak of surgical wound infection due to group A streptococci carried on the scalp. N Engl J Med 1990; 323:968.

May J, Chalmers JP, Loewenthal J, Rountree PM. Factors in the patient contributing to surgical sepsis. Surg Gynecol Obstet 1966; 122:28.

McCafferty EL, Lyons C. Supportive fasciitis as the essential feature of hemolytic streptococcal gangrene. Surgery 1948; 24:438.

Meleney FL. Hemolytic streptococcus gangrene. Arch Surg 1924; 9:317.

Meleney FL. Hemolytic streptococcal gangrene. J Am Med Assoc 1929; 92:2009.

Meleney FL. Bacterial synergism in disease processes with a confirmation of the synergistic bacterial etiology of a certain type of progressive gangrene of the abdominal wall. Ann Surg 1931; 94:961.

Rea WJ, Wyrick WJ. Necrotizing fasciitis. Ann Surg 1970; 172:957.

Strasberg SM, Silver MS. Hemolytic streptococcal gangrene: an uncommon but frequently fatal infection in the antibiotic era. Am J Surg 1968; 115:763.

Webb HE, Hoover NW, Nichols DR, Weed LA. Streptococcal gangrene. Arch Surg 1962; 85:969.

Streptococcal Toxic Shock Syndrome

Batter T, Dascal A, Carrol K, Curley FJ. "Toxic strep syndrome," a manifestation of group A streptococcal infection. Arch Intern Med 1988; 148:1421.

Cone LA, Woodard DR, Schlievert PM, Tomory GS. Clinical and bacteriologic observations of a toxic shock-like syndrome due to streptococcus pyogenes. N Engl J Med 1987; 317:146.

Crum NF, Gaylord TG, Hale BR. Group A streptococcal toxic shock syndrome developing in the third trimester of pregnancy. Infect Dis Obstet Gynecol 2002; 10:209.

Dotters DJ, Katz VL. Streptococcal toxic shock associated with septic abortion. Obstet Gynecol 1991; 78:549.

Jorup-Ronstrom C, Hofling M, Lundberg C, Holm S. Streptococcal toxic shock syndrome in a postpartum woman: case report and review of the literature. Infection 1996; 24:164.

Noronha S, Yue C, Sekosan M. Puerperal group A beta-hemolytic streptococcal toxic shock-like syndrome. Obstet Gynecol 1996; 89:729.

Schummer W, Schummer C. Two cases of delayed diagnosis of postpartum streptococcal toxic shock syndrome. Infect Dis Obstet Gynecol 2002; 10:217.

Stevens DL, Tanner MH, Winship J, et al. Severe group A streptococcal infections associated with a toxic shock-like syndrome and scarlet fever toxin A. N Engl J Med 1988; 148:1268.

Stollerman GH. Changing group A streptococci: the reappearance of streptococcal "toxic shock." Arch Intern Med 1988; 148:1268.

Whitted WR, Yeomans ER, Hankins GDV. Group A beta-hemolytic streptococcus as a cause of toxic shock syndrome: a case report. J Reprod Med 1990; 35:558.

Wood TF, Potter MA, Jonasson O. Streptococcal toxic shock-like syndrome: the importance of surgical intervention. Ann Surg 1993; 217:109.

Actinomyces israelii

INTRODUCTION

Actinomyces israelii is an anaerobic, gram-positive, branching filamentous bacterium whose filaments, by their radial attachment to the granule, give the organism its name: *actino* (radial), *myces* (mold like). The diameter of the branching filaments is comparable to that of other bacteria; however, the overall length of the hyphae resembles that of molds measuring hundreds of thousands of microns.

The organism is a common saprophyte of the oropharynx and the intestinal tract. Under normal circumstances, it is incapable of penetrating intact anatomic barriers.

A. israelii is a strict anaerobe. Its pathogenesis in a given host is determined by this characteristic. Disease, when it occurs, is a function of a synergistic association between the anaerobic microbes of the *Actinomyces* group and other bacteria. Cultures of exudates confirm the observation that most, if not all, cases of actinomycosis represent mixed or combined infection. When material is analyzed at necropsy using special stains, organisms other than *Actinomyces* almost invariably can be demonstrated.

FEMALE GENITAL TRACT INVOLVEMENT

Actinomycosis is a progressive inflammatory disease with local or systemic manifestations, or both, characterized by a tendency to produce multiple draining sinuses. Infection of the female genital tract is an unusual variant of abdominal, disseminated, or ascending actinomycosis. The principal ways in which the female genital tract may be involved include the following:

1. Direct dissemination from a contiguous area
2. Local lymphatic spread from contiguous areas (e.g., a ruptured appendix or inflamed colonic diverticula)
3. Hematogenous dissemination during systemic infection
4. Ascending infection associated with a contraceptive intrauterine device (IUD) (Fig. 1).

The interim between initial systemic seeding of the female genital tract and onset of disease may be prolonged. A case of tubo-ovarian involvement occurred 6 years and 11 months after a ruptured appendix. When involvement of the genital tract is secondary to widespread systemic disease, initial infection appears to occur within the distal portion of the fallopian tubes. In this respect, actinomycosis behaves very similarly to hematogenous seeding by *Mycobacterium tuberculosis*. Endometrial and ovarian involvement are usually secondary to tubal disease.

The initial pathologic process is abscess formation. Physical expansion of an encapsulated organ or inflammatory neuritis may make pain a prominent symptom. The abscesses tend to burrow, eventually resulting in tortuous

sinus tracts composed of dense fibrous connective and granulation tissue surrounded at the margins by a chronic inflammatory infiltrate. Within the lesions, aggregate colonies of the organism, known as "sulfur granules," can be demonstrated (Fig. 2). Infection is contingent on synergistic, facultative, anaerobic bacteria creating a low oxidation–reduction potential; consequently, contagion is not a major consideration.

A small percentage of women who choose the IUD as their mode of contraception develop a chronic polymicrobial infection of the endometrial cavity that ultimately becomes clinically manifested. Endometrial involvement appears to be due to an ascending infection. Burnhill (1974) described a syndrome of progressive endometritis characterized by foul-smelling intermenstrual leukorrhea, metrorrhagia, premenstrual bloating, and menorrhagia. Papanicolaou smears from such patients have often demonstrated collections of pseudomycelial bacteria that, by immunofluorescence, can be demonstrated to be *A. israelii*.

A significant number of these patients develop a unilateral abscess associated with IUD utilization or shortly after its removal. It is postulated that the development of a unilateral tubo-ovarian abscess is an expanded manifestation of anaerobic endometritis. The presence of *A. israelii* in the polymicrobial bacterial infection may be one of the factors predisposing to this complication.

DIAGNOSIS

Although used for taxonomic identification, serologic tests are devoid of diagnostic value. Both immediate and delayed types of skin reactions have been observed in actinomycotic patients; however, the nonavailability of antigenic material for cutaneous challenge limits the clinical usefulness of this procedure.

Diagnosis of actinomycosis is often inferred from a fresh smear or a simple Gram stain smear of exudate or aspirated material. A fresh smear of pus or exudate may reveal a tangled mass of wavy organismal threads, the so-called yellow "sulfur granules." These characteristic mycelia-like collections are often scanty. Their identification often depends on extensive searching of smears of histologic sections or necrotic material. Sulfur granules per se are not pathognomonic of actinomycosis. Both *A. israelii* and *Nocardia asteroides* may produce them. The two organisms can be distinguished on the basis of histochemical staining. Whereas *N. asteroides* is acid-fast, *A. israelii* is not (unless the Putt modification of the Ziehl-Neelsen acid-fast method is used). The sulfur granules of *A. israelii* are sometimes confused with clusters or colonies of other bacteria growing in an anaerobic environment. The greater affinity

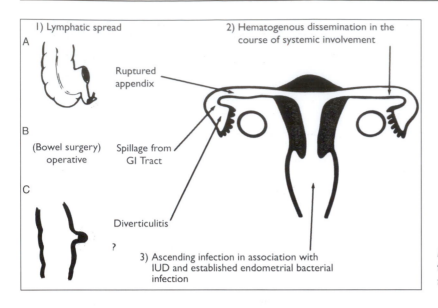

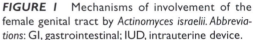

FIGURE 1 Mechanisms of involvement of the female genital tract by *Actinomyces israelii*. *Abbreviations*: GI, gastrointestinal; IUD, intrauterine device.

of *A. israelii* for silver stains provides one means of histologic differentiation between the two conditions.

A. israelii can be grown if appropriate anaerobic culture techniques and media are used. Culturing of the organism provides the definitive means of identifying it as the causative agent. Polymerase chain reaction testing is an alternative option for establishment of isolate identity.

THERAPY

Actinomyces species are sensitive to penicillin, ampicillin, the tetracyclines, chloramphenicol, clindamycin, and selected aminoglycosides. In dealing with deep-seated, soft-tissue infections of the female genital tract, chemotherapy is more than an adjunct to surgical resection of diseased tissue; it is a necessary prerequisite. Prior to an operative procedure, it is recommended that a patient receive penicillin, a new generation erythromycin, or doxycycline. The extent of the disease determines the drug dosage and its duration of administration.

When fallopian tube involvement is secondary to spillage from the gastrointestinal tract, maximum gastrointestinal shrinkage of an abscess should be attempted with antibiotics. If the disease is still evident after adequate therapy, or if a single relapse occurs, surgical removal of diseased tissue under antibiotic coverage is indicated.

Therapy for localized disease associated with IUDs requires a degree of individualization. If the patient with pseudomycelial clumps of bacteria is asymptomatic and the pelvic examination does not reveal cervical tenderness to motion or an adnexal mass, very often, mere removal of the IUD is sufficient to eradicate disease. If the IUD presents with either menstrual irregularities or Burnhill's syndrome, it has been the author's policy to place these patients on antibiotics prior to the removal of the IUD. If the pelvic examination is abnormal, aggressive antibiotic therapy should be implemented to eradicate the symbiotic polymicrobial infection, which frequently includes members of the *Bacteroides/Prevotella* species. If an adnexal

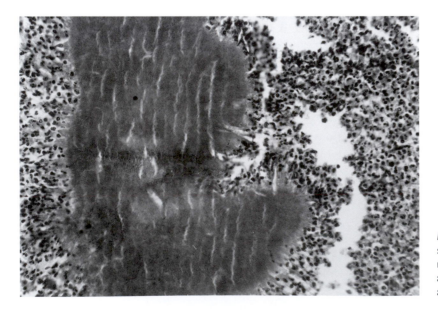

FIGURE 2 Sulfur granules of *Actinomyces israelii* showing the radial arrangement of branching filamentous organisms that stain positive with Gram and silver stains, surrounded by necrotic debris and acute inflammatory cells (H&E, ×140).

mass does not respond to antibiotic therapy and surgery is required, as conservative an operation as technically possible should be carried out.

SELECTED READING

Natural History of Infection
Cope A. Actinomycosis. New York: Oxford University Press, 1939.
Cummings JR, Beekley ME, Garley N. Abdominal actinomycosis. Ohio State Med J 1959; 55:340.
Curtis EM, Pine L. Actinomyces in the vaginas of women with and without intrauterine contraceptive devices. Am J Obstet Gynecol 1981; 140:880.
Duguid HDL. *Actinomyces*-like organisms and the IUD. Acta Cytol 1981; 25:66.
Duncan JA. Abdominal actinomycosis: changed concepts. Am J Surg 1965; 110:148.
Gupta PK, Luff RD, Spence MR, Frost JK. *Actinomyces* infection with IUD usage. Acta Cytol 1976; 20:582.
Neuhauser EB. Actinomycosis and botryomycosis. Postgrad Med J 1970; 48:59.
Peabody JW, Seabury JF. Actinomycosis and nocardiosis. Am J Med 1960; 28:99.
Waksman SA. The Actinomycetes: A Summary of Current Knowledge. New York: Ronald Press, 1967.
Zinsser H. Actinomycosis and actinomycetes. In: Smith DT, Conont MF, Willet HP, eds. Microbiology, 14th ed. New York: Appleton-Century-Crofts, 1968.

Female Genital Tract Involvement
Brenner RW, Gehring SW. Pelvic actinomycosis in the presence of an endocervical contraceptive device. Obstet Gynecol 1967; 29:71.
Burnhill MS. Syndrome of progressive endometritis associated with intrauterine contraceptive devices. Adv Plann Parent 1974; 9:144.
Dawson JM, O'Riordan B, Chopra S. Ovarian actinomycosis presenting as acute peritonitis. Aust N Z J Surg 1992; 62:161.
Farrior HL, Rathbun LS, Doolan J Jr, Turner FG. Pelvic actinomycosis. Am J Obstet Gynecol 1969; 103:908.
Ingall EG, Merendino KA. Actinomycosis of the female genitalia. West J Surg 1952; 60:476.
Loth MF. Actinomycosis of the fallopian tube. Am J Obstet Gynecol 1956; 70:919.
Spence MR, Gupta PK, Frost JK, et al. Cytologic detection and clinical significance of *Actinomyces israelii* in women using intrauterine contraceptive devices. Am J Obstet Gynecol 1978; 131:295.
Stevenson AEM. Actinomycosis of ovaries and fallopian tubes. Br J Obstet Gynaecol 1957; 44:365.
Sweeney DR, Blackwelder TF. Pelvic actinomycosis. Report of a case. Obstet Gynecol 1965; 25:690.

Actinomyces-IUD-Unilateral Tubo-Ovarian Abscesses
Gupta PK, Hollander DH, Frost JK. Actinomycetes in cervicovaginal smears: an association with IUD usage. Acta Cytol 1976; 20:295.
Henderson SR. Pelvic actinomycosis associated with an intrauterine device. Obstet Gynecol 1973; 41:726.
Paalman RJ, Dockerty MD, Mussey RD. Actinomycosis of the ovaries and fallopian tubes. Am J Obstet Gynecol 1949; 58:419.
Schiffer MA, Elguezabal A, Sultana M, Allen AC. Actinomycosis infections associated with intrauterine contraceptive devices. Obstet Gynecol 1975; 45:67.
Taylor ES, McMillan JH, Greer BE, et al. The intrauterine device and tubo-ovarian abscess. Am J Obstet Gynecol 1975; 123:338.

Bacteroidaceae/*Prevotella* 31

INTRODUCTION

The family Bacteroidaceae consists of gram-negative non–spore-forming anaerobic bacilli that constitute one of the major groups of anaerobes that function effectively as class III anaerobes (obligate anaerobes). These bacteria can be differentiated from other organisms of this schema by morphology, biochemical characteristics, and identification of metabolic end products by gas liquid chromatography. The *Bacteroides*, *Prevotella*, and the fusobacteria are the most commonly found organisms of this group. Because of shared characteristics, *Bacteroides* and *Prevotella* species are grouped together. Morphologically, *Bacteroides* and *Prevotella* appear as rods with rounded ends or as coccobacilli. Fusobacteria are generally characterized by long, thin fusiform shapes or extremely pleomorphic spherical forms. Therapeutically, the *Bacteroides/Prevotella* species can be subdivided for pragmatic purposes into the penicillin-sensitive and the non–penicillin-sensitive organisms.

The ability to function as an effective pathogen for the female genital tract is independent of the bacterium's relative sensitivity to penicillin. Originally, the *Bacteroides* were subdivided into bile-resistant and bile-sensitive organisms. The principal bile-resistant species were *B. fragilis*, *B. distasonis*, *B. vulgatus*, *B. ovatus*, *B. thetaiotaomicron*, and *B. uniformus*. The major bile-sensitive species included *B. bivius*, *B. disiens*, *B. capillosus*, *B. gracilis*, *B. ureolyticus*, *B. oralis*, *B. melaninogenicus*, and *B. asaccharolyticus*.

In recent years, the taxonomy of anaerobic gram-negative bacilli has been in a state of great change, and this trend will continue. The genus *Bacteroides* has been restricted to the *B. fragilis* group only (including *B. eggerthii*); the taxonomic positions of other species still included in the genus *Bacteroides* remain uncertain, but all of these species will ultimately be transferred to other genera. As currently constituted, the *B. fragilis* group includes *B. caccae*, *B. distasonis*, *B. eggerthii*, *B. fragilis*, *B. merdae*, *B. ovatus*, *B. stercoris*, *B. thetaiotaomicron*, *B. uniformis*, and *B. vulgatus*.

This bile-resistant *B. fragilis* group is the most commonly recovered anaerobe in clinical specimens and is more resistant to antimicrobial agents than are most other anaerobes. *B. fragilis* and *B. thetaiotaomicron* are of the greatest clinical significance.

The genera *Prevotella* (saccharolytic) and *Porphyromonas* (pigmented asaccharolytic organisms) were previously included in the genus *Bacteroides*. *Prevotella* species are the bile-sensitive, nonpigmented, saccharolytic, gram-negative bacilli. *Prevotella* species are found in the same settings as the pigmented gram-negative rods.

Porphyromonas (Bacteroides) melaninogenicus is a monomorphic (i.e., not pleomorphic) species, characterized by the formation of a black pigment on blood agar. *P. melaninogenicus* is part of the normal flora of mucous membranes and is commonly found in association with Peptostreptococci. The two organisms may act synergistically.

Bacteroidaceae are relatively common anaerobic female genital tract isolates. The bacteria have been cultured in the cervix, placenta, and/or amniotic fluid of gravidas with premature or prolonged rupture of the fetal membranes.

Anaerobic bacteria may colonize amniotic fluid in the absence of ruptured membranes. The frequency with which anaerobic bacteria enter amniotic fluid is significant, yet progression to disease, chorioamnionitis, or perinatal septicemia is not a common phenomenon. A potential explanation for this discrepancy between infection and disease rates may be inferred from the prerequisites for disease. Amniotic fluid preferentially supports the growth of class I (bacteria that replicate better in the presence of air than in its absence) over class II (microaerophilic) anaerobic bacteria. For the Bacteroidaceae to function effectively, some change must occur in its local microbiologic environment. Meconium enhances anaerobic replication by lowering the oxidation–reduction potential.

PATHOGENESIS

The *Bacteroides* and *Prevotella* species exist as microaerophilic constituents of the female genital tract, being present usually as class II anaerobes, which are defined as bacteria that are unable to initiate growth unless the oxidation–reduction potential of the medium is low or unless they are present in an extremely large number. The transformation from a state of colonization to a state of disease can be achieved by two major pathways:
1. The anaerobic progression
2. The immediate anaerobic syndrome
The mandatory prerequisite in each case is an alteration of the oxidation–reduction potential.

THE ANAEROBIC PROGRESSION

The anaerobic progression has its genesis in bacteria whose ability to replicate at different oxygen levels vary significantly. The polymicrobial infection present at the initiation of anaerobic disease undergoes selective changes as the consequence of the induced alterations in the microbiologic environment. As the oxidation–reduction potential is lowered, acidification of the local environment occurs and molecular oxygen is removed; the more aerobic bacteria, which are unable to replicate under these adverse conditions, undergo the process of autoelimination. Sequential samplings of what is ultimately to be an abscess due to *B. fragilis* might reveal *B. fragilis* present as a class II anaerobe with such bacteria as *Escherichia coli*, *Staphylococcus epidermidis*, the enterococci (group D streptococci), *Gardnerella vaginalis*, and the Peptostreptococci. When environmental requirements for anaerobic dominance are achieved and anaerobic progression has shifted from organisms of class II to class III, many of these cofacilitating bacteria undergo autoelimination so that *Bacteroides* and Peptostreptococci, either singly or in combination, predominate.

The ultimate result of anaerobic infection is abscess formation. In a well-established abscess, one rarely finds more than one or two types of bacteria. In an evolving abscess, a more polymicrobial representation of bacteria is to be anticipated. Factors that predispose to anaerobic infection include the following:

1. New tissue space, e.g., hematoma
2. Necrotic tissue, as might be present with incomplete abortions or retained products of conception, criminal abortions, degenerated tumor masses, crush injury, or devitalized previously healthy tissue
3. Penetration of the gastrointestinal tract with spillage of fecal material
4. Alteration of the microbiologic environment by *Neisseria gonorrhoeae*

Under these conditions, the probability of the Bacteroidaceae functioning as effective pathogens in the female genital tract is great.

Many of the *Bacteroides* strains elaborate beta-lactamases that can protect beta-lactamase–sensitive constituents, e.g., enterococci, until a critical oxidation–reduction potential is reached that allows the *Bacteroides* strain to function as a monomicrobial pathogen.

All members of the *B. fragilis* group appear to be able to encapsulate during an inflammatory process. Nonencapsulated strains can become encapsulated with the assistance of their aerobic counterparts in the anaerobic progression. These encapsulated strains are more virulent to the host than nonencapsulated strains. This increased virulence can be demonstrated by a higher rate of induction of bacteremia, and a greater enhancement of growth of other bacteria. Antimicrobial therapy directed only at the eradication of aerobic bacteria does not prevent encapsulation or reduce the number of *Bacteroides* species.

IMMEDIATE ANAEROBIC SYNDROME

The right microbiologic environment can be combined with the right bacteria to produce disease. This sequencing of events is called the immediate anaerobic syndrome, the classical example of which is either spontaneous or iatrogenic perforation of the gastrointestinal tract. The oxidation–reduction potential of feces is one of the lowest recorded. The bacterial flora of the gastrointestinal tract is predominantly anaerobic. The spillage of fecal material requires no intermediary events for the production of anaerobic infection.

CLINICAL CONSEQUENCES
Endomyometritis–Septic Thrombophlebitis–Septicemia
Under normal physiologic conditions, the endometrial cavity has no demonstrable bacterial flora. Even when organisms

are iatrogenically introduced, as with insertion of an intrauterine contraceptive device, bacterial replication (barring the presence of group A beta-hemolytic streptococci) is not sustained. Within a relatively short time after insertion of the device, transcervical cultures of the endometrial cavity are again sterile. In the postpartum period, the endometrium represents a functional tissue system whose normal defense mechanisms have undergone significant alteration. The loss of mucosal integrity and the presence of blood and a necrotic decidua sustain bacterial colonization. Transcervical aspiration almost invariably documents the occurrence of bacterial replication. When one is dealing with nonquantitative data, the major bacteriologic difference between infected and noninfected endometria (excluding infection due to *N. gonorrhoeae*, group A beta-hemolytic streptococci, and *Listeria monocytogenes*) is a shift toward the more obligate anaerobes.

What is impressive is the ability of the endometrial cavity to limit the number of instances in which bacterial replication progresses to infectious morbidity. Unless there are retained products of conception, or the mode of delivery has been a cesarean section, the presence of other synergistic or facilitating organisms is not sufficient to sustain anaerobic dominance by the *Bacteroides/Prevotella*. In these instances, *Bacteroides/Prevotella* may participate as part of a mixed aerobic/anaerobic low-grade endometritis that is usually not clinically discernible.

The situation is markedly altered when one is dealing with retained products of conception or with an infected uterus after cesarean section. In the former and as a consequence of the altered oxidation–reduction potential, the *Bacteroides* or *Prevotella* alone or in conjunction with the anaerobic streptococci and/or the anaerobic staphylococci produce disease. Patients present with fever, a foul-smelling lochia, and uterine tenderness. If the process is not arrested by surgical removal of the retained products of conception, it may progress to involve the maternal implantation site, in which case, septic thrombophlebitis and septicemia may develop. *Bacteroides* can spread in the clots within the thrombosed sinuses to the uterine and ovarian veins. More extensive spread involves the iliac veins, the inferior vena cava, and the renal vein. The patient develops chills and hectic fevers, which are often accompanied by rigors. Subsequent pleuritic chest pain and hemoptysis may indicate pulmonary emboli and segmental infarction of the pulmonary parenchyma. Careful inspection of the placenta is one of the most effective means of averting this sequence of events.

Puerperal Infection from Septic Abortion
In terms of fulfilling the major prerequisite for *Bacteroides/Prevotella* infection, namely, a low oxidation–reduction potential, septic abortion, whether spontaneous or induced by instrumentation, creates a condition analogous to that observed with retained products of conception. In the absence of more virulent pathogens within the vaginal flora, *E. coli*, group B beta-hemolytic streptococci, and enterococci are often the leading organisms. However, they may be subsequently superseded by the more obligate anaerobes. The amount of tissue available for bacterial replication and

the direct access to the maternal vascular compartment or the presence of peritonitis secondary to uterine perforation sets the stage for sustained septicemia, which in turn can be correlated with maternal morbidity and possibly mortality. The situation here is analogous to a patient's being administered a continuous intravenous infusion of bacteria. The key to therapy in this situation consists of surgically disconnecting the intravenous line while aborting potential metastatic complications with antibiotics.

Perinatal Septicemia

A subgroup of neonatal septicemia has been established, based on perceived differences in the events that combine to produce disease. Septicemia in the first 24 to 48 hours of life is termed perinatal septicemia, whereas that occurring after 48 hours is termed neonatal septicemia. Maternal factors such as chorioamnionitis, urinary tract infection, and prolonged and/or premature rupture of the fetal membranes predispose to perinatal septicemia. In contrast, neonatal septicemia, occurring after the first 48 hours, is primarily a nosocomial disease of infants who are debilitated or chronically ill (e.g., those with congenital anomalies, necrotizing enterocolitis) or who have been anatomically compromised (e.g., by surgical procedures or central line complications).

There are very few demographic factors that distinguish anaerobic perinatal septicemia (specifically that due to Bacteroidaceae) from its aerobic counterpart. Maternal chorioamnionitis, fetal distress, and perinatal respiratory difficulty are common to both. A foul-smelling neonate is evidence of anaerobic replication in utero. In the series of Chow and Guze (1974), eight of nine newborns with a foul smell at birth had *Bacteroides*. Both cases of *Bacteroides* perinatal septicemia reported by Keffer and Monif (1988) occurred in women who had intact fetal membranes until the immediate parturition period.

Foul-smelling amniotic fluid and/or a maternal history of prolonged labor with intact membranes, coupled with a potentially septic neonate, should alert the neonatologist to the possibility of anaerobic infection from a member of the Bacteroidaceae/*Prevotella*. Many of the Bacteroidaceae/ *Prevotella* are resistant to a penicillinaminoglycoside combination. In terms of perinatal outcome, failure to adequately cover for the penicillin-resistant isolates may be equivalent to delayed therapy.

DIAGNOSIS

The initial diagnosis of *Bacteroides/Prevotella* infection must emanate from the physician and not the clinical laboratory. By having insight into the pathogenesis of the anaerobic infections, one can often anticipate those clinical situations in which *Bacteroides/Prevotella* may represent a significant portion of the group of bacteria that have combined to produce disease. Certain clinical situations carry with them a high probability of organismic participation:

1. Postpartum endometritis associated with retained products of conception
2. Postpartum endomyometritis in patients who have undergone cesarean section

3. Septic abortion
4. Septic thrombophlebitis
5. Any abscess (irrespective of site), particularly one that had access to the vaginal flora or is the consequence of penetration of the gastrointestinal tract and spillage of fecal material

A prospective orientation to the problem is best. However, the diagnosis of *Bacteroides/Prevotella* infection is sometimes retrospectively suggested by the failure of infectious morbidity to respond to beta-lactam antibiotics.

The mortality rate due to perinatal septicemia is directly contingent on the interim between onset of disease and initiation of effective antibiotic therapy. Monif et al. demonstrated that when therapy was delayed for more than four hours, 80% of the infants died or had residual sequelae. The possibility of a penicillin-resistant strain should influence antibiotic selection.

If anaerobic collection containers are not available, Gram staining becomes the most important diagnostic tool next to the physician's ability to anticipate participation by Bacteroidaceae. As previously stated, the presence in smears from body fluids or abscesses of gram-negative pleomorphic rods that fail to grow in aerobic cultures should suggest the Bacteroidaceae/*Prevotella*.

THERAPY

Antibiotic selection significantly depends on whether the process is in evolution or whether the critical conditions for anaerobic dominance have been met. The contention of Gorbach and Bartlett (personal communication) that by treating the synergistic component, one can disrupt the anaerobic progression appears to be valid so long as it is restricted to the early phase of disease. Once obligate anaerobic dominance has been established, all the bacterial constituents in the synergism should be treated with appropriate antibiotics to effect a definitive cure (Table 1).

The *Bacteroides/Prevotella* pose a difficult problem to clinicians because of their ability to produce the enzyme beta-lactamase. The resistance of most anaerobic gram-negative bacteria to beta-lactam antimicrobial agents is primarily mediated by the production of beta-lactamases. A great variation in specific activity has been demonstrated among enzymes from different *Bacteroides/Prevotella* strains. Consequently, coverage in both categories I and II of the Gainesville Classification needs to be implemented. The drugs of choice are clindamycin, imipenem, and metronidazole.

There have been two major attempts to overcome resistance to beta-lactam drugs:

1. Coupling of semisynthetic penicillins with beta-lactamase inhibitors such as clavulanic acid, sulbactam, and tazobactam. The inhibitors produce a marked reduction in MIC_{50}s and MIC_{90}s for the companion penicillin.
2. The development of antibiotics that are more resistant to degradation by beta-lactamase enzymes. Some modifications including the 7-alpha-methoxy cephalosporins (cefoxitin, cefotetan, and moxalactam) and the 7-beta-methoxy aminoacetamide cephalosporins (cefotaxime

TABLE I Advocated antibiotic regimens in the treatment of infections due to the penicillin-resistant Bacteroidaceae/*Prevotella*

Degree of efficacy	Drug	In vitro susceptibility
Penicillin-resistant Bacteroidaceae/*Prevotella*	Chloramphenicol[a]	98%
	Metronidazole[a,b]	94–96%
	Clindamycin[a]	70–85%
	Doxycycline[c]	80–85%
	Cefoxitin	72–85%
	Ureidopenicillins	60–70%
Category designation	Ampicillin/sulbactam[d]	
	Chloramphenicol[a]	
	Clindamycin[a]	
	Imipenem	
	Metronidazole[a]	
Antibiotics with reasonable effectiveness	Cefoxitin	
	Doxycycline	
	Trovofloxacin[e]	
	Ureidopenicillin	

[a]Chloramphenicol, clindamycin, and metronidazole each carry an FDA black box indicating possible dangerous or lethal adverse drug reaction.
[b]The intravenous form of metronidazole has been released for the treatment of anaerobic infections; consequently, the correlation between in vitro and in vivo,while probably excellent, is not as well substantiated as for chloramphenicol and clindamycin.
[c]Must use 300 mg/day to achieve these precentages, which exceeds FDA recommendations but is commonly used.
[d]Other 'fifth generation' penicillin may also have category designation.
[e]Excellent in vitro data may well correlate with clinical data.

and cefmenoxime) have greatly enhanced the efficacy against Bacteroidaceae.

Neither of these two groups achieve category designation status.

Bacteroides/Prevotella and *Fusobacterium* do not produce beta-lactamase and consequently are sensitive to the penicillins.

Because of the increasing resistance to clindamycin and metronidazole and the rapid induction of resistance to imipenem, selective use of ampicillin–sulbactam and ticarcillin–clavulanic acid and possibly piperacillintazobactam provides some coverage.

Although metronidazole can be readily substituted for clindamycin in the context of triple therapy for category II coverage in the Gainesville Classification, its failure to cover the aerobic gram-positive bacteria of category I precludes its combination with just an aminoglycoside. Effective preliminary antibiotic coverage requires the concomitant administration of an antibiotic whose spectrum of susceptibility encompasses both gram-positive and gram-negative aerobic bacteria.

SELECTED READING

Aldridge KE, Sanders CV, Janney A, et al. Comparison of the activities of penicillin G and new beta-lactam antibiotics against clinical isolates of *Bacteroides* species. Antimicrob Agents Chemother 1984; 26:410.

Bawdon RE, Crane LR, Palchaudhuri S. Antibiotic resistance in anerobic bacteria: molecular biology and clinical aspects. Antimicrob Agents Chemother 1982; 17:629.

Beazley RM, Polakavetz SE, Miller RM. *Bacteroides* infections on a university surgical service. Surg Gynecol Obstet 1972; 135:742.

Bodner SJ, Koenig MG, Goodman JS. Bacteremic *Bacteroides* infections. Ann Intern Med 1970; 73:537.

Carter M, Jones CP, Ather RL, et al. *Bacteroides* infections in obstetrics and gynecology. Obstet Gynecol 1953; 1:491.

Chow AW, Guze LB. Bacteroidaceae bacteremia: clinical experience with 112 patients. Medicine (Baltimore) 1974; 53:93.

Eley A, Greenwood D. Characterization of beta-lactamases in clinical isolates of *Bacteroides*. J Antimicrob Chemother 1986; 18:325.

Fekete T, McGowen J, Cundy KR. Activity of cefazolin and two beta-lactamase inhibitors, clavulanic acid and sulbactam against *Bacteroides fragilis*. Antimicrob Agents Chemother 1987; 31:321.

Felner JM, Dowell VR. *Bacteroides* bacteremia. Am J Med 1971; 50:787.

File TM, Thomson RB Jr, Tan JS, et al. *In vitro* susceptibility of the *Bacteroides* fragilis group in community hospitals. Diagn Microbiol Infect Dis 1986; 5:317.

Gelb AF, Seligkman SJ. Bacteroidaceae bactermia. J Am Med Assoc 1970; 212:1038.

Henthorne JC, Thompson L, Beaver DC. Gram-negative bacilli of the genus *Bacteroides*. J Bacteriol 1936; 31:255.

Kagnoff MF, Armstrong D, Blevins A. *Bacteroides* bacteremia. Cancer 1972; 29:245.

Keffer G, Monif GRG: Perinatal septicemia due to Bacteroidaceae. Obstet Gynecol 1988; 71:403.

Keffer GL, Monif GRG. Perinatal septicemia due to the Bacteroidaceae. Obstet Gynecol 1988; 71:463.

Lamothe F, Fijalkowski C, Malouin F, et al. *Bacteroides fragilis* resistant to both metronidazole and imipenem. Antimicrob Agents Chemother 1986; 18:642.

Monif GRG, Baer H: The impact of coverage for the non-penicillin-sensitive and non-tetracycline sensitive Bacteroidaceae to doxycycline and minocycline. Current Therap Res 1982; 142:896.

Monif GRG, Hempling RE: The impact of coverage for the non-penicillin-sensitive Bacteroidaceae on infectious morbidity with Caesarian section. Obstet Gynecol 1981; 57:177.

Monif GRG, Hume R Jr, Goodlin RC: Neonatal considerations in the management of premature rupture of the fetal membranes. Am J Obstet Gynecol Surv 1986; 41:531.

Pearson HE, Anderson GV. *Bacteroides* infections and pregnancy. Obstet Gynecol 1970; 35:31.

Pearson HE, Anderson GV. Genital bacterial abscess in women. Am J Obstet Gynecol 1970; 107:1264.

Tally FP, Cuchural GJ, Jacobus NV, et al. Nationwide study of the susceptibility of the *Bacteroides fragilis* group in the United States. Antimicrob Agents Chemother 1985; 28:675.

Clostridium perfringens 32

INTRODUCTION

Clostridium perfringens is a gram-positive, anaerobic, non-motile, spore-forming rod that is capable of producing potent exotoxins. The bacterium is subdivided into five types based upon the production of four major lethal toxins: alpha, beta, epsilon, and iota. The most important toxin is alpha toxin, a lecithinase that destroys cell membranes, alters capillary permeability, destroys platelets, and causes severe hemolysis. In appropriate environmental conditions, vegetative forms of the histotoxic clostridia replicate and elaborate toxins that diffuse into adjacent soft tissue and promote local spread as well as extensive systemic effects. Despite its relatively high prevalence in the lower gastrointestinal tract bacterial flora, *C. perfringens* is a rare isolate from the female genital tract.

Two explanations have been advanced to explain the disassociation between bacterial isolation/infection and disease. The first is that of variability in the toxigenicity of individual strains of *C. perfringens*. The alternate hypothesis has to do with variability in the conditions necessary to produce disease. Holtz and Mauch (1962) postulated that primarily three conditions are necessary for the development of clostridium myonecroses:

1. The organism must be introduced into the uterus from an outside source or must be carried into the uterus from the vagina or cervix.
2. Dead tissue must be present at the time the organisms are introduced.
3. Injured tissue must remain in the uterus for sufficient time to permit incubation of the organisms.

One can readily visualize situations in which, despite vascular access, conditions necessary for toxic production might be transient; e.g., transient retention of a larger fragment of necrotic decidua. Neither theory is mutually exclusive.

The time over which *C. perfringens* can produce toxins influences both morbidity and lethality. In obstetric and gynecological patients, the severity of extrauterine manifestations of disease is a partial function of the extent of pelvic tissue necroses. Within necrotic tissue, the production of exotoxins requires approximately 24 to 28 hours of incubation. The exotoxins necrotize surrounding normal tissue, especially muscle, thereby creating a wide area for invasion by the proliferating organisms.

The exotoxins produce the full-blown syndrome of *C. perfringens* septicemia, characterized by hemolysis, hemoglobinemia, hemoglobinuria, hyperbilirubinemia, acute renal failure, hyperkalemia, and diffuse intravascular coagulation (DIC). The alpha toxin, a lecithinase, causes lysis of the red blood cell membrane. Hemoglobin is liberated and circulates as free hemoglobin in the plasma, producing the characteristic

port-wine–colored serum and urine. Acute renal failure is due to acute tubular necroses secondary to renal ischemia. Hyperkalemia is a result of the liberation of potassium from hemolyzed red blood cells compounded by an inability to excrete this overload in the presence of renal failure. DIC is due to both the action of alpha toxin on the vascular endothelium and the release of a thromboplastin-like substance.

CLINICAL MANIFESTATIONS

Clostridial Myonecrosis

The principal clinical setting for cases of clostridial myonecrosis (gas gangrene) due to *C. perfringens* is that of criminal abortion, retained products of conception, or endomyometritis. A wider clinical spectrum is observed with clostridial septicemia, ranging from a relatively benign course to septic toxemia with renal failure due to massive intravascular hemolysis and to death. Markedly less frequent is the occurrence of clostridial myonecrosis following a surgical procedure. The determining factor governing the severity of disease is the local oxidation-reduction potential. A sustained decreased oxidation-reduction potential promotes toxin production. With the exception of septic abortion, overwhelming sepsis is a relatively rare event. However, when serial blood cultures are done in cases of endomyometritis following cesarean section, an occasional case can be identified in which *C. perfringens* is isolated from the intravascular compartment; the clinical course is one that readily responses to antibiotic therapy.

With postabortion and puerperal uterine infections, *C. perfringens* can produce a low-grade endometritis. Patients present with vaginal discharge, uterine tenderness, and fever. There are no signs of systemic toxemia. The diagnosis is suggested by the identification of large gram-positive rods on Gram staining and confirmed by the growth of *C. perfringens* in culture specimens. Ramsey (1949) noted that in his series of 190 cases of postabortion sepsis in which clostridia were isolated from the cervix, 130 (66%) were mild infections localized to the uterus, and the response was rapid. In the 15% of postabortion clostridial infections with clostridial bacteremia, two-thirds had no clinical evidence of systemic infection.

The key to the induction of postabortal clostridial disease is the presence of necrotic tissue, which occurs with incomplete abortion or an intrauterine fetal demise. In these cases, clinical response to dilation and curettage, coupled with effective antibiotic therapy, is rapid. When the underlying causation is due to excessive tissue destruction, as would occur with abortions induced by caustic agents or injection of hypertonic saline into the myometrium during intra-amniotic infusion, or significant delay in therapy occurs, the patients develop severe endomyometritis, peritonitis, and septicemia.

Clinically, the patients usually present with fever and abdominal pain. On physical examination, an elevated temperature, uterine tenderness, and the presence of a foul-smelling discharge are usually demonstrable. The diagnosis may be inferred by the identification of large gram-positive, box-like rods on Gram-stained smears. With progression of clostridial disease, the consequence of alpha toxin production is manifest. Full-blown clostridia septic toxemia is characterized by intravascular hemolysis, hemoglobinemia, hemoglobinuria, hypotension, and renal failure. Depending upon the quality and timing of interventions, the ensuing mortality ranges from 21% to 85%.

Soft-Tissue Clostridial Infections

Soft-tissue clostridial infection in the gynecological patients requires, in addition to bacterial access to the site of infection and tissue necrosis, poor tissue perfusion. In the nonpregnant woman, clostridial myonecrosis tends to occur primarily in irradiated or diabetic patients or in patients with either benign (leiomyoma) or malignant genital tract tumors that have undergone significant necrosis. When clostridial myonecrosis complicates these types of cases, a higher than expected mortality rate occurs, owing primarily to the failure of recognizing clostridia superinfection after surgery. Postoperatively, the development of severe pain and systemic toxicity that is out of proportion to the physical finding should alert the clinician to the possibility of clostridial infection.

In the absence of extensive trauma to the operative site, surgical wound infections rarely develop clostridia myonecrosis. Clostridia may be isolated from a simple wound infection. However, unless there is an extensive area of tissue necrosis or hematoma formation, the process is limited, and the impact of alpha toxin production is relatively negligible.

DIAGNOSIS

The diagnosis is usually made in one of three ways:

1. Recovery of C. perfringens from a wound or blood culture
2. Visual or roentgenographic evidence of myocerosis with gas fermentation (Fig. 1)
3. Clinical picture suggestive of toxigenic clostridial sepsis

Pain, which is caused by the rapid infiltration of muscle by edema and gas, is the earliest symptom. When pain is the result of trauma, disease appears within 24 to 72 hours of the event. A tachycardia out of proportion to the temperature is characteristic. A subnormal temperature with a marked tachycardia is a grave prognostic sign.

When the site of myonecrosis is visible, the appearance of the wound is that of an edematous, purulent wound with brownish, bubbling exudate. Crepitation may be demonstrable in the adjacent tissues. The surrounding skin becomes edematous and has a brown discoloration, termed "brown erysipelas." Gram-stained smears reveal the presence of large, gram-positive rods.

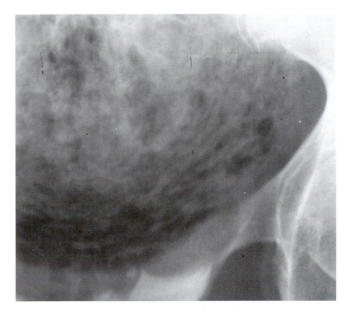

FIGURE 1 Gas formation in the pelvic tissues of a woman with postpartum endomyometritis due to *Clostridium perfringens*.

The full-blown syndrome of clostridial sepsis includes hypotension, intravascular hemolyses, hemoglobinemia, hemoglobinuria, jaundice, and renal failure. The skin exhibits a gray pallor, and profuse diaphoreses may be present. The patient may be apathetic and indifferent to her condition. X-ray films can usually demonstrate the spread of the gas in the involved tissues. A definite diagnosis is based on bacteriological identification of C. *perfringens*.

THERAPY

Most cases of postabortal or postpartum endometritis/endomyometritis without evidence of intravascular hemolysis do well with removal of necrotic tissue and appropriate antibiotic therapy. The isolation of *clostridium* from the uterus or bloodstream is not indicative, by itself, of a severe infection. The development of intravascular hemolysis in association with clostridial infection is a poor prognostic sign and delineates a group of patients with potentially lethal infections. Once clostridial organisms are identified on a Gram-stained smear from the site of infection in a septic patient, prompt surgical intervention is urged.

Better than 80% survival rates can be achieved with early aggressive therapy that includes antibiotics, prompt operative debridement of necrotic tissue with removal of the nidus of infection, which is the source of the exotoxins responsible for the clinical findings, and prompt medical therapy of acute renal failure. In severe uterine and pelvic infections, total abdominal hysterectomy and bilateral salpingo-oophorectomy may be required.

The most important component of therapy is prompt and extensive surgical removal of infected tissue when disease involves the uterus. Hysterectomy is indicated. With wound infection and myonecrosis, extensive surgical debridement with wide excision of involved muscle when the abdominal wall is involved needs to be carried out.

When available, antecedent hyperbaric oxygen therapy can facilitate surgery by increasing the visual demarcation between visible and dead tissue.

Early antimicrobial therapy is essential for optimal outcome. Penicillin G in large doses is advocated for severe infection. Alternative therapy includes metronidazole and clindamycin. Cefoxitin is less active against clostridia than most other cephalosporins and should be avoided. Antitoxin therapy is no longer available commercially. The high frequency of allergic reactions and a relative lack of efficacy were the reasons behind its discontinuation. The concomitant use of an aminoglycoside antibiotic is advocated. Antibiotics that impact on 50s ribosomes, and to a lesser degree 30s ribosomes, can be shown to alter the in vitro production of exotoxins.

The timing of hyperbaric oxygen continues to be controversial. If laparotomy or hysterectomy is indicated, the operation should not be delayed for hyperbaric oxygen therapy. Hyperbaric oxygen before surgery has the benefit of clearly demarcating involved tissue, and thus potentially sparing viable tissue while halting toxin production. If used, hyperbaric oxygen should be available within a one-hour or less time frame and used as a temporizing adjunct to therapy.

SELECTED READING

Alpern RJ, Dowell VR Jr. Non-histotoxic clostridial bacteremia. Am J Clin Pathol 1971; 55:717.

Altemeier WA, Fullen WD. Prevention and treatment of gas gangrene. J Am Med Assoc 1971; 217:806.

Borkowf HI. Bacterial gangrene associated with pelvic surgery. Clin Obstet Gynecol 1973; 16:40.

Brummelkamp WH, Boerema I, Hoogendyk L. Treatment of clostridial infections with hyperbaric oxygen drenching. A report on 26 cases. Lancet 1963; 1:235.

Butler HM. Bacteriological studies of Clostridium welchii infections in man. Surg Gynecol Obstet 1945; 81:475.

Caplan ES, Kluge RM. Gas gangrene: review of 34 cases. Arch Intern Med 1976; 136:788.

Cohen AL, Bhatnagar J, Reagan S, et al.: Toxic shock with Clostridium sordelli and Clostridium perfringens after medical and spontaneous abortions. Obstet Gynecol 2007; 110:1027.

Decker WH, Hall W. Treatment of abortions infected with Clostridium welchii. Am J Obstet Gynecol 1966; 95:394.

Eaton CJ, Peterson EP. Diagnosis and acute management of patients with advanced clostridial sepsis complicating abortion. Am J Obstet Gynecol 1971; 109:1162.

Holtz FO, Mauch EW. Gas gangrene of uterus. Survival following hysterectomy. Obstet Gynecol 1962; 19:545.

Kadner ML, Anderson GV. Septic abortion with hemoglobinuria and renal insufficiency with special reference to Clostridium welchii infection. Obstet Gynecol 1963; 21:86.

Lacey CG, Futoran R, Morrow CP. Clostridium perfringens infection complicating chemotherapy for choriocarcinoma. Obstet Gynecol 1976; 47:337.

Ledger WJ, Hackett KA. Significance of clostridia in the female reproductive tract. Obstet Gynecol 1973; 41:525.

O'Neill RT, Schwarz RH. Clostridial organisms in septic abortions. Obstet Gynecol 1970; 35:458.

Pritchard JA, Whalley PJ. Abortion complicated by Clostridium perfringens infection. Am J Obstet Gynecol 1971; 3:484.

Ramsey AM. The significance of Clostridium welchii in the cervical swab and bloodstream in post partum and post abortum sepsis. Br J Obstet Gynaecol 1949; 56:247.

Rathbun HK. Clostridia bacteremia without hemolysis. Arch Intern Med 1968; 122:496.

Slack WK, Hanson GC, Chew HE. Hyperbaric oxygen in the treatment of gas gangrene and clostridial infection: a report of 40 patients treated in a single-person hyperbaric oxygen chamber. Br J Surg 1969; 56:505.

Smith JW, Southern PM Jr, Lehmann JD. Bacteremia in septic abortion: complications and treatment. Obstet Gynecol 1970; 35:704.

Smith LDS. The Pathogenic Anaerobic Bacteria. Springfield, IL: CC Thomas, 1975.

Smith LP, McLean AH, Maughan GB. Clostridium welchii septicotoxemia. Am J Obstet Gynecol 1971; 110:135.

INTRODUCTION

Clostridium sordellii is a gram-positive, anaerobic, non-motile, spore-forming rod. Like *Clostridium perfringens*, it produces a variety of potent exotoxins. Until relatively recent times, *C. sordellii* was considered to be a common soil enteric bacterium that was rarely isolated from the vagina. Its ability to produce fulminant and lethal wound infections has radically altered that concept.

The clinicopathologic manifestations and significant morbidity and mortality described with *C. sordellii* infections have been linked to the elaboration of two unique exoproteins: edema-producing, or lethal, toxin (LT) and hemorrhagic toxin (HT). Strains with the capacity to produce LT and HT have been associated with puerperal wound infections that are accompanied by anasarca and a clinical picture of septic shock.

CLINICAL MANIFESTATIONS

The histotoxic exoproteins manufactured by *C. sordellii* result in localized fascial necrosis and myonecrosis, which can mimic gas gangrene. Characteristically, infections occur less than one week postpartum.

Each patient described in the literature has had a distinctive course characterized by sudden onset of clinical shock marked by severe and unrelenting hypotension associated with marked, generalized tissue edema and "third spacing" with increased hematocrit, presence of marked leukemoid reaction with total neutrophil counts of 84,000/mm^3, 66,000/mm^3, and 93,600/mm^3, absence of rash or fever, limited or no myonecrosis, and a rapid and potentially lethal course.

Low-grade fever, massive edema, subsequent vascular collapse due to extracellular sequestering of the fluid, and a very rapid progression from initial infection to death are characteristic for the course of events. Despite adequate debridement, most patients have died.

Infections with *C. sordellii* are most commonly associated with relatively "clean" incisions. They produce localized tissue damage characterized by a profound exotoxin-mediated systemic response with anasarca, refractory hypotension, and marked leukocytosis. The exotoxins (primarily LT) appear to disrupt the vascular integrity, producing extensive "third spacing" and, ultimately, cardiovascular collapse.

C. sordellii has been shown to cause puerperal infection as well as a distinctive toxic shock-like syndrome (Table 1). Recently, an association between *C. sordellii* septic shock and use of mifepristone in medical abortion was identified. Mifepristone appears to block both progesterone and glucocorticoid receptors and, by so doing, interferes with the controlled release and functioning of cortisol and cytokines, resulting in an impaired innate immune system response to organismal challenge.

The most common setting for *C. sordelli* toxic shock syndrome is after either medical or spontaneous abortions (Cohen et al., 2007). In this clinical situation, disease due to *Clostridium* species should be at the top of the list.

DIAGNOSIS

An early diagnosis of this or any necrotizing subcutaneous infection based on clinical grounds and an external examination alone can be exceedingly difficult. Once so identified, prompt surgical intervention and antibiotic therapy are advocated.

The presence of systemic toxicity and profound, rapidly progressive, widespread edema, leukocytosis, hemoconcentration, and lack of a predominant organism on tissue Gram stain in the presence of myonecrosis should suggest *C. sordelli* as the potential etiological agent. Confirmation of a presumptive diagnosis is predicated on culture recovery of the organism.

THERAPY

The management of puerperal infections with this clostridial species has been similar to the treatment of *C. perfringens* myonecrosis: surgical debridement of necrotic tissue, broad-spectrum antimicrobials because of the polymicrobic nature of perineal infections, high doses of beta-lactam antibiotics, hyperbaric oxygen therapy, and intensive supportive care. Surgical intervention involves the following:

1. Determination of the extent and nature of the soft-tissue damage
2. Removal of the source of toxin production and necrotic tissue
3. Obtaining tissue for histopathologic examination and culture confirmation

A theoretical argument can be made for using a combination of bacteriocidal and bacteriostatic antibiotics. Antibiotics that impact primarily on 30S or 50S ribosomes have been shown to abort or lessen toxin production.

TABLE I   *Clostridium sordellii* syndrome

Sudden onset of clinical shock
Severe unrelenting shock
Generalized edema progressing to anasarca
Rapid deterioration of cardiovascular status
Marked leukemoid reaction
Absence of rash or fever
Minimal purulent discharge from infected lesions

Source: Daly (1990).

Despite this aggressive therapy, most maternal infections have been fatal. Cardiovascular collapse secondary to marked "third space" sequestration of fluid has been the usual cause of death.

Since debridement and antibiotic therapy do not necessarily reverse the chain of events set in motion by the elaboration of toxins in this disease process, the use of exchange transfusion and hyperbaric oxygen should be considered.

SELECTED READING

Barnes P, Leedom IM. Infective endocarditis due to *Clostridium sordellii*. Am J Med 1987; 83:605.

Cohen AL, Bhatnagar J, Reagan S, et al.: Toxic shock with *Clostridium sordelli* and *Clostridium perfringens* after medical and spontaneous abortions. Obstet Gynecol 2007; 110:1027.

Centers for Disease Control and Prevention. *Clostridium sordelli* toxic shock syndrome after medical abortion with mifepristone and intravaginal misprosstol—United States and Canada 2001–2005. MMWR 2005; 54:724.

Daly JW. Infect Dis Lttr Obstet Gynecol 1990; 12:48.

Grimwood K, Evans GA, Govender ST, Woods DE. *Clostridium sordellii* infection and toxin neutralization. Pediatr Infect Dis J 1990; 9:582.

Hatheway CL. Toxigenic clostridia. Clin Microbiol Rev 1990; 1:66.

Hogan SF, Ireland K. Fatal acute spontaneous endometritis resulting from *Clostridium sordellii*. Am J Clin Pathol 1989; 91:104.

Martinez RD, Wilkins TD. Purification and characterization of *Clostridium sordellii* hemorrhagic toxin and cross-reactivity with *Clostridium difficile* toxin A (enterotoxin). Infect Immun 1988; 56:1215.

Martinez RD, Wilkins TD. Comparison of *Clostridium sordellii* toxins HT and LT with toxins A and B of *C. difficile*. J Med Microbiol 1992; 36:30.

McGregor JA, Soper DE, Lovell G, Todd JK. Maternal deaths associated with *Clostridium sordellii* infection. Am J Obstet Gynecol 1989; 161:987.

Miech RP. Pathophysiology of mifepristone-induced septic shock due to *Clostridium sordellii*. Ann Pharmacother 2005, 39:1483.

Popoff MR. Purification and characterization of *Clostridium sordellii* lethal toxin and cross-reactivity with *Clostridium difficile* cytotoxin. Infect Immun 1987; 55:35.

Sinave C, Le Templier G, Blouin D, et al.: Toxic shock syndrome due to *Clostridium sordelli*: a dramatic postpartum and postabortion disease. Clin Infect Dis 2002; 35:1441.

Sosolik RC, Savage BA, Vaccarello L. *Clostridium sordellii* toxic shock syndrome: a case report and review of the literature. Infect Dis Obstet Gynecol 1996; 4:31.

INTRODUCTION

Escherichia coli is a short, gram-negative bacillus. Most strains are motile. The organism is a facultative anaerobe and grows readily on most laboratory media, producing a characteristic fetid odor. Serologic identification is based on the antigen specificity of the O antigens. To date, more than 150 group O (somatic cell wall), at least 50 H (flagellar), and a similar number of K (capsular) antigens have been identified. Clinical studies indicate that certain O group antigens are more likely to be incriminated in disease than other strains; this finding suggests a correlation between pathogenicity and antigenic composition. Strains that are rich in K antigens are more resistant to destruction by antibody, complement, and phagocytosis and thus are more likely to circumvent host defense mechanisms than are other strains.

Although the gastrointestinal tract is the probable reservoir of organisms, recent studies have documented the existence of significant differences between fecal *E. coli* and those strains isolated from the female genital tract and cases of neonatal sepsis. Cook et al. (2001) examined 50 *E. coli* isolates from cases of vaginitis, 45 isolates from tubo-ovarian complexes, and 45 isolates from infants with neonatal sepsis for selected phenotypic and genetic virulence properties. Results were compared with fecal *E. coli* isolates not associated with disease. A statistically significant greater proportion of *E. coli* associated with infection exhibited D-mannose–resistant hemagglutination compared with fecal *E. coli*. This adherence phenotype correlated statistically with the presence of P fimbriae genes.

Selected strains termed "enteropathic *E. coli*" produce exotoxins. These strains function either by exotoxin production or by their tissue-invasive properties, which result in bacillary dysentery. Approximately 30% to 40% of diarrhea observed in U.S. travelers in developing countries is caused by these strains.

FEMALE GENITAL TRACT INVOLVEMENT

As part of the intestinal and vaginal flora endogenous to humans, *E. coli* is pervasive in its pathogenetic spectrum. Within obstetrics and gynecology, it can function as a monoetiologic pathogen to produce urinary tract infection or chorioamnionitis, or the organism can be a lead constituent of polymicrobial infection (i.e., septic abortion, postpartum endometritis, or wound infections). Both monoetiologic and polymicrobial infection may result in septicemia.

URINARY TRACT INFECTIONS

Maternal Infection

About 5% of all the serotypes (04, 06, and 075, and less frequently 01, 07, 02, and 050) account for almost 75% of *E. coli* urinary tract infections. Irrespective of the route of infection (hematogenous or ascending), the strains that are responsible for infection of the female genital tract almost invariably have as their reservoir the patient's own feces. The prevalence of *E. coli* in feces alone cannot account for its overwhelming predominance as a cause of urinary tract infection. Variables other than merely fecal contamination of the perineum must function to favor the establishment of *E. coli* colonization at the urethral introitus and its subsequent replication in the urine. Since the serotypes of *E. coli* that cause acute urinary tract infection are derived from the fecal flora, any factor that alters the predominant fecal serotype of *E. coli* may be of potential clinical significance. When a patient is hospitalized, considerable alterations in strain prevalence of *E. coli* may occur, with the acquisition of new strains, particularly following the use of broad-spectrum antibiotics. Once colonization occurs, the new strains persist. The newly acquired strains, having been selected predominantly by prior administration of antibiotics, are more likely to be resistant to multiple antibiotics. The high incidence of strains rich in K antigen in pyelonephritic gravidas suggests that although initial access to the genital tract may be due to mechanical transfer of *E. coli* by fecal contamination, the K strains, with their enhanced resistance to host defense mechanisms, may possess a greater capacity to invade the kidney. Although the concept of pyelonephritogenic strains of *E. coli* is still controversial, it is probable that antigenic differences among transported strains of *E. coli* may be important in the pathogenesis of urinary tract infections.

Fetal Impact

Urinary tract infection in pregnancy may not be without consequences to the fetus. Some evidence suggests that occasionally, neonates born to mothers who had urinary tract infections during pregnancy have immunoglobulin M (IgM) elevations for which other readily identifiable causes are not apparent. The concept of in utero immunologic stimulation has been reinforced by the demonstration of lymphocyte blast transformation in some neonates whose mothers had urinary tract infections in pregnancy when the cells of the neonates are incubated with specific *E. coli* antigens. Whether or not antigenic exposure of the fetus occurs and is responsible for fetal morbidity is an issue that is yet to be adequately elucidated.

E. COLI SEPTICEMIA SECONDARY TO ABORTION OR CHORIOAMNIONITIS

Several properties of *E. coli* organisms enhance their ability to function as pathogens. They can replicate both in aerobic and in partially anaerobic environments. Unlike the majority of bacteria present in the feces and vaginal flora, most strains of *E. coli* are motile. Motility per se is not the major determinant of disease. The organisms must be able not only to reach the site of infection, such as the intra-amniotic space or devitalized tissue, but also to replicate successfully. If a strain of *E. coli* has established a persistent pattern of replication in the urinary tract, its ability to produce uterine infection is markedly augmented. When cases of pyelonephritis are excluded, the major factor selecting for septicemia due to the Enterobacteriaceae, and *E. coli* in particular, is antecedent asymptomatic bacteriuria. The majority of patients with Enterobacteriaceae septicemia for which the uterus is clearly the portal of infection can be demonstrated to have concomitant asymptomatic bacteriuria. The strains of *E. coli* that produce asymptomatic bacteriuria appear to differ from nonnephrogenic isolates obtained from the vagina by virtue of their augmented ability to adhere to cell membranes. With premature rupture of the membranes, effective dissolution of the physiologic and anatomic barrier, represented by the cervical mucous plug and intact fetal membranes, occurs.

The nephrogenic *E. coli* concomitantly sustained within the vaginal flora now obtain potential access. Access to amniotic fluid does not necessarily correlate with ensuing infection unless the bacterium in question is an exogenous pathogen (i.e., group A streptococci, *Neisseria gonorrhoeae*, or an endogenous bacteria for which augmented virulence has been preselected). Once the organism either overwhelms the infant's defense mechanisms at the alveolar level or penetrates the chorioamnion of the placenta, fetal infection is initiated. Maternal infection is observed when the disease process extends through the placental tissue and reaches the maternal vascular channels at the implantation site. When infection due to *E. coli* is associated with retained products of conception, septicemia may occur. In contrast to most infections in which access to a vascular space occurs, in this case, the placental site cannot be completely thrombosed. The situation is analogous to a patient who receives an IV infusion of a potentially unlimited quantity of bacterial organisms. The focus of therapy is surgical removal of the source of organisms while instituting supportive measures to sustain the gravida. It is imperative that the antibiotic therapy be such that the divergent spectrum of Enterobacteriaceae is more than adequately covered. In the management of retained products of conception and criminal abortion, there is not one but a multitude of potential or functional pathogens; hence the necessity for broad-spectrum antimicrobials that will destroy both gram-positive and gram-negative organisms. With prolongation of the disease process, anaerobic organisms have a progressively larger representation in the pathogenetic flora, and there is a greater tendency for anaerobic streptococci and *Bacteroides* species to predominate and gain access to the maternal intravascular space.

Aggressive implementation of group B streptococcal prophylaxis has resulted in *E. coli* becoming the leading cause of perinatal septicemia. The characteristic antibiotic resistance pattern is that of community *E. coli* minus those isolates sensitive to first- and/or second-generation penicillins.

WOUND INFECTIONS

E. coli is not an infrequent isolate from infected wounds. Rarely is it isolated in pure culture. Although *E. coli* is important in initiating the disease, one almost never sees progressive wound infections and resulting septicemia due to *E. coli* per se. Once an appropriate anaerobic oxidation–reduction potential is achieved, the more obligatory anaerobes, such as anaerobic streptococci and *Bacteroides* species, emerge as the dominant organisms in the wound. Therapy directed against *E. coli* in the absence of early abscess formation may be effective in aborting the progression of the local process. In contrast to *E. coli* isolates from the patient with primary pyelonephritis, a higher incidence of organisms with resistance to broad-spectrum antibiotics is encountered.

POSTPARTUM ENDOMETRITIS

Barring obstetrical trauma or retained products of conception, postpartum endometritis following spontaneous vaginal delivery occurs in 2% to 3% of gravidas. In the great majority of patients, an exogenous pathogen can be isolated from the endometrium. In selected instances, a member of the Enterobacteriaceae can be isolated as the quantitatively dominant bacteria amidst a polymicrobial background. The majority of these patients have concomitant asymptomatic bacteriuria. The probability of ensuing postpartum endometritis due to *E. coli* is markedly enhanced when chorioamnionitis due to the bacteria in question anteceded parturition. When a woman is delivered by cesarean section, the need for a virulence factor to select for pathogenicity is obviated. In this setting, the Enterobacteriaceae can function as part of the anaerobic progression. *E. coli* is more prone to exhibit gas formation in the course of soft-tissue infection in diabetics. All that is crepitant is not *Clostridium perfringens*, but one is committed therapeutically to use a regimen effective against both organisms until a definitive bacteriologic diagnosis has been established.

THERAPY

Generally, the major consideration in the therapy of urinary tract infections (Chapter 68), legal termination of pregnancy (Chapter 64), chorioamnionitis (Chapter 60), and wound infections (Chapter 78) is whether the pathogenic strain of *E. coli* was acquired from the hospital or from a nonhospital environment. The acquisition of infection in the former milieu or infection in a patient who had received prior antibiotic therapy argues for the selection of an aminoglycoside or a fluoroquinolone.

SELECTED READING

Brody II, Oski FA, Wallach EE. Neonatal lymphocyte reactivity as an indicator of intrauterine bacterial contact. Lancet 1968; 1:136.

Brumfitt W, Reeves DS, Faiers MC, Dalta M. Antibiotic-resistant *Escherichia coli* causing urinary tract infections in general practice: relation to fecal flora. Lancet 1971; 1:315.

Cook SW, Hammill HA, Hull RA. Virulence factors of *Escherichia coli* isolated from female reproductive tract and neonatal sepsis. Infect Dis Obstet Gynecol 2001; 9:203.

Cooke CW, Hallack JA, Wurzel H, et al. Fetal maternal outcome in asymptomatic bacilluria of pregnancy. Obstet Gynecol 1970; 36:840.

Dalta M, Brumfitt W, Faiers MD, et al. R factors in *Escherichia coli* in feces after oral chemotherapy in general practice. Lancet 1971; 1:312.

Editorial. *Escherichia* serotypes and renal infection. Lancet 1971; 1:532.

Glynn AA, Brumfitt W, Howard CJ. K antigens of *Escherichia coli* and renal involvement of urinary tract infections. Lancet 1971; 1:514.

Gruneburg RN, Leigh DA, Brumfitt W. *E. coli* serotypes in urinary tract infections: studies in domiciliary, antenatal and hospital practice. In: O'Grady F, Brumfitt W, eds. Urinary Tract Infections. London: Oxford University Press, 1968:68.

Johnson JR. Virulence factors in *Escherichia coli* urinary tract infection. Clin Microbiol Rev 1991; 4:80.

Johnson JR. PapG alleles among *Escherichia coli* strains causing urosepsis: associations with other bacterial characteristics and host compromise. Infect Immun 1998; 66:4568.

O'Grady FW, Richards B, McSherry MA, Caltell WR. Introital enterobacteria, urinary infection and the urethral syndrome. Lancet 1970; 2:1208.

Wallach EE, Brody II, Oski FA. Fetal immunization as a consequence of bacilluria during pregnancy. Obstet Gynecol 1969; 33:100.

Gardnerella vaginalis

Bryan Larsen

OVERVIEW

Gardnerella vaginalis has had an interesting history that is fraught with some confusion. Despite confusion, it is an organism that is frequently a topic of discussion and research in obstetrics and gynecology, with more than 1100 papers cited by the MedLine database by the end of 2006.

The primary reason for interest in this organism relates to its key role in bacterial vaginosis (BV), a somewhat awkward neologism, but one that has gained common use in medical parlance. Although it plays a key role in BV, several decades of research focused on the organism has convinced most experts that it is improper to refer to *G. vaginalis* as the etiologic agent of BV. Indeed, it is equally improper to refer to the condition of BV as vaginitis. To physicians schooled in thinking of a single organism causing a specific infectious disease, the relationship of *Gardnerella* and BV may seem somewhat counterintuitive, which has led to many confusing statements in the medical literature.

The most proper understanding of the *Gardnerella* organism and BV requires recognition that BV represents a profound disruption of the microbial ecosystem of the vagina—a dysbiosis—in which *G. vaginalis* is present in increased abundance and its presence undoubtedly contributes to the altered ecosystem. Moreover, it is equally important to note the concomitant alteration of other bacterial species in the lower genital tract during BV episodes.

BV has gained a reputation as being a predisposing factor in a variety of other conditions (salpingitis, prematurity, and postpartum and postoperative morbidity), and these have also focused attention on *G. vaginalis* and other BV-related organisms over the past two decades.

THE ORGANISM

This organism shows a variable Gram-staining reaction, although analyses of the cell surface characteristics suggest that it is a gram-positive rod. The organism belongs to the Bifidobacteria family and is cultivated from clinical material principally by isolation on human blood Tween because of its ability to produce hemolysis on human but not sheep blood. It also grows on chocolate agar (an enriched medium containing thermally lysed blood), which led earlier observers to assign it to the genus *Haemophilus*. Chocolate agar makes heme (X factor) and nicotinamide adenine dinucleotide (Y factor) available to the organism, and these are essential for growth of members of the genus *Haemophilus*.

The biochemical reactions of this organism can be used in the clinical microbiology laboratory for confirming its identity (starch or hippurate hydrolysis), but these are rarely of practical value. Indeed, except for basic microbiological research, the organism is rarely even cultivated. Its presence in clinical specimens is frequently inferred from the appearance of Gram-stained smears. However, the preponderance of culture-based studies that took care to look for *G. vaginalis* suggests that it is often present in the absence of symptoms, suggesting that it probably is part of the normal flora in many women of reproductive age.

Molecular methods based on DNA hybridization or polymerase chain reaction (PCR) have become the more frequently used ones in relation to organisms that are difficult to cultivate and further underscore the frequent colonization of the female genital tract by *G. vaginalis*. Bradshaw et al. (2006) indicated that 99% of women with BV (by microscopic criteria) had positive PCR for *G. vaginalis* and 96% of women with BV were PCR positive for *Atopobium vaginae*. The latter organism has only recently been recognized as a common vaginal organism, and its role is still a matter of uncertainty. Fluorescent in situ hybridization represents an additional method for nonculture-based flora characterization.

G. vaginalis has been evaluated for virulence factors, and it possesses adherence properties, biofilm generation, and hemolysin activity that may each be postulated to have a role in virulence. Shubair et al. (1993) provided evidence that the *G. vaginalis* hemolysin may contribute to the lack of leukocytosis in BV, and Cauci et al. ()1998 found that sialidases that may diminish vaginal mucin content are more abundant when *Gardnerella*-positive women fail to produce anti-*Gardnerella* hemolysin antibody. However, these virulence factors (*i*) apparently are either not expressed or not expressed in abundance in women who are colonized by *Gardnerella* but who are not symptomatic for BV and (*ii*) do not seem to be so potent as to create a situation in which *Gardnerella* colonization always causes symptoms. For this reason, it may be appropriate to think of the organism as having a moderately benign virulence profile, which underscores the observation that its role as part of the entire microbiological content of the vagina is more important in creating the presence or absence of symptoms in the vagina, than are its individual traits.

VAGINAL DYSBIOSIS—BV

Prior to the classic paper of Gardner and Dukes in 1955, the term "nonspecific vaginitis" was applied to a condition characterized by a gray, malodorous homogeneous discharge with a pH greater than 5. Epithelial cells from such patients were stippled with coccobacilli (Clue cells), and these coccobacilli also appeared in the background besides being attached to cells. Pus cells were usually few or absent. In recognition of the work of Gardner, the organism isolated from cases of so-called nonspecific vaginitis was named "*Gardnerella vaginalis.*"

The early work of Gardner and Dukes contained the early seeds of our present understanding of BV. They sought to demonstrate that the organism was etiologic for vaginitis, but found that pure cultures instilled into the vaginas of human volunteers only rarely could produce symptoms of nonspecific vaginitis. However, the vaginal discharge from symptomatic women was far more effective in producing symptoms in the inoculated women than the pure *Gardnerella*. Our current view being that BV is a dysbiosis, it should not be surprising that the mixture of organisms and chemical milieu transmitted in the inoculum was effective in transmitting the clinical condition. But despite these early observations, physicians still struggled with the idea that this was something other than a monoetiologic infectious disease.

Careful documentation of symptoms, a search for common patterns among symptoms, improved care in differentiation of the *Gardnerella*-associated vaginal condition from specific vaginal mycosis or trichomoniasis, and more extensive use of microscopic observations, particularly in the research setting, led investigators to a set of symptoms that seemed pathognomonic for BV, the term that ultimately replaced the term "nonspecific vaginitis."

Significant research involving the vaginal flora seen in BV led to the recognition that the condition includes a decrease in lactobacillus and a concomitant relative increase in G. *vaginalis* and various strictly anaerobic bacteria, which sometimes include curved rods such as *Mobiluncus*. The impracticality of culture-based analysis of the flora and the realization that BV involves a change mainly in the proportion of bacteria already extant in the vagina led investigators to look to Gram staining of vaginal material to document the shift in flora.

Two sets of diagnostic criteria dominate the field today, and these focus more or less on two areas of BV. Observations may focus on the patient and her symptoms (Amsel criteria) or observations may focus on microscopic examination of the discharge (Nugent criteria). Interestingly, some clinicians have opined that one method is better than another on the basis of subjectivity versus objectivity, but it must be borne in mind that even microscopic observations require skill and judgment, just as clinical observations do. Papers continue to appear in the literature pitting one diagnostic method against the other to determine the sensitivity and specificity of individual elements of each method. As a practical matter, however, it would seem that a diligent clinician would use all observations available regardless of which set of criteria these observations meet.

As introduced above, the criteria that focus more on clinical observation are Amsel's criteria, in which three of four of the following are considered necessary for diagnosis of BV: thin homogeneous vaginal discharge, vaginal pH greater than 4.5, a positive "whiff test" (a fishy smell emanating from alkalinized discharge), and clue cells on wet mount. The result of the Amsel criteria is to categorize a patient as BV positive or negative.

The Nugent criteria are directed at noting the status of the flora on Gram stain, because the shift in flora associated with BV involves microscopic morphotypes that are readily identifiable to the trained observer. It should be noted, however, that to be accurate, microscopic observation identifies organisms consistent with certain microbial genera, but the observer should realize that this type of observation is not able to provide unequivocal identification of specific genera; such identification can only be done with detailed biochemical or molecular tests. The Nugent criteria scores smears from 0 to 10, with a score of 7 to 10 being considered BV. The Nugent criteria awards up to 4 points for decreases in *Lactobacillus* (large gram-positive rods), up to 4 points for morphotypes consistent with G. *vaginalis* (small gram-variable rods), and up to 2 points for *Mobiluncus*-like morphotypes (curved gram-negative rods). The Nugent criteria provides for a continuum of scores and allows for the possibility of categorizing patients as having BV even if they have few or no symptoms.

Naturally, with different evaluation systems, investigators have attempted to provide evidence of the value of each. In a 2004 report from Thailand, Chaijareenont et al. compared Amsel (as the gold standard) to Nugent criteria and showed the following results for Nugent: 65.6% sensitivity and 97.3% specificity; 80.8% positive predictive value and 94.2% negative predictive value. They also noted that pH and whiff test used together were sufficient to attain 100% sensitivity. In contrast, in a 2005 report from Chicago by Sha et al., the Nugent scoring (203 with scores 7–10; that is, positive for BV) was used as a gold standard. The report stated that only 75 of these were diagnosed by Amsel criteria as BV positive, providing a 37% sensitivity and 99% specificity, leading them to conclude the "Amsel criteria were poorly predictive" in their cohort.

The disparity between the above two reports is striking, but many differences might be at work. The reports involve different populations, different sample collection methods, and different patient selection approaches, and the observers may have had differing levels of facility with the methods employed. In addition to the potential confusion between different sets of characteristics that are believed to identify BV patients, it is possible that variant conditions may yet emerge that involve flora types that have been heretofore difficult or impossible to cultivate (such as A. *vaginae*) or may involve symptoms that are similar to BV, but are somehow distinct (aerobic vaginitis).

AEROBIC VAGINITIS

As physicians have become more cognizant of the value of proper differentiation between the major types of infectious vaginal conditions, researchers have become aware of variant forms of symptomatic vaginal conditions that do not seem to fit the pattern of vaginal candidiasis, vaginal trichomoniasis, or BV. Donders has been primarily responsible for suggesting the existence of a condition they describe as anaerobic vaginitis. In their groundbreaking report in 2002, they noted a condition that was characterized by diminished lactobacillus colonization, but no significant presence of clue cells and increased inflammatory and parabasal cells. Further characterization showed an absence of succinate (in contrast to BV) and increased levels of proinflammatory cytokines including interleukin-6 (Il-6) and Il-1β. The aerobic organisms most often associated with this condition were group B *Streptococcus* and *Escherichia coli*. Several subsequent reports have used the term "aerobic vaginitis," and in the future, it may become a more widely accepted term to describe a condition of dysbiosis that is clearly not BV. While not espousing the term "aerobic vaginitis," some researchers have noted that among patients initially categorized by positive BV status, there was a cluster who had elevated *E. coli* and *Enterococcus* in addition to the diminished *Lactobacillus* colonization.

BV-ASSOCIATED CONDITIONS

Gardnerella colonization of the vagina clearly should not be considered pathological as it occurs in more than half of women who have no vaginal symptoms. Even in BV in which *Gardnerella* populations are expanded relative to *Lactobacillus* spp., the symptoms, although clinically important and significant to the symptomatic woman, are not life threatening. The greatest concern expressed by experts involves conditions that are related to the presence of BV or exacerbated by it. These include an elevated risk of premature birth, an increased risk of postpartum febrile morbidity especially when delivery is by means of Cesarean section, an increased risk of postoperative febrile morbidity in gynecologic surgeries, and increased risk of salpingitis when there is preexisting BV.

The above concerns have been elaborated on the basis of epidemiologic findings and, for the most part, lack mechanistic underpinnings at present. It is not appropriate, therefore, to assume that the expanded microbial populations directly cause these epidemiological synergies. Some of the epidemiologic relationships noted come from the work of McGregor et al. (1994), who reported a 3.3-fold relative risk for premature birth when BV was diagnosed, and a 3.8-fold relative risk for premature rupture of the membranes when BV was present. With respect to specific organisms, there has been only a modest increase in risk of obstetrical and postpartum complications. Krohn et al. (1995) reported on intrauterine infection risk and indicated a 1.8-fold relative risk for *Gardnerella*-colonized women, 1.5-fold relative risk for those heavily colonized with *Bacteroides*, and a 1.7-fold risk with *Mycoplasma hominis* colonization. More profound was the postpartum risk of endometritis after cesarean section reported by Watts who found an unadjusted odds ratio of 6.1 among BV cases compared to non–BV-positive controls. From these various reports, it is

apparent that women with BV are at elevated risk for birth and postpartum complications, but the relationship to individual microorganisms is weak and is strengthened by a relationship to certain mixtures of organisms, and density of colonization.

Some evidence exists to implicate host inflammatory responses as in the case of prematurity. Andrews et al. (2006) reported a strong association of neutrophilic inflammation of the membranes and increased IL-6 with prematurity; others related an IL-10 mutation to extreme prematurity. The role of BV-related microorganisms directly causing prematurity was also brought into question when it was discovered that metronidazole prophylaxis was not beneficial in preventing premature birth.

Nevertheless, there are subsets of birth complications that more directly implicate the microbial species associated with BV. In 1988, Hillier et al. noted that bacteria were 3.2 times more likely to be found in the chorion–amniotic interface if BV was present compared to non-BV cases. Germain et al. (1994) only found a modest increase in odds ratio for intrauterine growth retardation for anaerobic bacteria, Trichomonas, Mycoplasma, and Ureaplasma (if colonized by all four groups of organisms, the relative risk for intrauterine growth restriction was 1.79). The studies of McGregor suggest that the role of BV flora may include increasing sialidase production by anaerobic species, and this enzyme may affect the integrity of the amniotic barrier, predisposing to infectious pregnancy complications.

In addition to an epidemiologic relationship of BV to obstetric and postpartum complications, its role in salpingitis risk and postoperative morbidity have been reported. Although salpingitis and related upper tract infectious processes are usually initiated by sexually transmitted pathogens, they often show evidence of upper tract invasion by cervical–vaginal organisms. The expansion of anaerobic species in patients with BV may expand the population of those organisms capable of causing serious upper tract inflammatory reaction. An expanded population of anaerobic flora may also predispose to postoperative morbidity following gynecologic surgery, although many additional factors could be in play in these, predominantly epidemiologic associations.

G. vaginalis has been occasionally listed as a cause of extragenital infections, although these are exceedingly rare. Various reports have included urinary tract isolation of *G. vaginalis*, abscesses in a male patient, and adult and neonatal bacteremias. A few reports of reactive arthritis secondary to *Gardnerella* infection have been mentioned in the literature (Francois et al., 1997; Schapira et al., 2002). Thus far, reports of extragenital *Gardnerella* seem attributable to vagaries of individual cases and serve as a reminder that virtually any microorganism, even if it is of limited virulence, can occasionally participate in infectious complications of the compromised host.

Because the topic of this chapter is *Gardnerella*, it would be appropriate to end this section by emphasizing that the complications that have been cited above have been more

linked to BV (as defined variously by multiple authors) and may only have a tangential relationship to *Gardnerella*. As will be noted in the next section, it may be useful to gauge the density of the *Gardnerella* population in the vagina, but primarily as a marker for an overall shift in the flora that may be associated with obstetrical and gynecologic risks.

DIAGNOSTIC TESTING

Because the presence of vaginal *Gardnerella* alone is not of clinical relevance, diagnostic testing for the presence of the organism is rarely employed except in the case of specific research protocols. The culture of *Gardnerella* is likewise not part of the BV diagnosis. High-density colonization with *Gardnerella* may be indicative of BV, but quantitative culture is not a practical diagnostic procedure, especially in view of the clinical and microscopic methods that have been described previously.

The primarily clinical criteria of Amsel and the primarily microbiological criteria of Nugent have both been used to identify women who have signs of BV. The clinician who seeks to help a patient with vaginal symptoms has an obligation to examine the patient, even though some physicians assert that they can diagnose vaginal conditions from a careful history by telephone. Interestingly, a recent study indicated that even with patient examination, misjudgments were made in symptomatic women. History and examination of the nature of the discharge with microscopic examination including KOH preparation can guide the physician. When candidiasis and trichomoniasis have been ruled out, attention to the characteristics of BV embodied in both the Amsel and the Nugent criteria can be brought to bear on the diagnostic evaluation, and notably, these observations can be made without a great deal of sophisticated diagnostic equipment. Physicians who frequently care for women with vaginal complaints are well served by a good microscope and familiarity with the appearance of vaginal smears both in wet mount and in Gram stain.

Not surprisingly, there is a desire to develop diagnostic methods for BV that are less subjective than clinical or microscopic examination. The elevated sialidase that can occur in cases of anaerobic overgrowth has been proposed as a diagnostic test and has even been commercialized. The commercial test (BV Blue) as been compared with Amsel and Nugent criteria and has an overall accuracy of greater than 90%. It should be remembered that broader application among different population groups may result in different degrees of accuracy than have thus far been recorded for this test. The current STD Treatment Guidelines published by the Centers for Disease Control and Prevention (CDC) state that a DNA hybridization test for high levels of *G. vaginalis* (Becton Dickinson's Affirm) may have clinical utility and that other tests now marketed (Quidel Quick Vue for triethylamine and elevated pH) or a prolineaminopeptidase card test (Quidel) might be useful for BV diagnosis.

Since BV is characterized by decreased *Lactobacillus* colonization with concomitant increases in *G. vaginalis* and anaerobic bacterial colonization, quantitative culture would seem informative, but such methods are impractical for clinical use. However, akin to quantitative culture are newer molecular methods such as quantitative real-time PCR that allow investigators the opportunity to quantitate the relative number of DNA copies of specific organisms. These techniques are not likely to supplant the straightforward clinical observations that experienced practitioners make and will certainly not be as cost effective. Nevertheless, greater use of molecular methods will undoubtedly occur in the future. A recent report by Fredricks et al. (2005) demonstrated the sensitivity and specificity of molecular-based diagnosis of BV, although many limitations exist, such as quantitating all relevant organisms, level of specificity needed (genus level or more specific identification), and cut-off points for significant levels of organisms.

Perhaps the more interesting area of molecular characterization is the discovery of the possible involvement of previously unknown species of microbes—some of which are not easily cultivated—in vaginal samples of healthy women and those with BV. The work of Hyman et al. (2005) used amplification and sequencing of 16s ribosomal RNA genes and found that both *Lactobacillus* and *Gardnerella* could predominate in the flora of healthy women, as could *Bifidobacterium*, *Prevotella*, *Pseudomonas*, and *Streptococcus*. New molecular methods applied to the vaginal flora have been responsible for the discovery that organisms such as *Atopobium* may be a dominant normal flora organism and that hitherto unrecognized and difficult-to-culture organisms may play a role in the flora and in BV.

There may be a cautionary tale in the recent history of vaginal flora, now being rewritten by molecular identification of bacteria. The emphasis on *G. vaginalis* has created a vast literature in which this particular organism seems to play an important role, but does not by itself represent the sole player in a clinical condition that many have tried to understand as an infection, but which probably should not be categorized as such. Moreover, it seems that we are now on the verge of discovering other interesting microbial players in vaginal colonization and vaginal dysbiosis.

THERAPEUTIC CONSIDERATIONS

As this chapter has tried to emphasize, *G. vaginalis* is not often an etiology of an infectious disease. Its involvement in BV has led antimicrobial treatment of the condition to focus on *Gardnerella*. Treatment is appropriately offered to women who have symptoms related to BV, but much more controversial is the altered flora that can be identified by Nugent score, but in which the patient is not sufficiently symptomatic to seek treatment. Because of the related conditions for which BV has been named a risk factor (premature delivery, postpartum endometritis, postsurgical morbidity), patients who show signs of BV may be candidates for treatment. The American College of Obstetricians and Gynecologists guidelines for prematurity indicate that screening for BV has not been demonstrated to be of predictive value in prematurity. The CDC states that because of the possible sequelae related to BV, including its asymptomatic form, physicians should "consider evaluation and treatment of high-risk pregnant women with asymptomatic BV."

Treatment of vaginal conditions such as BV can be approached with systemic or topical therapy, with their individual attendant advantages and disadvantages. The latest STD Treatment Guidelines from the CDC outline major options. These include a seven-day course of oral metronidazole (500 mg twice daily), metronidazole intravaginal gel (five days), or clindamycin cream (seven days). Clindamycin is contraindicated in the second half of pregnancy.

The lack of high levels of *Lactobacillus* in the vaginal environment suggests that a probiotic approach to BV may be appropriate in the future, using probiotic bacteria either to supplant the high numbers of BV-related organisms or as an inoculum to repopulate the vagina after antimicrobial therapy. This remains an active area of research and reviews are available elsewhere.

SELECTED READING

Agostini A, Beerli M, Franchi F, Bretelle F, Blanc B. Garnerella vaginalis basteremia after vaginal myomectomy. Eur J Obstet Gynecol 2003; 108:229.

Amaya RA, Al-Dossary F, Demmler GJ. J Perinatol 2002; 22:585.

Amsel R, Totten P, Spiegel C, Chen K, Eschenbach D, Holmes K. Nonspecific vaginitis: diagnostic criteria and epidemiologic associations. Am J Med 1983; 74:14.

Andrews WW, Goldenberg RL, Faye-Petersen O, Cliver S, Goepfert AR, Hauth JC. The Alabama Preterm Birth study: polymorphonuclear and mononuclear cell placental infiltrations, other markers of inflammation, and outcomes in 23- to 32-week preterm newborn infants. Am J Obstet Gynecol 2006; 195:803.

Bradshaw CS, Tabrizi SN, Fairley CK, Morton AN, Rudland E, Garland SM. The association of *Atopobium vaginae* and *Gardnerella vaginalis* with bacterial vaginosis and recurrence after oral metronidazole therapy. J Infect Dis 2006; 194:828.

Calvert LD, Collins M, Bateman JR. Multiple abscesses caused by *Gardnerella vaginalis* in an immunocompetent man. J Infect 2005; 51:E27.

Catalnotti P, Rossano F, de Paolis P, Baroni A, Buttini G, Tufano MA. Effects of *Cetyltrimethylammonium naproxenate* on the adherence of *Gardnerella vaginalis*, *Mobiluncus curtisii*, and *Lactobacillus acidophilus* to vaginal epithelial cells. Sex Transm Dis 1994; 21:338.

Cauci S, Driussi S, Monte R, Lanzafame P, Pitzus E, Quadrifoglio F. Immunoglobulin A response against *Gardnerella vaginalis* hemolysin and sialidase activity in bacterial vaginosis. Am J Obstet Gynecol 1998; 178:511.

Chaijareenont K, Sirimai K, Boriboonhirunsarn D, Kiriwat O. Accuracy of Nugent's score and each Amsel's criteria diagnosis of bacterial vaginosis. J Med Assoc Thai 2004; 87:1270.

Donders GG. Lower genital tract infections in diabetic women. Curr Infect Dis Rep 2002; 4:536.

Falagas ME, Betsi GI, Athanasiou S. Probiotics for prevention of recurrent vulvovaginal candidasis: a review. J Antimicrob Chemother 2006; 58:266.

Francois S, Guyadier-Souguieres G, Marcelli C. Reactive arthritis due to *Gardnerella vaginalis*. Rev Rhum Engl Ed 1997; 64:138.

Fredricks DN, Fiedler TL, Marrazzo JM. Molecular identification of bacteria associated with bacterial vaginosis. N Engl J Med 2005; 353:1899.

Fredricks DN, Marrazzo JM. Molecular methodology in determining vaginal flora in health and disease: its time has come. Curr Infect Dis Rep 2005; 7:463.

Gardner H, Dukes C. *Haemophilus vaginalis* vaginitis. Am J Obstet Gynecol 1955; 69:962.

Germain M, Krohn MA, Hillier SL, Eschenbach DA. Genital flora in pregnancy and its association with intrauterine growth retardation. J Clin Microbiol 1994; 32:2162.

Greenwood J, Pickett M. Transfer of *Haemophilus vaginalis* to a new genus, Gardnerella: *G. vaginalis* (Gardner and Dukes) comb nov. Int J Syst Bact 1980; 30:170.

Hillier SL, Martius J, Krohn M, Kiviat N, Holmes KK, Eschenbach DA. A case–control study of chorioamnionic infection and histologic chorioamnionitis in prematurity. N Engl J Med 1988; 319:972.

Hyman R, Fukushima M, Diamond L, Kumm J, Giudice L, Davis R. Microbes on the human vaginal epithelium. Proc Nat Acad Sci 2005; 22:7952.

Kerk J, Dordelmann M, Bartels D, et al. Multiplex measurement of cytokine/receptor gene polymorphisms and interaction between interleukin-10 (-1082) genotype and chorioamnionitis in extreme preterm delivery. Soc Gynecol Investig 2006; 13:350.

Krohn MA, Hillier SL, Nugent RP, et al. The genital flora of women with intraamniotic infection. Vaginal infections and prematurity study group. J Infect Disc 1995; 171:1475.

McGregor JA, French JI, Jones W, et al. Bacterial vaginosis is associated with prematurity and vaginal fluid mucinase and sialidase: results of a controlled trial of topical clindamyclin cream. Am J Obstet Gynecol 1994; 170:1048.

Myziuk L, Romanowski B, Johnson S. BVBlue test for diagnosis of bacterial vaginosis. J Clin Microbiol 2003; 41:1925.

Nugent R, Krohn M, Hillier S. Reliability of diagnosing bacterial vaginosis is improved by a standardized method of Gram stain interpretation. J Clin Microbiol 1991; 29:297.

Reid G, Kim SO, Kohler GA. Selecting, testing and understanding probiotic microorganisms. FEMS Immuno Med Microbiol 2006; 46:149.

Sha BE, Chen HY, Wang QJ, Zariffard MR, Cohen MH, Spear GT. Utility of Amsel criteria, Nugent score, and quantitative PCR for *Gardnerella vaginalis*, *Mycoplasma hominis*, and *Lactobacillus* spp. for diagnosis of bacterial vaginosis in human immunodeficiency virus-infected women. J Clin Microbiol 2005; 43:4607.

Schapira D, Braun-Moscovici Y, Nahir AM. Reactive arthritis induced by *Gardnerella vaginalis*. Clin Exp Rheumatol 2002; 20:732.

Schweirtz A, Taras D, Rusch K, Rusch V. Throwing the dice for the dignosis of vaginal complaints? Ann Clin Microbiol Antimicrob 2006; 5:4.

Shubair M, Snyder I, Larsen B. *Gardnerella vaginalis* hemolysin. I. Production and purification. Immun Infect Dis 1993; 3:135.

Sumeksri P, Koprasert C, Panichkul S. BVBLUE test for diagnosis of bacterial vaginosis in pregnant women attending antenatal care at Phramongkutklao Hospital. J Med Assoc Thai 2005; 3:S7.

Swindsinski A, Mendling W, Loening-Baucke V, et al. Adherent biofilms in bacterial vaginosis. Obstet Gynecol 2005; 106:1013.

Watts DH, Krohn MA, Hillier SL, Eschenbach DA. Bacterial vaginosis as a risk factor for post-cesarean endometritis. Obstet Gynecol 1990; 75:52.

Zhou X, Bent S, Schneider M, Davis C, Islam M. Characterization of vaginal microbial communities in adult healthy women using cultivation-independent methods. Microbiology 2004; 150:2565.

INTRODUCTION

Like *Escherichia coli*, *Klebsiella* and *Enterobacter* belong to the family Enterobacteriaceae, but are grouped under the tribe Klebsiellae. They are colonizers of the human gastrointestinal tract.

KLEBSIELLA

On Gram stains, *Klebsiella* appears as a large, gram-negative rod. Owing to its prominent polysaccharide capsule, it forms large mucoid colonies on agar media. Serotyping is done using predominantly the K capsular antigen. More than 70 K types have been identified. Although the capsule is an important virulence factor in preventing phagocytosis and helping to retard leukocyte migration, no specific K type is more pathogenic than another. Like most Enterobacteriaceae, *Klebsiella* produces endotoxin. The predominant species within obstetrics and gynecology is *Klebsiella pneumoniae*. Other species tend to be lumped together and reported just as *Klebsiella* species.

Clinical Manifestations

As a monoetiological pathogen in obstetrics and gynecology, *K. pneumoniae* functions as an important agent in urinary tract infection, chorioamnionitis, perinatal septicemia, and endometritis. When the organism functions as part of the anaerobic progression, it may be a constituent of a polymicrobial endomyometritis or the lead organism in a ruptured tubo-ovarian complex.

The incidence of disease is approximately 1/10 that due to *E. coli*. Clinically, disease due to *Klebsiella* species is identical to that described for *E. coli*.

Therapy

The *Klebsiella* are almost invariably resistant to all the penicillins. The antibiotics of choice for the *Klebsiella* are the cephalosporins, in particular the third-generation cephalosporins and the aminoglycosides.

ENTEROBACTER

Enterobacter consists primarily of *E. aerogenes*, *E. cloacae*, and *E. agglomerans*. Unlike *Klebsiella*, *Enterobacter* organisms are motile and tend to be less heavily encapsulated. They do not produce H_2S on triple sugar iron medium, are indole negative and methyl red negative, use citrate as the sole carbon source, and can ferment lactose. Simplified tests for decarboxylation of the diamino acids lysine, arginine, and ornithine differentiate *E. cloacae*, *E. aerogenes*, *E. agglomerans*, and *K. pneumoniae*.

The pathogenic spectrum is comparable to that described for *Klebsiella*. Their disease prevalence is 1/10 that observed

with *Klebsiella*, but it is of greater clinical significance, owing to their resistance to many of the penicillins and to all first-generation cephalosporins and some of the second- and third-generation cephalosporins. This lack of susceptibility to the commonly used antibiotics in obstetrics and gynecology underlines the importance of this group of bacteria.

Clinical Manifestations

E. cloacae, along with *E. agglomerans*, is a significant cause of hospital-acquired infections. These organisms are capable of horizontal spread in the hospital environment and, like many opportunistic Enterobacteriaceae, are spread through the hands of hospital personnel.

The three clinical areas in which the *Enterobacter* function as significant pathogens in obstetrics and gynecology are the following:

1. Nosocomial infections
2. Urinary tract infection
3. Maternal and perinatal septicemia/meningitis

E. cloacae is the species most frequently associated with nosocomial infections. Within a hospital setting, *Enterobacter* organisms can establish widespread colonization of patients, and as such, they represent an ongoing threat by a multiresistant bacteria to a vulnerable patient population.

The association of *Enterobacter* with contaminated intravenous fluids is somewhat predictable considering its aquatic lineage. *Enterobacter* species as the sole pathogen in the majority of blood cultures should suggest the possibility of parenteral introduction of *Enterobacter*-contaminated fluid or the presence of significant urinary tract infection.

Although all *Enterobacter* species are capable of causing disease, the three primary nosocomial pathogens are *E. aerogenes*, *E. cloacae*, and *E. agglomerans*.

The *Enterobacter* produce a spectrum of infection and/or disease of the genitourinary tract that is very similar to that induced by *E. coli*. The *Enterobacter* are the etiological agents for approximately 1% of the cases of asymptomatic bacteriuria, but 5% of the cases of pyelonephritis. This discrepancy is due to prior failure to eradicate identified asymptomatic bacteriuria. Most of the antibiotics used to treat urinary tract infection are ineffective against *Enterobacter* species.

Asymptomatic bacteriuria provides a reservoir of gram-negative aerobic bacteria of increased virulence within the vaginal flora. With prolonged rupture of the fetal membranes, the nephrogenic strains of *Enterobacter* ascend into the amniotic cavity from where they may induce chorioamnionitis, maternal septicemia, and/or perinatal septicemia. A woman with asymptomatic bacteriuria due to the Enterobacteriaceae has an eightfold increased probability of endometritis following vaginal delivery.

Therapy

The first-generation cephalosporins classically have little or no inherent anti-*Enterobacter* activity. Antimicrobials that have a high degree of activity against the *Enterobacter* are the third-generation cephalosporins, the fluoroquinolones, and the aminoglycosides. As in the case with *Klebsiella*, there have been increasing reports of aminoglycoside-resistant *Enterobacter* strains from across the country. In such situations, amikacin has remained the preferred aminoglycoside.

In the treatment of uncomplicated urinary tract bacteriuria, the carboxy penicillins and nalidixic acid are active against most *Enterobacter* species. Nitrofurantoin is reliable only against *E. agglomerans*.

SELECTED READING

Brenner DJ, Farmer JS III, Hickman FW, et al. Taxonomic and Nomenclature Changes in Enterobacteriaceae. Atlanta, GA: Centers for Disease Control, 1977.

Felts SK, Schaffner W, Melly MA, et al. Sepsis caused by contaminated intravenous fluids. Ann Intern Med 1972; 77:881–890.

Moellering RC, Wennersten C, Kunz LJ, et al. Resistance to gentamicin, tobramycin, and amikacin among clinical isolates of bacteria. Am J Med 1977; 62:873–881.

Toala P, Lee YH, Wilcox C, et al. Susceptibility of *Enterobacter aerogenes* and *Enterobacter cloacae* to 19 antimicrobial agents *in vitro*. Am J Med Sci 1970; 260:41–54.

Mobiluncus

Bryan Larsen

This curved, anaerobic, motile, rod-shaped gram-negative organism is primarily found in the vagina of women with bacterial vaginosis, although due to its refractoriness to cultivation on artificial media, it may be present in the vaginal flora in low concentrations more often than available reports indicate. Most reports in the literature report on the presence of *Mobiluncus* through Gram-stained vaginal smears (*Mobiluncus curtisii* being described as short, curved rods and *Mobiluncus mulieris* is described as long, curved rods), although it must be noted that the identification of an organism to the genus level is not technically possible with Gram stain only. Moreover, identification of the organism by Gram stain requires a certain degree of skill on the part of the microscopist; and such skill is not universally honed by the majority of gynecologists. This caveat must be applied to much of the information currently available on the organism that has observations based solely on microscopy.

Mobiluncus was originally described by Spiegel and Roberts (1984) and was divided into two species, *M. curtisii* and *M. mulieris*, with the former species subdivided into subspecies of *curtisii* and *holmsii*. Contemporary molecular methods have allowed taxonomists the opportunity to divide groups of organisms into species on the basis of sequence relatedness of DNA, particularly the sequences related to the 16s ribosomal genes. This has led to the conclusion that there should be two species, *curtisii* and *mulieris*, but that the subspecies designation for *M. curtisii* was not supported (Tiveljung et al., 1996). Despite this current level of taxonomic clarity, it is not apparent that there is any clinical significance to the difference in species.

Although the majority of the limited literature on *Mobiluncus* clearly presents it as a vaginal microbe, there are reports of its occurrence in other locations such as the rectum (Hallen et al., 1998) of women vaginally colonized by *Mobiluncus* (generally the same species as in the vagina) and has been reported as occurring in a breast abscess (Sturm, 1989), although its role as a solitary primary pathogen will probably require substantial additional corroborating information. Given its regular occurrence along with the vaginal flora, especially when the anaerobic population has expanded in cases of bacterial vaginosis, one may anticipate that reports in the future will find that this organism can be found in polymicrobial infections arising from the flora of the lower female genital tract. Such an as yet unproven role suggests that future studies that seek to characterize all microbial players in mixed anaerobic infections should make an effort to find *Mobiluncus* species among the other, more easily cultivated organisms.

As previously alluded to, most standard approaches to the analysis of the normal vaginal flora will meet with difficulty in cultivating this organism. Attempts have been made to develop media particularly suited to the growth of *Mobiluncus*, and in 2002, Taylor-Robinson and Taylor-Robinson reported that variable growth could be obtained in Columbia blood broth or peptone starch dextrose broth, each supplemented with horse serum. Their goal was not to enhance primary isolation, but rather to provide a medium that could be used to study antigens and toxins of this fastidious genus. Primary culture may be enhanced by using the method of Smith and Moore (1988), which employs specialized enriched media with antibiotic supplements coupled with a cold enrichment method that apparently diminishes the metabolism of the more rapidly growing flora and allows the *Mobiluncus* spp. an opportunity to compete among more abundant members of the polymicrobial environment.

In its most common context, *Mobiluncus* appears to be one of the many microorganisms that participate in the dysbiosis that is commonly referred to as bacterial vaginosis. Bacterial vaginosis is a concept that has developed a very large volume of literature since the original attempt of Gardner and Dukes (1955) to associate it with a specific etiologic agent. The complex history of the development of our current understanding of this condition will not be recited here, but most experts are generally agreed that bacterial vaginosis is an altered state of the lower genital tract flora characterized by a decreased quantity of lactobacilli with a concomitant increased abundance of anaerobic flora and *Gardnerella vaginalis*. Other clinical features include the presence of amine (fishy) odor in the vaginal secretion after alkalinization with KOH and the microscopic appearance of clue cells. These characteristics are mentioned here because two methods of scoring these clinical observations have been developed and these depend on either microscopy alone (Nugent et al., 1991) or microscopy combined with other clinical observations (Amsel et al., 1983).

Whenever Gram staining of the discharge from women with bacterial vaginosis is performed, there is a possibility that the skilled observer might find curved gram-negative rods among other bacteria in the smear. Thus, particularly when the 10-point Nugent scoring system is in use, the observer is required to search for curved rods and award points for the presence of *Mobiluncus*-like morphotypes. This scoring system considers scores of 3 or less to be associated with normal flora, scores of 4 to 6 as intermediate, and scores of 7 or greater as bacterial vaginosis. Because a score is given for curved gram-negative rods, those individuals with scores of 9 or 10 have to contain curved rods in their smears.

Thus, even if a publication reports only Nugent scores and not the prevalence of the factors that led to the score, it is possible to at least ascertain the minimum number of women in these studies whose smears were positive for curved rods. This said, it appears that elevated numbers of *Gardnerella* and gram-negative rods are most frequently contributors to Nugent scores consistent with bacterial vaginosis, and the curved rods consistent with *Mobiluncus* may or may not be present along with other microscopic and clinical qualities ascribed to bacterial vaginosis.

Establishing the importance of *Mobiluncus* independent of bacterial vaginosis is probably not feasible with our current level of knowledge. It is clear that bacterial vaginosis often, and perhaps usually, occurs without the presence of *Mobiluncus*. Smith and Moore (1988) obtained cultures from 201 women, and although their work involved changing methods during their research to maximize the recovery of *Mobiluncus*, only 24 positives were found. In the original Nugent et al. paper (1991), it appeared that fewer than one quarter of bacterial vaginosis cases had curved rods. DeLaney and Onderdonk (2001) reported that among pregnant patients they studied, approximately 25% had Gram stains (Nugent criteria) consistent with intermediate flora or bacterial vaginosis flora, and only 11/14 patients had Nugent scores of 7 or above, indicating that *Mobiluncus*-positive bacterial vaginosis was below 10% prevalence. Among the most useful recent studies that offer information regarding the prevalence of *Mobiluncus* in the lower female genital tract is the multicenter (three hospitals) study involving 1805 pregnant women (Culhane et al., 2006). The investigators noted that 44% had Nugent scores of 7 to 10, which was considered consistent with bacterial vaginosis. A subset of this population (265 vaginal smears from first prenatal visits) was evaluated more closely and stratified into *Mobiluncus*-positive (43%) and *Mobiluncus*-negative cases. They also noted that 97% of women concomitantly having bacterial vaginosis and *Mobiluncus* morphotypes had Nugent scores of 9 or 10. Although these numbers cannot be extrapolated to all populations, the study of Culhane et al. (2006), which was performed in the United States, suggests that *Mobiluncus* may be observed in about 18% of pregnant women.

While microscopic methods suggest that *Mobiluncus* may be present in one or two in five women with bacterial vaginosis, other methods have been employed to estimate the prevalence and significance of this organism independent of bacterial vaginosis. Schwebke et al. (1996) found a 75% prevalence of antibody against *M. mulieris* in the sera of pregnant women, but this finding did not correlate with a history of bacterial vaginosis. The authors concluded that this may have been related to a prior contact with the *Mobiluncus* organism (nonsexually active females did not have antibody) rather than current invasion by *Mobiluncus*. It must also be noted that studies such as that of Culhane et al. (2006) mentioned that among their subjects who had bacterial vaginosis by Nugent scores of 7 to 10, only 30% of their medical records indicated that their primary physician had noted bacterial vaginosis in their charts, suggesting that what researchers refer to as bacterial vaginosis may

not be as aggressively sought as a diagnosis in practices not engaged in research. In addition, it is possible that a substantial percentage of women may have had bacterial vaginosis without their physicians using that term, leading to a faulty history upon later inquiry. Together, these observations may indicate that a majority of sexually active women may encounter *Mobiluncus* some time during their reproductive years, but such encounters rarely lead to symptoms that lead to a clinic visit and diagnosis of bacterial vaginosis.

A more contemporary approach to assessing the presence of difficult-to-culture organisms in the lower female genital tract is DNA-based methods such as polymerase chain reaction (PCR). This technique can be used to amplify known sequences from specific organisms, including *Mobiluncus*. In a study reported by Obata-Yasuoka et al. (2002), a multiplex PCR technique (i.e., a PCR reaction that is able to amplify specific sequences from more than one species of microorganism in the same reaction) for several bacterial vaginosis–related organisms showed that 22% of bacterial vaginosis patients had positive reactions for *Mobiluncus*, although these same individuals had positive reactions for other organisms as well. Again, this report further corroborates the case for *Mobiluncus* being one of many species of microorganisms that increases in abundance in the event of lactobacillus colonization undergoing a decline.

Although the presence of *Mobiluncus* cannot be taken as a *sine qua non* of bacterial vaginosis, it does raise the question of whether bacterial vaginosis with *Mobiluncus* (M + BV) is different in some empirically demonstrable way compared to bacterial vaginosis without *Mobiluncus* (M − BV). This question is especially important, since there is little evidence to support pathogenic activity of *Mobiluncus* independent of other microorganisms in a polymicrobial environment. Culhane et al. (2006) have noted that with respect to a broad range of inflammatory indicators, the presence or absence of *Mobiluncus* in bacterial vaginosis patients was associated with differences in sialidase activity, with a higher level of this enzyme in M + BV than among M − BV patients. Higher levels of Il-1β and Il-8 were also noted in M + BV, but when the data were reevaluated with *Trichomonas vaginalis* coinfected patients removed from analysis, only sialidase remained as significantly higher in M + BV compared to M − BV.

The importance of sialidase in the lower female genital tract was suggested in the work of McGregor et al. (1994) and further investigated by Cauci et al. (2005), who found that both prolidase and sialidase elevations in the presence of vaginal pH of 5 or greater was associated with an increased risk of premature birth or low birthweight. Sialidase, or neuraminidase, is not known to be produced by *Mobiluncus*, or if it is, it is not necessarily produced solely by *Mobiluncus*. Most references indicate that sialidase is elevated in bacterial vaginosis cases, but this does not indicate which organism(s) are individually responsible for the elevation of this enzyme. Two studies of cultured *M. curtisii* and *M. mulieris* (Briselden et al., 1992; Puapermpoonsiri et al., 1996) failed to show the production of neuraminidase. These investigators, however, did not use precisely the same substrate as that employed in the initial study of McGregor (1994), and it is also possible that some strains of *Mobiluncus* are producers of sialidase while others are not. It may also be that *Mobiluncus* is able to produce sialidase in vivo, but not in an artificial medium. Despite these unanswered questions, a commercial sialidase test kit has been developed as an indicator of bacterial vaginosis (Myziuk et al., 2003).

The concept that *Mobiluncus* may somehow exacerbate adverse sequelae of bacterial vaginosis, particularly those ill-defined factors that related to premature birth or low birth weight, has been espoused by Hauth et al. (2003), who indicate that pregnant women with Nugent scores of 9 and 10 which, as noted earlier in this chapter, require that curved rods are observed on Gram stain, are more prone to premature delivery compared to women with scores of 7 and 8. There has been a long-standing recognition that among African-Americans, the rate of low birth weight and prematurity is significantly greater than among Caucasians (Ness et al., 2003), and although this may be partially related to a racial disparity in bacterial vaginosis itself, the study of Culhane et al. (2006) found a significantly higher rate of M + BV among women of black race compared to white women. This is consistent with a potential synergistic effect of *Mobiluncus* in bacterial vaginosis on prematurity and low birth weight, although it is insufficient evidence to establish the unique pathogenicity of the organism.

Some preliminary studies of the potential virulence attributes of *Mobiluncus* have been conducted. Taylor-Robinson et al. (1993) demonstrated the presence of an extracellular cytotoxin in spent liquid cultures of *Mobiluncus*. Necrotic damage to several cell lines were noted within three days of exposure of the cell lines to the toxin. Limited characterization of the properties of the toxin were reported. In a study that sought to evaluate the phagocytosis of two *Mobiluncus* species by human leukocytes in human serum, Moi et al. (1991) showed that chemiluminescence, an indicator of oxidative metabolism that is upregulated secondary to phagocytosis of the bacterium, was greater for *M. curtisii* than for *M. mulieris*, suggesting that the latter was less well phagocytized and hence may be considered more virulent with respect to phagocytic cell clearance. These studies were in accord with previous observations that suggested *M. mulieris* may be more aggressive and more likely to cause infection beyond the lower female genital tract. Nevertheless, these studies must be considered extremely preliminary, and methods for the evaluation of microbial virulence have advanced substantially since these studies were performed, making it appropriate to revisit the question of what virulence attributes are possessed by *Mobiluncus*.

In further characterizing the role of *Mobiluncus* as a contributor to bacterial vaginosis, it is important to realize that while bacterial vaginosis has been described in many geographical areas, ethnic or racial groups, the epidemiology of *Mobiluncus* is less well characterized. Bacterial vaginosis with *Mobiluncus* colonization was found to be more common among pregnant women over the age of 21 and among non-Hispanic black women in the large study of Pereira et al. (2005) than was bacterial vaginosis without *Mobiluncus*. Tolosa et al. (2002) noted that nearly four in five women from their study in Bogota, Columbia, were M + BV, whereas in Dublin, Ireland, none had M + BV. This again underscores the fact that the complex microflora dysbiosis described as bacterial vaginosis may occur without the presence of *Mobiluncus*, but the same researchers found that when *Mobiluncus* was present, patients were more likely to have clue cells and a positive "whiff test" for amines.

If research continues to establish a special role for *Mobiluncus* that will require offering therapy to those colonized and symptomatic, it will be important to understand the patterns of antibiotic susceptibility among clinical isolates of the species currently known. Spiegel (1987) evaluated the susceptibility of 22 *Mobiluncus* representing both species. Notable in her findings was the resistance of all *M. curtisii* strains and half of *M. mulieris* strains to metronidazole. However, clindamycin and beta-lactams showed more comprehensive inhibitory activity to her collection of strains. A Cochrane review (Okun et al., 2005) did not find evidence to support the use of bacterial vaginosis diagnosis, and treatment was not effective in reducing prematurity. This is essentially in consonance with the findings of the large national vaginal infections and prematurity study (Carey et al., 2000) in which metronidazole treatment was used to try to interdict prematurity and.

In summary, the curved rods that may be seen in Gram-stained smears by experienced observers, present in one-quarter to one-half of individuals with bacterial vaginosis, may represent a subset of bacterial vaginosis cases in which clinical indicators of the condition are somewhat more prominent, and adverse outcomes of pregnancy may be more likely and disproportionately found among non-Hispanic black women and among those who are above the age of 21. However, at present, the organism has not been recognized as a pathogen in its own right, but rather as one of many contributors to a disordered flora that may occur with or without symptoms recognized by the patient. Further research will be needed to delineate the specific and unique role of these organisms, but thus far, we have not found the evidence to suggest that this organism must be identified and treated separately from treatment for the underlying bacterial vaginosis. Successful approaches to vaginal dysbiosis may lie in rebalancing the flora in contradistinction to finding microbes to kill. Clinicians must anticipate that recommendations may change as further research attention is focused on this organism, as there are hints in the literature that suggest that this organism could be a marker for a subset of bacterial vaginosis cases that are more difficult to treat, but are more likely to be associated with adverse pregnancy outcomes. Further underscoring the importance of the continued development of our knowledge is the recognition that we may not yet be aware of all of the microbial participants in bacterial vaginosis. Recently, *Atopobium vaginae* was found to be present in some women with bacterial vaginosis, and our understanding of its role is even more rudimentary than our understanding of *Mobiluncus* and may remain that way for quite some time (Ferris et al., 2004).

REFERENCES

Amsel R, Totten PA, Spiegel CA, Chen KC, Eschenbach D, Holmes KK. Nonspecific vaginitis. Diagnostic criteria and microbial and epidemiologic associations. Am J Med 1983; 74:14.

Briselden AM, Moncla BJ, Stevens CE, et al. Sialidases (neuraminidases) in bacterial vaginosis-associated microflora. J Clin Micro 1992; 30:663.

Carey CJ, Klebanoff MA, Hauth JC, et al. National Institute of Child Health and Human Development Network of Maternal Fetal Medicine Units. Metronidazole to prevent preterm delivery in pregnant women with asymptomatic bacterial vaginosis. N Engl J Med 2000; 342:534.

Cauci S, McGregor J, Thorsen P, Grove J, Guaschino S. Combination of vaginal pH with vaginal sialidase and prolidase activities for prediction of low birth weight and preterm birth. Am J Obstet Gynecol 2005; 192:489.

Culhane JF, Nyirjesy P, McCollum K, Goldenberg RI, Gelber SE, Cauci S. Variation in vaginal immune parameters and microbial hydrolytic enzymes in bacterial vaginosis positive pregnant women with and without *Mobiluncus* species. Am J Obstet Gynecol 2006; 195:516.

Delaney ML, Onderdonk AB. Nugent score related to vaginal culture in pregnant women. Obstet Gynecol 2001; 98:79.

Ferris MJ, Masztal A, Aldridge KE, Fortenberry JD, Fidel PL Jr, Martin DH. Association of *Atopobium vaginae*, a recently described metronidazole resistant anaerobe, with bacterial vaginosis. BMC Infectious Diseases 2004; 4 (open access: online:http://www.biomedcentral.com/1471–2334/4/5).

Gardner HL, Dukes, CD. Haemophilus vaginalis vaginitis: a newly defined specific infection previously classified non-specific vaginitis. Am J Obstet Gynecol 1955; 69:962.

Hallen A, Pahlson C, Forsum U. Rectal occurrence of Mobiluncus species. Genitourin Med 1998; 64:273.

Hauth JC, MacPherson C, Carey C, et al. National Institute of Child Health and Human Development Maternal Fetal Medicine Units Network. Early pregnancy threshold vaginal pH and gram stain scores predictive of subsequent preterm birth in asymptomatic women. Am J Obstet Gynecol 2003; 188:831.

McGregor JA, French JI, Jones W, et al. Bacterial vaginosis is associated with prematurity and vaginal fluid mucinase and sialidase: results of a controlled trial of topical clindamycin cream. Am J Obstet Gynecol 1994; 170:1048.

Moi H, Fredlund H, Tornqvist E, Danielsson D. Mobiluncus species in bacterial vaginosis: aspects of pathogenesis. APMIS 1991; 99:1049.

Myziuk L, Romanowski B, Johnson SC. BVBlue test for diagnosis of bacterial vaginosis. J Clin Microbiol 2003; 41:1925.

Ness RB, Hillier S, Richter HE, et al. Can known risk factors explain racial differences in the occurrence of bacterial vaginosis? J Natl Med Assoc 2003; 95:201.

Nugent RP, Krohn MA, Hillier SL. Reliability of diagnosing bacterial vaginosis is improved by a standardized method of gram stain interpretation. J Clin Microbiol 1991; 29:297.

Obata-Yasuoka M, Ba-Thien W, Hamada H, Hayashi H. A multiplex polymerase chain reaction-based diagnostic method for bacterial vaginosis. Obstet Gynecol 2002; 100:759.

Okun N, Gronau KA, Hannah ME. Antibiotics for bacterial vaginosis or *Trichomonas vaginalis* in pregnancy: a systematic review. Obstet Gynecol 2005; 105:857.

Pereira L, Culhane J, McCullum K, Agnew K, Nyirjesy P. Variation in the microbiologic profiles in pregnant women with bacterial vaginosis. Am J Obstet Gynecol 2005; 193:746.

Puapermpoonsiri S, Kato N, Watanabe K, et al. Vaginal microflora associated with bacterial vaginosis in Japanese and Thai pregnant women. Clin Infect Dis 1996; 23:748.

Schwebke JR, Morgan SC, Hillier SL. Humoral antibody to *Mobiluncus curtisii*, a potential serological marker for bacterial vaginosis. Clin Diagn Lab Immunol 1996; 3:567.

Smith HJ, Moore HB. Isolation of *Mobiluncus* species from clinical specimens by cold enrichment and selective medium. J Clin Microbiol 1988; 26:1134.

Spiegel CA. Susceptibility of *Mobiluncus* species to 23 antimicrobial agents and 15 other compounds. Antimicrob Agents Chemother 1987; 31:249.

Spiegel CA, Roberts M. *Mobiluncus* gen nov, *Mobiluncus curtisii* subsp *curtisii* sp nov *Mobiluncus curtisii* subsp *holmsii* subsp nov and *Mobiluncus mulieris* sp nov, curved rods from the human vagina. Int J Syst Bacteriol 1984; 34:177.

Sturm AW. Mobiluncus species and other anaerobic bacteria in non-puerperal breast abscesses. Eur J Clin Microbiol Infect Dis 1989; 8:789.

Taylor-Robinson AW, Taylor-Robinson D. Evaluation of liquid culture medium to support the growth of Mobiluncus species. J Med Microbiol 2002; 51:491.

Taylor-Robinson AW, Borriello SP, Taylor-Robinson D. Identification and preliminary characterization of a cytotoxin isolated from Mobiluncus spp. Int J Exp Pathol 1993; 74:357.

Tiveljung A, Forsum U, Monstein H-J. Classification of the genus Mobiluncus based on comparative partial 16S rRNA gene analysis. Int J Systematic Bacteriol 1996; 46:332.

Tolosa J, Whitney C, Lyons MD, Andrews W, Win M. Worldwide variation in the prevalence of asymptomatic bacterial vaginosis in pregnancy. 50th Annual Meeting of the American College of Obstetrician Gynecologists. Obstet Gynecol 2002; 99.

Peptostreptococci

INTRODUCTION

In 1893, Veillon first described what is today recognized as the anaerobic *Streptococcus*. He recovered a strictly anaerobic *Streptococcus*, which he called *Micrococcus foetidus*, from a case of suppurative bartholinitis. The anaerobic streptococci are gram-positive cocci that grow in chains, clumps, pairs, or even tetrads. Because of the extent of heterogeneity within the group, there is no characteristic pattern of fermentation. With the exception of the microaerophilic group, the peptostreptococci do not produce beta-hemolysis. Because of their proteolytic properties, the bacteria often produce large amounts of hydrogen sulfide from sulfur-containing amino acids, resulting in a putrefactive odor. Taxonomically, the peptostreptococci and the peptococci have recently been grouped together under the peptostreptococci. Because of the similarity of their pathogenic spectrum, the clinical distinctions between the two had never been sharply delineated. Morphologically, the peptococci are distinct from the peptostreptococci and are more properly thought of as the anaerobic staphylococci. They are larger than the peptostreptococci and, rather than aggregating in chains, tend to form clusters similar to their more aerobic counterparts.

FEMALE GENITAL TRACT INVOLVEMENT

The peptostreptococci constitute part of the natural flora of humans. The presence of these organisms within the vaginal and alimentary tracts readily favors their conversion from commensal organisms to opportunistic pathogens. The peptostreptococci have been implicated in many infections, including chronic ulcers, the anaerobic form of gangrene, pelvic abscesses, septic abortion, pyogenic liver abscesses, septicemia, urinary tract infection, and subacute bacterial endocarditis. However, the disease entities affecting the female genital tract are often examples of synergistic bacterial growth. In its original definition by Meleney, bacterial synergism was described as not being a phenomenon in which one organism initiates a process and another takes over, but rather one in which there is a necessity for organisms to grow together intimately, implying the cross-utilization of intermediary products of metabolism. In obstetrics and gynecology, peptostreptococcal infections that deserve special attention include endometritis and septicemia, and progressive synergistic bacterial gangrene.

Endometritis and Septicemia

In as early as 1910, peptostreptococci had been isolated from cases of puerperal sepsis. The prerequisite for infection is a low oxidation–reduction potential, such as that provided by grossly traumatized or devitalized tissue. Not infrequently, a synergistic relationship exists with either *Gardnerella vaginalis* or the Bacteroidaceae. The *G. vaginalis*–peptostreptococci coinfection occurs more frequently in obstetric patients, whereas the *Bacteroides*–peptostreptococci are more common synergistic pathogens in gynecologic patients. Given the conditions permitting anaerobic growth, the initial infection is endometritis. The signs of infection include a foul-smelling lochia that is usually followed by pyrexia. If infection is the consequence of retained septic products of conception, the process spreads through the partially thrombosed sinuses at the placental site and gains access to uterine and ovarian veins. The process may not progress beyond this point, with resolution of the infection occurring gradually over several weeks.

In uncontrolled infection, more widespread thrombophlebitis occurs (Fig. 1). The process may involve the iliac veins, inferior vena cava, and left renal vein. Frequently, the thrombosis is discontinuous, so that both external iliac veins may be involved, whereas the common iliac veins remain patent. Septicemia is almost inevitable with extensive phlebitis of the pelvic veins. Its severity is influenced by the presence of a copathogen. Immediate sequelae of the bacteremia include implantation of the anaerobic streptococci on a previously damaged heart valve or hepatic localization in conjunction with a *Bacteroides/Prevotella* species, resulting in subacute bacterial endocarditis or hepatic abscess, respectively. The late sequelae of this disease process include septic embolization and the resultant abscess in the lungs and/or pulmonary infarcts. Septicemia associated with thrombophlebitis is characterized by repetitive, sudden febrile spikes, which lend a characteristic profile to the temperature chart. At necropsy, widespread pelvic thrombophlebitis and multiple lung abscesses are frequent findings. The morbidity and mortality seen with *Bacteroides*–peptostreptococci is far more significant than that observed with *G. vaginalis*–peptostreptococci alone.

Antibacterial therapy is best directed against both components in the synergism, although it is possible that the eradication of one of the two organisms and the surgical removal of the conditions favoring anaerobic growth will allow the condition to resolve itself. Penicillin, the drug of choice in the treatment of the peptostreptococci, is usually ineffective in eradicating *Bacteroides/Prevotella* species. The presence of thrombophlebitis is an indication for heparinization.

Progressive Bacterial Synergistic Gangrene

In 1926, Meleney first described a condition that he later termed "progressive synergistic gangrene," which was due to beta-hemolytic, microaerophilic streptococci in synergism with other organisms (e.g., *Staphylococcus aureus*, *Proteus*, etc.). The disease process usually begins around retention sutures after abdominal surgical repairs. The initial lesion is a small, very painful, superficial ulcer that gradually spreads. The central shaggy ulcerated area is surrounded by a rim of gangrenous skin. This in turn is surrounded by an outer

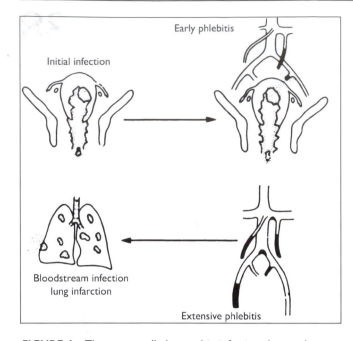

Early phlebitis

Initial infection

Bloodstream infection
lung infarction

Extensive phlebitis

FIGURE I The uncontrolled spread in infection due to the peptostreptococci. Frequently associated with severe injuries to the birth canal and with retained pieces of placenta, the infection is initially limited to these injured areas. Organisms tend to spread in the clot within thrombosed sinuses to the uterine and ovarian veins. Later, more widespread thrombophlebitis may involve the iliac veins, inferior vena cava, and renal vein. From these foci, septic emboli slough off, causing intermittent septicemia and abscesses in the lung. *Source*: From Gibberd (1966).

zone of peripheral erythema that infiltrates the adjacent pink edematous skin. The condition is distinct from the fulminating ulcer described by Meleney that is associated with group A hemolytic streptococci and which occurs without the synergistic action of other organisms. Meleney reproduced this lesion experimentally with · a mixture of microaerophilic anaerobic streptococci and *S. aureus*. If pure cultures of either organism were used, gangrenous ulcers did not develop. It should be noted that even in the preantibiotic period, this was a rare disease.

Therapy involves massive systemic administration of antibiotics, including penicillin, with a wide incision of the lesion. Conservative treatment has resulted in repetitive operations. The incisional line must go far beyond the area of redness and edema and bleed readily.

DIAGNOSIS AND THERAPY

The diagnosis and therapy of peptostreptococcal disease is that discussed in Chapter 3.

SELECTED READING

Bartlett JG, Louis TJ, Gorbach SL, Onderdonk AB. Therapeutic efficacy of 29 antimicrobial regimens in experimental intra-abdominal sepsis. Rev Infect Dis 1981; 3:535.

Bartlett JG, Onderdonk AB, Drude E. Quantitative microbiology of the vaginal flora. J Infect Dis 1977; 136:271.
Chow AW, Marshall JR, Guze LB. Anaerobic infections of the female genital tract: prospects and prospectives. Obstet Gynecol Surv 1975; 30:477.
Duma RJ, Weinberg AM, Medrek TF, Kunz LF. Streptococcal infections: a bacteriologic and clinical study of streptococcal bacteremia. Medicine 1969; 48:87.
Finegold SM. Infections due to anaerobes. Med Times 1968; 96:174.
Gorbach SL, Bartlett JG. Anaerobic infections: old myths and new realities. J Infect Dis 1974; 130:307.
Ledger WJ. Selection of antimicrobial agents for treatment of infections of the female genital tract. Rev Infect Dis 1983; 5(Suppl):98.
Sweet RL. Anaerobic infections of the female genital tract. Am J Obstet Gynecol 1975; 122:891.
Sweet RL. Treatment of mixed aerobic–anaerobic infections of the female genital tract. J Antimicrob Chemother 1981; 8(Suppl D):105.
Weinstein WM, Onderdonk AB, Bartlett JG, Gorbach SL. Experimental intra-abdominal abscesses in rats: development of an experimental model. Infect Immun 1974; 10:1250.
Weinstein WM, Onderdonk AB, Bartlett JG, et al. Antimicrobial therapy of experimental intra-abdominal sepsis. J Infect Dis 1975; 132:282.

Endometritis and Septicemia
Colebrook L. Infection by anaerobic streptococci in puerperal fever. Br Med J 1930; 2:134.
diZerega G, Yonekura L, Roy S, et al. A comparison of clindamycin-gentamicin and penicillin-gentamicin in the treatment of postcesarean section endomyometritis. Am J Obstet Gynecol 1979; 134:238.
Gibberd GF. Puerperal sepsis. J Obstet Gynaecol Br Commonw 1966; 73:1.
Gibbs RS, Jones PM, Wilder CJ. Antibiotic therapy of endometritis following cesarean section: treatment success and failures. Obstet Gynecol 1978; 52:31.
Harris JW, Brown JH. A clinical and bacteriological study of 113 cases of streptococcal puerperal infection. Bull Johns Hopkins Hosp 1929; 44:1.
Ledger WJ, Norman M, Gee C, Lewis W. Bacteremia on an obstetric/gynecologic service. Am J Obstet Gynecol 1975; 121:205.
Ramsey AM, Brown EH, Manners SM. Investigations and reactions of septic abortion. Br Med J 1955; 2:1239.
Rivett LC, Williams L, Colebrook L, et al. Puerperal fever—a report. Proc Roy Soc Med 1933; 26:1161.
Rotheram EB, Schick SF. Nonclostridial anaerobic bacteria in septic abortion. Am J Med 1969; 46:80.
Schwartz OH, Dieckmann WJ. Puerperal infections due to anaerobic streptococci. Am J Obstet Gynecol 1927; 13:467.
Swenson RM, Michaelson TC, Daly MJ, et al. Anaerobic bacterial infections of the female genital tract. Obstet Gynecol 1973; 42:538.

Progressive Synergistic Bacterial Gangrene
Cullen T. A progressive enlarging ulcer of the abdominal wall involving the skin and fat. Surg Gynecol Obstet 1924; 38:579.
de Jongh DS, Smith JP, Thoma GW. Postoperative synergistic gangrene. J Am Med Assoc 1967; 200:557.
Meleney FL. Bacterial synergism in disease processes. Ann Surg 1931; 94:361.
Meleney FL, Friedman ST, Harvey HD. The treatment of progressive bacterial synergistic gangrene with penicillin. Surgery 1945; 18:423.
Smith JG. Progressive bacterial synergistic gangrene: report of a case treated with chloramphenicol. Ann Intern Med 1956; 44:1007.
Williard AG. Chronic progressive postoperative gangrene in the abdominal wall. Ann Surg 1936; 104:227.

The *Proteus* Group

39

INTRODUCTION

The *Proteus* organisms are motile, gram-negative bacilli that exhibit significant variation in size and shape. Young cultures grown on solid agar are particularly pleomorphic. Short coccobacillary and long filamentous forms may be identified in cultures and exhibit rapid spread over the entire surface of the culture. Such "swarming" is due to the organism's very high motility. The spread is so rapid that, not infrequently, the presence of a *Proteus* strain as a component in a specimen may mask the presence of another pathogen. Such specimens should be reisolated by cultivation on relatively dry surfaces of 5% agar or on ordinary 1% to 2% agar containing 0.1% chloral hydrate. Urease production is characteristic of the *Proteus* group. Experimental evidence suggests that urease production may preferentially enhance bacterial replication within the renal medulla once infection is established. While urease production is a distinguishing metabolic characteristic, functional subdivision of the *Proteus* group is based on maltose fermentation and indole formation. The maltose-fermenting strains form indole; those that do not ferment maltose are indole negative. The relative ability or inability to form indole is important in antibiotic chemotherapy. Indole-positive strains, such as *P. vulgaris*, are resistant to ampicillin, whereas most of the indole-negative strains, such as *P. mirabilis*, are highly susceptible.

IMMUNOLOGY OF INFECTION

Motile strains of *Proteus* contain H (flagellar) antigens in addition to the somatic O antigens. Certain strains of *P. vulgaris* labeled OX share specific polysaccharide antigenic determinants with *Rickettsia prowazekii* (the organism of epidemic typhus) and other rickettsiae. The serologic cross-reactivity of the OX strains with certain rickettsial organisms has resulted in the recognition of three types: OX 2, OX 19, and OX K, by virtue of the Weil-Felix reaction. While these antigens are important in the diagnosis of typhus fever and other rickettsial diseases, they have little clinical bacteriologic applicability.

FEMALE GENITAL TRACT INVOLVEMENT

The *Proteus* group is part of the naturally occurring flora of the gastrointestinal tract and secondarily colonizes the genitourinary tract. Although *P. morganii* has been incriminated in summer diarrhea in children, it is only when the organisms leave their normal habitat in the gastrointestinal tract and are placed in a specific milieu where they do not have to compete with the predominant *Escherichia coli* and *Klebsiella* organisms that they produce infection in humans.

They are present in large numbers in the gastrointestinal or vaginal flora only when some abnormality occurs that facilitates their multiplication. By and large, the *Proteus* organisms do not function as prime pathogens in humans. Even though they cause genitourinary and gastrointestinal infections, they do so primarily after more drug-sensitive enteric pathogens have been eradicated. Urinary tract, wound, and neonatal infections are the predominant forms of *Proteus* infection encountered in obstetrics and gynecology.

Urinary Tract Infection

The indole-negative strains (i.e., *P. mirabilis*) account for 8% to 9% of isolates obtained from patients with asymptomatic bacteriuria in pregnancy. Their relative prevalence as isolates from cases of pyelonephritis is markedly decreased. The recovery of an indole-positive *Proteus* from a patient with urinary tract infection often reflects prior administration of antibiotic agents. Infections with urea-splitting bacteria are likely to be associated with or causally related to renal calculus formation. In rare instances, as a consequence of internal metabolic derangement resulting in a persistently alkaline pH, *Proteus* may be the initial pathogen of the female genital tract. Such an alteration of pH permits the clinical expression of an organism of a lower pathogenicity. The group does not flourish at an acidic pH. Therapeutic use of this biologic property may be an important adjunct to therapy for a given patient.

Wound Infection

The factors permitting replication of *Proteus* bacilli in the urinary tract are similar to those that function in local wound infection. The organism appears in large numbers in wound infections either by virtue of its ability to overgrow drug-sensitive species or because local growth conditions, such as pH, have had a selective influence on the bacterial flora at the site of infection. One of the important considerations is the fact that *Proteus*, at the site of wound sepsis, may be masking the identification of another pathogen—hence the necessity of reculturing either the wound or the original specimen on specific media that inhibit swarming before a cause-and-effect relationship is attributed to the organism.

Neonatal Infection

Neonatal infection due to *Proteus* organisms is rare. When it occurs, it tends to take the form of meningitis and meningoencephalitis. *Proteus* is the cause of acute neonatal meningitis in approximately 4% of reported cases. Even in adults and older children, *Proteus* meningitis is rare; it is limited to cases of severe otitis media with sinus thrombosis. *Proteus* does not frequently constitute a significant part of the maternal vaginal flora unless the patient has been exposed to extensive broad-spectrum antibiotic therapy prior to vaginal delivery. Neonatal acquisition of infection is rarely associated with parturition through an infected birth canal. The neonatal umbilical vessels constitute the primary portal of infection, and the disease occurs primarily in patients requiring extensive and prolonged hospital care. Just as with the *Pseudomonas* organisms, the presence of a large vascular channel permits the clinical expression of infection. The signs and symptoms of *Proteus* infection are those of respiratory and central nervous system involvement. The infants exhibit grunting, restlessness, pyrexia, and, in advanced cases, evidence of meningitis in the form of stiff neck. A not uncommon feature of neonatal infection is an erythematous rash, which occasionally may exhibit focal hemorrhage. At necropsy, the cranial cavity has a characteristically fetid smell, the cerebral hemispheres are soft and swollen, and various degrees of intracerebral hemorrhage can be identified. Microscopic identification of necrosis within cerebral tissue can be made. The blood vessels show a series of changes ranging from bacterial vasculitis unassociated with significant inflammatory infiltrate to fibroid necrosis of the vessel. Although an inflammatory reaction in the vessels may be absent despite an intensive bacterial infiltration of the wall, acute inflammatory cells are common within the meninges. The occurrence of *Proteus* meningitis and its extreme lethality in the neonate stress the necessity for compulsive care of the umbilical stump.

THERAPY

For clinical purposes, the *Proteus* group can be subdivided into indole-positive and indole-negative subgroups. The justification for this distinction based on a metabolic characteristic is the divergent pattern of antibiotic sensitivity in the two groups. Indole-positive strains of *Proteus* are resistant to ampicillin and selected cephalosporins, whereas most strains of the indole-negative organisms are highly susceptible to these agents. Indole-positive strains (e.g., *P. vulgaris*) and indole-negative strains (e.g., *P. mirabilis*) are susceptible to aminoglycosides such as gentamicin. The aminoglycosides and the fluoroquinolones are currently the drugs of choice against indole-positive *Proteus* whereas ampicillin is the drug of choice for *P. mirabilis*.

SELECTED READING

Brumfitt W, Percival A, Williams JD. Problems in the treatment of urinary tract infection. Br J Clin Pract 1964; 18:503.

Davis BD, Dulbecco R, Eisen HN, et al. Microbiology. New York: Harper & Row, 1968:773.

France DR, Markham NP. Epidemiological aspects of *Proteus* infections with particular reference to phage typing. J Clin Pathol 1968; 21:97.

Groover RV, Sutherland JM, Landing BH. Purulent meningitis of newborn infants. N Engl J Med 1961; 264:115.

Hewitt CB, Overholt EL, Finder RI, Patton JF. Gram-negative septicemia in urology. J Urol 1965; 93:299.

Kahs EH. Chemotherapeutic and antibiotic drugs in the management of infections of the urinary tract. Am J Med 1955; 18:764.

MacLaron DM. The significance of urease in *Proteus* pyelonephritis: a histological and biochemical study. J Pathol 1969; 97:43.

Morgao HR. The enteric bacteria. In: Dubos RJ, Hirsch JG, eds. Bacterial and Mycotic Infections of Man, 4th ed. Philadelphia: Lippincott, 1972:617.

Rosenblatt MB, Zizza F, Beck I. Nosocomial infections. Bull NY Acad Med 1969; 45:10.

Shortland-Webb WR. *Proteus* and coliform meningencephalitis in neonates. J Clin Pathol 1968; 21:422.

Turck M, Browder AA, Lindemeyer RI, et al. Failure of prolonged treatment of chronic urinary tract infections with antibiotics. N Engl J Med 1962; 267:999.

Staphylococci

40

INTRODUCTION

The staphylococci are large, gram-positive cocci that, in liquid or on solid media, aggregate in grape-like clusters. This morphologic pattern that typifies staphylococci is the consequence of random cell division in three planes. The staphylococci are covered with a carbohydrate surface slime that forms intracellular bridges linking the cocci together in this arrangement.

The organisms were first cultured in vitro by Louis Pasteur in the year 1880. Two years later, Ogston named this unique genus of spherical, cluster-forming microorganisms the *Staphylococcus*. By 1886, predicated on the pigment production or the lack of it, Rosenbach defined two distinct subspecies: *Staphylococcus pyogenes aureus* and *Staphylococcus pyogenes albus*. However, the criterion of pigment production, which originally separated the staphylococci into distinct genera, is now regarded as a minor criterion for identification.

S. AUREUS (COAGULASE POSITIVE)

The typical morphology of *S. aureus* is characterized by golden yellow, glistening colonies, 1 to 2 mm in diameter, which may be surrounded by a zone of beta-hemolysis when grown on 57% sheep blood agar. Individual strains may or may not be encapsulated. The enhanced virulence of the encapsulated strains is attributed to a polysaccharide capsular surface antigen that requires antibody adherence and coating for optimal phagocytosis. This antigen may block the coagulase reaction as well as phage attachment. Anaerobic fermentation of mannitol and production of coagulase and extracellular deoxyribonuclease (DNAse) are the principal features that distinguish *S. aureus* from *S. epidermidis*.

The staphylococci possess multiple type-specific antigens. Individual strains can be differentiated by antigen analysis using prototype-specific antisera. The antigenic complexity of *S. aureus* and the lack of common reagents restrict the usefulness of this immunologic serotyping. Phage typing is currently performed using bacteriophages (viruses that infect bacteria). This typing is based on the phage lysis of susceptible bacterial cells and the inability to lyse resistant ones. The patterns formed by lysis, or lack thereof, by 22 phages permit the classification of *S. aureus* into four major groups. Staphylococcal isolates that differ by their reactions to two or more phages are considered different.

S. aureus is etiologically responsible for a number of clinical entities, including wound infections, progressive synergistic bacterial gangrene, the anaerobic progression (see Chapter 31), urinary tract infection, septicemia, puerperal mastitis, and toxic shock syndrome.

Wound Infections and Synergistic Bacterial Gangrene

The coagulase-positive staphylococci, one of the important constituents of the microbiologic flora of the skin, may play an important role in wound infections. Infection may be both endogenous, arising from strains colonizing the patient's skin, upper respiratory tract, or female genital tract, and exogenous, being acquired from the environment or the microbiologic flora of another individual. The prevalence of *S. aureus* in the microbiologic flora of the skin is in contrast to its relatively low representation in the vaginal flora. When present in conjunction with an appropriate oxidation–reduction potential, *S. aureus* organisms can function as class I through class III anaerobes. Their ability to replicate under both aerobic and anaerobic conditions and to synthesize bacteriocins or bacteriocin-like substances enhances their clinical recognition as a cause of wound infections, while the more obligatory anaerobes, which may be concomitantly involved, often escape recognition. A foul-smelling discharge should suggest the presence of concomitant anaerobic infection, even though routine anaerobic cultures may reveal only *S. aureus*.

The clinical manifestations of wound infections are primarily local tenderness, edema, and erythema. The discharge from staphylococcal wound infections is purulent. Gram staining readily demonstrates the presence of large, gram-positive cocci in clusters. Unless systemic signs of infection are present, as evidenced by fever and leukocytosis, the primary mode of therapy comprises drainage, surgical debridement, and appropriate wound care. The persistence of a low-grade fever that never returns to baseline levels despite apparent adequate antimicrobial therapy should alert to the possibility of an undrained wound or collar-button abscess.

S. aureus functions as a copathogen in progressive synergistic bacterial gangrene. In this situation, microaerophilic streptococci combine with *S. aureus* to produce a progressive gangrenous cutaneous lesion. Diagnosis and therapy are discussed in the section on necrotizing wound infections.

Role in the Anaerobic Progression

Although rarely isolated from abscesses per se, *S. aureus*, like the Enterobacteriaceae, may be the trigger organism for the rupturing of a tubo-ovarian abscess. Whereas local care and debridement are the prime keys to the management of wound infections, infections in continuity with the vaginal mucosa in which *S. aureus* functions as a copathogen require eradicative antibiotic therapy.

Urinary Tract Infection

S. aureus is a potential causative agent of asymptomatic bacteriuria or pyelonephritis. However, its prevalence in either category of patients is of the order of 0.1%. Therapeutically, both conditions should respond to an effective antibiotic regimen. What singles out *S. aureus* pyelonephritis for special attention is that in about 20% of the cases, renal parenchymal involvement is due to hematogenous rather than ascending infection. In these instances, the correct diagnosis is not pyelonephritis, but rather focal embolic glomerulonephritis with parenchymal extension secondary to unrecognized bacterial endocarditis or osteomyelitis (the latter is rare in women of childbearing age). Refractory anemia, an inverted albumin–globulin (A/G) ratio, and a persistently elevated erythrocyte sedimentation rate, as well as evidence of focal embolic phenomena involving the retina or conjunctiva of the eye or appropriate cutaneous sites (petechial hemorrhages, Janeway lesions, Osler's nodes, etc.), may corroborate the diagnosis of hematogenous renal involvement. In pyelonephritis due to *S. aureus* in a drug addict, a presumptive diagnosis of bacterial endocarditis should be made until proved otherwise. In cases of acute staphylococcal endocarditis, the infected emboli within the glomeruli may develop into multiple renal abscesses. These abscesses may coalesce to form a renal carbuncle or extend beyond the capsular confines to create a perinephric abscess. The usual presenting features of a renal or perinephric abscess are rigors, spiking fever, and flank pain. Both of these conditions require surgical intervention.

Septicemia

The most challenging problem that *S. aureus* poses for obstetricians and gynecologists is that of septicemia. Although septicemia may complicate any of the previously described disease processes, the problem is usually iatrogenic, engendered by the infection of intravenous catheters by *S. aureus*. Once the appropriate blood cultures have been obtained, all intravenous catheters should be removed and the tips cultured and Gram stained. The bacterial strains, being of nosocomial origin, tend to be resistant to penicillin. A penicillinase-resistant semisynthetic penicillin should therefore be used until antibiotic sensitivity tests sanction or contraindicate the use of a cephalosporin or penicillin G in the case of sensitive strains. The duration of therapy is critical. Despite eradication of the septicemia by appropriate antistaphylococcal therapy, death may result from late sequelae. Depending on its duration and magnitude, staphylococcal septicemia may produce severe metastatic complications. Osteomyelitis or brain abscesses may not become clinically manifest for six to eight weeks following vascular invasion. To avert the possible metastatic complications, once staphylococcal septicemia has been documented, a minimum of four weeks of therapy is a must.

Catheter-associated septicemia is intermittent, in contrast to the continuous bacteremia of staphylococcal endocarditis. The diagnosis of bacterial endocarditis is inferred by demonstrating the persistence of septicemia after the removal of an infected intravenous line.

S. aureus may function as a systemic pathogen following hypertonic saline abortion. The frequency with which *S. aureus* is isolated from the intravascular compartment in this clinical situation argues for the use of antibiotic coverage that is effective against *S. aureus*.

Gel diffusion or countercurrent immunoelectrophoresis (CIE) may aid in the differentiation between well-established, prolonged staphylococcal septicemia and that of recent onset. Gel diffusion tends to be markedly less sensitive than CIE, demonstrating a cross-reaction with streptococci in a significant number of instances. Countercurrent electrophoresis is more sensitive; however, there is a higher rate of false positivity. If such sophisticated technology is available, one should first do a CIE. If a positive identification is established, then one should resort to gel diffusion for confirmation.

In rare instances, one can produce a transient septicemia as a consequence of a surgical procedure on a cutaneous staphylococcal abscess. To prevent spread either by bloodstream dissemination or by direct local extension, antibiotic prophylaxis is recommended prior to the cutaneous drainage of furuncles on the head or neck or of large lesions with evidence of peripheral extension. Antibiotic administration should be continued for a minimum period of three days.

Puerperal Mastitis

Puerperal mastitis is a disease of the postgravid female that has its genesis in the neonate. The newborn infant becomes colonized within the nursery by a nosocomial penicillin-resistant *Staphylococcus*. Approximately 50% to 75% of nursing personnel are probable *Staphylococcus* carriers and a permanent source of penicillin-resistant organisms within the hospital environment. The infant becomes the prime disseminator of the staphylococci to the mother. Maternal infection is almost invariably due to a hospital-acquired and not an endogenous strain, unless the mother had a staphylococcal cutaneous infection that antedated her hospital admission.

The determinants of disease, as opposed to colonization, are difficult to discern. At least one of these appears to be the strain virulence of the organisms. A high rate of breast infection occurs among nursing mothers when there is a concomitant epidemic of overt *S. aureus* infection in the newborn nursery. Even then, there is far from a one-to-one correlation between colonization of a neonate with a virulent strain of *S. aureus* and subsequent maternal puerperal mastitis. Given the colonization of newborn infants with an epidemic strain, a few mothers will develop puerperal mastitis, but the majority will not.

The disease occurs most commonly between the 11th and 30th day postpartum, with the greatest number of cases being identified in the second to third week. Infection is usually a unilateral phenomenon. With progressive engorgement of the ducts, the breast becomes engorged, resulting in a discrete, tender mass. Cutaneous erythema develops locally. With progression of the disease, the patient may experience chills, fever, headaches, and malaise.

The conversion of mastitis to abscess occurs extremely rapidly. If specific therapy is not instituted within the first 24 to 36 hours, abscess is the usual sequela of puerperal mastitis, particularly when due primarily to *S. aureus*. Antibiotic therapy, to be effective, must be administered within the first 24 hours. The critical factor is the time of administration, namely, prior to the establishment of an irreversible process, rather than the choice of antibiotics per se. Both cephalothin and erythromycin are effective in this clinical setting.

Methicillin-Resistant *S. aureus*

Methicillin-resistant *S. aureus* (MRSA) was initially detected in Europe in the 1960s, soon after the introduction of methicillin. Naturally resistant strains were isolated in some countries before the use of methicillin or related agents. These strains spread initially from one or more ancestral genetic clones in natural populations of *S. aureus* by horizontal transfer and recombination. These original strains then increased in numbers and diversity in hospitals as a result of selection by exposure to antibiotics and by cross-infection. The main mode of spread is person-to-person within a unit or hospital and subsequently to other hospitals.

To date, MRSA has not been a major problem in obstetrics and gynecology only because of patient predisposition to disease conversion. Risk factors for MRSA bacteremia include a higher frequency of severe underlying disease, poorer underlying prognosis, prior antibiotic therapy, prolonged hospitalization, intravascular catheterization, and intensive care unit location. Risk factors for developing MRSA postoperative wound infections include prior antimicrobial therapy, prolonged hospitalization, and severity of underlying disease. Few data are available to identify specific risk factors for colonization or infection of burn wounds by MRSA. Rapid detection of MRSA, prompt implementation of barrier precautions, and prospective surveillance are essential components of a successful control program. Eradicating nasal carriage of MRSA among patients and personnel can be useful during epidemics.

Resistance to methicillin is due to chromosomally mediated alteration in the penicillin-binding proteins (PBPs). Low-affinity PBP-2A encoded by *mecA* is closely related to methicillin resistance in staphylococci. The management and therapy of MRSA is included in Chapter 72.

Staphylococcal Bacteremia Associated with Infected Intravenous Lines

Resistance by *S. aureus* is mediated primarily through two mechanisms:

1. The elaboration of penicillinases
2. Mutational changes in the PBPs

Production of penicillinase negates the microbiological efficacy of the first four generations of the penicillins and necessitates the use of a penicillinase-resistant semisynthetic analog or penicillinase-resistant second- or third-generation cephalosporin. A change in the PBPs selects for broad cross-resistance and necessitates the use of vancomycin. Currently, the staphylococci are classified as members of the family Micrococcaceae. The staphylococci have three clinically important species: *S. aureus*, *S. epidermidis*, and *S. saprophyticus*. The teichoic acid antibody (TAA) assay measures the presence or absence of antibodies to the teichoic acid moiety in the wall of *S. aureus*. The major role of this assay is not only to diagnose *S. aureus* infection, but also to determine the duration of treatment for bacteremic patients. Patients with *S. aureus* metastatic abscesses will usually develop TAA two to three weeks after the onset of the bacteremia (Fig. 1). A titer of greater than or equal to 1:2 favors the presence of a deep-seated staphylococcal infection. The predictive value of a negative assay in someone who has experienced an episode of *S. aureus* bacteremia is high. The test is useful in ruling out metastatic disease. If TAA antibodies are absent and serial tests remain negative, the prognosis is good. Therapy can be limited to four weeks as opposed to six weeks. The interim between bacteremia and secondary sequelae is usually about two to three weeks.

Once having attained vascular access, *S. aureus* has the potential for the induction of secondary metastatic disease involving primarily the lungs, heart valves, brain, bone, and kidneys. The incidence of infectious endocarditis following bacteremia from an infected intravenous site ranges from 3% to 38%. Endocarditis is associated with high morbidity and moderate mortality.

The following is the protocol advocated for the evaluation of patients with documented bacteremia associated with infected intravenous lines. The protocol assumes that one is dealing with an individual with intact host defense mechanisms, and with no evidence of established metastatic staphylococcal disease.

1. Remove infected intravenous site.
2. Do a careful physical examination. Look for established disease, i.e., infectious endocarditis.
3. Place patient on oxycillin.
4. Obtain antibody titers to TAA using CIE. If TAA antibodies are to appear, they usually do so two to three weeks after the onset of disease. If TAA antibodies are already present, do quantitative measurements using gel diffusion. A titer greater than or equal to 1:2 favors the presence of deep-seated staphylococcal infection. One way to rule out aggressive metastatic disease is to obtain echocardiography, bone scans, and urine cultures. If TAA antibodies are absent and serial tests remain negative, the prognosis is good. Therapy can be limited to four weeks as opposed to six weeks.

METHICILLIN-RESISTANT *S. AUREUS*

Since the first reports of significant outbreaks of MRSA in hospitals in the United States, the prevalence of MRSA colonization and infection has increased not only in acute and chronic care facilities, but also in outpatient clinics that serve community-based populations (Table 1).

The emergence of resistance to antibiotics has not been accompanied by an alteration of virulence. MRSA strains cause life-threatening infections, but they are no more pathogenic than methicillin-sensitive strains (MSSA).

The problems posed by MRSA strains are threefold:

1. Incorrect or missed identification of MRSA and, hence, inappropriate or ineffective antibiotic therapy
2. Inappropriate antibiotic use despite adequate identification
3. Nosocomial spread within a healthcare unit

MRSA isolates contain what is termed *mecA* gene, a 2130 bp stretch of DNA of nonstaphylococcal origin that, together with a longer block of "foreign" DNA, is incorporated into the staphylococcal chromosome. The *mecA* gene encodes for the 78 KD PBP-2A, which has a very low affinity for beta-lactam antibiotics. It is generally assumed that PBP-2A acts as a surrogate enzyme that takes over the task

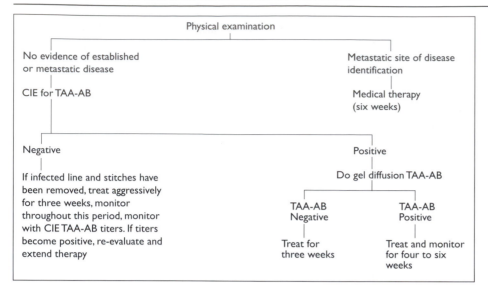

FIGURE 1 Protocol to determine the presence of metastatic staphylococcal infection following documented bacteremia. *Abbreviations*: CIE, countercurrent immunoelectrophoresis; TAA-AB, teichoic acid antibody.

of cell wall synthesis from the normal complement of staphylococcal PBPs.

An intact *mecA* gene component alone does not appear to fully account for phenotype resistance. Additional chromosomal sites outside of the *mecA* determinant locus appear to determine the minimum inhibitory concentration (MIC) value of an MRSA isolate. The auxiliary genes cofunction with the *mecA* gene in bringing about the high level beta-lactam resistance.

Microbiological Identification of MRSA
A number of conditions can affect the results of disk diffusion, broth dilution, and agar screening for MRSA. In the near future, DNA detection methodologies may replace susceptibility testing in the identification of MRSA.

Inappropriate Antibiotic Therapy
MRSA strains of the 1990s are significantly different from the MRSA strains of the 1960s and 1970s. The pattern of resistance is significantly broader and encompasses some antibiotics such as clindamycin, imipenem, the newer aminoglycosides, and some of the new generation tetracyclines. The only antibiotic for which efficacy can be projected with reasonable certainty is vancomycin.

Nosocomial Spread
Once MRSA is introduced into a healthcare unit and allowed to colonize patients, both sporadic and epidemic outbreaks may occur. When the units involved are newborn intensive

care units, postoperative care units, or intensive care units, the character of the patient population magnifies the morbidity and mortality of MRSA. Traditionally, cases of MRSA infection were due nosocomially to internal antibiotic pressures. Because of the aggressive use of antibiotics in nursing homes, this patient population, when subsequently hospitalized, has proved to be a significant vehicle for unit colonization. MRSA prevalence rates as high as 34% have been reported from long-care settings. Currently, MRSA is in the community.

Management of Wound Sepsis Due to MRSA
Once an MRSA isolate is identified, both active surveillance and control measures need to be implemented. Transmission occurs primarily from colonized or infected patients to others via the hands of healthcare personnel. Efforts to prevent the occurrence of new cases center on active surveillance to identify the existent patient reservoirs of MRSA and the institution of control measures to block further transmission from any reservoir. Therapy requires both local wound care and antibiotic therapy.

The following sequence is recommended:
1. Notify infection control of an MRSA isolate.
2. Institute hand care (povidone, iodine, or chlorhexidine) and barrier protection.
3. Isolate the patient from other individuals who may be at potential risk for localized infection.
4. Debride wound and institute appropriate local care.
5. Administer intravenous vancomycin; the end-titration point for parenteral administration should be a patient who is afebrile for 24 to 36 hours and has a negative wound culture for MRSA.
6. Infection control should (a) survey patients in the immediate vicinity and those cared for by nurses involved with the pilot case for nasal MRSA colonization and (b) survey all involved healthcare personnel for nasal carriage of MRSA.
7. Because the patient has both wound infection and wound sepsis (fever), parenteral vancomycin therapy should be implemented along with aggressive wound care.

If multiple patients are colonized, these individuals should be segregated together until all have been discharged.

TABLE 1 Patients at high-risk for colonization with MRSA

(1)	Patients recently discharged from the hospital requiring antibiotic therapy
(2)	Patients admitted from a nursing home or comparable chronic care facility
(3)	Patients who develop staphylococcal disease while in an intensive care unit
(4)	Patients admitted with obvious staphylococcal disease when MRSA is identified in the community

Abbreviation: MRSA, methicillin-resistant *Staphylococcus aureus*.

No new additional patients should be admitted to that unit or room. If healthcare personnel are nasally colonized, consideration should be given to local nasal treatment with mupirocin. Elimination of nasal carriage is critical to the success of any rational control policy.

Selective screening of "high-risk" groups will miss potential vectors of MRSA. The key to nosocomial control is not waiting until some arbitrary quota of MRSA isolates is identified but using the pilot case to address its existence with the same measures as if one were confronted with a mini-MRSA epidemic.

Mupirocin is a topical antimicrobial that appears to have some promise in dealing with MRSA colonization. The drug has been used to eliminate nasal carriage with local application. In a controlled trial, nasal carriage of S. aureus was eliminated in all subjects, and when recolonization eventually took place, only 29% relapse with the pretreatment strain was evidenced. Hill and Casewell (1990) reported an MRSA outbreak at a London hospital. Standard infection control means had failed to prevent colonization and infection of more than 200 patients. They achieved epidemiological control using mupirocin. Of the 40 patients and 32 staff studied, 98.6% and 90.1% respectively were free of nasal MRSA after treatment. With widespread use of nasal mupirocin ointment resistance develops. Miller et al. (1996) analyzed mupirocin resistance among MRSA over a four-year period in a large teaching hospital. Mupirocin resistance among MRSA increased markedly over this period (1990, 2.7%; 1991, 8.0%; 1991, 61.5%; 1993, 65%) in association with increased use of mupirocin ointment as an adjunct to infection control measures. Mupirocin is a valuable agent in the control of MRSA. The drug must be used judiciously.

Prevention

Monitoring for possible MRSA introduction into the hospital environment is the key to MRSA control. Patients at high risk for colonization with MRSA are listed in Table 4 of Chapter 73.

Nasal culturing for MRSA needs to be done on these individuals. Multiple studies have shown that nasal carriers of S. aureus are at higher risk for S. aureus bacteremia than are noncarriers in the setting of an MRSA outbreak. Colonization by methicillin-resistant strains represents a greater risk than does colonization by MSSA and strongly predicts the occurrence of MRSA bacteremia. In a prospective cohort study, Pujol et al. (1996) screened with nasal swabs 488 patients admitted to an intensive care unit. Nasal staphylococcal carriers were observed until the development of S. aureus bacteremia, ICU discharge, or death. Of the 488 patients, 147 (30.1%) were nasal S. aureus carriers; 84 patients (17.2%) harbored methicillin-sensitive S. aureus, and 63 patients had (12.9%) MRSA.

Nosocomial S. aureus bacteremia was diagnosed in 38 (7.7%) of 488 patients. Rates of bacteremia were 24 (38%) MRSA carriers, eight (9.5%) MSSA carriers, and six (1.7%) noncarriers. After adjusting for other predictors of bacteremia by means of a Cox proportional hazard regression model, the relative risk for S. aureus bacteremia was 3.9 (95% confidence interval, $1.6 - 9.8$; $p = 0.002$) for MRSA carriers compared with MSSA carriers.

S. EPIDERMIDIS

S. aureus alone has the capacity to produce coagulase. Most laboratories label all coagulase-negative isolates as "S. epidermidis," which results in the failure to differentiate S. epidermidis isolates from S. saprophyticus. S. saprophyticus is a significant cause of urinary tract infection in otherwise healthy young women who have no demonstrable abnormalities of the urinary tract. Unlike S. epidermidis, S. saprophyticus can function as a primary pathogen. Both coagulase-negative staphylococci are not only a cause of urinary tract infection, but also potential participants in the anaerobic progression.

Urinary Tract Infections

Coagulase-negative staphylococci are second only to the Enterobacteriaceae as a cause of significant urinary tract infection in young women of childbearing age with no renal abnormality. The fact that they are common inhabitants of the urethra has contributed to their presence in urine being regarded with skepticism. It should be stressed that coagulase-negative staphylococci have been isolated from urine obtained by suprapubic aspiration and by culture of renal biopsies. They are a significant cause of both upper and lower tract disease.

The wide variation in the reported incidence of gram-positive cocci in urinary tract infections is probably influenced by two important variables. If the bacteriologist does not accept coagulase-negative staphylococci as urinary tract pathogens, an isolate may be ignored. Also, effectiveness of McConkey's medium for urinary tract bacteriology is limited by its inability to support the growth of gram-positive cocci. Hence, 5% sheep blood agar plates should be used in parallel with McConkey's medium. A general rule of thumb to be used by the practitioner is that a coagulase–negative staphylococcus that is novobiocin resistant and is obtained from a young, healthy, ambulatory woman equates with S. saprophyticus, whereas urinary tract infection acquired within the hospital setting in an older patient usually equates with S. epidermidis. Although staphylococcal infection can be suspected on clinical grounds by the demonstration of more than 15 gram-positive cocci per high-power field in urinary sediment, definitive diagnosis emanates from the microbacteriology laboratory.

Septicemia

Coagulase-negative staphylococci are normal constituents of skin and most mucous membranes. Consequently, they are common contaminants in blood culture specimens obtained across intact cutaneous barriers. In recent years there has been a clear perception that coagulase-negative staphylococci can function as bonafide pathogens. They have become the most common organisms isolated from infectious prosthetic heart valves, cerebrospinal fluid shunts, peritoneal dialysis catheters, and indwelling intravenous catheters. In the presence of a foreign body, the staphylococci can be formidable pathogens.

For the obstetrician/gynecologist, the principal area of concern has been the newborn intensive care nursery. The technological advances necessary for the survival of low-birthweight infants have facilitated the emergence of coagulase-negative staphylococci as major pathogens in this setting. The infants with coagulase-negative staphylococcal bacteremia manifest with increased episodes of apnea and bradycardia, feeding intolerance, lethargy, irritability, temperature instability, abdominal distention, gastrointestinal disturbance, hypotension or poor perfusion, pallor and/or cyanosis, and tachycardia. Laboratory findings include a shift in the polymorphonuclear leukocyte count, resulting in leukocytosis or leukopenia, increase in immature granulocyte fraction, metabolic acidosis, and hypoglycemia. The clinical management of coagulase-negative bacteremia includes antibiotic therapy in combination with removal of the foreign body. Unlike the community-acquired isolates causing disease, the nosocomially acquired strains that cause septicemia are beta-lactam resistant.

Wound Infections and Anaerobic Progression

Regardless of the nature of the specimen, whether it is an exudate from an infected wound or blood from a patient with septicemia, the presence of coagulase-negative staphylococci is too frequently dismissed as being due to contamination or as being of little significance. It is estimated that 4% to 5% of wounds have coagulase-negative staphylococci as a significant component. The prime function of the organism is to alter the local microbiologic environment and render it more conducive to anaerobic replication. S. epidermidis may be present as a constituent of polymicrobial bacteremia and will undergo selective replacement by more anaerobic organisms. Although it is rare for this organism to function as a virulent pathogen in systemic infection, under appropriate conditions, it may be an effective pathogen for a damaged endocardium.

Neonatal Scalp Abscesses

S. epidermidis is a frequent isolate from neonatal scalp abscesses. In the series reported by Plavidal and Werch (1976), S. epidermidis accounted for 11 of the 19 positive cultures. In three of these abscesses, it was found with one or more other bacteria. In the majority of instances, there was a good correlation between Gram stains and culture data. In one of the two cases reported by Overturf and Balfour (1995), the organism was the apparent cause of osteomyelitis, which was seen as a direct sequel of scalp abscess at the site of previous fetal monitoring.

Methicillin-Resistant S. epidermidis

The traditional concept of S. epidermidis as a contaminant must be revised. It is now apparent that this bacteria can function as a major nosocomial pathogen. A physician can no longer dismiss the recovery of a coagulase-negative staphylococci as a mere contaminant. In many institutions, S. epidermidis is the most common causative agent of hospital-acquired infection. It is a major pathogen in catheter-related septicemia.

The major problem confronting clinicians is evaluating the significance of recovery of S. epidermidis obtained through central or peripheral venous lines of a patient who is potentially septic and distinguishing bacteremia from superficial cutaneous contamination. The significance of an isolate must be evaluated in the context of the clinical setting, clinical signs, total neutrophil count and, in the neonate, immature neutrophil to total neutrophil count ratio.

Nosocomial infection due to S. epidermidis is associated with clinical situations in which there is a foreign body implanted in the host, i.e., prosthetic cardiac valve, a cerebrospinal fluid shunt, or with prolonged use of an indwelling intravenous line.

The proper procedure for differentiating bacteremia from contamination is to obtain peripheral cultures and evaluate the patient for clinical symptoms or signs of sepsis. In adults, a good correlation exists between repeatedly positive central-line cultures, clinical symptoms of sepsis, and positive peripheral blood cultures. Clinical signs of associated coagulase- negative staphylococcal sepsis in infants are relatively nebulous. They include apnea, bradycardia, lethargy, or signs consistent with necrotizing enterocolitis.

The question as to whether removal of the catheter is mandatory for eradication of infection is controversial. If an alternative venous access is available, prompt removal is advocated. The probability of successful therapy without removing the catheter is markedly reduced.

Management

The methicillin-resistant strains of S. aureus are uniformly resistant to the semisynthetic, penicillinase-resistant penicillins and all the cephalosporins. Strains with this pattern of intrinsic resistance also acquire plasmid-mediated resistance to most other antimicrobials with antistaphylococcal activity. In vitro sensitivity to rifampin, trimethoprim–sulfamethoxazole, and the new generation tetracyclines may be demonstrated. Uniform susceptibility to vancomycin has also been demonstrated.

Therapeutic intervention for S. epidermidis is complicated by antibiotic resistance of most nosocomial strains. Between 5% and 40% of septicemic strains are methicillin or oxacillin resistant. Although strains will demonstrate susceptibility to cephalosporins in vitro, the response to this group of drugs is poor. Vancomycin is clearly the drug of clinical choice; however, a few vancomycin-resistant strains have been identified.

Vancomycin is active in a pH range of 6.5 to 8.0. Although effective in low concentrations in vitro against most gram-positive cocci and bacilli, the drug is bacteriostatic but not bactericidal for the enterococci in concentrations that can be safely achieved. There is no cross- resistance between vancomycin and other currently available antibiotics.

One of the unique problems associated with vancomycin administration is the so-called "red-neck syndrome." Rapid intravenous administration of vancomycin produces a histamine-like reaction characterized by flushing, tingling, pruritus, tachycardia, and an erythematous macular rash involving the face, neck, upper trunk, back, and arms but not the rest of the body. Systemic arterial hypotension may complicate the whole picture. The syndrome can be avoided by slow intravenous drug administration.

Once a strain of MRSA or methicillin-resistant *S. epidermidis* becomes established as an endemic nosocomial pathogen, eradication from the hospital environment is difficult.

S. SAPROPHYTICUS

In 1963, Baird-Parker developed a scheme that divided the gram-positive, catalase-positive, and coagulase-negative cocci into staphylococci and micrococci and then subdivided them further into subgroups and biotypes. What was termed *Micrococcus* subgroup 3 is now called *S. saprophyticus*. Separation of other staphylococci from *S. saprophyticus* is achieved by their different sensitivity to novobiocin; *S. saprophyticus* is generally resistant, while *S. epidermidis* is usually sensitive.

S. saprophyticus causes urinary tract infections more frequently in women without previous symptoms than among those with a history of recurrent urinary tract infection. *S. epidermidis* usually produces asymptomatic bacteriuria, while *S. saprophyticus* is usually associated with clinically overt disease. The magnitude of pyuria is comparable to that seen with other urinary tract pathogens.

The organism accesses to the female urinary tract from a fecal reservoir. Its prevalence in a given population varies significantly. A possible explanation is inferred from a Swedish study in which *S. saprophyticus* was recovered from a variety of food, which may function as the vehicle for gastrointestinal tract colonization. When recolonization occurs, it tends to be due to a different strain of *S. saprophyticus*.

THERAPY FOR STAPHYLOCOCCAL DISEASE

S. aureus

Therapy is predicated on whether one is dealing with monoetiologic disease such as that seen with *S. aureus* or urinary tract infection due to the coagulase-negative staphylococci or whether the organism is part of a polymicrobial infection. In dealing with a single microbe, the selection of an antibiotic is predicated on the drug-of-choice concept; for *S. aureus*, it must be presumed that the isolate is a penicillinase producer. At present, more than 90% of all isolates, whether nosocomial or community-acquired, are resistant to penicillin. Therefore, no patient suspected of having an infection with *S. aureus* should be started on a penicillinase-susceptible penicillin. Most staphylococci are susceptible to nafcillin and oxacillin. Usual doses of nafcillin and oxacillin are in the range of 6 to 12 g daily, and patients with endocarditis should receive between 9 and 12 g daily. In the penicillin-allergic individual, the cephalosporins can be used in the absence of a history of an anaphylactic type of penicillin hypersensitivity; however, the most effective alternative continues to be vancomycin. Vancomycin is used in a dose of 2 to 4 g per day parenterally and should be equal to the penicillins and cephalosporins in terms of therapeutic outcome. In dealing with staphylococcal septicemia, it is recommended that initial therapy involves one of the beta-lactamase–resistant

penicillins, e.g., nafcillin or oxacillin. Continued antimicrobial therapy is selected for by in vitro sensitivities. If the strain of *S. aureus* is sensitive to penicillin and methicillin, therapy is switched to penicillin G. If the strain is resistant to penicillin, but susceptible to methicillin, initial therapy is continued. If the strain is resistant to both antibiotics, the patient is switched to vancomycin.

Vancomycin hydrochloride is the treatment of choice for empiric treatment of both coagulase-negative staphylococci infection and those infections involving methicillin-resistant, coagulase-positive staphylococci. The fluoroquinolones may be effective against the mild-to-moderate infection due to methicillin-resistant staphylococci. Imipenem (a carbapenem) should probably not be used despite in vitro sensitivity. When vancomycin resistance is identified, a fall-back drug combination that may be effective is the coupling of sulfamethoxazole – trimethoprim and rifampin.

Coagulase-Negative Staphylococci

Along with the increased incidence of coagulase-negative staphylococci infections, a marked increase in antimicrobial resistance has been observed. Approximately 90% of clinically encountered strains produce beta-lactamase.

Another mechanism of resistance to beta-lactam antibiotics is the production of altered PBPs with low affinity for beta-lactam antibiotics. The detection of the methicillin-resistant phenotype can be difficult due to heterotypic expression. From 1980 to 1989, the incidence of methicillin-resistant, coagulase-negative staphylococci rose from 20% to 60%. Most methicillin-resistant isolates are also resistant to other multiple classes of antibiotics.

For the coagulase-negative staphylococci, it is indispensable to determine disc sensitivities or MIC for all coagulase-negative septicemic isolates. Due to the high prevalence of methicillin-resistant isolates, the use of vancomycin is advocated. Being methicillin-resistant equates with resistance to all beta-lactam antibiotics, regardless of in vitro data to the contrary, aminoglycosides, and most macrolides and tetracyclines.

The only available agents with consistent activity against multiresistant, coagulase-negative staphylococci are vancomycin and rifampin. Some strains remain susceptible to aminoglycosides, trimethoprim–sulfamethoxazole, clindamycin, minocycline, or fluoroquinolones, and therapy should be guided by susceptibility testing. Rifampin should never be used alone in the treatment of coagulase-negative staphylococci infection as resistant isolates rapidly emerge.

The optimum therapy of nosocomial coagulase-negative staphylococci requires the combination of two or three agents. Such agents as gentamicin, trimethoprim–sulfamethoxazole, clindamycin, minocycline, a fluoroquinolone, or various investigational drugs in combination with vancomycin and/or rifampin against susceptible isolates appear to be viable therapeutic options.

S. saprophyticus

S. saprophyticus readily responds to most urinary tract antimicrobials, except for nalidixic acid.

SELECTED READING

S. aureus

Aldridge KE. Methicillin-resistant *Staphylococcus aureus* clinical and laboratory features. Infect Control 1985; 6:461.

Barber M, Wilson BDR, Rippon JE, Williams REO. Spread of *Staphylococcus aureus* in a maternity department in the absence of severe sepsis. J Obstet Gynaecol Br Empire 1953; 60:476.

Bentley DW, Lepper MH. Septicemia related to indwelling venous catheter. J Am Med Assoc 1968; 206:1749.

Berger GS, Gibson JJ, Harvey RP, et al. One death and a cluster of female complications related to saline abortions. Obstet Gyencol 1973; 42:121.

Charles D, Klein TA. In: Charles D, Finland M, eds. Postpartum Infection in Obstetrics and Perinatal Infections. Philadelphia: Lea & Febiger, 1973:253–254, 268–270.

Cohen LS, Fekety FR, Cluff LE. Studies of the epidemiology of staphylococcal infection. IV. The changing ecology of hospital staphylococci. N Engl J Med 1962; 266:367.

Colbeck JC. Extensive outbreak of staphylococcal infections in maternity units. Can Med Assoc J 1949; 61:557.

Elck SD, Conen PE. The virulence of *Staphylococcus pyogenes* for man, a study of the problems of wound infection. Br J Exp Pathol 1957; 38:573.

Gibbard GF. Sporadic and epidemic puerperal breast infections. Am J Obstet Gynecol 1953; 65:1039.

Hare R, Cooke EM. Self-contamination of patients with staphylococcal infections. Br Med J 1963; 2:149.

Hartman B, Tomacz A. Altered penicillin binding proteins in methicillin-resistant strains of *Staphylococcus aureus*. Antimicrob Agents Chemother 1981; 19:726.

Kaplan MH, Tenenbaum MJ. *Staphylococcus aureus*: cellular biology and clinical application. Am J Med 1982; 72:248.

McCallum MF, Govan ADT. The bacteriology of surgical induction of labour. Br J Obstet Gynaecol 1963; 70:244.

MacDonald D, O'Driscoll MK. Intra-amniotic dextrose—a maternal death. Br J Obstet Gynaecol 1965; 72:452.

Musher DM, McKenzie SO. Infections due to *Staphylococcus aureus*. Medicine 1977; 56:383.

Oeding P. Antigenic properties of *Staphylococcus aureus*. Bact Rev 1980; 24:374.

Rammelkamp CH Jr, Lebovitz JL. The role of coagulase in staphylococcal infections. Ann NY Acad Sci 1956; 65:144.

Roodyn L. Epidemiology of staphylococcal infections. J Hyg 1960; 58:1.

Soltau DH, Hatcher GW. Some observations on the aetiology of breast abscess in the puerperium. Br Med J 1960; 1:1603.

Williams REO. Carriage of staphylococci in the newborn: a comparison on infants born at home with those born in hospital. Lancet 1961; 2:173.

S. epidermidis/S. saprophyticus

Archer GL. *Staphylococcus epidermidis* and other coagulase-negative staphylococci. In: Mandell GL, Bennett JE, Dolin R, eds. Principles and Practice of Infectious Disease. 4th ed. New York: Churchill Livingstone, 1995:1777–1784.

Christensen GD, Bisno AL, Parisi JT, et al. Nosocomial septicemia due to multiple antibiotic-resistant *Staphylococcus epidermidis*. Ann Intern Med 1982; 96:1.

Fidalgo S, Vasquez F, Mendoze MC, et al. Bacteremia due to *Staphylococcus epidermidis*: microbiologic, epidemiologic, and prognostic features. Rev Infect Dis 1990; 12:520.

Haley CE, Gregory WW, Donowitz LG, Wenzel RP. Neonatal intensive care unit bloodstream infections: emergence of gram-positive bacteria as major pathogens. In: Program and Abstracts of the 22nd Interscience Conference on Antimicrobial Agents and Chemotherapy. Washington, DC: American Society for Microbiology, 1982, Abstr 691.

Jordon PA, Iravani A, Richard GA, Baer H. Urinary tract infection caused by *Staphylococcus saprophyticus*. J Infect Dis 1980; 142:510.

Kloos WE, Bannerman TL. Update on clinical significance of coagulase-negative staphylococci. Clin Microbiol Rev 1994; 7:117.

Latham RH, Running K, Stamm WE. Urinary tract infections in young adult women caused by *Staphylococcus saprophyticus*. J Am Med Assoc 1980; 250:3063.

Lewis JF, Brake SR, Anderson DJ, Vredeveld GN. Urinary tract infection due to coagulase-negative staphylococcus. Am J Clin Pathol 1982; 77:736.

Nicolle LE, Hoban SA, Harding GKM. Characterization of coagulase-negative staphylococci from urinary tract infections. J Clin Microbiol 1983; 17:267.

Overturf CD, Balfour G. Osteomyelitis and sepsis: severe complications of fetal monitoring. Pediatrics 1995; 55:244.

Peters G, Locci R, Pulverer G. Adherence and growth of coagulase-negative staphylococci on surfaces of intravenous catheters. J Infect Dis 1982; 146:479.

Plavidal FJ, Werch A. Fetal scalp abscess secondary to intrauterine monitoring. Am J Obstet Gynecol 1976; 125:65.

Rupp ME, Archer GL. Coagulase-negative staphylococci: pathogens associated with medical progress. Clin Infect Dis 1994; 10:231.

Rupp ME, Soper DE, Archer GL. Colonization of the female genital tract with *Staphylococcus saprophyticus*. J Clin Microbiol 1992; 30:2975–2979.

Rupp MR, Han J, Goering RV. Repeated recovery of staphylococcus saprophyticus from the urogenital tracts of women: persistence vs. recurrence. Infect Dis Obstet Gynecol 1995; 2:218.

Sewell CM, Clarridge JE, Young EJ, Guthrie RK. Clinical significance of coagulase-negative staphylococci. J Clin Microbiol 1982; 16:236.

Sitges-Serra A, Puig P, Jaurrieta E, et al. Catheter sepsis due to *Staphylococcus epidermidis* during parenteral nutrition. Surg Gynecol Obstet 1980; 151:481.

Wallmark G, Arremark I, Telander B. *Staphylococcus saprophyticus*: a frequent cause of acute urinary tract infection among female outpatients. J Infect Dis 1978; 138:791.

Methicillin-Resistant Staphylococci

Abdo-RA, Araj-GF, Talhouk-RS. Methicillin resistant *Staphylococcus aureus* (MRSA): disease spectrum, biological characteristics, resistant mechanisms, and typing methods. J Med Liban 1996; 44:21.

Ayliffe GA. The progressive intercontinental spread of methicillin-resistant *Staphylococcus aureus*. Clin Infect Dis 1997; 24(Suppl 1)S74.

Boyce JM. Should we vigorously try to contain and control methicillin-resistant *Staphylococcus aureus*? Infect Control Hosp Epidemiol 1991; 12:46.

Boyce JM. Strategies for controlling methicillin-resistant *Staphylococcus aureus* in hospitals. J Chemother 1995; 7(Suppl 3):S81.

Chambers HF. Detection of methicillin-resistant staphylococci. Infect Dis Clin North Am 1993; 7:425.

de Lencastre H, de Jonge BL, Matthews PR. Molecular aspects of methicillin-resistance in *Staphylococcus aureus*. J Antimicrob Chemother 1994; 33:7.

Gould D, Chamberlaine A. *Staphylococcus aureus*: a review of the literature. J Clin Nurs 1995; 4:5.

Hill RL, Casewell MW. Nasal carriage of MRSA the role of mupiro-cin and outlook for resistance. Drugs Exp Clin Res 1990; 1(8):397.

Hosein IK. Wound infection. 2. MRSA. J Wound Care 1996; 5:388.

Martin MA. Methicillin-resistant *Staphylococcus aureus*: the persistent resistant nosocomial pathogen. Curr Clin Top Infect Dis 1994; 14:170.

Miller MA, Dascal A, Portnoy J, et al. Development of mupirocin resistance among methicillin-resistant *Staphylococcus aureus* after widespread use of nasal mupirocin ointment. Infect Control Hosp Epidemiol 1996; 17:811.

Mulazimoglu L, Drenning SD, Muder RR. Vancomycin-gentamicin synergism revisited: effect of gentamicin susceptibllity of methicllllin-resistant. Antimicrob Agents Chemother 1996; 40:1534.

Netto-dos-Santos KR, de-Souza-Fonseca L, Gontijo-Filho PP. Emergence of high-level mupirocin resistance in methicillin-resistant *Staphylococcus aureus* isolated from Brazilian university hospitals [see comments]. Comment in: Infect Control Hosp Epidemiol 1996; 17:775.

Perry C. Methicillin-resistant *Staphylococcus aureus*. J Wound Care 1996; 5:31.

Pujol M, Pena C, Pallares R, et al. Nosocomial *Staphylococcus aureus* bacteremia among nasal carriers of methicillin-resistant and methicillin-susceptible strains. Am J Med 1996; 100:509.

Group B Streptococci

INTRODUCTION

The group B beta-hemolytic streptococcus (*Streptococcus agalactiae*) is a gram-positive coccus that grows in chains in vitro and in vivo. On appropriate media, the colonies appear as smooth, shiny white mounds, about 1 to 1.5 mm in diameter, with a narrow zone of beta-hemolysis. The group B streptococcus (GBS) lacks the M protein that is characteristic of the group A organisms; consequently, its virulence and pathogenicity for humans differ markedly from those of *Streptococcus pyogenes*.

Originally isolated from cows with mastitis, the GBS was regarded as a bovine organism and not as a prime pathogen for humans; hence the original name *Streptococcus mastitidis*. Once Lancefield had provided a basis for classification that was independent of the type of hemolysis and metabolism of specific carbohydrate substrates, the GBS was found in the human nasopharynx and upper respiratory tract, as well as in the normal flora of the female genital tract. Occasionally, the organisms may also be found on the skin.

On the basis of divergent carbohydrate antigenicity, the GBS can be divided into nine serotypes: Ia, Ib/c, Ia/c, II, IIc, III, IIIc, IV, and V. Lancefield originally described two cell-wall polysaccharides:
1. The group B–specific immunogen common to all strains of the species
2. That of type-specific immunity which allowed subsequent subdivision into four serotypes: Ia, Ib, II, and III

The major antigenic determinant for the GBS is L-rhamnose. Type I strains have three antigenically distinct polysaccharide constituents designated Ia, Ib/c, and Ia/c. Specific anticarbohydrate antibodies confer passive protection to mice challenged with homologous streptococci. The classic virulence seen with group A streptococci is not found among GBS organisms. GBS functions as an opportunistic organism whose pathogenicity is usually linked to some alteration of strain virulence.

EPIDEMIOLOGY

The GBS organisms are normal constituents of the vaginal flora. The principal reservoir is the gastrointestinal tract. When single sites of prevalence are evaluated, the fecal colonization rate exceeds both the cervical–vaginal and the throat colonization rates. A family study was reported with the index case being an infant who died of group B sepsis. Both mother (vagina and cervix) and father (urethra) carried the same strain that was cultured from the child at autopsy. Despite aggressive antimicrobial therapy, the organism showed prolonged persistence in the gastrointestinal tracts of the parents and was responsible for intermittent recolonization of the genitalia.

Between 14% and 25% of pregnant women may be continually, intermittently, or transiently colonized. The overall incidence of vaginal colonization is relatively consistent. Preliminary data suggest that approximately one-third of bacterially colonized women are positive throughout pregnancy, another one-third have transient vaginal colonization, and the remaining gravidas have spontaneous clearance of the GBS at the time of delivery. The pattern of colonization is influenced by a number of factors. Women with two or more previous pregnancies tend to be more frequently colonized than primigravidas or secundigravida. Data emanating from the Vaginal Infections and Prematurity Study Group demonstrated that GBS colonization was more common among older women and women with multiple sexual partners.

The major reservoir of the GBS is the gastrointestinal tract. Its preferential growth in an aerobic environment leads to its potential, if not probable, dissemination by coitus. The bacteria can be cultured from the urethra of 50% of sexual consorts of vaginally colonized women. The rate of recovery of GBS is significantly lower in women with no history of sexual intercourse than in women with a history of sexual intercourse with one or more sexual partners. The incidence of bacterial isolation is increased among women of lower socioeconomic groups.

SPECTRUM OF DISEASE

Urinary Tract Infections
Urinary tract infections due to streptococci are caused almost exclusively by groups B and D. Of 205 streptococcal group B isolates from extrarespiratory infections, 32% were from urine. Feingold et al. (1996) noted a surprisingly high incidence of urinary tract infections due to GBS. They pointed out that the frequency of group B infection is probably underestimated. Even though pyelonephritis secondary to GBS is a definite entity, it accounts for only a very small percentage of the cases of pyelonephritis observed during gestation. Infection responds to ampicillin.

Asymptomatic Group B Bacteriuria and Pregnancy
The identification of GBS as a cause of asymptomatic bacteriuria (ABU) in pregnancy appears to select for a higher probability of maternal and/or neonatal infection. Persson et al. (1985) studied women with ABU, comparing void urine specimens with $\geq 10^5$ colony-forming units (cfu)/mL and the occurrence of bacteria in the urinary bladder detected by bladder puncture. The only infant who contracted early-onset septicemia was born to a patient with growth of GBS type III in voided urine. During pregnancy, the mother repeatedly voided specimens with $\geq 10^5$ cfu/mL. She was not treated with antibiotics.

Moller et al. (1984) identified 68 women out of a group of 2745 consecutive gravidas sampled who had ABU due to GBS. The incidence of primary rupture of the membranes and premature delivery was 35% and 20%, respectively, in contrast to 15% and 8.5% in gravidas without GBS ABU. The five cases of GBS neonatal sepsis (four of which died) occurred in the progeny of women with positive urine cultures. Greater than 10^5 cfu/mL of urine appears to be of more predictive value than quantitative studies of vaginal prevalence.

These data substantiate an earlier study by Wood and Dillon (1981) in which they prospectively followed 46 patients with bacteriuria. The only adverse fetal outcome following any bacteria was observed with asymptomatic GBS bacteriuria. Two pregnancies ended in intrauterine fetal death and one neonate developed GBS sepsis. They concluded that screening for GBS bacteriuria at or near delivery may be more meaningful than other GBS surveillance culture studies.

Genital Tract Infections

While they are endogenous bacteria for the female genital tract under selected conditions, GBS organisms can function as formidable adversaries. They are the second most common cause of septicemia in postpartum women, a fact largely overshadowed by their potentially devastating effect on the neonate. As causes of monoetiologic disease, they may produce chorioamnionitis, postpartum endometritis, and maternal septicemia. They can function in polymicrobial postpartum endometritis as a constituent of the anaerobic progression.

Sutton et al. (1985) pointed out that under selected conditions, the group B as well as the group A beta-hemolytic streptococci can produce necrotizing fasciitis. Acute endocarditis and pneumonitis have been observed following septic abortion or other forms of puerperal infection, resulting in sustained septicemia. Sexton et al. (1985) reported two fatal cases of acute endocarditis involving the aortic valve, which occurred in one woman after a normal pregnancy and delivery and in the second woman after a second trimester abortion. Both women were thought to have normal heart valves before onset of their infection.

Both women with acute aortic valvulitis due to the GBS went on to develop annular abscesses and then died.

The ability of the GBS to produce disease in gynecologic/oncologic patients is linked to certain predisposing factors: diabetes mellitus, carcinomatosis, or some form of debilitating chronic disease. The most frequent manifestation of disease in this patient population is an acute cellulitis.

Perinatal Colonization

Given a mother whose bacterial flora contains the GBS, what is the probability of early bacterial colonization of the offspring by either ascending infection from the vagina or delivery through an infected birth canal? At 36 hours of age, colonization of surface sites or mucous membranes among all infants has been detected in 26% to 37% of neonates. Approximately one-third of the isolates are type Ia, Ib/c, or Ia/c; one-third are type II or IIc; and one-third are type III. The almost complete concordance of identical serotypes among isolates from mothers and their progeny partially substantiates the hypothesis that early-onset syndrome is the consequence of vertical bacterial transmission from mother to neonate. The overall attack rate for the early-onset type of disease has varied from 3.0 to 4.2 per 1000 live births. The attack rate for colonized newborns is approximately 1 per 1000 live births. The mortality rate is of the order of 1 to 2 per 1000 live births. Attack rates for late-onset infection have been estimated to be between 1.5 and 2.0 per 1000 live births (Table 1).

Factors influencing the neonatal attack rate include:
1. Smallness-for-dates or prematurity
2. Premature rupture of the fetal membranes
3. Lack of passive immunity derived from the mother
4. Ability of a given isolate of GBS to adhere to cell surfaces

Infants born to culture-negative women may acquire the bacterium from the hospital environment. In one nursery studied, infant colonization was reported to have increased from 20% to 25% during the first 24 hours of life to 50% to 65% at the time of discharge. It is presumed that the mode of nosocomial transmission is the cross-colonization of the infants as a consequence of contact with nursery personnel. When prospectively

TABLE I Clinical comparison of early-onset and late-onset neonatal disease due to group B streptococci

Property syndrome	Early-onset syndrome	Late-onset syndrome
Definition	The onset of clinical disease in the first 5 days of life (75% identified in the first 24 hr)	The onset of clinical disease after the 10th day of life
Predominant site of involvement	Lungs	Central nervous system
Clinical presentation	Pulmonary—apnea, tachypnea, and low peak ventilatory pressure on mechanicalventilation	Meningeal—stiff neck, clouding of sensorium, failure to feed, bulging fontanelles
Serotypes	Proportionately distributed between types Ia–c, II, III; serotype matches that of the mother's vaginal flora	Greater than 90% due to type III; a significant number of infants culture negative at birth
Gestational or maternal factors	Small-for-dates or premature infant, premature rupture of membranes, postpartum maternal endometritis, maternal fever	Prematurity; nosocomial acquisition of type III in the newborn nursery
Morbidity/mortality	Slightly in excess of 50% mortality; sequelae[a]	Death less frequent (12–18%); neurologic
Attack rate	3.0–4.2/1000 live births	0.5–1.0/1000 live births

[a]Sequelae include retarded speech and language development, transient hemiparesis, retarded psychomotor development, seizure disorders, and hydrocephalus.
Source: Monif GRG. Infect Dis Letters Obstet Gynecol 1975; 1:25.

followed, those infants who became thus colonized have to date not developed late-onset GBS disease.

The problem of chronic carriage and its potential for an adverse perinatal impact in subsequent pregnancy has been studied by Dykes et al. (1985). They prospectively monitored for up to 38 months, eight women who had given birth to infants with early-onset or intrauterine infections caused by GBS. Seven of the eight exhibited persistent carriage of the same serotype in contrast to only 34 of 88 GBS carriers who had given birth to healthy infants. Examples of recurrent early-onset septicemia exist in the literature.

Neonatal Septicemia and Meningitis

The major problem that the GBS causes for the disciplines of obstetrics and pediatrics is that it has been the most common cause of neonatal septicemia in the United States for the past 10 years. Two factors select for a statistically significant increase in the anticipated attack rate of early-onset disease by the GBS:

1. Ability to establish urinary tract colonization (asymptomatic bacteriuria)
2. Ability to establish high-density replication with vaginal and rectal bacterial flora

EARLY-ONSET VERSUS LATE-ONSET NEONATAL DISEASE

The GBS produces two patterns of neonatal disease, which are predicated on the time of onset (Table 1).

Early-Onset Disease

Early-onset neonatal infection caused by streptococci of Lancefield group B has an incidence of approximately 2 to 3 cases per 1000 live births. Early-onset septicemia is defined as disease whose onset occurs when infants are less than five days old. It is characteristically associated with maternal factors [i.e., premature rupture of the membranes (PROM), cesarean section, etc.]. Bacterial access to the neonate is primarily a consequence of intrapartum transmission resulting from delivery through an infected birth canal. Once labor has occurred, the GBS may gain access to the amniotic fluid despite the presence of intact fetal membranes. Early-onset disease presents with predominantly pulmonary findings. The clinical manifestations include apnea and tachypnea. The prime differential diagnosis is that of early-onset versus respiratory distress syndrome. There are only a few diagnostic modalities which may be of assistance in differentiating the two, the principal one being roentgenography. A small percentage of patients present with shock. Mortality has been significantly reduced from 15–20% to 2–5% with aggressive therapy and early intervention. If serotyping is done, 18% to 28% of the cases are found to be due to type Ia, Ib/c, or Ia/c; 35% to 44% to type II or IIc; and 33% to 37% to type III. The timing of early-onset disease is such that the bulk of disease develops in the immediate neonatal period. About 52% of cases will be identified in the first six hours, almost 75% of cases will be identified in the first 24 hours.

Early-onset disease is primarily a complication of immature and premature neonates. The major risk factors for the induction of disease are the following:

1. Small-for-dates or premature infants
2. Pulmonary immaturity
3. PROM greater than 12 hours

Where one or more risk factors are present, incidence of disease is 7.6/1000 live births. If risk factors are absent, incidence is 0.6/1000 live births. The attack rate for newborns whose gestation was greater than 37 weeks and whose membranes were ruptured at less than 12 hours is approximately 1/1000 live births; however, if intrapartum fever occurs, the attack rate jumps to 130/1000 live births.

Late-Onset Disease

Late-onset syndrome is defined as disease that occurs after the tenth day of life. Maternal predisposing factors are infrequently present. Rather than presenting as a septicemia, the prime manifestation is a pure meningitis with or without concomitant septicemia. Whereas the serotype of the organisms responsible for early-onset disease parallels that found in the population, more than 90% of the cases of late-onset syndrome are due to type III bacteria. It is conjectured that in the majority of these cases, there was a lack of passively acquired immunity of maternal derivation. It is probable that with late-onset disease, a combination of host factors and nosocomial influences selects for disease. Although death is a less frequent outcome, the incidence of neurologic sequelae observed with the late-onset type varies from 22% to 50%.

Clinical Management

The drug of choice in the treatment of early- or late-onset disease is ampicillin, in a dosage of 100 to 150 mg/kg body weight/day administered intravenously. The reason for the selection of ampicillin over penicillin is the bioavailability of the antibiotic, in terms of its ability to traverse the blood–brain barrier. About 2% to 18% of infants with early-onset syndrome will die. The critical factor in determining outcome is the point at which drug therapy is initiated. If more than four hours have elapsed between the onset of disease and the institution of therapy, the probability of a good outcome is markedly diminished.

PREVENTION

For the infected neonate, however, the answer does not lie in therapy but rather in prevention. In this vein, three divergent tracks have been developed to negate neonatal mortality and morbidity due to the GBS:

1. Maternal vaccination
2. Eradication of the maternal carrier state by systemic antibiotic administration
3. Prophylactic antibiotics for the neonate

Maternal Vaccination

Current attempts at vaccine development may be a valid approach for late-onset syndrome. But for early-onset disease, it probably will not be effective in terms of either efficacy or cost, because five serotypes exist with early-onset disease as opposed to a single dominant serotype with the late-onset syndrome.

Significance of GBS Colonization

The administration of antibiotic to the maternal carrier presumes that colonization per se is a risk factor. Attempts at eradication of the maternal carrier state are complicated by the reintroduction of bacteria from the gastrointestinal reservoir or by the sexual consort. It has been shown that the maternal carrier state can be eradicated; however, it requires that antibiotics be administered at the time of parturition. Close analysis indicates that this approach is not a cost-effective one, and the risk of anaphylaxis to penicillin or its derivative products is real. There is not a one-to-one correlation between the maternal carrier and the ensuing neonatal disease. Approximately 15% to 25% of pregnant women will harbor the organism, yet the attack rate in their offspring is somewhere of the order of 3 to 4 per 1000 deliveries.

Bobitt et al. (1985) evaluated 718 prenatal patients with several cultures. Complications that occurred more frequently in prenatal GBS carriers were the following:
1. Collective morbidity
2. Low birthweight infant
3. PROM associated with low birthweight

Maternal pelvic infection and neonatal sepsis were increased in colonized women at delivery. Maternal colonization did not predict ensuing morbidity. The predictive value of a positive prenatal culture did not exceed 8% for any of the complications. Dillon et al. (1987) have shown that the degree of neonatal colonization does influence the attack rate. Infants with three or four heavily colonized sites have an attack rate of 50/1000 live births. Those who were lightly colonized needed approximately one-tenth of this rate.

McDonald et al. (1989) prospectively studied vaginal swabs from 692 women at approximately 24 weeks of gestation. GBS was detected in 91 (13.2%) women. The rate of preterm labor (PTL) was significantly higher in GBS-positive women than in GBS-negative women (18.7% vs. 5.5%). This association remained significant even when patients with other recognized factors predisposing to PTL were excluded. The rate of PROM was also significantly higher in GBS-positive women (9.9% vs. 2.7%) and also remained significantly higher when patients with other recognized risk factors were excluded. Pregnant women who are vaginal carriers of GBS have a significantly increased risk of PROM and PTL.

Newton and Clark (1991) noted that when they compared gravidas with and without GBS, GBS-positive patients had earlier rupture of membranes (30.7 vs. 31.6 weeks) and shorter latent periods (76.8 vs. 138.5 hours). Not surprisingly, chorioamnionitis and endometritis were more common in GBS-colonized gravidas.

Matorras et al. (1989) demonstrated that when one intrapartum vaginal culture obtained at delivery was positive, GBS could be isolated from amniotic fluid two hours after rupture of the membranes in 81% of cases. The newborns of intrapartum maternal carriers who delivered vaginally were colonized in 69.2% of cases while only 5.6% of newborns with negative cultures during delivery become colonized by GBS. In a subsequent study, the same investigators analyzed the impact of antibiotic therapy at the time of delivery. Patients who were found to be carriers received ampicillin during delivery (500 mg IV), and noncarriers received no chemoprophylaxis. Compared with the noncarriers, the carriers without prophylaxis had a significant increase in the mild puerperal infective morbidity (10.6% vs. 25%). Puerperal infective morbidity in the carriers was lower than in those without prophylaxis and very similar to that of noncarrier women.

A relationship between heavy colonization and infection was initially suggested by the observations of Eickhoff et al. (1964). They isolated "pure" cultures of GBS from the genital tract in 19 of 20 patients who were cultured because of suspected infection. In their study, the growth of either pure or predominant GBS in the vaginal cultures was similarly achieved from three of four mothers with chorioamnionitis. Of the 42 cultures taken from the genital tracts of infected females, Finn and Holden (1970) demonstrated a pure growth of GBS in 21 instances. Bobitt et al. (1985) showed heavy growth of GBS in six of seven cultures from mothers whose infants had documented early-onset septicemia. The dominance of GBS in the maternal vaginal flora may be an important if not critical factor in the ensuing infectious morbidity for the mother and her progeny. The incidence of disease is 50/1000 live births when observations are restricted to heavily colonized gravidas.

Gravidas with GBS aerobic dominance of the vaginal flora, with a preterm baby, prolonged rupture of the fetal membranes greater or equal to 18 hours, or maternal intra- or postpartum infection have a greater probability of delivering a neonate who will develop GBS disease. When one of these factors is present, the risk of early-onset disease is 7.6/1000 live births. When none of these factors are present, the incidence of disease is 0.6/1000 live births.

Prophylactic Antibiotics

In 1996, the Centers for Disease Control (CDC), American College of Obstetricians and Gynecologists, and the Academy of Pediatrics introduced two divergent approaches for the prevention of perinatal group B streptococcal disease. The first of these approaches was predicated on prenatal maternal screening for GBS colonization at 35 to 37 weeks of gestation and offering intrapartum chemoprophylaxis (Table 2). This approach was subsequently modified to include gravidas with GBS bacteriuria and women who had previously given birth to a GBS-infected neonate. The second approach was contingent on the identification of one or more risk factors including preterm deliveries, preterm or prolonged rupture of the fetal membranes, intrapartum fever, prior GBS neonatal disease, and GBS bacteriuria. Both approaches were initially recommended as equally acceptable.

Both approaches have been successful in altering GBS neonatal and maternal morbidity and mortality. Neither has completely eliminated the occurrence of GBS neonatal disease. The principal shortcoming of a risk-based approach was the fact that 20% of GBS neonatal disease occurred in women without demonstrable risk factors. With the bacteriological screening approach for maternal GBS, the problems inherent in culturing on appropriate media, the number of sites needed to exclude GBS, and the ultimate site/technique for obtaining the screening culture assured less than 85% GBS detection.

Schrag et al. (2002) did a multistate retrospective cohort study involving 5144 births in which they compared the efficacy of the two officially recommended approaches. In the screened group, 18% of all gravidas with GBS did not present with an identifiable maternal risk factor. These found that the risk of early-onset GBS disease was significantly lower among infants of screened women than among infants in the risk-based group by approximately 50%. Both strategies were initially considered as equivalent.

In December 2002, the Committee on Obstetrical Practice of The American College of Obstetricians and Gynecologists adopted the new CDC recommendation that obstetrical providers adopt a culture-based strategy in newborns. The risk approach is deemed by the CDC to be no longer an acceptable alternative except for circumstances where culture results are not available before delivery. Laboratories must process GBS cultures correctly using recommended selective broth media

TABLE 2 CDC algorithms for prevention of early-onset GBS disease in neonates using prenatal screening at 35–37 wk

Risk factors: Previous infant who had invasive GBS disease; GBS bacteriuria during pregnancy; delivery at < 37 wk gestation[a]

| NO | | YES
Give intrapartum penicillin |

Collect rectal and vaginal swab for GBS culture at 35–37 wk gestation

| GBS
negative | Not done,
incomplete,
or results
unknown | | GBS
positive

Offer intrapartum
penicillin |

Risk factors:
Intrapartum temperature
≥ 100.4°F (≥ 38.0°C)
Membrane rupture ≥ 18 hr

| | NO | | YES
Give intrapartum
penicillin[b] |

No intrapartum prophylaxis needed

[a]If membranes ruptured at <37 wk of gestation, and the mother has not begun labor, collect GBS culture and administer either (a) antibiotics only when positive cultures are available, or (b) antibiotics if risk factor develops. No prophylaxis is needed if the culture obtained at 35–37 wk of gestation was negative.
[b]Broader-spectrum antibiotics may be considered at the physician's discretion, based on clinical indications.
Abbreviation: GBS, group B streptococcus.
Source: From Schuchat et al. (1996).

(Todd-Hewitt broth supplemented with either gentamicin and nalidixic acid or colistin and nalidixic acid). Culture specimens should be collected by swabbing the vaginal introitus, followed by the rectum, using either the same swab or two separate swabs. A speculum should not be used for culture collection. Swabs should be inserted into a nonnutritive transport medium.

Prior to 1996, it had been demonstrated that the universal administration of penicillin to all neonates would profoundly alter, but not totally eliminate, the incidence of ensuing neonatal group B streptococcal disease. The switch from a pediatric-directed approach for GBS early-onset disease to an obstetrical-directed approach was justified argumentatively by the significant maternal morbidity caused by GBS at parturition.

In terms of risk–benefit analysis, the justification has been less clear. Both penicillin and ampicillin carry with their administration the risk of anaphylaxis. The risk of fatal anaphylaxis has been estimated at 1 per 100,000. The risk of nonlethal allergic reactions is a concomitant consideration. Some researchers have contended that, unlike in pregnant women, anaphylaxis has not been described in a newborn.

Wendel et al. (2002) have used combined intrapartum antibiotics based on both risk factors and culture surveillance with universal neonatal penicillin administration effectively. These investigators contend that almost 1400 neonates could receive single-dose prophylaxis for the cost of a single successful treatment of one GBS-affected baby. If society's mandated goal on zero cases of early-onset GBS is to be met, it will require such a combined pediatric and obstetrical approach.

DIAGNOSIS

A presumptive identification of the organism can be made if a Gram smear reveals gram-positive cocci growing in chains. A definitive diagnosis of maternal infection is contingent on laboratory procedures.

The group B organisms are characterized by their ability to
1. hydrolyze sodium hippurate,
2. grow on 40% bile agar,
3. produce pH of 4.2 to 4.8 when grown in 1% glucose broth,
4. be partially resistant to bacitracin, and
5. produce hemolysis on blood agar plates.

In contrast to the group A streptococci, they do not dissolve human fibrin. The organisms are distinguished from group D streptococci by their in vitro sensitivity to methicillin. Nevertheless, despite these diverse biologic characteristics, the ultimate identification of the organisms is contingent on the demonstration of a positive precipitant reaction by group B anticarbohydrate antiserum.

The highest incidence of GBS can be achieved when a selective medium such as Todd-Hewitt broth with sheep blood, nalidixic acid, and gentamicin is used. Commercially available options include Trans-Vag broth supplemented with 5% defibrinated sheep blood or Lim broth. When nonselective culture plates are used for bacterial isolates, colonization rates as low as

4% to 5% are observed. With the use of selective media that eliminate endemic overgrowth, colonization rates of 14% to 24% are identified.

When a diagnostic laboratory is not available, transport media need to be employed. Comparison of direct inoculation of swab specimens unto a selective Todd-Hewitt media versus Todd-Hewitt broth versus delayed inoculation from transport medium resulted in a progressive decrease in the positive cultures identified. The literature suggests that the occurrence of false-negative culture becomes meaningful if the delay time exceeds two hours. A culture derived from a swab specimen inoculated into transport media may have built into the results a 4% to 8% false-negative rate.

The probability of identifying GBS is influenced by the site of bacteriological sampling. Cervical cultures are not ideal. When attempting to identify the presence or absence of GBS, samples from the vaginal introitus and the rectum should be obtained. Patients with high GBS replication ($>10^8$ cfu) will have both vaginal and rectal colonization. Positive vaginal and rectal or urine cultures for GBS potentially identify a gravida at significantly augmented risk for neonatal and/or maternal infection complications.

Several rapid diagnostic tests have been developed to make a presumptive diagnosis based on detection of group B or type-specific polysaccharide antigens in serum, urine, or cerebrospinal fluid by means of monoclonal antibodies or hyperimmune antisera. These tests include countercurrent immunoelectrophoresis, latex particle agglutination, staphylococcal coagglutination, and enzyme immunoassay. The specificity and sensitivity of these tests are significantly enhanced if specimens are preincubated for 4 to 12 hours before utilization. Using latex agglutination or enzyme-linked immunosorbent assay (ELISA) significantly reduces the time required for definitive diagnosis of the GBS. Concentrated urine is a valuable specimen for the detection of specific group B antigens in neonates.

Neonatal clues to the possibility of early-onset disease include the following:
1. Identification of gram-positive cocci in gastric aspirates
2. A low peak ventilatory pressure on mechanical ventilation
3. Repeated episodes of transient apnea or shock in the first 24 hours

A definitive diagnosis of neonatal disease is again contingent upon bacteriologic identification.

The principal shortcoming of most rapid diagnostic tests has been their sensitivity. Skoll et al. (1991) compared the sensitivity of a latex agglutination assay (Striptex) and a solid-phase immunoassay (Equate Strept B test) and found these sensitivities to be 15.1% and 21.5%, respectively. Both tests were highly specific. In general, for a rapid diagnostic test to be positive, at least 5×10^6 cfu need to be present. These tests have their value in identifying gravidas with heavy colonization. To increase sensitivity, it is advocated that specimens be incubated in appropriate broth culture media for four to six hours and then tested. The vaginal Gram stain lacks sensitivity, specificity, positive predictive value, and negative predictive value.

Confronted with a gravida with labor or rupture of membranes before 37 weeks of gestation at significant risk of preterm delivery, it is recommended that vaginal and rectal GBS cultures be obtained and appropriate antimicrobial prophylaxis be initiated. If at 48 hours, GBS is not identified, the antibiotic therapy can be terminated.

THERAPY

Penicillin is the drug of choice for both maternal and neonatal disease when the pathogen is the group B streptococci; however, in cases in which risk factors dictate antibiotic administration, because of the bacterial pathogenic spectrum that can function under these circumstances, ampicillin or, in selected cases, a cephalosporin becomes the drug of choice under best fit for spectrum doctrine. Large initial doses of ampicillin (2 g loading dose followed by 1 g every four to six hours) are frequently required because of the necessity for the drug to traverse the placental or blood–brain barrier.

If the mother is allergic to penicillin, two alternate prophylactic regimens have been advocated: clindamycin, 900 mg IV every eight hours until delivery, or erythromycin, 500 mg IV every six hours until delivery. Unfortunately, neither clindamycin nor erythromycin achieves category coverage for GBS.

The placenta is composed of ectodermal cells, a basement membrane, mesodermally derived tissue, another basement membrane, and fetal endothelial cells. The only other embryologic structure in the human body derived from ectoderm and mesoderm as opposed to mesoderm and endoderm is the choroid plexus. Not surprisingly, the antibiotic transports across these two membranes strongly parallel each other. The factors governing antibiotic transport across the placenta are the following:
1. Molecular size
2. Degree of ionization
3. Lipid solubility
4. Degree of protein binding

Both penicillin G ($pK_a = 2.8$ for its free carboxylic acid group) and ampicillin ($pK_a = 2.5$ for its free carboxylic acid group and $pK_a = 7.2$ for its free amino group) are highly ionized ($>99.9\%$) under physiologic conditions.

Both penicillin and ampicillin antibiotics exhibit only moderate lipophilicity. The oil/water partition coefficients ($K_{o/w}$) are 0.55 and 0.16 for penicillin G and ampicillin, respectively (isobutanol vs. pH 7.4 aqueous buffer).

Penicillin G is moderately bound to albumin in the sera of normal and pregnant subjects (65% bound compared with ampicillin's 20%). To be pharmacologically active, an antibiotic must exist in its unbound state. The amount of antibiotic available for transport in a given time is a direct function of the concentration of free drug. Once the antibiotic is removed by transport, the equilibrium between bound and unbound drug is reestablished. The free drug entering the fetal vascular compartment and amniotic fluid is once again subjected to similar protein-binding interactions, which reduces the amount of antibiotic available for biologic activity. One of the keys to effective in utero therapy involves how much pharmacologically active antibiotic appropriate to the bacteria in question can be delivered in a relatively limited time.

Penicillin G is slightly superior to ampicillin for the beta-hemolytic streptococci; however, this superior minimal inhibitory concentration (MIC) for the beta-hemolytic streptococci does not necessarily translate into biological significance. Both drugs have been highly effective against GBS in clinical trials. The clear difference between penicillin G and ampicillin is the latter's extended spectrum for gram-negative bacteria, specifically *Escherichia coli*, *Proteus mirabilis*, *Salmonella* species, enterococci, *Listeria monocytogenes*, and *Haemophilus influenzae*.

One of the reasons advanced for preferring penicillin over ampicillin is the statement that ampicillin selects for resistant bacteria. The concept of ampicillin's selecting for resistance emanates from a case series published by McDuffie et al. (1993). These authors reported four cases of Enterobacteriaceae chorioamnionitis in gravidas who had received ampicillin prophylaxis for premature rupture of the fetal membranes and GBS carriage. Three of the isolates were *E. coli*. The fourth case was due to *Klebsiella pneumoniae*. Two of the resultant neonates died with fulminant perinatal septicemia. The use of ampicillin identified resistant bacteria, but did not induce that resistance. Had penicillin been used, the same bacteria would have been isolated.

If an antibiotic is used against a bacterium whose spectrum of susceptibility is not encompassed by that drug, one cannot anticipate having a true biologic effect. Approximately 35% to 40% of all current *E. coli* isolates are resistant to ampicillin. This resistance is mediated primarily by the presence of significant quantities of beta-lactamases within the periplasmic space. More than 95% of all *K. pneumoniae* isolates are similarly inherently resistant to ampicillin. When isolated instances of disease due to Enterobacteriaceae occur in the face of ampicillin therapy, the probability is that the same pattern of disease would have been observed had penicillin been given.

If high-risk criteria are used to determine whether or not prophylactic antibiotic is given, ampicillin, owing to its partial coverage for the Enterobacteriaceae, should be used. The risk factors that select for perinatal septicemia due to Enterobacteriaceae are virtually identical to those that select for GBS septicemia (prolonged rupture of fetal membranes, urinary tract infection, maternal fever, prematurity).

If amnionitis or chorioamnionitis is suspected, broad-spectrum antibiotic therapy that includes an agent effective against GBS should replace GBS prophylaxis.

Group B Streptococcal Impact on Perinatal Septicemia

Effective implementation of the CDC guidelines has dramatically reduced the incidence of GBS perinatal septicemia as well as perinatal septicemia in general. Along with GBS, *L. monocytogenes* and the penicillin-Enterobacteriaceae (*P. mirabilis* and selected *E. coli*) and *H. influenzae* are theoretically eradicated by ampicillin prophylaxis. The net effect is that those bacteria now responsible for perinatal septicemia will be predominantly bacteria resistant to the first- and second-generation penicillins.

Group B Streptococcal Vaginitis

Group B streptococci are normal constituents of the bacterial flora of the female genital tract; however, if they obtain microbiological dominance such that they are the sole bacteria present, they will induce a unique type of vulvaginitis. Clinically, the individuals present with intense erythema not too dissimilar to that observed with candidiasis. The vaginal tissues are very tender to touch. Gram staining of the vaginal exudates will reveal just gram-positive cocci. The entity responds well to ampicillin therapy.

Recommended Antimicrobial Regimens

Penicillin is the preferred choice for intrapartum prophylaxis. For the reasons delineated, the alternative use of ampicillin is advocated (Table 3).

Therapy of gravidas with a history of penicillin hypersensitivity is complicated by the presence of significant resistance to both clindamycin and erythromycin. Up to 155 of GBS isolates are resistant to clindamycin. Resistance to erythromycin can be as high as 25%. An isolate resistant to erythromycin, but susceptible to clindamycin, may still have inducible resistance to clindamycin. The severity of the hypersensitivity reaction to penicillin needs to be carefully evaluated; penicillin-allergic gravidas who have experienced immediate hypersensitivity to penicillin, gravidas with asthma, and gravidas with beta-adrenergic–blocking agents are candidates for vancomycin prophylaxis. For gravidas with a history of other than that of an immediate hypersensitivity reaction, cefazolin is preferred over vancomycin.

In the future, greater emphasis will be placed on antibiotic selection that maximizes fetal/neonatal therapy. Intravenous administration of penicillins in high doses is advocated in order to achieve higher intra-amniotic drug concentrations. Erythromycin does not effectively traverse the placental barrier. Selected second- and third-generation cephalosporins penetrate into amniotic fluid in higher effective concentrations than cefazolin.

SELECTED READING

Urinary Tract Infection
Duma RJ, Weinberg AN, Medrek TF, Kunz LJ. Streptococcal infections: a bacteriologic and clinical study of streptococcal bacteremia. Medicine 1969; 48:87.

TABLE 3 Recommended antimicrobial prophylaxis regimens for perinatal GBS disease prevention

■ *Recommended*:
Penicillin G 5 million units IV initial dose, *then* 2.5 million units IV every 4 hr until delivery
■ *Alternative*:
Ampicillin 2 g IV initial dose, *then* 1 g IV every 8 hr until delivery
■ *Penicillin-allergic gravidas*:
GBS-susceptible isolate: clindamycin 900 mg IV every 8 hr until delivery; *or* erythromycin 500 mg IV every 6 hr until delivery
Clindamycin/erythromycin-resistant GBS: vancomycin 1 g IV every 12 hr until delivery; vancomycin is reserved for women at high risk for anaphylaxis. For gravidas with other than immediate hypersensitivity reactions, cefazolin 2 g IV initial dose, *then* 1 g every 8 hr until delivery is advocated

Abbreviation: GBS, group B streptococcus.

Hood M, Janney A, Dameron G. Beta-hemolytic streptococci group B associated with problems of the perinatal period. Am J Obstet Gynecol 1961; 82:809.

Mead PJ, Harris RE. The incidence of group B beta-hemolytic streptococcus in antepartum urinary tract infections. Obstet Gynecol 1978; 51:412.

Moller M, Thomsen AC, Borch K, Dimesen K, et al. Rupture of fetal membranes and premature delivery associated with GBS in urine of pregnant women. Lancet 1984; 2:69.

Persson K, Christensen KK, Christensen P, et al. Asymptomatic bacteriuria during pregnancy with special reference to GBS. Scand J Infect Dis 1985; 17:195.

White CP, Wilkins EG, Roberts C, Davidson DC. Premature delivery and GBS bacteriuria. Lancet 1984; 2:586.

Wood EG, Dillon HE Jr. A prospective study of GBS bacteriuria in pregnancy. Am J Obstet Gynecol 1981; 140:515.

Bacterial Colonization

Bobitt JR, Damato JD, Sakakini J Jr. Perinatal complications in GBS carriers: a longitudinal study of prenatal patients. Am J Obstet Gynecol 1985; 151:711.

Chaisilwattana P, Monif GRG. In vitro ability of the group B streptococci to inhibit gram-positive and gram-variable constituents of the bacterial flora of the female genital tract. Infect Dis Obstet Gynecol 1995; 3:91.

Boyer KM, Gadzala CA, Burd LI, et al. Selective intrapartum chemoprophylaxis of neonatal GBS early-onset disease. I: epidemiologic rationale. J Infect Dis 1983; 148:795.

Desa DJ, Trevenen CL. Intrauterine infections with group B beta-hemolytic streptococci. Br J Obstet Gynaecol 1984; 91:237.

Dillon HC, Hastings MJG, Neill J, et al. GBS carriage and disease: a 6-year prospective study. J Pediatr 1987; 110:31.

Dykes AK, Christensen KK, Christensen P. Chronic carrier state in mothers of infants with GBS infections. Obstet Gynecol 1985; 66:84–88.

Matorras R, Garcia-Perea A, Madero R, Usandizaga JA. Maternal colonization by group B streptococci and puerperal infection; analysis of intrapartum chemoprophylaxis. Eur J Obstet Gynecol Reprod Biol 1991; 38:203.

Matorras R, Garcia-Perea A, Usandizaga JA, Omenaca F. Natural transmission of group B streptococcus during delivery. Int J Gynaecol Obstet 1989; 30:99.

McDonald H, Vigneswaran R, O'Loughlin JA. Group B streptococcal colonization and preterm labour. Aust NZ J Obstet Gynaecol 1989; 29:291.

Papapetropoulou M, Kondakis XG. A study of risk factors of vaginal colonization with group B streptococci in pregnancy. Eur J Epidemiol 1987; 3:419.

Regan JA, Klebanoff MA, Nugent RP. The epidemiology of group B streptococcal colonization in pregnancy: Vaginal Infections and Prematurity Study Group. Obstet Gynecol 1991; 77:604.

Stapleton RD, Kahn JM, Evans LE, et al. Risk factors for group B streptococcal genitourinary tract colonization in pregnant women. Obstet Gynecol 2005; 106:1246.

Genital Tract Infection

Clark LR, Atendido M. Group B streptococcal vaginitis in postpubertal adolescent girls. J Adolest Health 2006; 36:437.

Feingold DS, Stagg NL, Kunz LJ. Extrarespiratory streptococcal infections: importance of the various serologic groups. N Engl J Med 1966; 275:356.

Finn PD, Holden FA. Observations and comments concerning the isolation of Group B beta-hemolytic streptococci from human sources. Can Med Assoc J 1970; 103:249.

Fry RM. Fatal infection by hemolytic streptococcus group B. Lancet 1938; 1:199.

Gallagher PC, Watanakunakorn C. GBS bacteremia in a community teaching hospital. Am J Med 1985; 78:795.

Hood M, Janney A, Dameron G. Beta-hemolytic streptococci group B associated with problems of the perinatal period. Am J Obstet Gynecol 1961; 82:809.

Ledger WJ, Norman M, Gee C, Lewis W. Bacteremia on an obstetric-gynecologic service. Am J Obstet Gynecol 1975; 121:205.

McKenna DS, Iams JD. Group B streptococcal infections. Semin Perinatol 1998; 22:267.

Pass MA, Gray BM, Dillon HC. Puerperal and perinatal infection with GBS. Am J Obstet Gynecol 1982; 143:147.

Ramsay AM, Gillespie M. Puerperal infection associated with hemolytic streptococci other than Lancefield's group A. Br J Obstet Gynaecol 1941; 48:569.

Reid TMS. Emergence of GBS in obstetric and perinatal infections. Br Med J 1976; 2:533.

Reid TMS. GBS endocarditis. Scott Med J 1977; 22:13.

Reinarz JA, Sanford JP. Human infection caused by nongroups A or D streptococci. Medicine 1965; 44:81.

Sexton DJ, Rockson SG, Hempling RE, Cathey CW. Pregnancy-associated GBS endocarditis: a report of two fatal cases. Obstet Gynecol 1985; 66:448.

Sutton GP, Smlirz LR, Clark DH, Bennett JE. GBS necrotizing fasciitis arising from an episiotomy. Obstet Gynecol 1985; 66:733.

Yow MD, Leeds LJ, Thompson PK, et al. The natural history of GBS colonization in the pregnant woman and her offspring. Am J Obstet Gynecol 1980; 137:34.

Ampicillin Vs. Penicillin for Prophylaxis

Allen UD, Navas L, King SM. Effectiveness of intrapartum penicillin prophylaxis in preventing early-onset group B streptococcal infection: results of a meta-analysis. Can Med Assoc J 1993; 149:1659.

Amstey MS, Gibbs RS. Is penicillin a better choice than ampicillin for prophylaxis of neonatal group B streptococcal infections? Obstet Gynecol 1994; 84:1058.

Eleck E, Ivan B, Arr M. Passage of the penicillins from mother to fetus in humans. Int J Clin Pharmacol Ther Toxicol 1972; 63:223.

Garland SM, Fliegner JR. Group B streptococcus and neonatal infection: the case for intrapartum chemoprophylaxis. Aust NZ J Obstet Gynaecol 1991; 31:119.

Glass NE, Schulkin J, Chamany S, et al. Opportunities to reduce overuse of antibiotics for perinatal group B streptococcal disease prevention and management of preterm premature rupture of membranes. Infect Dis Obstet Gynecol 2005; 12:5.

Glover DD, Lalka D, Monif GRG. Ampicillin vs. penicillin for in utero therapy. Infect Dis Obstet Gynecol 1996; 4:43.

Heim K, Alge A, Marth C. Anaphylactic reaction to ampicillin and severe complication in the fetus. Lancet 1991; 337:859.

MacAulay MA, Abour-Sabe M, Charles D. Transplacental transfer of ampicillin. Am J Obstet Gynecol 1966; 96:943.

McDuffie RS, McGregor JA, Gibbs RS. Adverse perinatal outcome and resistant Enterobacteriaceae after antibiotic usage for premature rupture of the membranes and group B streptococcus carriage. Obstet Gynecol 1993; 82:487.

Mercer BM, Ramsey RD, Sibai BM. Prenatal screening for group B streptococcus. II. Impact of antepartum screening and prophylaxis on neonatal care. Am J Obstet Gynecol 1995; 173:842.

Nau H. Clinical pharmacokinetics in pregnancy and perinatology II. Penicillins. Dev Pharmacol Ther 1987; 10:176.

Pyatl SP, Plides RS, Jacobs NM, et al. Penicillin in infants weighing two kilograms or less with early onset GBS disease. N Engl J Med 1983; 308:1383.

Williams DA. pK_a values for some drugs and miscellaneous organic acids and bases. In: Foye WO, Lemke TL, Williams DA, eds. Principles of Medicinal Chemistry. 4th ed. Media, PA: Williams & Wilkins, 1995:948.

Yow MD, Mason ED, Leeds LJ, et al. Ampicillin prevents intrapartum transmission of group B streptococcus. J Am Med Assoc 1979; 241:1245.

Neonatal Septicemia/Meningitis

Aber RC, Allen N, Howell JT, et al. Nosocomial transmission of GBS. Pediatrics 1976; 58:346.

Baker CJ, Barrett FF. GBS infections in infants: the importance of the various serotypes. J Am Med Assoc 1974; 230:1158.

Baker CJ, Edwards MS. Group B streptococcal infections. In: Remington TA, Klein JO, eds. Infectious Diseases of the Fetus and Newborn Infant. 4th ed. Philadelphia: WB Saunders, 1995:980.

Baker CJ, Kasper DL. Correlation of maternal antibody deficiency with susceptibility to neonatal GBS infection. N Engl J Med 1976; 294:753.

Barton LL, Feigin RD, Lins R. Group B beta-hemolytic streptococcal meningitis in infants. J Pediatr 1973; 82:719.

Bergqvist G, Hurvell B. Neonatal infections caused by Streptococcus agalactiae (Lancefield B). Acta Pathol Microbiol Scand 1970; 78:270.

Bergqvist G, Hurvell B, Malmborg AS, et al. Neonatal infections caused by group B streptococcus. Scand J Infect Dis 1971; 3:157.

Bergqvist G, Hurvell B, Thal E, Vaclavinkovo V. Neonatal infections caused by group B streptococcus: relation between the occurrence in the vaginal flora of term pregnant women and infection in the newborn infant. Scand J Infect Dis 1971; 3:209.

Bobitt JR. The group B beta-hemolytic streptococcus. Semin Perinatol 1977; 1:51.

Edwards MS. Group B streptococcal infections. Pediatr Infect Dis J 1990; 9:778.

Eickhoff TC, Klein JO, Daly AK, et al. Neonatal sepsis and other infections due to group B beta-hemolytic streptococci. N Engl J Med 1964; 271:1221.

Helmig R, Halaburt JT, Uldbjert N, et al. Increased cell adherence of group B streptococci from preterm infants with neonatal sepsis. Obstet Gynecol 1990; 76:825.

Hood M, Janney A, Dameron G. Beta-hemolytic streptococcus group B associated with problems of perinatal period. Am J Obstet Gynecol 1961; 82:809.

Jones DE, Kanarek KS, Lim DV. GBS colonization patterns in mothers and their infants. J Clin Microbiol 1984; 20:438.

Regan JA, Klebanof MA, Nugent RP, et al. Colonization with group B streptococci in pregnancy and adverse outcome. Am J Obstet Gynecol 1996; 174:1354.

Weisman LE, Stoll BJ, Cruess DF, et al. Early-onset group B streptococcal sepsis: a current assessment. J Pediatr 1992; 121:428.

Yancey MD, Duff P, Clark P, et al. Peripartum infection associated with vaginal group B streptococcal colonization. Obstet Gynecol 1994; 84:816.

Diagnosis

Armer T, Clark P, Duff P, Saravanos K. Rapid intrapartum detection of group B streptococcal colonization with an enzyme immunoassay. Am J Obstet Gynecol 1993; 168:39.

Carey JC, Klebanoff MA, Regan JA. Evaluation of the Gram stain as a screening tool for maternal carriage of group B beta-hemolytic streptococci: The Vaginal Infections and Prematurity Study Group. Obstet Gynecol 1990; 76:693.

Greenspoon JS, Fishman A, Wilcox JG, et al. Comparison of culture for group B streptococcus versus enzyme immunoassay and latex agglutination rapid tests: results in 250 patients during labor. Obstet Gynecol 1991; 77:97.

Lugenbill C, Clark RB, Fagnant RJ, et al. Comparison of the cervicovaginal Gram stain and rapid latex agglutination slide test for identification of group B streptococci. J Perinatol 1990; 10:403.

Monif GRG. Media selection for the identification of group B streptococcus. Infect Med 2004; 21:492.

Philipson EH, Palermino DA, Robinson A. Enhanced antenatal detection of group B streptococcus colonization. Obstet Gynecol 1995; 85:437.

Skoll MA, Mercer BM, Baselski V, et al. Evaluation of two rapid group B streptococcal antigen tests in labor and delivery patients. Obstet Gynecol 1991; 77:322.

Towers CV, Garite TJ, Friedman WW, et al. Comparison of a rapid enzyme-linked immunosorbent assay test and the Gram stain for detection of group B streptococcus in high-risk antepartum patients. Am J Obstet Gynecol 1990; 163:965.

Wang E, Richardson H. A rapid method for detection of group B streptococcal colonization: testing at the bedside. Obstet Gynecol 1990; 76:882.

Yancey MK, Schuchat A, Brown LK, et al. The accuracy of late antenatal screening cultures in predicting genital group B streptococcal colonization at delivery. Obstet Gynecol 1996; 88:811.

Therapy/Prevention

ACOG Committee Opinion. Prevention of early-onset group B streptococcal disease in newborns. 1996; 173:1.

ACOC Committee Opinion. Prevention of early-onset group B streptococcal disease in newborns. 2002; 279:1405.

Boyer KM, Gotoff SP. Prevention of early-onset neonatal GBS disease with selective intrapartum chemoprophylaxis. N Engl J Med 1986; 314:1665.

Boyer KM, Gotoff SP. Alternative algorithms for prevention of perinatal group B streptococcal infections. Pediatr Infect Dis J 1998; 17:973.

Boyer KM, Gadzala CA, Burd LI, et al. Selective intrapartum chemoprophylaxis of neonatal GBS early onset disease. I: epidemiologic rationale. J Infect Dis 1983; 148:795.

Boyer KM, Gadzala CA, Kelly PD, et al. Selective intrapartum chemoprophylaxis of neonatal GBS early onset disease. II: predictive value of prenatal cultures. J Infect Dis 1983; 148:802.

Boyer KM, Gadzala CA, Kelly PD. Selective intrapartum chemoprophylaxis of neonatal GBS early onset disease. III: interruption of mother-to infant transmission. J Infect Dis 1983; 148:810.

Committee on Infectious Diseases and Committee on Fetus and Newborn. Guidelines for prevention of group B streptococcal (GBS) infection by chemoprophylaxis. Pediatrics 1992; 90:776.

Dooley S, Larsen J. Universal antepartum screening for maternal GBS not recommended: ACOG recommendations. ACOGNewsletter 1993; 37:1.

Edwards RK, Clark P, Duff P. Intrapartum antibiotic prophylaxis 2: positive predictive value of antenatal group B streptococci cultures and antibiotic susceptibility of clinical isolates. Obstet Gynecol 2002; 100:540.

Edwards RK, Clark P, Sistrom CL, Duff P. Intrapartum antibiotic prophylaxis 1: relative effects of recommended antibiotics on gram-negative pathogens. Obstet Gynecol 2002; 100:534.

Gigante J, Hickson GB, Entman SS, Oquist NL. Universal screening for group B streptococcus: recommendations and obstetricians' practice decisions. Obstet Gynecol 1995; 85:440.

Katz VL, Moos MK, Cefalo RC, et al. Group B streptococci: results of a protocol of antepartum screening and intrapartum treatment. Am J Obstet Gynecol 1994; 170:521.

Minkoff H, Mead P. An obstetric approach to the prevention of early-onset group B beta-hemolytic streptococcal sepsis. Am J Obstet Gynecol 1986; 154:973.

Monif GRG. Neonatal group B streptococcal disease prevention. Infect Med 2004; 21:42.

Newton ER, Clark M. Group B streptococcus and preterm rupture of membranes. Obstet Gynecol 1991; 77: 322.

Ohlsson A, Myhr TL. Intrapartum chemoprophylaxis of perinatal group B streptococcal infections: critical review of randomized controlled trials. Am J Obstet Gynecol 1994; 170:910.

Pylipow M, Gaddis M, Kinney JS. Selective intrapartum prophylaxis for group B streptococcus colonization: management and outcome of newborns. Pediatrics 1994; 93:631.

Rouse DJ, Goldenberg RL, Cliver SP, et al. Strategies for the prevention of early-onset group B streptococcal sepsis: a decision analysis. Obstet Gynecol 1994; 83:483.

Sanders TR, Roberts CL, Gilbert GL. Compliance with a protocol for intrapartum antibiotic prophylaxis against neonatal group B streptococcal sepsis in women with clinical risk factors. Infect Dis Obstet Gynecol 2002; 10:223.

Schrag S, Gorwitz R, Fultz-Butts K, Schuchat A. Prevention of perinatal group B streptococcal disease: revised guidelines from CDC. MMWR Recomm Rep 2002; 51:(RR-11)1.

Schrag SJ, Zell ER, Lynfield R, et al. A population-based comparison of strategies to prevent early-onset group B streptococcal disease in neonates. N Engl J Med 2002; 347:233.

Schrag SJ, Zywicki S, Farley MM, et al. Group B streptococcus disease in the era of intrapartum antibiotic prophylaxis. N Engl J Med 2000; 342:15.

Schuchat A, Whitney C, Zangwill K. Prevention of perinatal group B streptococcal disease: public health perspective. MMWR 1996; 45:1.

Spaetgens R, DeBella K, MA D, et al. Perinatal antibiotic usage and changes in colonization and resistance rates of group B streptococcus and other pathogens. Obstet Gynecol 2002; 100:525.

Wendel GD Jr, Leveno KJ, Sanchez PJ, et al. Prevention of neonatal group B streptococcal disease: a combined intrapartum and neonatal protocol. Am J Obstet Gynecol 2002; 188:618.

42

Group C Beta-Hemolytic Streptococci (*Streptococcus milleri*)

INTRODUCTION

Streptococci of the milleri group are part of the normal flora of human mucous membranes. These streptococci have also been reported to be significant pathogens. Like other mucosal streptococci, they may cause infective endocarditis; unlike other mucosal streptococci, however, they have also been repeatedly associated (more frequently in men than in women) with serious suppurative infections. Evidence for the pathogenicity of the *Streptococcus milleri* group is scattered and mainly circumstantial. Although the organisms are found in a high proportion of certain suppurative infections, other bacteria are often present as well. Successful treatment of these infections with surgery and broad-spectrum antibiotics is not indicative of any specific etiology. "*Streptococcus milleri*" is an unofficial name that has been applied to a group of streptococci which, although basically similar, show various hemolytic, serological, and physiological characteristics. Head and neck infections and pneumonia are most often associated with beta-hemolytic strains, and bacteremia and gastrointestinal and urogenital tract infections with alpha-hemolytic strains. The species name *Streptococcus anginosus* has recently been recognized as the approved name for these organisms. Streptococci known as *S. milleri* have been implicated as etiologic agents in a variety of serious purulent infections, but because of their heterogeneous characteristics, these organisms may be unrecognized or misidentified by clinical laboratories.

S. milleri is unique among the streptococci because it produces abscesses. An infection caused by *S. milleri* often has its genesis in the gastrointestinal tract. Its isolation from pus or blood cultures is clinically relevant. The identification of *S. milleri* from blood cultures suggests the possibility of serious purulent infection, whose source may lie in the gastrointestinal tract. *S. milleri* differs from other group C beta-hemolytic streptococci and, in particular, *Streptococcus equisimilis* by the appearance of human Fc (gamma) receptors. The majority of hemolytic strains of *S. milleri* produce hyaluronidase. There is a strong positive correlation between hyaluronidase production and isolation of the strain from internal abscesses. Strains isolated from patients with endocarditis tend to be uniformly nonproducers of hyaluronidase. Demonstration of hyaluronidase production in isolates from blood cultures should alert the physician to the possibility of deep-seated abscess.

DIAGNOSIS

Definitive diagnosis is based upon bacteriological isolate. The presence or absence of beta-hemolysis and hyaluronidase production is important. Latex agglutination will identify 94 to 96 isolates of group C beta-hemolytic streptococci. Alpha-hemolytic streptococci in this group tend to be discarded as "normal flora."

Microbiologists and physicians need to become aware of the group C streptococci. The heterogeneous nature of this group of streptococci means that laboratories will have to use a combination of antigenic, physiologic, and hemolytic characteristics to identify them.

CLINICAL SPECTRUM IN OBSTETRICAL AND GYNECOLOGICAL PATIENTS

S. milleri functions both as a class II and as a class III anaerobe. In gynecological patients, *S. milleri* has produced tubo-ovarian abscess and spontaneous necrotic cutaneous infections. The bacterium is frequently isolated in patients with active perineal suppurative hidradenitis. Its presence is significantly associated with disease activity and its disappearance significantly correlates with clinical improvement. In this clinical setting, *S. milleri* frequently cofunctions with anaerobic bacteria or *Staphylococcus aureus*. When a bacteremia is induced, metatastic hepatic abscesses may ensue. *S. milleri* can function as a significant perinatal pathogen. A number of fatal perinatal septicemias due to this bacteria have been described.

THERAPY

Streptococci milleri strains have minimal inhibitory concentration for penicillin G between 0.015 and 0.12 µg/L. Treatment consists of drainage by laparotomy or percutaneous aspiration combined with approximately six weeks of penicillin administration. Patients with liver abscesses who receive metronidazole may not respond if *S. milleri* is the infecting organism. Physicians need to recognize that these microorganisms as a group are able to cause serious infections that may require prolonged treatment and/or surgical drainage of abscesses.

SELECTED READING

Barnham H, Xerby J, Chandler RS, Hillar MR. Group C streptococci in human infections: a study of 305 isolates with clinical correlations. Epidemiol Infect 1989; 102:3798.

Chua D, Reinhart HH, Sobel JD. Liver abscess caused by *Streptococcus milleri*. Rev Infect Dis 1989; 11:197.

Cox RA, Chen K, Coykendall AL, et al. Fatal infection in neonates of 26 weeks' gestation due to *Streptococcus milleri*: report of two cases. J Clin Pathol 1987; 40:190.

Gelfand HS, Hodgkiss T, Simmons BP. Multiple hepatic abscesses caused by *Streptococcus milleri* in association with an intrauterine device. Rev Infect Dis 1989; 11:983.

Gossling J. Occurrence and pathogenicity of the *Streptococcus milleri* group. Rev Infect Dis 1988; 10:257.

Hocken DB, Dussek JE. *Streptococcus milleri* as a cause of pleural empyema. Thorax 1985; 40:626.

Lebrun L, Guibert M, Wallet P, et al. Human Fe (gamma) receptors for differentiation in throat cultures of group C "*Streptococcus equisimilis*" and group C "*Streptococcus milleri*." J Clin Microbiol 1986; 24:705.

Peck G, Coe PR, Allen B. Fatal infection in neonates caused by *S. milleri*. J Clin Pathol 1987; 40:1386.

Ruoff KL. Streptococcus anginosus ("*Streptococcus milleri*"): the unrecognized pathogen. Clin Microbiol Rev 1988; 1:102.

Singh KP, Morris A, Lang SD, et al. Clinically significant *Streptococcus anginosus* (*Streptococcus milleri*) infections: a review of 186 cases. NZ Med J 1988; 101:813.

Spertini F, Baumgartner JD, Bille J. Clinical spectrum of a common and insidious pathogen: *Streptococcus milleri*. Schweiz Med Wochenschr 1988; 118:1393.

Steel A. An unusual case of necrotizing fasciitis. Br J Oral Maxillofac Surg 1987; 25:328.

Unsworth PP. Hyaluronidase production in *Streptococcus milleri* in relation to infection. J Clin Pathol 1989; 42:506.

Wu CJ, Tsung SH. Meningitis due to *Streptococcus milleri* (*Streptococcus*) C. South Med J 1983; 76:1322.

Enterococcus

Bryan Larsen

43

INTRODUCTION

Enterococcus has become one of the major nosocomial pathogens, rivaling *Escherichia coli* and *Staphylococcus aureus* for prominence in the hospital environment. Historically, the organism may not have been recognized as prominently as it is today because of its occurrence in polymicrobial infections where other organisms were present that were more likely to be implicated as the primary pathogen. In addition, its prevalence in infections is increasing because of its profound resistance to many antibiotics that are used empirically in polymicrobial infections. While some of the microbial participants in a polymicrobial infection are suppressed by the antibiotics used for first-line therapy, the resistant enterococci may persist and emerge as dominant microbes (Berger-Bachi, 2002).

The enterococci, like many of the pathogens encountered in compromised individuals, are frequently found in a commensal relationship with the host in the intestinal tract and other mucosal sites. As with most opportunistic infections, host compromise is usually the precipitating event that results in these colonizing species becoming involved in a pathologic process. Although many infections arise from the normal host biota, the enterococci have been shown also to spread among hospitalized individuals by fomites or through person-to-person contact (Jett et al., 1994). Further, in the hospital environment, strain replacement (whereby an endogenous strain of *Enterococcus* is replaced by one acquired in the hospital) may play a role in nosocomial infections involving the *Enterococcus* (Dobbs et al., 2006). As will be elaborated subsequently, among the most troubling problems related to enterococcal infections involves the frequency of resistance to antibiotics, at times even to antibiotics of last resort such as vancomycin.

While the majority of an extensive literature related to this organism focuses on specific infections such as bacteremias, urinary tract infections, endocarditis, and postsurgical infections, this chapter will focus more directly on the role of these organisms in relation to obstetrical and gynecologic infections that tend to include the enterococci along with other organisms derived from the lower female genital tract. The importance of the enterococcal role in complications that can occur with neonatal sepsis will also be considered as a sequel to maternal infections.

MICROBIOLOGY AND TAXONOMY

The enterococci are gram-positive organisms that contain the same Lancefield antigen as group D *Streptococcus*, and as a result, they were for many years categorized as Group D streptococci if typing was done; or if categorized by bile resistance and resistance to elevated salt concentration, they were categorized presumptively as Group D *Streptococcus*. Indeed, in Gram stains, the microscopic morphology of the organism is identical to the streptococci. Molecular taxonomic methods indicated that it was appropriate to separate the enterococci from the genus *Streptococcus* (Schleifer and Kilpper-Balz, 1984). In the older literature, speciation was not commonly undertaken when these organisms were isolated from mixed flora sites. Numerous species of enterococci exist in animals and in nature, but *Enterococcus faecalis* and *Enterococcus faecium* are the two species most commonly involved in human infections, with the former being responsible for about 80% of cases (Huycke et al., 1998). Despite this discrepancy in significance between the two major human enterococcal species, this chapter will generally not make a distinction between the species unless such specificity is required. One distinction that must be made at the outset is *E. faecalis* tends to be less likely than *E. faecium* to show resistance to ampicillin or vancomycin, but is more abundant in gut flora than *E. faecium* and appears to have a more extensive panoply of virulence attributes (Pillar and Gilmore, 2004).

The enterococci, as suggested by the genus name, are associated with gut flora and have long been notable among medically important organisms for their resistance to bile salts, their acid tolerance, thermotolerance, and their ability to grow in the presence of 6.5% sodium chloride. Bile-esculin agar is used as a laboratory medium to provide putative identification of *Enterococcus* because they are able to grow in the presence of bile while degrading esculin to produce a dark-colored split product. Primary culture media may also be supplemented with 6 µg/mL of vancomycin to select for vancomycin-resistant strains, since these are currently of great clinical importance. Early investigators found that enterococci survived exposure to soaps, detergents, and other disinfectants, and as new antibiotics have become available, the enterococci tend to show intrinsic tolerance to drugs and develop frank resistance with alarming frequency. This hardiness may underlie some of the persistence of enterococci in the hospital environment.

PATHOGENIC ATTRIBUTES OF *ENTEROCOCCUS*

In recent years, efforts to understand the pathogenicity of *Enterococcus* have accelerated as its importance as a nosocomial pathogen has developed. Thorough reviews of the mechanisms of various virulence attributes of the enterococci are published elsewhere, and in this section, only a brief summary will be presented (Pillar et al., 2004; Koch et al., 2004; Tendolkar et al., 2003). As with other commensal organisms that occasionally participate in pathologic processes, particularly as part of a polymicrobic infectious complication of a primary compromising condition such as surgery, the

Enterococcus does not appear to have a single major and devastatingly potent virulence factor. Rather, several factors seem to participate in concert, allowing this normally low-virulence organism to participate in infectious processes. Some of the putative virulence attributes are mentioned below.

Antimicrobial resistance, such a prominent feature of enterococcal physiology, allows this organism to emerge from among other commensal organisms in the course of antibiotic treatment. The concern that developed during the decades of the 1970s and 1980s focusing on gram-negative enteric organisms complicating clean-contaminated surgeries, was met with the use of second- and third-generation cephalosporins for their broad spectrum of coverage when single-drug empirical therapy for postoperative infections was desired. In addition, when clean-contaminated cases are undertaken, i.e., cases that involve incisions through normally colonized tissues, prophylactic application of second-generation cephalosporins has commonly been employed to obtain coverage for both the gram-negative facultative organisms and gram-negative strictly anaerobic bacteria that commonly participate in mixed postsurgical soft tissue infections and abscesses. Because the *Enterococcus* is generally resistant to cephalosporins, its presence may be enhanced during administration of antimicrobial prophylaxis and during therapy of postoperative infections as well. Aminoglycoside antibiotics, used to obtain coverage for gram-negative opportunistic organisms, are generally unable to inhibit the enterococci unless an additional cell wall damaging drug is included to enhance migration of the aminoglycoside into the *Enterococcus*. Enterococcal emergence has consequently become a rather common occurrence in clinical settings.

Colonization factors including pH resistance (Svensater et al., 1997) and adherence factors (Johnson, 1994) are probably most responsible for enterococcal persistence in the host to begin with, and can subsequently participate in infectious processes. Enterococci are found in the oral cavity and will naturally move through the gut. The ability of the enterococci to persist in the presence of acidic pH suggests that the organism could survive passage through the stomach, and there is evidence to suggest that enterococci can upregulate their pH tolerance by exposure to sublethal hydrogen ion concentrations (Flahaut et al., 1997). This adaptation may also play a role in the replacement of a community strain for a hospital strain as the organism passes through the gut.

Adherence to the epithelia where persistent colonization occurs is of primary importance in maintaining enterococci as part of the flora. Studies have focused more on the adherence to gut epithelium than to the vaginal epithelium, but it may be anticipated that vaginal colonization is dependent on microbial adherence as in the gut. In addition, once the organism migrates beyond its normal locus of colonization, it may require a different repertoire of adhesins to attach to such diverse tissues as bladder epithelium heart valves. The finding that exposure of *E. faecalis* to serum increased its adherence to heart cells (Guzman et al., 1991) suggests that some adhesion molecules may be regulated by environmental cues. Evidence has been presented for the existence of multiple adhesins comprising protein or carbohydrate, which in turn suggests a multiplicity of adherence mechanisms (Guzman et al., 1991).

Despite the presumed importance of stable colonization of the host by enterococci coupled with the recognition that these colonizing organisms can participate in endogenously derived infections, there is nevertheless information to suggest that some cases of nosocomial infection display clonality (Baldassari et al., 2005); i.e., infecting organisms in multiple patients appearing to be genetically identical. Such a finding hints that enterococcal infections may, at least in some instances, be due to acquired organisms that possess a special repertoire of virulence factors and that these exogenous strains supplant or at least coexist with endogenous strains. One factor that could play a role in certain strains obtaining ecological dominance is superoxide, which is expressed extracellularly more by invasive than by commensal strains (Huycke et al., 2001). Superoxide may be produced by *E. faecium*, but is predominantly a product of *E. faecalis*.

A number of enterococcal substances that either cause damage to host cells or interfere with host defenses have been described as potential virulence mechanisms, and these have been more comprehensively reviewed elsewhere (Lempianen et al., 2005). Among the virulence factors that seem to play a key role is the enterococcal cytolysin. This substance produces beta-hemolysis on certain blood cells (human, not sheep) and has bacteriocin-like activity (Cox et al., 2005). Although not all strains produce the cytolysin, the hemolytic factor has been associated with organ damage and increased mortality in various animal infection studies.

Aggregation substance is an interesting factor with multiple activities (Waters et al., 2004). The aggregation of bacterial cells may alter the ability of phagocytes to ingest the bacterial complexes, and this substance may also enhance intraphagocytic survival. Less well established is the possibility that aggregation substance has super antigen activity that could be responsible for systemic effects related to enterococcal infections (Schlievert et al., 1998). Finally, bacteria expressing this particular surface substance also display increased cell surface hydrophobicity (Tendolkar et al., 2004), which is believed to enhance adhesion to certain cell types such as gut epithelium.

Additional research will help to better define the specific role of these and other potential virulence factors such as the zinc metalloproteinase (Hancock and Perego, 2004), antiphagocytic capsules (Hufnagel et al., 2005), and antiphagocytic surface proteins with similar roles as the M protein, which is better known as a dominant virulence attribute in the Streptococci, and perhaps by analogy, may be significant for enterococcal virulence (Shankar et al., 2001). Much of the information relating microbial factors to virulence has necessarily been derived from animal studies that, while instructive, do not clearly portray the importance of these factors in humans. As researchers continue to focus more on clinical infections involving *Enterococcus*, they will undoubtedly gain a clearer picture of the significance of particular virulence factors.

MAJOR CLINICAL PROCESSES

It should first be emphasized that because the enterococci are abundant colonizers of the human intestinal tract and the vagina, they are frequently present without causing any untoward consequences. At the same time, it is important to note that because these organisms are prominent commensals, they will be present in patients who undergo surgical or other invasive procedures and may emerge postoperatively as a result of both their intrinsic virulence attributes and selection by antibiotics to which they are resistant. Infections related to manipulations of the gastrointestinal tract will frequently involve the enterococci, alone or in conjunction with other organisms. For example, infection of biliary stents by *Enterococcus* may relate to the resistance of the organism to bile (Basoli et al., 1999).

Translocation of microorganisms from the gastrointestinal tract into the bloodstream is a phenomenon that has been known for many years, but its mechanism remains poorly understood (Berg, 1995). Individuals who are significantly stressed, as in the case of traumatic injury or major surgery, can experience a movement of intestinal organisms across the gut epithelium to the mesenteric lymphatic drainage and on to the bloodstream. Irrespective of whether this process is the result of general physiologic stresses as in trauma patients, increased bacterial load in the gut, nutritional disturbance, epithelial secretory dysfunction, or inflammatory mediators (or a combination of these potential mechanisms), the enterococci are able to participate in this process of translocation, leading to bacteremic events (Wells et al., 1990). Although still a matter of informed speculation, translocation may provide a possible explanation of some bloodstream infections of unknown origin. Endocarditis mostly involving native valves and, to a lesser extent, artificial valves, pleural infection, urinary tract infection, and meningeal invasion are all possible consequences of the translocation process.

In addition to dissemination of enterococci through translocation, a frequent source of metastatic infection is direct spread from a surgical site, including the female genital tract. Even in the older literature, evidence can be found that independent of antibiotic selection, surgical procedures increase the bacterial burden in colonized sites for at least five days postoperatively (Ohm and Galask, 1976). Given this expanded reservoir of organisms, it is not surprising that postoperative infections would develop with regularity even in the absence of exogenous contamination.

Cases of cystitis due to enterococci in adult women are fairly uncommon (Gupta et al., 1999), usually less than 5%, with *E. coli* still predominating among this group, although in cases of catheterization or other instrumentation of the urinary tract, enterococcal cystitis may develop and can progress to pyelonephritis. It appears that urinary tract infection may be either an antecedent or a sequel of bacteremia involving enterococci.

Wound infections represent another source of morbidly involving the enterococci, and are probably most often the result of direct contamination of the operative site with the patient's own flora. Wound infections and other enterococcal infections are more likely to occur in individuals who are otherwise debilitated. Thus, the frail elderly who undergo surgical procedures are especially susceptible (Mouton et al., 2001). In addition, those who have been exposed to antibiotics in the preoperative period may have experienced a shift in their flora that favors resistant bacteria such as the enterococci.

As will be noted below, infections that arise as a result of the spread of enterococci from colonized tissues to otherwise sterile sites are likely to contain multiple species of microbes, since colonized sites such as the gut and the lower female genital tract possess a flora that is polymicrobic.

ENTEROCOCCUS IN THE LOWER FEMALE GENITAL TRACT

A flurry of descriptive microbiology took place during the decades of the 1970s and 1980s, resulting in many reports describing the vaginal flora of healthy women or women of various demographic groups or with specific pathologies (Larsen and Galask, 1980). During this time, there was a great deal of variability in the quality of the microbiological methods employed, some taxonomies were in flux, and an apparent wide variation in the relative experience and technical expertise of the investigators was embedded into this literature. Some studies included culture of strict anaerobes, while others did not. Some investigators used several kinds of primary culture media to increase the likelihood of cultivating certain hard-to-isolate organisms, while others used only one type of medium. Many other differences in these early studies made it difficult to get to a firm idea of the prevalence of individual organisms, although this seemed to be the major goal of many studies in that era. This history suggests that a cautious approach to interpreting the older literature is warranted. In the more recent decades, studies have turned away from cataloging the prevalence of organisms to more hypothesis-driven research and research into the molecular mechanisms of pathogenesis and antimicrobial drug resistance.

Despite the limitations of older culture-based studies, the preponderance of this older literature suggests that the natural prevalence of vaginal enterococci is in the range of 25% to 40% of asymptomatic women, and it may be added that, in general, culture methods were sufficiently reliable with respect to the enterococci to consider such estimates as valid (Larsen, 1985). More recent literature support a similar estimate, but suggest at the same time that enterococcal colonization and *E. coli* colonization seem to track together, suggesting that, not surprisingly, the ultimate source of the flora that contains *E. coli* and *Enterococcus* may be the gut. In fact, a report (Ness et al., 2005) suggests there may be two types of flora in *Lactobacillus*-depleted individuals, namely a bacterial vaginosis type flora (*Gardnerella*, *Mobiluncus*, gram-negative anaerobic rods, and *Mycoplasma*) or an enteric-dominated one (gram-negative enterics plus enterococci).

At present, it is not clear what factors are responsible for the development of a vaginal flora that is tilted in the direction of enteric organisms, but continued studies of the dynamics of the flora are yielding new insights. A potentially useful finding on the dynamics of the vaginal flora is that women with recurrent urinary tract infection may rather consistently harbor enteric organisms at the vaginal vestibule and introitus and at the same time display a paucity of *Lactobacillus* (Stapleton and Stamm, 1997). It has been hypothesized that the dearth of lactobacilli is related to insufficient estrogenic stimulation of the vagina, which ordinarily encourages *Lactobacillus* colonization and discourages introital colonization by *E. coli* and similar organisms. A practical application of this concept is the use of vaginal estrogen preparations as a relatively successful adjunct to cystitis treatment.

Another finding that helps explain the dynamics of vaginal flora is the ability of bacteriocins produced by the enterococci to inhibit lactobacilli isolated from vaginal cultures. This, like the superoxide production by enterococci, could have an effect on regulation of other species within the ecosystem (Cintas et al., 1998; Huycke et al., 1998).

While it appears that some inverse relationship between benign *Lactobacillus* and *Enterococcus* may exist, such a general observation should not be construed as indicating that the presence of enterococci in the lower genital flora is somehow abnormal or even potentially dangerous per se, especially in view of the high frequency of colonization by these organisms among asymptomatic women. In those individuals who do not experience symptoms when colonized by enterococci, it is probably appropriate to view enterococci as commensals, albeit commensals that can participate in infectious complications. Specifically, enterococcal colonization may have more austere connotations if it is accompanied by an apparent suppression of the vaginal lactobacilli or if the flora undergoes strain replacement by hospital strains having a high degree of antibiotic and antiseptic resistance, although such a viewpoint requires specific investigation and confirmation.

OBSTETRICAL AND GYNECOLOGIC IMPLICATIONS

Salpingitis
It is a complex infectious process that is frequently initiated by gonococcal or chlamydial infections, but the ascent of organisms from the lower genital microflora may create a mixed infection after contiguous spread of bacteria across the endometrium, resulting in transient endometritis and inflammation within the fallopian tubes. As mentioned previously, much attention has been given to a flora consistent with bacterial vaginosis (elevated levels of *Gardnerella*, *Mobiluncus*, gram-negative anaerobic bacteria, and *Mycoplasma*) as predisposing to the upper tract involvement that can create a significant salpingitis and, in some instances, tubo-ovarian abscess or peritoneal involvement. While bacterial vaginosis may be statistically identified as predisposing to complicated upper tract infections (Quan, 1994), the enteric organisms including *E. coli* and *Enterococcus* can likewise contribute to upper tract invasion.

Although any combination of organisms might participate in upper tract invasion, it is difficult, and consequently rare, to obtain clinical samples that will document the organisms involved in salpingian infection. Even if such information

were readily available, it would be unlikely and probably inappropriate to incriminate just one microbial species. Generally, in cases of salpingitis, antibiotic coverage sufficient to address many of the potential species that may be involved is administered in addition to the drugs directed at the *Chlamydia* and gonococcus (Workowski and Berman, 2006), but due to its resistance characteristics, the *Enterococcus* may be persistent, requiring a change in antibiotics. Often, a history of cephalosporin use precedes the emergence of *Enterococcus* as a major player in an infected site, and such a history may help guide a change in therapy even when the site is not readily accessible to sampling for culture and susceptibility testing.

Postpartum Endometritis
The microorganisms from the lower genital tract can infect the endometrium after delivery, and the probability that symptomatic infection will occur is related to a broad range of risk factors (Faro, 2005). In cases of vaginal delivery, the risk is generally low (2–4% of women experiencing signs of endometritis). An expansion of the flora that will increase numbers of organisms present or shift the flora from a dominance of benign organisms to those with greater virulence as well as the presence of retained products of conception in the uterus will provide conditions suitable for endometrial infection. Because the vaginal flora contains a mixture of organisms that have virulence potential, postpartum endometritis is usually associated with multiple species, although intrauterine culture is not routinely employed to document the nature of the infectious agents. In those studies where intrauterine culture was obtained, the intrauterine bacteria generally reflect the more virulent among vaginal flora organisms, which includes the enterococci (Eschenbach et al., 1986).

Since culturing intrauterine bacteria is not routinely done, therapy is usually administered on the basis of anticipated content of the uterine cavity rather than culture results. The bacteria associated with endometritis include Streptococci, Enterococci, and gram-negative facultative and anaerobic organisms in the infected uterus. *Enterococcus* may be found in a significant proportion of the cases, especially when cephalosporins are used prophylactically (Newton and Wallace, 1998). As noted before, the enterococcal population may be expanded as a result of developing infection, as can occur with prolonged rupture of the membranes, chorioamnionitis, or prolonged labor. Multiple vaginal examinations have been named by some as a predisposing factor, but its importance as a risk factor has been questioned. Cephalosporin use can also be a predisposing factor. One of the most significant risk factors is cesarean section, which increases the likelihood of postpartum endometritis about 10-fold over the rate following vaginal delivery (Ledger, 2003). Regardless of the predisposing condition, endometritis will be a polymicrobic infection and will often involve *Enterococcus* as one of the infecting species.

The fact that a substantial number of individuals who have infection risk factors and undergo cesarean section will develop infection that can be quite serious raises the question as to the appropriateness of prophylactic antibiotics. Although there is no evidence to support prophylaxis in the absence of risk factors, some experts use prophylactic antibiotics after cord clamping. Although cephalosporins may be used in this context, they may allow for a breakthrough of the enterococci. Graham et al. (1993) studied rate of pre-cesarean section vaginal colonization (almost 40%) and concluded that a single dose of ampicillin did not alter the postpartum colonization rate. Resnik et al. (1994) did not find that PVP iodine prep of the vagina influenced postpartum fever or endometritis.

Peritoneal Infections and Intra-abdominal Abscess

These usually arise after abdominal surgery or another primary event, and enterococcal infection is usually part of more complicated enteric organism collection. Gynecologic procedures can lead to peritoneal infections that involve the enterococci, but peritonitis is more frequently secondary to other surgical conditions including intestinal perforations, fistulae, and necrotizing colitis. Coates et al. (2005) reported that about one-quarter of each intra-abdominal infection harbored *Enterococcus*, but it was not the predominant organism in most cases. However, Sotto et al. (2002) also indicated that when *Enterococcus* was involved as part of a mixed infection, a greater likelihood of death within 30 days of peritonitis was observed, which they speculated may relate to a particular proinflammatory property of the organism. Enterococcal involvement in intra-abdominal infections is not limited to adults, as reported by Brook (2004), who has noted that *S. aureus* and *Enterococcus* are the most common aerobic bacteria in pediatric intra-abdominal abscesses.

In addition to secondary peritonitis as described above, spontaneous infection with enterococcal strains has been identified in persons with liver cirrhosis (Brann, 2001). Peritoneal dialysis represents an additional predisposing factor in intra-abdominal enterococcal infection (Piraino, 2000). Because of its particular resistance to bile acids, biliary infections and infections arising secondary to gall bladder infection should be considered a likely source of enterococcal participation in intra-abdominal infections. It must also be borne in mind that irrespective of whether the source of infection is gut or genital tract, the enterococcal population may undergo expansion in tissue infections, but spread to the bloodstream. Information from the Centers for Disease Control and Prevention has indicated that *Enterococcus* is among the most common nosocomial infection agents (Jarvis et al., 1996), and when in the bloodstream, as noted already, this organism my have a propensity for attaching to valvular tissue in the heart.

ANTIMICROBIAL RESISTANCE AND THERAPY

The enterococci are intrinsically hardy microorganisms, as mentioned earlier. As with their resistance to elevated temperature, osmolarity, and bile, they also seem to display intrinsic resistance to antimicrobial drugs. True resistance to antibiotics is a more pronounced feature of *E. faecium* than *E. faecalis*, and this is fortunate, because the latter is the species more commonly involved in clinical infections

(Huycke et al., 1998). With *E. faecium*, however, it has been shown that prolonged hospital stay and increased morbidity can be documented when the organism is vancomycin resistant and reaches the bloodstream (Edmond et al., 1996; Linden et al., 1995).

Enterococci may possess the markers *vanA*, *vanB*, *vanC*, *vanD*, or *vanE*. The *vanA* and *vanB* markers are associated with acquired resistance and the most worrying in clinical practice (Grayson et al., 1991). Although clinical laboratories do not generally employ techniques to screen for these genetic markers specifically, they may use bile-esculin-azide agar with 6 μg/mL vancomycin on which putative vancomycin-resistant enterococci will form black colonies to establish the presence of vancomycin-resistant *Enterococcus* (VRE).

Since the *Enterococcus* is a gram-positive organism, the use of beta-lactam drugs would seem intuitive. A 22-year study by Grayson et al. (1991) showed a rise in penicillin and ampicillin resistance among clinical strains of *E. faecium*. However, *E. faecalis* is usually susceptible to penicillin, although it can develop resistance by acquiring a beta-lactamase gene and by overexpression of penicillin-binding proteins. Federal surveillance programs have indicated that in a short period of active surveillance, the rate of ampicillin resistance in *E. faecium* increased from 69% to 83% and vancomycin resistance in this study increased from 28% to 52% (Jarvis et al., 1996). A commensurate increase was not seen in *E. faecalis*, but this may not and probably should not be taken as an overly comforting sign that it will not ever happen.

The availability of synergistic combinations of beta-lactam drugs and beta-lactamase inhibitors has been viewed as an alternative to beta-lactams alone. Recently, DiNubile et al. (2005) reported that while on tazobactam piperacillin, 1.6% developed VRE in gut flora and on ertapenem, 6.4% developed VRE.

Vancomycin is usually thought of as the "last line" compound for serious gram-positive infections, and while *E. faecalis* tends to be more susceptible to antimicrobial drugs, it too has been subject to acquisition of vancomycin resistance. Among most experts, the concern is not so much the presence of VRE but the possibility that the resistance gene could jump to *S. aureus*, particularly methicillin-resistant *S. aureus*, a possibility that has been confirmed through in vitro observation (DeSousa and deLencastre, 2004). The increasing prevalence of VRE is worrying, because it was first found in Europe in 1987 and by 1993, it was present in 14% of enterococci in intensive care units in the United States, and now it is present in more than a quarter of ICU patients.

The enterococci are intrinsically resistant to cephems and tend not to show susceptibility to aminoglycosides unless these are combined with a beta-lactam that causes sufficient disruption of the cell wall structure to allow the aminoglycoside access to the interior of the microorganism. Not surprisingly, the use of this combination has resulted in increases in aminoglycoside resistance, though it remains in frequent use.

Linezolid has been used as an alternative in VRE. However, several reports of linezolid resistance have been published, and resistance was found in both *E. faecalis* and

E. faecium and has been seen without prior exposure to linezolid (Bonora et al., 2006).

Because of the dire-sounding state of antimicrobial resistance and apparently increasing importance of enterococci in clinical infections, it may be natural to consider providing early and aggressive therapy in empirical treatment of infections that arise from sites with a mixed flora. However, most infectious-disease experts encourage caution in procedures that can lead to overuse of antibiotics and early resort to agents that should be reserved. Blot and De Waele (2005) do not recommend *Enterococcus* coverage in primary peritonitis treatment unless septic shock develops, when *Entercoccus* coverage would be appropriate. Harbarth and Uckay (2004) suggested that it should be considered as part of empiric therapy in compromised individuals such as those with bacteremias or endocarditis superimposed on severely diminished immunity as in neutropenic patients. Prudent and cautious use of vancomycin is advocated by most experts in the field.

It should be noted here that a much greater focus on hygiene and careful techniques is being emphasized in the hospital environment as a result of the challenge of VRE and multiply-resistant enterococci, because the promise of potent new antibiotics may not fully meet the clinical needs in the near future and the exuberant use of antibiotics in the past has led to surprisingly rapid emergence of resistant strains.

If an infecting enterococcal strain is multiple-drug resistant, a very challenging situation exists in which various combinations have been employed (but controlled trials are currently lacking). Some of the combinations reported include penicillin plus vancomycin, ampicillin plus ciprofloxacin, novobiocin plus doxycycline, and chloramphenicol alone. Among the concerns for therapy are whether drugs and drug combinations are bacteriostatic or bactericidal, a significant issue when host defenses are defective. Newer drugs on the horizon include streptogramins (dalfopristin/quinupristin), glycopeptide drugs, newer fluoroquinolones (clinafloxacin), and oxazolidones.

While the presence of *Enterococcus* in a mixed infection in a person without significant host defense compromise should not sound alarm bells, multiple-drug resistant *Enterococcus* in a critical site such as the bloodstream in a compromised host may be an appropriate candidate for special therapeutic regimens. It is important to know if the infectious agent is *E. faecium* and if it is vancomycin resistant. This information will help clarify therapeutic options. The current parlance among infectious-disease specialists is "VRE" and "VREF" (vancomycin-resistant *E. faecium*), with the latter being by definition multiple drug resistant.

Obstetricians and gynecologists will primarily deal with peritoneal infections and urinary infections involving *Enterococcus*. Although other serious conditions (e.g., bacteremia, endocarditis, meningitis) may occur, they will probably require the involvement of an infectious-disease consultant, and detailed treatment options will be based on knowledge of local conditions and on susceptibility patterns if available. For the purposes of this chapter, it may be noted that most uncomplicated urinary tract infections can be treated with penicillin or ampicillin unless the organism is a known beta-lactamase producer. Nitrofurantoin is a useful alternative in uncomplicated urinary tract infections. For intra-abdominal infections when acquired in the community, therapy aimed specifically at *Enterococcus* is not generally indicated. However, nosocomial infections involving *Enterococcus* that is strongly beta-lactam resistant may require therapy with aminoglycosides. Glycopeptides, linezolid or quinupristin dalfopristin may be considered according to guidelines promulgated by the Infectious Disease Society of America (Solomkin et al., 2003).

SUMMARY

The enterococci are challenging organisms, emerging in importance and having an ever-expanding role in nosocomial and, less commonly, community-acquired infections. Most often, these organisms participate as components of a polymicrobial infection, but due to their hardiness and antimicrobial resistance, they are often selected for by prior antibiotic therapy. The most significant problem on the horizon is advancing antimicrobial resistance and the possibility that resistance genes will be transferred to even more virulent organisms. Currently, most resistance is centered in the species *E. faecium*, while *E. faecalis* is the more commonly encountered organism in clinical infections. Of greatest importance is to note the level of compromise among patients, as this may be one of the most important predisposing factors to enterococcal infection.

Secondarily, it is important to know the species of the *Enterococcus* involved and its antimicrobial resistance pattern. Because of the dynamic nature of the resistance of these organisms, clinicians will have to obtain the most accurate and current information about the enterococci they encounter in their patients, because generalities will remain true only until the organisms adapt to changing environmental conditions.

SELECTED READING

Baldassari L, Bertuccini L, Creti R, et al. Clonality among *Enterococcus faecium* clinical isolates. Microb Drug Resist 2005; 11:141–145.
Basoli A, Fiocca F, DiRosa R, Baldassarri L, Donelli G. Biliary stent occlusion: a microbiological and scanning electron microscopy (SEM) investigation. In: Zanella E, ed. Advances in Abdominal Surgery. Kluwer 1999:69–80.
Berg RD. Bacterial translocation from the gastrointestinal tract. Trends Microbiol 1995; 3:149–154.
Berger-Bachi B. Resistance mechanisms of gram positive bacteria. Int J Med Microbiol 2002; 292:27–35.
Blot S, De Waele JJ. Critical issues in the clinical management of complicated intra-abdominal infections. Drugs 2005; 65:1611–1620.
Bonora MG, Solbiati M, Stepan E, et al. Emergence of linezolid resistance in the vancomycin-resistant *Enterococcus* facecium multi-locus sequence typing CI epidemic lineage. J Clin Micro 2006; 44:1153–1155.
Brann OS. Infectious complications of cirrhosis. Curr Gastroenterol Rep 2001; 3:285–292.
Brook I. Intra-abdominal, retroperitoneal and visceral abscesses in children. Eur J Pediatr Surg 2004; 14:265–273.
Cintas LM, Causas P, Holo H, Hernandez PE, Nes IF, Havarstein LS. Enterocins L50A and L50B: two novel bacteriocins from Enteococcus faecium L50 are related to staphylococcal hemolysins. J Bacteriol 1998; 180:1988–1994.
Coates EW, Karlowicz MG, Croitoru DP, Buescher ES. Distinctive distribution of pathogens associated with peritonitis in neonates

with focal intestinal perforation compared with necrotizing enterocolitis. Pediatrics 2005; 116:241–246.

Courvalin P. Vancomycin resistance in gram positive organisms. Clin Infect Dis 2006; 42:25–34.

Cox CR, Coburn PS, Gilmore MS. Enterococcal cytolysin: a novel two-component peptide system that serves as a bacterial defense against eukaryotic and prokaryotic cells. Curr Protein Pept Sci 2005; 6:77–84.

DeSousa AM, deLencastre H. Bridges from hospitals to the laboratory: genetic portraits of methicillin-resistant *Staphylococcus aureus* clones. FEMS Immunol Med Microbiol 2004; 40:101–111.

DiNubile MJ, Chow JW, Satishchandran V, et al. Acquisition of resistant bowel flora during a double-blind randomized clinical trial of ertapenem versus piperacillin-tazobactam therapy for intraabdominal infections. Antimicrob Agents Chemother 2005; 49:3217–3221.

Dobbs TE, Patel M, Waites KB, Moser SA, Stamm AM, Hoesley CJ. Nosocomial spread of *Enterococcus* faecium resistant to vancomycin and linezolid in a tertiary care medical center. J Clin Microbiol 2006; 44:3368–3370.

Edmond MB, Ober JF, Dawson JD, Weinbaum DL, Wenzel RP. Vancomycin-resistant enterococcal bacteremia: natural history and attributable mortality. Clin Infect Dis 1996; 23:1234–1239.

Eschenbach DA, Rosene K, Tompkins LS, Watkins H, Gravett MG. Endometrial cultures obtained by a triple-lumen method from afebrile and febrile postpartum women. J Infect Dis 1986; 153:1038–1045.

Faro S. Postpartum endometritis. Clin Perinatol 2005; 32:803–814.

Flahaut S, Hartke A, Giard J, Auffray Y. Alkaline stress response in *Enterococcus* faecalis: adaptation, cross-protection, and changes in protein synthesis. Appl Environ Microbiol 1997; 63:812–814.

Graham JM, Blanco JD, Oshiro BT, Magee KP, Monga M, Eriksen N. Single-dose ampicillin prophylaxis does not eradicate *Enterococcus* from the lower genital tract. Obstet Gynecol 1993; 81:115–117.

Grayson ML, Eliopoulos GM, Wennersten CB, et al. Increasing resistance to beta-lactam antibiotics clinical isolates of *Enterococcus* faecium: a 22-year review at one institution. Antimicrob Agents Chemother 1991; 35:2180–2184.

Gupta K, Hooton TM, Wobbe CL, Stamm WE. The prevalence of antimicrobial resistance among uropathogens causing acute uncomplicated cystitis in young women. Int J Antimicrob Agents 1999; 11:305–308.

Guzman CA, Pruzzo C, Plate M, Guardati MC, Calegari L. Serum dependent expression of *Enterococcus* faecalis adhesins involved in the colonization of heart cells. Microb Pathog 1991; 11:399–409.

Hancock LE, Perego M. The *Enterococcus* faecalis fsr two-component system controls biofilm development through production of gelatinase. J Bacteriol 2004; 186:5629–5639.

Harbarth S, Uckay I. Are there patients with peritonitis who require empirical therapy for *Enterococcus*? Eur J Clin Microbiol Infect Dis 2004; 23:73–77.

Hufnagel M, Kropec A, Theilacker C, Huebner J. Naturally acquired antibodies against four *Enterococcus* faecalis capsular polysaccharides in healthy human sera. Diagn Lab Immunol 2005; 12: 930–934.

Huycke MM, Sahm DF, Gilmore MS. Multiple-drug resistant enterococci: the nature of the problem and an agenda for the future. Emerg Infect Dis 1998; 4:239–249.

Huycke MM, Moore D, Joyce W, et al. Extracellular superoxide production by *Enterococcus* faecalis requires demethylmenaquinone and is attenuated by functional terminal quinol oxidases. Mol Microbiol 2001; 42:729–740.

Jarvis WR, Gaynes RP, Horan TC, et al. Semi-annual report aggregated data National Nosocomial Infections Surveillance (NNIS) system. CDC 1996:1–27.

Jett BD, Huycke MM, Gilmore MS. Virulence of enterococci. J Clin Microbiol 1994; 7:462–478.

Johnson AP. The pathogenicity of enterococci. J Antimicrob Chemother 1994; 33:1083–1089.

Koch S, Hufnagel M, Huebner J. Treatment and prevention of enterococcal infection—alternative and experimental approaches. Expert Opin Biol Ther 2004; 9:1519–1531.

Larsen B. Normal genital microflora. In: Keith LG, Berger GS, Edelman DA, eds. Common Infections. Lancaster, England: MTP Press, 1985; 1:3–31.

Larsen B, Galask RP. Vaginal microbial flora: practical and theoretical relevance. Obstet Gynecol 1980; 55:100–113.

Ledger WJ. Post-partum endomyometritis diagnosis and treatment: a review. Am J Obstet Gynecol Res 2003; 29:364–373.

Lempianen H, Kinnunen K, Mertanin A, von Wright A. Occurrence of virulence factors among human intestinal enterococcal isolates. Lett Appl Microbiol 2005; 41:341–344.

Linden PK, Pasculie AW, Manez R, et al. Differences in outcomes for patients with bacteremia due to vancomycin-resistant *Enterococcus* faecium or vancomycin-susceptible E. faecium. Clin Infect Dis 1995; 22:663–670.

Mouton CP, Bazaldua OV, Pierce B, Espino DV. Common infections in older adults. Am Fam Phys 2001; 63:257–268.

Ness RB, Kip KE, Hillier SL, et al. A cluster analysis of bacterial vaginosis-associated microflora and pelvic inflammatory disease. Am J Epidemiol 2005; 162:585–590.

Newton ER, Wallace PA. Effects of prophylactic antibiotics on endometrial flora in women with postcesarean endometritis. Obstet Gynecol 1998; 92:262–268.

Ohm MJ, Galask RP. The effect of antibiotic prophylaxis on patients undergoing abdominal hysterectomy II: alterations of microbial flora. Am J Obstet Gynecol 1976; 125:448–454.

Pillar CM, Gilmore MS. Enterococcal pathogenicity island of E. faecalis. Front Biosci 2004; 9:2335–2346.

Piraino B. Peritoneal infections. Adv Ren Replace Ther 2000; 7:280–828.

Quan M. Pelvic inflammatory disease: diagnosis and management. J Am Board Family Pract 1994; 7:110–123.

Resnik E, Harger JH, Kuller JA. Early postpartum endometritis. Randomized comparison of ampicillin/sulbactam vs. ampicillin, gentamicin and clindamycin. J Reprod Med 1994; 39(6):467–472.

Schleifer KH, Kilpper-Balz R. Transfer of *Streptoccus faecalis* and *Streptococcus* faecium to the genus *Enterococcus* nom rev as *Enterococcus* faecalis comb nov and *Enterococcus* faecium comb nov. Int J Syst Bact 1984; 34:31–34.

Schlievert PM, Gahr PJ, Assimacopoulos AP, et al. Aggregation and binding substances enhance pathogenicity in rabbit models of *Enterococcus* faecalis endocarditis. Infect Immun 1998; 66:218–223.

Shankar N, Lockatelle CV, Baghdyan AS, Drachenberg C, Gilmore M, Johnson DE. Role of *Enterococcus* facalis surface protein ESP in the pathogenesis of ascending urinary tract infection. Infect Immun 2001; 69:4366–4372.

Solomkin JS, Jazuski JE, Baron EJ, et al. Guidelines for the selection of anti-infective agents for complicated intraabdominal infections. Clin Infect Dis 2003; 37:997–1005.

Sotto A, Lefrant JY, Fabbro-Peray P, et al. Evaluation of antimicrobial therapy management of 120 consecutive patients with secondary peritonitis. J Antimicrob Chemother 2002; 50:569–576.

Stapleton A, Stamm WA. Prevention of urinary tract infection. Infect Dis Clin North Am 1997; 11:719–733.

Svensater G, Larsson UB, Greif EC, Cvtlkovitch DG, Hamilton IR. Acid tolerance responses and survival by oral bacteria. Oral Microbiol Immunol 1997; 12:266–273.

Tendolkar PM, Baghdayan AS, Shankar N. Pathogenic enterococci: new developments in the 21st century. Cell Mol Life Sci 2003; 60:2622–2636.

Tendolkar PM, Baghdayan AS, Gilmore MS, Shankar N. Enterococcal surface protein, Esp, enhances biofilm formation by *Enterococcus* faecalis. Infect Immun 2004; 72:6032–6039.

Waters CM, Hirt H, McCormick JK, Schlievert PM, Wells CL, Dunny GM. An amino-terminal domain of *Enterococcus* faecalis aggregation substance is required for aggregation, bacterial internalization by epithelial cells and binding to lipoteichoic acid. Mol Microbiol 2004; 52:1159–1171.

Wells CL, Jechorek RP, Erlandsen SL. Evidence for the translocation of *Enterococcus* faecalis across the mouse intestinal tract. J Infect Dis 1990; 162:82–90.

Workowski KA, Berman SM. Sexually transmitted disease treatment guidelines 2006. MMWR Recomm Rep 2006; 5:1–94.

The group F streptococci belong to the *Streptococcus milleri* group, which includes *S. anginosus*, *S. constellatus*, and *S. intermedius*. The *S. milleri* have a property that differs from classical streptococcal infections. They produce suppurating lesions. They have been isolated from Bartholin's gland abscesses and wound infections as well as from brain and hepatic abscesses. Inflammatory diseases such as arthritis and meningitis have been described as a consequence of hematogenous metastatic spread.

The group F streptococci tend to be primarily constituents of bowel and oropharyngeal bacterial flora. Of 279 bacterin-resistant streptococci obtained from children and adolescents with pharyngitis, 35 were group F. The group F beta-hemolytic streptococci are not a common cause of disease, but when disease induction occurs, its consequences are often significant. Bacteremia due to the group F streptococci may produce disease in distal organ systems. DeAngelo et al. (2001) reported a case of bacteremia in a patient following manipulation of a three-day-old vulvar abscess.

During the decade 1970 to 1980, group F streptococcal bacteremia accounted for 2% of the beta-hemolytic streptococci isolated from all patients hospitalized with bacteremia at Mayo Clinic–affiliated hospitals.

Almost all isolates of group F streptococci are extremely sensitive to the penicillin antimicrobials (<0.1 μg of penicillin/mL). This sensitivity to penicillin coupled with its rarity as a constituent of the genital flora may have masked the perception of the group F streptococci as a potential perinatal pathogen.

Wells and Kenney in 1980 reported a case of prolonged rupture of membranes that occurred at 37 weeks of gestational age in which the ensuing progeny developed subsequent perinatal pneumonia. Group F streptococci were isolated from skin, cord, blood cultures, nasopharynx, throat, stomach, tracheal aspirates, and fetal surface of the placenta. Hill et al. (1992) reported a case of perinatal bacteremia/septicemia in a premature infant with prolonged rupture of the fetal membranes and anaerobic amnionitis.

SELECTED READING

Beasley GR, Marsh EJ, Sottile WS. Acute osteomyelitis/pyoarthritis caused by Lancefield group B beta-hemolytic streptococcus. J Am Osteopath Assoc 1982; 81:797.

Butler KM, Barker CJ. Group F streptococcus: an unusual cause of arthritis. Clin Ortho 1988; 228:261.

Crawford I, Russell C. Streptococci isolated from the bloodstream and gingival crevice of man. J Med Microbiol 1983; 16:163.

DeAngelo AJ, Dooley DP, Skidmore PJ, Kopecky CT. Group F streptococcal bacteremia complicating a Bartholin's abscess. Infect Dis Obstet Gynecol 2001; 9:55.

Gallis HA. Streptococcus. In: Wolfgana J, Willet HP, Bernard AD, eds. Zinsser Microbiology, 18th ed. Norkalk, CT: Appleton Century Crofts, 1984:463.

Hill WC, Armor SA, Monif GRG. Perinatal bacteremia due to group F streptococci. Am J Perinatol 1992; 9:337.

Libertin CR, Hermans PE, Washington JA II. Beta-hemolytic group F streptococcal bacteremia. A study and review of the literature. Rev Infect Dis 1985; 7:498.

Lopez-Zeno JA, Ross E, O'Grady JP. Septic shock complicating drainage of a Bartholin gland abscess. Obstet Gynecol 1990; 76:915.

Matsubayashi T, Fugimoto S, Katoh I, et al. A case of meningoencephalitis caused by group F streptococcus anginosus. Kansenshogaku Zasshi 1987; 61:368.

Molina J-M, Leport C, Bure A, et al. Clinical and bacterial features of infections caused by *Streptococcus milleri*. Scand J Infect Dis 1991; 23:659.

Poole PM, Wilson G. Occurrence and cultural features of *Streptococcus milleri* in various body sites. J Clin Pathol 1979; 32:764.

Schwartz RH, McCoy P, Hayden GF, Hallas G. Group F streptococci in the pharynx: pathogens or innocent bystanders? South Med J 1986; 79:952.

Wells DW, Kenney GT. Group F streptococcus associated with intrauterine pneumonia. Pediatrics 1980; 66:820.

Wort AJ. Observations on group F streptococci from human sources. J Med Microbiol 1975; 8:455.

Group G Beta-Hemolytic Streptococci

In 1933, Rebecca Lancefield, by means of a precipitin reaction, serologically identified and grouped the streptococci according to their cellular carbohydrates. Initially, she identified five antigenically distinct streptococcal groups and designated them A, B, C, D, and E. Since these earlier observations, 18 groups, A through H and K through T, have been identified. The groups A, B, C, D, and G are the principal groups associated with human disease.

Like the group A beta-hemolytic streptococci, the group G streptococci appear to function as exogenous pathogens for the female genital tract. Structurally and pathophysiologically, both groups are similar to the group A streptococci. Immunofluorescent techniques have demonstrated cross-reactivity between the cell membranes of groups A, C, and G, implying antigenic similarities. All three groups share the propensity for involving the skin, the respiratory tract, and the female genital tract. Despite these similarities, infection with group G streptococci is not followed by nonsuppurative complications (acute rheumatic fever and acute glomerulonephritis). The group G streptococcus is considered a normal constituent of the female genital tract bacterial flora.

With the exception of cutaneous disease superimposed upon pregnancy or occurring in a gynecologic oncologic patient, the principal clinical manifestation is postpartum endometritis. Although most cases of puerperal sepsis with group G streptococci are described as mild, several deaths have been reported. The typical pattern of onset is that of a spiking temperature rising to 39.5°C to 41°C. Like the group A streptococcus, the group C and G streptococci are extremely sensitive to penicillin G. The anticipated response to effective therapy is a rapid defervescence over a 24- to 48-hour period.

The group G streptococci are recognized as a cause of perinatal septicemia. Infection occurs primarily in premature or low-birthweight infants and in the setting of prolonged rupture of the fetal membranes. Early aggressive therapy is the principal factor selecting for outcome. Once complications such as progressive respiratory distress, shock, and disseminated intravascular coagulation occur, the prognosis is almost invariably poor.

Disease due to the group G streptococcus can occur as a complication of gynecologic surgery. Recurrent cellulitis has been reported as a rare complication of radical hysterectomy and radiation therapy. Auckenthaler et al., in 1983, described five patients with gynecologic malignancies treated with radiation therapy who developed cellulitis and bacteremia due to group G streptococci. The initial surgical wound and impaired lymphatic drainage were thought to be predisposing factors.

SELECTED READING

Appelbaum PC, Freidman Z, Fairbroher PF, et al. Neonatal sepsis due to group G streptococci (case report). Acta Paediatr Scand 1980; 69:559.

Auckenthaler R, Hermans PE, Washington JA. Group G streptococcal bacteremia: clinical study and review of the literature. Rev Infect Dis 1983; 5:196.

Baker CJ. Unusual occurrence of neonatal septicemia due to group G streptococcus. Pediatrics 1974; 53:568.

Carstensen H, Pers C, Pryds O. Group G streptococcal neonatal septicaemia: two case reports and a brief review of the literature. Scand J Infect Dis 1988; 20:407.

Chmel H, Hamdy M. Recurrent streptococcal cellulitis complicating radical hysterectomy and radiation therapy. Obstet Gynecol 1984; 63:862.

Elill AM, Butler HM. Haemolytic streptococcal infection following childbirth and abortion. Med J Aust 1940; 1:293–300.

Feingold DS, Stagg NL, Kunz LJ. Extrarespiratory streptococcal infections. N Engl J Med 1966; 275:356–361.

Filker RS, Monif GRG. Postpartum septicemia due to the group G streptococci. Obstet Gynecol 1979; 53:283.

Gaunt PN, Seal DV. Group G streptococcal infections. J Infect 1987; 15:5.

Krishna MVK, Tilton RC, Raye JR, et al. Fatal group G streptococcal sepsis in a preterm neonate. Am J Dis Child 1980; 134:894.

MacDonald I. Fatal and severe human infections with haemolytic streptococci group G (Lancefield). Med J Aust 1939; 2:471.

Ramsay AM, Gillespie M. Puerperal infection associated with haemolytic streptococci other than Lancefield's group A. Br J Obstet Gynaecol 1941; 48:569–585.

Rolston KVI. Group G streptococcal infections. Arch Intern Med 1986; 146:857.

Vartian C, Lerner PI, Shales DM, et al. Infections due to Lancefield group G streptococci. Medicine 1985; 64:75.

Chlamydia trachomatis

INTRODUCTION

Members of the genus *Chlamydia* are obligatory intracellular gram-negative parasites. The infectious particles form elementary bodies and have an overall diameter of 325 mm. Pinocytosis of the infectious elementary bodies by a cell results in their transformation into initial bodies, which in turn congregate to form actively dividing inclusions (reticular bodies). These reticular bodies, visible under light microscopy, appear to divide by a simple pinching-off process similar to that observed with other gram-negative organisms. Both RNA and DNA have been identified in them. Biochemical analysis reveals the presence of muramic acid, which is an important mucoprotein of bacterial cell walls. Chlamydial particles parasitize their host cells for the adenosine triphosphate required for metabolic activity and transformation of the initial/reticular bodies into infectious elementary bodies. Chlamydial infection of the host cell finally leads to cell death and release of the newly synthesized elementary bodies.

Chlamydia organisms can be segregated into subgroups (A and B) on the basis of whether or not the intranuclear inclusion bodies produced in tissue culture cells will stain with iodine. *Chlamydia psittaci* (subgroup B) organisms, which are responsible for ornithosis, do not stain with iodine, in contrast to those of the A subgroup (Fig. 1). The *Chlamydia trachomatis* (subgroup A) strains that infect humans can be differentiated into lymphogranuloma venereum strains (LGV or L strains) and the trachoma-inclusion conjunctivitis (TRIC) agents. Most of the ocular infections due to the TRIC agents, in regions where trachoma is epidemic, belong to the serologic types A, B, BA, and C. In those areas where trachoma is endemic, trachoma infections are due to serotypes D through K. These latter serotypes primarily infect the female genital tract and appear to be sexually transmitted. However, the eye occasionally is infected from the female genital tract. A great deal of confusion exists concerning nomenclature. The TRIC delineates primarily ocular strains. The genital strains tend to be referred to by the genus name *Chlamydia*.

FEMALE GENITAL TRACT INVOLVEMENT

The name "chlamydia" is derived from the Greek work "chlamys" which means "to cloak." The major focus has been on the strains of *C. trachomatis* that cause genital tract infection. In contrast to men with nongonococcal urethritis or postgonococcal urethritis, women with cervicovaginal infection rarely present with specific symptoms or signs. The spectrum of clinical disease attributed to the genital strains of *C. trachomatis* that impact on women and their progeny is listed in Table 1.

Asymptomatic Carriage

In the United States, chlamydial genital infection is the most frequently reported sexually transmitted disease (STD). *C. trachomatis* can be isolated from 12% to 28% of women attending clinics for STD, exclusive of those women who either have gonorrhea or are the female sexual

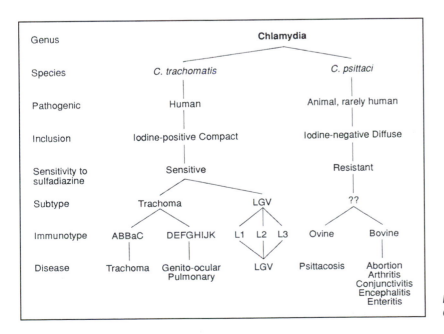

FIGURE 1 Summary of the characteristics of *Chlamydia*.

TABLE I The spectrum of clinical disease attributable to D, E, F, G, H, I, and K strains of *Chlamydia trachomatis*

Females	Neonates
I. Mucopurulent cervicitis	I. Inclusion conjunctivitis
II. Abacterial urethritis	II. Pneumonia
III. Acute salpingitis (stages I and II)	
IV. Curtis–Fitz Hugh syndrome	
V. Ectopic pregnancy	
VI. Endometritis	
VII. Preterm deliveries ??	
VIII. Adult inclusion conjunctivitis	

contacts of men with nongonococcal urethritis. These figures are in contradistinction to the 1% to 4% isolate rate achieved in control populations. The genital strains of *Chlamydia* can be isolated from 4% to 7% of women who have cervical dysplasia or are attending a women's health clinic. Less than 1% of women of advanced age undergoing selective cancer screening appear to harbor the organism.

Among *Chlamydia*-positive women identified from women attending gynecological clinics, 55% to 75% will be subjectively asymptomatic. In the absence of appropriate antimicrobial therapy, the organism may persist for months and provide a continuing reservoir for chlamydial infection. Latency has long been recognized as a common state in chlamydial infection. *Chlamydia* utilizes cellular metabolites, amino acids, and nucleotides. The failure to supply the agent with essential growth factors may lead to a state of latency.

The prevalence of infection caused by *C. trachomatis* now exceeds that caused by *Neisseria gonorrhoeae*. In the United States, about three million individuals are infected annually. The changes with the sexual revolution and the availability of alternate forms of contraceptives other than the condom have resulted in *Chlamydia* becoming the most important STD for women. Its importance is in part due to the fact that occult or subacute forms of infection are fully capable of destructive sequelae.

Wide disparity in the rate of chlamydial infection has been observed in different populations. Certain groups of women are at apparently higher risk. Women who come from a disadvantaged socioeconomic background and have multiple sexual partners are at highest risk. Age is also a risk indicator but only insofar as it connotes the high risk factors involving augmented sexual activity. The anticipated incidence of positive cultures of single, unmarried, teenage gravidas may approach 14%. The incidence of gravidas over the age of 35 coming to chorionic villus sampling because of age is less than one-half of 1%. A 4% to 9% incidence is about average in most balanced obstetrical populations.

Mucopurulent Cervicitis

When clinically overt, the most common presentation of chlamydial infection is mucopurulent cervicitis. Mucopurulent cervicitis is defined as the presence of mucopus at the endocervix in a female with a vaginal discharge and/or the demonstration of 10 or more polymorphic neutrophils per field at a magnification of 100 per cervical mucus. Approximately 20% of the women with mucopurulent cervicitis will be demonstrated to have infection with *C. trachomatis*. Speculum examination of the cervix reveals the presence of inflamed ectopions that readily bleed to the touch. Particularly in patients who had previously been on low-dose progestational oral contraceptives, patients with a history of chlamydial endometritis will persist with a history of intramenstrual bleeding with or without pelvic pain suggestive of Krettek's Syndrome (Fig. 2). In retrospect, it is probable that some of the intramenstrual symptomatology associated with the intrauterine contraceptive device (IUD) was probably also due to *C. trachomatis* endometritis and not necessarily to IUD-related chronic anaerobic endometritis. One-third of women with mucopurulent cervicitis will have a second STD pathogen identified.

The cervicitis may be sufficiently extensive so as to mimic vulvovaginitis. Among couples seen in STD clinics, it is not uncommon to have the male in one room with nongonococcal urethritis while, in another room, the woman presents with a clinically significant vaginal discharge for which none of the traditional vulvovaginal pathogens can be discerned or isolated.

Although both *C. trachomatis* and *N. gonorrhoeae* can cause mucopurulent cervicitis, in most cases, neither

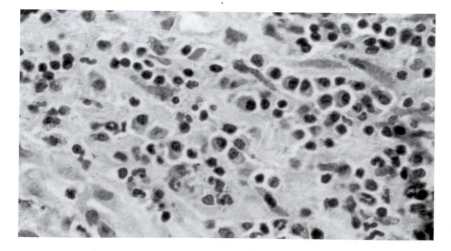

FIGURE 2 Endometrial biopsy from a patient with breakthrough bleeding demonstrating a mononuclear cell stromal infiltrate composed of both lymphocytes and plasma cells within the inflammatory infiltrate (hematoxylin and eosin, × 400).

organism can be isolated. The sexual consorts of women with mucopurulent cervicitis should be evaluated for STDs and managed appropriately.

Abacterial Urethritis

C. trachomatis has been proposed as one of the etiologic agents for a bacterial urethritis, the so-called "urethral syndrome." Women with positive cervical cultures for *C. trachomatis* frequently have concomitant urethral colonization. These women with positive isolations of *C. trachomatis* from the urethra more often have urethral symptoms of dysuria and frequency compared with those women with positive isolations from the cervix alone. Urethral involvement seldom occurs in the absence of cervical infection. It is frequently silent, producing no signs or symptoms of urethritis.

Chlamydial Salpingitis

Chlamydial salpingitis has always been part of the venereal disease spectrum. In 1732, John Astruc wrote in his book based upon observations of Parisian prostitutes of a chronic form of salpingitis which:

> occurs in women whose uterus is thrown into contractions by lascivious ticklings and by excess of prostitution. Many have no pain but their infection in time injures the internal surface of the uterus and its tube.

In contrast to gonococcal salpingitis, chlamydial tubal infection appears to be a true chronic infection. Intracellular chlamydial organisms may persist in the genital tissues for extremely long periods of time and continue to produce silent progressive tubal damage unless treatment with appropriate antibiotics is instituted. When infertile patients with chlamydial antibodies are evaluated with laparoscopy, frequently no history of an illness or procedure can be elicited which could explain the presence of postinflammatory tubal damage.

Cultural and serologic data have built an extensive case for *C. trachomatis* as both an etiologic agent and a potential copathogen in acute salpingitis. As in the male with gonococcal urethritis, chlamydial cervicitis is not infrequently concomitantly present in patients with gonococcal endometritis–salpingitis. Mardh et al. (1981) have recovered *C. trachomatis* from 6 out of 20 specimens from fallopian tube aspirations from women with acute endometritis salpingitis compared with none from the 12 controls.

Thirty percent of women with acute salpingitis from whom *C. trachomatis* is recovered have concomitant gonococcal endocervicitis. Ripa et al. (1980) demonstrated that 86 of 143 patients (62%) with acute salpingitis had significant chlamydial immunoglobulin G (IgG) antibodies in their serum. The magnitude of antibody correlated with the staging of disease, the highest geometric mean titers being found in women with the most severe grade of salpingitis.

In contrast to "classical pelvic inflammatory disease," *Chlamydia* disease tends to be more occult. Often only vague peritoneal pain precipitated by jarring movements is the prime motivating factor for the patient to seek medical attention. Characteristically, the temperature is less than 38°C, and the only significant finding on pelvic examination is cervical motion tenderness and varying degrees of cervicitis.

The role of *Chlamydia* in acute salpingitis is poorly understood. Can *C. trachomatis* initiate infection and pave the way for bacterial superinfection or does it work synergistically with other bacteria?

IUD-Associated Chlamydial Salpingitis

In retrospect, some of the structural morbidity attributed to IUD-associated chronic anaerobic endometritis is probably due to concurrent chlamydial infection. Guderian and Trobough (1986) evaluated by laparoscopy or laparotomy 245 infertile patients for inflammatory residues; 176 patients had not used an IUD and 69 had used this form of contraception. Chlamydial antibody titers were performed on all patients. Although users had a higher overall prevalence of inflammatory residues than nonusers, there was no difference in residue prevalence for either group at the same titer level. "Residues of pelvic inflammatory disease" included a spectrum of postinfectious pelvic abnormalities ranging from severe periadnexal adhesions and tubal occlusion to mild adhesions and minimal tubal epithelial damage. No specific type of device appeared to be associated with either an increased or a decreased residue frequency. "Silent" chlamydial infections occurred with equal frequency in both users and nonusers. They conclude that inflammatory residues and tubal infertility in IUD users is more probably due to either overt or silent chlamydial infections.

Similarly, Chow et al. (1986) have demonstrated that while patients using IUDs have a higher prevalence of inflammatory residues than nonusers, they also have a higher prevalence of chlamydial antibodies.

The increased frequency of chlamydial salpingitis in users may be a function of either increased exposure rate or increased attack rate. The IUD may increase the prevalence of upper tract disease after chlamydial exposure (increased attack rate) by modification of host defenses. On the other hand, IUD users may be exposed to *C. trachomatis* and other STDs with greater frequency than nonusers (increased exposure rate).

Endometritis

The increased prevalence of a late-onset postpartum endometritis in *Chlamydia*-positive gravidas who undergo cesarean section or voluntary termination of pregnancy has been focused upon the ability of *Chlamydia* to produce disease in this clinical setting.

The possibility that chlamydial endometritis is a distinct entity has been suggested from the studies of pelvic inflammatory disease, which have included histopathological analyses of endometrial biopsies. In one study, severe plasma cell endometritis and lymphoid follicles with transformed lymphocytes were significantly more common in those patients with recovery of *C. trachomatis* from their endometrial biopsies than in the nonchlamydial group.

A poorly recognized variant of *Chlamydia* endometritis is Krettek's syndrome. Krettek et al. (1993) described breakthrough midcycle bleeding in women on oral contraceptives.

Classically, these patients responded to a seven- to ten-day course of tetracycline or doxycycline much in the same way as did women with menstrual irregularities secondary to IUD-associated chronic anaerobic endometritis. When done, biopsies of the endometrium have revealed the presence of a mononuclear cell infiltrate in 30% to 40% of patients with endocervical chlamydial infection.

Osser and Persson (1995) note a 23.2% and 14.5% incidence of endometritis and salpingitis among *Chlamydia*-positive women in contrast to 5.7% and 0.6% in *Chlamydia*-negative women during the first postoperative month following legal abortion by vacuum aspiration. These differences were highly significant and suggested that *C. trachomatis* may be an etiologic agent in postabortion endometritis.

Curtis–Fitz Hugh syndrome

The Curtis–Fitz Hugh syndrome is an inflammation process due to an STD pathogen that involves the supra- or intrahepatic portion of the capsule of the liver. Both Fitz Hugh and Curtis were of the opinion that the condition occurred only in women. Disease has been postulated to result from either direct extension, passage of infecting organisms up the paracolic gutters, or lymphatic drainage to the liver surface. The rare occurrence of this syndrome in males has led to a focus on the probable existence of an additional mechanism for hepatic involvement. More than half of the reported cases of Curtis–Fitz Hugh syndrome in males occurred in individuals who had experienced hematogenous dissemination. In these cases, rather than being a perihepatitis, true parenchymal involvement probably occurs.

The initial symptom is that of a dramatic, excruciating, sharp pain most intense at the level of the right lower rib margin and over the area of the gallbladder. With the suprahepatic variant, the pain may be referred to the right shoulder or the inside of the right arm. The pain is pleuritic in character, being exaggerated by coughing, deep inspiration, laughing, and rotational movements of the torso. Hiccups and nausea frequently accompany the pain. Vomiting may be present. The clinical presentation may also involve chills, fever, night sweats, headache, and general malaise.

Initially *N. gonorrhoeae* had been etiologically deemed the sole cause of Curtis–Fitz Hugh syndrome. Subsequently, through serological and culture studies, *C. trachomatis* has been documented to be an etiological agent for this entity. Wolner-Hanssen et al. (1983) have isolated the organism from the liver capsule. The Curtis–Fitz Hugh syndrome associated with *C. trachomatis* tends to occur most frequently in women who have had relatively recent insertion of the IUD.

OBSTETRICAL SPECTRUM OF DISEASE

The role of *C. trachomatis* as an STD and a relatively incomplete knowledge base concerning the natural history of female genital tract involvement have largely obscured the perinatal, as opposed to neonatal, impact of this organism.

Ectopic Pregnancy

Fragmentary data purport that endocervical chlamydial infection is associated with a 30% to 40% probability of concomitant endometrial infection. Should conception occur, chlamydial fallopian tube and/or endometrial infection appears to have the potential to adversely impact on blastocyst implantation. Brunham et al. (1992) studied 50 women with ectopic pregnancies for serological evidence of chlamydial infection. Histological analysis of fallopian tube tissue distant from the site of ectopic implantation was available in 41 cases. The histopathologic finding of plasma cell salpingitis in approximately one-third of women without an identified cause of ectopic pregnancy was interpreted as being consistent with the hypothesis that tubal infection was an underlying cause in this group of women.

Preterm Labor

Postconceptional acquisition has been associated in some, but not all, studies with a statistically significant increase in premature rupture of the fetal membranes (PROM) and/or preterm labor. The exact mechanism by which these consequences are induced remains speculative.

Berman et al. (1987) studied 1204 Navajo women enrolling for prenatal care for the endocervical presence of C. trachomatis, *Mycoplasma hominis*, and *Ureaplasma urealyticum* cultures. Serum samples were taken at enrollment and, when possible, after 30 weeks. Although women with recent *C. trachomatis* infection (IgM titer >1:32 on either sample or IgG seroconversion) were at greater risk of low birthweight (19% [3/16]) than women with chronic infection (4.5% [6/133]; relative risk, 4.2%), this subgroup at risk was too small for valid statistical analysis.

Gravett et al. (1986) studied 534 gravid women for the presence of endocervical chlamydial infection. In this study, *C. trachomatis* infection was documented in 47 (9%) of the women. Cervical infection with *C. trachomatis* was independently associated with preterm PROM, preterm labor, and low birthweight. Unfortunately, the other microbiological variables and cofactors that might have contributed to adverse pregnancy outcome were poorly controlled.

In their study of pregnant women, Harrison et al. (1983) suggested that only the subset of women with recently acquired *C. trachomatis* infection are at risk for premature events. Only IgM-seropositive patients with *C. trachomatis* were at increased risk of preterm PROM and low neonatal birthweight.

When Sweet et al. (1987) reexamined the patient population reported by Schachter et al. (1986) and compared it with a matched controlled subject group, subjects being matched for age, race, and socioeconomic status, there was no statistical difference noted in terms of PROM, preterm delivery, amnionitis, intrapartum fever, small-for-gestational-age babies, postpartum endometritis, and neonatal septicemia. In the subset of women with recent or invasive chlamydial infection indicated by the presence of IgM antibodies against *C. trachomatis*, preterm delivery occurred in 13 of 64 IgM-positive individuals versus 8 of 99 IgM-negative individuals. The same statistics applied to PROM.

The studies published to date are less than perfect in terms of the experimental design. Too many uncontrolled variables that potentially impact on outcome exist in all studies that have purported a positive relationship between endocervical infection with *C. trachomatis*, adverse pregnancy outcomes, and those that demonstrate no difference. Incomplete demographic and microbiological profiling and flawed experimental designs allow one to choose those studies which appeal to a priori biases.

NEONATAL CHLAMYDIA INFECTION

Heggie et al. (1986) demonstrated that, despite failure to detect chlamydial infection in exposed infants, lymphocyte-proliferative responses are greater in neonates born to infected mothers than in infants born to uninfected mothers. Such data suggest that neonatal cellular immune responses to *Chlamydia* antigens are increased in infected mothers and that infants may acquire chlamydial cell-mediated immunity transplacentally.

The predominant focus of analysis to date has been on the periparturitional neonatal acquisition of infection. Chlamydial infections in the neonate are almost invariably the consequence of delivery through an infected birth canal.

Conjunctivitis and pneumonia are the principal two manifestations of neonatal chlamydial infection. Up to two-thirds of infants born to mothers with chlamydial genital infection will become infected and develop one or both of these sequelae.

Schachter et al. (1986) prospectively followed 5531 pregnant women. In this study population, they identified 262 (4.7%) of women who had positive cervical cultures for *C. trachomatis*. From the ensuing progeny, 131 were prospectively followed to ascertain the outcome of chlamydial exposure during the birth process. Culture-confirmed inclusion conjunctivitis was seen in 23 (18%) of the infants. Chlamydial pneumonia was diagnosed in 21 (16%) at risk. *C. trachomatis* was recovered from 47 (36%) of the infants; however, 79 (60%) had serological evidence of infection. Subclinical rectal and vaginal infections were detected in 14% of the infants. Of the infants with serological evidence of perinatal chlamydial infection, half of these developed either chlamydial pneumonia or conjunctivitis.

Neonatal Conjunctivitis

In contradistinction to gonococcal ophthalmia neonatorum, which usually appears within five days, chlamydial conjunctivitis usually has its onset between the fifth and fourteenth day postpartum. PROM or heavy vaginal colonization appears to select for an earlier onset of disease. Unlike the gonococcus, *C. trachomatis* is not affected by silver nitrate ophthalmic drops. The effective utilization of Crede prophylaxis has rendered the inclusion of conjunctivitis due to *C. trachomatis* the most common cause of infectious neonatal conjunctivitis. It is currently estimated that 1.1 to 4.4 cases occur per 1000 live births.

Approximately 44% of the progeny born to gravidas who, at the time of parturition, harbor *C. trachomatis* as a constituent of their vaginal flora will develop laboratory-proven inclusion conjunctivitis, characterized by a mucopurulent exudate. Without therapy, the disease tends to resolve spontaneously several weeks to a month after onset. In isolated instances, pseudopannus may form in the conjunctiva, resulting in permanent scarring. Early therapy appears to abort any late sequelae such as scar formation or corneal vascularization. The majority of neonates with inclusion conjunctivitis will have the organism present in the tracheobronchial tract and nasopharynx. Although tetracyclines are the drugs of choice for chlamydial infections, they should not to be used in a pediatric population when alternative effective therapy such as erythromycin is available. Since treatment failures will occur with topical therapy, systemic administration of antibiotics is advocated.

Topical therapy for neonatal ocular infection is not recommended. While it may eradicate ocular chlamydial infection, nasopharyngeal carriage persists, which can act as a source for pulmonary disease or ocular reinfection.

Occasionally, rhinitis, nasopharyngitis, tracheitis, and otitis media may be associated with chlamydial infections of the eye.

Postnatal Pneumonia

C. trachomatis is responsible for 20% to 60% of all pneumonias during the first six months of life. Typically, the symptoms begin in the second or third week of life and gradually worsen. Characteristic presentation of chlamydial pneumonia among infants is that of a repetitive staccato cough with tachypnea. The age at diagnosis of pneumonia is typically six weeks. The infants are afebrile and without malaise. Partial nasal obstruction and mucoid discharge are often noted. Respiratory signs are usually those of tachypnea and pertussis-like cough. The chest X ray tends to demonstrate a combination of hyperexpansion, with diffuse interstitial and focal alveolar infiltrates. Auscultation reveals fine inspiratory crepitant rales. About 50% of infants with chlamydial pneumonia have a prior history of concomitant chlamydial conjunctivitis.

The cough and tachypnea may require weeks to clear. The rales and X-ray findings may persist for more than a month. Approximately one-half of the affected children will have a prior history or concomitant demonstration of conjunctivitis.

Specimens should be collected from the nasopharynx for chlamydial testing. Tissue culture remains the definitive standard for chlamydial pneumonia; nonculture tests can be used; however, it should be noted that nonculture tests of nasopharyngeal specimens produce lower sensitivity and specificity than nonculture tests of ocular specimens. Tracheal aspirates and lung biopsy specimens, if collected, should be tested for *C. trachomatis*. An acute IgM antibody titer ≥1:32 is strongly suggestive of *C. trachomatis*.

The therapy of choice is erythromycin 50 mg/kg/day orally divided into four doses. The effectiveness of erythromycin treatment is approximately 80%; a second course of therapy may be required.

C. trachomatis is capable of replicating on any mucosal surface, including that of the gastrointestinal tract. Schachter et al. (1986) have demonstrated Chlamydia in the vagina of female neonates.

DIAGNOSIS OF CHLAMYDIAL INFECTION

Culture

Although culture is the most definitive means of making the diagnosis of Chlamydia, it is costly and takes at least two to three days before results are available. Although published methods are fairly standard, in practice, many laboratories introduce variations that alter the sensitivity and specificity of the test.

Two major components are needed to culture for C. trachomatis: (i) a cell-culture system, and (ii) a method to identify inclusions growing in cell culture. The cell line of choice is McCoy. Alternatively, a particular strain of HeLa cells (HeLa 229) can be used. Specimen material is centrifuged onto the cells for one hour and then incubated for two to three days in a medium containing cycloheximide. Incubation can take place in individual vials with cover slips at their base or on flat-bottomed wells in plastic microtiter plates. The choice between these methods is generally dictated by the number of specimens a laboratory has to process; the vial method is slightly more sensitive and less susceptible to cross-contamination, but is more time consuming and expensive.

For identification, either iodine stain or fluorescent antibody (FA) stain is usually used. FA stain offers the advantages of higher sensitivity and shorter processing time (two to three days) but requires a fluorescence microscope. The standard method for iodine staining requires one blind passage, which increases the processing time to four to six days. In microtiter plates, FA staining without passage appears equivalent to iodine staining with one blind passage. The most sensitive culture method currently available involves using cycloheximide-treated McCoy cells in vials in the presence of fluorescent monoclonal antibodies.

In collecting any specimen for chlamydial culture, it is imperative to avoid sampling mucopurulent exudate. C. trachomatis is an obligatory intracellular organism. The specimen must contain endocervical cells. Cotton swabs are not to be used because of the possible presence of cytotoxic material. Use of a Dacron or nylon swab with plastic or wire shaft is advocated.

Compared with other diagnostic tests for C. trachomatis, the major advantage of tissue culture is its specificity. With this method, the organism can also be positively identified or saved for other marker studies such as immunotyping. Thus, culture is clearly the method of choice for research studies. It is estimated that culture has a sensitivity of 80% to 90%, and a specificity of 100%.

There is limited value in obtaining routine urethral cultures to aid in the diagnosis of chlamydial infections. Dunlap et al. (1985) used triple culture tests at each site in the evaluation of 112 women with C. trachomatis infection. Organisms were recovered from the cervical material from 110, urethral material from 32, and rectal material from 19. Triple swabs provided 89 (81%) of the 110 diagnoses of cervical infection; the first swab yielded 65 (59%); the second swab 15 (14%); and the third an additional 9 (8%). Three sets of cervical scrapings provided 102 (93%) of 110 diagnoses of cervical infection, the first scraping yielding 76 (69%), the second 22 (20%), and the third another 4 (4%). These data are very similar to those documented for N. gonorrhoeae. They clearly demonstrate that the use of a single swab underestimates the prevalence of chlamydial infection.

Cytologic Methods

Cytologic identification of chlamydial infections—the only method available in the period 1909 to 1957—is an examination of epithelial cell scrapings (e.g., conjunctival, cervical, urethral) on the stained smear. A modified Giemsa stain is most often used, although Wright stain and other standard tissue stains can be used. Infection is identified by visualizing characteristic intracytoplasmic inclusions. Alternatively, cell scrapings can be examined using FA stains (Fig. 3).

The advantage of cytologic examination is clearly the simplicity of the process, particularly if light microscopy is used. The disadvantage is the poor sensitivity for diagnosing chlamydial infection. The sensitivity of cytologic methods in identifying chlamydial adult conjunctivitis is 45% for Giemsa and 85% for FA. In tests for cervical infection, the two stains have sensitivities of only 40% and 65%, respectively, and for urethral infection, 15% and 60%. Moreover, these upper levels of sensitivity can only be obtained with good specimens (many epithelial cells) and an experienced observer. Standard cytology is of little practical value as a diagnostic aid for genital chlamydial infection.

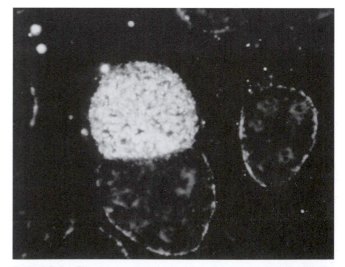

FIGURE 3 Fluorescent antibody stains for Chlamydia trachomatis.

Antigen Detection
The four principal methods of chlamydial antigen detection are (Table 2; also see Appendix V) the following:

1. FA examination of a direct smear
2. Enzyme immunoassay (EIA)
3. DNA probes
4. Polymerase chain reaction (PCR)

Commercially available nonculture methods of detecting *C. trachomatis* in general have sensitivities greater than 70% and specificities greater than 95% compared to culture. Continued revision of these tests takes place even after they become available commercially. Consequently, initial published data on efficacy may be outdated, so the most recent reference should be used.

Fluorescent Antibody
Compared with culture, the sensitivity of the direct-smear FA test is greater than or equal to 90% in most published studies, and the specificity is greater than or equal to 98%. The positive predictive value of this test has ranged from approximately 80% in populations with a *Chlamydia* prevalence of 10%, to 95% in populations with a *Chlamydia* prevalence of 30%. Lower sensitivities and specificities are often encountered in situations in which specimens are less than optimal or individuals reading the slides are relatively inexperienced. In these instances, assessment of the proficiency of laboratory techniques is essential.

Enzyme Immunoassay
The EIA test measures antigen–antibody reactions through an enzyme-linked immunoabsorbent assay (ELISA) and requires a spectrophotometer. Processing time for specimens is approximately four hours.

Questions continue to be raised about the reliability of EIAs for *C. trachomatis*. The sensitivity of the test has varied from 67% to 90%, the specificity from 92% to 97%, and the positive predictive value from 32% to 87%, depending on the population studied. Much of the observed disparity has been attributed to variable sensitivities of the tissue culture systems against which the EIA has been compared.

Probes
The use of DNA probes has been recently introduced for the diagnosis of chlamydial infection. Nucleic acid hybridization tests are based on the ability of complementary nucleic acid strands to specifically align and associate to form stable double-stranded complexes. The probe uses a chemiluminescent labeled, single-stranded DNA probe that is complementary to the ribosomal RNA of the target organism. After the ribosomal RNA is released from the organism, the labeled DNA probe combines with the target organism's ribosomal RNA to form a stable DNA:RNA hybrid (Appendix VII). The labeled DNA:RNA hybrid is separated from the nonhybridized probe and measured. The principal advantage of the DNA probes is the ability to concomitantly screen for *N. gonorrhoeae*. The benefits derived from the detection of additional positive specimens for *N. gonorrhoeae* outweighs the additional cost over the more standard diagnostic techniques.

Polymerase Chain Reaction
The PCR or ligase chain reaction (LCR) or transcription-mediated amplification (TMA) test has extremely high sensitivities and specificities when compared with culture PCR test and can be used for not only organismal detection, but also serotyping of infecting serovars. One of the great advantages of techniques such as PCR is the ability to detect *C. trachomatis* DNA in urine samples.

Noninvasive Specimen Collections
Urine as a Test Vehicle for Chlamydia Detection
Because of the frequency of concomitant urethral colonization, copies of target DNA within a urine sample can be detected by nucleic acid amplification tests. Lee et al. (1995) demonstrated that LCR testing on urine obtained from women gave sensitivities and specificities of 95.7% and 100%, respectively.

The urine to be tested should ideally meet the following criteria.

1. It should be the first 10 to 25 mL of urine voided.
2. It should be collected between one and two hours after previous urination.
3. It should be stored at 2°C to 8°C prior to testing.

Vaginal Introitus Sampling
DNA, PCR, or LCR testing of vaginal introitus specimens may provide an incidence of identification reasonably comparable to cervical sampling. Vaginal introitus specimens can be self-collected.

Specimen Collection for Culture
Endocervical
A Dacron cotton, calcium agliate-type swab should be used to obtain specimens from the endocervix. Swabs with wooden shafts may cause toxicity to cell cultures. The swab

TABLE 2 Test systems selection for identification of *Chlamydia trachomatis*

Clinical situation	Test procedure of choice
Low-prevalence screening	DNA hybridization probe (ultimately amplified DNA probe technologies)
Sexually transmitted disease clinic	DNA hybridization probe (ultimately amplified DNA probe technologies) PCR
Sexual assault/abuse	Culture only method recommended[a]
Test-of-cure:	
If <3 wk	Posttherapy culture
If >3 wk	Posttherapy culture or DNA hybridization probe

[a]If culture obtained within 48 hr after exposure, it is recommended that a second culture be obtained in 2 wk in the absence of preventative therapy. *Abbreviation*: PCR, polymerase chain reaction.

should be inserted past the squamocolumnar juncture about 2 cm and rotated for 15 to 30 seconds. If a Papanicolaou smear is to be collected, it should be done so before endocervical sampling. The pooling of a urethral swab specimen with endocervical swab specimens increases culture sensitivity. The likelihood of isolation is optimized if specimens are refrigerated immediately after collection and kept at 2°C to 8°C until transported to a testing facility. If greater than 48 hours elapse between collection and specimen processing, freezing at −70°C is an option. Freezing specimens at −70°C is associated with a 20% to 30% loss of viability. Freezing of specimens at −20°C is to be avoided.

Specimen Collection for Nonculture Tests
Once vaginal secretions are removed, collection of specimens for commercially licensed nonculture tests should be performed as per instructions.

Serology
Currently, *Chlamydia* serology has little value in routine clinical management and basically remains a research tool. Although some serologic tests are commercially available, they have not been shown to be useful in routine diagnosis.

There are two standard methods—complement fixation and microimmunofluorescence (MIF). ELISA tests have been developed, but none are recommended for wide use. The only valid clinical uses of serologic tests are in infant pneumonia, where specific IgM MIF serology, when available, is the diagnostic test of choice; and in occasional cases of suspected LGV. The difficulties in preparing the antigen and conducting the test restrict the use of the test to a limited number of research laboratories.

Proficiency in specimen collection and transport is paramount to accuracy in diagnostic testing for *C. trachomatis*. Both the sensitivity and the specificity of diagnostic tests for *C. trachomatis* are directly related to the adequacy of specimen collection. The choice of test system for the identification of *C. trachomatis* is a partial function of availability and clinical setting (Table 2).

Concurrent Gonococcal and Chlamydial Infections
Depending upon the study population and methodology used, 20% to 40% of women with documented endocervical gonorrhea are concomitantly infected with *C. trachomatis*. Asymptomatic women with lower tract chlamydial infection have a low rate of coinfection. Most estimates have been between 1% and 5%. Women with one STD warrant a study to exclude others.

Test of Cure
Historically, a routine test of cure during the immediate posttherapy period is not recommended. The Centers for Disease Control and Prevention (CDC) states that patients do not need to be retested for *Chlamydia* after completing treatment with doxycycline or azithromycin unless symptoms persist or reinfection is suspected, because these therapies, if taken, are highly efficacious. A test of cure should be considered three weeks after completion of treatment with erythromycin. With noncultured tests, residual chlamydial antigen and nucleic acid in the absence of viable organisms may result in a positive test. Such a positive result can be misinterpreted as a treatment failure. False-positive tests can occur for up to three weeks after doxycycline therapy.

Since the prevalence of infection in a test of cure is very low, tests with the highest positive predictive value, e.g., culture, are advocated. After three weeks, nucleic acid amplification tests, such as PCR and LCR, which have high predictive values, can be utilized. The use of combined *N. gonorrhoeae/C. trachomatis* for a test of cure is an uneconomical use of technology when culture is available. Use of DNA probe as a test of cure is warranted only if both organisms were initially identified or no other means of documenting eradication is available.

ADULT THERAPY

Nonpregnant Women
The therapies of choice for nongravid women with endocervical or urethral infection are (Table 3): azithromycin 1 g orally in a single dose; or doxycycline hyclate, 100 mg, by mouth twice daily for seven days.

Alternate regimens available for patients for whom tetracyclines are contraindicated or are not tolerated are: erythromycin base, 500 mg, by mouth four times a day for seven days; or erythromycin ethylsuccinate, 800 mg, by mouth four times a day for seven days; or ofloxacin 300 mg orally twice daily for seven days; or levofloxacin 500 mg orally once for seven days.

Doxycycline, ofloxacin, and levofloxacin are contraindicated in pregnant and lactating women.

Infected patients with concomitant HIV should receive the same treatment regimen as those who are HIV negative.

In populations with erratic health-seeking behavior, poor drug compliance, or little follow-up, azithromycin may be more cost effective as it provides single-dose, directly observed therapy. Doxycycline has a longer history of extensive use and the advantage of lower cost. Erythromycin is less efficacious than azithromycin or doxycycline. Its gastrointestinal side effects frequently discourage patients from complying with this regimen. The indicated fluoroquinolones are similar in efficacy to doxycycline and azithromycin.

To maximize compliance with recommended therapies, medications for chlamydial infections should be dispensed on site. To minimize further transmission of infection, patients treated for *Chlamydia* should be instructed to abstain from sexual intercourse for seven days after single-dose therapy or until completion of a seven-day regimen. Patients should also be instructed to abstain from sexual intercourse until all of their partners are cured, to minimize the risk of infection.

Pregnant Women
The teratogenic and/or embryopathic effects of the tetracycline and fluoroquinolones preclude drug utilization in pregnancy.

TABLE 3 CDC recommended regimens for *Chlamydia trachomatis* (2006)

Adults
- *Recommended regimen*
  Azithromycin 1 g orally in a single dose[a] *or* doxycycline 100 mg orally twice a day for 7 days[a]
- *Alternative regimen*
  Erythromycin base 500 mg orally 4 times a day for 7 days *or* erythromycin ethylsuccinate 800 mg orally 4 times a day for 7 days *or* ofloxacin 300 mg orally twice a day for 7 days *or* levofloxacin 500 mg orally once for 7 days

Pregnant women
- *Recommended regimen*
  Azithromycin 1 g orally in a single dose
  Amoxicillin 500 mg orally 3 times daily for 7 days[b]
- *Alternative regimen*
  Erythromycin base 500 mg orally 4 times daily for 7 days *or* erythromycin base 250 mg orally 4 times daily for 14 days *or* erythromycin ethylsuccinate 800 mg orally 4 times daily for 7 days *or* erythromycin ethylsuccinate 400 mg orally 4 times daily for 14 days

[a]While azithromycin and doxycycline have shown equal efficacy in studies to date, these clinical trials have primarily been done in populations where follow-up has been strongly encouraged and compliance with a 7-day regimen has been good.
[b]The author strongly disagrees with the recommendation for amoxicillin; the penicillin will push *Chlamydia* into latency but some isolates may regain their infectious form in time.
Abbreviation: CDC, Centers for Disease Control and Prevention.

Schachter et al. (1986) treated 65 gravidas with erythromycin ethylsuccinate (400 mg four times a day for seven days). Five of the ten women who had gastrointestinal disturbances discontinued therapy. Of the 60 women and 59 infants who completed the entire protocol, 55 (92%) of the women had negative cultures for *Chlamydia* at follow-up. The introduction of an azithromycin 1 g bolus dose has significantly impacted on *Chlamydia* therapy in pregnancy. Despite its higher cost, achieving patient compliance and effective therapy with a single administration clearly overshadows the consequences of failed therapy.

Because the *Chlamydia* cell wall is different from bacteria, beta-lactam antibiotics such as penicillins lack bacterial activity in vitro against these microorganisms. Nevertheless, the penicillins appear to drive *Chlamydia* into latency from which some will ultimately escape in time. The cephalosporins and aminoglycosides have no effect on *C. trachomatis*.

Management of Sex Partners

Patients should be instructed to refer their sex partners for evaluation, testing, and treatment. Because exposure intervals have received limited evaluation, the following recommendations are somewhat arbitrary. Sex partners whose last sexual contact with the index patient was within 60 days of onset of the index partner's symptoms or of diagnosis, which ever is later, should be evaluated, tested, and treated.

PREVENTION

Sexually active women aged 18 to 25 years should be screened for chlamydial infection annually. Similarly, any women with a new sex partner or multiple sex partners should be screened as frequently as warranted by her risk factors. Women who have had chlamydial infection should be rescreened three to four months after treatment.

All pregnant women should be screened for chlamydial infection in the first trimester or at the first clinic visit. Serious consideration should be given to rescreening women with high risk factors again at 36 weeks.

SELECTED READING

Alexander ER, Harrison HR. Role of *Chlamydia trachomatis* in perinatal infection. Rev Infect Dis 1983; 5:713.

Alger LS, Lovchik JC. Comparative efficacy of clindamycin versus erythromycin in eradication of antenatal *Chlamydia trachomatis*. Am J Obstet Gynecol 1991; 165:375.

Bass CA, Jungkind DL, Silverman NS, et al. Clinical evaluation of a new polymerase chain reaction assay for detection of *Chlamydia trachomatis* in endocervical specimens. J Clin Microbiol 1993; 31:2648.

Bell TA, Stamm WE, Kuo C-C, et al. Delayed appearance of *Chlamydia trachomatis* infections acquired at birth. Pediatr Infect Dis J 1987; 6:928.

Berman SM, Harrison HR, Boyce WT, et al. Low birth weight, prematurity, and postpartum endometritis: association with prenatal cervical *Mycoplasma hominis* and *Chlamydia trachomatis* infection. J Am Med Assoc 1987; 257:1189.

Brunham RC, Peeling R, MacLean I, et al. *Chlamydia trachomatis* associated with ectopic pregnancy: serological and histological correlates. J Infect Dis 1992; 165:1076.

Cates W Jr, Wasserhert JN. Genital chlamydial infections: epidemiology and reproductive sequelae. Am J Obstet Gynecol 1991; 164:1771.

Centers for Disease Control and Prevention. Recommendations for the prevention and management of Chlamydia trachomatis infections. MMWR Weekly 1993; Rep 42(RR-12):1.

Centers for Disease Control and Prevention. 2002 Guidelines for treatment of sexually transmitted diseases. MMWR 1998; 51(RR-6):1.

Center for Disease Control and Prevention. 2006 Guidelines for Sexually Transmitted Diseases. MMWR 2006; 55:RR-11.

Donders GGG. Treatment of sexually transmitted diseases in pregnant women. Drugs 2000; 59:480.

Dunlap EM, Goh BT, Darougan S, Woodland R. Triple culture test for diagnosis of chlamydial infection of the female genital tract. Sex Transm Dis 1985; 12:68.

Faro S. *Chlamydia trachomatis*: female pelvic infection. Am J Obstet Gynecol 1991; 164:1767.

Giertz G, Kallings I, Nordenvall M, Fuchs T. A prospective study of *Chlamydia trachomatis* infection following legal abortion. Acta Obstet Gynecol 1987; 66:107.

Gravett MG, Nelson HP, Derower T, et al. Independent association of bacterial vaginosis and *Chlamydia trachomatis* infection with adverse pregnancy outcomes. JAMA 1986; 256:1899.

Guderian AM, Trobough GE. Residues of pelvic inflammatory disease in intrauterine device users: a result of intrauterine device or *Chlamydia trachomatis* infection. Am J Obstet Gynecol 1986; 154:497.

Harrison HR, Alexander ER, Weinstein L, et al. Cervical *Chlamydia trachomatis* and mycoplasmal infections in pregnancy; epidemiology and outcome. JAMA 1983; 250:1721.

Heggie AD, Wyrich PB, Chase PA, Sorensen RU. Cell-mediated immune response to *Chlamydia trachomatis* in mothers and infants. Pros Soc Exp Biol Med 1986; 181:586.

La Scolea LJ, Paroski JS, Burzynski L, Faden HS. *Chlamydia trachomatis* infection in infants delivered by cesarean section. Clin Pediatr 1984; 23:118.

Mardh PA, Ripa T, Svensson L, et al. *Chlamydia trachomatis* in patients with acute salpingitis. N Engl J Med 1977; 296:1377.

Mardh PA, Moller BR, Paavonen J. Chlamydial infection of the female genital tract with special emphasis on pelvic inflammatory disease: a review of the Scandinavian studies. Sex Transm Dis 1981; 6:140.

McMillan JA, Weiner LB, Lamberson HV, et al. Efficacy of maternal screening and therapy in the prevention of chlamydial infection of the membranes. Infection 1985; 13:263.

Ripa KT, Svensson L, Tracharne JD et al. *Chlamydia trachomatis* in patients with laparoscopically verified acute salpingitis; results of isolation and antibody determination. Am J Obstet Gynecol 1980; 138:960.

Robinson AJ, Ridgwy GL. Concurrent gonococcal and chlamydial infection. Drugs 2000; 59:801.

Schachter J, Grossman M, Sweet RL, et al. Prospective study of perinatal transmission of *Chlamydia trachomatis*. J Am Med Assoc 1986; 255:3374.

Stagno S, Brasfield DM, Brown MB, et al. Infant pneumonitis associated with cytomegalovirus, chlamydia, pneumocystis, and ureaplasma: a prospective study. Pediatrics 1981; 68:322.

Sweet RL, Landers DV, Walker C, Schachter J. *Chlamydia trachomatis* infection and pregnancy outcome. Am J Obstet Gynecol 1987; 156:824.

Workowski KA, Lampe MF, Wong KG, et al. Long term eradication of *Chlamydia trachomatis* genital infection after antimicrobial therapy. Evidence against persistent infection. J Am Med Assoc 1993; 270:2071.

World Health Organization. Management of sexually transmitted diseases. WHO/GPA/TEM 1997; 94:1.

Diagnosis

Barnes RC. Laboratory diagnosis of human chlamydial infections. Clin Micro Rev 1989; 2:119.

Bauwens JE, Clark AM, Stamm WE. Diagnosis of *Chlamydia trachomatis* endocervical infections by a commercial polymerase. J Clin Microbiol 1993; 31:3023.

Black CM. Current methods of laboratory diagnosis of *chlamydia trachomatis* infections. Clin Microb Rev 1997; 10:1.

Blanding J, Hirsch L, Stranton N, et al. Comparison of the Clearview Chlamydia, the PACE 2 Assay, and culture for detection of *Chlamydia trachomatis* from cervical specimens in a low-prevalence population. J Clin Microbiol 1993; 31:1622.

Chow WH, Daling JR, Weiss NS, et al. The IUD and subsequent tubal ectopic pregnancy. Am J Public Health 1986; 76:536.

Clarke L, Sierra M, Daidone B, et al. Comparison of the Syva Microtrak enzyme immunoassay and Gen-Probe PACE 2 with cell culture for diagnosis of cervical *Chlamydia trachomatis* infection in a high-prevalence female population. J Clin Microbiol 1993; 31:968.

Kellog JA. Clinical laboratory considerations of culture vs antigen assays for detection of *Chlamydia trachomatis* from genital specimens. Arch Pathol Lab Med 1989; 113:453.

Krettek JE, Arkin SI, Chaisilwattana P, Monif GRG. *Chlamydia trachomatis* in patients who use oral contraceptives and had intermenstrual spotting. Obstet Gynecol 1993; 81:728.

LeBar W, Herschmann W, Jemal C, Pierzchalia J. Comparison of DNA probe, monoclonal antibody enzyme immuno assay and all culture for the detection of *Chlamydia trachomatis*. J Clin Microbol 1989; 27:826.

Lee HL, Chernesky MA, Schachter J et al. Diagnosis of *Chlamydia trachomatis* genitourinary infection in women by ligase chain reaction assay of urine specimens. Lancet 1995; 345:213.

Lefevre J, Laperione H, Rousseau H, Masse R. Comparison of three techniques for detection of *Chlamydia trachomatis* in endocervical specimens from asymptomatic women. J Clin Microbiol 1988; 26:726.

Limberger RJ, Biega R, McCarthy EL, et al. Evaluation of culture and the Gen-Probe PACE 2 Assay for detection of *Neisseria gonorrhoeae* and *Chlamydia trachomatis* in endocervical specimens transported to a state health laboratory. LJ Clin Microbiol 1992; 30:1162.

Loefferholz MJ, Lewinski CA, Silver SR, et al. Detection of *Chlamydia trachomatis* in endocervical specimens by polymerase chain reaction. J Clin Microbiol 1992; 30:2847.

Osser S, Persson K. Chlamydial antibodies in women who suffer miscarriages. Br J Obstet Gynaecol 1995; 103:137.

Twen PC, Blair TMH, Woods GL. Comparison of the Gen-Probe PACE 2® System, direct fluorescent antibody and all culture for detecting *Chlamydia trachomatis* in cervical specimens. Clin Microbiol Clin Chem 1991; 36:578.

Witkin SS, Jeremias J, Toth M, Ledger WJ. Detection of *Chlamydia trachomatis* by the polymerase chain reaction in the cervices of women with acute salpingitis. Am J Obstet Gynecol 1993; 168:1438.

Wölner-Hanssen P, Mardh PA, Svensson L, et al. Laparoscopy in women with chlamydial infection and pelvic pain: A comparison of patients with and without salpingitis. Obstet Gynecol 1983; 61:299.

Woods GL, Young A, Scott JC, et al. Evaluation of nonisotopic probe for detection of *Chlamydia trachomatis* in endocervical specimens. J Clin Microbiol 1990; 28:370.

Yang LI, Panke ES, Leist PA, et al. Detection of *Chlamydia trachomatis* endocervical infection in asymptomatic and symptomatic women: comparison of deoxyribonucleic acid probe test with tissue culture. Am J Obstet Gynecol 1991; 165:1444.

FEMALE GENITAL TRACT INVOLVEMENT

Lymphogranuloma venereum (LGV), a rare disease in the United States, is caused by the invasive serovars L1, L2, and L3 of *Chlamydia trachomatis*. Although its distribution is worldwide, LGV is more common in tropical and semitropical climates. The mode of transmission is believed to be through coitus or intimate physical contact. A number of small endemic foci have been traced to a specific prostitute. The disease may also be disseminated by close nonsexual contact as well as by autoinoculation. Disease has occurred in laboratory workers.

Classically, if the primary lesion occurs on the external genitalia, LGV presents as a transient herpetiform lesion. Although a grippe-like syndrome characterized by fever, malaise, headache, and anorexia may occur, it is rarely the chief presenting complaint in patients with LGV. Fever is present in over 50% of cases and tends to correlate primarily with severity of illness. Patients usually seek medical care because of acute inflammatory changes within lymph nodes or bloody proctocolitis. Manifestations of neglected disease are either consequences of lymphatic blockage draining the primary infection (elephantiasis) or scar tissue.

The most common clinical manifestation of LGV among heterosexuals is tender inguinal and/or femoral lymphadenopathy that is most commonly unilateral. Women and homosexually active men may have proctocolitis or inflammatory involvement of perirectal or perianal lymphatic tissues, resulting in fistulas and strictures.

LGV in its initial presentation may occur as one of two syndromes—inguinal or genitorectal.

Inguinal Syndrome

The initial genital lesion that develops varies from a slight erosion to a small cutaneous herpetiform lesion. It may either disappear or develop into an ulcer. The lesion is painless and only slightly tender to palpation. It exhibits ill-defined shallow margins and a fibrogranular base. The fourchette, urethral meatus, and medial surface of the labia are the usual sites of primary lesions. Clinical recognition of infection at this stage is the exception, not the rule. When multiple lesions are present, the adjacent labia or clitoris is often edematous. In the absence of secondary infection, most of the lesions will have healed prior to the onset of lymph node enlargement.

More than 50% of infected patients manifest no clinical symptoms. While most male patients develop inguinal adenopathy during the course of disease, this manifestation is relatively unusual in females (Table 1). The adenopathy may vary from shoddy nodes to fluctuant masses often associated with draining sinuses. Involvement of the inguinal and femoral lymph nodes may result in masses on either side of the inguinal ligament (so-called groove sign).

Lymph node involvement is indicative of lymphatic drainage from the primary lesions, and consequently unilateral adenopathy is not uncommon. The regional glands draining the primary site of infection, particularly in the male, enlarge dramatically and may appear as a series of buboes. Sixty percent of the buboes rupture, discharging a copious watery to purulent granular exudate.

The early histologic appearance of lymph nodes is that of diffuse reticular and lymphocytic hyperplasia. In the more advanced lesion, macrophages appear in significant numbers prior to the development of central necrosis. The macrophages assume a palisade-like arrangement around the central focus of necrotic cellular debris. Plasmacytosis is one of the important supplementary criteria in the histologic diagnosis of LGV. Healing is associated with fibroblastic proliferation and (ultimately) with the replacement of the diseased foci by fibrous connective tissue. Extensive cutaneous scarring may suggest the diagnosis in a patient seen for the first time late in the course of the disease.

If urethral involvement occurs, it exhibits the same sequential pattern—first ulceration and then destructive lesions with healing by fibrosis. Patients with partial urethral destruction may remain continent as long as the distal portion of the urethra is intact. Partial obstruction may cause difficulty in voiding. The resultant symptoms are those of urethral obstruction. Complete urethral destruction represents a difficult therapeutic challenge, necessitating surgical reconstruction.

Genitorectal Syndrome

The second syndrome, genitorectal, accounts for 25% of the cases seen in the early stage, and occurs predominantly in women. In the male, lymphatic drainage from the initial lesion is primarily to the inguinal lymph nodes. In the female, the perirectal and pelvic lymph nodes are the primary sites of drainage.

Rectal involvement occurs by contiguous spread from the perirectal lymph nodes. Initially proctocolitis develops, characterized by mucopurulent discharge and bloody diarrhea. Secondary bacterial infection of the ulcerated lesions and adjacent mucosa contributes significantly to the disease process. The proctitis is most severe at the anorectal ring. The regional mucosa is edematous, hemorrhagic, and friable. Neither adenopathy nor systemic signs and symptoms comparable to those attending the inguinal syndrome are commonly observed with this form of the disease. If treated with antibiotic agents and a low-residue diet, this stage of the disease can be cured, leaving no residual stigmata. No sharp clinical demarcation exists between late-stage proctitis and early stricture formation. The perirectal and rectal tissues become secondarily involved by contiguous spread;

TABLE I Differential diagnosis of inguinal adenopathy associated with a presumed venereal disease

Disease	Genital lesion	Nodal involvement	Cutaneous lesions
Granuloma inguinale	Extensive in males, less evident in females	Involvement of lymph nodes; draining cutaneous sinuses; late in the course of the disease; nodes become tender	Primary skin infection with superficial ulceration
Lymphogranuloma venereum	Occurs but is extremely transient in nature	Bilateral node involvement is determined by site of primary lesion	Multiple sinus tracts draining a thick, creamy exudate
Chancroid	Usually present	Primarily unilateral with limited involvement of lymph nodes	Acute, with crater-like slough
Genital tuberculosis	None	Bilateral inguinal adenopathy	Pleomorphic, often with sinus tract draining scanty thick exudate
Syphilis	Usually present	Bilateral; firm, rubbery nodes	Protean in its clinical manifestations

consequently, with healing, induration of the lower third of the posterior vagina and scarring of the rectovaginal septum are frequent findings. Extensive disease may result in strictures as far as the rectosigmoid junction.

Rectal stricture may then cause additional symptoms, namely, those of chronic obstruction of the distal colon. Occasionally, the infection culminates in intestinal obstruction sufficiently acute to necessitate colostomy. Once significant fibrosis with stricture formation has occurred, surgical incision of the stricture is the prime therapeutic modality.

A physiologically significant rectal stricture is important in the pathogenesis of a rectovaginal fistula. Almost invariably, rectovaginal fistulas occur in patients with stricture. The site of the fistula is fairly constant: at or below the level of the stricture in the midline about 2.54 to 3.81 cm from the fourchette.

Lesions in the late stages may not exhibit active inflammation or ulceration. There is no sure way of distinguishing burned-out cases from those that are still active and for which systemic therapy should be initiated prior to any attempt at repair or plastic procedures.

Laboratory results, with the exception of complement fixation or microimmunofluorescent and polymerase chain reaction tests for LGV, are inconclusive. Abnormalities in the white blood cell count include mild-to-marked leukocytosis, with a relative lymphocytosis. Biologically false-positive serologic tests for syphilis not infrequently occur. In longstanding disease, the albumin–globulin ratio is inverted.

LGV and Vulvar Carcinoma

LGV is often cited as a predisposing factor in vulvar carcinoma. This circumstantial association is based largely on the coexistence of the two diseases and on the observation that with a history of LGV, cancer of the vulva occurs at a significantly earlier age. If vulvar carcinoma develops in a patient with previous or concomitant LGV, the latter disorder appears to influence the natural history of the disease. Metastases through the lymphatics appear to be delayed, presumably because of inflammatory or postinflammatory alterations of the lymphatics.

LGV in Pregnancy

LGV may complicate pregnancy as a consequence of the inflammatory lesions and subsequent scar tissue formation

involving the vagina and rectum, which may impede normal vaginal delivery.

The disease process may result in vulvar elephantiasis esthiomene and produce a soft tissue outlet dystocia. In this circumstance, the management of delivery is similar to that in other types of soft tissue outlet dystocia.

A significant impediment to the descent of the presenting part as a consequence of extensive fibrosis is seen in the chronic stages of the disease. The obstruction reflects reparative fibrosis, which follows the retrograde spread of infection into both the bases of the broad ligament and the soft tissues of the pelvic wall. Rupture of the rectum or uterus is a potentially lethal complication of vaginal delivery in such cases. In rectal rupture, the pelvic portion, if fixed to the vagina, is torn away from the segment above the pouch of Douglas, where it is adherent to the sacrum by scar tissue. Kaiser and King (1947), in their compendium on the subject, recommend that the mode of delivery be based on the evaluation of the soft tissues of the pelvis prior to delivery. The extent of involvement can be ascertained under anesthesia in terms of

1. the presence of rectal stricture,
2. fixation in the region of the pouch of Douglas,
3. adnexal thickening, and
4. the presence of fistula formation.

When a trial of labor appears to be justified, it should be borne in mind that failure of descent of the presenting part is an indication for cesarean section rather than trial of forceps or version, regardless of the degree of cervical dilation. Version and extraction or any form of forceps delivery is contraindicated. If vaginal delivery is achieved, the patient must be carefully monitored for signs of rectal or uterine rupture. Postpartum shock, associated with lower abdominal pain and peritoneal irritation, necessitates immediate laparotomy following rapid expansion of the intravascular compartment and antibiotic therapy.

DIAGNOSIS

Disease in women is difficult to diagnose. The female patient is more likely to present with the genitorectal than with the inguinal syndrome or with inguinal adenopathy in a subclinical form.

With primary infection, she may complain of a small boil on the vagina or a slight discharge or irritation. Most often, the small shallow red ulcers with flat margins due to LGV escape clinical detection.

The second stage of disease, in which adenitis predominates, may pass unnoticed until a late phase in which fibrosis or tissue destruction has developed. Symptoms of disease are the result of destruction and secondary fibrosis involving the rectum, urethra, or lymphatic drainage of the labia. The patient may complain of urinary or fecal incontinence, or both, diarrhea, dyspareunia, or discomfort due to swelling of the vulva (vulvar elephantiasis). Rectal lesions are likely to draw the attention of gynecologists when either a rectovaginal fistula develops or repeated straining at stool leads to uterine prolapse. LGV must be considered in the differential diagnosis of any fistulous tract involving the perineum.

The chlamydial complement fixation test is used to confirm exposure to C. trachomatis. Titers equal to or greater than 1:64 are regularly present in the serum of women with LGV and can support the diagnosis.

Initially developed for serotyping strains of C. trachomatis, the microimmunofluorescence test effectively measures antibody response to the selective serotypes in its pool. It is of considerable value in documenting infection due to L serovars. Serologic confirmation of prior and/or concurrent antigenic experience with chlamydia organisms, coupled with a characteristic disease clustering, makes the diagnosis of LGV. Serovar-specific serological tests for C. trachomatis are not widely available.

Bubo aspirates or lesion swabs can be submitted for culture, direct immunofluorescence, or nucleic acid detection. Nucleic acid amplification tests for C. trachomatis have not been FDA cleared for testing of rectal specimens.

THERAPY

Therapy is directed not only at curing infection/disease, but also at preventing or limiting healing complications of scarring and chronic lymphatic blockage. In nonpregnant women, doxycycline is the preferred treatment (100 mg orally twice daily for 21 days). Doxycycline is contraindicated in pregnant and lactating women. The alternative regimen consists of erythromycin base 500 mg orally four times a day for 21 days. An erythromycin regimen is preferred when clinical ambiguity exists between LGV and chancroid (Haemophilus ducreyi).

Erythromycin is the drug of choice in pregnant and lactating women (500 mg orally four times a day for 21 days). The activity of azithromycin against C. trachomatis suggests it may be effective in multiple doses over two to three weeks, but substantial clinical data are lacking.

Aspiration of fluctuant nodes can be implemented as a therapeutic adjunct in adenitis. Aspiration of suppurative nodes in lieu of spontaneous rupture has been advocated and appears free of significant complications. Aspiration is best achieved with a No 20 needle, inserting it through adjacent noninvolved skin rather than aspirating the lesion directly through skin overlying the node.

A patient with significant disease must be monitored for possible development of vulvar carcinoma. Biopsy of any suspicious lesion is mandatory.

Women with both LGV and HIV infection should receive the same treatment regimens as those who are not HIV positive. Prolonged therapy may be required to achieve resolution of disease.

Management of Sex Partners

Persons who have had sexual contact with a patient who has LGV within 30 days before onset of the patient's symptoms should be examined, tested for urethral chlamydial infection, and treated.

SELECTED READING

Female Genital Tract Involvement

Abrams A. Lymphogranuloma venereum. J Am Med Assoc 1968; 205:199.

Centers for Disease Control. 2006 Guidelines for sexually transmitted diseases. MMWR 2006; 55: RR-11.

Centers for Disease Control. Sexually transmitted diseases treatment guidelines 2002. MMWR 2002; 51(RR-6):1.

Chandra M, Jain AK. Fine structure of *Calymmatobacterium granulomatis* with particular reference to the surface structure. Indian J Med Res 1991; 93:225.

Chandra M, Jain AK, Ganguly DD. An ultrastructural study of donovanosis. Indian J Med Res 1989; 89:158.

Douglas CP. Lymphogranuloma venereum and granuloma inguinale of the vulva. Br J Obstet Gynaecol 1962; 69:871.

Faro S. Lymphogranuloma venereum, chancroid, and granuloma inguinale. Obstet Gynecol Clin North Am 1989; 16:517.

Kampmeier RH. Granuloma inguinale. Sex Transm Dis 1984; 11:318.

Lee HL, Chernesky MA, Schachter J, et al. Diagnosis of *Chlamydia trachomatis* genitourinary tract infections in women by ligase chain reaction assay of urinary specimen. Lancet 1995; 345:213.

Megran DW. Quinolones in the treatment of sexually transmitted diseases. Clin Invest Med 1989; 12:50.

Schachter J. Lymphogranuloma venereum and other nonocular *Chlamydia trachomatis* infections. In: Hobson D, Holmes KK, eds. Nongonococcal Urethritis and Related Infections. Washington, DC: American Society for Microbiology, 1977.

Sigel MM, ed. Lymphogranuloma Venereum. Coral Gables, FL: University of Miami Press, 1962.

World Heath Organization. Management of sexually transmitted diseases. WHO/GPA/TEM/ 1997; 94:1.

LGV and Vulvar Carcinoma

Hoosen AA, Draper G, Moodley J. Granuloma inguinale of the cervix: a carcinoma look-alike. Genitourin Med 1995; 5:380.

Rainey R. The association of lymphogranuloma inguinale and cancer. Surgery 1954; 35:221.

Saltzstein SL, Woodruff JD, Novak ER. Postgranulomatous carcinoma of the vulva. Obstet Gynecol 1956; 7:80.

Turell R. Colorectal lesions in pregnancy. In: Guttmacker AF, Rovinsky JJ, eds. Medical, Surgical and Gynecological Complications of Pregnancy. Baltimore: Williams & Wilkins, 1960.

White BH, Miller JM. Lymphogranuloma inguinale complicated by carcinoma. Am J Syph 1953; 37:177.

LGV in Pregnancy

Finn W. Lymphogranuloma venereum in pregnancy. Am J Obstet Gynecol 1944; 48:696.

Kaiser IH, King EL. Lymphopathia venereum complicating labor. Am J Obstet Gynecol 1947; 54:219.

Mycoplasma

Newton G. Osborne

INTRODUCTION

The mycoplasmas are small (0.2–0.3 milicrons) membrane-bound, pleomorphic, free-living procaryotes. They are the smallest organisms capable of independent self-replication. They belong to the class of Mollicutes, which is a taxon that contains small procaryotic organisms bounded by a single cell membrane. Mollicutes have no known relationship to bacteria, but because of their filamentous shape, star shape, or spherical appearance, they can be confused with cell wall–deficient L-forms.

Mycoplasmatales is the only order in the class Mollicutes. The order Mycoplasmatales has four families: Mycoplasmataceae, Acholeplasmataceae, Spiroplamataceae, and Anaeroplasmataceae. There are no known species among the Spiroplasmataceae nor among the Anaeroplasmataceae that are capable of colonizing or infecting humans. Ten of the twelve species that are recovered from humans are in the genus *Mycoplasma: M. buccale, M. faucium, M. fermentans, M. genitalium, M. hominis, M. lipophilum, M. orale, M. pneumoniae, M. primatum,* and *M. salivarium.* The two other organisms among the Mycoplasmataceae found in humans are *Ureaplasma urealyticum* and *Acheloplasma laidlawii.* However, only *M. genitalium, M. hominis, M. pneumoniae,* and *U. urealyticum* have been associated with disease in humans. *M. hominis, M. genitalium,* and *U. urealyticum* are urogenital tract pathogens.

M. pneumoniae is a known agent of serious respiratory infections in humans, and it has also been recovered from patients with pericarditis and those with otitis media, from the joint fluid of patients with chronic arthritis, and in cases of meningitis, among infections at sites other than the respiratory tract.

Mycoplasmas do not stain with Gram reagent. They stain poorly with Giemsa stain. Colonies are recognized on special solid media either by a characteristic "fried egg" configuration or by the formation of small golden spherules. Although unlike viruses they are capable of growing on cell-free media, the mycoplasmas are fastidious in their growth requirements. It is necessary to provide them with enriched media containing peptone, yeast extract, and serum. These materials provide a source for urea, nucleic acids, and cholesterol. Members of the class can be identified by their ability to hydrolyze urea (*U. urealyticum*), utilize arginine (*M. hominis* and *M. fermentans*), or ferment glucose (*M. fermentans* and *M. genitalium*). *U. urealyticum* is unique among bacteria in its requirement for urea even when inoculated into complex media.

The absence of a cell wall makes mycoplasmas insensitive to penicillin and other antibiotics whose action depend on interference with cell wall synthesis.

GENITAL STRAINS

Four strains can be recovered from the genital tract: *U. urealyticum, M. hominis, M. fermentans,* and *M. genitalium.*

M. hominis and *U. urealyticum* are recovered frequently from the cervix and vagina of sexually experienced women. Carriage of *M. hominis* and *U. urealyticum* is so common in women that it has been considered normal flora by some. Both organisms have been isolated from the blood of patients with puerperal and postabortal low-grade fever.

M. genitalium is a common cause of persistent urethritis among men treated with doxycycline for nongonococcal urethritis. Recent reports suggest that *M. genitalium* is more common than *Chlamydia trachomatis* in these patients. Eradication of *M. genitalium* with doxycycline or erythromycin from patients with persistent or recurrent urethritis appears to be less efficient than with azithromycin.

Like with other sexually transmitted organisms, the probability of mycoplasmal recovery from the lower genital tract is directly related to the number of sexual partners either the patient or her sexual partner have been exposed to. However, the presence of mycoplasmas in the lower genital tract of women is not necessarily associated with clinical infection.

LABORATORY DIAGNOSIS

The proper handling of specimens is critical for the recovery of these fastidious microorganisms. Specimens taken on swabs should be received in the laboratory within an hour of collection. Plastic shafted swabs are preferable to wooden ones since they are less likely to contain toxic chemicals that may interfere with optimum growth. Because the microorganisms are in a natural environment, specimens such as semen or urine can be kept for several hours following collection prior to culturing. Two specimens from each patient are recommended in order to ensure the best possible chance of isolation. A cervical swab and urine from the female, semen, urethral swab, and urine from the male are the most readily available, involve the least discomfort, and at the same time yield reproducible information as to the presence of *U. urealyticum* and *M. hominis.*

If the specimens are to be mailed, immediate freezing in dry ice is essential, followed by shipping in dry ice. Freezing results in a loss of microorganisms and is not recommended unless absolutely necessary. There may be a loss of at least two logs in the colony count when samples are frozen and subsequently defrosted for culture.

Considerable experience is necessary for isolation. A solid agar, Shepard's A7, and a broth medium are inoculated simultaneously. Both media are observed daily. The broth is observed for a color change, from yellow to pink. This change indicates that urease, characteristic of *U. urealyticum*, is present. The solid medium demonstrates the presence of actual colonies. The colonies are very small and usually cannot be visualized by the naked eye. Under the low power of the microscope, *U. urealyticum* appear as dark-brown, accretion colonies. Classical mycoplasmas appear as almost colorless, film-like colonies with obvious central cores. The classical mycoplasmas, unlike bacterial colonies, accept the Dienes stain.

No further identification of *U. urealyticum* is required beyond demonstration of the presence of urease and the typical colonial morphology on A7 agar. *M. hominis*, however, requires further identification. The standard means of identification is the use of known antisera for growth inhibition of a subculture of the original isolate. Recently, special methods of identification such as DNA extraction to identify biotypes by polymerase chain reaction direct sequence methods have been used to identify mycoplasmas in urine and urogenital swab specimens and have become the methods of choice for research with mycoplasmas.

Specimens other than genital swabs, semen, and urine have been found positive for the genital mycoplasmas. Isolations of *U. urealyticum* have been made from the placenta, amniotic fluid, and the nasopharynx of neonates and adults, and from the lungs of infants dying in the perinatal period. *M. hominis* has also been isolated from the lungs of infants dying in the perinatal period, the nasopharynx of neonates and adults, and most recently, from the brain abscess of a neonate, and an infected knee joint following total knee replacement.

Because of the observation that tetracycline-resistant strains of *U. urealyticum* and *M. hominis* make up 10% to 15% of patient isolates, a simple, direct, broth-disk method for antibiotic susceptibility testing was developed by Kundsin et al. (1984). The test utilizes urine sediment as the inoculum and impregnated paper disks as the source of antibiotic. Antibiotic levels that approximate attainable serum levels are used. Combinations of antibiotics can be tested in this fashion.

GYNECOLOGICAL INFECTION

M. hominis and *U. urealyticum* have been isolated from both the lower and upper genital tracts of women with classical symptoms of pelvic inflammatory disease (PID). In 1937, Dienes and Edsall isolated *mycoplasma* in pure culture from a Bartholin abscess. In 1954, Shephard reported the recovery of *U. urealyticum* from men with nongonococcal urethritis. Since then, Kundsin et al. (1984) have demonstrated that there is a female counterpart to nonspecific urethritis in males. Kundsin et al. (1984) demonstrated that 80% of women with symptoms of genitourinary infection attending the genital infectious disease clinic at Brigham and Women's Hospital had *U. urealyticum* in their urine as opposed to 2% of nuns in a teaching order in Boston.

Mardh et al. (1981) have reported isolation of mycoplasmas from the fallopian tubes of patients with a diagnosis of salpingitis verified by laparoscopy. Mardh et al. went on further to report that in no cases where there were normal tubes seen through the laparoscope were mycoplasmas isolated from the pouch of Douglas. Others, however, have reported the recovery of mycoplasmas from these areas in some patients without laparoscopic evidence of salpingitis. Other investigators have reported the presence of specific hemagglutination inhibition (HAI) antibodies in patients with acute salpingitis. All patients with HAI antibodies had *M. hominis* in the genital tract and over half of those patients had a fourfold or greater rise in titer.

The recovery of mycoplasmas and ureaplasmas in pure culture from infected fallopian tubes, the demonstration of elevated immunoglobulin M (IgM)–specific for *M. hominis* in patients with acute salpingitis, and the correlation of indirect hemagglutination antibodies against *M. hominis* with the isolation of *M. hominis* in patients with salpingitis are strong evidence that mycoplasmas are pathogenic in at least a percentage of patients with salpingitis.

The literature on mycoplasmas and infertility is obviously controversial. *M. hominis* and *U. urealyticum* are reported to be cultured more frequently from women attending infertility clinics, particularly if tubal or cervical abnormalities are detected or if there is an abnormal vaginal discharge. In addition, subtle endometrial changes have been described in as many as 55% of patients with urine cultures positive for *U. urealyticum*. However, double-blind studies have not yet demonstrated a relationship between the presence of mycoplasmas in the lower genital tract and secondary infertility. Although *M. hominis* and *U. urealyticum* have been demonstrated to be capable of attaching to human spermatozoa in infertile patients, the mechanism for infertility presumably caused by the mycoplasmas has not been established. Experiments carried out with *U. urealyticum* serotype 4 suggest the production of diffusible, relatively heat-stable factors responsible for inhibition of sperm penetration of hamster eggs. Since the effects on sperm may be delayed, it is possible that for postcoital tests to be valid, they should be performed after eight hours, even if excellent results are obtained at two hours.

Gump et al. (1984) presented a study of 205 couples with infertility in whom ovulatory dysfunction was ruled out. The results indicated that in the women studied, isolation of *M. hominis* was more common in patients with a history of PID. However, no relationship could be established between positive cultures and hysterosalpingographic or laparoscopic evidence of previous tubal infection. They could not establish a relationship between the presence of mycoplasmas, and cervical inflammation or postcoital testing. Their conclusion was that, in their series, no association between the presence of genital mycoplasmas and infertility could be demonstrated. They, however, did not do an eight-hour postcoital test. In addition, they used wooden handles on their cotton-tipped applicators for sample collection, they did not collect samples from urine, and some of their cultures were obtained from frozen endometrium that was thawed.

Another study of infertile women by Horne (1974) and Kundsin (1970) found that of 99 consecutive patients, 64 (65%) had genital mycoplasmas. They also noted that antibodies to *C. trachomatis* were significantly associated with the presence of genital mycoplasmas. Of 23 patients with elevated antibody titers to *C. trachomatis*, 20 (87%) had genital mycoplasmas. Of 76 patients with no *C. trachomatis* antibody titers, 44 (58%) had genital mycoplasmas. This was a statistically significant difference (chi square 6.52, $p = 0.01$). What this means is that essentially most women with *C. trachomatis* antibody titers also have genital mycoplasmas. The role of each microorganism in infertility must therefore be evaluated. This can only be done if cultures for both genital mycoplasmas and chlamydia antibody titers are obtained from each patient evaluated for infertility and matched with suitable controls.

OBSTETRIC INFECTION

M. hominis is found in association with *U. urealyticum* in the genitourinary tract of approximately 10% to 15% of patients. Both of these mycoplasmas, separately or in combination, have been found in human placentas, and their presence has been significantly associated with perinatal morbidity and mortality. Mycoplasmas can be isolated from approximately 15% of pregnant women during the first trimester and this increases to approximately 20% during the last trimester. More than 11% of women who have afebrile abortions have mycoplasmas present in their cervix. This number is not significantly different from patients who do not abort. In contrast, if fever is considered, 39% of patients who have febrile spontaneous abortions have *M. hominis* isolated from the cervix, and the percentage is even higher if stricter criteria for febrile abortion are applied.

Harwick et al. (1967) reported mycoplasmemia associated with these infected abortions. This observation demonstrates the invasive potential of mycoplasmas. Their conclusion was that in the febrile cases, mycoplasmas might act as opportunistic microorganisms invading only traumatized or previously infected tissues. But there is also the possibility, of course, that they initiate an infectious process that results in fetal wastage.

U. urealyticum is a common commensal of the urogenital tract of sexually mature humans. While its etiologic significance in many aspects of adverse pregnancy remains controversial, recent evidence indicates that *U. urealyticum* in the absence of other organisms is a cause of chorioamnionitis. Furthermore, ureaplasmal infection of the chorioamnion is significantly associated with premature spontaneous labor and delivery. In at least some cases, it appears to be causal. Present evidence indicates that *U. urealyticum* is a cause of septicemia, meningitis, and pneumonia in newborn infants,

particularly those born prematurely. There is strong but not definitive evidence that ureaplasmal infection of the lower respiratory tract can lead to development of chronic lung disease in very-low-birthweight infants. Although risk factors for colonization of the lower genitourinary tract have been identified, little information is available concerning risk factors for intrauterine infection and host immune responses to invasive infection.

Isolation of *U. urealyticum* from the placentas of infants born at the Boston Lying-in Hospital also showed a documented increase in morbidity and mortality for those infants whose placentas harbored this microorganism.

Kundsin et al. (1984) have reported a relationship between *U. urealyticum* and infertility as well as with spontaneous abortion and ectopic pregnancy. Another phase of their investigation dealt with diethylstilbestrol (DES)-exposed women having problems of infertility. Cultures from this population of women revealed a high rate of isolation of *U. urealyticum* from the genitourinary tract. Furthermore, the incidence of ectopic pregnancy and spontaneous abortion was significantly higher than in non–DES-exposed women. Analysis of the data, however, suggested that pregnancy wastage in DES-exposed women is related more to *U. urealyticum* colonization than to DES exposure in utero.

Mycoplasmas have been shown to cause chromosomal alterations in cultured human diploid fibroblasts. Reportedly, they can produce lesions on the short arm of chromosomes 21 and 22. Structural alterations in chromosomes have also been reported in human peripheral lymphocyte cultures infected with *U. urealyticum*. *U. urealyticum* has been identified as a pathogen associated with chorioamnionitis, premature delivery, and neonatal pneumonia. It is suggested that since some strains can induce chromosomal change in vitro, it is possible that these organisms can also produce chromosomal alterations in the zygote and be responsible for some cases of spontaneous abortion associated with lower genital tract infections with mycoplasmas.

Several studies have demonstrated that genital mycoplasmas, especially the strains of *U. urealyticum*, are isolated more frequently in the lower genital tract of women who deliver placentas with histologic evidence of chorioamnionitis when they are compared with the placentas of women who have no manifestations of inflammation. Most of the studies correlating chorioamnionitis with the presence of mycoplasmas have had poor controls and lack the results of serologic antibodies in the mother and the neonate to demonstrate an adverse effect of colonization by these organisms.

The literature therefore does not support unequivocally the theory that a direct relationship exists between sexual activity in pregnancy and isolation of mycoplasmas from the lower genital tract of women who develop chorioamnionitis.

An association between *M. hominis* in the genital tract and low birthweight has been postulated. A report by McCormack et al. (1987) indicated that patients treated four times daily with erythromycin for six weeks in a randomized, double-blind study gave birth to infants with heavier mean birthweights when compared with infants born to placebo-treated women. Erythromycin treatment had no effect when administered in the second trimester. In contrast, women whose treatment with erythromycin was initiated in the third trimester had babies with heavier mean birthweight than the babies born to the placebo-treated women. The incidence of infants weighing 2500 g or less was 3% while women treated with placebo gave birth to babies at or below this weight 12% of the time. This difference was statistically significant. The data suggested that treatment with erythromycin during the third trimester prevented low birthweight in *mycoplasma*-colonized pregnant women. It was not certain, however, whether the erythromycin effect was also due to an action on *U. urealyticum*.

Postpartum fever has been associated with *M. hominis* infection confirmed by blood culture and with a significant elevation in antibody titer. The possibility that mycoplasmas can be responsible for postpartum morbidity should always be considered in postpartum patients with cryptogenic fever. This is especially true if there have been no abnormalities during the labor or any operative intervention.

Mycoplasmas are ubiquitous in the genitourinary tract of pregnant women. Local changes in the genital tract associated with the pregnant state may favor recovery of *U. urealyticum* and *M. hominis* from the genital tract. It is almost certain that mycoplasmas are at least synergistic organisms in the development of fever in some parturient and postpartum females. It is most likely that they do represent in some cases primary true pathogens involved in the infectious process.

In summary, both *U. urealyticum* and *M. hominis* have been incriminated in sexually transmissible disease in adults, in infertility and reproductive wastage, in postpartum and postabortal maternal infection, and in neonatal morbidity and mortality. Definitive proof is still lacking.

The controversy regarding the significance of *U. urealyticum* and *M. hominis* infections demands that any studies on the association of these microorganisms with human infection be done by competent individuals thoroughly familiar with appropriate methodology for securing specimens, transporting them, culturing them on appropriate media, and with identification of isolates.

If mycoplasmas are shown unequivocally to be related to reproductive morbidity and mortality, the resolution of the health problems caused by these microorganisms will depend on the application of reliable techniques for isolation, identification, and determination of antibiotic susceptibilities of the offending strains. Appropriate and effective therapy will depend on these factors.

THERAPY

M. hominis is susceptible to the tetracyclines, but quickly develops resistance. It responds to clindamycin, but is resistant to erythromycin. *U. urealyticum* can be treated with erythromycin.

Simple carriage of these organisms in the vagina does not warrant therapy.

SELECTED READING

Mycoplasmas and Infertility
Busolo F, Zanchetta R, Bertoloni G. Mycoplasmic localization patterns on spermatozoa from infertile men. Fertil Steril 1984; 42:412.
Cassell GH, Waites KB, Watson HL, et al. *Ureaplasma urealyticum* intrauterine infection: role in prematurity and disease in newborns. Clin Microbiol Rev 1993; 6:69.
Cassell GH, Younger JB, Brown MB, et al. Microbiologic study of infertile women at the time of diagnostic laparoscopy: association of *Ureaplasma urealyticum* with a defined subpopulation. N Engl J Med 1983; 308:502.
Eschenbach DA. *Ureaplasma urealyticum* respiratory disease in newborns. Clin Infect Dis 1993; 17(suppl 1):243s.
Gump DW, Gibson M, Ashikaya T. Lack of association between genital mycoplasmas and infertility. N Engl J Med 1984; 310:937.
Horne HW Jr, et al. The role of mycoplasma infection in human reproductive failure. Fertil Steril 1974; 25:380.
Horne HW Jr. Genital mycoplasma infections in infertile patients and their conceptuses. Ann NY Acad Sci 1988; 549:65.
Kundsin RB. Mycoplasma in genitourinary tract infection and reproductive failure. Prog Gynecol 1970; 5:275.
Miettinen A, Heinonen PK, Teisala k, et al. Serologic evidence for the role of *Chlamydia trachomatis*, *Neisseria gonorrhoeae*, and *Mycoplasma hominis* in the etiology of tubal factor infertility and ectopic pregnancy. Sex Transm Dis 1990; 17:10.
Rusolo F, Zanchetta R. The effect of *Mycoplasma hominis* and *Ureaplasma urealyticum* on hamster egg in vitro penetration by human spermatozoa. Fertil Steril 1985; 43:110.
Tredway DR, Wortham JWE, Condon-Mahony M, et al. Correlation of postcoital evaluation with in vitro sperm cervical mucus determinations and ureaplasma cultures. Fertil Steril 1985; 43:286.

Mycoplasmas in Gynecology
Falk L, Fredlund H, Jensen JS. Symptomatic urethritis is more prevalent in men infected with Mycoplasma genitalium than with Chlamydia trachomatis. Sex Transm Infect 2004; 80:289–293.
Ginsburg KS, Kundsin RB, Walter CW, Schur PH. *Ureaplasma urealyticum* and *Mycoplasma hominis* in women with systemic lupus erythematosus. Arthritis Rheum 1992; 35:429.
Glatt AE, McCormack WM, Taylor-Robinson D. Genital mycoplasma. In: Holmes KK, Marrdh PA, Spaulding PF, et al., eds. Sexually Transmitted Diseases. New York: McGraw-Hill, 1990:279.
Iwasaka T, Wada T, Kidera Y, Sugimori H. Hormonal status and mycoplasma colonization in the female genital tract. Obstet Gynecol 1986; 68:263.
Jensen JS, Bjornelius E, Dohn B, Lidbrink P. Comparison of first void urine and urogenital swab specimens for detection of Mycoplasma genitalium and Chlamydia trachomatis by polymerase chain reaction in patients attending a sexually transmitted disease clinic. Sex Transm Dis 2004; 31:499–507.
Osborne NG. Tubo-ovarian abscess: pathogenesis and management. J Natl Med Assoc 1986; 78:937.
Osborne NG, Grubin L, Pratson L. Vaginitis in sexually active women: relationship to nine sexually transmitted organisms. Am J Obstet Gynecol 1982; 142:962.
Rissi GF Jr, Sanders CV. The genital mycoplasmas. Obstet Gynecol Clin North Am 1989; 16:611.
Taylor-Robinson D, Gilroy CB, Thomas BJ, Hay PE. Mycoplasma genitalium in chronic gonococcal urethritis. Int J STD AIDS 2004; 15:21–25.
Taylor-Robinson D, McCormack WM. Medical progress: the genital mycoplasmas. N Engl J Med 1980; 302:1003, 1063.
Wikstrom A, Jensen JS. Mycoplasma genitalium: a common cause of persistent urethritis among men treated with doxycycline. Sex Trans Infect 2006; 82:276–279.

Mycoplasmas in Obstetrics

Braun P, Lee Y-H, Klein JO, et al. Birth weight and genital mycoplasmas in pregnancy. N Engl J Med 1971; 284:167.

Embree JE. *Mycoplasma hominis* in maternal and fetal infections. Ann NY Acad Sci 1988; 549:56.

Embree JE, Krause VW, Embil JA, et al. Placental infection with *Mycoplasma hominis* and *Ureaplasma urealyticum*: clinical correlation. Obstet Gynecol 1980; 56:475.

Foulon W, Naessens A, Dewaele M, et al. Chronic *U. urealyticum* amnionitis associated with abruptio placentae. Obstet Gynecol 1986; 68:280.

Harada K, Tanaka H, Tsuji Y, Koyama K. Analysis of the relationship between ureaplasmal infection and premature delivery. Amer J Reprod Immunol 2006; 55(6):398.

Harwick HJ, Iuppa JB, Purcell RH, et al. *Mycoplasma hominis* septicemia associated with abortion. Am J Obstet Gynecol 1967; 99:725.

Kass EH, McCormack WM, Lin J-S. Genital mycoplasmas as a cause of excess premature delivery. Trans Assoc Am Physicians 1981; 94:261.

Klein JO, Buckland D, Finland M. Colonization of newborn infants by mycoplasmas. N Engl J Med 1969; 280:1025.

Kundsin RB, Driscoll SG, Monson RR, et al. Association of *U. urealyticum* in the placenta with perinatal morbidity and mortality. N Engl J Med 1984; 310:941.

Lamey JR, Eschenbach DA, Mitchell SH, et al. Isolation of mycoplasmas and bacteria from the blood of postpartum women. Am J Obstet Gynecol 1982; 143:104.

Madan E, Meyers MP, Amortegui AJ. Histologic manifestations of perinatal genital mycoplasmal infection. Arch Pathol Lab Med 1989; 113:465.

Mardh PA, Lind I, Svensson L, et al. Antibodies to *Chlamydia trachomatis*, *Mycoplasma hominis*, and *Neisseria gonorrhoeae* in sera from patients with acute salpingitis. Br J Vener Dis 1981; 57:125.

McCormack WM, Rosney B, Lee Y-H, et al. Effect on birth weight of erythromycin treatment of pregnant women. Obstet Gynecol 1987; 69:202.

McDonald HM, O'Loughlin JA, Jolley P, et al. Prenatal microbiological risk factors associated with preterm birth. Br J Obstet Gynaecol 1992; 99:190.

Minkoff HL, Grunebaum AN, Schwarz RH, et al. Risk factors for prematurity and premature rupture of membranes: a prospective study of the vaginal flora in pregnancy. Am J Obstet Gynecol 1984; 150:965.

Naessens A, Foulon W, Breynaert J, Lauwers S. Postpartum bacteremia and placental colonization with genital mycoplasmas and pregnancy outcome. Am J Obstet Gynecol 1989; 160:647.

Platt R, Lin JS, Warren JW, et al. Infection with *Mycoplasma hominis* in postpartum fever. Lancet 1980; II:1217.

Romero R, Mazor M, Oyarzun E, et al. Is genital colonization with *Mycoplasma hominis* or *Ureaplasma urealyticum* associated with prematurity/low birth weight? Obstet Gynecol 1989; 73:532.

The Johns Hopkins Study of Cervicitis and Adverse Pregnancy Outcome. Association of *Chlamydia trachomatis* and *Mycoplasma hominis* with intrauterine growth retardation and preterm delivery. Am J Epidemiol 1989; 129:1247.

Watts DH, Eschenbach DA, Kenny GE. Early postpartum endometritis: the role of bacteria, genital mycoplasmas, and *Chlamydia trachomatis*. Obstet Gynecol 1989; 73:52.

Borrelia recurrentis (Relapsing Fever)

49

INTRODUCTION

Borrelia is a genus of spirochetes belonging to the Spirochaetaceae. Morphologically, the typical organism is composed of five to ten loosely wound, irregular coils measuring 10 to 35 μ in length and 0.3 to 0.5 μ in width. Although susceptible to desiccation and to many chemical agents, the organisms are able to survive in citrated blood for as long as three months at 2°C to 3°C. Disease caused by these spirochetes may be divided into two forms:

1. An epidemic form, in which the body louse, *Pediculus humanus corporis*, is usually the principal vector
2. An endemic form, in which infection is mostly transmitted through ticks of the *Ornithodoros* genus

Louse-borne relapsing fever is rare and occurs primarily by importation. Tick-borne disease usually occurs in the spring and summer, primarily in the western mountainous states in the United States. The clustering of cases is not unusual.

In the natural life cycle, arthropod infection is acquired when lice feed on a patient during an attack of relapsing fever. Only about 12% to 17% of lice feeding on patients experiencing an attack of relapsing fever transmit infection. A louse ingests up to 1 mg of blood during a single feed. This meal must contain at least one to two organisms per oil immersion field to be infective. The spirochetes enter the midgut of the louse, disappearing therefrom in about one day. A "negative phase" ensues in which borreliae are present as granules that can be distinguished only by fluorescent microscopy. After five to six days, short, corkscrew-like metacyclic forms appear in the coelomic cavity of the louse. Thereafter, the louse is infected for its lifetime.

Since the infection does not involve the parasite's salivary or coxal glands and the microorganisms are not found within the louse's gastrointestinal tract or feces, transmission of relapsing fever necessitates the crushing of the lice, permitting coelomic fluid containing borreliae to contaminate the site of the bite. It is believed that the organisms are capable of penetrating either very small abrasions or, if ingested, intact intestinal mucosa. No animal reservoir exists.

In contrast, the host–parasite relationship between *Borrelia* and its endemic arthropod vector, the tick, is far more sophisticated. Spirochetes persist in saliva, coxal gland fluid, and feces, thus facilitating human infection independent of being crushed into the bite lesion. Ticks, in feeding, not only permit saliva to reach open capillary beds, but toward the end of the meal, they also evacuate the contents of the gut as well as excreting coxal fluid. A single spirochete is sufficient to initiate disease. Unlike other tick-borne diseases such as Lyme disease, inoculation of *Borrelia* organisms occurs within minutes of fever.

Regardless of the mode of transmission, *Borrelia* organisms invade the endothelium and produce an initial low-grade disseminated intravascular coagulopathy and thrombocytopenia. The relapse phenomenon occurs because of programmed shifting of outer surface proteins that allows a new clone to circumvent the now established host defense mechanisms. Tick-borne disease tends to have more relapses compared with louse-borne disease.

Relapsing fever develops abruptly 3 to 18 days after organism acquisition. Myalgias and chills occur in approximately 90% of cases. Headache is even more common. The pulse rate is rapid in proportion to the fever.

Spirochetemia that persists for several weeks ultimately results in metastatic infection of the central nervous system, eyes, and visceral organs. *Borrelia burgdorferi* is able to achieve prolongation of its phase of spirochetemia by multiphasic antigenic variation.

Louse-borne disease is usually associated with conditions of overcrowding, poor housing, malnutrition, and lack of sanitation, circumstances that may attend prolonged disaster. On the other hand, tick-borne *Borrelia* infections most often reflect disease in individuals who are newly arrived within an endemic setting.

Although tick- and louse-borne diseases induce the same syndrome in humans, variations exist in incubation periods, in severity of clinical manifestations, and in recurrences of febrile episodes. In general, louse-borne relapsing fever has a longer incubation period (9–14 days) tick-borne *Borrelia* infection. In both forms of *Borrelia* infection, disease is heralded by chills, fever, nausea, vomiting, myalgia, arthralgia, and photophobia. Patients frequently complain of nausea, vomiting, and upper abdominal pain due to liver and spleen involvement. In malnourished populations, mortality rates of 30% to 70% have been reported in untreated patients during epidemics of louse-borne disease. With therapy, the mortality rate falls to 5%. The mortality rate for patents with tick-borne relapsing fever who are treated is less than 1%.

The temperature may reach 42°C to 43°C and is almost always significantly elevated. In the louse-borne variant, the first episode of unremitting fever lasts three to six days and is followed by a single, less-severe episode. Tick-borne relapsing fever is characterized by multiple temperature spikes of one to three days. The interval between febrile periods ranges from 4 to 14 days.

Tracheobronchitis, meningeal involvement, erythematous macular rashes, and petechiae are not uncommon, particularly with louse-borne *Borrelia*. With tick-borne borreliae, severe ophthalmologic and neurologic involvement is characteristic. These manifestations may appear late in the disease and leave permanent sequelae.

The first febrile episode terminates in crisis in which the patient exhibits hyperthermia, shaking chills, and hypertension. The crisis is followed by profuse diaphoresis and hypotension. Maternal and fetal death most commonly occur during the crisis or shortly thereafter.

Relapses are contingent on the selection and replication of antigenic variants of the original *Borrelia* strain. Each relapse clinically emulates the preceding episodes, only in a more attenuated form. The pyrexial attacks become shorter and the intercalary periods longer.

For untreated relapsing fever, the eventual eradication of the organisms is contingent on the synthesis of lysins and immobilizins with a sufficiently broad antigenic spectrum to cover all significant antigenic variants.

Therapy per se introduces an added risk factor. Up to 90% of patients with louse-borne relapsing fever and 40% of those with tick-borne relapsing fever experience a Jarisch-Herxheimer reaction. Within one to two hours, the patient experiences intense shaking chills, elevation of an already elevated temperature, and apprehensiveness. In a minority of patients, the reaction is life threatening.

FEMALE GENITAL TRACT INVOLVEMENT

Pregnant women are at a higher risk of more severe disease and adverse pregnancy outcomes.

Acute infection with either form of relapsing fever may result in adverse effects on the conceptus. Abortion is not an infrequent consequence of an acute attack during gestation. Although most cases are probably secondary to the maternal response to systemic illness, a number of late abortions may be due to direct involvement of the products of conception. It has been clearly demonstrated that, as with *Treponema pallidum*, congenital infection occurs. Whether or not transplacental transmission occurs is not contingent on the severity of maternal infection. Attenuated maternal disease does not preclude fetal involvement. The diagnosis of congenital infection necessitates both the onset of neonatal disease prior to the third day of life and demonstration of spirochetes in peripheral blood smears. Hyperbilirubinemia and evidence of meningoencephalitis predominate. In necropsy material, the principal pathologic findings involve the central nervous system and the spleen. The meninges are thickened due to predominantly mononuclear cell infiltration. Scattered neutrophils are present in areas of cellular necrobiosis. Macroscopically, the cut surface of the spleen usually reveals scattered yellow miliary lesions that, on histologic examination, are seen to be composed of focal areas of coagulative necrosis. Touch preparations of spleen or meninges, stained with Giemsa's or Wright's stain, or silver impregnation stains of fixed tissue reveal spirochetes with large irregular spirals characteristic of the *Borrelia* genus.

DIAGNOSIS

Definite diagnosis of *Borrelia* is made by demonstration of spirochetes in blood, cerebral spinal fluid, or tissues. Blood samples for diagnostic analysis should be obtained with the onset of fever and before its zenith. Once the temperature is declining uninfluenced by antipyretics, visual detection of spirochetes in blood is markedly diminished. Thin and thick smears of blood need to be obtained. Direct identification of spirochetes in blood correlates with approximately 100,000 organisms/mL of blood. Centrifugation of the blood and examination of the buffy coat and overlying plasma increase the sensitivity of direct microscopy. Spirochetes are found in the same fraction as are platelets.

When the diagnosis of relapsing fever is strongly suspected but the spirochetes have not been directly visualized, inoculation of blood into weanling mice can demonstrate the presence of a *Borrelia* species. Stain smears of tail blood are examined for spirochetes one to four days later. In vitro culturing of blood on selected media is an alternative to animal inoculation. These latter techniques are applicable in the latter phase of a febrile episode or between fever spikes.

Borrelia can be stained with most aniline or acid dyes. Dehemoglobinization of slides with 6% acetic acid and 95% ethyl alcohol for five seconds, followed by staining with carbol fuchsin for one minute, provides a simple procedure applicable to both thin and thick smears.

An alternative method for demonstrating the organism is prolonged (10–12 hours) staining of ethyl alcohol–fixed smears with Wright's stain followed by the application of 1% crystal violet solution for 10 to 30 seconds.

Serological tests can provide indirect evidence of infection. Because of antigenic variability, these tests are not highly specific. Enzyme-linked immunoabsorbent assay (ELISA) or indirect fluorescent antibody tests are of value when acute and convalescent maternal sera are available. For ELISA results to be considered diagnostic, the Western blot assay for Lyme disease and reagin-based and treponema-specific assays for syphilis should be negative. A polymerase chain reaction test can detect *Borrelia* species antigen in blood, cerebrospinal fluid, and tissues.

THERAPY

Although erythromycin, tetracyclines, doxycycline, and chloramphenicol are all effective oral medications, penicillin and tetracyclines constitute the parental drugs of choice for relapsing fever. The minimal inhibitory concentrations of these antibiotics for *Borrelia* species tends to be less than 0.1 mg/mL. *Borrelia* species are also susceptible to cephalosporins, chloramphenicol, other macrolides, and vancomycin. In the nulligravid female, the tetracyclines constitute the drug of choice (Table 1). Both tetracyclines and chloramphenicol are contraindicated in pregnancy.

The effectiveness of antibiotic therapy can be monitored by the clearance of spirochetes from the blood. Within eight hours following the administration of an effective antibiotic, spirochetes are no longer demonstrable in the blood. The current recommendation is seven days of antibiotic therapy.

Drugs that immobilize or destroy borreliae may give rise to a Jarisch-Herxheimer–like reaction, similar to that observed with *T. pallidum*. Because of a high probability of a Jarisch-Herxheimer reaction, initial therapy should be

TABLE I   Parental antibiotic regimens in the treatment of acute infection with *Borrelia*

	Febrile phase
Penicillin	Procaine penicillin G (800,000 units; route of administration: IM/single dose) for 7 days *or* 600,000 units IU IV once a day for 7 days
Tetracycline	250 mg IV followed by 250 mg every 6 hr for 7 days *or* 500 mg every 12 hr for 7 days
Erythromycin stearate/base	500 mg IV every 6 hr for 7 days
Doxycycline	200 mg PO/IV followed by 100 mg bid for 6 days
Alternate beta-lactam antibiotic	Ceftriaxone 1 g bid; oral/10 days

Source: Adapted from Harrison's Principles of Internal Medicine. 16th ed. 2004:994, as cited by the Centers for Disease Control and Prevention.

done in a controlled environment. A central venous line should be in place as well as a means of increasing oxygenation and controlling hyperthermia. Core body temperature can be reduced with tepid water, sponge baths, and/or acetaminophen.

Attempts have been made to decrease the incidence of the Jarisch-Herxheimer reaction by reducing the cytokine response. Fekade et al. (1996) intravenously administered antitumor necrosis factor-alpha antibodies to patients with louse-borne relapsing fever immediately before intramuscular injection of penicillin. They were able to reduce the incidence of a reaction by almost 50%. For pregnant women, a comparable reduction can be achieved by initiating parental therapy with a dose of erythromycin which is then followed several hours later by parenteral penicillin.

PREVENTION

Personal hygiene and reduction of crowding greatly decrease the potential for louse-borne disease. Once an infestation is identified, delousing of patients and household becomes essential.

When tick exposure occurs on an occasional basis, prophylaxis with tetracycline 500 mg orally qid for two to three days will reduce the risk of infection if taken within two days of exposure.

Antimicrobial drugs can be utilized prophylactically in epidemics. However, the key to prevention of louse-borne relapsing fever is the reinforcement of those conditions destructive to lice, notably regular personal hygiene, cleanliness, and disinfection of louse-infested clothing.

SELECTED READING

Barbour A. Antigenic variation of a relapsing fever *Borrelia* species. Ann Rev Microbiol 1990; 44:155.

Barbour AG. Linear DNA of *Borrelia* spp. and antigenic variation. Trends Microbiol 1994; 1:236.

Borgnolo G, Haliu B, Ciancarelli A, et al. Louse-borne relapsing fever. A clinical and an epidemiological study of 389 patients in Asella Hospital, Ethiopia. Trop Geogr Med 1993; 45:66.

Caldwell HG. A case of congenital relapsing fever. E Afr Med J 1936; 12:347.

Correa P, Baylet RJ, Bourgoin P. A propos d'un cas de fievre recurrente a *Borrelia duttoni* chez un noveau-ne l'infection par voie transplacentaire parait peu contestable. Bull Soc Med Afr Noire Lang Fr 1964; 9:215.

Dworkin MS, Schwan TG, Anderson DE Jr. Tick-borne relapsing fever in North America. Med Clin North Am 2002; 86:417.

Felsenfeld O. Borreliae, human relapsing fever, and parasite- vector-host relationships. Bacteriol Rev 1965; 29:46.

Fekade D, Knox K, Hassein K, et al. Prevention of Jarisch-Herxheimer reactions by treatment with antibodies against tumor necrosis factor alpha. N Engl J Med 1996; 335:311.

Fuchs PC, Oyama AA. Neonatal relapsing fever due to transplacental transmission of *Borrelia*. J Am Med Assoc 1969; 208:690.

Hasin T, Davidovitch N, Cohen R, et al. Postexposure treatment with doxycycline for the prevention of tick-borne relapsing fever. N Engl J Med 2006; 355:148.

MacDonald AB. Human fetal borreliosis, toxemia of pregnancy, and fetal death. Zentralbl Bakteriol Mikrobiol Hyg 1986; 263:189.

Montanes MRL. Fievre recurrente congenital. Rev Esp Pediat 1949; 5:1.

Morrison SK, Parsons L. Relapsing fever: report of three cases, one in a 6-day-old infant. J Am Med Assoc 1941; 116:220.

Negussie Y, Remick D, DeForge L, et al. Detection of plasma tumor necrosis factor, interleukins 6 and 8 during the Jarisch-Herxheimer reaction of relapsing fever. J Exp Med 1992; 175:1207.

Paul WS, Maupin G, Scott-Wright AO, et al. Outbreak of tick-borne relapsing fever at the north rim of the Grand canyon: evidence for effectiveness of preventive measures. Am J Trop Med Hyg 2002; 66:71.

Ras NM, Lascola B, Postic D, et al. Phylogenesis of relapsing fever *Borrelia* spp. Int J Syst Bacteriol 1996; 46:859.

Thorstein G. Relapsing fevers. In: Beeson PB, McDermott W, eds. Cecil-Loeb Textbook of Medicine, 13th ed. Philadelphia: WB Saunders, 1971:675.

Wang CW, Lee CU. Malaria and relapsing fever following blood transfusion, including the report of a case of congenital transmission of relapsing fever. Chin Med J 1936; 50:241.

INTRODUCTION

Lyme disease, first described in 1977, is initially characterized by a distinctive skin lesion, erythema chronicum migrans (ECM), which starts as a red macule at the site of a tick bite and expands to become an annular erythema with central clearing. Late Lyme disease is a multisystem disorder that is characterized in various stages by dermatologic, neurologic, cardiac, and rheumatic manifestations.

Borrelia burgdorferi is the cause of this disorder. Ticks are the best documented vectors of the spirochete. *B. burgdorferi* has been isolated from *Ixodesscapularis* and *Ixodes pacificus*. Lyme disease is now the most commonly reported tick-borne illness in the United States. Infection of greater than 20% of ticks with *B. burgdorferi* generally occurs in parts of New England, the Mid-Atlantic sates, Minnesota, and Wisconsin, but not in most other locations in the United States.

CLINICAL MANIFESTATIONS

Early cases of Lyme disease are characterized by the presence or the history of the skin lesion (ECM). This lesion is the earliest and most specific observable manifestation of the disorder. ECM that occurs within approximately 30 days after exposure in an endemic area is virtually diagnostic of Lyme disease. If no exposure to ticks is recognized, ECM followed by other neurologic, cardiac, or joint involvement suggests the diagnosis. Other cases that occur within the endemic areas may be suspected because of typical organ involvement, despite the absence of ECM and the lack of recognized exposure to ticks. Of all the patients with Lyme disease in Connecticut, 83% of the patients studied had erythema migrans; 24% had arthritis; 8% had neurologic manifestations; and 2% had cardiac involvement. For those with arthritis, affected joints were the knee (89%), hip (9%), shoulder (9%), ankle (7%), and elbow (2%). Persons under 20 years of age were 1.6 times more likely to have arthritis than persons over 20 (7/100,000 compared with 4/100,000), while both groups were equally likely to develop ECM (13/100,000). Seventy-nine percent of patients with arthritis did not report antecedent erythema migrans.

The clinical manifestations of Lyme disease occur in stages that roughly parallel their chronologic appearance. Stage 1 is characterized by ECM and nonspecific influenza-like symptoms that occur 3 to 32 days after exposure to ticks. ECM itself begins as an erythematous papule or macule, which gradually becomes an annular lesion that can be many centimeters wide. Some lesions are less distinctive. Secondary lesions may occur at a distance from the original tick bite. Stage 2 often occurs weeks to months after stage 1. Neurologic or cardiac abnormalities develop in 15% and 8% of cases, respectively. Patients may have signs of meningitis, encephalitis, cranial neuritis, motor or sensory radiculoneuritis, and possibly myelitis. Either tachycardia or bradycardia may occur, in association with variable degrees of atrioventricular nodal block. Rarely is there evidence of pericarditis or myocarditis. Stage 3, typified by arthritis, occurs in about 60% of cases. Synovitis may first be manifested weeks to years after ECM. Characteristically, the synovitis affects the knees, but other large joints may be involved as well.

At each stage, symptoms and signs frequently wax and wane. Some symptoms are self-limited regardless of therapy.

LYME DISEASE IN PREGNANCY

Transplacental transmission of the vector, *B. burgdorferi*, has been documented: the patient, a pregnant woman with Lyme disease who did not receive antimicrobial therapy, delivered an infant with a congenital heart defect. More cases are likely to be reported that will delineate the organism's potential for an adverse impact on the developing fetus.

DIAGNOSIS

The diagnosis of early Lyme disease remains primarily clinical. The Centers for Disease Control and Prevention's original case definition is presented in Table 1.

The erythrocyte sedimentation rate is often mildly elevated. Likewise, the serum concentration of immunoglobulin M (IgM) may be elevated, and IgM- or IgG-containing cryoglobulins may be detected. The patient may have lymphopenia. Serum transaminase activity may be increased if mild hepatic involvement is present.

During the later stages of Lyme disease, characteristic changes occur in the cerebrospinal fluid. None of these abnormalities, however, is diagnostic.

Serologic studies have been developed for measuring the antibody response to the infecting spirochete. These tests include the indirect immunofluorescence assay (IFA) and enzyme-linked immunosorbent assay (ELISA). The IFA for the Lyme disease spirochete is analogous to the fluorescent treponemal antibody assay for detection of antibodies to *Treponema pallidum*. *B. burgdorferi* spirochetes from a known source are fixed to a microscope slide. The patient's serum is incubated on the slide. The slide is washed, overlayered with fluorescent antihuman immunoglobulin, and washed again. Then it is examined by fluorescence microscopy. If the patient's serum contains antibody to the spirochete, the latter will fluoresce. The ELISA for Lyme disease uses an extract of the *B. burgdorferi* spirochete. The extract is bound in an assay-well to which the patient's serum is added. After a brief incubation, the well is washed, and alkaline phosphatase conjugated with antihuman immunoglobulin is added. It is washed again to remove unbound immunoglobulin, and any antibody from the patient's serum that specifically binds is detected by a colorimetric assay for alkaline phosphatase activity.

Physicians should be aware of the marked limitations of current tests. Sensitivities of the IFA and the ELISA are relatively low during stage 1, and the antibody response can be curtailed or aborted by early treatment with antibiotics. In contrast, some research laboratories have reported sensitivities >95% for tests of patients with stage 2 or 3 Lyme disease. False-positive results have been reported in Lyme disease assays. Serum samples from patients with treponemal diseases, including syphilis, yaws, and pinta, have considerable cross-reactivity in the tests for antibody to *B. burgdorferi*.

Serologic tests, when positive, can help support the clinical suspicion of Lyme disease in atypical late cases, such as those without ECM or those occurring outside recognized endemic areas. However, serologic tests are often negative, particularly early in Lyme disease. Therefore, a negative result does not exclude the diagnosis early in the course of the illness.

THERAPY

Because antimicrobial therapy decreases the morbidity from Lyme disease, it is important that cases be recognized early and patients treated.

If a patient presents with an attached tick which, based upon the degree of its engorgement, has been attached less than 36 hours or if less than 72 hours have elapsed from when the tick was removed, the 2006 Infectious Disease Society of America recommends the administration of a single dose of doxycycline be offered to nonpregnant women in these circumstances. The time limit of 72 hours is suggested because of the absence of data on the efficacy of chemoprophylaxis for tick bites following tick removal after longer time intervals. Doxycycline is relatively contraindicated in pregnant or lactating women.

If a portion of the tick's mouth remains embedded in the skin after removal with fine-tip forceps, topical disinfection is recommended.

Persons who have had attached ticks removed should be closely monitored for signs or symptoms of tick-borne disease for up to 30 days. Development of a skin lesion or a viral infection–like illness within one month after tick removal need to have Lyme disease ruled in or out.

For adults with erythema migrans and local or early disseminated Lyme disease, doxycycline (100 mg twice a day for 14–21 days), amoxicillin (500 mg three times a day for 10–21 days), or cefuroxime axetil (500 mg twice a day for 10–21 days) is recommended.

Macrolide antibiotics (azithromycin 500 mg orally daily for 7–10 days; clarithromycin 500 mg orally twice a day; or erythromycin 500 mg orally four times a day) are not recommended as first-line therapy for early Lyme disease. They are reserved for patients who should not take amoxicillin, cefuroxime, or doxycycline. First-line cephalosporins are ineffective for the treatment of Lyme disease and should not be used.

For patients with Lyme meningitis or other manifestations of neurologic disease, ceftriaxone (2 g once a day intravenously for 10–28 days) is recommended. Parenteral therapy with cefotaxime (2 g intravenously every eight hours) or penicillin G (200,000–40,000 units/kg/day, 18–24 million units maximum, for patients with normal renal function, divided into doses given every four hours) may be a satisfactory alternative.

Pregnant and lactating women may be treated similarly to nonpregnant patients with the same disease manifestations, except that doxycycline should be avoided.

PREVENTION

The best currently available method to prevent infection with *B. burgdorferi* is to avoid tick-infested areas. If exposure is unavoidable, using protective clothing (long-sleeved shirts tucked into pants and long pants tucked into socks) increases the time required for ticks to find exposed skin. Wearing light-colored clothing makes it easier to identify ticks on clothing. Tick repellents containing *N,N*-diethyl-3-methylbenzamide applied to skin or clothing provide additional protection.

SELECTED READING

Benach JL, Bosler EM, Hanrahan JP, et al. Spirochetes isolated from the blood of two patients with Lyme disease. N Engl J Med 1983; 308:740–742.

Centers for Disease Control and Prevention. Lyme disease surveillance—United States, 1898–1990. MMWR 1991; 40:417.

Ciesielski CA, Markowitz LE, Horsley R, et al. Lyme disease surveillance in the United States, 1983–1986. Rev Infect Dis 1989; 11:S1435.

Eichenfield AH. Diagnosis and management of Lyme disease. Pediatr Ann 1986; 15:583–587.

Johnson RC, Schmid GP, Hyde FW, et al. *Borrelia burgdorferi* sp. nov.: etiologic agent of Lyme disease. Int J Syst Bacteriol 1984; 34:496–497.

Johnston YE, Duray PH, Steere AC, et al. Lyme arthritis: spirochetes found in synovial microangiopathic lesions. Am J Pathol 1985; 118:26–34.

IDSA Guidelines. The clinical assessment, treatment, and prevention of Lyme disease, human granulocytic anaplasmosis and babesiosis: clinical practice guidelines by the Infectious Disease Society of America. Clin Infect Dis 2006; 43:1089–1134.

Markowitz LE, Steere AC, Benach JL, et al. Lyme disease during pregnancy. J Am Med Assoc 1986; 255:3394.

Russell H, Sampson JS, Schmid GP, et al. Enzyme-linked immunosorbent assay and indirect immunofluorescence assay for Lyme disease. J Infect Dis 1984; 149:465–470.

Schlesinger PA, Duray PH, Burke BA, et al. Maternal-fetal transmission of the Lyme disease spirochete, *Borrelia burgdorferi*. Ann Intern Med 1985; 103:67.

Shrestha M, Grodzicki RL, Steere AC. Diagnosing early Lyme disease. Am J Med 1985; 78:235–240.

Steere AC, Grodzicki RL, Kornblatt AN, et al. The spirochetal etiology of Lyme disease. N Engl J Med 1983; 308:733–740.

Steere AC, Hutchinson GJ, Rahn DW, et al. Treatment of the early manifestations of Lyme disease. Ann Intern Med 1983; 99:22–26.

Steere AC, Malawista SE, Bartenhagen NH, et al. The clinical spectrum and treatment of Lyme disease. Yale J Biol Med 1984; 57:453–461.

Steere AC, Pachner AR, Malawista SE. Neurologic abnormalities of Lyme disease: successful treatment with high-dose intravenous penicillin. Ann Intern Med 1983; 99:767–772.

Update. Lyme disease—United States. MMWR 1984; 33:268–270.

Wharton M, Chorba TL, Vogt RL, et al. Case definitions for public health surveillance. MMWR 1990; 39:19.

Wilkinson HW. Immunodiagnostic tests for Lyme disease. Yale J Biol Med 1984; 57:567–562.

Leptospira

INTRODUCTION

Leptospira organisms are slender, round, active, and mobile spirochetes with one or both ends bent in the form of a hook. They are generally between 5 and 15 μm long and, unlike *Treponema pallidum*, they are readily cultured on relatively simple bacteriologic media. Virtually all of the pathogenic leptospires are represented in the *L. interrogans* group. Although there are over 100 serotypes of *L. interrogans*, the great majority of infections in humans are from the following serotypes: *L. icterohaemorrhagiae, L. canicola, L. grippotyphosa, L. pomona, L. hebdomidis, L. mitis, L. bovis, L. autumnalis,* and *L. kasman*.

Leptospirosis is an infection of worldwide distribution. In the United States, the disease is observed within certain occupations that involve contact with animals or as a consequence of recreational activities such as hiking, swimming, canoeing, etc.

Leptospiral infection is common among many wild and domestic animals including rodents, livestock, wild mammals, dogs, and cats. Human infection occurs either through direct contact with an infected animal or indirectly through contact with water or soil contaminated by the urine of infected animals (Fig. 1). The spirochetes can survive in untreated water for months. Person-to-person contact is at best rare.

Leptospirosis is endemic in the tropics. *Leptospira* proliferate in fresh water, damp soil, vegetation, and mud. The occurrence of flooding after heavy rainfall facilitates the spread of the organism because, as water saturates the environment, *Leptospira* present in the soil pass directly into surface waters.

Leptospires are thought to enter the host through abrasions in healthy skin or directly through intact mucosal membranes.

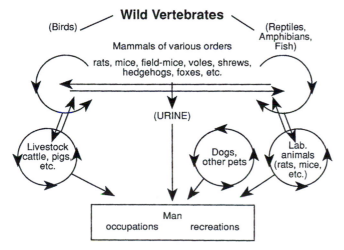

FIGURE 1 Relationships of the principal reservoir hosts of *Leptospira. Source:* From Turner (1967).

The incubation period is said to vary from 7 to 12 days (range 2–20 days). This variation in the incubation period is in part a function of the inoculum size and host defense mechanisms. Leptospires are thought to multiply in small-blood-vessel endothelium, resulting in vasculitis. Intravascular leptospiral replication results in a prolonged leptospiremia, with widespread dissemination of the spirochetes through the body. There is a tendency for preferential localization within kidneys, adrenals, liver, meninges, and lungs.

In the United States, clinically recognized illness exhibits a seasonal pattern in which the majority of cases occur in the months of July through October. The ensuing pattern of infection can be subdivided into two distinct phases, the first characterized by leptospiremia and the second by leptospiruria, which is associated with the development of immunity.

Only a minority of patients for whom occupational data were available had apparent job-related illness. Most individuals acquire their infection when engaged in nonvocational activities. The most probable sources of infection were surface water (ponds, creeks, or sewage systems), which accounted for 29%, dogs (22%), rodents (11%), and cattle or swine (8%).

The phase of leptospiremia is characterized by clinical manifestations of an acute systemic infection that persists for seven to eight days. Two distinct clinical presentations occur.

(i) *Anicteric leptospirosis:* The vast majority of patients present with a mild anicteric febrile illness. The septicemic phase of disease manifests with the abrupt onset of high fever and rigors. Myalgia, commonly involving the calf muscles, occurs as do headache, abdominal pain, nausea, vomiting, and diarrhea. Conjunctival suffusion is prominent. The septicemic phase is followed by one to three days without fever and then progresses to 4 to 30 days of the delayed phase of the illness.

At the time of onset, clinically predicting if a mild or severe form of the disease will ensue is not possible.

(ii) *Icteric leptospirosis:* Approximately 5% to 10% of infected individuals develop full-blown Weil's syndrome, with jaundice, fever, rigors, severe myalgias, severe conjunctivitis, diarrhea, and skin rashes. Manifestations of more severe disease may include renal failure, pulmonary hemorrhage, and hemodynamic collapse. The spirochetes are initially demonstrable within the blood and cerebrospinal fluid (CSF). This phase of the disease leads either to death or to defervescence and symptomatic improvement during the immune phase of disease (10–30 days).

Localization within renal tubules can produce an interstitial nephritis with tubular necrosis and impaired capillary permeability terminating in renal failure. If properly supported with dialysis, normal renal function is ultimately restored.

In the immune phase, the leptospires are no longer demonstrable in either blood or CSF. Because of the multiplicity of potentially involved organ systems, a wide spectrum of clinical signs and symptoms may be elicited. Characteristic is the marked prostration, which tends to override other clinical signs. Engorgement of the small conjunctival vessels is very common. Jaundice may occur while the patient is febrile and in a period of clinical deterioration. The anticipated case fatality is of the order of 2% to 4%.

With the appearance of specific antibodies, leptospiral organisms are removed from blood and tissues by phagocytosis. The one exception to this appears to be the kidney, where organismal replication within the renal medulla persists, resulting in prolonged shedding of the organisms, first into the urine and then into the extracorporeal environment. This carrier–shedder convalescent phase persists for one or two months.

Fever and earlier symptoms may reoccur in some patients. These patients are prone to exhibit signs of central nervous system involvement, such as headaches, photophobia, and nuchal rigidity. Complications such as optic neuritis, uveitis, iridocyclitis, chorioretinitis, and peripheral neuropathy may occur during the phase of leptospiruria.

INVOLVEMENT OF THE PRODUCTS OF CONCEPTION/FETUS

It is not uncommon for a gravida to abort during leptospiremia. The high rate of abortion and miscarriages in certain rice-growing areas of China where leptospirosis is an occupational hazard is frequently cited in the literature. Chang (1973) has demonstrated that intrauterine infection of the human fetus can occur. He isolated leptospires from the liver and kidney of a five-month abortus of a patient suffering from leptospirosis due to serotype *L. kasman*.

Lindsay and Luke (1949) reported a fatal case of leptospirosis occurring within hours of parturition, presumably due to intrauterine infection. Histologic analyses revealed extensive hepatocellular necrosis with relative sparing of the periportal areas. Sections of the kidneys demonstrated extensive tubular epithelial cell degeneration involving particularly the proximal and distal convoluted tubules. Leptospires were demonstrated in both organs. Of note was the fact that the maternal illness was subclinical. Apparently, attenuation of maternal infection did not impair the ability of the organism to traverse the placental barrier.

The diagnosis of congenital disease necessitates the presence of illness at birth or within the first 48 hours. Although congenital infection occurs, it is probable that the bulk of fetal wastage observed is secondary to maternal disease and not fetal involvement per se.

DIAGNOSIS

Laboratory studies are used for two purposes: (*i*) to establish the diagnosis of leptospirosis and (*ii*) to determine the extent of organ involvement.

A definitive diagnosis of leptospirosis is contingent upon laboratory identification of the spirochete. The laboratory criteria for leptospirosis are: (*i*) isolation of *Leptospira* from a clinical specimen, (*ii*) fourfold or greater increase in serological titer between acute and convalescent serum obtained at least two weeks apart and run in the same test, and/or (*iii*) demonstration of *Leptospira* in tissue specimens by immunohistochemistry or immunofluorescence.

During leptospiremia, the organisms may be demonstrated by dark-field microscopic analysis of blood samples (including the clot) and the CSF within the first 7 to 10 days of the illness. Thin and thick blood smears should be obtained before meals to avoid lipemic samples.

Isolation can be achieved using weanling mice or special semisolid, protein-supplemented media such as Fletcher, Stuart, or polysorbate 80–albumin media. Blood, CSF, and tissues provide the highest yields in the first two weeks of illness. Thereafter, urine becomes the testing specimen of choice.

Even in the hands of the experienced worker, dark-field microscopy results in failure or misdiagnosis so frequently that it should never be used as the sole diagnostic test.

The microscopic antileptospiral agglutination test is the most commonly used immunologic method for the detection of specific antibodies. Testing requires acute and convalescent sera obtained at least two weeks apart. Other tests include enzyme-linked immunosorbent assays, immunofluorescent antibody test, and indirect hemagglutination test. The Centers for Disease Control and Prevention can be requested to perform a microscopic agglutination test (MAT) using 23 leptospire antigens. A single MAT titer of 1:800 or identification of spirochetes in urine on dark-field microscopy, when accompanied by the appropriate clinical scenario, is highly suggestive of the diagnosis.

Fluorescein-labeled antileptospiral globulins afford a means of establishing a definitive diagnosis for organisms identified in tissue, blood, urine, or bacteriologic cultures. The only limiting factor is the relatively narrow range of serotypes encompassed.

A potential, but rarely used, ancillary procedure is biopsy of the patient's gastrocnemius muscle during the acute phase of illness. The spirochetes can occasionally be demonstrated by use of the Levaditi staining method. Muscle necrosis and a mononuclear cell infiltration associated with perivascular cuffing may aid in suggesting the diagnosis.

THERAPY

Penicillin is the antibiotic of choice (Table 1). The dosage depends on the duration of the illness, its severity, and the general condition of the patient.

In the nonpregnant patient, doxycycline 100 mg twice a day for seven days constitutes an alternate effective therapy.

As with any of the treponemal diseases, antibiotic therapy may result in the production of a Jarisch-Herxheimer reaction, resulting in a sharp rise in temperature, hypotension, and precipitation and aggravation of the prevalent signs and symptoms. The probability of such a reaction can be diminished by using either a tetracycline or an erythromycin as the initial dose, prior to instituting intravenous penicillin therapy. When possible, the initial antibiotic dose should be given by

TABLE I Advocated antibiotic regimens in the treatment of severe infection with *Leptospira*

Drug	Dosage	Duration of therapy (days)
Penicillin[a]	2.4 to 3.6 million units IV in divided doses (probenecid can increase the effects of penicillin)	7
Doxycycline[b]	100 mg bid	7

[b]The use of doxycycline is contraindicated in pregnancy.
[a]In pregnant patients allergic to penicillin, erythromycin 500 mg IV q6 h can be used initially and then switched to 500 mg orally qid.

the intravenous route using either a central line catheter or multiple intravenous lines in place. Facilities to increase blood oxygenation, combat hypotension, and counter hyperthermia should be available.

The earlier the treatment is started, the more likely it is that complications and existing symptoms will be modified. Specific impairment of hepatic and renal function requires individualization of therapy. Analgesics and hot compresses are effective in relieving the myalgia and arthralgia so common during leptospiremia.

Supportive therapy is indicated for treating dehydration, hypotension, hemorrhage, and renal failure.

Care needs to be given to antibiotic dosing. With the icteric variant of leptospirosis, either renal or hepatic failure may necessitate dosing adjustments.

Oral doxycycline (200 mg weekly) may provide effective chemoprophylaxis for persons with short-term exposure in environments associated with increased risk for infection.

Nonpregnant women with known exposure can be treated with doxycycline 100 mg daily for seven days. Persons participating in recreational water activities in areas where leptospirosis is endemic may be at increased risk for the disease, particularly during periods of flooding, and should consider preventive measures such as wearing protective clothing, minimizing contact with potentially contaminated water, and disinfection of contaminated work area.

SELECTED READING

Ashe WF, Pratt-Thomas HR, Kumper CW. Weil's disease. Medicine 1941; 20:145.

CDC. Leptospirosis—United States. MMWR 1995; 44:841.

CDC. Outbreak of acute febrile illness and pulmonary hemorrhage—Nicaragua. MMWR 1977; 26:21.

CDC. Outbreak of leptospirosis among white-water rafters. MMWR 1997; 46:577.

CDC. Brief report: leptospirosis after flooding of a university campus-hawaii 2004. MMWR 2006; 55:125.

Chang RS. Leptospirosis. In: Hoeprich PD, ed. Infectious Diseases. Hagerstown: Harper & Row, 1973:654.

Doudier B, Garcia S, Quennee V. Prognostic factors associated with severe leptospirosis. Clin Microbiol Infect 2006; 12:299.

Everard JD. Leptospirosis. In: Cox FEC, ed. Illustrated History of Tropical Diseases. London: Welcome Trust, 1996:110.

Farr RW, Leptospirosis. Clin Infect Dis 1995; 21:1.

Farrar WE. *Leptospira* species (Leptospirosis). In: Mandell GL, Bennett JE, Dolin R, eds. Principles and Practice of Infectious Diseases. 4th ed. New York: Churchill Livingstone, 1995.

Felsenfeld O. Borrelias, human relapsing fever and parasite-vector-host relationships. Bacteriol Rev 1965; 29:46.

Galton MM. Methods in the laboratory diagnosis of leptospirosis. Ann NY Acad Sci 1962; 98:675.

Galton MM, Menges RW, Shotts EB, et al. Leptospirosis epidemiology, clinical manifestations in man and animals, and methods in laboratory diagnosis. U.S. Dept of Health, Education and Welfare, Public Health, Service Publication No. 951, 1962.

Heath CM Jr, Alexander AD, Galton MM. Leptospirosis in the United States. N Engl J Med 1965; 273:857, 915.

McClain JB, Ballou WR, Harrison SM. Doxycycline therapy for leptospirosis. Ann Intern Med 1984; 100:696.

Moore GE, Guptill LF, Glickman NW. Canine leptospirosis, United States, 2002–2004. Emerg Infect Dis 2006; 12:501.

Palmer MF, Waitkins SA, Wanyangu SW. A comparison of live and formized leptospiral microscopic agglutination test. Int Med Microbiol Virol Parasitol Infect Dis 1987; 265:151.

Turner LH. Leptospirosis. I. Trans R Soc Trop Med Hyg 1967; 61:842.

Turner LH. Leptospirosis. II. Serology. Trans R Soc Trop Med Hyg 1968; 62:880.

Turner LH. Leptospirosis. Br Med J 1969; 1:231.

van Crevel R, Speelman P, Gravekamp ESJ, et al. Leptospirosis in travelers. Clin Infect Dis 1994; 19:132.

Vance SF III. Leptospirosis—methods in the laboratory diagnosis. VA Med 1969; 96:335.

Congenital Leptospirosis

Das Guptas BM. On the intrauterine infection of the fetus with *Leptospira* icterohemorrhagiae. Ind M Gaz 1939; 74:28.

Hiyeda G. On the fetal infection by Spirocheta icterohemorrhagiae (abstr). Tocyo Iji-Shinshi, No. 2537. Trop Dis Bull 1928; 25:610, Jpn Med World 1928; 8:15.

Lindsay S, Luke IW. Fatal leptospirosis in a newborn infant. J Pediatr 1949; 34:90.

Takagi S. Passage of the spirocheta of Akiyami-Fever and Weil's disease through the placenta (abstr). Aichi Med Soc 34(6). Trop Dis Bull 1928; 25:610.

Zaki SR, Shieh WJ. Epidemic Working Group at the Ministry of Health in Nicaragua. Leptospirosis associated with the outbreak of acute febrile illness and pulmonary hemorrhage. Nicaragua. Lancet 1995; 347:535.

INTRODUCTION

Treponema pallidum is an elongated spiral organism, the morphology of which differs markedly from that of other bacteria. The spirochete is 5 to 20 μm long and approximately 0.2 μm thick. Electron microscopy reveals an outer enveloping membrane, the periplast, contoured to give between 4 and 14 spirals. Within the underlying protoplasmic cylinder is an axial filament composed of several fibrils. The outer envelope is between 70 and 90 μm thick, lying between two membrane bundles of fibrils that are stretched from one end of the treponeme to the other and wind in helical coils. The marked thinness of the organism renders it relatively nondetectable by light microscopy. The presence of muramic acid suggests the existence of a cell wall component, which is thought to be the reason for the therapeutic effectiveness of penicillin. *T. pallidum* grows best at 34°C to 35°C both in vitro and in vivo. The sensitivity of the organism to elevated temperature [*T. pallidum* is destroyed at 105°F (40.5°C)] had long been clinically noted and constituted the basis for the efficacy of artificial fever therapy in the treatment of tertiary syphilis.

IMMUNOLOGY OF INFECTION

The initial response to infection with *T. pallidum* results in the synthesis of predominantly immunoglobulin M (IgM) antibodies early in the disease. Within two weeks, antibodies of the IgG type are produced. They appear to be the prime mediator of immunity. With early eradication of disease, there is loss of immunity to infection. In contrast, the development of latency is associated with relative immunity to reinfection.

What causes the ultimate destruction of *T. pallidum* is controversial. It is currently postulated that the destruction of the organisms occurs extracellularly. The histologic lesions caused by *T. pallidum* suggest that both humoral immunity (immobilizing antibodies, plasma cells) and cellular immunity (lymphocytes) play important roles in its eradication.

The seroresponse of women treated for primary or secondary syphilis is such that the VDRL should decline approximately fourfold at three months and eightfold at six months. Failure of the VDRL to change significantly with time should alert the physician to possible treatment failures or reinfection.

NATURAL HISTORY OF THE DISEASE

Syphilis is an infection of mucous membranes. Transmission of the spirochete is predominantly the result of coitus. In the female, the primary lesion may occur on the labia, vaginal wall, or cervix. Extragenital sites, depending on sexual proclivities, are not uncommon.

Adequate sexual exposure is not the sole determinant of infection. Infection develops in only 10% of human volunteers from a single sexual encounter. In clinical situations, almost two-thirds of individuals intensively exposed to syphilis in its infectious stage will acquire infection. It is probable that *T. pallidum* breaches the mucous membrane barrier, but it is equally probable that minute breaks in the membrane in many instances provide the true portal of infection. Treatment during incubation is almost 100% effective and should be considered mandatory in the management of persons exposed to infectious syphilis. The time required for the development of the primary lesion is partly a function of the number of organisms establishing the initial infection and their subsequent replication at the portal of entry. Infections with a large inoculum (e.g., 107 organisms) may cause a chancre in five to seven days. The inoculation of 50 to 100 organisms is followed by an incubation period of about three weeks. The longest incubation period appears to be approximately five weeks. The prolonged incubations reflect the fact that the division time of *T. pallidum* is about 33 hours, compared to minutes for other bacteria.

Primary Syphilis

Once *T. pallidum* has penetrated the epithelial layer, the organisms replicate locally. During this period, proliferation of treponemes is associated with stimulation of cell-mediated and humoral immunity. Sensitized thymus-dependent lymphocytes appear in primary syphilitic lesions. Ingestion of the treponemes initially by polymorphic neutrophils and later by macrophages leads to antigen processing. In the presence of specific antibodies, the number of viable organisms declines. The presence of a variety of antibodies can be demonstrated in the serum of most (≥80%) but not all patients seeking medical attention for syphilis.

By the time the primary lesion is detected, both humoral and cell-mediated immune mechanisms have been activated. Classical chancres are solitary lesions (Fig. 1). However, multiple chancres have been identified in up to 40% of individuals with primary syphilis. Genital chancres are frequently atypical. A high index of suspicion is required for their diagnosis. Regional adenopathy normally accompanies the chancre of primary syphilis. The adenopathy usually develops a week after the appearance of the initial lesions. Untreated, a chancre will persist for two to eight weeks and then spontaneously disappear.

Macroscopically, the primary lesion consists of a small papule, which breaks down to form a superficial, painless ulcer with a clean granular base and firm scrolled margins. A histologic analysis reveals, in the absence of secondary infection, an extensive plasma cell and lymphocytic infiltration (Fig. 2). Characteristic of the lesion is the effect of *treponema* on the small blood vessels. Extensive endothelial proliferation in association with a significant plasma cell infiltrate should suggest a diagnosis of primary syphilis on histologic grounds alone.

The organism is not detectable by conventional staining techniques that utilize the ability of silver salts to delineate the organism's contours or by dark-field microscopy of a wet preparation from the primary lesion.

Most frequently, dissemination from the portal of infection to the regional lymph nodes occurs during the primary phase of the disease, with the result being "satellite" buboes. Physical examination reveals enlarged, firm, but tender lymph nodes, reflecting both organismal replication and reticular and lymphocytic cellular proliferation.

Irrespective of the subsequent clinical course, the chancre heals spontaneously. In approximately 30% of the cases, disease is limited to replication at the portal of entry, and even without therapy, eradication of the infection may occur in conjunction with the disappearance of serologic evidence of syphilitic infection as measured by nontreponemal tests.

From the regional lymph node drainage of the portal of infection, hematogenous dissemination characteristic of the secondary phase of the disease occurs.

Secondary Syphilis

The interim between the primary and secondary phases is in part a function of the time required for the development of the primary lesion and its satellite buboes. The secondary stage of syphilis usually manifests three to six weeks after the primary chancre has occurred. The lesions of secondary syphilis are the consequence of

1. hematogenous dissemination and
2. selective replication of treponemes at sites of slightly reduced body temperature that afford more optimal conditions for replication, i.e., skin and mucous membranes.

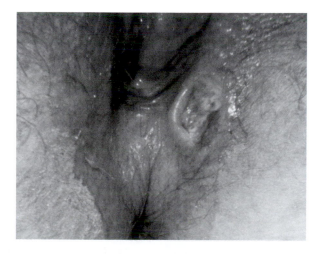

FIGURE I   Classical chancre.

The secondary phase is characterized by a generalized eruption, primarily on mucous membranes, the palms of the hands, and the soles of the feet. Cutaneous involvement is merely a reflection of widespread organ colonization. Clinically recognizable lesions have been observed in almost every organ system. Nevertheless, signs and symptoms referable to this extensive involvement are uncommon. An individual, during the secondary phase of syphilis, may exhibit bone tenderness when pressure is applied. In rare instances, iritis and alopecia occur.

The cutaneous lesion of the secondary stage of syphilis is a papular lesion, except in intertriginous areas where it is condylomatous. In the latter areas, the papules are circumscribed, flat, and moist and tend to become confluent (Fig. 3A and B). The lesions contain large numbers of spirochetes. The patient is again capable of transmitting disease and must be regarded as highly infectious to those in the immediate environment. A mucous membrane in which lesions are present is a potential locus for infection and dissemination. This predilection for cutaneous and mucous membranes appears to reflect T. pallidum's ability to replicate more rapidly at a temperature slightly below that of the internal body. It is in the late phase of primary illness and the second stage of the disease, during which hematogenous dissemination is occurring, that T. pallidum is afforded the opportunity to traverse the placenta and infect the conceptus. The depression of cellular immune responses to T. pallidum may in some way be involved in recrudescence of active lesions in secondary syphilis. The character of the lesions is partially governed by the induced systemic immunity. Rather than appearing like primary chancres, the appearance is that of a localized inflammatory lesion. If systemic immunity fails to develop, a florid type of infection called malignant secondary syphilis occurs, in which the secondary lesions resemble the primary chancre. The small multiple lesions of the disseminated stage of acquired syphilis persist for weeks to months. Patients with this stage of disease have high antibody titers to both specific treponemal and nontreponemal antigens. Circulating antigen–antibody complexes can be detected at this stage of infection and may lead to immune complex deposition in the kidneys. While the host is unable to contain the initial infection, intradermal rechallenge with T. pallidum is unlikely to induce a chancre. This situation in which the host resists rechallenge but is unable to clear the initial infection is called premunition.

Latency

The third stage, latency, is a stage of disease in which the systemic immunity of the host is sufficient to suppress all morphological evidence of treponemal replication. Whether subsequent disease (tertiary syphilis) develops is a partial function not only of combined cell-mediated immunity and humoral immunity but also of organismal virulence. Virulent treponemes display a remarkable capacity to resist attempts of both humoral and cellular host responses to eradicate them. Termination of active systemic infection probably requires the interaction of both types of immunity.

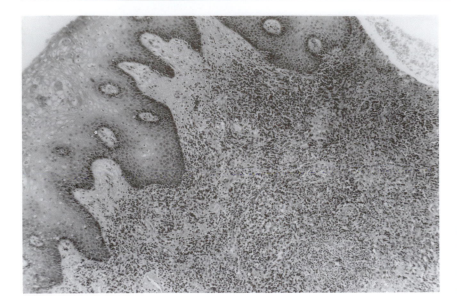

FIGURE 2 Histologic section of biopsy, revealing extensive lymphocytic and plasma cell infiltration of the underlying connective tissue. Marked endothelial proliferation is present (H&E, × 260).

Secondary relapses during latency occur in 25% of untreated patients, primarily in the first year of latency. In the remaining cases, relapse occurs in the ensuing five years. This first-year period is called early latency. Tertiary syphilis appears 1 to 20 years after the induction of latency. The sites of lesions are no longer influenced by temperature considerations. Gumma appear in soft tissue and viscera. The relative absence of or the difficulty of demonstrating intact treponemes has suggested that these lesions are the partial consequences of the immune state. Although visceral involvement tends to be the rule, gumma may appear subcutaneously. They have a predilection for areas of trauma such as the elbows and knees. The most common problem encountered is how to handle the asymptomatic patient with untreated syphilis of more than one year's duration. Wiesel (1985) compared treatment with 7.2 million units of penicillin G benzathine with and without performing a lumbar puncture. Based on subsequent cerebrospinal fluid (CSF) analysis, both strategies resulted in a cure rate of at least 99.7%. Lumbar puncture offers little or no additional benefits and is not cost effective in patients with asymptomatic late syphilis provided that therapy is that for neurosyphilis.

DIAGNOSIS

Confirmation of a syphilitic chancre depends on the demonstration of *T. pallidum* on dark-field microscopic examination. The lesion should be cleansed and abraded with gauze to induce superficial bleeding, and the blood blotted away. Once the serum begins to ooze, a small aliquot is placed on a glass slide and a cover slide applied. Dark-field analysis should be completed before the slide dries. If a specimen must be transported a short distance, the serum specimen should be collected in a relatively large-bore capillary tube and one end temporarily sealed

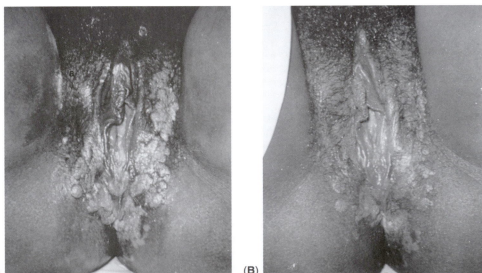

(A)   (B)

FIGURE 3 Secondary syphilis: (**A**) Manifestations of secondary syphilis (extensive condylomata lata) in intertriginous areas. (**B**) Same patient after five days of penicillin therapy.

with clay. Dark-field examination and direct fluorescent antibody tests of lesion exudates are the definitive methods for diagnosing early syphilis.

A presumptive diagnosis is possible with the use of two types of serological tests for the detection of *T. pallidum*: nontreponemal (flocculation and complement-fixation tests) and treponemal tests [e.g., *T. pallidum*-particle agglutination (TP-PA), fluorescent treponemal antibody (FTA) tests].

The complement-fixation tests are serologic assays for antibodies that react with cardiolipin, a nonspecific antigen; the latter, by using *T. pallidum* or an avirulent strain of *T. pallidum*—known as the Reiter treponeme—as the test antigen, detect specific antibodies.

The flocculation tests for syphilis utilize a cardiolipin–lecithin complex chemically extracted from beef heart. Cardiolipin constitutes about 15% of treponemal lipids and is present in mammary tissues. It is not clear whether the antibodies detected are directed against altered mammillary tissue or against treponeme-incorporated mammillary lipids.

The flocculation tests represent the combination of cardiolipin antigen with antibodies directed against comparable antigenic determinants (reagin); the combination precipitates grossly so as to form a visible aggregate. These tests tend to be highly sensitive for the late primary and the secondary stages of infection and are utilized for rapid screening.

Nontreponemal test antibody titers usually correlate with disease activity. A fourfold change in titer is considered necessary to demonstrate a clinically significant difference between two nontreponemal tests using the same serological test. The VDRL and raped plasma reagin (RPR) are equally valid assays, but quantitative results from the two tests cannot be compared directly. RPR values are frequently higher than the VDRL titers. The nontreponemal test should become nonreactive with time after successful therapy; however, some patients develop what is termed a serofast reaction in which a low titer persists for an indefinite period of time.

Since both the flocculation and complement-fixation tests are nontreponemal, there are clinical cases in which positive test results may be detected in the absence of syphilitic infection. These biologic positive tests are due to substances in the patient's serum that react like the reagin antibody and result in positive flocculation or complement-fixation reactions. Biologic false-positive reactions have been identified in patients with evidence of drug abuse, malaria, leprosy, vaccinia, infectious mononucleosis, and certain other viral infections. However, any febrile disease or immunization procedure may be associated with a false-positive serologic test. Biologic false-positive reactions of long duration have been identified in collagen disorders [such as rheumatoid arthritis and systemic lupus erythematosus (SLE)], sarcoid, and lymphomas.

The significance of a positive nontreponemal test should be confirmed by a treponemal test. The use of only one type of serological test is insufficient for diagnosis because false-positive nontreponemal tests can result with various medical conditions unrelated to syphilis.

Treponemal tests normally remain reactive for the remainder of a patient's life; however, 15% to 25% of patients treated during the primary stage of disease will revert back to being serologically nonreactive after two to three years.

Persons with a positive treponemal screening test should have a nontreponema test with titer done to guide patient management decisions. If the nontreponemal test is negative, a different nontreponemal test should be done to confirm the initial test results.

Currently, some clinical laboratories and blood banks are using treponemal enzyme-linked immunosorbent assay tests. These tests identify persons with previous treatment for syphilis as well as untreated or incompletely treated syphilis. False-positive results can occur.

False-Positive VDRL Test

The identification of a positive VDRL test necessitates

1. determining whether it is causally related to infection with *T. pallidum* and
2. evaluating the stage of the disease process.

Biologic false-positives occur in roughly 1% of patients. These VDRL tests are usually of low titer and not associated with a positive FTA test except in patients with SLE. Approximately 10% of SLE patients exhibit an atypical fluorescent pattern in which the usual homogeneous pattern of fluorescence is replaced by the organism assuming a beaded appearance. Unless the characteristic pattern of fluorescence can be identified, an alternative explanation for a positive test must be sought. A positive VDRL test in conjunction with a negative FTA-ABS test is not indicative of infection with *T. pallidum*.

THERAPY

Once a causal relationship is inferred, clinical staging of the disease process in terms of primary, secondary, latent tertiary, or neurosyphilitic stages should be attempted, since the clinical staging has therapeutic implications; that is, the patient is treated according to the stage of the disease (Table 1). In primary or secondary syphilis, fetal as well as maternal indications for therapy are applicable. Analysis of the CSF to identify those patients with already established neurosyphilis is imperative since the dosage and duration of therapy are different for neurosyphilis than for other stages. A gravida with a positive low-titer VDRL and a positive FTA-ABS test, in the absence of clinical evidence of infection, should be treated as if she had late latent syphilis (Table 2). If a diagnostic lumbar puncture is not performed, the patient needs to be treated as an asymptomatic neurosyphilitic. No single test can be used to diagnose neurosyphilis. The VDRL test done on CSF is highly specific, but it is not sensitive. CSF cell count and protein levels can be used to support a presumptive diagnosis and/or measure the effectiveness of therapy.

The key to successful therapy is as much the time interval during which antibiotics are administered as it is the actual dosage.

TABLE I Advocated antibiotic regimen for the treatment of syphilis in pregnancy

Drug of choice	Dosage	Route of administration	Duration of therapy (days)
Primary or secondary (infectious): benzathine penicillin G[a] session	2.4 million units total (1.2 million units in each buttock) in a single dose	IM	—
Primary or secondary[b] (infectious) syphilis in third trimester: benzathine penicillin G	2.4 million units followed by 1.2 million units at each of the next 3 clinic visits, 4 days apart	IM	12 days
Latent syphilis of less than 1 yr duration: benzathine penicillin G[a]	50,000 units/kg up to the adult dose of 2.4 million units in a single session	IM	—
Latent syphilis or unknown duration indeterminant: benzathine penicillin G[c]	50,000 units/kg up to the adult dose of 2.4 million units as 3 doses at 1 wk intervals	IM	3 wk

[a]Benzathine penicillin G is the drug of choice because it provides effective treatment in a single visit.
[b]Not a CDC recommendation.
[c]Cerebrospinal fluid examination is recommended in any patient with syphilis of >1 yr duration or with neurologic signs to exclude asymptomatic neurosyphilis.
Abbreviation: CDC, Centers for Disease Control and Prevention.

Clinical staging of the disease becomes more important when the physician is confronted with a patient who has a documented reaction to penicillin. The alternate drugs of choice, namely, erythromycin and tetracycline, have limited applications in the gravida. Erythromycin traverses the placental barrier, but inefficiently. Fetal plasma levels are about 6% to 20% of maternal plasma levels. Adequate maternal therapy may not abort infection in the fetus. As was previously stated, tetracycline is contraindicated in the gravida. The experimental evidence that tetracycline is a teratogen if it is given during the period of osseous organogenesis is almost as incriminating as that which existed for thalidomide. Its therapeutic use in the second and third trimesters, the periods of growth and differentiation, results in retardation and hypoplasia of the deciduous teeth and inhibition of bone growth.

For a gravida in the first trimester with either primary or secondary syphilis, early latent syphilis, or a high VDRL and documented penicillin hypersensitivity, it is advocated that she be brought into a controlled environment (preferably hospitalized) and treated by desensitization and penicillin therapy. If infection in the second or third trimester is treated with an erythromycin, the infant must be retreated in the neonatal period with penicillin. Even inadequate therapy, while not aborting infection, can retard its progression.

The reversion to seronegativity of the nontreponemal type of test is a function of the stage of the disease as well as of the efficacy of therapy. A serologic cure will be achieved sooner in the early stage of syphilis, whereas for patients in the late stages, a serologic cure may never be realized.

In a patient who has primary syphilis and a dark-field–positive ulcer, a positive nontreponemal test may not develop until after the initiation of therapy. The test

reverts, usually within three months, unless reinfection or relapse occurs. Six to nine months may pass before the patient's serum becomes negative. Any patient whose serum fails to become negative nine months after treatment should be retreated.

THERAPEUTIC FAILURE

Up to a 2% incidence of therapeutic failures can be anticipated with one course of adequately administered penicillin in the treatment of primary syphilis. Patients in the secondary stage of syphilis invariably have positive reagin tests. Immediately after treatment, the serologic titer usually rises and then pursues a downward pattern. Within one year, about 98% of patients will become seronegative. The remaining 2% should become seronegative during the second year. As with primary syphilis, if the expected serologic response is not observed, the patient should receive a lumbar puncture and then be retreated within one year after the initial treatment. The CSF should be examined for cell count and protein; a VDRL test should also be performed. If any of the CSF tests are abnormal, the patient should be treated for neurosyphilis.

Patients should be reexamined clinically and serologically 6 and 12 months after treatment.

PENICILLIN DESENSITIZATION DURING PREGNANCY

Parenteral penicillin G is the only therapy with documented efficacy for syphilis during pregnancy. No proven alternatives to penicillin are available for treating congenital syphilis or syphilis in pregnancy. An estimated 10% of persons who report a history of allergic reaction to penicillin remain reactive. With the passage of time, a significant number of persons who have had a severe reaction to penicillin stop repressing penicillin-specific IgE. According to the Centers for Disease Control and Prevention (CDC), skin testing with the major and minor determinants of penicillin can reliably identify individuals at risk for an adverse reaction. Testing with only

TABLE 2 Therapy for latent or indeterminant syphilis of more than 1 yr duration in pregnancy

Benzathine penicillin G
7.2 million units total; 2.4 million units weekly for 3 successive weeks; route of administration: IM

the major determinant of penicillin G identifies 90% to 97% of currently allergic individuals. Skin testing without the minor determinant can miss 3% to 10% of allergic patients.

The presence of allergy to penicillin in a gravida with syphilis presents a major therapeutic problem. This clinical situation has been successfully addressed by oral or intravenous penicillin desensitization. Ziaya et al. (1986) described a woman with an allergy against both major and minor determinants of penicillin in whom syphilis was diagnosed on routine obstetric screening. The patient underwent desensitization utilizing graduated intravenous doses of penicillin followed by treatment with a constant infusion for eight days. She experienced no serious allergic reactions requiring alteration of therapy. Wendel et al. (1985) reported on 15 pregnant women with histories of penicillin allergy confirmed by positive immediate wheal-and-flare skin tests (Table 3). Thirteen women had syphilis, one *Listeria* sepsis, and one *Streptococcus viridan*'s endocarditis. Each patient was desensitized over four to six hours by oral administration of increasing doses of penicillin V. At the completion of the procedure, bolus dose parenteral therapy with penicillin G or ampicillin was instituted. Five of the subjects (33%) experienced either pruritus (three) or urticaria (two). No interruption of desensitization or therapy was necessary. All clinically apparent maternal infections were cured. The pregnancy complicated by listeriosis aborted in the first trimester. No cases of congenital syphilis were identified. These studies indicate that oral or intravenous desensitization is an acceptable, safe approach to therapy of syphilis in gravidas with documented hypersensitivity to penicillin and should be initiated in an intensive care unit with staff for intubation and management of anaphylaxis.

The method of Van Arsde was utilized by Ziaya et al. (1986). In this regimen, aliquots of 50 mL were infused, each containing a tenfold increase in the concentration of penicillin G beginning at 0.01 U/mL and reaching 100,000 U/mL (Table 4). Each aliquot was administered over a period of 30 minutes. Once desensitization was achieved, a continuous infusion of aqueous penicillin G at 25,000 U/hr was given to maintain a blood level to cover at least three replications (more than 30 hours per replication) of *T. pallidum*.

Although intravenous and oral therapy have not been compared, the CDC regards oral desensitization as safer and easier to perform (Table 5).

Using the oral desensitization protocol of Wendel et al. (1985), the procedure can be completed in approximately four hours, after which the first dose of penicillin can be administer. After desensitization, patients must be maintained on penicillin continuously for the duration of therapy.

Irrespective of which desensitization protocol is used, the procedures must be done in a hospital setting in the event that a serious IgE-mediated allergic reaction occurs during desensitization.

Pregnant women with syphilis in any stage who have penicillin allergy should be desensitized and treated with penicillin according to the CDC Recommended Guidelines.

IMPACT OF HIV INFECTION ON SYPHILIS

Patients with AIDS represent only a minority of the total number of T-cell–deficient patients with HIV disease. The T-cell deficiency has caused severe complications when live-virus vaccines are inadvertently administered to recipients with impaired immunologic function due to HIV.

All patients with syphilis should be tested for HIV infection. In geographic areas or specific populations in which the prevalence of HIV is high, patients with primary syphilis should be retested for HIV three months after the first HIV test was negative.

Several investigators have reported the subsequent development of neurologic complications following standard penicillin therapy in patients infected with HIV. These reports have suggested that standard penicillin therapy alone is probably not adequate to eradicate infection in the absence of a vigorous host response. According to the CDC, neurosyphilis has developed in only a limited number of patients after standard treatment with penicillin regimens

TABLE 3 Oral desensitization regimen for the patients with positive skin test

Penicillin V suspension dose[a]	Amount (units/mL)[b]	mL	Units	Cumulative dose (units)
1	1,000	0.1	100	100
2	1,000	0.2	200	300
3	1,000	0.4	400	700
4	1,000	0.8	800	1,500
5	1,000	1.6	1,600	3,100
6	1,000	3.2	3,200	6,300
7	1,000	6.4	6,400	12,700
8	10,000	1.2	12,000	24,700
9	10,000	2.4	24,000	48,700
10	10,000	4.8	48,000	96,700
11	80,000	1.0	80,000	176,700
12	80,000	2.0	160,000	336,700
13	80,000	4.0	320,000	656,700
14	80,000	8.0	640,000	1,296,700

Observation period: 30 min before parenteral administration of penicillin.
[a]Interval between doses: 15 min; elapsed time: 3 hr and 45 min; and cumulative dose: 1.3 million units.
[b]The specific amount of drug was diluted in approximately 30 mL of water and then administered orally.
Source: Wendel et al. (1985).

TABLE 4 Regimen of Van Arsde for incremental intravenous penicillin G infusion

Concentration (U/mL)	Volume (mL)	Duration (min)
0.01	50	30
1	50	30
10	50	30
100	50	30
1,000	50	30
10,000	50	30
100,000	50	30

Source: Ziaya et al. (1986).

recommended for primary and secondary syphilis. The immunologic response of the patient appears to be important in controlling the infection, even in the presence of adequate antibiotic therapy. What is implied is that everyone with HIV infection who contracts syphilis must be treated with higher doses of antibiotics for prolonged periods. The antibiotic therapy for neurosyphilis appears to be the minimal acceptable regimen (2.4 million units aqueous penicillin IV for 8–10 days).

JARISCH-HERXHEIMER REACTION

The issue of therapy is further complicated by the potential adverse host response to penicillin at the placental level. The Jarisch-Herxheimer reaction is an acute febrile reaction that usually occurs within the first 24 hours after any therapy for syphilis. Klein et al. monitored 33 gravidas with syphilis for 24 hours after treatment with benzathine penicillin G. Fifteen (40%) of the women had a Jarisch-Herxheimer reaction, and 12 of the 15 patients had secondary syphilis. The incidence of a Jarisch-Herxheimer reaction among the 20 gravidas with secondary syphilis monitored was 60%. The most common symptoms were fever (73%), uterine contractions (67%), and decreased fetal movement (67%). The signs or symptoms began 2 to 8 hours after treatment; fevers peaked at 6 to 12 hours posttherapy, and the events usually abated by 16 to 24 hours after treatment. Uterine contractions and decreased fetal activity began concurrent with maternal fever in eight of ten women reporting contractions. Transient late decelerations were detected in 3 of 11 monitored patients. Three of the women with Jarisch-Herxheimer reactions delivered infants with congenital syphilis, including one stillbirth, but none of those without a detectable reaction had fetal treatment failures. The Jarisch-Herxheimer reaction that is sometimes induced by therapy may not be limited to the maternal host.

Approximately 10% to 25% of pregnant women with secondary syphilis in whom a Jarisch-Herxheimer reaction develops will experience an intrauterine demise within one to four weeks. Why these fetuses subjected to a Jarisch-Herxheimer reaction die is a matter of conjecture. Induction of acute placental insufficiency by additional compromise of the placental vasculature is a distinct possibility. The sustained hyperthermia associated with Jarisch-Herxheimer reaction may be either a significant cofactor or the principal catalyst in these late gestational fetal deaths.

About 9% of patients with secondary and early latent syphilis will exhibit a Jarisch-Herxheimer reaction several hours after the first injection of penicillin. The reaction is characterized by chills, fever, headaches, myalgia, and arthralgia. The syphilitic lesions become prominent, edematous, and more brilliant in color. The reaction lasts only a few hours and can be controlled by mild sedation. The rash begins to fade within 48 hours and is usually gone by the 14th day. The reaction does not occur after a second injection. Reduction of the initial dose of penicillin does not prevent the Jarisch-Herxheimer reaction. In no case should treatment be withheld or discontinued because of it. Management of a Jarisch-Herxheimer reaction involves effective control of the hyperthermia and the immediate administration of oxygen to the mother.

For patients at high risk for a Jarisch-Herxheimer reaction, the author has given, in a controlled environment, an erythromycin antibiotic the day before administration of the benzathine penicillin in an attempt to avert such a reaction.

TABLE 5 Alternative therapy advocated for a gravida with secondary syphilis[a]

Medication and route	Rationale
I. 10 million units of penicillin G (intravenous)	40% to 60% of pregnant patients with secondary syphilis will exhibit a Jarisch-Herxheimer reaction. A comparable phenomenon may occur involving the placenta, causing acute placental insufficiency and possible abortion. If the reaction occurs, diminish but do not discontinue infusion, and administer oxygen and antipyretic drugs; intravenous route of administration is chosen to give better drug control. If no reaction occurs, discontinue intravenous therapy
II. 2.4 million units of slowly released the CDC	Standard treatment of the nonpregnant female benzathine penicillin zas advocated by
III. Ampicillin 2 g q 12 hr × 10 days (oral) Despite in utero treatment standard therapy	Penicillin traverses the placental barrier poorly. T. pallidum may not be eradicated. To treat fetus, as opposed to mother, the placental drug gradient must be stacked. Ampicillin traverses the placental barrier more effectively than penicillin. Replication time for T. pallidum is 33–36 hr. Because of nonsynchronous replication, the fetus should be treated for a minimum of 7 days

[a]This therapy differs significantly from that advocated by the CDC and is not FDA approved.
Abbreviations: CDC, Centers for Disease Control and Prevention; FDA, Food and Drug Administration.

It is strongly advocated that gravidas with high VDRLs, secondary syphilis, or early latent syphilis have therapy administered in a setting in which hyperthermia and fetal need for supplemental oxygenation can be effectively handled.

ADEQUACY OF CURRENT MATERNAL THERAPY FOR PREVENTION OF CONGENITAL SYPHILIS

During pregnancy, in the absence of appropriate therapy, early untreated syphilis gives rise to significant loss by spontaneous abortion, stillbirth, or perinatal demise. Among the survivors of such infected pregnancies, about 40% of the offspring exhibit various stigmata of congenital syphilis.

The therapy of syphilis in pregnancy has been that of syphilis of the nonpregnant woman. The CDC recommends 2.4 million units of benzathine penicillin G for the management of early syphilis (disease of less than one year's duration). The clinical study that best focuses on the problem of therapeutic failures is that of Mascola et al. (1984). In 1982, 50 of the 159 cases of congenital syphilis reported to the CDC occurred in Texas. Of the 50 cases analyzed, 39 could have been prevented by appropriate prenatal care with adequate clinical diagnosis and treatment. Of the remaining 11 cases, seven women were incubating syphilis at the time of delivery and had negative serological results at the time of parturition. What was disturbing was the fact that four women who received the recommended treatment with benzathine penicillin went on to deliver congenitally infected infants. Ricci et al. published a series of 56 cases of congenital syphilis. In this series, seven of the gravidas were treated during pregnancy. Five received benzathine penicillin G (2.4 million units) and two received erythromycin. Most of the treatment failures occurred after therapy in the second or third trimester. Benzathine penicillin G therapy in these cases failed to eradicate apparently established fetal disease. Like congenital rubella, fetal infection in utero is not a time-limited event. Fetuses with congenital syphilis have a continued organism–cell interaction such that morbidity is cumulative with time.

Wendel et al. (1985) have reported on the impact of maternal therapy with syphilis during pregnancy. Theirs is one of the few studies in the literature which identified the stage of maternal syphilis and in so doing provided some insight as to the actual level of efficacy of maternal therapy on infants with established fetal infection. When pregnant women with secondary syphilis were treated with greater than 2.4 million units of benzathine penicillin G, 5.3% of neonates were born infected.

There have been very few, if any, adequate studies on therapy for syphilis in pregnancy and on the ability of maternally administered antibiotics to eradicate established disease in utero. Good demographic and therapeutic studies analyzing the frequency of therapeutic failure for a given stage of maternal disease are lacking. What is known is that penicillin per se does not readily traverse the placental barrier. To achieve therapeutic drug levels in amniotic fluid for bacterial disease, it is necessary to "stack" the maternal–fetal gradient by administering large doses of the antibiotic. Penicillin can be demonstrated within amniotic fluid after 24 hours following administration or 2.4 million units of benzathine penicillin. The inability of traditional benzathine penicillin therapy (advocated by the CDC) to preclude the occurrence of congenital syphilis may be a partial function of the low levels of penicillin demonstrable in serum after intramuscular injections of 2.4 million units of benzathine penicillin, the difficulty with which penicillin enters the fetal compartment, and the dosage required to abort incipient viruses and eradicate established disease.

PROPOSED MATERNAL THERAPY OF SECONDARY SYPHILIS IN PREGNANCY

The major therapeutic considerations in the treatment of gravidas with advanced active disease are

1. avoidance of fetal death in utero and
2. effective eradication of maternal and fetal disease.

Because of the possibility of adverse fetal consequences from the Jarisch-Herxheimer reaction, Monif (1983) has advocated a policy of initiating penicillin therapy through a controllable vehicle (Table 4). Five million units of penicillin G in a liter of 5% dextrose are administered by a slow intravenous drip. If a Jarisch-Herxheimer reaction occurs, the infusion is temporarily discontinued. Oxygen is given by a Venture mask with the patient lying on her left side. Antipyretics are given to maintain the temperature below 38.5° C. The fetal heart rate is monitored. If nonstress tests remain positive and good fetal heart rate variability persists, the infusion is cautiously reinstated. If evidence of fetal distress is identified, the situation is discussed with the mother and an individualized program of therapy is instituted.

The conversion from intravenous penicillin to oral ampicillin is predicated upon fetal considerations. The difference in lipid solubility and ionic binding between benzathine penicillin and ampicillin is such that ampicillin more readily traverses the placental barrier. The level of penicillin in cord and amniotic fluid is governed by the maternal/fetal gradient. The maternal levels attainable with benzathine penicillin are low and vary from individual to individual.

The use of benzathine penicillin assures compliance and effective maternal therapy, which is a cornerstone of public health policy.

Without a collaborative multiple institutional double-blinded comparative study spanning at least a five- to ten-year period, documentation of the superiority or otherwise of this regimen will be wanting.

CONGENITAL SYPHILIS

Congenital syphilis is primarily a reflection of inadequate prenatal care. In a review of 54 cases of congenital syphilis in the state of Massachusetts, 18 mothers had received no prenatal care, 23 had received inadequate prenatal care, 10 cases resulted from maternal infection or reinfection following initial prenatal examination, and three were due to the failure of the physician to obtain the appropriate tests. Now, a significant number of congenital syphilis cases have been identified in which the mother had received adequate maternal therapy during gestation.

An analysis of infant therapeutic failures after maternal treatment for syphilis in pregnancy has documented the significance of proximity to maternal spirochetemia and probably the magnitude of its occurrence. Sheffield et al. (2002) identified 43 gravidas who had received antepartum therapy for syphilis according to the CDC guidelines and who were delivered of a newborn with congenital syphilis. The majority of these women had been treated for secondary or early latent syphilis. Thirty-five percent of these women were treated within 30 days of delivery. Fifty-six percent of the infants were delivered before 36 weeks and 26% of them were stillborn. The majority of failures occur in women with either secondary or early latent syphilis.

Why did these therapeutic failures occur, and is there a relationship of therapy to preterm delivery?

The incidence of occult neonatal infection or disease does not parallel the incidence of syphilis in pregnancy. Maternal therapy given early in the infection is often adequate to eradicate spirochetal replication prior to spirochetemia. If the occurrence of spirochetemia antedates the establishment of pregnancy, the probability of subsequent metastatic spread to the products of conception in the face of an established maternal immune response is near nonexistent.

Penicillin concentrations as low as 0.018 mg/mL sustained for seven days result in nearly 100% treponemicidal activity. Idsoe et al. (1972) demonstrated that this drug concentration can be achieved with a single dose of 2.4 mU of benzathine penicillin in nonpregnant adults. The physiology of pregnancy alters penicillin pharmacokinetics such that the majority of pregnant women administered a single dose of 2.4 mU of benzathine penicillin do not attain a level of 0.018 mg/mL in fetal blood for the time required to eradicate the organism.

The risk of an adverse fetal/neonatal outcome is theoretically a function of the magnitude of the maternal spirochetemia, the effectiveness and safety of antimicrobial therapy, and the magnitude of fetal involvement.

The placenta, like the conceptus, is involved in the disease process. As with organ pathology, the mass of *treponema* organisms determines the extent of fetal pathology. In its most overt form, syphilitic placentitis is manifested by a marked increase in placental weight such that the placental–fetal weight ratio is in the range of 1:3 or even 1:2. The increase in weight reflects the presence of a dense stroma beneath the chorionic layer of the villus, in which a compensatory increase in the number of vascular channels may be identified. The overall effect is an increase in connective tissue and cellular mass between the maternal and fetal circulation, analogous to an alveolar capillary block in the lungs. With advanced disease, placental erythroblastosis may be present.

The chorionic villi show inflammation, with proliferative vasculitis, perivasculitis, or endovasculitis. The net effect of these alterations of placental architecture is probably reflected in an alteration of function resulting in low-birth-weight babies and stillborn infants. Owing to the lengthy division time of *T. pallidum* compared to that of most bacteria, infection of the products of conception does not tend to result in immediate abortion. However, extensive involvement of the fetus may result in its demise prior to parturition.

The demonstration on ultrasonograms of a thickened placenta should alert the clinician to the possibility, if not probability, that with the institution of penicillin therapy, the mother will experience a Jarisch-Herxheimer reaction. The accompanying hyperthermia may be sufficient, when added to an already compromised maternal/fetal exchange, to terminate life.

Congenital syphilis following hematogenous dissemination results in multiple organ involvement, with characteristic lesions occurring in the placenta, lungs, bone marrow, liver, and spleen. Tissue response is markedly similar to that observed in the adult except that parenchymal growth seems to be retarded, a condition that may reflect the predilection for and pathologic effect on small blood vessels. The main histologic features are extensive proliferation of fibrous connective tissue in association with mononuclear cell infiltration and small-vessel endothelial proliferation. The principal difference between this pattern and that observed in adult tissues is that plasma cell infiltration, which is so characteristic in adult tissue, is markedly less conspicuous.

Despite the fact that a target organ is the site of spirochetal replication (as demonstrated by appropriate staining techniques), prior to the fifth month of gestation, there is an absence of a significant host response to *T. pallidum* by the fetal organs. The absence of morphologic stigmata of infection had provided the basis for the contention that fetal involvement did not occur until the fourth month of gestation. *T. pallidum* does cross the placenta and can involve fetal organs at any time during gestation; however, inflammatory lesions indicative of a host response with plasmacytoid or plasma cells do not occur until the 20th week of gestation in congenital syphilis.

Widespread organ involvement may be responsible for a hemolytic anemia, thrombocytopenia, and hepatosplenomegaly. These manifestations of disease may or may not be associated with cutaneous and mucous membrane lesions. In very advanced cases, the diagnosis may be inferred and documented by placental examination.

Congenital syphilis is rarely diagnosed in the neonatal period. If clinical signs are present at birth, 50% of the infants will die in the neonatal period. In the first month of life, fewer than 10% of the cases are identified. That organ pathology is not full blown at birth emphasizes the necessity for early diagnosis and therapy. Owing to the rising incidence of infection since the 1950s, more and more cases of infection in the terminal stages of gestation will occur and will result in the delivery of infants with no overt manifestation of spirochete replication. The probability of the acquisition of disease between initial serologic surveillance and parturition is approximately 0.6 to 2 per 1000 live births. It becomes increasingly apparent that in high-risk populations, serologic surveillance at parturition needs to become part of comprehensive prenatal care.

Diagnosis

An infant born to a mother whose pregnancy was complicated with syphilis will have within its intravascular compartment IgG antibody of maternal origin. These antibodies quantitatively and qualitatively may mask a fetal response to infection, which is predominantly IgM in character. The cord VDRL and FTA-ABS titers correspond to those determined for the maternal serum. If intrauterine infection has occurred, cord blood or neonatal serum will contain a composite of IgG of maternal derivation and endogenous fetal IgM. If the infant is born at term, the VDRL titer tends to be slightly higher than the maternal value. Since maternal IgM does not cross the placenta, the detection of specific IgM in cord or newborn serum indicates that there has been exposure in utero of the developing embryo or fetus to the antigenic determinants of *T. pallidum*. Depending on the severity and duration of the disease, IgM levels within cord or neonatal serum may be markedly elevated above the anticipated value. Congenital infection can be documented by the IgM FTA-ABS test or IgM immunoblots. Cardiolipin tests, such as the VDRL test and the usual treponemal test, are of little value in the diagnosis of congenital syphilis. The application of the IgM FTA-ABS test may be useful for the identification of congenital syphilis in infants who have few or no symptoms at birth, or for confirmation of the diagnosis in the more overt form. Because both false-positive and false-negative results have been reported with the IgM FTA-ABS test, serial follow-up is still indicated when nonspecific IgM antibodies are demonstrable in the cord serum of a neonate born of a seropositive gravida. Low levels of IgM specific for *T. pallidum* may be present at birth—even though the mother may have received adequate treatment—and represent a serologic scar similar to that of the FTA in the adult. Children born of a seropositive mother must be periodically monitored for as long as three months for FTA-IgM antibody in order to exclude the possibility of delayed onset of infection.

An underutilized means of confirming congenital syphilis is the application of polymerase chain reaction testing directly to placental tissues. This procedure is particularly applicable to the establishment of a diagnosis in stillborn fetuses.

At birth, neonates with congenital syphilis may present a spectrum from full-blown syndrome to a normal-appearing infant. *Forme fruste* of the disease may present with unexplained hepatomegaly, usually associated with anemia.

Therapy for Congenital Syphilis

Infants with congenital syphilis should have a CSF examination before treatment, since the findings will influence therapy. If the CSF is abnormal, the neonate should receive aqueous crystalline penicillin G 50,000 units/kg IV every 12 hours for the first seven days and every eight hours thereafter for a total of 10 days. Other antibiotics are not recommended for neonatal congenital syphilis. In the more severely affected newborn infants, a Jarisch-Herxheimer reaction often occurs in the course of penicillin therapy. Infected neonates may be seronegative if maternal infection occurred late in gestation.

Infants who have a normal physical examination and a serum quantitative nontreponema titer equal or greater than that of their mothers should receive a full course of therapy, particularly if (*i*) maternal therapy was inadequate, (*ii*) material treatment is unknown, (*iii*) drugs other than a penicillin were given, or (*iv*) adequate follow-up of the infant cannot be assured.

SELECTED READING

Syphilis and Pregnancy
Alexander JM, Sheffeld JS, Sanchez PJ, et al. Efficacy of treatment for syphillis in pregnancy. Obset Gynecol 1999; 93:5.
Centers for Disease Control. Sexually transmitted diseases treatment guidelines 2002. MMWR 2002; 51:RR-6.
Centers for Disease Control. Sexually transmitted diseases treatment guidelines 2006. MMWR 2006; 55:RR-11.
Chapel TA, Prasad P, Chapel J, Lekas N. Extragenital syphilitic chancres. J Am Acad Dermatol 1985; 13:582.
Fiumara NJ. The treatment of syphilis. N Engl J Med 1964; 270:1185.
Holder WR, Know JM. Syphilis in pregnancy. Med Clin North Am 1972; 56:1151.
Ingraham NR. The value of penicillin alone in the prevention and treatment of congenital syphilis. Acta Derm Venereol 1951; 31:60.
Jackson FR, Vanderstoep EM, Knox JM. Use of aqueous benzathine penicillin G in the treatment of syphilis in pregnant women. Am J Obstet Gynecol 1983; 83:1389.
Kampmeier RH. Prenatal syphilis and syphilis in pregnancy. South Med Bull 1965; 53:35.
Liljestrand J, Bergstrom S, Nieuwenhuis F, Hederstedt B. Syphilis in pregnant women in Mozambique. Genitourin Med 1985; 61:355.
Monif GRG. Infectious Disease in Obstetrics, 1982. Gainesville: Infectious Diseases Inc., 1982:115.
Monif GRG. Maternal syphilis and pregnancy. Infect Dis Lttrs Obstet Gynecol 1983; 5:25.
Nelson NA, Struve VR. Prevention of congenital syphilis by treatment of syphilis in pregnancy. J Am Med Assoc 1956; 161:689.
Pickering LK. Diagnosis and therapy of patients with congenital and primary syphilis. Pediatr Infect Dis 1985; 4:602.
Philipson A, Sabath LD, Charles D. Transplacental passage of erythromycin and clindamycin. N Engl J Med 1973; 288:1219.
Philipson A, Sabath LD, Charles D. Erythromycin and clindamycin absorption and elimination in pregnant women. Clin Pharmacol Ther 1976; 19:68.
Sparling PF. Diagnosis and treatment of syphilis. N Engl J Med 1971; 284:642.
Tanaka M, Katayama H, Sakumoto M, et al. Trends of sexually transmitted diseases and condom use patterns among commercial sex workers in Fukuoka City, Japan 1900–93. Genitourin Med 1996; 72:358.
Trujillo L, Munoz D, Gotuzzo E, et al. Sexual practices and prevalence of HIV, HTLV-I/II and *Treponema pallidum* among clandestine female sex workers in Lima, Peru. Sex Transm Dis 1999; 26:115.
Wiesel J, Rose DN, Silver AL, et al. Lumbar puncture in asymptomatic late syphilis. An analysis of the benefits and risks. Arch Intern Med 1985; 145:465.

Immunology of Infection
Aiuti F, Ungari S, Turbessi G, Serra GB. Immunologic aspects of congenital syphilis. Helv Paediatr Acta 1966; 21:66.
Alford CA Jr, Polt SS, Cassady GE, et al. Gamma-M fluorescent treponemal antibody in the diagnosis of congenital syphilis. N Engl J Med 1969; 280:1086.
Baker-Zander SA, Hook EW 3d, Bonin P, et al. Antigens of *Treponema pallidum* recognized by IgG and IgM antibodies during syphilis in humans. J Infect Dis 1985; 151:264.
Bradford LL, Tuffanelli DL, Puffer J, et al. Fluorescent treponemal absorption and *Treponema pallidum* immobilization tests in

syphilitic patients and biologic false-positive reactors. Tech Bull Regist Med Tech 1967; 37:59.

Brown ST, Zaidi A, Larsen SA, Reynolds GH. Serological response to syphilis treatment. A new analysis of old data. J Am Med Assoc 1985; 253:1296.

Deacon WE, Lucas JB, Price FV. Fluorescent treponemal antibody-absorption (FTA-ABS) test for syphilis. J Am Med Assoc 1966; 198:624.

Hart G. Syphilis tests in diagnostic and therapeutic decision making. Ann Intern Med 1986; 104:368.

Kaufman RE, Olansky DC, Wiesner PJ. The FTA-ABS (IgM) test for neonatal congenital syphilis: a critical review. J Am Vener Dis Assoc 1974; 1:79.

Merlin S, Andre J, Alacoque B, Paris-Hamelin A. Importance of specific IgM antibodies in 116 patients with various stages of syphilis. Genitourin Med 1985; 61:82.

Sato T, Kubo E, Yokota M, et al. *Treponema pallidum* specific IgM hemagglutination test for sero-diagnosis of syphilis. Br J Vener Dis 1984; 60:364.

Scotti AT, Logan BS, Caldwell JC. Fluorescent antibody test for neonatal congenital syphilis: a progress report. J Pediatr 1969; 75:1.

Wicher K, Horowitz HW, Wicher V. Laboratory methods of diagnosis of syphilis for the beginning of the third millennium. Microbes Infect 1999; 1:1093.

Wigfield AS. Immunological phenomena of syphilis. Br J Vener Dis 1965; 41:275.

Congenital Syphilis

Ackerman BDL. Congenital syphilis: observations on laboratory diagnosis of intrauterine infection. J Pediatr 1969; 74:459.

Al-Salihi FL, Curran JP, Shteir OS. Occurrence of fetal syphilis after a non-reactive early gestational serologic test. J Pediatr 1971; 78:121.

Bakkes PM. An unusual case of congenital syphilis. Dermatologica 1966; 133:430.

Blodi FC, Hervouet F. Syphilitic chorioretinitis. An histologic study. Arch Ophthalmol 1968; 79:294.

Brown JW, Moore BM. Congenital syphilis in the United States. Clin Pediatr (Phila) 1963; 2:220.

Chawla V, Gupta K, Raghu MB. Congenital syphilis: a clinical profile. J Trop Pediatr 1983; 31:204.

Epstein H, King CR. Diagnosis of congenital syphilis by immunofluorescence following fetal death in utero. Am J Obstet Gynecol 1985; 152:689.

Ewing CI, Roberts C, Davidson DC, Arya OP. Early congenital syphilis still occurs. Arch Dis Child 1985; 60:1128.

Fiumara NJ. Clinical syphilis in Massachusetts. N Engl J Med 1953; 245:634.

Fiumara NJ, Lessel S. Manifestations of late congenital syphilis and analysis of 271 patients. Arch Dermatol 1970; 102:78.

Garner MF. Clinical value of the IgM FTA-ABS test tor congenital syphilis in the newborn. Aust NZ J Obstet Gynaecol 1975; 15:104.

Genest DR, Choi-Hong SR, Tate JE, et al. Diagnosis of congenital syphilis from placental examination: comparison of histopathology, Steiner stain, and polymerase chain reaction for *Treponema pallidum* DNA. Hum Pathol 1996; 27:366.

Hallock J, Tunnessen WW. Congenital syphilis in an infant of a seronegative mother. Obstet Gynecol 1968; 32:336.

Harter CA, Benirshke K. Fetal syphilis in the first trimester. Am J Obstet Gynecol 1976; 124:705.

Hira SK, Bhat GJ, Patel JB, et al. Early congenital syphilis: clinico-radiologic features in 202 patients. Sex Transm Dis; 1985; 12:177.

Hollier LM, Harstad TW, Sanchez PJ, et al. Fetal syphilis: clinical and laboratory characteristics. Obstet Gynecol 2001; 97:947.

Mascola L, Pelosi R, Blount JH, et al. Congenital syphilis revisited. Am J Dis Child 1985; 139:575.

Saxoni F, Lapatosanis P, Pantelakis P. Congenital syphilis: a description of 18 cases and reexamination of an old but ever present disease. Clin Pediatr 1967; 6:687.

Scotti AT, Logan L. A specific IgM antibody test in neonatal congenital syphilis. J Pediatr 1968; 73:242.

Shaffer LW, Courville CHJ. Effect of penicillin in the prevention of congenital syphilis. Arch Dermatol 1951; 63:91.

Sheffield JS, Sanchez P, Wendel GD Jr, et al. Placental histopathology of congenital syphilis. Obstet Gynecol 2002; 100:126.

Wilkinson RW, Helles RM. Congenital syphilis: resurgence of an old problem. Pediatrics 1971; 47:27.

Woody MC, Sistrunk WF, Platou RV. Congenital syphilis: a laid ghost walks. J Pediatr 1964; 64:63.

Adequacy of Maternal Therapy to Prevent Congenital Syphilis

Alford CA Jr. Discussion of paper by Scotti et al. J Pediatr 1956; 75:1133.

Dunlop EM. Survival of treponemes after treatment: comments, clinical conclusions, and recommendations. Genitourin Med 1985; 61:293.

Goldman JN, Girard KF. Intraocular treponemes in treated congenital syphilis. Arch Ophthalmol 1967; 78:47.

Hardy JB, Hardy PH, Oppenheimer EH, et al. Failure of penicillin in a newborn with congenital syphilis. J Am Med Assoc 1970; 212:1345.

Harris WD, Cave VG. Congenital syphilis in the newborn. Diagnosis and treatment. J Am Med Assoc 1965; 194:1312.

Laird SM. Failure to prevent congenital syphilis. Br Med J 1956; 1:768.

Mamunes P, Budell JW, Stewart RE, et al. Early diagnosis of neonatal syphilis. Am J Dis Child 1970; 120:17.

Mascola L, Pelosi R, Alexander CE. Inadequate treatment of syphilis in pregnancy. Am J Obstet Gynecol 1984; 150:945.

Mascola L, Pelosi R, Blount JH, et al. Congenital syphilis: why is it still occurring? J Am Med Assoc 1984; 252:1719.

Scotti A, Logan L, Caldwell JG. Fluorescent antibody tests for neonatal congenital syphilis: a prognosis report. J Pediatr 1959; 75:1129.

South MA, Short DH, Knox JM. Failure of erythromycin estolate therapy for in utero syphilis. J Am Med Assoc 1964; 190:70.

Penicillin Desensitization

Idsoe O, Guthe T, Willcox RR. Penicillin in the treatment of syphilis: the experience of three decades. Bull World Health Organ 1972; 47:1.

Wendel GD, Stark BJ, Jamison RD, et al. Penicillin allergy and desensitization in serious infections during pregnancy. N Engl J Med 1985; 312:1229.

Ziaya PR, Hankins DV, Gilstrap LG, et al. Intravenous penicillin desensitization and treatment during pregnancy. J Am Med Assoc 1986; 256:2561.

Entamoeba histolytica (Amebiasis)

INTRODUCTION

Entamoeba histolytica is a pseudopod-forming, nonflagellate protozoan parasite. Based on isoenzyme analysis, typing by monoclonal antibodies to surface antigens, and restriction length polymorphism, *E. histolytica* has been reclassified into two species that are morphologically identical: *E. histolytica*, an invasive disease-causing organism, and *E. dispar*, a noninvasive parasite.

The subspherical cyst form of *E. histolytica* ranges from 10 to 20 nm in diameter and is surrounded by a hyaline-like cyst wall. This form of the organism is present only within the lumen of the colon and in the feces. It is uninucleated and contains within its cytoplasm a large glycogen vacuole and chromatoidal bodies. The cyst undergoes binary fissions, resulting ultimately in a quadrinucleated cyst. With the series of divisions, the chromatoidal bodies and glycogen vacuole are lost. The morphologic diagnosis of amebiasis often rests on the identification of the quadrinucleated cyst form. *E. histolytica* undergoes distinct morphologic alterations during its natural life cycle within the gastrointestinal tract.

Dissemination of the organism and infection are due to ingestion of contaminated water, vegetables, or other food containing the cyst form. Asymptomatic cyst passers comprise the main reservoir for infection and disease. Cysts may remain viable for months in an appropriate moist environment. It is probable that dirt and houseflies are important intermediaries in the dissemination of the organism.

The active trophozoites are liberated by enzymatic digestion of the cyst wall within the small intestine. Organism replication is optimal under anaerobic conditions. Bacterial multiplication, by reducing the oxidation–reduction potential within areas of fecal stasis, creates an environment favorable for *E. histolytica*. Consequently, the concentrations of trophozoites are greatest at sites of maximum fecal stasis, such as the cecum, sigmoid colon, and rectum. The sites of mucosal invasion parallel the sites of greatest concentration of the organism.

The amebic trophozoites are present at the sites of tissue invasion as well as within feces. Trophozoites are characterized by granular cytoplasm in which phagocytized red blood cells can frequently be demonstrated. The erythrophagocytosis by the trophozoites is deemed a pathognomonic characteristic of *E. histolytica*.

The incidence of *E. histolytica* in a given population depends on the sources of contamination and the hygienic standards governing the environment. Infection is predominantly asymptomatic (90–99%). Only a small percentage of individuals harboring the organism experience an acute diarrheal syndrome characterized by cyclical bouts of diarrhea and constipation or, occasionally, bloody diarrhea associated with colicky abdominal pains. Most individuals eliminate the organism from the gut in 12 months.

The tissue invasiveness of the trophozoites is reflected in the organism's ability to produce ulcerated lesions associated with extensive undermining of the mucosal margins, resulting in a flask-shaped submucosal abscess. Pathogenic *E. histolytica* exerts a lytic effect on tissue. Nevertheless, unless secondary bacterial infection occurs, there is a relative paucity of an inflammatory response in the adjacent tissue. Precysts are formed as the trophozoites migrate toward the rectum.

Extraintestinal infection occurs. The prime target organs are liver, lung, brain, and spleen. The major organ of extraintestinal infection is by and large the liver. It is thought that microemboli containing trophozoites may occur as the result of thrombosis of vessels in the submucosa, particularly of the ileum. The microemboli are carried to the liver by the portal circulation. Cerebral abscesses are rare, are almost always associated with hepatic involvement, and are thought to be due to hematogenous spread.

Approximately 4% of patients with clinically overt amebiasis develop extraintestinal complications; however, the true incidence of amebic hepatic abscesses exceeds this figure. In endemic areas, more than 50% of patients with hepatic involvement give no history of amebic diarrhea or dysentery and have no demonstrable amebae in the feces.

The ability of *E. histolytica* to adhere to epithelial cells appears to be a prerequisite for disease. Amebic adherence to mammalian cells and human erythrocytes in vitro appears to be mediated by at least two amebic receptors. Amebic microfilament function and possibly intracellular calcium flux are necessary for adherence to occur. Amebae are able to lyse target cells only after adherence has occurred. Cytolysis requires intact amebic microfilament and calcium flux to function.

Host factors such as age, species specificity, bacterial flora, nutrition, iron availability, and cholesterol levels may be relevant to occurrence of disease. High-carbohydrate, low-protein diets produce more severe amebiasis in laboratory animals. A high incidence of amebic dysentery as well as extraintestinal amebiasis is documented in populations subsisting on diets of this nature.

In the United States, women at greatest risk for developing clinically overt amebiasis are immigrants from and travelers to countries where infection is endemic. Infection usually manifests within a year of immigration to the United States. Travelers returning from endemic areas are at a low but definite risk of acquiring amebic infection. In a study of 2700 German citizens returning from tropical areas, Weinke et al. (1990) documented a 4% incidence of *E. histolytica/E. dispar* infection. Diarrhea occurred in 80%

of travelers with *E. histolytica*. Only 5% of travelers with diarrhea and amebic infection had *E. dispar* infection.

AMEBIASIS AND PREGNANCY

Malnutrition and the immunosuppression of pregnancy may convert asymptomatic intestinal or vaginal carriage into clinically overt disease or magnify the resultant morbidity of disease. Amebiasis occurring in a gravida tends to be more severe and is associated with a higher incidence of complications. Abioye (1973) noted that 68% of fatal cases of amebiasis in females occurred in association with pregnancy. On the other hand, only 17.1% of fatal typhoid cases and 12.5% of other fatal enterocolitis cases among females occurred during pregnancy. Czeizel et al. (1966) noted that women with spontaneous abortions had a significantly higher incidence of positive stool cultures for *E. histolytica*, as compared to women having term births.

As a rule, more severe disease is seen in the very young and old, the malnourished, and pregnant women.

FEMALE GENITAL TRACT INVOLVEMENT

Two syndromes that can be attributed to *E. histolytica* are encountered in the nonpregnant female and involve the female genital tract. They are

1. amebic vulvovaginitis and
2. amebic vulvar ulcers (cutaneous amebiasis).

Although extraintestinal amebiasis is thought to be caused by blood-borne microemboli from the intestines, involvement of the female genital tract is more likely due to metastatic mechanical spread from feces or anorectal involvement, or both. Characteristically, the patient complains of a serosanguineous or seropurulent vaginal discharge, soreness of the vagina, and dyspareunia. The character of the vaginal discharge may be so sanguinous that a patient complains of menstruating every day or, in postmenopausal women, of recurrence of menses.

Amebic penetration of the vaginal mucosa is associated with cell necrosis. In general, the edge of the resultant ulcer is relatively shallow compared to those in the gastrointestinal tract. Secondary bacterial infection is primarily responsible for purulent sloughing of the overlying mucosa and severe inflammatory reactions in the submucosa.

Colonization or mild diarrhea with *E. dispar* rarely requires medical intervention as these ameba have not been identified as the etiology of colitis or hepatic abscess. In contrast, women colonized by *E. histolytica* are at risk months and even possibly years later for the development of invasive disease.

DIAGNOSIS

Patients with amebic colitis characteristically present with a history over several weeks of gradual abdominal pain and diarrhea which may be overtly bloody. Fever is present in the minority of patients with amebic colitis and absent in women with vulvovaginal disease.

The initial diagnostic dilemma is distinguishing diarrhea that contains blood due to amebiasis from that caused by *Shigella, Salmonella, Campylobacter, Clostridium difficile*, and enteroinvasive/enterohemorrhagic *Escherichia coli*. The diagnosis of amebic colitis may be difficult as the presentation may be insidious. Bleeding may occur without diarrhea. Fever is an unusual finding. A single stool examination for parasites is insensitive and nonspecific. The identification of motile trophozoites with engulfed red blood cells in test material is relatively specific, but not sensitive for determining the presence of *E. histolytica*. The sensitive for microscopy can be as low as 30%. The diagnosis of amebiasis is made by identifying trophozoites or cysts in vaginal discharge or ulcer exudate. Only the trophozoites are present in the exudate. Scraping of the ulcer edge or of discharge should be examined for motile erythrocyte-containing amebae by direct mount in saline on a warm microscope stage. The characteristic motility is that of a directed, linear movement across the microscope stage. Microscopic examination is not species specific. Erythrophagocytic ameba are more likely to be *E. histolytica* than *E. dispar*. Because a single stool examination identifies only one-third of infected patients, at least three specimens should be examined for amebic cysts and trophozoites before excluding the diagnosis of amebiasis.

In vitro culture and isoenzyme analysis can be done; however, none of the existing culture methods are selective for *E. histolytica*. Isoenzyme analysis is the current gold standard for diagnosis. The test requires one to two weeks to complete, which renders it impractical as a clinical tool.

In biopsy material stained with conventional hematoxylin and eosin, the amebae are not readily identifiable except by experienced viewers. It is necessary to utilize periodic acid-Schiff stain, which causes the amoebae to stand out as bright red rounded bodies. Histologic confirmation of infection on a biopsy specimen may miss a diagnostic lesion.

The diagnostic gold standard is culture confirmation with isoenzyme analysis. Advances in technology [strain-specific DNA probes and polymerase chain reaction (PCR)] have made direct detection of *E. histolytica* antigens in serum and feces possible. Using enzyme-linked immunosorbent assay (ELISA) or epitope-specific monoclonal antibodies, one can further differentiate nonpathogenic from pathogenic *E. histolytica*. Demonstration of galactose adhesion in serum is highly specific for infection by pathogenic *E. histolytica*. PCR and antigen-detection tests have comparable sensitivities, identifying approximately 85% of *E. histolytica* identified by the gold standard.

Several ELISA and indirect hemoagglutination (IHA) tests have been developed that identify the presence of antibodies to *Entamoeba*. Serological tests for *E. histolytica* tend to remain positive for years after initial infection. These may be of limited value in distinguishing current disease from a prior invasive event. Eighty-five percent of patients with biopsy-proven invasive intestinal amebiasis have a positive serologic study by various techniques. The elevation of specific antibody titers does not correlate with severity of disease. The prime value of serologic testing is in enhancing or supporting a tentative diagnosis of extraintestinal (hepatic) amebiasis.

In cases of amebic vulvovaginitis or cutaneous ulcers, the possibility of concomitant amoebic complications must be ruled out.

THERAPY

The key to therapy of amoebic vulvovaginitis is the eradication of the intestinal reservoir of the organism. Local vulvar lesions will respond to systemic therapy for amebiasis. Drug therapy for genital involvement is contingent on the extent of the disease process elsewhere. Metronidazole (Flagyl) coupled with luminal therapy is the regimen intestinal for amebiasis. Side effects with metronidazole include anorexia, nausea, metallic taste, disulfiram-like reaction to alcohol, and peripheral neuropathy. In rare cases, seizures have occurred following administration of metronidazole in large doses. Treatment with metronidazole should be followed with a luminal agent to avoid the risk of relapse. Tinidazole and omidazole are as effective as, if not more effective than, metronidazole and are better tolerated.

Simple colonization with *E. histolytica* can be treated with a luminal agent alone. Drugs effective against uncomplicated gastrointestinal infection include paromomycin and iodoquinol. The recommended duration of administration with paromomycin is seven days, and with iodoquinol, it is 20 days. The dosage for iodoquinol is 650 mg tid.

Paromomycin has been used in pregnancy. Given as 5 to 35 mg/kg/day in thee divided doses, it has the advantage in pregnancy of being better tolerated. Cure rates as high as 92% have been achieved. Sigmoidoscopic studies indicate that trophozoites are no longer in the feces, and the ulcers heal by the end of the fifth or sixth day of treatment. Because therapy is only 90% to 95% effective, follow-up cultures of both genital sites of infection and stool are generally warranted.

SELECTED READING

Abd-Alla MD, Jackson TFGH, Gatherim V, et al. Differentiation of pathogenic from nonpathogenic *Entamoeba histolytica* infection by detection of galactose-inhibitable adherence protein antigen in sera and feces. J Clin Microbiol 1993; 31:2845.

Acuna-Soto R, Samuelson J, de Girolami, et al. Application of polymerase chain reaction to the epidemiology of pathogenic and nonpathogenic *Entamoeba histolytica*. Am J Trop Med 1993; 48:58.

Armon PJ. Amoebiasis in pregnancy and the puerperium. Br J Obstet Gynaecol 1978; 85:264.

Gonzalez-Ruiz A, Haque R, Aguirre A, et al. Value of microscopy in the diagnosis of dysentery associated with invasive *Entamoeba histolytica*. J Clin Pathol 1994; 47:236.

Gonzalez-Ruiz A, Haque R, Rehman T, et al. Diagnosis of amebic dysentery by detection of *Entamoeba histolytica* fecal antigen by an invasive strain-specific, monoclonal antibody-based enzyme linked immunoabsorbent assay. J Clin Microbiol 1994; 32:964.

Kobiler D, Mirelman D. Adhesion of *Entamoeba histolytica* trophozoites to monolayers of human cells. J Infect Dis 1981; 144:539.

Li E, Stanley SL Jr. Protozoa. Amebiasis. Gastroenterol Clin North Am 1996; 25:471.

McAuley JB, Juranek DD. Paromomycin in the treatment of mild-to-moderate intestinal amoebiasis. Clin Infect Dis 1992; 15:551.

Patterson M, Healy GR, Shabot JM. Serologic testing for amoebiasis. Gastroenterology 1980; 78:136.

Petri WA Jr. Recent advances in amebiasis. Crit Rev Clin Lab Sci 1996; 33:1.

Petri WA Jr, Clark GC, Mann BJ, et al. International seminar on amoebiasis. Parasitol Today 1993; 9:73.

Phillips SC, Mildvan D, William DC, et al. Sexual transmission of enteric protozoa and helminths in a venereal-disease-clinic population. N Engl J Med 1981; 305:603.

Ravdin JI. Intestinal disease caused by *Entamoeba histolytica*. In: Ravdin JI, ed. Amebiasis: Human Infection by Entamoeba histolytica. New York: Churchill Livingstone 1988:495–510.

Ravdin JI, Guerrant RL. Role of adherence in cytopathogenic mechanisms of *Entamoeba histolytica*. J Clin Invest 1981; 68:1305.

Amebiasis and Pregnancy

Abioye AA. Fatal amoebic colitis in pregnancy and the puerperium: a new clinico-pathological entity. J Trop Med Hyg 1973; 76:97.

Armon PJ. Amoebiasis in pregnancy and the puerperium. Br J Obstet Gynaecol 1978; 85:264.

Atlay RD, Weekes AR. The treatment of gastrointestinal disease in pregnancy. Clin Obstet Gynaecol 1986; 13:335.

Constantine G, Menon V, Luesley D. Amoebic peritonitis in pregnancy in the United Kingdom. Postgrad Med J 1987; 63:495.

Czeizel E, Hancsok M, Palkowich I, et al. Possible relation between fetal death and *E. histolytica* infection of the mother. Am J Obstet Gynecol 1966; 96:264.

Grandien M, Sterner G, Kalin M, Engardt L. Management of pregnant women with diarrhea at term and of healthy carriers of infectious agents in stools at delivery. Scand J Infect Dis 1990; 71:9.

Haddock DW. Treatment of parasitic infestations and exotic disease in pregnancy. Clin Exp Obstet Gynecol 1986; 13:368.

Kerrigan KR. Fulminant amoebic colitis in pregnancy. Trop Doctor 1991; 21:46.

McCahill ME, Braff DL. Atypical postpartum psychosis possibly associated with metronidazole therapy. J Fam Pract 1988; 27:323.

Miltra S. Tropical diseases and pregnancy. In: Holland E, Bourne O, eds. British Obstetrical and Gynecological Practice, 2nd ed. London: Heineman, 1959.

Reinhardt MC. Effects of parasitic infections in pregnant women. In: Perinatal Infections. Ciba Foundation Symposium 77. Amsterdam: Excerpta Medica, 1980:149.

Wagner VP, Smale LE, Lischke JH. Amebic abscess of the liver and spleen in pregnancy and the puerperium. Obstet Gynecol 1975; 45:562.

Weingerz Mehl S, Perez Torres JF, Moran Cruz JJ. The incidence of amebiasis in abortion. Ginecol Obstetr De Mexico 1988; 56:251.

Weinke T, Fredrich-Janicke B, Hopp P, et al. Prevalence and clinical importance *Entamoeba histolytica* in two high-risk groups: travelers returning from the tropics and male homosexuals. J Infect Dis 1990; 161:1029.

Wig JD, Bushnurmath SR, Kaushik SP. Complications of amoebiasis in pregnancy and puerperium. Indian J Gastroenterol 1984; 3:37.

Genital Tract Amebiasis

Adams EB, MacLeod N. Invasive amebiasis. I. Amebic dysentery and its complications. Medicine 1977; 56:315.

Moghraby AS. A case of amoebic vaginitis. J Obstet Gynecol Br Commonw 1960; 67:332.

Seldom RE. Pseudo-malignant cutaneous amoebiasis. Am J Trop Med Hyg 1972; 21:18.

Weinstein BB, Weed JC. Amoebic vaginitis. Am J Obstet Gynecol 1948; 56:180.

Wilmot AJ. Clinical Amoebiasis. Philadelphia: Davis, 1962.

Plasmodial Infections (Malaria) 54

INTRODUCTION

Malarial infection in humans results from the bite of an infected female *Anopheles* mosquito in which the sporogenic cycle of development of the malarial parasite has taken place. Schizogony, or the asexual cycle (Fig. 1), begins within the parenchymal cells of the liver. The exo-erythrocytic cycles within the liver result in the production of merozoites. This form of the malarial parasite then enters red blood cells where it develops and multiplies asexually. This is termed the schizogenic erythrocytic cycle. The end product is a new crop of merozoites, which are released through rupture from the cells and recommence the cycle. During the erythrocytic cycle, a few parasites become differentiated into male and female gametocytes and are present within the intravascular compartment awaiting ingestion by blood-sucking female *Anopheles* mosquitoes to complete their life cycle. Within the mosquitoes, fertilization occurs, with the production of the zygote. The zygote then undergoes successive stages of differentiation into an ookinete, which then penetrates the stomach wall of the mosquito to form an oocyst. From the mature oocyst, sporozoites are liberated; these ultimately migrate

to and reside within the salivary gland of the mosquito. They are then injected with the saliva into the human host at the time of a blood meal.

The incubation period from the infective bite by the *Anopheles* mosquito and onset of symptomology varies between 7 and 30 days. The shorter incubation periods are observed most frequently with *Plasmodium falciparum* and the longer ones with *Plasmodium malariae*.

Four different species of *Plasmodium* infect humans: *P. vivax*, *P. ovale*, *P. malariae*, and *P. falciparum*. Although basically similar in their life cycles, they differ significantly in pathogenic potential, relapse rate, chronicity, and development of resistance to drugs.

IMMUNOLOGY OF INFECTION

An understanding of female genital tract involvement in malaria is almost inseparable from an understanding of the immunology of infection. Plasmodial infection, owing to an intravascular cycle and access to the reticuloendothelial (RE) system, represents an intense form of antigenic stimulation. Marked immunoglobulin synthesis occurs, resulting in greatly

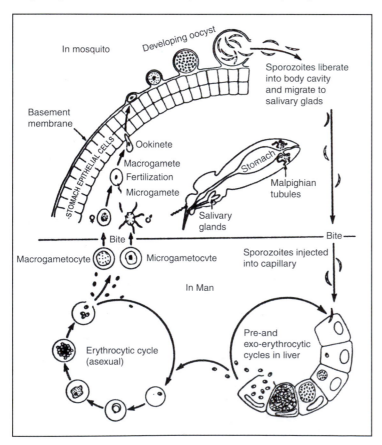

FIGURE 1 Life cycle of *Plasmodium vivax*. *Source:* Adam MG. In: Medical and Veterinary Protozoology. Edinburgh: Livingstone, 1971:89.

increased levels of serum immunoglobulins. Shortly after parasitemia appears, there is a marked increase in immunoglobulin G (IgG), IgM, and IgA antibodies, with IgG rising to the highest levels and persisting the longest. The end result is a hypergammaglobulinemia, the major component of which is IgG. Only 1% to 5% of the IgG appears to be specific antibodies. IgG and IgM antibodies, principally the former, can afford some protection apparently, mainly against the merozoite stage of the parasite.

Immunity to infection usually requires repeated exposure to the parasite to become long-lasting. The malarial organisms have the ability to vary major target antigens. Antibody-dependent immunity is mediated primarily by cytophilic IgG antibodies, which activate cytotoxic and phagocytic effector functions of neutrophils and monocytes. Malarial infection also results in the production of IgE-specific antibodies. IgE immune complexes, by cross-linking IgE receptors on monocytes, elicit a local overproduction of tumor necrosis factor (TNF). Elevated production of TNF is associated with increased risk of severe disease and death due to P. falciparum infection.

The major cells controlling blood-stage infection are the TH1 and TH2 subsets of CD4 cells. Interferon-gamma production plays a key role in antimalarial defense.

Antibodies to the malarial parasites tend to be basically species and strain specific. This can be strongly inferred from clinical studies. The administration of 2.5 g hyperimmune gamma-globulin to children results in both a dramatic drop in parasitemia and, within one week, a progressive regulation of disease. This phenomenon is not observed with nonimmune gamma-globulin nor with that prepared from an endemic area where different strains of Plasmodium predominate. The effectiveness of passively acquired specific antibody from mother to fetus also suggests the importance of humoral immunity. Even when parasitemia occurs at birth, its clinical expression is suppressed.

Parasitemia results in hypertrophy of the RE system, as reflected by hepatosplenomegaly and by bone marrow alterations. The importance of this, as can be shown experimentally, is that nonspecific activation of phagocytosis can greatly increase the rate of parasitic removal. The importance of the RE system in controlling erythrocytic infection can be inferred from the effects of splenectomy, which, in essence, constitutes a significant reduction in the size of the RE pool. Splenectomy decreases immunity to all malarial parasites and may result in relapse and recrudescence of infection.

Phagocytosis of the parasites is often opsonin mediated. The antigens on the surface of the parasitized erythrocytes are important in terms of opsonization and phagocytosis of infected erythrocytes. Destruction of the parasite is predicated on intracellular digestion by macrophage elements. The immune destruction of red blood cells may produce a serious folic acid deficiency, which not infrequently is superimposed on a microcytic hypochromic iron-deficiency anemia.

Malaria is a worldwide problem of massive scale that has been compounded by the development of drug-resistant P. falciparum. About 40% of the world's population is at risk of acquiring malaria. The annual occurrence of malaria is estimated to be 500 million cases. Deaths from malaria range up to 3 million cases per year. The majority of deaths involve children under five years of age and pregnant women.

In the United States, over 1000 cases of malaria are reported by health officials annually. The majority of cases occur among immigrants and travelers to endemic malaria regions. They are imported from regions in the world where malaria transmission is known to occur. However, each year, congenital infection and infection resulting from exposure to blood or blood products are reported in the United States. In rare instances, infection has occurred through local mosquito-borne transmission. More than 80% of imported malaria cases occurred in persons who were either not taking or taking nonrecommended chemoprophylaxis.

MALARIA IN PREGNANCY

Malarial infection in pregnancy is associated with significant maternal and perinatal mortality. Pregnant women are three times more likely to develop severe disease than nonpregnant women acquiring infection in the same area. Malarial parasitic sequestration and replication within the placenta adds an additional adverse element to fetal well-being. Malaria in pregnancy can lead to miscarriage, premature delivery, low birthweight, congenital infection, and/or neonatal mortality. When pregnancy is concomitantly complicated by malaria and HIV infections, the consequences in terms of morbidity and mortality are enhanced proportional to the degree of immunocompromise present.

Malaria is said to be exacerbated by pregnancy. Women with little or no immunological experience with the parasite prior to the first pregnancy are particularly vulnerable to infection. Ensuing disease tends to be more virulent.

Mechanisms by which organisms, especially P. falciparum, produce added morbidity include: (i) collection of infected erythrocytes within proteoglycan matrix of the placenta, (ii) infected erythrocytes sequestered throughout the placenta, (iii) stimulation of pancreatic beta cells leading to hyperinsulinemia and subsequent hypoglycemia, and (iv) cerebral involvement.

Parasites have been shown to adhere to the surface of the trophoblastic villi, eliciting local inflammation and necrosis of adjacent placental tissue. Histologically, placental malaria is characterized by the presence of parasites and leucocytes within the intervillous spaces, proliferation of cytotrophoblastic cells, and thickening of trophoblastic basement membrane. In holoendemic areas, both placental infection and poor pregnancy outcomes decrease in frequency with successive pregnancies.

It has long been noted that women residing in areas endemic for malaria appear to lose some of their acquired resistance during pregnancy and may experience severe malarial attacks. A theoretic basis for this clinical impression seems to exist. For many strains of P. falciparum, maturation of the schizonts occurs within the bloodstream in what are termed "internal organs" or "deep sinuses," for example, the spleen. Sequestration results from adhesive interaction between parasite-derived proteins expressed on the surface of red blood cells and host molecules on the surface of endothelial and cytotrophoblastic cells. Parasite-encoded adhesion molecules prevent the circulation of parasitized erythrocytes. The maternal vascular compartment within the placenta constitutes an additional site for parasitic replication. The greatest degree of placental infestation is observed in highly immune patients. While maternal symptomatology is relatively mild, fetal wastage is disproportionately increased. Experimental data tend to point to a decreased maternal response in terms of cellular immunity and a possible decrease in RE system clearance during pregnancy. Should such data be applicable and substantiated in human subjects, they might provide a partial mechanism for the clinical deterioration observed in pregnancy.

Severe attacks of malaria not infrequently result in second-trimester abortion, intrauterine death with macerated stillbirths, fresh stillbirths due to intrapartum asphyxia, or premature labor and delivery. The predominantly hypochromic microcytic anemia caused by the plasmodial organisms may be of sufficient severity to induce congestive heart failure. If the disease remains untreated, both maternal and fetal demise may occur. In hyperendemic areas, gravidas may exhibit severe anemia and marked hepatosplenomegaly at the time of parturition. The enlarged spleen may protrude into the pelvis and, on a mechanical basis, cause dystocia.

Potential maternal complications include severe anemia, thrombocytopenia, hypoglycemia, lactic acidosis, renal failure, cardiopulmonary failure, cerebral involvement, and postpartum hemorrhage.

Fetal consequences of malaria are due primarily to the magnitude of placental involvement and the severity of maternal disease. These include intrauterine growth retardation, preterm delivery, low-birthweight newborns, and higher rates of infant mortality.

CONGENITAL MALARIA

Detectable malarial parasitemia in newborn babies from areas highly endemic for malaria is strikingly rare. In contrast, infants from nonindigenous infected mothers may have clinically overt congenital malaria. The importance of passive transfer of immunity is suggested by the initial rarity of disease in neonates and infants in an endemic area. Congenital malaria is exceptional in babies of immune mothers, even though the placenta is not infrequently—and sometimes heavily—infected. With increasing degrees of immunity to malaria, the frequency of placental infection rises. The intervillous space in the placenta may be packed with parasitized cells and macrophages. More severe infestation tends to occur in gravida with established immunity.

Well-immunized patients through prior exposure to the parasites tend to have minimal clinical symptoms of malaria, but have significant fetal wastage. Placental infection with *P. falciparum* is associated with low-birthweight babies on the presumed basis of impaired placental circulation.

The relatively common occurrence of congenital malaria in babies born to nonimmune but infected mothers indicates that in the majority of cases, the parasites often attain access in utero to the fetal circulation. It is presumed that the levels of specific protective maternally derived antibodies prevent parasitic multiplication. Even when parasitemia is present at birth, the disease process is usually not manifested until the second or third month, at a time when the bulk of maternally acquired specific antibodies has undergone degradative elimination.

DIAGNOSIS

The signs and symptoms of malaria are variable. The majority of patients present with fever. Other common symptoms include headache, back pain, chills, increased sweating, myalgia, nausea, vomiting, diarrhea, and cough. These first symptoms of malaria are often not specific and are common to a number of other infectious diseases.

Uncomplicated malaria: The initial malaria attack lasts 6 to 10 hours. It consists of a cold stage characterized by shivering, which is followed then by fever, headache, and vomiting. With the onset of significant sweating, the temperature returns to a normal range. Classically, such an attack occurs every second day with *P. falciparum, P. vivax, and P. ovale*, and every third day with *P. malariae*.

Severe malaria: Severe malaria occurs most often in individuals who have no prior immunity, particularly to *P. falciparum*, or whose immunity to the parasite has decreased. The manifestations of severe malaria include abnormal behavior, impaired consciousness, seizures, severe anemia, hemoglobinuria, and pulmonary edema, or adult respiratory distress syndrome, thrombocytopenia, and cardiovascular collapse. Severe malaria is a medical emergency and should be treated urgently and aggressively.

In *P. vivax* and *P. ovale* infections, patients who have recovered from the first episode of illness may suffer several additional attacks after months or even years without symptoms. Relapses occur because *P. vivax* and *P. oval* leave dormant liver-stage hypnozoites that may reactivate.

Malaria needs to be included in the differential diagnosis of illness in a febrile person with a recent history of travel to a malarial area. Clinicians should ask febrile patients for a travel history, particularly when evaluating febrile illnesses in international visitors, immigrants, refugees, migrant laborers, and international travelers.

The presence of detectable parasitemia almost always accompanies a clinical malaria attack; however, parasitemia may occur in the absence of significant symptoms.

The diagnosis of acute, active malaria is based on the identification of asexual stages in the erythrocytes. Diagnosis of acute malaria depends on the identification of the parasites in the peripheral blood or in bone marrow. Usually, when the organisms are not readily demonstrable in the blood, bone marrow examination is also likely to be unproductive.

Demonstration of gametocytes, while confirming malarial infection, is not diagnostic of acute infection. Gametocytes may be found in the peripheral blood weeks and even months after an overt attack has subsided or been cured.

Both thick and thin blood smears should be made. The thick blood smear is made by touching a drop of blood with a clean slide. Using the corner of another slide, spread the blood drop into the shape of a circle or a square of about 1 cm². Gently squeeze the patient's finger again and touch the end of a clean slide to the newly formed drop of blood. Take this slide and hold the edge that has the drop of blood at a 45° angle against the surface of the first slide. Wait until the blood has completely spread along the edge of the second slide. While holding the second slide at the same angle, rapidly and smoothly push the slide forward to make the thin smear. Air dry the thin film slide, fix it with methyl alcohol, and stain with Giemsa's stain. *Plasmodium* parasites are always intracellular. If properly stained, they appear with blue cytoplasm with a red chromatin dot.

Persons suspected of having malaria but whose blood smears do not show the presence of the parasite should have blood smears repeated every 12 to 24 hours for three consecutive days. The numbers of parasites in peripheral blood smears may vary significantly during a given day. Consequently, repeated examination may be necessary to establish the diagnosis of active malaria.

As a rule, all stages of the erythrocytic cycle can be found in peripheral blood smears of subjects with active vivax, malariae, and ovale malaria. Only the ring forms usually occur in falciparum malaria during the first 10 days of the clinical attack. If no parasites are found on the thin film, wait until the thick film is dry and examine it for organisms that might not have been detected on the thin film preparation.

Rapid diagnostic tests (RDTs) and polymerase chain reaction tests have been developed. Although currently, RDTs are not approved by the U.S. Food and Drug Administration for use in the United States, the World Health Organization (WHO) does provide information on commercially available RDTs, at http://www.wpro.who.int/rdt/.

THERAPY

Since the clinical manifestations of acute malaria are the consequence of the erythrocytic cycle of the parasite, therapy is directed at eradicating this phase of infection. Drugs that destroy the erythrocytic forms of the parasites are termed schizonticides. They include 4-aminoquinolines, quinine, chloroguanide (proguanil), and pyrimethamine. Of these, only the 4-aminoquinolines are commonly used. To achieve a radical cure in *P. vivax*, *P. ovale*, and *P. malariae* infections, chloroquine has been combined with an 8-aminoquinoline such as primaquine. The destruction of the persistent exoerythrocytic parasites in the liver is achieved only by the latter group of drugs, the 8-aminoquinolines.

Any patient receiving primaquine should ideally be tested for glucose-6-phosphate dehydrogenase (G6PD) deficiency to avoid the possibility of hemolysis in susceptible individuals. The drug is given to destroy the exoerythrocytic forms of the parasite which persist within the parenchymal cells of the liver and from which the relapse-provoking parasites

emerge. If the enzymatic deficiency cannot be tested for, it is suggested that patients receive a dose one-quarter of that normally administered and be closely observed.

The choice of chemotherapy is influenced by three considerations, including the species of *Plasmodium*, the immunologic status of the individual, and the susceptibility or resistance of the infecting parasite to antimalarial therapy. Chloroquine-resistance of *P. falciparum* is a significant therapeutic problem. In *P. falciparum* infections, eradication of the erythrocytic cycle is the prime objective of therapy. In the relapsing malarias, eradication of both the erythrocytic and the exoerythrocytic cycle necessitates individualized therapy.

Some of the prophylactic drugs have been shown to alter glutathione levels, and in so doing, they may exacerbate the oxidation–reduction potential attendant in HIV infection. The potential for antimalarial agents to cause problems when combined with other drugs needs careful evaluation.

For pregnant women diagnosed with uncomplicated malaria caused by *P. malariae*, *P. vivax*, *P. ovale*, or chloroquine-sensitive *P. falciparum*, prompt treatment with chloroquine using the treatment schedule for nonpregnant adults is recommended by the Centers for Disease Control and Prevention (CDC). As a second-line alternative for treatment, hydroxychloroquine may be given. For pregnant women diagnosed with uncomplicated malaria caused by chloroquine-resistant *P. falciparum*, prompt treatment with quinine sulfate and clindamycin is recommended. Quinine treatment should be continued for seven days for infections acquired in Southeast Asia and for three days for infections acquired in Africa or South America. Clindamycin treatment should be for seven days regardless of where the infection was acquired.

Chloroquine, a category C drug, appears to be safe in all trimesters. It is used as first-line therapy except when *P. falciparum* resistance has been documented. The drug can be administered orally or by intravenous infusion.

Atovaquone/proguanil is classified as a pregnancy category C drug. It is generally not indicated for use in pregnancy because no adequate, well-controlled clinical trials exist for atovaquone and/or proguanil hydrochloride in pregnant women. For women diagnosed with uncomplicated malaria caused by chloroquine-resistant *P. falciparum* infection, atovaquone/proguanil may be used if other treatment options are not available or are not being tolerated. The potential benefit needs to outweigh projected risks.

Mefloquine is another category C drug that, although not generally indicated for treatment in pregnant women, has been used in the therapy of chloroquine-resistant parasites. Mefloquine has not been associated with an increased risk of congenital abnormalities; however, a possible association between mefloquine treatment in pregnancy and an increase in stillbirths has been reported. The CDC recommends mefloquine only when no other treatment options are available and if the potential benefit is judged to outweigh the potential risks.

For *P. vivax* and *P. ovale* infections, primaquine phosphate for radical treatment of hypnozoites *should not be given during pregnancy.* Pregnant patients with *P. vivax* or *P. ovale* infections should be maintained on chloroquine prophylaxis (300 mg base PO once per week) during their pregnancy. After delivery, infected individuals who do not have G6PD deficiency should be aggressively treated with primaquine (category C drug).

Severe *P. falciparum* Infection

Complicated *P. falciparum* infection is a medical emergency and requires aggressive medical care. An essential component of the management of severe *P. falciparum* infection is the prompt parenteral administration of a rapidly acting drug that kills the asexual erythrocytic stages of the parasite (a schizonticidal drug). Equally important is counteracting the presence of significant anemia.

Quinidine, the dextrorotatory diastereoisomer of quinine, is widely available in the United States as parenteral quinidine gluconate. It is primarily used in the treatment of persons with cardiac arrhythmias; however, it has also long been recognized as a potent antimalarial. On an equimolar basis, quinidine is a more active antimalarial than quinine for *P. falciparum*.

WHO has recommended that an individual with malaria should be treated parenterally if (*i*) vomiting is prominent and oral fluids and medication are not retained, (*ii*) there are signs or symptoms of neurologic dysfunction, or (*iii*) the peripheral asexual parasitemia is at a level of >5% of erythrocytes infected.

Quinidine administered by slow intravenous infusion is generally well tolerated, even by critically ill patients, individuals with underlying cardiac disease, and children. Close attention to electrocardiographic changes, such as prolongation of the QT-interval and widening of the QRS complex, may be an accurate indicator of both plasma concentration and incipient cardiotoxicity. Continuous-infusion quinidine gluconate produces effective drug concentrations. A loading dose of 10 mg of quinidine gluconate salt (equivalent to 6.2 mg of quinidine base)/kg of body weight is given over one to two hours, followed by a constant infusion of 0.0125 mg of quinidine gluconate base/kg/min (0.02 mg salt/kg/min). Plasma quinidine levels >6 mg/mL, QT interval >0.6S, or QRS widening beyond 25% of baseline are indications for slowing infusion rates.

Persons with hypoglycemia, which may be a manifestation of *P. falciparum* malaria and which is exacerbated by quinine/quinidine-induced hyperinsulinemia, should be treated with intravenous dextrose.

Parenteral therapy should continue until parasitemia is <1% (generally, within 48 hours) and/or until oral medication can be tolerated. When patients with cerebral malaria are treated, clinical improvement is usually observed within 72 hours. If improvement does not occur, drug resistance or inadequate drug delivery, complications of malaria, or other etiologies for the illness should be investigated. Treatment is continued (usually with oral quinine) for a total of three or seven days, depending on the geographic origin of the infecting parasite (seven days for Southeast Asia, three days for Africa and South America).

The course of the parasitemia must be assessed at 12-hour intervals. Failure to reduce parasitemia in the first 24 to 48 hours of treatment should raise the possibility of parasitic resistance to that treatment. No sexual parasite should be detectable on smears four to five days after the course of chloroquine is completed. Persistence after the fifth day indicates drug failure. Gametocytes may persist in the blood for weeks after asexual forms have been successfully eliminated; however, these gametocytes do not cause disease. Their presence should not be indicative of partial treatment failure.

In the nonimmune subject who is unlikely to be reexposed, the objective of therapy may be complete parasitic eradication. In patients in endemic areas, the goal of therapy is to suppress rather than to eradicate infection. Complete eradication would lead to a loss of immunity and probably reinfection. In general, chemotherapeutic agents are administered orally. The parenteral route is indicated only when oral administration is impossible or when parasitemia is severe and rapid control is essential.

The CDC recommends that exchange transfusion be considered for individuals with a parasite density of more than 10% or if a complication such as cerebral edema, nonvolume overload pulmonary edema, or renal complications exists.

MALARIA PROPHYLAXIS

WHO recommends malaria prevention and control during pregnancy in areas of stable transmission with the use of intermittent preventive treatment (IPT) and insecticide-treated bed nets. Sulfadoxine–pyrimethamine has been used for IPT.

Chemoprophylaxis against malaria in pregnancy has included chloroquine, mefloquine, proguanil, pyrimethamine, and pyrimethamine–sulfadone. Use of these agents has been based primarily on risk–benefit criteria.

CDC recommends mefloquine (Lariam) alone for malaria prevention for nonimmune travelers to areas with drug-resistant *P. falciparum* malaria. Based on accumulating experience with this drug, the prophylactic dosing regimen has been revised to a single dose of mefloquine to be taken every week. The first dose should be taken one week before travel. It should be continued weekly during the entire period of travel in malarious areas and for four weeks after departure from such areas.

Mefloquine is well tolerated when used for prophylaxis. No serious adverse reactions to mefloquine prophylaxis (i.e., psychoses and convulsions) have been observed among persons enrolled in most prophylactic drug trials and surveys of travelers who were taking mefloquine weekly. However, serious adverse reactions have been reported, especially when mefloquine was used for treatment of patients with malaria. The drug is not recommended for use by travelers with known hypersensitivity to mefloquine, pregnant women, travelers using beta blockers, travelers involved in tasks requiring fine coordination and spatial discrimination, such as airplane pilots, and travelers with histories of epilepsy or psychiatric disorder.

Travelers to areas of risk where chloroquine-resistant *P. falciparum* is endemic and for whom mefloquine is contraindicated may elect to use daily doxycycline alone or chloroquine alone. If chloroquine is used, the traveler needs to be aware of the need to seek medical attention for febrile episodes and to carry a treatment dose of pyrimethamine–sulfadoxine (Fansidar®) to be used if medical care is not available within 24 hours. Because of the ever-changing guidelines, consultation should be obtained from CDC's Malaria Branch, Division of Parasitic Diseases, Center for Infectious Diseases (Table 1).

The use of doxycycline in pregnancy is contraindicated owing to the potential induction of thalidomide-like anomalies if given in the period of osseous organogenesis or subsequent adverse impact on bone and dental development.

Malarial chemoprophylaxis with chloroquine phosphate during pregnancy presents the problem of potential embryopathy. Retinopathy, auditory nerve injury, and central nervous system disturbances have been noted with the use of chloroquine. Hart (1983) and Nauton reported on a patient who had taken excessive amounts of chloroquine during four of her seven pregnancies. One pregnancy terminated in miscarriage at four months. The remaining three pregnancies resulted in two children with evidence of eighth nerve damage. One child had concomitant posterior column disease and was severely mentally retarded. The remaining child had neonatal convulsions.

Although Fansidar also presents theoretical problems, the drug has yet not been shown to be teratogenic in humans. At the time of parturition, sulfonamides may increase the risk of hyperbilirubinemic neonates because of displacement of unconjugated bilirubin from albumin. Short-acting sulfonamides should not be used close to term. Reinstitution of their use is contraindicated in a nursing mother.

Despite the potential induction of an embryopathy, combined maternal and fetal considerations may argue for chloroquine prophylaxis for gravidas visiting malarial endemic areas. The suggested prophylactic dose is 500 mg chloroquine phosphate (300 mg chloroquine base) orally once a week. Medication should be initiated one week prior to entry into the endemic area and continued for six weeks after departure. Nursing infants are thought to develop adequate drug levels provided the mother is on full-dose chemoprophylaxis.

SELECTED READING

Malaria in Pregnancy
Archibald HM. Influence of maternal malaria on newborn infants. Br Med J 1958; 2:1512.
Blacklock DB, Gordon RM. Malaria infection as it occurs in late pregnancy. Am J Trop Med 1925; 19:326.
Edozien JC, Gilles HM, Udeozo IOK. Adult and cord-blood gammaglobulin and immunity to malaria in Nigerians. Lancet 1962; 2:951.
Hart WA. Chemoprophlaxis of malaria in Africa. Br Med J 1983; 286:978.
Lewis R, Lauersen WH, Birnbaum S. Malaria associated with pregnancy. Obstet Gynecol 1973; 42:696.
Louis CF. Malaria occurring during the puerperium and in the neonate. Med J Aust 1965; 1:223.
Nguyen-Dinh P, Steketee RW, Greenberg AE, et al. Rapid spontaneous clearance of *Plasmodium falciparum* in African Women. Lancet 1988; 2:751.
Phillips RE, Looareesuwan S, White NJ, et al. Quinine pharmacokinetics and toxicity in pregnant and lactating women with falciparum malaria. Br J Clin Pharmacol 1986; 21:677.
Sankar D, Richards A, Moodley J, Moodley SC. Malaria in pregnancy. S Afr Med J 1985; 67:403.
Shaw LM. Malaria reactivated by pregnancy. Practitioner 1985; 229:197.
Silver HM. Malarial infection in pregnancy. Infect Dis Clin North Am 1997; 11:99.
Torpin R. Malaria in pregnancy. Am J Obstet Gynecol 1941; 41:882.
Wickramsuriya GAW. Some observations on malaria occurring in association with pregnancy. Br J Obstet Gynecol 1935; 42:861.
Wolfe MS, Cordero JR. Safety of chloroquine in chemosuppression of malaria during pregnancy. Br Med J 1985; 290:1466.

Congenital Malaria
Ahmed A, Cerilli LA, Sanchez PJ. Congenital malaria in a preterm neonate: case report and review of the literature. Am J Perinatol 1998; 15:19.
Anagnos D, Lanoie LO, Palmieri JR, et al. Effects of placental malaria on mothers and neonates from Zaire. Z Parasitenkd 1986; 72:57.
Bass MH. Congenital malaria. Arch Pediatr 1914; 31:251.
Brabin BJ. Congenital malaria—a recrudescent problem? Papua New Guinea Med J 1985; 28:229.
Brabin BJ. An analysis of malaria in pregnancy in Africa. Bull World Health Organ 1983; 61:1005.
Cannon DWH. Malaria and prematurity in W. Nigeria. Br Med J 1958; 2:877.
Covell G. Congenital malaria. Trop Dis Bull 1950; 47:1147.
CDC. Congenital malaria as a result of *Plamodium malariae*—North Carolina. MMWR 2002; 51:164.
Dodge JS. A case of congenital malaria. Trans R Soc Trop Med Hyg 1971; 65:689.
Edozien JC, Gilles HM, Udeozo IOK. Adult and cord-blood gammaglobulin and immunity to malaria in Nigerians. Lancet 1962; 2:951.
Gammin RP. Congenital malaria in England. Lancet 1944; 2:375.
Garnham PCC. The placenta in malaria. Trans R Soc Trop Med Hyg 1938; 32:13.
Gouyon JB, Aujard Y, Jacqu E, et al. A Parisian case of congenital malaria. Arch Fr Pediatr 1986; 43:201.

TABLE 1 CDC sources for malaria prophylaxis and treatment recommendations

Type of information	Source	Contact
Prophylaxis	CDC Traveler's Health Voice Information System	877-394-8747
Prophylaxis	CDC Traveler's Health Internet Home page	www.cdc.gov/travel
Prophylaxis	Health Information for International Travel (The "Yellow Book")	800-545-2520
Treatment	CDC Malaria Epidemiology Branch	404-639-2888 (request Malaria Epidemiology Branch)

Abbreviation: CDC, Centers for Disease Control and Prevention.

Hubert TV. Congenital malaria in the United States: a case report and review. Clin Infect Dis 1992; 14:922–926.

Jones BS. Congenital malaria. Br Med J 1950; 2:459.

Louis CF. Malaria occurring during the puerperium and in the neonate. Med J Aust 1965; 1:223.

McQuay RM, Silberman S, Mudork P, Keith LE. Congenital malaria in Chicago: a case report and review of published reports (USA). Am J Trop Med Hyg 1967; 16:258.

Meerstadt PW. Congenital malaria. Clin Exp Obstet Gynecol 1986; 13:78.

Mendoza JB, Ongkiko B. Congenital malaria: a case report. J Philipp Med Assoc 1954; 30:398.

Okereke CS. Management of HIV-infected pregnant patients in malaria-endemic areas: therapeutic and safety considerations in concomitant use of antiretroviral and antimalarial agents. Clin Ther 1999; 21:1456.

Orbeck H, Ragnhildstveit E. Congenital malaria in Scandinavia. Scand J Infect Dis 1986; 18:79.

Procop GW, Jessen R, Hyde SR, Scheck DN. Persistence of *Plasmodium falciparum* in the placenta after apparently effective quinidine/clindamycin therapy. J Perinatol 2001; 21:128.

Schuurkamp GJ, Paika RL, Spicer PE, Kereu RK. Congenital malaria due to *Plasmodium vivax*: a case study in Papua, New Guinea. Papua New Guinea Med J 1986; 29:309.

Singh SC, Tandon PL. Congenital malaria. Indian Pract 1965; 19:359.

Watkinson M, Rushton DI, Lunn PG. Placental malaria and fetoplacental function: low plasma oestradiols associated with malarial pigmentation of the placenta. Trans R Soc Trop Med Hyg 1985; 79:448.

Therapy

Centers for Disease Control. Health information for international travel. U.S. Public Health Service, Department of Health and Human Services [publication no. (CDC) 87–8280], 1987.

Centers for Disease Control. Malaria Surveillance—United States, 1998. MMWR 2001; 50/No. SS-5:1.

Drugs for parasitic infections. Med Lett Drugs Ther 1990; 32:23.

Miller KD, Greenberg AE, Campbell CC. Treatment of severe malaria in the United States with a continuous infusion of quinidine gluconate and exchange transfusion. N Engl J Med 1989; 321:65.

Miller KD, Lobel HO, Pappaioanou M, et al. Failures of combined chloroquine and Fansidar prophylaxis in American travelers to East Africa. J Inf Dis 1986; 154:689.

Nosten F. The effects of mefloquine treatment in pregnancy. Clin Infect Dis 1999; 28:808.

Rudnitsky G, Miller KD, Pudua T, Stull TL. Continuous-infusion quinidine gluconate for treating children with severe *Plasmodium falciparum* malaria. J Infect Dis 1987; 155:1040.

Swerdlow CD, Yu JO, Jacobson E, et al. Safety and efficacy of intravenous quinidine. Am J Med 1983; 75:36.

Warrell DA, Molyneux ME, Beales PF, eds. Severe and complicated malaria, 2nd ed. Trans R Soc Trop Med Hyg 1990; 84(Suppl)2:28.

White NJ, Plorde JJ. Malaria. In: Wilson JD, Braunwald E, Isselbacher KJ, et al., eds. Harrison's Principles of Internal Medicine. 12th ed. New York: McGraw-Hill, Inc., 1990:782.

World Health Organization Malaria Action Programme. Severe and complicated malaria. Trans R Soc Trop Med Hyg 1986; 80(Suppl):1.

World Health Organization. Severe falciparum malaria. World Health Organization, Communicable Diseases Cluster. Trans R Soc Trop Med Hyg 2000; 94(Suppl):11s.

Zucker JR, Campbell CC. Malaria. Principles of prevention and treatment. Infect Dis Clin North Am 1993; 7:547.

Prophylaxis

Centers for Disease Control. Recommendations for the prevention of malaria among travelers. MMWR 1990; 39(no. RR-3).

Centers for Disease Control. Health information for international travel, 1990. Atlanta: U.S. Department of Health and Human Services, Public Health Service, 1990, DHHS publication no. (CDC) 90–8280.

Centers for Disease Control. Revised dosing regimen for malaria prophylaxis with mefloquine. MMWR 1990; 39:630.

Lackritz EM, Lobel HO, Howell J, et al. Imported *Plasmodium falciparum* malaria in American travelers to Africa: implications for prevention strategies. J Am Med Assoc 1991; 265:383.

Lobel HO, Bernard KW, Williams SL, et al. Effectiveness and tolerance of long-term malaria prophylaxis with mefloquine: need for a better dosing regimen. J Am Med Assoc 1991; 265:361.

MacArthur JR, Holtz TH, Jenkins J, et al. Probable locally acquired mosquito-transmitted malaria in Georgia. Clin Infect Dis 2001; 32e:124.

Zucker JR. Changing patterns of autochthonous malaria transmission in the United States: a review of recent outbreaks. Emerg Infect Dis 1996; 2; 1:37.

Toxoplasma gondii (Toxoplasmosis) 55

INTRODUCTION

Toxoplasma gondii derives its specific name from the gundii, a North African rodent from which this protozoon was first isolated in 1908. The organism's distribution is ubiquitous. *T. gondii* possesses the capacity to traverse species lines and establish infection not only in humans' domestic animals, but in humans themselves. In the United States, an estimated 23% of adolescents and adults have laboratory evidence of infection with *T. gondii*.

Toxoplasma exists in nature in three forms, the trophozoite, the cyst, and the oocyst. The most important mode of transmission of infection to humans is through the ingestion of poorly cooked meat containing encysted organisms. While the trophozoitic form of the protozoon is particularly sensitive to enzymatic digestion, the encysted form can survive trypsin or acid pepsin for prolonged periods. The presence of viable organisms within striated muscle has incriminated meat as the prime mode of dissemination among carnivores but has failed to explain the widespread prevalence in herbivores. The oocysts are the probable mechanism for the dissemination of infection to sheep, horses, and cattle. Carnivores such as cats will excrete oocysts in their feces for two to three weeks following acute infection (Fig. 1). Once excreted, the oocysts undergo further maturation for three to four days after which they are infectious, and in warm moist soil, they may remain infectious for more than one year. Human or animal contact with soil, grass, or other objects contaminated with oocysts and subsequent gastrointestinal processing results in an additional mode of dissemination. Flies can contaminate food with viable oocysts for up to 48 hours after contact with cat feces.

A susceptible cat devoid of antibodies to *T. gondii* will become infected after ingestion of food containing encysted organisms and will excrete oocysts for several weeks. Approximately 50% of felines subsequently challenged with cyst feeding will again excrete oocysts, indicating the probability that a cat may be infectious several times during a lifetime. Cats that hunt or eat raw meat contaminate their environment by fecal excretion of oocysts. Contact with contamenated faces may constitute a potential hazard to gravidas.

The principal ways a gravida acquires toxoplasmosis is by ingestion of raw or inadequately cooked meat or ingestion of oocysts acquired through exposure to cat litter or contaminated soil (e.g., from gardening or unwashed fruits or vegetables). Once infected by *T. gondii*, an infected pregnant woman can potentially pass the organism transplacentally to her fetus.

MATERNAL INFECTION

Approximately 20% to 25% of women of childbearing age in the United States exhibit serologic evidence of previous *T. gondii* infection. Although the prevalence of prior infection increases with age, at no time does it attain the high incidence observed for a comparable population in certain tropical countries and France. In a study from Norway, Kapperud et al. (1996) found significant maternal risk factors to be, in order of decreasing probability, eating raw or undercooked minced meat products, undercooked mutton, and eating raw or undercooked pork; cleaning the cat litter box; and washing the kitchen knives infrequently after preparation of raw

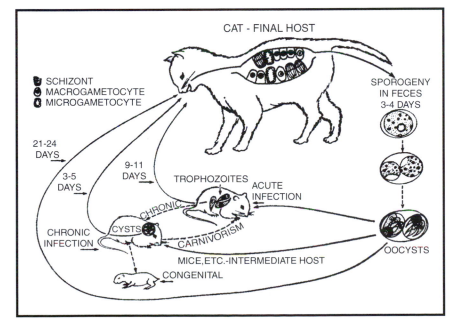

FIGURE I Postulated life cycle of *Toxoplasma gondii* showing means of transmission by oocysts from cat feces and by ingestion of trphozoites or cysts from intermediate hosts. Days indicated represent time from ingestion of *Toxoplasma* by cat to the excretion of oocysts. Mice are shown to represent the many mammals and birds that can serve as facultative intermediary hosts among which infection may spread, usually by carnivorism. Congenital transmission may take place during chronic infection as in mice, or during acute infection as in humans.

meat, prior to handling another food item. In the United States, two to six women per thousand serosusceptible women will acquire the infection during pregnancy. Approximately one-third of the females who acquire toxoplasmosis during pregnancy transmit the infection to their offspring. The later in gestation maternal infection is acquired, the greater the probability of fetal involvement.

When infection occurs during the first trimester of pregnancy, approximately 14% of the offspring will be infected; the figures for infection acquired during the second and third trimesters are 29% and 59%, respectively. The earlier the infection occurs in pregnancy, the more severe the disease is in the newborn. Almost all infected infants born to mothers who acquire the infection in the third trimester will appear normal at birth and only months or years later develop any clinical manifestations of the infection.

It is probable that the magnitude of the infective dose is an important determinant of whether an embryopathy ensues and what its pathogenic expression may be. A single oocyst contains eight sporozoites, in contrast to a single cyst, which may contain up to several thousand organisms. The impact of maternal infection with *T. gondii* in terms of fetal wastage and perinatal mortality appears to be directly related to the effects of the organism on the products of conception and is not due to the induced maternal reaction. The protozoa have been recovered or identified from aborted products of conception and stillbirths. Maternal parasitemia during gestation may result in a wide spectrum of fetal involvement, ranging from seropositivity to full-blown congenital toxoplasmosis.

Infection with *T. gondii* in adults is not often symptomatic. Less than 10% of infection clinically manifests as disease. *T. gondii* produces a spectrum of disease that includes *toxoplasma* lymphadenopathy, chorioretinitis, myocarditis, meningoencephalitis, and any whose clinical presentation resembles that of typhus. Overt disease is a poor indicator of the true prevalence of infection.

Within an obstetric population, the most commonly recognized manifestation of acute toxoplasmosis is lymphadenopathy. The lymphadenopathy may be the sole presenting sign or there may be an associated febrile response. The nodal enlargement may focally involve the cervical, supraclavicular, or inguinal regions, and is frequently unilateral. The principal histologic characteristic of these lymph nodes is marked reticulum cell hyperplasia. This feature, in conjunction with the absence of significant lymphadenitis, accounts for the firm, nontender, enlarged lymph nodes commonly observed. Any significant tenderness weakens the diagnosis of acute toxoplasmosis. The lymphadenopathy ordinarily is asymptomatic, but occasionally it may be associated with an infectious mononucleosis-like syndrome. Fatigue is the most common presenting symptom in more severe infection. It may be associated with headache, mental depression, myalgia, and a low-grade intermittent fever. A migratory polyarthritis and various types of predominantly macular rashes have also been described. In rare instances, abdominal pain secondary to mesenteric lymph node involvement may be the principal presenting complaint. In more pronounced instances of

systemic infestation, symptoms such as myalgia, myositis, and sustained fever are observed. Hepatosplenomegaly indicative of reticuloendothelial involvement can often be demonstrated. The severest manifestations of systemic disease are myocarditis, meningoencephalitis, or both.

The encysted forms begin to appear about the eighth day after infection (Fig. 2). Viable residual cysts are demonstrable in muscle, intestinal mucosa, alveolar macrophages, brain, kidney, and uterus. Although they are regarded as dormant because of the absence of a host cellular response, it is postulated that such encysted forms may periodically be responsible for reactivation of infection. Although most cases of congenital toxoplasmosis are probably the result of hematogenous dissemination, the finding of toxoplasma cysts in the uteri of normal females at hysterectomy, as well as postpartum in uterine curettage of gravidas who miscarried or aborted, suggested the possibility of an alternate route of transmission for congenital toxoplasmosis. Should implantation coincide with or impinge on a nidus of chronic infection, dissemination of the protozoon to the conceptus could occur by direct continuity.

With the exception of an augmented index of suspicion associated with unexplained lymphadenopathy, there are no pathognomonic clinical features for toxoplasmosis. The disease cannot be definitively diagnosed on clinical grounds because it may mimic a variety of other diseases.

CONGENITAL INFECTION

Although congenital toxoplasmosis is not a nationally reportable disease in the United States and no national data are available regarding its occurrence, extrapolation from regional studies indicates that an estimated 400 to 4000 cases occur each year in the United States. The projected incidence of congenital infection with *T. gondii* varies from 1 in 500 deliveries to 1 in 1300, depending upon geographic location.

The first case of congenital toxoplasmosis was described in 1927. In the classic full-blown syndrome, the infant is usually premature or small for age, with microcephaly, intracranial calcification, abnormal cerebrospinal fluid (CSF) findings, and possible internal hydrocephaly (Fig. 3), chorioretinitis, hepatosplenomegaly, jaundice, fever, and thrombocytopenia. The intracranial calcification, like that observed in first-trimester congenital cytomegalovirus infection, involves primarily the lateral ventricles (Fig. 4).

At necropsy, multisystem involvement can be demonstrated, with chorioretinitis, perimyoendocarditis, meningoencephalitis, interstitial pneumonitis, nephritis, and focal adrenal necrosis. The trophozoite or its encysted form may be identified within virtually all of the major organ systems. Extramedullary hematopoiesis is usually marked.

The spectrum of neonatal involvement runs the gamut from the classic overt congenital toxoplasmosis to subclinical infection. The probability of congenital infection increases proportionally with respect to when in gestation maternal infection occurs. During the first, second, and third trimesters, approximately 15%, 30%, and 60%, respectively, of the fetuses are estimated to become infected in utero.

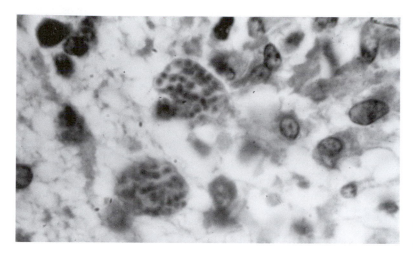

FIGURE 2 Encysted form of *Toxoplasma gondii* within glial cells (H&E, ×400).

There is a strong inverse correlation between time of infection acquisition and the severity of the ensuing infection in the fetus. The TORCH baby due to *T. gondii* is usually infected during the first trimester of pregnancy.

Second-trimester fetal infection more probably results in *formes frustes* of the disease, which are more common than the full-blown syndrome. These clinical presentations are unexplained hepatomegaly or hepatosplenomegaly, disseminated intravascular coagulopathy present at birth, or jaundice in the first 24 hours of life. In these instances, the serum immunoglobulin M (IgM) level tends to be greater than 20 mg/mL. Elevation of the IgM level is a crude gauge of the infection's chronicity.

SUBCLINICAL CONGENITAL TOXOPLASMOSIS

Subclinical infection is documented by the demonstration of IgM antitoxoplasma antibodies in cord or neonatal serum, of encysted organisms within placental tissue, or of persistence of a significant antibody titer beyond six months of age. The incidence of asymptomatic congenital toxoplasmosis versus overt toxoplasmosis is approximately three or four to one. The significance of subclinical toxoplasmosis has been a matter of speculation. Glasser and Delta (1965) identified *T. gondii* in the chorionic villi, amnion, and umbilical cords of

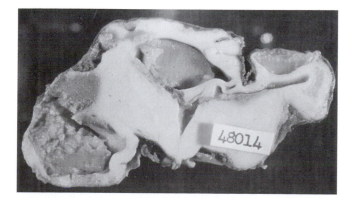

FIGURE 3 Marked distortion of the normal brain architecture (sagittal section) owing to massive tissue necrosis and secondary hydrocephaly. *Source:* Courtesy of M. Kuschner, MD. Stony Brook, NY.

two monozygotic twins. The infants were normal at birth. At seven months, both infants (under clinical observation) developed intracranial calcification, strabismus, and active chorioretinitis. As more information has become available, it is apparent that subclinical congenital toxoplasmosis has significant delayed morbidity (mental retardation or epilepsy in adulthood) and possibly mortality. In one study, by the age of 3½ years, 92% of such infants had untoward sequelae. Most cases of *toxoplasma* chorioretinitis are probably due to congenital infection. That organ pathology, in most instances, is not complete at birth stresses the need for recognition of congenital infection in the immediate neonatal period and the institution of appropriate therapy.

CHRONIC OR RECURRENT MATERNAL PARASITEMIA

Although congenital transmission of *T. gondii* occurs in chronically infected animals, it has long been presumed that primary maternal infection with *T. gondii* had to occur during gestation in order to involve the conceptus. This concept is no longer held to be valid. Remington (1964) cultured 34 gravidas who exhibited serologic evidence of chronic toxoplasmosis and whose pregnancy terminated in abortion, stillbirth, or neonatal death. He recovered the organism in two cases of abortion and in one case of neonatal death.

Gravidas do not have to acquire primary infection during gestation to transmit the organism to the conceptus. While studying another infant with congenital disease, Remington isolated *T. gondii* from maternal blood at one, four, and five months after birth. The mother was asymptomatic. Persistent parasitemia occurred despite high antitoxoplasma antibody levels.

Recurrent toxoplasmosis in severely immunocompromised individuals with CD4+ T-cell counts less than 50 to 100 cells/mm^3 is a well-documented phenomenon.

Congenital infection in successive offspring may occur as a very rare event. Although the risk of a second infected infant appears to be infinitesimally small, it nonetheless exists. Langer recovered the organisms from the brains of two successive stillborn infants. Similarly, Garcia (1968) identified the organism in a conceptus, a live-born premature

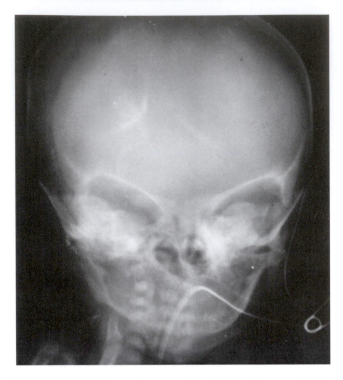

FIGURE 4 Skull X-ray demonstrating significant intracranial dystrophic calcification in the area of the lateral ventricles due to *Toxoplasma gondii*.

infant, and a six-month abortus, which comprised successive pregnancies in a given female. An additional well-documented case was recorded in Switzerland in which a congenitally infected infant was born to a woman who apparently acquired the infection approximately 8 to 12 weeks prior to gestation. Following birth of a congenitally infected infant, it may be prudent for the mother to use some form of contraceptive for at least one year. The question of whether to administer chemotherapeutic agents to the mother is very controversial. If therapy is instituted, it is for potential fetal and not for maternal considerations.

DIAGNOSIS

Maternal

Quantitative studies of the immunoglobulin (antibody) profile reveal that the initial response in acute acquired toxoplasmosis is the elaboration of IgM and IgA antibodies.

IgM-specific antibodies appear early in the course of the disease. IgM can be detected by immunofluorescence antibody test (IFA), enzyme-linked immunosorbent assay (ELISA), or the immunosorbent agglutination assay. The presence of antinuclear antibodies in sera may yield false-positive results. If available, the double-sandwich IgM-ELISA is a more sensitive and specific test than the IgM-IFA test or the standard IgM-ELISA test. Persistence of detectable IgM antibodies varies, depending on the testing methodology. Most commercial kits for detection of IgM antibodies to *T. gondii* are not completely reliable according to the Food and Drug Administration Public Health Advisory of July 25, 1997. A report of a positive IgM titer (in the United States) should be confirmed using an accredited reference laboratory such as that of the Palo Alto Foundation Research Division.

The positive predictive value of a positive IgM antibody test is lower than anticipated owing to its prolonged persistent acute infection. Gorgievski-Hrisoho et al. (1996) have contended that while the positive predictive value is lower, the negative predictive value (absence of IgM- and IgA-specific antibodies) is 100%. The presence of a high *toxoplasma*-specific IgM antibody titer combined with a high IgG titer probably indicates an acute infection within the previous three months. A low-to-medium IgM titer and a high IgG titer might indicate an acute infection three to six months previously. IgM antibodies have been detected as long as 18 months after initial infection. An IgM-IFA titer of 1:160 or greater or an IgM-ELISA titer of 1:256 or greater is considered diagnostic of recently acquired *T. gondii* infection. Because of false-positive titers achieved with some commercial kits for *toxoplasma*-specific antibodies, IgM-positive test results should be confirmed by a *toxoplasma* reference laboratory.

In chronic toxoplasmosis, the antibody is exclusively IgG; thus the possibility exists of distinguishing acute from chronic infection on the basis of the immunoglobulin profile.

Specific maternal IgG antibodies develop within 7 to 10 days. These antibodies are long lived and, in the absence of sequential specimens, may indicate only previous exposure to the organism. A positive test for IgG antibodies and a negative test for IgM antibodies early in pregnancy indicate infection prior to gestation.

Fetal

The fetal response to the protozoon is sequentially comparable to that of the adult. However, the qualitative relationships are different. The fetus in utero responds to infection with *T. gondii* by elaborating IgM antibodies. This response may result in an overall elevation of the IgM level in the cord serum as well as the presence of specific IgM antibodies. This type of immunoglobulin predominates in the neonatal period and during the first few months of life. Fetal infection early in gestation may not elicit a demonstrable IgM response.

The diagnosis of congenital toxoplasmosis in the neonate depends on either the demonstration of specific IgM or IgA antibodies or recovery of the protozoan. The persistence of specific antitoxoplasma antibody beyond the first six months of life usually reflects active infection. Whereas only approximately 25% of congenitally infected infants will be positive by the IgM-IFA test, 80% will be positive by the IgM-ELISA test. The demonstration of specific IgA in fetal or neonatal serum appears to be more sensitive than IgM for the diagnosis of congenital infection. Its diagnostic use to date has been limited by the availability of testing facilities.

Infants first infected near to or at the time of delivery may have an IgM response only after several weeks. The presence of high levels of maternal IgG antibody in the fetus before exposure to the organism may suppress the ability of the infant to produce IgM antibodies.

In the study reported by Grover et al. (1990), detection of specific IgM antibodies correctly identified only three of the ten positive fetuses. Because of these considerations, repeat testing of an infant's serum should be performed in any infant suspected on clinical grounds of having congenital infection but in whom initial testing does not show an IgM-specific antibody.

A rapid diagnostic test using polymerase chain reaction has been developed to detect the presence of specific antigens in lysed, pelleted amniotic fluid cell samples. Grover et al. (1990) used this technique to correctly diagnose four cases of congenital infection in utero. In this study of 43 documented cases of acute maternal infection during gestation, there were no false-positive diagnoses. This technique will probably supplant the more time-consuming methodology of mouse inoculation with amniotic fluid and fetal blood. The antigens of the organism are detectable not only in amniotic fluid, CSF, and blood, but also in urine.

Newer tests for diagnosis of congenital toxoplasmosis are in development. Enzyme-linked immunofiltration assay and immunoblot have better sensitivities than conventional IgM immunosorbent agglutination assay, IgM-ELISA, IgM-IFA test, in vitro culture, and mouse inoculation.

T. gondii is an obligate intracellular parasite. All methods to cultivate it on synthetic media have been unsuccessful. However, it grows readily in a variety of tissue culture lines. The alternate isolation system for the recovery of the organism utilizes a biologic indicator system, by injecting infected material into the peritoneal cavity of seronegative mice. Isolation of tachyzoites from blood or other body fluids is proof of acute infection. Histological demonstration of tachyzoites in cytological preparations of body fluids or tissue sections is diagnostic of acute infection. Histological findings in lymph nodes obtained at biopsy are usually sufficient to document the infection.

In isolated instances, ultrasound studies may identify a fetus with advanced disease. The sonographic finding of significant ventriculomegaly usually correlated with significant neurological problems in life.

THERAPY

Therapy for Maternal Indications

Chemotherapy is indicated for individuals who have severe forms of toxoplasmosis or immunologic impairment of the host defense mechanisms.

The standard treatment in adults consists of pyrimethamine (Daraprim) and sulfadiazine. The combination of pyrimethamine and sulfonamides is synergistic against trophozoites.

Pyrimethamine is a folic acid antagonist that selectively inhibits dihydrofolate reductase. The usual adult dose is 25 to 50 mg/day for three to four weeks. Megaloblastic anemia and/or pancytopenia may result from induced folic acid deficiency.

Thrombocytopenia, agranulocytosis, or megaloblastic anemia may develop as a consequence of therapy. Baker's yeast 5 to 7 g daily or folinic acid 10 to 20 mg daily should be given concurrently to obviate hematologic toxicity.

Women undergoing therapy should be closely followed with leukocyte assays, platelet counts, and hematocrit determinations biweekly.

Sulfadiazine (Microsulfon) interferes with microbial growth through competitive antagonism. The usual adult diose is 2 to 4 g initially followed by 2 to 4 g daily in three to six equally divided doses. The drug can cause renal failure secondary to crystallization within renal tubules and severe epidermal necrolysis. Individuals receiving this drug need to drink plenty of fluids and avoid dehydration.

Because of concern of possible teratogenic consequences, the drug should not be administered in the first trimester in the absence of overriding maternal considerations. The safety of pyrimethamine and sulfadiazine use during pregnancy has not been definitively established.

There is no effective therapy currently available against the encysted form of *T. gondii*.

Therapy for Fetal Indications

There are reservations about instituting therapy for an asymptomatic gravida with acute infection during gestation. The indications for therapy are those of potential fetal involvement and not of maternal derivation. Only 25% to 35% of women whose gestation is complicated by acute toxoplasmosis will give birth to a congenitally infected neonate. Current data indicate that in utero chemotherapy with sulfadiazene and pyrimethamine has the ability to alter the observed incidence of congenital *toxoplasma embryopathy*.

Wallon et al. (1994) reported on the effectiveness of therapy. They studied 490 infants whose mothers were treated during gestation. At one year of age, 77% of the infants were seronegative. Of the remaining 116 infants, 27% had cerebral calcification or ocular lesions. None had overt neurological impairment.

Therapy for maternal infection has shown that in fetuses that become infected despite maternal treatment, the clinical manifestations are greatly attenuated. With a normal antenatal sonogram and appropriate subsequent infant therapy, the long-term neurological outlook for infected infants appears to be quite favorable.

An alternate approach to empiric therapy was that proposed by Daffos et al. (1988) which focuses on establishing documentation of fetal infection in utero. Once acute infection is documented by serological conversion and/or the presence of specific IgM antitoxoplasma antibodies, at some time after 20 weeks of gestation, under ultrasonographic guidance, a minimal amount of blood was aspirated from the umbilical cord. At amniocentesis, 15 to 20 mL of amniotic fluid was obtained for intraperitoneal inoculation into seronegative mice. An additional parameter used to augment the probability of diagnosing in utero diseases was the finding of ventricular dilation on ultrasonography. In their prospective study of the documented cases of maternal *toxoplasma* infection, they were able to diagnose antenatally 39 of the 42 congenitally infected infants. Of 15 fetuses who carried to term, all but two who had chorioretinitis remained clinically well. The organism was isolated from fetal blood in 64% of the 42 cases and from amniotic fluid in 52%. Specific fetal IgM was found in only 21% of cases. Unilateral or bilateral dilation of the ventricles occurred in 17 cases. In these cases, one pregnancy resulted in dizygotic twins. One died of congenital toxoplasmosis; the second had neither clinical nor serological evidence of disease.

In general, documented maternal infection is an indication for therapy irrespective of signs and symptoms of systemic disease. The therapeutic focus is aimed at attempting to avert or limit future organism–cell interaction.

An informed consent should be obtained that clearly states not only that the gravida is aware of the potential problems associated with drug therapy but also that she will not benefit per se from therapy. There should be a willingness on the part of the mother to share the responsibility of drug therapy. For first-trimester maternal infection, it is recommended that therapy be withheld during the period of organogenesis. Only one-third of the fetuses will actually require therapy, yet 100% of the fetuses will be subject to drug exposure during the critical periods of organogenesis.

In Europe, the use of spiramycin has been advocated as soon as the diagnosis of maternal infection is established. Once organogenesis is completed, a combination treatment regimen using pyrimethamine and sulfadiazine is implemented, because spiramycin does not reliably cross the placenta.

Pyrimethamine should not be used in the first 16 weeks of pregnancy because of concern for teratogenicity (in this circumstance, sulfadiazine should be administered alone).

Sulfonamides should be discontinued two to three weeks prior to the expected date of confinement to avert the problem of competitive antagonism with bilirubin in the postpartum period. The sulfonamides successfully compete with bilirubin for the albumin-binding site. Extensive displacement of bilirubin from albumin-binding sites can be responsible for the induction of kernicterus in the neonate.

Comparative tests have shown that sulfapyrazine, sulfamethazine, and sulfamerazine are about as effective as sulfadiazine. Sulfathiazole, sulfapyridine, sulfadimetine, and sulfisoxazole are much less effective and are not recommended. The usual dosage of sulfadiazine or triple sulfonamides is 50 to 100 mg/kg of body weight every 24 hours in two to four equal doses by mouth.

Pyrimethamine, being a folic acid antagonist, will cause a reversible and gradual depression of the bone marrow. Although toxicity is dose related, absorption of the drug is not uniform in all patients. Platelet depression, with its associated bleeding tendency, is the most serious consequence of toxicity. Both leukopenia and anemia may occur as well. Other side effects are gastrointestinal distress, headaches, and a bad taste in the mouth. All patients treated with pyrimethamine should have a peripheral blood cell and platelet count ideally twice a week. Folinic acid (in the form of leucovorin calcium) has been used to lessen the effects of the drug on platelets (5–15 mg/day intramuscularly). Baker's yeast 5 g daily has been used in lieu of leucovorum.

MANAGEMENT IN PREGNANCY

Routine serological screening for toxoplasmosis is probably not cost effective; however, limited screening of gravidas who like raw or poorly cooked meat, who have significant contact with animals, or who do extensive gardening is advocated. IgG-specific antibodies will be present in a significant number of these patients. Gravidas with a concomitant specific IgM titer definitely need further evaluation and management.

All gravidas who are immunologically compromised or immunosuppressed should be screened for the presence of antitoxoplasma antibodies. Seropositive women need to be carefully monitored for potential reactivation of disease.

PREVENTION

Toxoplasma infection of the pregnant female is preventable. This is accomplished by avoidance of the ingestion of cysts or sporulated oocysts by the seronegative woman. Cysts are rendered noninfective by heating meat to 66° C or by smoking or curing it. Freezing is less reliable since it requires temperatures (−20° C) not achieved by most home freezers. Raw fruits and vegetables should be thoroughly washed and specific steps taken to prevent access of flies, cockroaches, and other insects to animal feces. Hands should be washed thoroughly after handling raw meat or vegetables. The handling of cat feces should be avoided altogether. If this is not possible, disposable gloves should be worn when disposing of cat litter and when gardening out of doors. Treatment of the cat litter pan with nearly boiling water for five minutes will kill potentially infective oocysts.

In a study of risk factors, frequent contact with soil may be more important a risk for maternal infection than the household presence of a cat. The key elements in preventing maternal toxoplasmosis include cooking meat until it is well done, washing fruits and vegetables, and wearing gloves when working in the garden (if cats frequent the area) or disposing of cat litter.

There are no drugs to kill *T. gondii* tissue cysts in human or animal tissues. Freezing to −20° C, cooking to an internal temperature of 66° C, or gamma irradiation (0.5 kGy) can kill tissue cysts in meat.

SELECTED READING

Maternal Infection
Alford CA. An epidemiologic overview of intrauterine and perinatal infections of man. Mead Johnson Symp Perinat Dev Med 1982; 21:3.
Alger LS. Toxoplasmosis and parvovirus B19 infection. Infect Dis Clin North Am 1997; 11:55.
Beazley DM, Egerman RS. Toxoplasmosis. Semin Perinatol 1998; 4:332.
Couvreur J, Thulliez PH, Daffos F. In utero treatment of toxoplasmic fetopathy with the combination of pyrimethamine—sulfadiazine. Fetal Diagn Ther 1993; 8:45.
Daffos F, Forestier F, Capella-Pavlovsky M, et al. Prenatal management of 746 pregnancies at risk for congenital toxoplasmosis. N Engl J Med 1988; 318:271.
Decavalas G, Papapetropoulou M, Giannoulaki E, et al. Prevalence of *Toxoplasma gondii* antibodies in gravidas and recently

aborted women and study of risk factors. Eur J Epidemiol 1990; 6:223.

Desmonts G, Couvreur J. Congenital toxoplasmosis: a prospective study of 378 pregnancies. N Engl J Med 1974; 290:1110.

Desmonts G, Thulliez P. The toxoplasma agglutination antigen as a tool for routine screening and diagnosis of toxoplasma infection in the mother and infant. Dev Biol Stand 1985; 62:31.

Djurkovic-Djakovic O. Toxoplasma infection and pathological outcome of pregnancy. Gynecol Obstet Invest 1995; 40:36.

Dubey JP. Strategies to reduce transmission of *Toxoplasma gondii* to animals and humans. Vet Parasitol 1996; 64:65.

Eckerling B, Neri A, Eylan E. Toxoplasmosis; a cause of infertility. Fertil Steril 1986; 19:883.

Frenkel JK. Toxoplasmosis testing during pregnancy. J Am Med Assoc 1991; 265:211.

Gaafar T, el-Fakahany AF. Assessment of IgG & IgM, ELISA and IFAT in diagnosis of toxoplasmosis in pregnancies at risk. J Egypt Soc Parasit 1990; 20:817.

Grose C, Itani O, Weiner CP. Prenatal diagnosis of fetal infection: advances from amniocentesis to cordocentesis—congenital toxoplasmosis, rubella, cytomegalovirus, varicella virus, parvovirus and human immunodeficiency virus. Pediatr Infect Dis J 1989; 8:459.

Hofgartner W, Swanzy S, Bacina R, et al. Detection of immunoglobulin G (IgG) and IgM antibodies to *Toxoplasma gondii*: evaluation of four commercial immunoassay systems. J Clin Microbiol 1997; 35:3313.

Holliman RE, Barker KF, Johnson JD. Selective antenatal screening for toxoplasmosis and the latex agglutination test. Epidemiol Infect 1990; 105:409.

Kapperud G, Jenum PA, Stray-Pedersen B, Melby KK. Results of a prospective case-control study in Norway. Am J Epidemiol 1996; 144:405.

Klapper PE, Morris DJ. Screening for viral and protozoal infections in pregnancy: a review. Br J Obstet Gynaecol 1990; 97:974.

Lebech M, Joynson DH, Seitz HM, et al. Classification system and case definition of *Toxoplasma gondii* infection in immunocompetent pregnant women and their congenitally infected offspring. Eur J Clin Microbiol Infect Dis 1996; 15:799.

Lynfield R, Guerina NG. Toxoplasmosis. Pediatr Rev 1997; 18:75.

Naot Y, Desmonts G, Remington JS. IgM enzyme-linked immunosorbent assay test for the diagnosis of congenital toxoplasma infection. J Pediatr 1981; 98:32.

Newton ER. Diagnosis of perinatal TORCH infections. Clin Obstet Gynecol 1999; 42:59.

Remington JS. Spontaneous abortion and chronic toxoplasmosis: report of a case with isolation of the parasite. Obstet Gynecol 1964; 24:25.

Remington JS. Toxoplasma and chronic abortion. Obstet Gynecol 1964; 24:155.

Remington JS, Melton M, Jacobs L. Chronic toxoplasma infection in the uterus. J Lab Clin Med 1960; 56:879.

Sever JL. The importance of considering clinical usefulness in the evaluation of medical laboratory tests. Am J Obstet Gynecol 1990; 163:678.

Stepick-Biek P, Thulliez P, Araujo FG, Remington JS. IgA antibodies for diagnosis of acute congenital and acquired toxoplasmosis. J Infect Dis 1990; 162:270.

Weinman D. Toxoplasma and abortion: a field for further investigation. Fertil Steril 1960; 11:525.

Wilson M, McAuley JB. Toxoplasma. In: Murray P, ed. Manual of Clinical Microbiology, 7th ed. Washington, DC: ASM Press, 1999:1374.

Congenital Infection

Alford CA. Clinical findings, laboratory diagnosis and treatment of chronic congenital and perinatal infections. Mead Johnson Symp Perinat Dev Med 1982; 21:27.

Baron J, Youngblood L, Siewers CMF, Medearis D. The incidence of cytomegalovirus, herpes simplex, rubella and toxoplasma antibody in microcephalic mentally retarded and normocephalic children. Pediatrics 1969; 44:932.

Centers for Disease Control. Preventing congenital toxoplasmosis. MMWR 2000; 49 (RR02):57.

Chumpitazi BF, Boussai A, Pellous H, et al. Diagnosis of congenital toxoplasmosis by immunoblotting and relationship with other methods. J Clin Microbiol 1995; 33:1479.

Daffos F, Capella-Pavlovsky M, Forestier F. Fetal blood sampling during pregnancy with use of a needle guided by ultrasound: a study of 606 consecutive cases. Am J Obstet Gynecol 1985; 153:655.

Desmonts G, Daffos F, Forestier F, et al. Prenatal diagnosis of congenital toxoplasmosis. Lancet 1985; 1:500.

D'Ercole C, Boubli L, Frank J, et al. Recurrent congenital toxoplasmosis in a woman with lupus erythematous. Prenat Diag 1995; 15:1171.

European Collaborative Study and Research Network on Congenital Toxoplasmosis. Low incidence of congenital toxoplasmosis in children born to mothers infected with human immunodeficiency virus. Eur J Obstet Gynecol Reprod Biol 1996; 68:93.

Fuentes I, Rodriguez M, Domingo CJ, et al. Urine sample used for congenital toxoplasmosis diagnosis by PCR. J Clin Microbiol 1996; 34:2368.

Garcia AG. Congenital toxoplasmosis in two successive sibs. Arch Dis Child 1968; 43:705.

Gorgievski-Hrisoho M, Germann D, Matter L. Diagnostic implications of kinetics of immunoglobulin M and A antibody responses to *Toxoplasma gondii*. J Clin Microbiol 1996; 34:1506.

Grover CM, Thulliez P, Remington JS, Boothroyd JC. Rapid prenatal diagnosis of congenital toxoplasma infection by using polymerase chain reaction and amniotic fluid. J Clin Microbiol 1990; 28:2297.

Hohlfeld P, Daffos F, Thulliez P, et al. Fetal toxoplasmosis: outcome of pregnancy and infant follow-up after *in utero* treatment. J Pediatr 1989; 115:765.

Kimball AC, Kean BH, Fuchs F. Congenital toxoplasmosis; a prospective study of 4,048 obstetric patients. Am J Obstet Gynecol 1971; 111:211.

Langer H. Repeated congenital toxoplasmosis gondii. Obstet Gynecol 1963; 21:318.

Mitchell CD, Erlich SS, Mastrucci MT, et al. Congenital toxoplasmosis occurring in infants perinatally infected with human immunodeficiency virus 1. Pediatr Infect Dis J 1990; 9:512.

Remington JS. The tragedy of toxoplasmosis. Pediatr Infect Dis J 1990; 9:762.

Robert-Gangneux F, Gavinet MF, Ancelle T, et al. Value of prenatal diagnosis and early postpartum diagnosis of congenital toxoplasmosis; retrospective study of 110 cases. J Clin Microbiol 1999; 39:2893.

Wallon M, Gandihon F, Peyron F, et al. Toxoplasmosis in pregnancy. Lancet 1994; 334:540.

Wilson CB. Treatment of congenital toxoplasmosis during pregnancy. J Pediatr 1990; 116:1003.

Wilson CB, Remington JS. What can be done to prevent congenital toxoplasmosis? Am J Obstet Gynecol 1980; 138:357.

Wilson CB, Remington JS, Stango S, Reynolds DW. Development of adverse sequelae in children born with subclinical congenital toxoplasma infection. Pediatrics 1980; 66:767.

Wong S-Y, Remington JS. Toxoplasmosis in pregnancy. Clin Infect Dis 1994; 18:853.

Placental Infection

Elliott WG. Placental toxoplasmosis; report of a case. Am J Clin Pathol 1970; 53:413.

Foulon W, Naessens A, de Catte L, Amy JJ. Detection of congenital toxoplasmosis by chorionic villus sampling and early amniocentesis. Am J Obstet Gynecol 1990; 163:1511.

Glasser L, Delta BG. Congenital toxoplasmosis with placental infection in monozygotic twins. Pediatrics 1965; 35:276.

Trichomonas vaginalis   56

David S. Bard and Gilles R. G. Monif / *Revised by* Paul Summers

INTRODUCTION

Donne, in 1830, observed organisms on slides of purulent discharges from the genital tracts of men and women and named them *Trichomonas vaginale*. The name *Trichomonas vaginalis* was suggested two years later by Ehrenberg. Since then, over 100 separate species of the genus *Trichomonas* have been reported, but only three have been isolated in humans. *T. vaginalis* is the only species of the trichomonads that is pathogenic for humans. *T. tenax* and *T. hominis* infect the human gastrointestinal tract, but as harmless commensals.

Although it is primarily a sexually transmitted disease (STD), the demography of disease suggests that it may be transmitted by an alternate mode. Prevalence studies have demonstrated two peaks: one in young sexually active women and the second in older women who have no evidence of sexually transmitted infection.

T. vaginalis is a tetraflagellated, motile protozoon with an anterior nucleus, an anterolateral undulating membrane, and a prominent axostyle (Fig. 1). Usually, the organism's shape is oval or fusiform and its size is slightly larger than that of the average leukocyte (15Ê). However, under adverse conditions or with certain strains, its shape may be round or pear shaped, and its size considerably smaller (7Ê–13Ê) or larger (20Ê–30Ê) (Fig. 2). An oval nucleus, which appears more dense than the surrounding cytoplasm, is located toward the flagellated pole and is usually 1/3 to 1/2 the length of the organism. The cytoplasm is basically clear but frequently contains varying amounts of cytoplasmic particles, vacuoles, debris, and bacteria. Rarely, intracytoplasmic leukocytes or erythrocytes may be identified. Reproduction is by mitotic division of the nucleus and longitudinal fission into two daughter cells. The organism is believed to exist only in the trophozoite form; a cyst form has not been found.

The viability and growth of *T. vaginalis* are supported when its milieu is moist, the pH is 4.9 to 7.5, and the temperature is 35°C to 37°C. The more robust and usually smaller organisms are observed in the pH range of 5.5 to 5.8, and the less motile and often larger organisms are encountered when the pH is higher or lower than optimum. It is believed that *T. vaginalis* is a facultative anaerobe because it forms lactic acid and carbon dioxide from sugars and starches, but excessive oxygen reduces carbohydrate metabolism and depresses growth. Culture media should contain cysteine, peptone, proteolysed liver, maltose, serum, and antibiotics. Estrogen has no effect on growth in culture.

The organism is killed on drying or after prolonged exposure to sunlight, and it will not survive more than five days at 0°C, 30 minutes in tap water, four minutes at 50°C, or six hours in warm saline.

NATURAL HISTORY OF THE DISEASE

Humans are the only known host of *T. vaginalis*. In women, the organism usually infests the vagina and urethra but may involve the endocervix, Bartholin's glands, Skene's glands, or the bladder. Isolated cases have been reported in which the protozoon was recovered from the uterus, fallopian tubes, and renal pelvis. In men, the organism usually colonizes the lower urethra, but occasionally it infests the prostate gland, seminal vesicles, or epididymis.

Prevalence

The prevalence of *T. vaginalis* is unknown, but it is worldwide in distribution and has been demonstrated in every society and subculture in which it has been sought. As a global estimate, approximately 15% to 20% of all women and 3% to 10% of all men harbor the organism.

Sources of Infection

T. vaginalis is ordinarily transmitted through sexual intercourse, with the female being the primary reservoir and the male the vector. When chronically infected, the male may also act as a reservoir. Once the female is infected, spontaneous eradication of the disease is extremely rare and, if it is untreated, the organism appears to survive indefinitely in the lower urogenital tract. In recent studies of male consorts of infected females, the organism was cultured from the

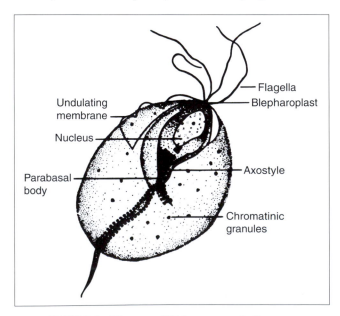

FIGURE I Diagram of *Trichomonas vaginalis*.

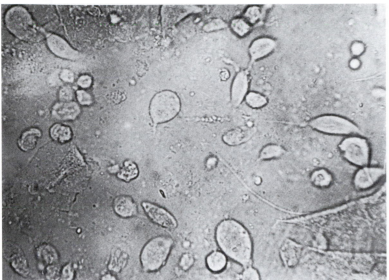

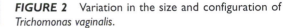

FIGURE 2 Variation in the size and configuration of *Trichomonas vaginalis*.

lower urethra in over 90% of the cases. However, in the male, spontaneous decolonization of the lower urinary tract occurs within three weeks unless reinoculation intervenes or there is chronic trichomonad infestation of the prostate, seminal vesicles, or epididymis.

Neonates and infants may develop trichomonad infection in the vagina and lower urinary tract when delivered vaginally of an infected mother. Since the vagina of a young girl is not optimally suited for growth of the organism, inoculation at birth has been postulated as leading to a latent, low-grade colonization during prepubescence. With the onset of puberty, optimal growth conditions for the trichomonad develop in the vagina, and thereafter the disease begins its clinical manifestations.

Numerous studies suggest the possible transmission of *T. vaginalis* through public toilets, saunas, swimming pools, washcloths, bath towels, and nonsterile pelvic examination techniques. Under the appropriate conditions, each of the foregoing may transmit infection, but in reality, its occurrence is probably rare.

The mechanism by which *T. vaginalis* evokes clinical infection remains an enigma. Under experimental conditions, induction of clinical disease in a healthy human vagina requires inoculation of large numbers of organisms and an incubation period of several weeks, but intravaginal inoculation of one viable trichomonad may, under ideal growth conditions, induce colonization.

Several physiologic and pathologic states of the vagina or of the host appear to enhance the viability and growth of *T. vaginalis* and perhaps activate its pathogenicity. These environmental conditions are interrelated and often additive in their effects on the protozoon's growth. However, in individual cases of trichomoniasis, it is not uncommon to encounter a single, predisposing growth factor that predominates over other factors known to inhibit *T. vaginalis*.

Mature Vaginal Epithelium

Owing to stimulation by circulating estrogen, the mucosa of the healthy adult vagina consists of mature, glycogenated, squamous epithelium, and the vaginal cavity contains free, glycogen-derived glucose, which is essential for the growth of *T. vaginalis*. Clinically symptomatic trichomoniasis occurs most frequently during the reproductive years when ovarian output of estrogen is maximal, the epithelium of the vagina is most mature, and the vagina contains large amounts of glucose. Prepubescent girls and estrogen-deficient women (castrates or postmenopausal) harboring the trichomonad are usually asymptomatic. Exacerbation of trichomoniasis is not uncommon soon after starting estrogen replacement therapy in an estrogen-deficient menopausal patient.

Elevated Vaginal pH

The healthy adult vagina contains large numbers of *Lactobacillus acidophilus*, which metabolize the free glucose into lactic acid, thereby maintaining the vaginal pH at 3.5 to 4.5 and creating an unfavorable environmental pH for the growth of most vaginal pathogens, including *T. vaginalis* (optimal pH 5.5–5.8).

Certain conditions, however, may temporarily elevate the vaginal pH and encourage the growth and colonization of *T. vaginalis*. These include

1. progesterone-dominant states such as pregnancy,
2. the presence of intravaginal secretions such as menstrual blood, excessive cervical mucus, or exudate from cervical or vaginal lesions, and
3. the more alkaline vaginal milieu engendered by pathologic alterations of the vaginal flora such as certain bacterial overgrowths (*Staphylococcus aureus*, alpha-streptococcus), with a consequent reduction in lactobacilli.

Studies in human volunteer have demonstrated that induction of trichomoniasis is faciliated when an abnormal vaginal flora, characterized by a diminished number of absense of aerobic lactobacilli, is present.

As significant colonization and multiplication of *T. vaginalis* ensues, a corresponding and directly related rise in vaginal pH may occur—initially due solely to the trichomonad population. This encourages bacterial overgrowth, inhibits lactobacillus production, and establishes the infestation of the organism. Specific eradication of the trichomonad with metronidazole promptly returns the pathologic process (the reduced lactobacilli, the altered bacterial flora, and the elevated vaginal pH) to normal.

Preexisting Vaginal or Cervical Lesions

Any vaginal or cervical lesion capable of weakening or destroying the surface epithelium may allow access of *T. vaginalis* to either the deeper epithelium or the submucosa, thereby creating more intense inflammation, discharge, and other symptoms. Some of these lesions include trauma (from tampons or chemicals), certain bacterial infections, cervicitis, candidiasis, genital herpes, and certain neoplastic lesions (carcinoma and condyloma acuminatum).

HISTOPATHOLOGY

The histologic findings of acute *T. vaginalis* infection are nonspecific and similar to other superficial, inflammatory reactions of the vagina and urethra. There is diffuse or patchy blood vessel dilation and proliferation in the surface epithelium and submucosa. Tufts of capillaries (double-crested) permeating the epithelium may be observed. This results in the double, or paired, punctuation noted on the cervix with colposcope in active *Trichomonas* infection as well as the cervical changes described as "strawberry" cervix. Postcoital bleeding and mild cervical bleeding when collecting Papanicolaou (Pap) smear samples result from this increased vascularity.

This vascular engorgement, combined with a variable degree of polymorphonuclear leukocyte infiltration and elongation of the papillae, may resemble an acute papillitis. In severe infections, the outer portions of the surface epithelium may become detached and replaced with an inflammatory exudate. In chronic trichomoniasis, the inflammation is less severe, with lymphocyte and plasma cell infiltration, but the surface epithelial cells often show intracellular edema, vacuolization, and a perinuclear halo or "chicken wire" effect. The nuclei of these cells may be enlarged, hyperchromatic, and irregular. However, the outward maturation of the epithelial cells progresses normally. True tissue invasion or involvement of endocervical glands by the trichomonad is extremely rare.

Cytopathology

Although *T. vaginalis* may be identified in only 15% (range 7–30%) of Pap smears in large, unselected, cervical cancer-screening programs, approximately 30% to 40% of all abnormal cytologic smears are associated with the identification of *T. vaginalis*. In patients with urogenital trichomoniasis, 2% to 8% will have an abnormal cytologic smear, which is usually interpreted as an atypical smear (ASCUS), but not infrequently a low-grade smear (LGSIL) or even a high-grade smear (HGSIL) (usually over interpreted) may be attributes of cytologic alterations induced by *T. vaginalis*.

Characteristically, the smear is "dirty," with large numbers of leukocytes, necrotic cells, clumped bacteria, cellular debris, and occasionally *Leptothrix* in the background. Clusters of leukocytes overlying squamous cells are common but nonspecific. The trichomonad appears as a gray-green, round, or fusiform "blob" with an eccentrically located, slightly denser nucleus. The flagella are not usually seen.

Of clinical importance is the curiosity that, in premenopausal woman, trichomoniasis tends to increase the number of intermediate and parabasal cell types, thereby yielding a falsely low estrogen activity, whereas in postmenopausal patients, the organism tends to induce the growth of the more mature intermediate and superficial cells, yielding a falsely high level of estrogen activity. These trichomonad-induced alterations of the epithelial cells make the estimation of estrogen activity on cytologic smears in patients with trichomoniasis of dubious value.

An abnormal cytologic smear due to *T. vaginalis* infestation will revert to normal within 6 to 12 weeks after eradication of the organism with metronidazole therapy, but even if a previously abnormal cytologic smear returns to normal, these patients should have repeat smears performed every four months for at least one year. If the cytologic abnormality persists after metronidazole, and there is no evidence of recurrent or persistent trichomonad infestation, appropriate colposcopy-directed biopsies of the cervix and endocervix should be obtained for histologic diagnosis of the cytologic changes.

CLINICAL PATTERNS OF TRICHOMONIASIS

In women, urogenital trichomoniasis is one of the major causes of vulvovaginitis and abnormal cervicovaginal cytology. In men, *T. vaginalis* produces a mild, transient, and usually asymptomatic urethritis. Trichomonad infestations of the prostate gland, seminal vesicles, and epididymis occur but are uncommon.

The symptomatology of vulvovaginitis is nonspecific and consists of variable degrees of vaginal discharge, perineal odor, itching, burning, vulvar swelling, introital tenderness, dyspareunia, dysuria, and urinary frequency. Trichomoniasis alone accounts for about 15% to 20% of vulvovaginitis, but in another 10% to 20% of cases, the trichomonad coexists with one or more additional vaginal pathogens. *T. vaginalis* frequently coexists with bacterial vaginosis to such a degree that symptomology characteristic of the latter is often attributed to trichomoniasis.

The clinical patterns of urogenital trichomoniasis in women consist of

1. asymptomatic trichomoniasis,
2. symptomatic trichomoniasis, acute and chronic forms,
3. recurrent or persistent trichomoniasis after metronidazole therapy, and
4. neonatal and prepubescent trichomoniasis.

Asymptomatic

Approximately 70% of women harboring *T. vaginalis* are asymptomatic carriers of the organism. In a study of inner-city gravidas who presented for prenatal care, 9.4% were infected with *T. vaginalis*. Only 18.2% of infected women had vaginitis-related symptoms prior to the pelvic examinations.

Characteristically, the patient fails to experience any symptom usually associated with the disease. The pelvic examination shows no objective signs of tissue reaction. The vaginal pH is normal. Lactobacilli are present. It is postulated that in these women, either the vaginal environment is temporarily unfavorable for progressive growth of *T. vaginalis* or the particular organism is a less virulent strain incapable of evoking significant tissue response and symptoms.

Since all women with asymptomatic trichomoniasis are capable of transmitting the disease, and many will eventually become symptomatic, therapy is indicated.

Symptomatic—Acute Form

The symptoms of acute urogenital trichomoniasis are variable. The patient may exhibit profuse, frothy, gray, and malodorous vaginal discharge, which is often associated with severe itching, redness, swelling, and tenderness of the introitus; and complain of dyspareunia, dysuria, and urinary frequency (Figs. 3 and 4). Uterine tenderness may be present. But this classic syndrome accounts for only 10% of cases. Usually, the symptoms are less severe.

Patients with the acute form may have copious watery vaginal discharge requiring a perineal pad for control. Others, with scanty discharge, may complain of severe introital tenderness, swelling, dyspareunia, or dysuria. An occasional patient may have postcoital spotting, menorrhagia, or dysmenorrhea due to increased pelvic vascularity wrought by extensive trichomoniasis. Rarely, inguinal adenopathy is observed. Pregnancy may exacerbate the symptoms.

The examination usually discloses moderate erythema, edema, and tenderness of the introitus and lower side walls of the vagina. The erythema and edema of the upper vagina and ectocervix are usually diffuse. There is often a mild cervicitis. Small areas of subepithelial hyperemia of the vaginal mucosa and cervix can be demonstrated with colposcopy. When grossly discernable, punctate submucosal hemorrhages are often referred to as the "strawberry" cervix or vagina. Frequently, the vaginal fornices contain slightly raised, coarsely nodular, and often indurated patches of submucosal edema and inflammation ("cobblestone" vagina). The character of the discharge is nonspecific. It may be thin, thick, or mucoid, and its color may be white, gray, yellow, or green. It usually has a disagreeable odor and sometimes contains small bubbles, but these findings may be associated with other vaginal infections, such as vaginal bacteriosis. Characteristically, lactobacilli are absent, and the vaginal pH is above 5.5.

Wet mount examination reveals, in addition to the presence of trichomonads, a significant number of white blood cells and a disruption of the vaginal bacterial flora. Between 30% and 60% of women with acute symptomatic disease have a positive volatile amine test and demonstrate the presence of clue cells.

Symptomatic—Chronic Form

The most frequent type of symptomatic trichomoniasis is the chronic form. Usually women with the chronic form of the infection have a long history of intermittent vulvovaginitis, with many having been treated repeatedly with various topical preparations. Some patients choose to endure the symptoms, whereas others temporarily alleviate them by self-medication with douches, perfumes, and other proprietary preparations.

The complaints vary but are usually mild. There may be slight-to-moderate malodorous vaginal discharge, perineal itching, or dyspareunia.

Pelvic examination usually reveals mild introital erythema and tenderness, and white, gray, or slightly yellow mucoid discharge that may be malodorous and contain a few bubbles. The mucosa of the vagina and cervix usually shows no gross evidence of significant inflammation, but despite this, abnormal Pap smears are relatively frequent in patients with chronic trichomoniasis. Lactobacilli are reduced in number, and the vaginal pH is usually over 4.5.

NEONATAL AND PREPUBESCENT TRICHOMONIASIS

The neonatal infant or the prepubescent female may asymptomatically harbor *T. vaginalis* or may develop symptomatic vaginal discharge, itching, sleeplessness, or pyuria. Most cases in the newborn infant are transmitted during vaginal delivery in a trichomonad-infected mother.

Symptomatic trichomoniasis in young girls is encountered most frequently in the first few months of life and one to two years prior to menarche. A somewhat higher level of circulatory estrogen and a relatively more mature vaginal epithelium, which occur during these periods,

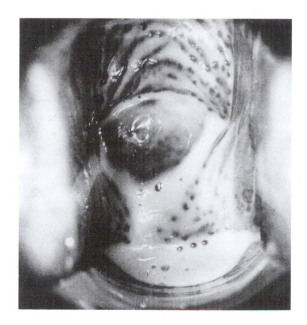

FIGURE 3 Trichomoniasis with a "strawberry vagina." While diagnostic when present, this finding is seen in only a few of the patients with the infection.

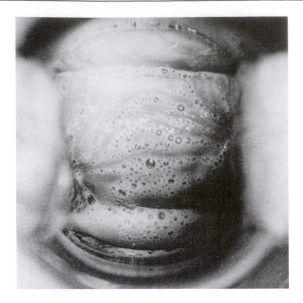

FIGURE 4 Marked frothiness, when present, is usually a sign of trichomoniasis, but frothiness is usually minimal and present in only about 10% of the patients with trichomonal infections.

appear to augment the growth and the subsequent symptomatology of the trichomonad.

Symptomatic trichomoniasis is less common in the one-to nine-year age group, when maternally derived estrogen is no longer present and when the ovarian output of estrogen is minimal. However, a latent or asymptomatic phase of *T. vaginalis* infestation may exist during these early years.

TRICHOMONIASIS IN PREGNANCY

Several studies have suggested that pregnant women infected with *T. vaginalis* may be at increased risk of an adverse perinatal outcome. In a multi–university-affiliated hospital study of 13,816 patients, Cotch et al. (1991) found that pregnant women infected with *T. vaginalis* at midgestation were statistically significantly more likely to have a low-birthweight infant and to deliver preterm. Compared to in whites and Hispanics, *T. vaginalis* infection accounts for a disproportionately larger share of the low-birthweight rate in blacks. In contrast, a smaller study by the National Institute of Child Health and Human Development Maternal–Fetal Medicine Units Network of 2929 gravidas at 10 centers failed to detect a significant association between infection with *T. vaginalis* and preterm births.

Neither study subdivided gravidas with trichomoniasis into acute versus chronic and with or without concomitant vaginal bacteriosis. Meis et al. (1995) and McGregor et al. (1996) have demonstrated that the presence of vaginal bacteriosis at 22 and 28 weeks of gestation was statistically associated with an increased risk of spontaneous preterm births. McGregor et al. (1991) have similarly demonstrated that orally administered clindamycin treatment was associated with a 50% reduction of bacterial vaginosis–linked preterm birth and preterm premature rupture of membranes. There is a growing movement to screen all gravidas

at risk for preterm births for bacterial vaginosis or common genital tract infections.

The Vaginal Infections and Prematurity Study Group (Meis et al., 1995), who evaluated the relationship between frequent sexual intercourse, preterm delivery, and vaginal colonization with specific microorganisms, found that frequent sexual intercourse by itself was not associated with an increased risk of preterm birth. However, women who were colonized with *T. vaginalis* and *Mycoplasma hominis* and who engage in frequent intercourse are at increased risk for preterm delivery.

DIAGNOSIS

The diagnosis of all types of vulvovaginitis, including urogenital trichomoniasis, is considerably more accurate and conclusive if the patient has been instructed not to douche or use any form of topical vaginal preparation (contraceptives or antivaginitis creams, foams, or suppositories) for 48 hours prior to examination.

After a careful history, the external genitalia are examined. The urethra, periurethral glands, and Bartholin's glands are milked, and the vagina and cervix are visualized with a dry unlubricated sterile speculum. Appropriate cultures, a wet smear, a cytologic cancer smear, and often certain biopsies are necessary to determine the presence or absence of other common vaginal and cervical diseases that may cause vulvovaginitis or that may coexist with urogenital trichomoniasis, such as candidiasis, *Gardnerella vaginalis* infection, gonorrhea, genital herpes, chronic cervicitis, condyloma acuminatum, or cervical carcinoma.

Urogenital trichomoniasis cannot be diagnosed with any reasonable degree of accuracy on the basis of the history and the objective signs found on pelvic examination. The only acceptable methods of diagnosis are wet smear and/or cultural identification of the viable trichomonad.

Wet Smear

The wet smear identification of *T. vaginalis* is rapid and inexpensive and, in symptomatic patients, at least 80% to 90% reliable. A fresh specimen of vaginal discharge or urine sediment is mixed with a drop of warm saline on a slide, topped with a coverslip, and examined quickly with a microscope (light phase or dark-field). Under low power, the organism usually moves actively in a jerky and twisting fashion due to the lashing and waving motions of the anterior flagella and the undulating membrane. If no obvious activity is apparent, higher-power observation and some experience are necessary to identify the action of the undulating membrane or the inconspicuous ameboid movement of sluggish organisms.

Culture

The inoculation of a suitable transport medium (Stuart or thioglycollate) with the subsequent culture, incubation, and microscopic identification of viable *T. vaginalis* is expensive and time consuming. It is the most sensitive and accurate means of detecting *T. vaginalis* in cases of suspected male trichomoniasis, in cases of refractory, undiagnosed vulvovaginitis, and in most investigational studies of the protozoon. The commercially available Feinberg-Whittington or Kupferberg (simplified trypticase serum) culture media are both satisfactory for clinical practice, but Diamond or Lowe media are more sensitive.

Cytological Smears

The Pap cancer smear is not a reliable method for the detection of *T. vaginalis* since most cytopathology laboratories report considerable errors, both false positives and false negatives, in the identification of the organisms. Therefore, confirmatory identification of viable organisms by the wet smear or culture techniques is essential before treatment of any patient with "trichomonads" initially identified on cytological smear.

The Gram or Giemsa staining methods of *T. vaginalis* are somewhat more time consuming and probably of no greater accuracy than the wet smear preparation.

Although identification of the trichomonad is the basic starting point in the diagnosis and the subsequent therapy of urogenital trichomoniasis, the true etiology of the patient's symptoms and pelvic findings must always be regarded as uncertain until all signs and symptoms, including an abnormal Pap smear, have been completely resolved after specific management.

Test Kits

An enzyme-linked immunoabsorbent assay (ELISA) based test kit for private practice use (Genzyme Corp., Cambridge, MA) is commercially available for *Trichomonas* identification. Sensitivity is stated to be superior to microscopy and almost equal to culture. Other test kits are in development.

THERAPY

Eradication of organisms from the genital or urinary system depends upon the administration of a systemic agent.

Metronidazole and tinidazole are the only agents from the imidazole antibiotic group approved for treatment of trichomoniasis in the United States. No vaginal medication will eradicate organisms from Skene's duct and urinary tract. Instillation of topical trichomonacidal drugs into the urethra and bladder of either sex is ineffective. Metronidazole and tinidazole are the only effective agents available that eradicate trichomonads from the host. Metronidazole is usually less expensive, having been accepted in the United States as a generic drug.

The remarkable success of oral metronidazole is due to its antitrichomonal activity in the urine, serum, glands, and other tissues, enabling it to treat those trichomonad-infested anatomical areas of the genitourinary tract (urethra, bladder, periurethral glands, Bartholin's glands, endocervix, prostate, and seminal vesicles) inaccessible to topical preparations. Imidazoles diffuse well, even into poorly perfused tissues. Metronidazole in a single 2 g dose produces peak serum levels of 40 g/mL. Its serum half-life is approximately eight hours. Levels of metronidazole in breast milk equal the serum concentration. Approximately 20% of an ingested dose is excreted unchanged in the urine. The pharmacodynamics of tinidazole are similar, except for a longer tinidazole half-life of approximately 13 hours.

Imidazole antibiotics are unstable electron receptors that readily donate the electron to oxidize various *Trichomonas* proteins and DNA in an anaerobic (low oxidation–reduction potential) protozoal environment. Spontaneous reduction to an unstable imidazole nitro group oxidizes the protozoal DNA, which results in cell death. Human DNA is resistant to the harmful effects of imidazoles because of the higher oxidation–reduction potential of normal human physiology. In vitro, trichomonads are rendered nonviable when in contact with metronidazole for approximately four hours.

The dosage schedules of metronidazole most widely employed are the following:

- 250 mg three times a day for five to seven days
- 500 mg three times a day for three days
- 500 mg every 12 hours for five to seven days
- 2 g single stat bolus

The typical dosage schedule for tinidazole is a 2 g single oral bolus dose.

If the patient can swallow the larger pills, four 500 mg pills are more economical than eight 250 mg pills. Bolus administration and five- to seven-day regimens are equally effective in the treatment of uncomplicated trichomoniasis. Higher cure rates are achieved when the male consort is concomitantly treated. Posttherapy vulvovaginal candidiasis (ping-pong vaginitis) is more common in association with the multiday therapy.

The clinical response to treatment with imidazoles is often dramatic. Symptoms abate in a few days and local tissue alterations usually resolve in three to six weeks.

Imidazole-induced complications are usually mild and occur in less than 10% of cases. Most are orally or gastrointestinally related, such as dry mouth, metallic or bitter taste, glossitis, stomatitis, furry tongue, anorexia, nausea, epigastric or abdominal pain, vomiting, or diarrhea. A metallic taste may be the most frequent adverse complaint and is associated with imidazole in the saliva. The "furry tongue" sensation occasionally persists for several weeks after therapy. Central nervous system (CNS) reactions are rare, but headache, dizziness, vertigo, ataxia, confusion, and depression have been reported. A few patients have developed a drug-related rash or urticaria, and a dark urine has been ascribed to a metabolite of metronidazole. A transient, mild, and reversible neutropenia has been reported, and patients receiving frequent courses of metronidazole therapy should have blood count monitoring before, during, and after therapy. Because of a disulfiram-like effect, ingestion of alcohol during or immediately following metronidazole therapy may induce an annoying clinical syndrome comprising many of the gastrointestinal and CNS symptoms. Tinidazole generally demonstrates a more favorable efficacy profile than metronidazole and possibly fewer side effects.

Fetal Considerations

Animal studies have demonstrated the ability of metronidazole to function as a mutogen. To date, no recognizable teratogenic or adverse neonatal effect has been demonstrated. Nevertheless, drug administration during the first 16 weeks is best delayed for theoretical reasons.

Sexual Partner Therapy

To prevent reinfection, treatment of a patient's sexual consorts is imperative. Therapy of the male partner may reduce transmission of infection to other females. Males refusing therapy should use a condom for four weeks after initial treatment of the female.

Trichomonas Therapy During Pregnancy

Unanswered questions remain regarding the treatment of *Trichomonas* infection during therapy. It would appear natural to treat any case of trichomoniasis during pregnancy. Some studies have suggested that active *Trichomonas* infection in pregnancy may increase the risk of preterm labor and contribute to other pregnancy-related morbidities. The risk of preterm birth is most evident when bacterial vaginosis coexists.

As a general principle, infections during pregnancy are treated at the first opportunity; however, speculative concerns of mutogenesis cause some reluctance to administer imidazoles during the first trimester of pregnancy. To date, treatment of asymptomatic *T. vaginalis* in pregnancy has not been found to lower the risk for preterm delivery. Klebanoff et al. (2001) found an even greater risk of mid-third trimester preterm birth if trichomoniasis is treated with metronidazole during pregnancy (relative risk of 1.78). It is postulated that toxins released from dying trichomonads may activate the labor mechanisms. In Klebanoff's review, *Trichomonas* therapy had no adverse effect or beneficial impact upon extreme prematurity prior to 32 weeks. The decision to treat *Trichomonas* infection during pregnancy remains a case-by-case matter, potentially based upon the severity of the patient's vaginal symptoms and the status of fetal development.

METRONIDAZOLE-RESISTANT *T. VAGINALIS*

Induction of resistance of *T. vaginalis* to metronidazole can be demonstrated both in vitro and in vivo. With serial passage in vitro of an initially moderately resistant strain to increasing concentrations of metronidazole, the minimal lethal concentration of metronidazole will increase from <0.2 µg/mL to >50 mg/mL. With repeated passage of the organism in mice treated with suboptimal doses of metronidazole, the activity of metronidazole will be 14 to 48 times less than that of the original strain.

There are no well-established protocols for the therapy of metronidazole-resistant *T. vaginalis*. The majority of cases have relative, rather than absolute, resistance.

Most patients who fail to respond to bolus or 500 mg b.i.d. for five to seven days represent a composite of individuals with either poor compliance, reinfection, or relative resistance.

Management of a patient with persistent *Trichomonas* following metronidazole therapy involves initially doubling the prescribed therapeutic dose, prolonging the duration of administration, and having the patient refrain from sexual activities and/or douching (Table 1). Tinidazole has a longer half-life than metronidazole as well as significantly lower minimal inhibitary concentration (MIC) values than metronidazole. Approximately 1/3 of metronidazole-resistant strains may show decreased sensitivity to tinidazole. Using the therapy of resistant trichomoniasis involves the standard dose administered over twice the established duration.

Failure to respond to increased dosing and prolonged duration of therapy warrants obtaining metronidazole susceptibility testing. A prewarmed culture tube should be inoculated and mailed by overnight delivery service to a reference laboratory capable of performing susceptibility testing. The patient may be placed on intravaginal clotrimazole in an attempt to ameliorate her symptoms while awaiting the results of the *T. vaginalis* susceptibility testing.

Therapy of metronidazole-resistant *T. vaginalis* involves aggressive use of metronidazole or tinidazole. Concomitantly, 1 g of metronidazole in an appropriate vehicle can be administered intravaginally at bedtime. Five grams of metronidazole gel (37.5 mg of metronidazole) may be used intravaginally b.i.d. as an adjunct to high-dose oral therapy in highly resistant cases. Dosages of metronidazole required for cure are not approved by the Food and Drug Administration and may be associated with a high incidence of adverse drug reactions. Administration of 4 to 6 g or more daily has been associated with seizures and a potentially disabling peripheral neuropathy. Sobel et al. (2001) have reported well-tolerated successful therapy for documented metronidazole-resistant *Trichomonas* infection with daily oral doses of tinidazole ranging from 500 mg orally four times a day to 1 g orally three times a day, combined with insertion of 500 mg tinidazole (oral) tablet vaginally two to three times daily for 14 days.

How long oral therapy should persist is speculative. Many clinicians will do daily wet mounts. As soon as the wet mount becomes negative, the dosage is reduced and therapy is continued for two to four additional days.

TABLE I Suggestions for the treatment of metronidazole-resistant trichomoniasis

Resistance to metronidazole is relative, not an all-or-none phenomenon

Mild-to-moderate resistance
Most cases can be cured by increased dosages of metronidazole or tinidazole. As a rule of thumb, doubling the initial recommended dose and extending the duration of therapy by 2 days is usually all that is required

Moderate-to-severe resistance
Select to treat patient in midcycle. Have patient use saline douches twice a day for at least 3 days prior to the initiation of therapy. Prior to the first insertion of intravaginal imidazole treatment, mechanically cleanse the vagina with initially H_2O_2 and then paint with gentian violet. Initiate tinidazole therapy using concomitantly oral and intravaginal portals of administrations. Patients must be *very* closely monitored for adverse drug reaction

PROPHYLAXIS FOR VULVOVAGINAL TRICHOMONIASIS

Postcoital douching with an acid preparation soon after intercourse, contraceptive creams, jellies and foams with trichomonadal properties (if used before and after intercourse), condoms, and prophylactic use of metronidazole have all been advocated for the prevention of reinfection. Only condoms are effective.

SELECTED READING

Diagnosis
Caliendo AM, Jordan JA, Green AM et al. Real-time PCR improves detection of *Trichomonas* vaginalis infections compared with culture using self-collected vaginal swabs. Infect Dis Obstet Gynecol 2005; 13:145.

Cotch MF, Pastorek JG, Nugent RP, et al. Demographic and behavioral predictors of *Trichomonas vaginalis* infection among pregnant women. Obstet Gynecol 1991; 6:1067.

Donne A. Animalcules observes dans les matieres purulentes et le produit des secretions des organes genitaux de l'homme et de la femme. Compt Rend Acad Sci 1836; 3:38.

Fouts Ac, Kraus SJ. *Trichomonas vaginalis*: re-evaluation of its clinical presentation and laboratory diagnosis. J Infect Dis 1990; 141:137.

Franklin TL, Monif GRG. *Trichomonas vaginalis* and bacterial vaginosis in wet mount examinations of pregnant women. J Reprod Med 2000; 45:131.

Hammill HA. *Trichomonas vaginalis*. Obstet Gynecol Clin North Am 1989; 16:531.

Heine RP, McGregor JA, Patterson E, et al. *Trichomonas vaginalis*: diagnosis and clinical characteristics in pregnancy. Infect Dis Obstet Gynecol 1994; 1:228.

Krieger JN, Tam MR, Stevens CE, et al. Diagnosis of trichomoniasis: comparison of conventional wet mount examination with cytological studies, cultures, and monoclonal antibody staining of direct specimens. J Am Med Assoc 1988; 259:1223.

McCann JS. Comparison of direct microscopy and culture in the diagnosis of trichomoniasis. Br J Vener Dis 1974; 50:450.

McLennan R, Spence MR, Brockman M, et al. The clinical diagnosis of trichomoniasis. Obstet Gynecol 1982; 60:30.

McMillian A. Laboratory diagnostic methods and cryopreservation of trichomonads. In: Honigberg BM, ed. Trichomonads Parasitic in Humans. New York: Spring Hill, 1990:297.

Perl G. Errors in the diagnosis of *Trichomonas vaginalis* infection as observed among 1199 patients. Obstet Gynecol 1972; 39:7.

Rein MF. Clinical manifestations of urogenital trichomoniasis in women. In: Honigberg BM, ed. Trichomonads Parasitic in Humans. New York: Spring Hill, 1990:225.

Spence MR, Hollander DH, Smith JL, et al. The clinical and laboratory diagnosis of *Trichomonas vaginalis* infection. Sex Transm Dis 1980; 7:168.

Therapy
Ahmed-Jushuf IH, Murray AE, McKeown J. Managing *Trichomonas vaginalis* refractory to conventional treatment with metronidazole. Genitourin Med 1988; 641:25.

Chang JH, Ryang YS, Morio T, Chang EJ. *Trichomonas vaginalis* inhibits pro-inflammatory cytokine production in macrophages by suppressing NF-kappaB activation. Mol Cells 2004; 18:177.

Crowell AL, Sanders-Lewis KA, Secor WE. *In vitro* metroniidazole and tinidazole activities against metronidazole-resistant strains of *Trichomonas vaginalis*. Antimicrob Agents Chemother 2003; 47:1407.

Cudmore SL, Delgaty KL, Hayward-McClelland SF, et al. Treatment of infections caused by metronidazole-resistant *Trichomonas* vaginalis. Clin Microbiol Rev 2004; 17:783.

Lossick JG, Kent HL. Trichomoniasis: trends in diagnosis and management. Am J Obstet Gynecol 1991; 165:1217.

Lumsden WH, Robertson DH, Heyworth R, Harrison C. Treatment failure in *Trichomonas vaginalis* vaginitis. Genitourin Med 1988; 64:217.

Mammen-Tobin A, Wilson JD. Management of metronidazole-resistant *Trichomonas* vaginalis—a new approach. Int J STD AIDS 2005; 16:488.

McClean AN. Treatment of trichomoniasis in the female with a 5-day course of metronidazole (Flagyl). Br J Vener Dis 1971; 47:36.

Metronidazole (Flagyl) box warning. FDA Drug Bull 1976; 6:22.

Nanda N, Michael RG, Kurdgelashvilv G, Wendel KA. *Trichomonas* and its treatment. Expert Rev Anti Infect Ther 2006; 4:125.

Sobel JD, Nyirjesy P, Brown W. Tinidazole therapy for metronidazole-resistant vaginal *Trichomonas*. Clin Infect 2001; 33:1341.

Thomason JL, Gelbart SM. *Trichomonas vaginalis*. Obstet Gynecol 1989; 74:536.

Thomason JL, Gelbart SM, James JA, Broekhuizen FF. Vaginitis in reproductive-age women. Curr Opin Obstet Gynecol 1989; 1:35.

Neonatal and Prepubescent Trichomonas
Binder SS. Vaginal trichomoniasis in a 2-month-old child. Obstet Gynecol 1963; 21:354.

Blattner RJ. *Trichomonas vaginalis* infection in a newborn infant. J Pediatr 1967; 71:608.

Feo LG. The incidence of *Trichomonas vaginalis* in the various age groups. Am J Trop Med 1956; 5:786.

Soper DE. Bacterial vaginosis and trichomoniasis: epidemiology and management of recurrent disease. Infect Dis Obstet Gynecol 1994; 2:242.

Trichomoniasis and Pregnancy
Cotch MF, Pastorek JG II, Nugent RP, et al. *Trichomonas* vaginalis associated with low birth weight and preterm delivery. The Vaginal Infections and Prematurity Study Group 1997; 24:353.

Klebanoff MA, Carey JC, Hauth JC, et al. Failure of metronidazole to prevent preterm delivery among pregnant women with asymptomatic *Trichomonas* vaginalis infection. N Engl J Med 2001; 345:487.

Mcgregor JA, French JI. Bacterial vaginosis and preterm birth. N Engl J Med 1996; 334:1337.

McGregor JA, French JI, Seo K. Adjunctive clindamycin therapy for preterm labor: results of a double-blind, placebo-controlled trial. Am J Obstet Gynecol 1991; 165:867.

Meis PJ, Goldenbury RL, Mercer B. The preterm prediction study; significance of vaginal infections. Amer J obstet Gynecol 1995; 183:1231.

Meis PJ, Goldenburg RL, Mercer B. The preterm prediction study: significance of vaginal infections. National Institute of Child Health and Human Development Maternal Fetal Medicine Units Network. Am J Obstet Gynecol 1995; 183:1231.

Murphy PA, Jones E. Use of oral metronidazole in pregnancy, risks, benefits and practice guidelines. J Nurse Midwifery 1994; 39:214.

Nadisauskiene R, Bergstrom S, Stankeviciene I, et al. Endocervical pathogens in women with preterm and term labour. Gynecol Obstet Invest 1995; 40:179.

Okun N, Gronau KA, Hannah ME. Antibiotics for bacterial vaginosis or *Trichomonas vaginalis* in pregnancy: a systematic review. Obstet Gynecol 2005; 105:857.

Read JS, Klebanoff MA. Sexual intercourse during pregnancy and preterm delivery: effects of vaginal microorganisms. Am J Obstet Gynecol 1993; 168:514.

INTRODUCTION

Candida albicans is a dimorphic, gram-positive fungus that exhibits both yeast and filamentous growth. Growth of the organism either on surfaces or in biologic fluids results in an over-budding yeast-like form, measuring 2–3 × 4–6 mm (Fig. 1). When the organism invades tissue, both hyphae and pseudohyphae develop (Fig. 2). They are common in infected tissue.

The female genital tract is a sophisticated microbiological environment. The microbiological presence of an organism does not necessarily equate with the disease. Depending upon age group, geographical location, and socioeconomic status, up to 41% of women may harbor one or more species of *Candida* as a "normal" constituent of the vaginal flora. Greater than 400 strains of *Candida* have been identified. There is no evidence of vaginotropism. The distribution of strains is comparable between
1. vaginal versus nonvaginal sites and
2. patients with candidal vulvovaginitis and with asymptomatic carriage.

Among women who harbor a strain of *Candida* in the vaginal flora, 45% will have more than one additional strain of *Candida* present.

While the point prevalence of candidal organisms as constituents of the vaginal flora is significant, it is probable that the principal reservoir for the organism is the gastrointestinal tract. *C. albicans* can be recovered from 65% of gastrointestinal tract fecal samples in a random population. Patients with vaginal colonization invariably have intestinal carriage of the same organism. Studies in healthy adults suggest that *C. albicans* can be recovered from the oropharynx in 30% of normal adults, from the jejunum in 50%, the ileum in 50%, and the rectum in 60%. Horowitz et al. (1985) found that the species of yeast found in the vagina of women with recrudescence of vulvovaginal candidiasis is likely to be the same species found in the oral cavity of both partners and in the male ejaculate. In this study, cultures of the oral cavity of the male partner were positive in 36%, ejaculate cultures were positive in 15%, and rectal cultures were positive in 33%. Prostatic cultures failed to reveal a single positive culture. The absence of yeast in prostatic fluid and its presence in seminal ejaculate suggests that an untreated reservoir for recolonization exists in the seminal vesicles.

Asymptomatic penile yeast carriage occurs in 5% to 25% of male partners of women with vulvovaginitis candidiasis. The organism can be isolated primarily from the coronal sulcius. The absence of circumcision may not be a critical factor. Horowitz et al. observed comparable rates of penile carriage in circumcised and uncircumcised males.

Oropharyngeal cultures from women with recurrent candidiasis were positive for mycotic organism in 36% of the patients. The oral cavity of the female may be a source for male colonization and subsequent reintroduction of the organism into the vaginal flora. While the incidence of rectal isolation in women with chronic vulvovaginitis is comparable to that in controlled populations, both oral and vaginal carriage of the organism is elevated in those who have chronic or recurrent disease compared to control groups.

Despite the large number of strains, the spectrum of candidal strains causing vulvovaginitis is limited. The majority of cases are due to *C. albicans*. One-third of the cases are due to *C. tropicalis*, *C. pseudotropicalis*, *C. stellatoidea*, *C. krusei*, and *C. guilliermondi*. To cause disease, a given strain of *Candida* must have the ability to attach to squamous epithelial cells. Adhesion can be made between candidal organisms and nonbiological materials, such as catheters, by electrostatic forces or by complementary receptors and ligands. Nonalbicans *Candida* have reduced ability to attach to vaginal epithelial cells.

PATHOGENESIS OF DISEASE

When isolates from patients with recurrent and/or chronic vulvovaginitis candidiasis are compared with isolates from patients with asymptomatic colonization, no differences in attachment avidity have been demonstrated. The principal factors determining disease are the availability of the organism and some change in the local microbiological environment that permits attachment and organismal replication.

Vulvovaginal candidiasis is rarely a sexually transmitted disease. In more than 85% of the cases, the organism is of endogenous origin. In less than 10% of the cases, sexual intercourse is the probable mode of dissemination.

A demonstrable difference between asymptomatic colonization and vulvovaginal candidiasis is the magnitude of organism replication. Asymptomatic colonization is associated with $10^2 – 10^5$ cfu/mL of vaginal fluid. The emergence

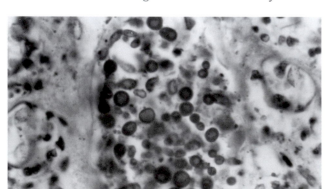

FIGURE 1 *Candida albicans* yeast-like forms. Oval, budding yeast-like form growing within the lumen of a renal tubule (PAS ×630).

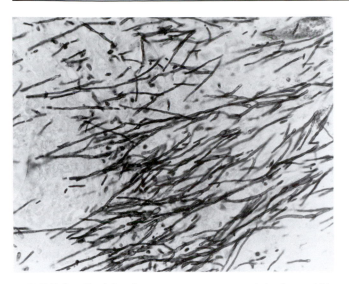

FIGURE 2 *Candida albicans* growing as pseudohyphae within infected tissue (PAS ×320).

of disease from a state of prior colonization is accompanied by a quantitative change in the magnitude of organism replication (>10^{6}cfu/mL of vaginal fluid).

Candidal vulvovaginitis is rare in premenarchal and postmenopausal women. The most common predisposing factors are the glycogen content of vaginal secretions, especially in pregnancy, and moisture. Disease is highest among women living in tropical areas with prolonged high temperature and humidity.

The concept is slowly evolving that for patients with recurring candidiasis who do not have a demonstrable etiological factor; i.e., minor impairment of T-cell functions, the key to reducing the degree of recrudescence of vulvovaginal candidiasis is the reduction of the degree or the eradication of the potential reservoirs. Studies have suggested that by attacking the individual reservoirs, whether oral, seminal, vesical, or intestinal, one can begin to impact on the incidence of recurrence in this group of patients who do not have genesis III type of vulvovaginitis. Both intermittent, short-term monthly therapy and persistent low-dose daily therapy have reduced the frequency of recurrences in these kinds of patients. Exactly which therapeutic strategy is most effective awaits scientific confirmation.

VULVOVAGINAL CANDIDIASIS

Pruritus vulvae is easily the most prominent symptom of the patient with vulvovaginal candidiasis. Frequently, the itching is intense. Relief may occur during menstrual periods, perhaps due to the alkalinity of menstrual blood. Dyspareunia is a common complaint. Dysuria may result from the passage of urine over the irritated areas. Vaginal discharge is a variable finding; when present, it is practically always preceded by pruritus. Premenstrual exacerbation is characteristic.

Vulvovaginal candidiasis is more a vulvitis rather than a vaginitis. The presence of noncharacteristic discharge should alert one to the probability that the etiology

of disease may be due to *Trichomonas vaginalis* and not *C. albicans*. When discharge indicative of significant concomitant vaginitis is present, it tends to be relatively sparse in quantity and has a characteristic cottage cheese–like appearance (Fig. 3). Vaginitis predominating over vulvitis is more characteristic of antibiotic-induced disease.

Pruritus or perineal itching is the symptom of a patient presenting with vulvovaginal candidiasis. The localization of perineal itching is of diagnostic importance. Pruritus limited to the labia majora suggests either cutaneous candidiasis or the presence of ectoparasites. Perineal and vaginal pruritus can be due to either *T. vaginalis*, human papilloma viruses, or *C. albicans*. Determination of pH and examination of KOH and saline wet mounts are often diagnostic.

The reason for the exacerbation or amelioration of clinical disease in relation to the menstrual cycle is again primarily a function of pH. The pH of menstrual blood is 7.2. *T. vaginalis* thrives on an alkaline milieu whereas *C. albicans* is relatively inhibited.

Other symptoms may include vaginal soreness, vulvar burning, dyspareunia, and external dysuria. None of these symptoms are specific.

OMAHA CLASSIFICATION OF VULVOVAGINAL CANDIDIASIS

Although candidiasis of the female genital tract is a monoetiological disease, the pathways to pathogenic expression are significantly divergent to constitute a classification scheme for vaginal candidiasis (Table 1).

The classification of vulvovaginal candidiasis is composed of three distinct geneses as shown in Table 1.

Primary Candidiasis

Primary candidiasis has a spectrum of disease whose dipoles are a vulvitis on one hand and a vaginitis on the other. The presence of a clinically significant vulvitis is more characteristic of this group. Augmented moisture/humidity is its principal catalytic factor. In these cases, therapy must concomitantly treat the labia as well as the vaginal reservoir.

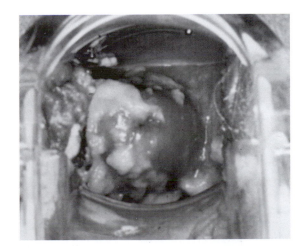

FIGURE 3 Characteristic cottage cheese–like appearance.

TABLE I Omaha classification of vulvovaginal candidiasis

Genesis I	Primary vulvovaginal candidiasis
	A. Vulvitis
	B. Vulvovaginitis with predominant vulvar involvement
	C. Vaginitis with relatively minimal vulvar involvement
Genesis II	Antibiotic-associated vulvovaginal candidiasis
	A. Secondary to systemic therapy for nonvulvovaginal condition
	B. Ping-pong vaginitis
Genesis III	Systemically influenced vulvovaginal candidiasis
	A. Pregnancy, high-dose estrogen contraceptives
	B. Steroids
	C. Diabetes mellitus
	D. T-cell dysfunction
	1. Congenital
	2. Acquired

Antibiotic-Activated Candidiasis

Antibiotic-activated candidiasis results from a different alteration of the microbiological environment that is achieved by the eradication of bacterial attachment to mannan and mannoprotein surface antigens. Eradication of the bacteria attached to mannan receptors frees these sites for attachment by *Candida* yeast cells.

Just as *Candida* is susceptible to bacteriocins, it is also capable of elaborating bacteriocins that are effective only at an acid pH. Vaginitis is more characteristic of this group than is vulvovaginitis. The major therapeutic goal in treating antibiotic-induced disease is the eradication of the disease in the vaginal reservoir. Some preference is given to the tablet form of therapy owing to better patient compliance.

Ping-Pong Vaginitis

Ping-pong vaginitis is a variant of antibiotic-induced candidiasis in which antimicrobial therapy is given for antecedent genital tract infections rather than infections involving another organ system. The classic history of ping-pong vaginitis is that of a patient improving significantly for a short period of time and then reexperiencing symptoms. A complete reevaluation of the patient is required in order not to continue prescribing pharmacologically similar drugs which, if anything, aggravate the situation. The most common setting for "ping-pong" vaginitis is a patient with bacterial vaginosis who is treated with oral metronidazole. In those patients with bacterial vaginosis who subsequently develop vulvovaginal candidiasis, wet mount analyses have shown that *C. albicans* is already present and is present in its pseudohyphae form prior to therapy for bacterial vaginosis.

Systemically Induced Candidiasis

The principal critical factor selecting for systemically induced candidiasis is an increase in the glucose substrate available in the local microbiological environment or in the presence of T-cell dysfunction for patients with systemically induced candidiasis due to steroids, diabetes mellitus, or immunodeficiency involving T-cell function. Intravaginal/vulvar therapy with anticandidal creams applied topically coupled with perioral fluconazole is preferred.

Pregnancy

Approximately 30% of gravidas have positive vaginal cultures for *Candida* as compared with 16% of nongravid individuals. Pregnanediol, a steroid hormone produced in large quantities during pregnancy, enhances the growth of *C. albicans* in vitro. Following delivery, the retrogression of the vaginal epithelium and disappearance of glycogen remove the factors enhancing fungal growth. These changes are reflected in a rapid disappearance of *Candida* from the postpartum vagina. Only topical azole therapies, applied for seven days, are recommended for use in pregnant women.

Oral Contraceptives

Diddle et al. (1969) reported on a large series of patients studied over a prolonged period to determine the relationship between oral contraceptives and vaginal candidiasis. They concluded that the incidence of candidal vulvovaginitis was more common in women using oral contraceptives for one or more years than in women abstaining from antibirth pills or those taking the medication for less than one year. It should be pointed out, however, that only a limited number of investigators are convinced that a specific relationship exists between oral contraceptives and vaginal candidiasis.

Diabetes Mellitus

Diabetes mellitus is usually considered to be one of the conditions that predispose to infection by *Candida*. There is a higher frequency of positive vaginal cultures for *Candida* and a greater incidence of vulvovaginitis due to this organism in diabetic than in nondiabetic women.

Diabetes mellitus is thought to act by increasing the glucose substrates available in the local microbiological environment. Although it is an important factor in determining the severity of disease and the incidence of colonization, increased glucose in body excretion or secretion is probably not the critical factor selecting for disease in a given patient. Other than vulvovaginitis, no other form of candidiasis is more common in the diabetic person.

Women with poorly controlled diabetes and/or receiving corticosteroids do not respond well to short-term therapies. Prevention of recurrent candidiasis necessitates rectifying where possible the underlying predisposing condition.

Adrenal Steroids

Administration of adrenal glucocorticoids enhances experimental infections due to a variety of microbial agents. Corticosteroids predispose to host cell destruction by stabilizing the lysosomal membrane, thus preventing the release of catabolic enzymes that ordinarily digest phagocytized organisms. This alteration of a primary host defense mechanism results in an increased incidence of both local and systemic candidiasis.

Immunologic Disorders

Certain conditions pathogenic for humans underscore the importance of cell-mediated immunity in the resistance of *C. albicans*. Cutaneous or systemic candidiasis is more likely to develop in subjects with congenital maldevelopment of the thymus (e.g., thymic dysplasia, thymic alymphoplasia, the fourth pharyngeal syndrome, and retrovirus infection with HIV-1 and HIV-2). Certain families with a genetically determined defect in cellular immunity (characterized in vivo by the absence of delayed hypersensitivity and a failure to reject homograph transplants, and in vitro by a lack of lymphocyte transformation by *Candida* antigens and the elaboration of a serum factor inhibiting the proliferative response to normal antigen-stimulated lymphocytes) exhibit an exaggerated susceptibility to the organisms. Iatrogenic drug impairment of normal cellular immunity, as reflected by in vitro suppression of lymphocyte transformation in response to specific antigenic stimulation, predisposes to candidiasis. Although depression of humoral immunity plays a role in the host's defenses, it is of secondary importance compared to cellular immunity. Disorders of phagocytic function or quantity, defects in phagocytic chemotaxis, phagocyte-killing capacities, and intraleukocytic metabolism predispose to candidiasis. Among the presenting manifestations of patients with acquired immune deficiency syndrome (AIDS) are vaginal and oropharyngeal candidiasis.

The Centers for Disease Control and Prevention (CDC) has recently adopted a new classification of vulvovaginal candidiasis, based not on pathogenesis, but on potential antifungal selection, which divides cases into uncomplicated and complicated. Uncomplicated vuluovaginal candidiasis defines mild to moderate, sporadic, non-recurring disease. Patients with intact host defense mechanisms can be anticipated to respond to azole therapy (even single dose) in less than seven days.

DIAGNOSIS

Speculum examination reveals variable amounts of a thick, white, curd-like or flocculent discharge that is loosely adherent to the vaginal mucosa. The character of the discharge has often been likened to cottage cheese. This type of discharge, while suggestive, is not diagnostic of candidal vulvovaginitis. Such a discharge may be physiological. Vaginal and vulvar findings can vary from complete normality of the parts to diffuse vaginal, cervical, and vulvar erythema. In the latter circumstance, the vagina may bleed easily on contact, and slight edema of the vulva is common. Cutaneous lesions as an extension from the vagina are not common, but when seen, they consist of small reddish macules and vesicopustules that may rupture and become secondarily infected. Such "satellite" lesions are a clue to the etiology of the attendant vaginitis. Excoriation is common due to the intense pruritus.

Determination of pH is one of the most important diagnostic aids (Table 2). Patients with candidal vulvovaginitis have a pH of 4.2 to 4.4. Disease usually occurs in the absence of a significant inflammatory response. The presence of >5 WBC/hpf should alert the physician to the possible presence of an additional disease entity. The principal organisms associated with an acid pH are *C. albicans* and group B

streptococci (the latter usually functions with a member of the Enterobacteriaceae). Although the diagnosis of vulvovaginal candidiasis is suggested clinically by pruritus and erythema in the vulvovaginal area and, in some cases, by the presence of a white, curdy discharge, the diagnosis is made when a wet preparation or Gram stain of vaginal discharge demonstrates yeasts or pseudohyphae, or when a culture or other test yields a positive result for a yeast species.

In deep-seated candidiasis, the presence of pseudohypae necessitates special fungal stains such as the Grocott-Gomori methenamine–silver nitrate stain or periodic acid Schiff (PAS) staining.

HIV–ASSOCIATED CANDIDIASIS

Candidal oropharyngitis/esophagitis is often one of the early AIDS-defining events in women. A women presenting with oropharyngeal candidiasis needs to be evaluated for possible retrovirus infection.

Recurrent vulvovaginal candidiasis is also a potential early marker of disease. The definition for recurrent vulvovaginal candidiasis is four documented episodes in a 12-month period. Vaginal colonization rates are higher among HIV-positive women. Symptomatic vulvovaginal candidiasis tends to correlate with the degree of immunodeficiency. Prior systemic azole therapy appears to select for subsequent colonization and infection with nonalbicans *Candida* species.

Long-term prophylactic therapy with fluconazole at a dose of 200 mg weekly is reserved primarily for HIV-infected women who experience recurrent vulvovaginal candidiasis.

CANDIDA-RELATED RECURRENT ALLERGIC VAGINITIS

There is a small group of women with recurrent vaginitis in whom there is an association between coitus and the initiation of pruritus and discharge. The induction of disease may vary depending on the specific male partner. Recent evidence suggests that recurrent vaginitis can arise as a consequence of a transient and localized inhibition of cell-mediated immunity. Lymphocytes from many women with this disorder manifest a reduced in vitro proliferative response to *C. albicans*. The inhibition appears to be due to increased production by the patient's macrophages of prostaglandin E, which inhibits interleukin-2 production and thereby blocks lymphocyte proliferation. When lymphocyte responses are impaired, *C. albicans* can readily proliferate and initiate a clinical infection. Prostaglandin E2 production can arise as a consequence of a vaginal allergic response inducing immunoglobulin E (IgE) antibodies to *C. albicans*, ryegrass, contraceptive spermicides, and seminal fluid. Medications or

TABLE 2 Characteristics of candidal vulvovaginitis

Clinical presentation	Discharge	pH	KOH wet mount
Pruritus	Sparse, curd-like (cottage cheese appearance)	4.0–4.5	Budding yeast pseudohyphae

chemicals ingested by the male and present in his semen may be transmitted to sensitized females by coitus. Male-specific allergic responses may be induced in females through the seminal transfer of specific IgE antibodies.

The increased realization that recurrent vaginitis may be related to sexual exposure to a specific male will necessitate that semen from the affected woman's partner should be cultured for *Candida* and tested for IgE antibodies reactive with components in his semen or his partner's vaginal secretions.

DISSEMINATED CANDIDIASIS

In obstetrics and gynecology, disseminated candidiasis occurs primarily in the context of two clinical situations:
1. Indwelling vascular catheters
2. Parenteral nutrition

Indwelling Vascular Catheters and Needles
The weight of evidence suggests that most systemic candidal infections arise from iatrogenic creation of a vascular access through intravenous catheters. A minority of hematogenous infections are secondary to blood vessel invasion from the gastrointestinal tract. Not infrequently, the fungus has been demonstrated in the center of blood clots in thrombosed veins through which infusions had been administered. In reported cases, all obstetric and gynecologic patients developing disseminated candidiasis had received IV therapy, and the majority of these had been managed with large indwelling plastic catheters.

Parenteral Nutrition
C. albicans septicemia is a recognized complication of total parenteral nutrition (TPN) therapy. In a recent summary of the incidence of sepsis complicating TPN, candidemia was found in 3% to 25% of patients receiving such therapy. Several factors may be involved in the development of fungal sepsis in patients receiving TPN:
1. Many of the conditions that predispose patients to fungal septicemia (e.g., broad-spectrum antibiotic therapy, radiation, steroid therapy, immunosuppressant therapy) are also present in patients chosen to receive TPN. It is possible that prolonged central venous catheterization coupled with these other variables favors fungal proliferation.
2. *Candida* proliferates more rapidly than most common bacterial pathogens in TPN solutions.
3. Several clinical trials have suggested that ointments containing antibacterial substances applied to polyethylene catheter sites predispose patients to colonization with *Candida*. Since these ointments have been used liberally in the maintenance of TPN catheters, it is conceivable that they have contributed to the increased incidence of fungal septicemia.

CANDIDAL URINARY TRACT INFECTION

The increasing use of corticosteroids, immunosuppressive drugs, antineoplastic agents, and the urinary catheter has led to a significant increase in the prevalence of genitourinary fungal infections. The majority of fungal genitourinary tract infections are either caused by *C. albicans*, one of the other *Candida* species, or by *Torulopsis glabrata*.

Cystitis
Candidal cystitis usually occurs in a setting of diabetes mellitus or because of the indwelling use of a Foley catheter associated with antibiotic therapy. Symptoms include nocturia, constant burning and discomfort, and an unusual degree of frequency. The urine may be turbid or even bloody. The bladder capacity can be severely compromised. If candidal cystitis is suspected, a suprapubic aspirate should be done to rule out fungal infection of the more proximal part of the urinary tract.

Pyelonephritis
Renal involvement may present either as pyelonephritis or with obstructive symptomatology. Candidal infections frequently occur in conjunction with chronic pyelonephritis. There is a tendency for fungal infiltrations of the tip of the papillae, which may result in obstruction of the collecting tubules. A bezoar formation with secondary obstructive uropathy may also occur. A temporary diuresis in the course of an otherwise progressive oliguria is said to be diagnostic. Renal or urethral colic may occur with the passage of fungus balls. Other symptoms may be indistinguishable from those of bacterial pyelonephritis. While candidal infection may coexist with concomitant bacterial infection, coinfection with *Proteus* spp. or *Pseudomonas* spp. does not occur.

Evaluation of Funguria
Renal involvement occurs in up to 90% of the patients with sustained candidal septicemia. The spectrum of genitourinary candidiasis runs the gamut from asymptomatic candiduria to candidal cystitis to primary renal candidiasis. The major problem is distinguishing true parenchymal involvement from superficial colonization, which usually occurs in association with the use of antibiotics and a urinary catheter. In general, the genitourinary tract appears to have a considerable ability to rid itself of fungus in the absence of deep-seated infection. The real problem is distinguishing asymptomatic ascending disease from seeding of the urine by established renal disease. Prolonged use of catheterization often delineates a patient who has other potential portals, such as central venous lines or hyperalimentation sites, that provide excellent alternate sites of infection for candidal septicemia.

The diagnosis of genitourinary fungal infection is inferred by the recovery of the agent. When catheterized or suprapubically aspirated specimens in the female are obtained, the incidence of positive urine falls dramatically. A urine culture that is positive for fungus always calls for confirmation by a properly collected specimen. The definition of funguria is growth of the organism on culture of urine sediments collected on two occasions with an interval of one or more days using proper collection techniques. Cultures of sediment of 10 mL urine centrifuged at 3000 revolutions per minute for three minutes are much more sensitive than ordinary urine cultures and are preferred for diagnosis and the evaluation of therapeutic results. The quantitative colony counts are of little interest and may be misleading since there is no absolute correlation between the degree of funguria and the site or severity of the infection.

To determine the significance of a positive urine culture, blood cultures must be obtained. Renal functions should be evaluated and, if abnormal, an intravenous pyelogram should be done to assess the condition of the upper tract.

Agglutinin titers are of relatively little value because of their inability to distinguish between superficial and deep infections and their frequent cross-reaction with other infections. The *Candida* precipitin titers greater than 1:1 are suggestive of parenchymal infection; however, there is a 7% to 13% false-positive rate. The majority of patients with these false-positive reactions have had mucocutaneous candidiasis associated with autoimmune hypoparathyroidism or hypoadrenalism. The incidence of false-negative reactions is approximately 12%. These are thought to be due to terminal anergy or the lag phase between the onset of infection and development of precipitin antibodies.

CONGENITAL AND NEONATAL INFECTION

Neonatal candidal infection has been documented and studied extensively for many years. While it has only been recently that intrauterine-acquired candidiasis of the fetus and placenta have been recognized, it was not until 1968 that an association between spontaneous abortion and intrauterine fetal infection by *Candida* was first suggested.

Candidiasis Acquired in Utero

Candidal infection acquired in utero and clinically manifested at birth is rare.

The most important question to be answered in considering the pathogenesis of intrauterine-acquired *Candida* infection is how the fungus gains access to the fetus and fetal adnexa. Three mechanisms have been postulated.

1. The most obvious explanation is direct invasion of *Candida* from the vagina to the amniotic fluid following premature rupture of the membranes (PROM). Of the 16 cases reported, however, only four were associated with PROM. In 10 cases, the membranes ruptured during labor or parturition and the infant subsequently evidenced disease that was clearly established well before the onset of labor. In two cases of documented intrauterine-acquired infection, the infant had been delivered by cesarean section with membranes intact at the time of the procedure. Thus the association of PROM with placental and fetal candidiasis cannot be documented in the majority of cases reported in the literature.

2. Benirschke and Raphael (1958) postulate the existence of subclinical, self-healing ruptures in the membranes through which *C. albicans* may enter the amniotic sac. The difficulty of unequivocally proving this mechanism is obvious.

3. Penetration of *C. albicans* through intact membranes is the third possibility. It has been shown that *C. albicans* is able to penetrate and infect the chick chorioallantoic membrane and to kill the embryo by invading its internal organs. It is also conceivable that local areas of inflammation or other insidious pathologic changes may render the intact fetal membranes more permeable to fungi. The report of two cases of congenital candidiasis following repeated amnioscopy suggests that trauma to intact membranes may play a role as well.

Regardless of the primary mechanism of the fetal membrane invasion, once the amniotic fluid is infected with *C. albicans*, involvement of the fetal skin, surface of the umbilical cord, fetal bronchi, and fetal gastrointestinal tract becomes almost inevitable.

The lesions resulting from intrauterine-acquired candidal infection have been well described by Aterman (1968). The gross appearance of the umbilical cord is normal to cursory inspection, but upon careful examination, barely perceptible discrete, variable, yellowish white lesions are seen irregularly scattered over the epithelial surface. They are flat and mostly of pinpoint size. Histologically, the surface of the cord may be covered by a mycelium of hyphae, or hyphae may have penetrated the substance of the cord. Penetration into the substance of Wharton's jelly is never deep, according to Aterman (1968), owing to the intense inflammatory response elicited by the invading *Candida*. As a result of the invasion of the cord by *Candida*, an effusion of fetal leukocytes through the large vessels occurs, and the so-called *Candida* granulomas develop. They are characterized by foci of necrotic Wharton's jelly containing much nuclear debris, surrounded by pyknotic cell nuclei belonging to polymorphonuclear leukocytes and mononuclear cells within and around the granuloma. At the periphery is a gradual transition toward otherwise normal jelly permeated by varying numbers of migrating inflammatory cells. Interestingly, there appears to be an inverse relationship between the ease with which *Candida* organisms can be seen and the stage of development of the inflammatory response.

Gross pathologic findings in infants contracting candidiasis in utero consist of multiple petechial hemorrhages in the thymus, heart, and adrenals. Histologically, yeast forms without an associated inflammatory reaction have been described in the alveolar spaces. Both yeast and mycelial elements have been demonstrated in the lumen of the bowel. Pathologic findings may be confined exclusively to the skin (congenital cutaneous candidiasis), with widespread, diffuse, macular, papular, vesicular, and pustular eruptions and exfoliation. Microabscesses of the skin and paranychia have been reported.

Prematurity is a common finding in infants acquiring candidal infection in utero.

SPONTANEOUS ABORTION AND FETAL CANDIDIASIS

In 1968, Schweid and Hopkins (1968) reported the first case of spontaneous abortion associated with fetal candidal infection. Their patient was a 19-year-old primipara who had had an intrauterine contraceptive device (IUD) (Lippe's loop) in place for 13 months. She spontaneously aborted a 69-mm fetus at 13 weeks of gestation. There was no history of maternal candidiasis or other infection. Examination of the conceptus revealed an inflammatory exudate in the chorionic plate that did not extend into the amniotic sac, chorionic villi, or decidua. The inflamed chorion adjacent to the amniotic sac contained a heavy growth of blastospores and pseudohyphae characteristic of *Candida*. No other organisms were demonstrated.

Another case report associating fetal candidal infection with spontaneous abortion is that of Ho and Aterman (1970). Their patient was a 32-year-old multigravida who had had an IUD in place for 15 months. At 14 weeks of gestation, she spontaneously aborted a 75 g fetus, 11 hours after rupture of the membranes had occurred. Microscopic examination revealed fungi and typical lesions in the fetal membranes, lungs, and gastrointestinal tract.

The source of infection in these two cases is obscure, but the same possibilities seem to exist as were previously described for intrauterine-acquired neonatal candidiasis. It is known that in cattle, in which fungi have also been implicated as a rare cause of abortion, it is possible to isolate organisms previously injected into the maternal circulation from calves or abortuses postpartum. This raises the further possibility of a hematogenous source of infection.

That both patients had IUDs in place for more than a year is intriguing. Schweid and Hopkins (1968) have suggested that the altered local environment induced by the IUD might well have fostered the infection caused by this opportunistic fungus. It is also interesting to speculate on the relationship between the candidiasis and the occurrence of the abortion. The common occurrence of premature labor in cases of intrauterine-acquired candidal infection has already been mentioned. Ho and Aterman (1970) argue that, if candidal infection can precipitate premature labor, it may occasionally provoke abortion as well.

SIGNIFICANCE OF CANDIDEMIA

One of the most difficult problems is determining the biological significance of the recovery of *Candida* from the intravascular compartment of seriously ill patients.

Recovery of a *Candida* species from the blood requires the differentiation of self-limited infection associated with an intravenous cannula from systemic candidiasis. Factors suggesting the latter condition are the following:

1. Development of macronodular skin lesions in a febrile patient
2. Concomitant demonstration of candiduria
3. Development of endophthalmitis
4. Presence of classic physical findings of infectious endocarditis
5. Embolization to medium-sized arteries of the extremities, brain, lungs, or mesentery
6. Persistent candidemia after removal of all intravenous arteries

7. Use of oral hyperalimentation in a patient with some underlying defect in the gastrointestinal tract or in host defense mechanisms
8. Development of osteomyelitis, meningitis, pyelonephritis, or arthritis
9. Occurrence in an intravenous drug abuser or immunosuppressed individual receiving intravenous hyperalimentation

Although a presumptive diagnosis may be inferred from one of the above, a definitive diagnosis requires demonstration of the organism within at distant organ system. Biopsy and culture of the macronodules should prove the presence of *Candida* species. About 5% of patients develop an endophthalmitis within one to six weeks following candidemia. These patients complain of orbital or periorbital pain, blurred vision, and scotoma. On ophthalmoscopic examination, white glistening exudates, sometimes with a ray-like appearance involving the retina and choroid, can be visualized if embolization to medium-sized arteries has occurred. The key to the diagnosis of disseminated candidiasis is either persistent candidemia after removal of an intravenous catheter or the presence of candidal precipitins in serum. A titer of candidal precipitins exceeding 1:8 by counter-immunoelectrophoresis or a rising titer suggests the diagnosis of disseminated candidiasis.

THERAPY OF VULVOVAGINAL CANDIDIASIS

Genesis I—Primary

Primary candidal vulvovaginitis is not a totally homogenous disease entity. It is a spectrum of disease whose dipoles are a vulvitis on one hand and a vaginitis on the other. The distinction between those situations in which vulvitis is greater than vaginitis from those cases in which vaginitis is greater than vulvitis is of more than academic importance. Total reliance on intravaginal medication in cases with significant vulvitis is associated with frequent therapeutic failures. If vulvitis is clinically significant, simple eradication of the vaginal reservoir will not afford relatively prompt relief of symptoms nor a 1 standard deviation probability of a microbiological cure. The physician must concomitantly treat for vulvitis. This is best achieved through direct application of medication to the perineum and vulva and restriction of undergarments to loose-fitting cotton pants.

If there is anorectal extension of disease, this is one situation where the topical use of perioral nystatin may be warranted. It is not necessary in primary vulvovaginal candidiasis to attempt eradication of the intestinal reservoir. Although it is the probable source of initial vaginal colonization, the presence of the organism in the gastrointestinal tract is not the cause of a disease state. A critical change in the microbiological environment must occur for colonization to become a disease state. Increased moisture appears to be the most important catalytic factor in genesis I type of disease.

Current effective therapies for genesis I and II are listed in Table 3.

Preparations for intravaginal administration of butoconazole, clotrimazole, miconazole, and tioconazole are now

TABLE 3 CDC 2002 regimens for candidal vulvovaginitis

Oral agent
Fluconazole 150 mg oral tablet, one tablet in single dose
or
Intravaginal agents (one of the following):
Butoconazole 2% cream 5 g intravaginally for 3 days[a,b]
Butoconazole 2% sustained release cream 5 g intravaginally, single application
Clotrimazole 1% cream 5 g intravaginally for 7–14 days[a,b]
Clotrimazole 100 mg vaginal tablet for 7 days[a,b]
Clotrimazole 100 mg vaginal tablet, two tablets for 3 days[a]
Clotrimazole 500 mg vaginal tablet, one tablet in a single application[a]
Miconazole 2% cream 5 g intravaginally for 7 days[a,b]
Miconazole 200 mg vaginal suppository, one suppository for 3 days[a,b]
Miconazole 100 mg vaginal suppository, one suppository for 7 days[a,b]
Nystatin 100,000-U vaginal tablet, one tablet for 14 days
Tioconazole 6.5% ointment 5 g intravaginally in a single application[a,b]
Terconazole 0.4% cream 5 g intravaginally for 7 days[a]
Terconazole 0.8% cream 5 g intravaginally for 3 days[a]
Terconazole 80 mg vaginal suppository, 1 suppository for 3 days[a]

[a]These creams and suppositories are oil based and may weaken latex condoms and diaphragms. Refer to product labeling for further information.
[b]Over-the-counter (OTC) preparations.
Abbreviation: CDC, Centers for Disease Control and Prevention.

available over-the-counter (OTC), and women with vulvovaginal candidiasis can choose one of those preparations. The duration of treatment with these preparations may be one, three, or seven days. Self-medication with OTC preparations should be advised only for women who have been diagnosed previously with vulvovaginal candidiasis and who experience a recurrence of the same symptoms. Any woman whose symptoms persist after using an OTC preparation should be counseled to seek medical care.

Genesis II–Antibiotic-Associated Candidal Vaginitis

Why do antibiotics induce candidiasis? The antibiotic, to induce candidiasis, must alter the microbiological environment through the eradication of the principal anaerobic bacteria that govern pH. The inhibitory effects of bacteriocins and bacteriocin-like products are pH dependent. The eradication of selective bacteria, especially anaerobes, in selected cases, frees *Candida* from its replicative constraints. Administration of antibiotics per se does not cause vulvovaginal candidiasis unless the proper prerequisites for disease induction are present.

Antibiotic-associated vulvovaginal candidiasis manifests as primarily a vaginitis when the magnitude of replication exceeds 10^6 cfu/mL of vaginal fluid and the *Candida* revert to their tissue-invasive dimorphic form. Vaginitis is more characteristic of this group than is vulvitis.

In antibiotic-associated disease, the major goal is the eradication of the vaginal reservoir. If the vaginal reservoir is eliminated, unless a concomitantly significant vulvitis is present, the problem will cure itself.

Genesis III—Systemically Influenced Candidiasis

The critical factor selecting for systemically induced candidiasis is an increase in the glucose substrate available in the local microbiological environment or T-cell dysfunction.

Patients with chronic candidiasis appear to have reduced responsiveness to candidal antigen. Hyporesponsiveness may be induced by the disease itself and may not be due to a pre-existing condition. For patients with systemically induced vulvovaginal candidiasis due to steroids, diabetes mellitus, or immunodeficiency involving T-cell function, intravaginal/vulvar therapy with anticandicidal creams topically applied coupled with fluconazole is preferred. It is imperative to treat the underlying condition aggressively or change the physiological status, i.e., pregnancy. Candidiasis associated with poorly controlled diabetes will relapse unless the problem in carbohydrate metabolism is brought under control.

Fluconazole, itraconazole, and ketoconazole are oral antimycotic agents that are effective against candidal vulvovaginitis. They are thought to affect sterol metabolisms in yeast and fungal cells, resulting in the accumulation of 14 alpha-methyl sterols that are known to disturb membrane and cell properties. There is an intracellular build-up of peroxide that is thought to contribute to cell death.

The use of oral antimycotics for vulvovaginal candidiasis has been somewhat blunted by the potential adverse drug reactions associated with ketoconazole. Systemic hepatotoxicity occurs in 1/10,000 to 1/15,000 of patients taking ketoconazole. Transient minor elevation of levels of liver enzymes occurs in 5% to 10% of patients taking the drug. At least four fatal cases have been reported that occurred despite discontinuation of ketoconazole to inhibit adrenal steroidogenesis, which may result in gynecomastia and in rare instances, hypoadrenalism.

Clinically important interactions may occur when some of the oral agents are administered with other drugs, including astemizole, calcium channel antagonists, cisapride, coumarin-like agents, cyclosporin A, oral hypoglycemic agents, phenytoin, protease inhibitors, tacrolimus, terfenadine, theophylline, trimetrexate, and rifampin.

CONSEQUENCES OF VULVOVAGINAL CANDIDIASIS FOR THE MALE

Two types of disease occur in male consorts. One group develops a specific candidal balanoposthitis. The second group presents with an allergic balanoposthitis presumably due to hypersensitivity to *Candida* antigens. The condition may be more common than is generally recognized. Diddle et al. (1969) found balanoposthitis in more than 10% of the husbands of the 225 women with candidal vaginitis in their series.

Hypersensitivity reaction is distinguished from balanitis in that the reaction begins within hours after sexual intercourse. Itching is most commonly the initial manifestation. The goal is to eliminate penile carriage as well as to eradicate the reservoirs of the oral cavity and seminal vesicles. Postcoital suppressive prophylaxis is indicated for the male when institution of personal hygiene is not accepted or chronic candidal seminal vesicle involvement is documented.

Preventive treatment of the sexual partners of women with candidiasis is not recommended, with the possible exception of women with recurrent vulvovaginal candidiasis.

RECURRENT CANDIDIASIS

Recurrent vulvovaginal candidiasis is defined as four or more episodes of vulvovaginal candidiasis in one year. The pathogenesis is poorly understood owing primarily to the number of distinct entities that can mimic vulvovaginal candidiasis. Each episode must be documented by culture and gross quantitative organismal assessment by wet mount. The most common confounding conditions tend to be human papilloma virus infection, allergic candidal vulvitis, *C. glabrata*, nonalbicans *Candida* species, and trichomoniasis. *C. glabrata* and other nonalbicans *Candida* species account for 10% to 20% of patients with recurrent vulvovaginal candidiasis. Conventional antimycotic therapies are not as effective against these species as they are against *C. albicans*.

Episodes that are due to enhanced organismal replication respond well to short-duration oral or topical azole therapy. The problem is that insufficient changes are induced to prevent recolonization and disease induction at a later date. For the small percentage of women with recurrent vulvovaginal candidiasis, individual episodes of candidiasis are treated longer (e.g., 7 to 14 days of topical therapy or a 100 mg, 150 mg, or 200 mg oral dose of fluconazole every third day for a total of three doses) to achieve clinical and microbiologic control before initiating a maintenance antifungal regimen.

Maintenance regimens: Oral fluconazole (i.e., 100 mg, 150 mg, or 200 mg dose) weekly for six months is deemed the first-line treatment by the CDC. Alternate regimens include topical clotrimazole 200 mg twice weekly or clotrimazole 500 mg vaginal suppositories once weekly. Boric acid 600 mg in a gelatin capsule administered vaginally once daily for one to two weeks has been used effectively in cases of nonalbicans strains that fail to respond to oral or topical azole therapy.

Although the maintenance prophylaxis is often effective in preventing recurrent episodes of vulvovaginitis, relapse was extremely common after the withdrawal of drugs; 30% to 50% of women will have recurrent disease after maintenance therapy is discontinued.

C. GLABRATA (TORULOPSIS)

C. glabrata is a small oval yeast belonging to the family Cryptococcaceae. Like *C. albicans*, it may be a constituent of the biological flora of skin, oropharynx, genitourinary tract, and gastrointestinal tract of humans. It grows preferentially in the presence of air and in so doing produces blastospores rather than pseudohyphae or ascospores.

The organism is thought to be a symbiont of humans; however, similar factors that select for disease with *C. albicans* also permit *C. glabrata* to function as an opportunistic pathogen. Certain conditions have been found in association with the pathogenic potential of the organism. These include

1. previous antibiotic therapy,
2. indwelling intravenous catheter and/or hyperalimentation therapy,
3. radiotherapy,
4. chemotherapy,
5. immunosuppressive therapy including steroids, and
6. diabetes mellitus.

C. glabrata can function as both a local and a systemic pathogen. Both fungicemia and endocarditis have been reported. The organism can produce a histological pattern that resembles *Histoplasma capsulatum*.

Vulvovaginitis

Vaginal torulopsis does not compare in intensity with the discomfort induced by vulvovaginal candidiasis Fig. 4. The pruritus or burning tends to be markedly less. Because of its minimal cytotoxic effect, leukorrhea tends to be scant. There is no tendency to clumping or creation of vaginal plaques. Rarely is dyspareunia or burning on the initiation of micturition present. The vaginal pH remains acidic, varying between 4.0 and 4.5. The lactobacilli associated with a simplified bacterial flora are usually present in cases of vaginal torulopsis. Mixed infections are rare.

Diagnosis

Examination of wet mount preparations reveals spores of variable size (two to eight microns) with unilateral germination that occur singly or group in cumuli. Gram staining reveals gram-positive spores of variable size with unilateral germination that tend to form small cumuli in the form of brancus. In contradistinction to *C. albicans*, the leukocytes may exhibit a tendency to phagocytize the spores of *C. glabrata*. In cases of *C. glabrata* fungicemia, the organism can occasionally be identified in smears of buffy coat of blood.

The organism grows readily on Sabouraud's dextrose agar where it produces smooth, glistening, pasty-white colonies. With time, they become grayish-brown. An Indian-ink preparation fails to demonstrate a capsule. Neither pseudohyphae nor ascospores are identifiable. Blastospores can be demonstrated on rice plates. A definitive diagnosis is achieved by demonstrating fermentation of glucose and tre-

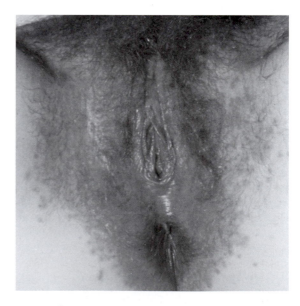

FIGURE 4 Cutaneous extension of vulvovaginal candidiasis due to *Candida albicans* hypersensitivity reaction.

halose and not maltose, sucrose, lactose, galactose, urea, and potassium nitrate.

Therapy

Drugs such as clotrimazole achieve their fungistatic efficacy primarily by inhibition of demethylation of 4,4,14-trimethyl steroids. When the imidazoles are used in the therapy of *C. albicans*, the ersosteril precursor accumulates, whereas with *C. glabrata*, lanosterol accumulation occurs. Apparently in *C. glabrata*, side-chain alkylation proceeds after demethylation reactions. The variable success attained with intravaginal imidazoles effective against *C. albicans* is thought to be due to the failure to eradicate coinfection of the urinary tract and subsequent reinfection from this source.

SELECTED READING

Pathogenesis

Auger P, Joly J. *Microbial flora* associated with *Candida* albicans vulvovaginitis. Obstet Gynecol 1980; 55:397.

Curuso LJ. Vaginal moniliasis after tetracycline therapy. Am J Obstet Gynecol 1964; 90:374.

Center for Disease Control and Prevention. 2006 Guidelines for Sexually Transmitted Diseases. MMWR 2006; 55:RR-11.

Davidson F. Yeasts and circumcision in the male. Br J Vener Dis 1977; 53:121.

Diddle AW, Gardner WH, Williamson PJ, O'Connor KA. Oral contraceptive medications and vulvovaginal candidiasis. Obstet Gynecol 1969; 34:373.

Goldman DA, Make DG. Infection control in total parenteral nutrition. J Am Med Assoc 1973; 223:1360.

Hilton AL, Warnock DW. Vaginal candidiasis and the role of the digestive tract as a source of infection. Br J Obstet Gynaecol 1975; 82:922.

Lapan B. Is the "pill" a cause of vaginal candidiasis? NY State J Med 1970; 70:949.

Mathur S, Koistinen GV, Horger E, et al. Humoral immunity in vaginal candidiasis. Infect Immun 1977; 15:287.

Meinhof W. Demonstration of typical features of individual *Candida albicans* strains as a means of studying sources of infection. Chemotherapy 1982; 28:51.

Monif GRG. Classification and pathogenesis of vulvovaginal candidiasis. Am J Obstet Gynecol 1985; 152:935.

Morton RS, Rashid S. Candidal vaginitis: natural history, predisposing factors and prevention. Proc R Soc Med 1977; 70 (suppl 4):3.

Oriel JD, Waterworth PM. Effect of minocycline and tetracycline on the vaginal yeast flora. J Clin Pathol 1975; 28:403.

Spellacy WM, Zaias N, Buhi WC, Burk SA. Vaginal yeast growth and contraceptive practices. Obstet Gynecol 1971; 38:343.

Suther RL, Brown WJ. Sequential vaginal cultures from normal young women. J Clin Microbiol 1980; 11:479.

Thin RN, Leighton M, Dixon MJ. How often is genital yeast infection sexually transmitted? Br Med J 1977; 93:9.

Warnock DW, Speller DCE, Day JK, et al. Resistogram method for differentiation of strains of *Candida* albicans. J Appl Bacteriol 1979; 46:571.

Warnock DW, Speller DCE, Milne JD, et al. Epidemiological investigation of patients with vulvovaginal candidosis. Br J Vener Dis 1979; 55:356.

Immunology of Candidal Vulvovaginitis

Hobbs JR. Immunological aspects of candidal vaginitis. Proc R Soc Med 1977; 70 (suppl 4):11.

Mathus S, Koistinen GV, Horger EO, et al. Humoral immunity in vaginal candidiasis. Infect Immun 1977; 15:287.

Rosedale N, Browne K. Hyposensitization in the management of recurring vaginal candidiasis. Ann Allergy 1979; 43:250.

Schulkind ML, Adler WH III, Altemeier WA III, Ayoub EM. Transfer factor in the treatment of a case of chronic mucocutaneous candidiasis. Cell Immunol 1972; 3:606.

Stoney VC, Hurley R. *Candida* precipitins in pregnant women: validity of the test systems used. J Clin Pathol 1974; 27:66.

Syverson RE, Buckley H, Gibian J, Ryan GM Jr. Cellular and humoral immune status in women with chronic *Candida* vaginitis. Am J Obstet Gynecol 1979; 134:624.

Valdimarsson H, Higgs JM, Wells RS, et al. Immune abnormalities associated with chronic mucocutaneous candidiasis. Cell Immunol 1973; 6:348.

Waldman RH, Cruz JM, Rowe DS. Immunoglobulin levels and antibody to *Candida albicans* in human cervicovaginal secretions. Clin Exp Immunol 1972; 10:247.

Witkin SS, Yu IR, Ledger WJ. Inhibition of *Candida albicans* induced lymphocyte proliferation by lymphocytes and sera from women with recurrent vaginitis. Am J Obstet Gynecol 1983; 147:809.

Candidal Vulvovaginitis

Carroll CJ, Hurley R, Stanley VC. Criteria for diagnosis of *Candida* vulvovaginitis in pregnant women. J Obstet Gynaecol Br Commonw 1973; 80:258.

Davidson F. Yeasts and circumcision in the male. Br J Vener Dis 1977; 53:121.

Elegbe IA, Botu M. A preliminary study on dressing patterns and incidence of candidiasis. Am J Public Health 1982; 72:176.

Felman YM, Nikitas JA. Genital candidiasis. Cutis 1983; 31:369.

Fleury FJ. Adult vaginitis. Clin Obstet Gynecol 1981; 24:407.

Odds FC. *Candida* and Candidosis. Baltimore: University Park Press, 1979.

Oriel JD, Oartrudge BM, Denny MJ, Coleman JC. Genital yeast infections. Br Med J 1972; 4:761.

Rodin P, Kolator B. Carriage of yeasts on the penis. Br Med J 1976; 1:1123.

Rohatiner JJ. Relationship of *Candida albicans* in the genital and anorectal tract. Br J Vener Dis 1966; 42:197–200.

Recurrent Candidiasis

Davidson F, Mould RF. Recurrent genital candidiasis in women and the effect of intermittent prophylactic treatment. Br J Vener Dis 1974; 54:176.

Davidson F, Hayes JP, Hussein S. Recurrent genital candidosis and iron metabolism. Br J Vener Dis 1977; 53:123.

Eliot BW, Howat RCL, Mack AE. A comparison between the effects of nystatin, clotrimazole and miconazole on vaginal candidiasis. Br J Obstet Gynaecol 1979; 86:572.

Eschenbach DA, Hummel D, Grayett MG. Recurrent and persistent vulvovaginal candidiasis: treatment with ketoconazole. Obstet Gynecol 1985; 66:248.

Fleury FJ. Recurrent *Candida* vulvovaginitis. Chemotherapy 1982; 28:48.

Hurley R. Recurrent *Candida* infection. Clin Obstet Gynecol 1981; 8:209.

Miles MR, Olsen L, Rogers A. Recurrent vaginal candidiasis. J Am Med Assoc 1977; 238:1836.

Milne JD, Warnock DW. Effect of simultaneous oral and vaginal treatment on the rate of cure and relapse in vaginal candidosis. Br J Vener Dis 1979; 55:362.

Milson I, Forssman L. Repeated candidiasis: reinfection or recrudescence? A review. Am J Obstet Gynecol 1985; 152:956.

Sobel JD. Recurrent vulvovaginal candidiasis: what we know and what we don't (editorial). Ann Intern Med 1984; 101:390.

Sobel JD. Epidemiology and pathogenesis of recurrent vulvovaginal candidiasis. Am J Obstet Gynecol 1985; 152:956.

Trumbore DF, Sobel JD. Recurrent vulvovaginal candidiasis: vaginal epithelial cell susceptibility to *Candida albicans* adherence. Obstet Gynecol 1986; 67:810.

Congenital/Neonatal Infection

Aterman K. Pathology of *Candida* infection of the umbilical cord. Am J Clin Pathol 1968; 49:798.

Benirschke K, Raphael SL. *Candida albicans* infection of the amniotic sac. Am J Obstet Gynecol 1958; 75:200.

Delprado WJ, Baird PJ, Russell P. Placental candidiasis: report of three cases with a review of the literature. Pathology 1982; 14:191.

Ho C-Y, Aterman K. Infection of the fetus by *Candida* in a spontaneous abortion. Am J Obstet Gynecol 1970; 106:705.

Hopsu-Havu VK, Gronroos M, Punnoren R. Vaginal yeasts in parturients and infestation of the newborns. Acta Obstet Gynecol Scand 1980; 59:73.

Johnson DE, Thompson TR, Ferrieri P. Congenital candidiasis. Am J Dis Child 1981; 135:273.

Kozinn PJ, Taschdjian CL, Wiener H. Incidence and pathogenesis of neonatal candidiasis. Pediatrics 1958; 21:421.

Levin S, Zaidel L, Bernstein D. Intrauterine infection of fetal brain by Candida. Am J Obstet Gynecol 1978; 130:597.

Lopex E, Aterman K. Intrauterine infection by *Candida*. Am J Dis Child 1968; 115:663.

Nagata K, Nakamura Y, Hosokawa Y, et al. Intrauterine *Candida* infection in premature baby. Acta Pathol Jpn 1981; 31:695.

Patriquin H, Lebowitz R, Perreault G, Yousefzadeh D. Neonatal candidiasis: renal and pulmonary manifestations. Am J Roentgenol 1980; 135:1205.

Schweid AI, Hopkins GB. Monilial chorionitis associated with an intrauterine contraceptive device. Obstet Gynecol 1968; 31:719.

Seebacher C, Bottger D. Intrauterine *Candida albicans* infection of fetus after repeated amnioscopy. Stsch Gesundheitsw 1973; 28:835.

Whyte RK, Hussain Z, Desa D. Antenatal infections with *Candida* species. Arch Dis Child 1982; 57:528.

Disseminated Candidiasis

Anderson AO, Yardby JH. Demonstration of *Candida* in blood smears. N Engl J Med 1972; 286:108.

Cantrill HL, Rodman WP, Ramsay RC, Knobloch WH. Postpartum *Candida* endophthalmitis. J Am Med Assoc 1980; 243:1163.

Chilgren RA, Quie PG, Meuwissen HJ, Hong R. Chronic mucocutaneous candidiasis, deficiency of delayed hypersensitivity, and selective local antibody defect. Lancet 1967; 2:688.

Chilgren RA, Hong R, Quie PG. *Candida*-serum interactions in six patients with chronic candidiasis. Fed Proc 1967; 26:699.

Davis JB, Whitaker JD, Ding LK, Kiefer JH. Disseminated fatal, postpartum candidiasis with renal suppuration: case report. J Urol 1956; 75:930.

Dennis D, Miller MJ, Peterson DF. *Candida* septicemia. Surg Gynecol Obstet 1964; 119:520.

Dobias B. Specific and nonspecific immunity in *Candida* infections: experimental studies of role of *Candida* cell constituents and review of literature. Acta Med Scand 1964; (Suppl)176:1.

Ellis CA, Spivack ML. The significance of candidemia. Ann Intern Med 1967; 67:511.

Fox LP. Fatal superinfection with monilia in gynecological surgery. Am J Obstet Gynecol 1971; 110:285.

Goldman JA, Eckerling B, Bassat MB. Fatal *Candida* infection developing after hysterectomy and transfusion. Am J Obstet Gynecol 1967; 98:885.

Hart PD, Russell E Jr, Remington JS. The compromised host and infection. II. Deep fungal infection. J Infect Dis 1969; 120:169.

Hutter RVP, Collins HS. The concurrence of opportunistic fungus infections in a cancer hospital. Lab Invest 1962; 11:1035.

Louria DB. Pathogenesis of candidiasis. Antimicrob Agents Chemother 1965; 5:417.

Smith JM, Mason AB, Meech RJ. Serological procedures in the diagnosis and monitoring of invasive candidosis. NZ Med J 1984; 97:155.

Tami M. Acute fulminating moniliasis. RI Med J 1967; 50:29.

Urinary Tract Candidiasis

Roy JB, Geyer JR, Mohr JA. Urinary tract candidiasis: an update. Urology 1984; 23:533.

Seneca H, Longo F, Peer P. The clinical significance of *Candida albicans* in urine cultures. J Urol 1968; 100:266.

Treatment

Brown D, Binder GL, Gardner HL, Wells J. Comparison of econazole and clotrimazole in the treatment of vulvovaginal candidiasis. Obstet Gynecol 1980; 56:121.

Buch A, Christensen J. Treatment of vaginal candidosis with natamycin and effect of treating the partner at the same time. Acta Obstet Gynecol Scand 1982; 61:393.

Centers for Disease Control. Sexually transmitted disease treatment guidelines 2002 51(RR-6):1.2002.

Cho N, Saito CN, Fukadem J, et al. Clinical statistics in clotrimazole as anti-fungal therapy in obstetrics and gynaecology. Curr Med Res Opin 1974; 2:1.

Codish SD, Tobias JS. Managing systemic mycoses in the compromised host. J Am Med Assoc 1976; 235:2132.

Dennerstein GJ, Langley R. Vulvovaginal candidiasis: treatment and recurrence. Aust NZ J Obstet Gynaecol 1982; 22:231.

Heel RC, Brogden RN, Carmine A, et al. Ketoconazole: a review of its therapeutic efficacy in superficial and systemic fungal infections. Drugs 1982; 23:1.

Horowitz BJ, Edelstein SW, Lippman L. *Candida tropicalis* vulvovaginitis. Obstet Gynecol 1985; 66:229.

Hurley R, de Louvois J. *Candida* vaginitis. Postgrad Med J 1979; 55:645.

Masterson G, Napier IR, Henderson JN, et al. Three-day clotrimazole treatment in candidal vulvovaginitis. Br J Vener Dis 1977; 53:126.

McNellis D, McLeod M, Lawson J, Pasquale SA. Treatment of vulvovaginal candidiasis in pregnancy, a comparative study. Obstet Gynecol 1977; 50:674.

Milne JD, Warnock DW. Effect of simultaneous oral and vaginal treatment on the rate of cure and relapse in vaginal candidiasis. Br J Vener Dis 1979; 55:362.

Milsom I, Forssman L. Treatment of vaginal candidiasis with a single 500 mg clotrimazole pessary. Br J Vener Dis 1982; 58:124.

Nystatin Multicenter Study Group. Therapy of candidal vaginitis: the effect of eliminating intestinal *Candida*. Am J Obstet Gynecol 1986; 155:651.

Odds FC. Cure and relapse with anti-fungal therapy. Proc R Soc Med 1977; 70(suppl 4):24.

Oriel JD, Partridge BM, Denny MJ, et al. Genital yeast infections. Br Med J 1972; 4:761.

Robertson WH. A concentrated therapeutic regimen for vulvovagnal candidiasis. J Am Med Assoc 1980; 244:2549.

Rodin P, Kolator B. Carriage of yeasts on the penis. Br Med J 1976; 1:1123.

Sobel JD. In: Eliot BV, ed. Pathogenesis of Vaginal Candidosis, Oral Therapy in Vaginal Candidosis. Oxford: The Medicine Publishing Foundation, 1984:1–3.

Sobel JD. Epidemiology and pathogenesis of recurrent vulvovaginal candidiasis. Am J Obstet Gynecol 1985; 152:924.

Sobel JD. Management of recurrent vulvovaginal candidiasis with intermittent ketoconazole prophylaxis. Obstet Gynecol 1985; 65:435.

Swate TE, Weed JC. Boric acid treatment of vulvovaginal candidiasis. Obstet Gynecol 1974; 43:893.

Thin RN, Leighton M, Dixon MJ. How often is genital yeast infection sexually transmitted? Br Med J 1977; 93:9.

Van Der Pas H, Peeters F, Janssens D, et al. Treatment of vaginal candidosis with oral ketoconazole. Eur J Obstet Gynecol Reprod Biol 1983; 14:399.

Van Slyke KK, Michel VP, Rein MF. Treatment of vulvovaginal candidiasis with boric acid powder. Am J Obstet Gynecol 1981; 141:145.

Wolfson N, Samuels B, Riley J. A three-day treatment regimen for vulvovaginal candidiasis. J LA State Med Soc 1982; 134:28.

58

Coccidioides immitis and Coccidioides posadasil

INTRODUCTION

Coccidioides immitis and *Coccidioides posadasil* are saprophytic fungi with a dimorphic mode of growth in humans and in the soil. The organisms are endemic to arid regions in the southwestern United States, Mexico, Central America, and South America. *C. immitis* is geographically limited to the San Joaquin valley region in California. *C. posadasil* is found in the desert region of the southwestern United States, Mexico, and South America. With the significant population growth in the Sunbelt states, coccidioidomycosis has become a well-defined endemic cases of coccidioidomycosis. An estimated 100,000 cases of coccidioidomycosis occur annually in the United States. Disease is a tip-of-the-iceberg phenomenon compared to the true incidence of infection. Even when disease occurs, the great majority of cases are not properly diagnosed.

Coccidioidomycosis is an occupational hazard for anyone working outdoors in endemic regions. The peak incidence of infection often has a seasonal distribution and coincides with those months in which rainfall is lowest (late summer and fall). Anything disturbing the soil conditions, either natural (wind) or manmade (agricultural plowing, construction, etc.) increases the potential for aerosol dissemination. The respiratory tract functions as the portal for infection. In areas of highest endemicity, the infection rate is approximately 2% to 4% per year.

The Coccidioides organisms grow as mycelial forms in soil. As the mycelial structure matures, arthrocondia are produced. The arthrocondia are the infectious particles of coccidioidomycosis. When the soil is disturbed, the arthrocondia become airborne. If inhaled by a susceptible host, they produce disease. The fungus reproduces in host tissues by endosporulation, and consequently person-to-person transmission from this source does not occur. In rare instances, skin abrasions have permitted the establishment of infection.

After an 8- to 14-day incubation period, disease, if it is to be manifested, occurs. In approximately 30% to 50% of infected individuals, a clinical pattern evolves that ranges from a mild influenza-like syndrome to one characterized by chills, fever, malaise, myalgia, a cough that often has a pleuritic component, and night sweats. Approximately 25% of infected individuals will develop erythema nodosum.

In approximately 0.2% of infected individuals, systemic dissemination occurs. Extrapulmonary lesions characteristically develop as a late-phase event in the progression of the initial infection. All organ systems are potential sites of involvement, although there seems to be a predilection for skin, the reticuloendothelial system, bone, and the central nervous system. The tissue response is one of granuloma formation in which typical endosporulating spherules may be identified within a multinucleated giant cell.

The probability of dissemination and consequently of morbidity and mortality is greater in dark-skinned individuals, African Americans, Hispanics, Filipinos, and Asians. They are at greater risk of serious infection with both pulmonary and disseminated disease.

Immunity to the Coccidioides organisms is mediated by cell-mediated immunity. T-cell activation and inflammatory cytokines are central to the killing of the organisms. Dissemination is more common in immunocompromised individuals with diminished cell-mediated immunity or those receiving immunosuppressive therapies. The probability of overt coccidioidomycosis in patients with AIDS is similarly significantly increased. Pregnant women in their third trimester constitute an additional population at enhanced risk for disseminated disease.

Like tuberculosis, both disease and female genital tract involvement may be due to reactivation of previously disseminated infection.

DIAGNOSIS

Direct Examination

The diagnosis can be made by direct examination of sputum, smears, or biopsy material. In exudative lesions, the organisms exist in a spherical, thick-walled endospore as spherules. The spherule measures 40 to 70 µm in diameter. Organismal identification from smears can be made using calcofluor white or cytological stains. For biopsy material, the organisms can be identified using hematoxylin and eosin or silver or periodic acid-Schiff stains.

Cultures

In culture, the fungus develops a mole-like configuration identical to its growth in soil. The fungus grows within five days well on most common laboratory media. A definitive diagnosis of culture isolates is achieved using ribosomal RNA gene probes. The resultant arthroconida are infectious; consequently, the laboratory should be warned in advance if coccidioidomycosis is suspected.

Skin Testing

Cultivation of the fungus in a liquid medium results in the elaboration of an immunologically specific polysaccharide, coccidioidin, which may be used as the source of antigen for

1. skin testing,
2. immunodiffusion, and
3. complement fixation.

A delayed type of hypersensitivity reaction appears 2 to 21 days after the onset of symptoms. Cutaneous assessment of reactivity to coccidioidal antigens is of limited sensitivity and specificity in endemic areas. Healthy individuals may have a positive reaction because of prior infection.

The development of a delayed type of hypersensitivity can be demonstrated by a tuberculin-like reaction secondary to the intradermal injection of coccidioidin. When the area of induration exceeds 5 mm in diameter, the reaction is interpreted as being indicative of prior antigenic stimulation. The onset of delayed hypersensitivity occurs within a few days to two weeks after the onset of disease and usually before serological evidence of infection occurs. Once delayed hypersensitivity to the organism is acquired, the individual (barring significant changes in immunologic status) is basically immune to exogenous reinfection. There is a low degree of cross-reactivity with antigens derived from *Histoplasma capsulatum* and *Blastomyces dermatitidis*. Anergy is common in disseminated coccidioidomycosis.

Serological Testing

Antibodies against the mycelial phase antigen develop in response to acute infection with *C. immitis* within one to three weeks after the onset of disease and disappear within four months. Specific serological tests applicable to establishing a definitive diagnosis of coccidioidomycosis include complement fixation, immunodiffusion, and enzyme-linked immunosorbent assay tests. False-negative tests can occur in the early stages of disease. Immunoglobulin M (IgM)–specific antibody is detectable using the tube-precipitation method; however, false-positive results are a significant problem.

A serum complement-fixation titer of 1:32 or higher is usually indicative of disseminated disease. In general, the antibody titer parallels the activity of the disease. A rising titer when a patient is on therapy is a poor prognostic sign.

FEMALE GENITAL TRACT INVOLVEMENT

Female genital tract involvement is a rare manifestation of disseminated coccidioidomycosis. Coccidioidomycosis of the female genital tract is usually manifested as granulomatous endometritis and/or granulomatous tubo-ovarian disease with peritonitis. The patient usually presents with secondary infertility, recurrent pelvic pain, or a history of repeated pelvic infection refractory to conventional therapy. The last presentation usually occurs in conjunction with fever or a significant vaginal discharge.

With advanced disease, in addition to fever and leukocytosis, the patient may exhibit, on a pelvic examination, marked tenderness involving the adnexa and above all the cul-de-sac. Disease is usually bilateral. Not infrequently, a tubo-ovarian complex is present. At laparotomy, miliary granulomatous nodules can be discerned involving the omentum, peritoneum, and serosa.

As in genital infection with *Mycobacterium tuberculosis*, the fallopian tube is the probable site of initial metastatic infection and bears the brunt of the disease process. While pelvic coccidioidomycosis is usually associated with coccidioidal peritonitis, fallopian tube disease can result in both endometrial disease and serosal involvement. Histologic analysis reveals a diffuse chronic interstitial inflammatory response, with focal areas of granulomatous involvement characterized by epithelial cells, rare giant cells, and Coccidioides spherules. The occurrence of coagulative necrosis is not uncommon.

There is usually no evidence of disease elsewhere. Chest roentgenograms are negative or may indicate old disease. The absence of concomitant disease has implied the probability that, as with *M. tuberculosis* infection, genital involvement is the consequence of hematogenous dissemination at the time of the initial pulmonary infection and subsequent endogenous activation at a later date. The latent period during which endogenous reinfection may occur may be up to 8 to 10 years.

Pelvic coccidioidomycosis appears to be a distinct entity and not merely a concomitant involvement associated with systemic dissemination. Huntington et al. (1967) in a review of 142 autopsy cases of acute fatal coccidioidomycosis, could not identify a single instance of involvement of the female genital tract. Similarly, there were no documented cases of pelvic infection due to *C. immitis* in the study of 40 cases of disseminated coccidioidomycosis seen at Kern General Hospital from 1965 to 1972. These patients may not have survived long enough for genital tract disease to have evolved. Saw et al. (1974) demonstrated the presence of granulomatous coccidioidal endometritis at six weeks postpartum in a 22-year-old Mexican woman with disseminated coccidioidomycosis. She had delivered a premature baby who died at three weeks of age from disseminated coccidioidomycosis.

Of the 11 patients described by Bylund et al. (1986), seven had tubo-ovarian coccidioidomycosis and coccidioidal peritonitis; two of the seven had concomitant coccidioidal endometritis. The other four patients had coccidioidal endometritis, two as part of generalized coccidioidomycosis and two as apparently localized endometritis.

The seven patients with tubo-ovarian coccidioidomycosis and coccidioidal peritonitis all had chronic abdominopelvic pain. Three patients without endometritis had vaginal discharge; the two patients with concomitant endometritis had palpable adnexal or cul-de-sac disease.

Since the spherules are noninfectious for humans, infection of the sexual consort is not a clinical consideration.

The prerequisite for diagnosis of pelvic coccidioidomycosis is a knowledge concerning potential genital tract involvement and a high index of suspicion in patients from endemic areas presenting with some combination of fever, recurrent pelvic pain, vaginal discharge, infertility, menstrual aberration, or a history of recurrent pelvic inflammatory disease (refractory to the usual mode of therapy). The finding of nodularity in the cul-de-sac in association with evidence of an acute inflammatory process may alert one to the possibility of pelvic coccidioidomycosis.

Not infrequently, the diagnosis is not suspected until laparotomy. The presence of widespread miliary involvement of the omentum, serosa, and peritoneum, in conjunction with significant adnexal pathology, renders the process indistinguishable from that due to *M. tuberculosis*. The need to make the diagnosis at the operating table is underscored by the fact that therapy for genital tuberculosis is medical, whereas pelvic coccidioidomycosis is best dealt with by surgical resection. Wet mounts of the peritoneal fluid can usually demonstrate the spherules of C. immitis. Confirmation can be achieved with culture techniques or histologic analysis. Serum organism-specific antibodies are demonstrable. A serological test for C. immitis should be a routine part of any infertility work-up in an endemic area. The value of the test is not in its being positive, but rather in its use for excluding the disease entity from the differential diagnosis.

The magnitude of disease and the age and condition of the patient may influence the extent of surgical resection. In most cases, the operative procedure of choice is total abdominal hysterectomy and bilateral salpingo-oophorectomy.

COCCIDIOIDOMYCOSIS COMPLICATING PREGNANCY

Coccidioidomycosis affects one in every 1000 pregnancies in endemic areas of the southwestern United States.

Pregnancy alters the natural history of coccidioidomycosis. Pregnant patients with infection/disease manifesting in the third trimester develop more serious disease than the general population. Whereas the incidence of dissemination in immunocompetent individuals is markedly less than 1%, that observed in pregnant women has been 40 times the rate observed in the general population. Caldwell et al. (2000) reported 32 cases of infected women who delivered live-born infants or aborted in the 1993 California epidemic. Disseminated disease occurred in 3 of the 32 cases. Based on their review of 61 cases of coccidioidomycosis in pregnancy, Arsura et al. (1998) have contended that the occurrence of erythema nodosum is a salient marker of a positive outcome for pregnant women. In endemic areas, coccidioidal infection may be a significant cause of maternal mortality.

Manifestation of coccidioidomycosis in pregnancy may include pain and swelling of knees, ankles, or wrists. In pregnant patients, both the incidence of dissemination and its resultant mortality rise markedly.

Women who have a history of resolved prior infection do not have a significant rate of recrudescence in a subsequent pregnancy.

THERAPY

Prior to amphotericin B, there was no effective therapy for coccidioidomycosis. When systemic dissemination occurred in nonpregnant patients, 50% mortality was not uncommon.

Most infections resolve with little or no therapy. Cases with mild-to-moderate pulmonary involvement are often treated with azoles such as fluconazole or itraconazole; however, amphotericin B remains the treatment of choice, either in the amphotericin B deoxycholate formulation or as a lipid formulation for severe infection.

Because of the enhanced maternal mortality in pregnancy with disseminated disease, it is recommended that pregnant women be evaluated for treatment with amphotericin B.

Amphotericin B causes regression and healing of disseminated foci. C. immitis appears to be uniformly susceptible in vitro to amphotericin B. Evidence suggests that amphotericin B may prevent dissemination in severe primary cases. However, amphotericin B therapy carries a significant risk of death. Smale and Waechter (1970) observed two deaths associated with kidney disease from the nephrotoxicity of amphotericin B. Amphotericin B can cause up to a 40% reduction in glomerular filtration rate. This phenomenon is dose dependent and usually reversible. By gradual escalation of dosage and by careful monitoring of renal function, the adverse nephrotoxic effect of drug therapy can be markedly reduced.

The effectiveness of therapy can often be measured by a decreasing complement-fixing antibody titer. The decrease is usually preceded by improvement both in the patient's clinical condition and in the changes in chest X rays. Because of the narrow therapeutic index, systemic therapy should be carried out only by skilled clinicians with prior experience and in a carefully controlled environment.

Nondisseminated disease occurring before the third trimester has been handled using itraconazole or fluconazole. Itraconazole (200 to 400 mg PO qid) and fluconazole (400 mg PO/IV qid) have been shown to be efficacious in managing the most progressive nonmeningeal forms of coccidioidomycosis. A prolonged course of antifungal therapy is usually advocated. Even after 12 months of therapy, relapse rates of 15% to 30% have been observed after discontinuation of therapy.

The indications for prolonged and/or changing treatment are as follows:

1. Persistent fever, prostration, elevated blood sedimentation rate, with considerable pulmonary involvement and hilar adenopathy
2. Unstable serology; that is
    (a) a rising titer of a primary pulmonary focus,
    (b) evidence of spread including invasion of lymphatic, cutaneous, skeletal, cardiac, genitourinary, and meningeal systems, or the pleuroperitoneal space
3. Weak or negative skin reaction to coccidioidin

Fully effective therapy for disseminated coccidioidal disease requires not only the use of antimicrobial therapy, but also the application of established surgical principles—drainage of abscesses, removal of infected bone, excision of sinuses, etc. Pre- or postoperatively, the patient should be treated with antifungal therapy and should be monitored with serial complement-fixation tests for C. immitis.

In deciding the drug of choice for a particular woman, one should take into account her race, age, immunological status, preexisting vital organ dysfunction, and serum complement-fixation titer. Taking the help of an infectious-disease consultant is again highly recommended.

The interim between initial infection and dissemination may be prolonged; this circumstance, however, tends to be the exception, not the rule. About 10% of patients with nondisseminated coccidioidomycosis (even if acquired several months prior to conception) may have subsequent dissemination during pregnancy. In its usual nondisseminated form, infection during gestation does not significantly alter the pregnancy outcome. Maternal mortality is related primarily to whether or not the disease becomes disseminated.

INVOLVEMENT OF THE PRODUCTS OF CONCEPTION/CONGENITAL INFECTION

Placental Coccidioidomycosis

Placental coccidioidomycosis without necessarily fetal involvement is well documented. Harris (1966) reported seven cases of placental involvement of coccidioidomycosis. Smale and Waechter (1970) identified three additional cases in which placental involvement occurred during systemic dissemination. In this series, only one probable case of congenital coccidioidomycosis was identified. The infant was born prematurely and died of coccidioidomycosis when 29 days old. A matter of speculation is whether the infrequency of congenital infection is a reflection of the probable limitations of infection to the placenta because of either

1. the size of the coccidioidal spherules, resulting in their physical exclusion from the fetal circulation, or
2. the severity of the host reaction, resulting in thrombosis of the adjacent vascular spaces and an acute inflammatory response.

Nickisch et al. (1993) demonstrated normal umbilical artery velocimetry in the only case of coccidioidal placentitis appropriately studied to date.

Congenital Coccidioidomycosis

Congenital disease does occur but is rare. In Smale and Waechter's series of 15 cases of disseminated coccidioidomycosis during gestation, fetal loss approached 50%. This loss was primarily due to prematurity or fetal death in utero secondary to maternal death. The women with nondisseminated disease who proceeded to term did not usually experience excessive fetal loss.

The prime obstetric problem is how to treat the gravida who develops nondisseminated coccidioidomycosis. Because of the 10% chance of dissemination, which carries the risk of maternal mortality, these patients must be closely followed for

1. a rising antibody titer, and
2. roentgenographic development of progressive pulmonary involvement.

Changes in either of these parameters argues for changing therapy.

The finding of placental coccidioidomycosis at parturition is deemed prima facie evidence of dissemination and hence argues for the institution of systemic therapy.

The regimen of amphotericin B is the same as that for the nonpregnant woman. The fetal outcomes of women with disseminated disease treated with amphotericin B have been reasonably good.

SELECTED READING

Female Genital Tract Involvement

Arsura EL, Kilgore WB, Ratnayake SN. Erythema nodosum in pregnant patients with coccidioidomycosis. Clin Infect Dis 1998; 27:1201.

Bylund DJ, Nanfro JJ, Marsh WL Jr. Coccidioidomycosis of the female genital tract. Arch Pathol Lab Med 1986; 110:232.

CDC. Coccidioidomycosis: Arizona, 1990–1995. MMWR 1996; 45:1069.

Catanzaro A, Galgiani JN, Levine BE, et al. Fluconazole in the treatment of chronic pulmonary and nonmeningeal disseminated coccidioidomycosis. Am J Med 1995; 98:249.

Collins MS, Pappagianis D. Uniform susceptibility of various strains of Coccidioides immitis to amphotericin B. Antimicrob Agents Chemother 1997; 11:1049.

Crum NF, Lederman ER, Stafford CM. Coccidioidomycosis: a descriptive survey of emerging disease. Clinical characteristic and current controversies. Medicine 2004; 83:149.

Drutz DF, Catanzaro A. Coccidioidomycosis. Am Rev Respir Dis 1978; 117:559.

Einstein HE, Johnson RH. Coccidioidomycosis: new aspects of epidemiology and therapy. Clin Infect Dis 1993; 16:349.

Galgiani JN, Catanzaro A, Cloud GA et al. Comparison of oral fluconazole and itraconazole for progressive nonmeningeal coccidioidomycosis. A randomized, double-blinded trial. Ann Intern Med 2000; 133:676.

Galgiani JN, Ampel NM, Catanzaro A. Practice guidelines for the treatment of coccidioidomycosis. Clin Infect Dis 2000; 30:658.

Hart W, Prinns RP, Tsai JC. Isolated coccidioidomycosis of the uterus. Hum Pathol 1976; 7:235.

Hassani M, Tanowitz HB, Levi MH, et al. Extrapulmonary nonmeningeal coccidioidomycosis. Infect Med 2004; 21:245.

Huntington RW, Jr., Waldman WJ, Sargent JA, et al.: Coccidioidomycosis. Proceedings 2nd Coccidioidomycosis symposium. Tucson, University of Arizona Press, 1967; pp. 143–167.

Jacobsen HP. Coccidioidal granuloma: further observation with report of seven additional cases. Med J Rec 1929; 130:424.

Page EW, Boyers LM. Coccidioidal pelvic inflammatory disease. Am J Obstet Gynecol 1945; 50:212.

Parker P, Adcock IL. Pelvic coccidioidomycosis. Obstet Gynecol Surv 1981; 36:225.

Peterson CH, Schuppert K, Kelley PC. Coccidioidomycosis and pregnancy. Obstet Gynecol Surv 1993; 48:149.

Rutala PJ, Smith JW. Coccidioidomycosis in potentially compromised hosts: the effect of immunosuppressive therapy in dissemination. Am J Med Sci 1978; 275:283.

Salgia K, Bhatia L, Rajashekaraiah KR, et al. Coccidioidomycosis of the uterus. South Med J 1982; 75:614.

Saw EC, Huntington RW Jr, Shields S, et al. Granulomatous peritonitis due to coccidioidomycosis immitis. Arch Surg 1974; 108:369.

Saw EC, Smale LE, Einstein H, Huntington RW Jr. Female genital coccidioidomycosis. Obstet Gynecol 1975; 45:199.

Stevens DA (ed). Coccidioidomycosis. New York: Plenum Publishing Corp, 1980.

Walker MPR, Brody CZ, Resnik R. Reactivation of coccidioidomycosis in pregnancy. Obstet Gynecol 1992; 279:815.

Wormley LC, Manoil L, Rosenthal M. Coccidioidomycosis of female adnexa. Am J Surg 1950; 80:958.

Coccidioidomycosis and Pregnancy

Arsura EL, Kilgore WB, Ratnayake SN. Erythema nodosum in pregnant patients with coccidioidomycosis. Clin Infect Dis 1998; 27:1201.

Baker RL. Pregnancy complicated by coccidioidomycosis: report of 2 cases. Am J Obstet Gynecol 1955; 70:1033.

Caldwell JW, Arsura EL, Kilgore WB, et al. Coccidiomycosis in pregnancy during an epidemic in California. Obstet Gynecol 2000; 95:263.

Charlton V, Ramsdell K, Sehring S. Intrauterine transmission of coccidioidomycosis. Pediatr Infect Dis 1999; 18:561.

Harris RE. Coccidioidomycosis complicating pregnancy. Obstet Gynecol 1966; 28:3.

Harrison HN. Fatal maternal coccidioidomycosis: a case report and review of sixteen cases from the literature. Am J Obstet Gynecol 1958; 75:813.

Mendenhall JC, Black WC, Pottz GE. Progressive (disseminated) coccidioidomycosis during pregnancy. Rocky Mount Med J 1948; 45:472.

Pappagianis D. Coccidioidomycosis. In: Samter M, ed. Immunological Diseases, 3rd ed. Boston: Little Brown & Co Inc, 1978:681–691.

Peterson CM. Coccidioidomycosis and pregnancy. Obstet Gynecol Surv 1993; 48:149.

Peterson CM, Johnson SL, Kelly PC. Coccidiodal meningitis and pregnancy: a case report. Obstet Gynecol 1989; 28:835–836.

Smale LE, Birsner JW. Maternal deaths from coccidioidomycosis. J Am Med Assoc 1949; 140:1152.

Smale LE, Waechter KG. Dissemination of coccidioidomycosis in pregnancy. Am J Obstet Gynecol 1970; 107:356.

Smith CE, Pappagianis D, Levine HB, Saito M. Human coccidioidomycosis. Bacteriol Rev 1961; 25:31.

Vaughan JE, Ramirez H. Coccidioidomycosis as complication of pregnancy. Calif Med 1951; 74:121.

Wack EE, Ampel NM, Galiani JN, Bronnimann DA. Coccidioidomycosis during pregnancy. Chest 1988; 94:376.

Walker MPR, Brody CZ, Resnik, R. Reactivation of coccidioidomycosis in pregnancy. Obstet Gynecol 1992; 79:815.

Congenital Infection

Bernstein DI, Tipton JR, Schott SF, Cherry JD. Coccidioidomycosis in a neonate: maternal infant transmission. J Pediatr 1981; 99:752.

Christian JR, Sarre SC, Peers JH, Salazar E. Pulmonary coccidioidomycosis in a 21-day-old infant. Am J Dis Child 1956; 92:66.

Larwood TR. Maternal fetal transmission of coccidioidomycosis. In: Wayne LE, ed. Transactions of the Seventh Annual Meeting of the Veterans Administration. Armed Forces coccidioidomycosis study group. Veterans Administration, 1978:28–29.

Linsangan LC, Ross LA. *Coccidiodes immitis* of the neonate: two routes of infection. Pediatr Infect Dis J 1999; 18:171.

McCaffree MA, Altshuler G, Benirschke K. Placental coccidioidomycosis without fetal disease. Arch Pathol Lab Med 1978; 102:512.

Nickisch, SA, Izquierdo, L, Vill, MA. Coccidioidal placentitus with normal umbilical artery velocimetry. Infect Dis Obstet Gynecol 1993; 1:144.

Shafai T. Neonatal coccidioidomycosis in premature twins. Am J Dis Child 1978; 132:634.

Spark RP. Does transplacental spread of coccidioidomycosis occur? Arch Pathol Lab Med 1981; 105:347.

Mycobacterium tuberculosis and *Mycobacterium bovis*

James W. Daly and Gilles R. G. Monif   /   *Revised by* Mahmoud Ismail

59

INTRODUCTION

The tubercle bacilli of the genus *Mycobacterium* are thin, straight rods measuring approximately $0.4\,\mu m \times 3\,\mu m$. They are characterized by their acid-fast staining, which is contingent on the fact that, once stained by basic dyes, they cannot be decolorized by alcohol. The mycobacteria are obligatory aerobes. In contrast to most bacteria, their replicating cycle is of the order of 17 to 24 hours. The tubercle bacilli are relatively resistant to desiccation and may survive for long periods in dry sputum.

The bacilli produce no endotoxin. Their gross and microscopic lesions represent the summation of the proliferation of mycobacteria and the cellular reaction of the host. The initial reaction of the human host to either *Mycobacterium tuberculosis* or *Mycobacterium bovis* is characterized by a polymorphonuclear neutrophilic inflammatory exudate. The polymorphonuclear neutrophils are transient and are replaced within 48 hours by monocytes and lymphocytes. Prior to the development of resistance and hypersensitivity by the host, the prime sites of tubercle replication become intracellular within monocytes and reticuloendothelial (RE) cells.

The advent of cellular immunity markedly influences the ability of the tubercle bacillus to replicate at these intracellular sites. The lesions undergo precipitous change. The intracellular destruction of the bacilli is enhanced, and caseation necrosis within fixed tissue tends to be the rule. Rechallenge with exogenous *M. tuberculosis* or reactivation of endogenous infections in an individual in whom immunity has developed results in a markedly different lesion. Rather than being exudative, the lesion elicits a proliferative granulomatous response, which in its most classic form is characterized by centrally located caseation necrosis surrounded by concentric layers of epithelial and giant cells, and finally a peripheral zone of lymphocytes, monocytes, and fibroblasts.

The portal of infection determines the mechanism by which the female genital tract is involved. Tuberculosis is primarily an infection of the respiratory tract. Female genital tract involvement can develop from a pulmonary nidus of infection or by hematogenous dissemination of organisms and their subsequent localization within the fallopian tube. When the gastrointestinal tract is the portal of infection, involvement of the ileocecal region permits lymphatic spread—primarily to the right fallopian tube.

Dissemination of disease from the fallopian tube occurs by continuous spread to potentially involve the ovary and retrograde into the uterus. Uterine extension involves primarily the endometrium with, at maximum, a 20% incidence of myometrial involvement. The involvement of the ovary is usually in the form of a perioophoritis. In some instances, the hilus of the ovary is invaded by direct hematogenous spread. The cervix can be involved either by extension from the endometrium or as part of the hematogenous infection.

Tuberculosis of the vagina and the vulva is extremely uncommon. This type of involvement is more common in a woman with tuberculosis of another organ who excretes tubercle bacilli in her stool, urine, or sputum. When in contact with the external genitalia, these secretions may result in tuberculosis of the vulva or vagina (particularly if the epithelium has been broken or damaged).

Tuberculous peritonitis is a variant of genital tract tuberculosis. Disease occurs as a consequence of an initial miliary dissemination during the primary bacillemia or secondarily during reactivation of extrapulmonary disease. Fallopian tube/uterine disease and tuberculous peritonitis can and does coexist in up to 50% of the cases. The female genital tract may become infected with either *M. tuberculosis* (human) or *M. bovis* (bovine) strains. Although it is a rare cause of genital tuberculosis in the United States, bovine tuberculosis is not an uncommon etiologic agent of genital tuberculosis in underdeveloped countries lacking facilities for pasteurization of milk. It is probable that some of the photochromogens, such as *M. kansasii*, may eventually be shown to be pathogens of the female genital tract. Irrespective of whether human or bovine strains of *Mycobacterium* are involved, both are pathogenic for humans.

FEMALE GENITAL TRACT INVOLVEMENT

Morgagni, in the mid-eighteenth century, was probably the first investigator to describe genital tuberculosis. In modern society, genital tuberculosis is almost invariably the result of seeding of the pelvic organs during tuberculous bacillemia from an extragenital focus. Involvement of the female genital tract is usually insidious and manifested late in the course of infection. Symptoms referable to the genital tract do not tend to appear immediately following colonization. An interim of 1 to 10 years may elapse between actual seeding and clinical manifestations. Once the disease is established, it tends to pursue a slow, indolent course. For reasons yet to be explained, the nearer a female is to menarche at the time of primary infection, the greater the likelihood of genital involvement.

Primary pulmonary infection is the consequence of the inhalation of tubercle bacilli. Because of aerosol transmission, the initial sites of infection are the lower lobes and in particular the right lower lobe. The initial host response is an acute exudative lesion. The bacilli ultimately disseminate through the lymphatics to the regional nodes. With the advent of both cellular and humoral immunity, the exudative lesion at the portal of infection (whether lung or intestines) resolves. Lymph nodes undergo caseation necrosis and possible dystrophic calcification at a later date. Calcification in tuberculous foci indicates that necrosis has previously taken place. Dystrophic calcification is not evidence of healing. The combination of primary tissue lesion (whether in lung or intestines) and involved regional nodes constitutes the Ghon complex.

A certain number of organisms, having once attained access to the intravascular compartment via the efferent lymphatics and thoracic duct, may, by hematogenous dissemination, be distributed to multiple organ systems. These organisms are responsible for the "Simon's foci" in the apical and/or posterior segments (or their equivalents) and possible deposition in the fallopian tubes. Thus, infection of the female genital tract may be caused by either acute or subacute hematogenous dissemination in an individual with active pulmonary tuberculosis. These foci can cause endogenous infection at a later date, although in most cases, they become quiescent after the development of tuberculin hypersensitivity and are of no further clinical significance.

The external portions of the perineum or vulva may on rare occasions be primary sites of infection. In these instances, genital tract involvement is via direct inoculation of infectious material. The pathogenesis is analogous to that of cutaneous tuberculosis at nongenital sites. External genital tract infection results in superficial ulcers, which may have an associated development of sinus tracts. Even partial healing is characterized by fibrosis and scar formation.

CLINICAL PRESENTATIONS

In the developed countries, the clinical presentation of genital tract tuberculosis is altered. Disease is being diagnosed in an older age group that, not infrequently, may be perimenopausal. The most common presentation in this group is menstrual irregularity. In developing countries, the principal manifestations are abdominal pain and infertility. When menstrual disturbances occur, primary amenorrhea is the most common presentation. Disease occurs primarily between the ages of 20 and 40 years.

Infertility
Infertility is the most common presenting complaint. Its incidence within a given population depends directly on the prevalence of extragenital tuberculosis and ranges from 2% to 5% of all cases of infertility. In most cases, there are no concomitant physical findings that provide a clue to the possible

relationship between presenting complaint and etiology. The Mantoux intradermal skin test should be a standard part of every clinical examination for infertility. A positive reaction should alert the physician to the possibility of genital tuberculosis and argues for a culture and histologic analysis of the endometrium. A high index of suspicion is required in an infertility evaluation if the patient is a recent immigrant from the "third world," or is the prime prerequisite for diagnosing the incipient stages of genital infection or disease. Menstrual irregularities and/or dysmenorrhea may be secondary to endometrial involvement. Derangement of the menses is not an uncommon clinical manifestation in women with genital tuberculosis. Although secondary amenorrhea or oligomenorrhea is uncommon, the menstrual pattern is unpredictable. Early in the infection, an increase in menstrual flow or irregular bleeding between menses may occur. Primary amenorrhea and postmenopausal bleeding have been observed in patients with tuberculous endometritis.

Pain
About 35% of women with genital tuberculosis complain of chronic lower abdominal pain, with an incidence roughly proportional to the number of women with abnormal physical findings on pelvic examination. It is not uncommon to elicit a history of recent appendectomy or actual laparotomy performed for chronic discomfort. Pelvic pain associated with inflammatory masses that does not improve with conventional therapy should raise the suspicion of genital tuberculosis.

Ascites
A common clinical presentation is ascites secondary to peritoneal tuberculosis (Fig. 1). The development of ascites presents a real diagnostic challenge, particularly when the patient is past the age of 20 years. In adolescent girls, the origin of ascitic abdominal swelling is frequently tuberculous. The swelling is often accompanied by pain and low-grade fever. Peripheral edema, which is characteristic of cardiovascular-related ascites, is not present with tuberculous peritonitis and ascites unless there is concomitant gastrointestinal involvement and resultant protein depletion.

The diagnosis of peritoneal tuberculosis can rarely be made on Ziehl-Neelsen staining of centrifuged sediment from ascitic fluid. In approximately 50% of patients, the organism can be isolated by appropriate cultures. With peritoneoscopy and biopsy, the probability of establishing the diagnosis approaches 85%; with laparotomy, 100%. Characteristic of tuberculous ascites is its failure to recur following laparotomy. Analysis of the ascitic fluid may suggest that one is dealing with an exudate rather than a transudate. Protein content greater than 3.5 g/100 mL or specific gravity greater than 1.015 are characteristic of the former. However, the specific gravity is in part a function of the density of peritoneal lesions and may vary considerably. A specific gravity less than 1.010 probably excludes tuberculosis from consideration. In general, there is a better correlation between protein content and causative factors than between specific gravity and etiology.

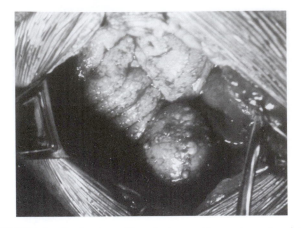

FIGURE 1 Coalescing miliary lesions, at laparotomy, involving the serosa, omentum, and peritoneal surfaces in a 16-year-old nulligravida who presented with ascites.

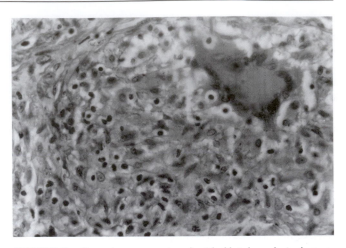

FIGURE 2 Granuloma associated with *M. tuberculosis* demonstrating epithelioid cells and a single Langhans' giant cell associated with *M. tuberculosis*.

Physical Signs of Genital Tuberculosis

Female genital tract organs infected with *M. tuberculosis* may appear entirely normal on physical examination. In only about 50% of the cases does bimanual examination reveal physical findings indicative of pelvic disease, such as enlargement or fixation of appendages, pyosalpinx, or abdominal swelling secondary to tuberculous peritonitis. Extensive adhesions in pelvic tuberculosis reflect the previous occurrence of tuberculous peritonitis. Even at laparotomy, unless tuberculous peritonitis with serosal seeding of the peritoneum or pyosalpinx is present, the diagnosis may not be evident on gross examination of the fallopian tubes and may be contingent on tubal biopsy or culture.

The fallopian tubes, like their embryologic male homolog, the epididymis, are the initial sites of pelvic involvement following hematogenous dissemination of the bacilli, with the distal portions appearing to be infected first. Infection then takes a more central path, with the uterus being ultimately involved. In a significant number of cases, endometrial biopsy fails to reveal the bacilli or histologic evidence of infection, even though the disease process is entrenched in the fallopian tubes. In approximately one-quarter of the cases of genital tuberculosis, the fallopian tubes are patent. Within the endometrium and the interstitium of the fallopian tubes, the tissue response to *M. tuberculosis* is that of epithelioid cell granulomas with or without scattered Langhans' giant cells (Fig. 2). Fibrosis marginal to the granuloma is usually present, as is lymphocytic infiltration. Caseation necrosis is rare and tends to be a late feature.

The endometrial glands frequently exhibit underdeveloped secretory patterns or a pattern of glandular hyperplasia. Epithelial hyperplasia may be so striking, with respect to fallopian tube lesions, as to be misinterpreted as a coexistent, well-differentiated adenocarcinoma. The presence of numerous plasma cells, as well as of lymphocytes, within the endometrial stroma is indicative of secondary infection.

TUBERCULOSIS OF THE BREAST

Tuberculous mastitis usually presents in the third decade of life. The patients usually present with a unilateral painful breast mass arising over weeks or a painless, nonfriable lump of short duration. The latter presentation is usually with lymphadenopathy. Occasionally, a draining sinus is presented. Rarely is tuberculous etiology postulated. The prebiopsy diagnoses are usually equally divided between breast abscess and carcinoma. The diagnosis of tuberculosis is based on the histopathological demonstration of tubercles, caseation, and a granulomatous inflammation with acid-fast bacilli. The differential diagnosis includes duct ectasia, a foreign-body giant-cell reaction with fat necrosis, foreign-body abscess, granulomatous mastitis, fungal mastitis, sarcoidosis, and a syphilitic gumma. The diagnosis is usually made by cultures of breast aspirate or by histological analysis of the biopsy sample. Treatment involves complete surgical excision of the lesion and at least six months of postoperative antituberculous chemotherapy.

DIAGNOSIS

Purified Protein Derivative Intradermal Skin Test (Mantoux)

The diagnosis of infection due to *M. tuberculosis* is contingent upon the demonstration of a positive purified protein derivative (PPD) tuberculin skin test. Based on the sensitivity and specificity of the PPD skin test, three different cut-points have been recommended for defining a positive tuberculin reaction.

When intermediate-strength PPD in a dose of 0.1 mL [5 tuberculin units (TU)] is injected into the dermis over the forearm of a tuberculous patient, a positive tuberculin reaction, characterized by an area of induration more than 10 mm in diameter, develops within 48 hours. Reactions less than 5 mm in diameter are read as negative and those in between 5 mm and 10 m as indeterminant. For persons who are at the highest risk for developing active disease if they become infected by *M. tuberculosis*, a 5 mm or greater induration is considered positive. This group includes persons with HIV infection, persons receiving immunosuppressive therapy, persons who have had close contact with an active case, and persons who have chest radiographs consistent with previous tuberculosis (Table 1).

A positive reaction indicates infection but does not necessarily correlate with active disease at the time of testing.

About 10% of patients with bacteriologically confirmed tuberculosis may fail to respond to 5 TU of PPD as well as to several purified protein products containing polysorbate 80 (Tween 80). Such individuals tend to react to second-strength PPD. A tuberculin test should not sensitize a noninfected person, but it can stimulate or enhance remotely established hypersensitivity. To circumvent the problem of the "booster effect," retesting should be done one week later. If the second test is positive, it is probably due to magnification of subclinical hypersensitivity to prior infection more than to new infection. Patients with miliary tuberculosis or overwhelming pulmonary tuberculosis may exhibit anergy.

The value of the skin test in infertility cases is to increase the index of suspicion and identify that population in whom culture techniques should be applied. Otherwise, its real value lies not in identifying those individuals with previous infection but in excluding tuberculosis from the differential diagnosis. A nonreactive skin test does not exclude infection in cases of tuberculous peritonitis or miliary tuberculosis.

Tuberculin reactivity caused by bacillus Calmette-Guerin (BCG) vaccination generally wanes with time. It can be boosted by the tuberculin skin test. Although no reliable method exists to distinguish tuberculin reactivity caused by vaccination with BCG from those caused by natural infection, reactions of 20 mm or greater of induration are not likely to be caused by BCG.

Histology and Microbiological Culturing

The diagnosis may be established on the basis of the histopathologic features of a premenstrual endometrial

TABLE 1 Criteria for a positive tuberculin test

A reaction of ≥15 mm is classified as positive in all individuals

A reaction of ≥10 mm is classified as positive in the following groups:
   Foreign-born individuals from high-prevalence areas, e.g., Asia
   Intravenous drug users
   Medically underserved–low-income populations
   Residents of long-term care facilities
   Individuals with medical risk factors, e.g., chronic renal disease,
      corticosteroids, lymphomas, leukemias, silicosis, gastrectomy,
      jejunoileal bypass, diabetes mellitus, weight loss of 10% of
      ideal bodyweight

A reaction of ≥5 mm is classified as positive in the following groups:
   HIV-positive individuals
   Individuals receiving immunosuppressive therapy
   Individuals with recent contact with active case of tuberculosis
   Individuals with chest X ray consistent with old healed
      tuberculosis
   Interpretation of PPD in HIV-infected persons is as follows:
      50% of HIV-positive individuals are anergic. A nonreactive
      PPD does not preclude the presence of *M. tuberculosis*
      Positive skin test is positive if the induration is 5 mm in diameter

Abbreviation: PPD, purified protein derivative tuberculin skin test.

biopsy or curettage fragments. Classically, one-half of endometrial fragments are sent for culture and the other half for histologic examination. The diagnosis is generally established by the presence of characteristic granulomas in the material analyzed. Failure to demonstrate the acid-fast bacilli by the Ziehl-Neelsen technique does not invalidate the diagnosis except in the absence of evidence of delayed hypersensitivity (i.e., a negative PPD).

Occasionally, histologic examination of the endometrial curettement alone does not reveal the disease process (due to sampling errors or to noninvolvement of the endometrium when the fallopian tubes are the prime sites of infection). Bacteriologic examination is important and should be done. Menstrual blood collected in a Tassette cup provides additional material for culture. At some future date, the current rapid culture techniques such as radiometric and biphasic methods and microcolony morphology will give way to DNA probes and high-performance liquid chromatography.

Hysterosalpingograms may reveal closed tubes with a "tobacco-pouch" deformity of the ampullary end or a rigid "pipe-stem" pattern (Fig. 3). In contrast to the morphologic changes in chronic salpingitis, the fimbriae are uninvolved. Some of the infected tubes demonstrate multiple fistulas.

Targeted scanning of the uterus and fallopian tubes is possible with high-resolution transvaginal sonography.

Once the diagnosis of genital tuberculosis is established, the patient's evaluation should include the following:

1. Chest X-ray
2. Three sputum collections for tubercle bacilli
3. IV pyelogram
4. Three urine cultures for tubercle bacilli

Although renal involvement will not alter therapy, these cultures are important as an additional source for culture material to ensure a bacteriologic diagnosis and specimens for sensitivity testing. About 10% of women with genital involvement have renal tuberculosis, and vice versa. All positive cultures need to be tested against a primary susceptibility test panel of five drugs; isoniazid (INH), pyrazinamide (PZA), ethambutol (EMB), streptomycin (STM), and rifampin.

Targeted tuberculin testing of populations at risk for acquisition of infection or its progression to disease is a strategic component of tuberculosis control.

Treatment of Latent Tuberculosis

A number of regimens have been recommended for the treatment of latent tuberculosis. The INH daily regimen for nine months is recommended. Before beginning treatment for latent tuberculosis, active disease should be ruled out by history, physical examination, chest radiography, and, when indicated, bacteriologic studies.

For pregnant, HIV-negative women, INH given daily or twice a week for six or nine months is recommended. For women at risk for progression to disease, especially those who are infected with HIV or who have likely been infected recently, initiation of therapy should not be

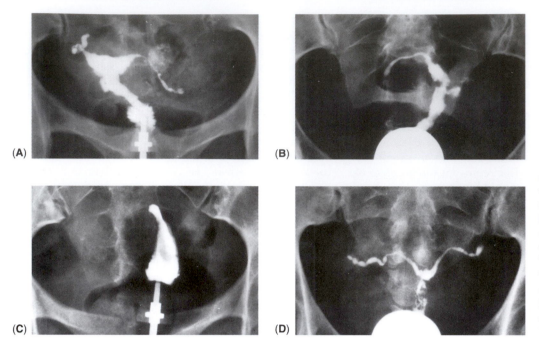

FIGURE 3 Patterns of tubal disease due to *M. tuberculosis* demonstrated by hysterosalpingograms. (**A**) Irregularity of the endometrial cavity. (**B**) Rigid "pipe-stem" pattern. (**C**) "Tobacco-pouch" deformity. (**D**) Beading within the tubal lumens. *Source*: Courtesy of Thomas Klein, MD, Bethesda, MD.

delayed on the basis of pregnancy alone, even in the first trimester. For women whose risk for active tuberculosis is lower, waiting until after delivery or at least the first trimester should be evaluated on an individual basis.

Twice-weekly treatment with rifampin and PZA for two or three months may be considered when INH cannot be given. To avert drug resistance, it is recommended that this regimen be given as five observed and two self-administered doses each week. In situations such as HIV-infected persons receiving protease inhibitors, in which rifampin cannot be used, rifabutin may be substituted.

A patient once identified should receive appropriate follow-up surveillance at least monthly. Baseline evaluation of pregnant women, women with HIV, women within three months of delivery, and women with hepatitis B, hepatitis C, or alcoholic hepatitis includes measurements of serum aspartate aminotransferase or alanine aminotransferase and bilirubin.

CONGENITAL TUBERCULOSIS

Congenital tuberculosis is a rare but well-defined entity. With the notable exception of miliary tuberculosis, there is no predictable correlation between maternal disease and the probability of infection of the conceptus. Fetal infection may take place when the maternal lesions are minimal. This lack of correlation reflects the fact that tuberculous bacillemia may occur at any time during the activity of an existing focus of infection. Fetal infection results primarily as a consequence of maternal bacillemia. If a thrombus containing mycobacteria forms in the intervillous spaces and if the inflammatory process proliferates so as to involve the adjacent placental area, embolization of infectious material to the fetus may occur.

Placental involvement attending maternal hematogenous bacillemia occurs far more frequently than infection of the fetus. Limitation of infection to the placenta may be in part a function of maternal immunity. Thrombosis of fetal vessels draining a nidus of infection is more likely to occur when placental involvement is the consequence of chronic hematogenous dissemination from a mother with longstanding disease rather than from one with miliary tuberculosis. When placental involvement is grossly discernible, examination of the umbilical cord may occasionally reveal multiple tuberculous granulomas around the umbilical vein.

With congenital disease, the primary complex develops in the liver or regional lymph nodes, or both. In contrast to adult tuberculosis, in which hepatic involvement is usually limited to small granulomas in the portal area, extensive and progressive destruction is observed in the fetal liver. This preferential growth within hepatic tissue in utero may reflect the dependence of *M. tuberculosis* on an oxygen-rich environment, which in fetal life is supplied by the umbilical vein. Although hepatic involvement is probably caused by secondary hematogenous spread of tubercle bacilli from a placental focus, extensive nodal involvement of the porta hepatis can conceivably be the result of lymphatic spread from an infected placental focus to the regional lymph nodes.

A second mechanism for congenital infection occurs in women with tuberculous endometritis. The majority of such women are sterile owing to prior fallopian tube involvement; this circumstance accounts for the rarity of congenital tuberculosis based on this mode of dissemination. By direct extension, the tuberculous process may either involve the placenta—from which there is subsequent dissemination to the fetus—or erode directly into the amniotic fluid, with subsequent fetal aspiration of infected material. In those cases in which the latter mode of transmission appears to be reasonably documented, the infants quickly succumb to tuberculous bronchopneumonia. When the degree of aspiration is relatively small, a successful response to antituberculosis therapy may be achieved.

At necropsy, infants with congenital tuberculosis usually exhibit macromiliary lesions of spleen, liver, and lungs. Microscopic examination reveals tuberculous granulomas with characteristic epithelial, mononuclear, and Langhans' giant cells and caseation necrosis. Occasionally, the lesions show only caseation necrosis with very little reaction. When the lesion has extended to a free surface, the response is predominantly one of mononuclear cells. This is most pronounced in tuberculous pneumonia in which endotracheal spread has occurred. In "fixed tissue" (intra-alveolar walls, spleen, liver), the more characteristic epithelioid response is observed. Both reactions may be seen in the same infant and are primarily related to the site of the lesion.

In aspiration-type congenital tuberculosis, the lungs are the sole organ of involvement. The disease process is confined to the alveoli, with an intra-alveolar exudate composed predominantly of macrophage and alveolar-lining cells with an accompanying alveolitis.

Fetal tuberculous bacillemia results in the dissemination of the organisms primarily to the liver, bone marrow, spleen, lung, and renal cortex. Less frequent sites of involvement include brain, skin, and adrenal glands. The distribution of the lesions parallels that of the RE cells and reflects the fact that *M. tuberculosis* behaves like particulate matter in the intravascular compartment.

Clinicopathologic Correlations

Although a few cases of congenital tuberculosis have been documented shortly after birth, in most instances, the symptoms evolve insidiously during the first months of life. The infants refuse to eat, with ensuing weight loss. Splenomegaly and eventually hepatosplenomegaly develop. Obstructive jaundice may develop as a result either of extensive hepatic involvement or, more frequently, of impingement on the biliary system by enlarged nodes in the porta hepatis. In more than half of the cases reported, the infants died within three to four weeks after the first sign of illness. Others, primarily those with pulmonary aspiration tuberculosis or extensive miliary dissemination, developed respiratory distress. These infants died early with tuberculous bronchopneumonia. Oddly enough, tuberculous meningitis is not common in cases of congenital involvement. The short interim between diagnosis and death stresses the necessity for prompt diagnosis and institution of therapy, despite an anticipated high mortality.

Diagnosis

Congenital tuberculosis essentially requires that certain criteria be met:

1. The primary tuberculous complex must be present in the liver.
2. Extrauterine acquisition of infection must be definitely excluded.
3. The tuberculous lesions must be present at birth.

The diagnosis of congenital tuberculosis should be actively sought in the progeny born to mothers with active cavitary, pelvic, or miliary tuberculosis who are not receiving therapy.

Placental examination is of limited value in the identification of congenital tuberculosis. Tuberculous involvement of the placenta is a more frequent phenomenon than congenital infection. Negative histologic examination of the placenta does not exclude the possibility of hematogenous dissemination. The likelihood that congenital tuberculosis will occur in any particular case cannot be predicted either by consideration of the mother's lesions or by the presence of foci of infection in the placenta.

Management of Neonates Born to Tuberculous Mothers

Infants born to mothers with active tuberculosis represent a real challenge in clinical therapeutic management. If disease has been established in utero, there is the necessity of instituting immediate therapy if the baby is to survive. Equally important is the need to institute prophylaxis, which may guard the neonate against subsequent acquisition of infection.

The infants of mothers being treated for active tuberculosis whose cultures are negative for *M. tuberculosis* merely need to be tuberculin tested between the second and fourth week of life with 5 TU 0.1 mL (intermediate strength) PPD and thereafter at two-month intervals during the first year of life. Infants born to mothers with active tuberculosis and sputum that is positive for *M. tuberculosis* "should be treated with INH for two to three months or at least until the mother is smear and culture negative and known to be complying with therapy. If after three months of therapy, the mother has a negative sputum smear and the infant is tuberculin negative and has a normal chest X ray, INH may be stopped." When the maternal disease is either miliary tuberculosis or tuberculous meningitis, owing to the 30% risk of congenital infection, the infant is immediately placed on INH therapy, 10 mg/kg/day, after baseline gastric and cerebrospinal fluid cultures, hepatic transaminase determinations, chest X rays, and tuberculin skin tests have been obtained. If the tuberculin test is positive or congenital infection is documented by isolation of the tubercle bacillus, the INH dosage can be increased to 20 mg/kg/day and rifampin 10 to 20 mg/kg PO each day for nine months can be added. Maternal antibacterial therapy during pregnancy may have an adverse fetal effect (Table 2). Ethionamide and rifampin are best avoided during pregnancy when possible.

If the neonate exhibits any evidence of an infectious process, antituberculosis therapy should be instituted despite a negative PPD test. Not infrequently, an infant with extensive disease may exhibit a transient anergy; however, failure of the PPD test to become positive after three to four weeks of therapy would be evidence against the diagnosis of congenital tuberculosis.

It is not always possible to obtain the organism for determination of sensitivities to antituberculous chemotherapeutic drugs. Use of the organism isolated from the mother is an acceptable alternative.

Therapy

Infants born to mothers with active pulmonary tuberculosis require the same baseline studies. The critical point in

TABLE 2 Potential fetal adverse drug reactions due to antituberculous therapy

Drug	Potential adverse effects on fetus/neonate
Cycloserine (Seromycin®)	Safety not established
Ethambutol (Myambutol®)	Not known—teratogenic in animals
Ethionamide (Treacator-SC®)	Teratogenic in animals
Isoniazid (INH and others)	Embryotoxic in animals
Pyrazinamide	Unknown
Rifampin (Rifadin®; Rimactane®)	Teratogenic in animals

their management is determining whether the tuberculin test is positive or negative. If the tuberculin test is positive, the infant is given the therapeutic regimen for congenital tuberculosis. If the tuberculin tests obtained in the second and fourth weeks of life are negative, three methods of management are available:

1. *INH prophylaxis*: The child may receive INH for six months to one year and be tuberculin tested every two months during chemoprophylaxis. The effectiveness of INH prophylaxis is dependent upon patient compliance. Whenever the tuberculin test becomes positive or culture evidence of infection with *M. tuberculosis* is obtained, the child is treated with the full therapeutic regimen.
2. *Cultural, roentgenographic, and tuberculin surveillance for one year*: This requires adequate health facilities and full parental cooperation. In addition, the mother's sputum should be culture negative and the infant's chest X ray normal, with no exposure of the infant to active tuberculosis in the immediate family.
3. *BCG vaccination*: Prior to BCG vaccination, the patient's roentgenogram should be normal and the tuberculin test negative.

BCG is advocated in cases involving poor or indifferent parental motivation, a socioeconomic impediment to surveillance or therapy, or inadequate health facilities. Kendig (1970) made a follow-up study of 105 infants born to tuberculous mothers. Of the 30 who received BCG vaccine, none contracted tuberculosis. Of the 75 nonvaccinated infants, 38 became infected. In this study, the known inadequacy of an imperfectly followed regimen of culture surveillance and chemoprophylaxis combined to make BCG vaccination the method of choice for noncompliant individuals. Neonates born to mothers with currently active tuberculosis should be treated with INH for two to three months or at least until the mother is smear and culture negative and known to be compliant with therapy. If the infant's tuberculin reaction is significant at three months, a posterior–anterior and a lateral radiograph are required.

PREVENTIVE THERAPY OF TUBERCULOUS INFECTION

A single drug, INH, is used for preventive therapy in a dose of 300 mg/day for adults and 10 mg/kg bodyweight/day, not to exceed 300 mg/day for children, to be administered in a daily single dose over a period of 6 to 12 months. INH is inexpensive, administered orally, and easy to take. Mild hepatic dysfunction, evidenced by elevation of serum aminotransferase (transaminase) activity, occurs in 10% to 20% of persons taking INH. This abnormality usually occurs in the first four to six months of treatment but can occur at any time during therapy. In most instances, enzyme levels return to normal and there is no necessity to discontinue medication. Occasionally, progressive liver damage occurs and presents symptoms; the drug should be discontinued immediately in these cases. The frequency of progressive liver damage increases with age. It is rare in individuals under the age of 20 years. The observed frequency in other age groups is as follows: ages 20 to 34 years, up to 0.3%; ages 35 to 49 years, up to 1.2%; 50 years and more, up to 2.3%. Pregnant and postpartum Hispanic women may have a twofold increase in morbidity.

Persons for Whom Preventive Therapy Is Recommended

Priorities must be set for preventive therapy, taking into consideration not only the risk of developing tuberculosis compared with the risk of INH toxicity, but also the ease in identifying and supervising persons for whom preventive therapy is indicated, and their likelihood of infecting others. The following groups are listed in order of priority:

1. *Household members and other close associates*: Household members and other close associates of patients with newly discovered tuberculous disease are at high risk of having been recently infected and of developing disease. The risk is approximately 2.5% for the first year. However, the risk is approximately 5.0% for those already infected (tuberculin positive) at the time of the initial examination. Contacts of patients should be examined and those diagnosed as having tuberculous disease should be treated with multiple drug therapy. All other contacts with Mantoux tuberculin skin test readings of 5 mm or more should receive preventive therapy, since in this group, such reactions are likely to be due to infection with *M. tuberculosis*.
2. *Positive tuberculin skin test reactor with abnormal chest roentgenogram*: Persons with past tuberculous disease not previously treated by adequate chemotherapy and tuberculin skin test reactors with roentgenographic findings consistent with nonprogressive tuberculous disease should receive preventive therapy. The rate of reactivation in such groups, if untreated, has been observed to range between 1.0% and 4.5% per year.
3. *Newly infected persons*: The risk of developing tuberculous disease for the newly infected is about 5.0% during the first year after infection. Because this excess risk is concentrated in the first year or so, the term "newly infected persons" should be applied only to those who have had a tuberculin skin test conversion within the past two years.

Preventive therapy is mandatory for positive reactors from the age of six years and highly recommended up to the age of 35 years, unless there are contraindications to the use of INH, as listed below.

Among positive tuberculin reactors aged 35 years and more, the risk of hepatitis precludes the routine use of preventive therapy unless an additional risk factor (such as contacts or converters) is present. Thus, persons aged 35 years and more who have normal chest roentgenograms and no other risk factors are not, as a group, recommended for preventive therapy. Rather, they should be considered for preventive therapy on an individual basis in situations where there is a likelihood of serious consequences to contacts who may become infected.

Screening Procedures
Before INH for preventive therapy is started, the following screening procedures should be carried out:

1. Rule out bacteriologically positive or progressive tuberculous disease. Every person who is a positive reactor should have a chest roentgenogram taken. If there are findings consistent with pulmonary tuberculous disease, further studies—medical evaluation, bacteriologic examinations, and comparison with previous roentgenographic findings—should be made to rule out progressive disease. This is because persons with progressive or bacteriologically confirmed tuberculous disease require more intensive chemotherapy than is given for preventive therapy.
2. Question for a history of INH administration to exclude those who have had an adequate course of the drug.
3. Ascertain the presence of contraindications to administration of INH for preventive therapy, which are
   (a) previous INH-associated hepatic injury,
   (b) severe adverse reactions to INH, such as drug fever, chills, and arthritis,
   (c) acute liver disease of any etiology.
4. Identify patients for whom preventive therapy is not contraindicated but in whom special attention is indicated by the following:
   (a) Concurrent use of any other medication on a long-term basis (in view of possible drug interactions).
   (b) Use of diphenylhydantoin, the dosage of which may need to be reduced to avoid diphenylhydantoin toxicity. This is because in some individuals, INH may decrease the excretion of diphenylhydantoin or may enhance its effect.
   (c) Daily use of alcohol, which may be associated with a higher incidence of INH hepatitis.
   (d) Previously discontinued INH because of possible but not definitely related side-effects (e.g., headaches, dizziness, nausea).
   (e) Possibility of current chronic liver disease.

INH Toxicity
INH toxicity usually manifests with biochemical evidence of hepatic dysfunction. Approximately 10% to 20% of patients taking the drug will have some elevation of transaminase activity. This abnormality usually occurs in the first four to six months of treatment, but can occur at any time during therapy. In most instances, the enzymatic abnormalities return to normal despite continued drug therapy. Unless there is progressive evidence of hepatic decompensation, discontinuation of the medication is not necessary.

Monitoring Individuals for INH Toxicity
Individuals receiving preventive therapy should be questioned carefully at monthly intervals for the following:

1. Symptoms consistent with those of liver damage or other toxic effects; i.e., unexplained anorexia, nausea, or vomiting of greater than three days duration, fatigue or weakness of greater than three days duration, persistent paresthesia of the hands and feet
2. Signs consistent with those of liver damage or other toxic effects; i.e., persistent dark urine, icterus, rash, unexplained elevated temperature of greater than three days duration

Monitoring by routine laboratory tests [e.g., serum glutamic oxaloacetic transaminase (SGOT), serum glutamic pyruvic transaminase, serum bilirubin, and alkaline phosphatase] is not useful in predicting hepatic disease in INH recipients and therefore is not recommended. However, in evaluating signs and symptoms, such tests are mandatory. Preventive therapy should be reinstituted only if biochemical studies are normal and signs and symptoms are absent.

In some instances, an SGOT may be obtained for some reason other than the presence of signs or symptoms. If the result of this test does not exceed three times the normal and no signs or symptoms have developed, the drug may be continued with caution and careful continued observation. If the level exceeds three times the normal, the decision to continue INH should be based on careful evaluation for liver damage and the reason for preventive therapy.

MANAGEMENT OF NEWLY ACQUIRED TUBERCULIN REACTIVITY IN PREGNANCY

If preexisting disease is treated prior to gestation, pregnancy does not appear to reactivate or aggravate it. The problem occurs when a gravida becomes tuberculin positive during pregnancy. All four of the first-line drugs (INH, EMB, rifampin, and STM) have apparent reasonable margins of safety when used during pregnancy. The American Thoracic Society, American Lung Association, and the Centers for Disease Control and Prevention (CDC) identify the relative safety of INH for the fetus. It is their recommendation to prescribe only therapeutically necessary medication during pregnancy. This position is not universally accepted.

Pregnancy is not without its effect on disease due to *M. tuberculosis*. Women in whom tuberculosis is discovered during pregnancy tend to fare much worse than do women in whom the diagnosis is made prior to conception. When disease occurs in the third trimester or the immediate postpartum period, fulminating disease (e.g., miliary dissemination or meningitis) is more characteristic than it is in the nonpregnant female or the gravida in the first trimester. These observations tend to confirm the concept that late in gestation, a significant depression in cell-mediated immunity occurs. Responsiveness to lymphocytoblast mitogens as measured by blast transformation or delayed cutaneous hypersensitivity is markedly depressed in the third trimester.

THERAPY

Risk of Developing Tuberculosis

The probability of developing tuberculosis can be crudely approximated by using two factors: tuberculin reactivity and roentgenographic evaluation of the chest. If a woman has a positive PPD test and a normal chest X ray, the risk of tuberculosis relapse is between 0.03% and 0.08% per year. If the chest X ray film is abnormal, the incidence of relapse becomes 0.8% to 2% per year. In selected populations such as the Vietnamese and Haitian refugees, the risk of relapse per year can be as high as 6.7%.

Pulmonary Tuberculosis

When primary drug resistance is unlikely, the combination of INH and EMB for a period of 18 to 24 months has been standard therapy for mild or moderately severe disease (Table 3). Triple therapy with the addition of STM has been used for advanced cavitary disease. INH (300 mg), EMB (15 to 18 mg/kg for outpatients and 25 mg/kg for inpatients), and STM are used for the first three months or until sputum is negative for advanced cavitary disease. After a two-month course, a twice-weekly schedule of INH (15 mg/kg) plus EMB (50 mg/kg) or STM (25 to 28 mg/kg) has been administered. This regimen can be used for intermittent therapy to ensure patient compliance.

Relatively comparable therapeutic results have been obtained with regimens containing both INH and rifampicin (RIF) over nine months. The combination of INH (300 mg) and RIF (600 mg) taken once daily by mouth on an empty stomach for nine months is now an established therapy for all forms of pulmonary and extrapulmonary disease. An alternate therapy is RIF, INH, and PZA for two months. A variation has INH and RIF administered daily for one or two months followed by 900 mg of INH and 600 mg of RIF given twice weekly. The more recent CDC recommendations are summarized in Table 4.

Patients receiving INH and RIF together may develop a rapidly progressive toxic hepatitis. Individuals receiving INH and especially STM and RIF need to be monitored by liver function tests since minor enzymatic changes are common.

Pending sensitivity studies, EMB (15 mg/kg) or STM (1 g) is often added to the early stages of therapy. The problem of the emergent drug resistance during therapy is usually linked to prior erratic antituberculous treatment. This problem is common in immigrants from Southeast Asia.

Genital Tuberculosis

The principles of chemotherapy for tuberculosis that has extended beyond the lung are the same as those for pulmonary tuberculosis. Two or more drugs, each individually effective, must be given to reduce the chance of emergence of resistant organisms; treatment must be prolonged for 18 to 24 months.

Many advanced cases will exhibit marked resolution of the abnormal physical findings under multiple drug therapy. However, surgical intervention is necessary if there is persistence or recurrence of

1. adnexal masses after at least six months of drug therapy,
2. pain, or
3. drug-resistant infection.

Surgical treatment should at minimum involve removal of both tubes; in some European clinics, this is standard procedure. The ovaries are infected in only about 5% of the cases. Even though the ovary is extremely resistant to tuberculous involvement, for technical reasons, it can seldom be preserved. The ovaries are almost invariably trapped in a mass of scar tissue, and the best surgical resolution is bilateral salpingo-oophorectomy and hysterectomy. Because of the possibility of inducing chronic fistulas, drains should not be used where possible.

TABLE 3 *Mycobacterium tuberculosis*: Drugs commonly used in therapy

Drug	Dose	Duration	Side effects
Isoniazid (INH)	5 mg/kg/day: max 300 mg	9 mo	Gastrointestinal distress, hepatitis, seizures, peripheral neuritis, hypersensitivity reactions
Rifampin (RIF)	10 mg/kg: max 600 mg	9 mo	Gastrointestinal distress, hepatitis, headache, purpura, febrile, reaction, orange secretions
Pyrazinamide (PZA)[a]: max 2 g/day	15–30 mg/kg: max 4 g	8 wk or until cultures are sensitive to INH/RIF	Hepatitis, hyperuricemia, arthralgias, gout
Ethambutol (EMB)	5–25 mg/kg: max 2.5 g/day	8 wk or until cultures are sensitive to INH/RIF	Altered visual acuity, red-green disturbance, optic neuritis, skin rash

[a]To be started initially only if resistance to INH is likely or in individuals infected with HIV.
Source: Adapted from MMWR 1993; 42/No. RR-7:1.

TABLE 4 Regimen options for the initial treatment of TB in adults without HIV infection

■ *TB without HIV infection*
Option 1: Daily isoniazid, rifampin, and pyrazinamide for 8 wk followed by 16 wk of isoniazid and rifampin daily or 2–3 times weekly (see text).[a] Ethambutol or streptomycin should be added to the initial regimen until sensitivity to isoniazid and rifampin is demonstrated. Continue treatment for at least a total of 6 mo and 3 mo beyond culture conversion. Consult TB medical expert if patient remains smear or culture positive after 3 mo
Option 2: Daily isoniazid, rifampin, pyrazinamide, and streptomycin or ethambutol for 2 wk followed by twice-weekly[a] administration of the same drugs for 6 wk, and subsequently twice-weekly isoniazid and rifampin for 16 wk. Consult TB medical expert if patient remains smear or culture positive after 3 mo
Option 3: Treat with directly observed therapy 3 times weekly,[a] with isoniazid, rifampin, pyrazinamide, and ethambutol or streptomycin for 6 mo. Consult TB medical expert if patient remains smear or culture positive after 3 mo
■ *TB with HIV infection*
Option 1, 2, or 3 can be utilized, but treatment regimens must continue for a total of 9 mo and at least 6 mo beyond culture conversion

[a]All regimens administered twice weekly or thrice weekly should be monitored by directly observed therapy.
Abbreviation: TB, tuberculosis.
Source: MMWR 1992; 41/No. RR-10.

Early detection and therapy for gravidas with active disease can probably abort or prevent the majority of cases of congenital tuberculosis. Women with active tuberculosis require therapy with two or more drugs. INH, EMB, and RIF are the most commonly used antituberculous drugs in pregnancy.

Although neurotoxicity has not been noted among neonates whose mothers received INH during pregnancy, maternal treatment with the drug during gestation is thought to cause retarded psychomotor activity and, in some instances, mental retardation in the progeny. This phenomenon presumably is due to interference with pyridoxine metabolism by degradation compounds from INH. To counter-balance this possibility, when INH is administered during pregnancy, it is advocated that vitamin B6, 50 mg daily, be given for possible fetal as well as maternal indications.

Patients with pulmonary tuberculosis during pregnancy should be treated with INH and EMB in the prescribed dosages for 18 to 24 months. In cases of open cavitary tuberculosis or for advanced disease, rifampin (RMP) may be added.

Tuberculosis in Pregnancy

For pregnant women, the treatment regimen must be adjusted. STM may cause congenital deafness. STM is the only licensed antituberculosis drug documented to have harmful effects on the fetus. Routine use of PZA also is not recommended during pregnancy because the risk of teratogenicity has not been determined. In addition, since the six-month treatment regimen cannot be used and a minimum of nine months of therapy is recommended, the preferred initial treatment is INH, RIF, and EMB. If resistance to other drugs is likely and susceptibility to PZA also is likely, the use of PZA should be considered and the risks and benefits of the drug carefully weighed. Because the small concentrations of antituberculosis drugs in breast milk do not produce toxicity in the nursing newborn, breastfeeding should not be discouraged. Further, because these drug levels are so low in breast milk, they cannot be relied upon for either prophylaxis or therapy for nursing infants.

Postmenopausal Tuberculosis

In the postmenopausal woman, several additional factors influence treatment. If a curettage reveals endometrial tuberculosis and an adnexal mass is palpable, one cannot be certain whether the mass is malignant, and hence surgery is indicated after a short course of chemotherapy. STM should be avoided in the elderly patient because of possible damage to both auditory and vestibular functions of the eighth nerve. Several days of continued administration, after symptoms appear, may result in irreversible damage.

For the postmenopausal woman with endometrial tuberculosis and other pelvic pathology, either uterine or adnexal, an effective regimen is INH and RIF for two months followed by total abdominal hysterectomy and bilateral salpingo-oophorectomy. INH and RIF are then continued for seven months. For the postmenopausal patient in whom no adnexal masses are found, whose medical condition precludes major surgery, or who is noncompliant, the following schedule is suggested: 30 mg INH and 600 mg RIF for one month and then 900 mg INH and 600 mg RIF twice weekly for eight months. Concomitant use of PZA can reduce the duration of therapy to six months.

Genital Tract Tuberculosis Discovered at Operation

If endometrial tuberculosis is discovered at curettage, the patient should immediately be given INH 300 mg and RIF 600 mg. EMB should be added if the possibility of resistance exists. The concurrent use of PZA can shorten the treatment time to six months. The patient should be examined at monthly intervals and, if no adnexal masses are palpable, therapy should be continued for a minimum of nine months. After six months, a curettage should be performed and repeated after one year. If no recurrence has occurred, no further therapy is necessary. A search for extragenital lesions of tuberculosis should be done at the inception of treatment.

Disease is occasionally first discovered postoperatively after removal of one or both tubes. If a total abdominal hysterectomy and bilateral salpingectomy were performed, the patient should receive INH, RIF, and EMB drug therapy—INH, RIF, and EMB for two months and then INH and RIF for two months. EMB should be added if resistance is demonstrated. Thereafter, the patient should receive INH and RIF for an additional seven months. EMB cannot be substituted for RIF in the shortened course of therapy. If EMB is used with INH, the duration of postoperative therapy should be for 18 months. If only one tube was removed, drug therapy should be started with the remaining tube removed after two months and INH and RIF continued for seven months.

TUBERCULOSIS AND HIV

Individuals with recently acquired *M. tuberculosis* infection are at a relatively high risk of developing active tuberculosis; in general, 5% to 10% of persons develop active disease within two years of primary infection. Individuals who have tuberculosis infection and subsequently acquire HIV infection are more likely to progress to tuberculosis disease than those who are HIV negative. Furthermore, persons who are HIV infected and subsequently are exposed to tuberculosis are more likely to progress from infection to disease than those who are HIV negative—and they are likely to have a rapid, severe progression of illness. Approximately 10% of the 1 million persons in the United States infected with HIV are also infected with tuberculosis. The prevalence of HIV infection among patients with tuberculosis disease varies around the country but may exceed 40% in some areas.

For HIV-infected persons, the higher disease attack rate and the shorter incubation period associated with newly acquired tuberculous infection and the high mortality rate associated with tuberculosis disease reinforce the rationale for the use of preventive therapy. In HIV-infected persons who become newly infected with *M. tuberculosis*, the use of drug therapy should be considered treatment of incubating or subclinical disease. A significant percentage of HIV-positive cases will be infected with multidrug-resistant strains.

MULTIDRUG-RESISTANT M. TUBERCULOSIS (MDR-TB)

The most potent factor that increases the probability that a person infected with *M. tuberculosis* will develop active tuberculosis is coinfection with HIV. The next most predictive factor for MDR-TB in newly infected individuals is exposure to a source with multidrug-resistant strains.

Resistance emerges from chromosomal mutations in specific genes. MDR-TB does not have any plasmids. Resistance genes are not chromosomally linked. MDR-TB is defined as resistant to at least INH and RIF and, in some instances, to as many as seven antituberculosis agents.

Because the administration of a single drug often leads to the development of a bacterial population resistant to that drug, effective regimens for the treatment of tuberculosis must contain multiple drugs to which the organisms are susceptible. When two or more drugs are used simultaneously,

each helps prevent the emergence of tubercle bacilli resistant to the others. However, when the in vitro susceptibility of a patient's isolate is not known—which is generally the case at the beginning of therapy—selecting two agents to which the patient's isolate is likely to be susceptible can be difficult. Improper selection of drugs for the treatment of drug-resistant tuberculosis (i.e., providing only one drug to which most organisms are susceptible) may subsequently result in the development of additional drug-resistant organisms.

The treatment options for MDR-TB are limited, since the majority of effective antituberculosis agents are compromised. The principles of treating tuberculosis are to start therapy with at least four drugs (INH, RIF, PZA, and either EMB or STM) unless the incidence of INH resistance in the area is <4% (EMB or STM can be omitted). The physician should modify the regimen once susceptibility results are available (about six to eight weeks). If the strain is susceptible, treatment should be continued such that the total treatment course is at least six months.

When adherence to the regimen is assured, the four-drug regimen is highly effective even for INH-resistant organisms. Based on the prevalence and characteristics of drug-resistant organisms, at least 95% of patients will receive an adequate regimen (at least two drugs to which their organisms are susceptible) if this four-drug regimen is used at the beginning of therapy. Even with susceptible organisms, sputum conversion is accomplished more rapidly from positive to negative with a four-drug regimen than with a three-drug regimen.

SELECTED READING

Female Genital Tract Involvement
Burnie JC. The age of onset of genital tuberculosis in women. Br J Obstet Gynaecol 1956; 63:96.
Carter JR. Unusual presentations of genital tract tuberculosis. Int J Gynaecol Obstet 1990; 33:171.
D'Costa GF, Nagle SB. Tuberculous endometritis—a histopathological study. J Postgrad Med 1988; 34:7.
de Vynck WE, Kruger TF, Joubert JJ, et al. Genital tuberculosis associated with female infertility in the Western Cape. S Afr Med J 1990; 77:630.
Dhillon SS, Gosewehr JA, Julian TM, et al. Genital tuberculosis. Case report and literature review. Wis Med J 1990; 89:14.
Earn AA. Living births following drug therapy for infertility associated with proven genital tuberculosis. Br J Obstet Gynaecol 1958; 65:739.
Ekengren K, Ryden ABV. Roentgen diagnosis of tuberculosis salpingitis. Acta Radiol 1950; 34:193.
Genell (cited by Jedberg H). Acta Obstet Gynaecol Scand 1950; 31:1.
Goyan ADT. Tuberculosis endometritis. J Pathol Bacteriol 1962; 83:363.
Haines M. Genital tuberculosis in the female. Br J Obstet Gynaecol 1952; 59:721.
Hok TT, Loen LK, Tijat NT, et al. The isolation of tubercle bacilli from endocervical mucus of infertile women. Am J Obstet Gynecol 1967; 99:397.
Jindal UN, Jindal SK, Shall GI. Short course chemotherapy for endometrial tuberculosis in infertile women. Int J Gynaecol Obstet 1990; 32:75.
Kendig EL Jr. Prognosis of women born of tuberculous mothers. Pediatrics 1960; 26:97.
Klein TA, Richmond JA, Mishell DR Jr. Pelvic tuberculosis. Obstet Gynecol 1976; 48:99.

Lackner JE, Schiller W, Tulsky AS. The coincidence of tuberculosis of the endometrium with tuberculosis of the lung. Am J Obstet Gynecol 1940; 40:429.

Lewit N, Thaler I, Rottem S. The uterus: a new look with transvaginal sonography. J Clin Ultrasound 1990; 18:331.

Merchant R. Endoscopy in the diagnosis of genital tuberculosis. J Reprod Med 1989; 34:468.

Millar WG. Investigation and treatment of female genital tuberculosis. Br J Obstet Gynaecol 1954; 61:372.

Millar WG. Tubal pregnancy after treatment of genital tuberculosis. Br J Obstet Gynaecol 1958; 65:747.

Myers JA. The natural history of tuberculosis in the human body. III. Tuberculous women and their children. Am Rev Respir Dis 1961; 84:558.

O'Donohoe NV. Congenital tuberculosis and maternal sarcoidosis. Arch Dis Child 1963; 38:83.

O'Herlihy C. Early successful pregnancy following TB endometritis. Acta Obstet Gynaecol Scand 1979; 58:57.

Oosthuizen AP, Wessels PH, Hefer JN. Tuberculosis of the female genital tract in patients attending an infertility clinic. S Afr Med J 1990; 77:562.

Pagel W, Hall S. Aspiration type of congenital tuberculosis. Tubercle 1946; 27:153.

Pagel W, Hall S. Aspiration type of congenital tuberculosis. Further communication. Tubercle 1948; 29:32.

Palomby L. Congenital tuberculosis. *Minerva Med* 1960; 51:3316.

Rabau E, Halbrecht I, Casper J. Endometrial tuberculosis as a cause of sterility. J Am Med Assoc 1943; 122:801.

Ramos AD, Hibbard LT, Craig JR. Congenital tuberculosis. Obstet Gynecol 1974; 43:61.

Reiss HE. Primary amenorrhoea as a manifestation of pelvic tuberculosis. Br J Obstet Gynaecol 1958; 65:734.

Rich AR. *The Pathogenesis of Tuberculosis.* Springfield, IL: CC Thomas, 1944:72.

Riechle HS, Wheelock MC. Aspiration type of congenital tuberculosis. Arch Pathol 1939; 28:799.

Robertson HE, Sullivan CF. Congenital tuberculosis. Can Med Assoc J 1950; 63:361.

Sakeena KC, Arora MM. Endometrial tuberculosis. Ind J Med Sci 1966; 20:543.

Schaefer G, Douglas RG, Dreishpeen IH. Extrapulmonary tuberculosis and pregnancy. Am J Obstet Gynecol 1954; 67:605.

Siegel M, Singer B. Occurrence of tubercle bacilli in the blood of the umbilical cord and in the newborn infants of tuberculous mothers. Am J Dis Child 1935; 50:636.

Stallworthy J. Genital tuberculosis in the female. Am J Obstet Gynecol 1952; 59:729.

Stephanopoulos C. The development of tuberculous meningitis during pregnancy. Am Rev Tuberc 1959; 76:1079.

Sutherland AM. Genital tuberculosis in women. Am J Obstet Gynecol 1960; 79:486.

Tans LC, Cho HK, Wong Taam VC. A typical presentation of female genital tract tuberculosis. Eur J Obstet Gynecol Reprod Biol 1984; 17:355.

Todd RMcL. Congenital tuberculosis: report of a case with unusual features. Tubercle 1960; 51:71.

Tripathy SN, Tripathy SN. Endometrial tuberculosis. J Indian Med Assoc 1987; 85:136.

Tripathy SN, Tripathy SN. Laparoscopic observations in pelvic organs in pulmonary tuberculosis. Int J Gynaecol Obstet 1990; 32:129.

Turneer M, Van Vooren JP, De Bruyn J, et al. Humoral immune response in human tuberculosis: immunoglobulins G, A, and M directed against the purified P32 protein antigen of *Mycobacterium bovis* bacillus Calmette-Guerin. J Clin Microbiol 1988; 26:1714.

Voyce MA, Hunt AC. Congenital tuberculosis. Arch Dis Child 1966; 41:299.

Warthin AS, Cowie DM. A contribution to the casuistry of placental and congenital tuberculosis. J Infect Dis 1994; 1(1):140.

Whitman RC, Greene LW. A case of disseminated miliary tuberculosis in a stillborn fetus. Arch Intern Med 1922; 29:261.

Ylinen O. Genital tuberculosis in women: clinical experience with 348 proved cases. Acta Obstet Gynaecol Scand 1961; 40:1.

Tuberculosis and Pregnancy

Anderson GD. Tuberculosis in pregnancy. Semin Perinatol 1997; 21:328.

Black PB. Tuberculosis: maternal infection of the newborn. Med J Aust 1969; 1:1055.

Durukan T, Urman B, Yarali H, et al. An abdominal pregnancy 10 years after treatment for pelvic tuberculosis. Am J Obstet Gynecol 1990; 163:594.

Flanagan P, Heusler NM. The course of active tuberculosis complicated by pregnancy. J Am Med Assoc 1959; 170:783.

Goodwin RH, Kenler MD. Miliary tuberculosis developing during pregnancy. N Engl J Med 1952; 246:572.

Hinds MW. Pregnancy and tuberculosis. Am Rev Respir Dis 1972; 196:785.

Kronick M. Successful post-mortem caesarian section following death from pulmonary tuberculosis. N Engl J Med 1950; 243:853.

Riley L. Pneumonia and tuberculosis in pregnancy. Infect Dis Clin North Am 1997; 11:119.

Schaefer G, Zervoudakis IA, Fuchs FF, et al. Pregnancy and pulmonary tuberculosis. Obstet Gynecol 1975; 46:706.

Smythe AR, Gallery GP Jr, Kraynack B. Assessment of severe pulmonary disease in pregnancy with Swan-Ganz monitoring. A report of two cases. J Reprod Med 1985; 30:133.

Snider D. Pregnancy and tuberculosis. Chest 1984; 86:10S.

Wilson EA, Thelin TJ, Dilts PV. Tuberculosis complicated by pregnancy. Am J Obstet Gynecol 1973; 115:526.

Management of Neonates Born to Tuberculous Mothers

Anttolainen I. Late prognosis of children born into tuberculous households. The effect of isolation and simultaneous BCG-vaccination. Acta Paediatr Scand 1972; 230:1.

Avery ME, Wolfsdorf J. Diagnosis and treatment: infants of tuberculous mothers. Pediatrics 1968; 43:519.

Committee on Drugs, American Academy of Pediatrics. Infants of tuberculous mothers: further thoughts. Pediatrics 1968; 42:393.

Curry FJ. Prophylactic effect on isoniazid in young tuberculin reactors. N Engl J Med 1967; 277:562.

Jacobs RF, Abernathy RS. Management of tuberculosis in pregnancy and the newborn. Clin Perinatol 1988; 15:305.

Kendig EL. The place of BCG vaccine in the management of infants born of tuberculous mothers. N Engl J Med 1970; 281:520.

Weinstein L, Murphy T. The management of tuberculosis during pregnancy. Clin Perinatol 1974; 1:395.

Congenital Tuberculosis

Amick FE, Alden MA, Sweet LK. Congenital tuberculosis. Pediatrics 1950; 6:384.

Arthur L. Congenital tuberculosis. Proc R Soc Med 1967; 60:15.

Asensi F, Otero MC, Perez-Tamarit D, et al. Congenital tuberculosis, still a problem (letter). Pediatr Infect Dis J 1990; 9:223.

Baumgartner W. Congenital TB. Monatsschrift fur Kinderheilkunde 1980; 128:563.

Beitzke H. Uber die angeborene tuberkulose infektion. Ergebn ges Tuberk Forsch 1935; 7:1.

Blackall PB. Tuberculosis: maternal infection of the newborn. Med J Aust 1969; 2.1055.

Corner BD, Brown NJ. Congenital tuberculosis: report of a case with necropsy findings in mother and child. Thorax 1955; 10:99.

Davin-Power M. Transplacental tuberculous infection. Br Med J 1941; 1:13.

Davis SF, Finley SC, Hare WK. Congenital tuberculosis. J Pediatr 1960; 57:221.

Debre R, Furiet-Láforet, Royer P. Tuberculose congenitale transplacentaire a forme icterique. Arch Fr Pediatr 1948; 5:225.

Dische MR. Congenital TB in a twin of immigrant parentage. Can Med Assoc J 1978; 119:1068.

Govan ADT. Tuberculous endometritis. J Pathol Bacteriol 1962; 83:363.

Hageman JR. Congenital and perinatal tuberculosis: discussion of difficult issues in diagnosis and management. J Perinatol 1998; 18:389.

Hamne B, Gellerstedt N. Zur kenntnis der kongnitalen tuberkulose. Acta Paediatr 1938; 20:380.

Harris EA, McCullough GC, Stone JJ, Brock WM. Congenital tuberculosis: review of disease with report of a case. J Pediatr 1948; 32:311.

Hertzog AJ, Chapman S, Herring J. Congenital pulmonary aspiration-tuberculosis: report of a case. Am J Clin Pathol 1949; 19:1139.

Horley JF. Congenital tuberculosis. Arch Dis Child 1952; 27:167.

Hudson FP. Clinical aspects of congenital tuberculosis. Arch Dis Child 1956; 31:136.

Hughesdon MR. Congenital tuberculosis. Arch Dis Child 1946; 21:121.

Imerslund O, Krohn J, Ringsted J. Congenital tuberculosis in premature twins. Acta Tuberc Scand 1962; 42:45.

Jones HS. Intrauterine tuberculosis as a complication of early pregnancy. Br J Clin Pract 1985; 39:39.

Jordan JW, Spencer H. A case of congenital tuberculosis. Br Med J 1949; 1:217.

Kaplan C, Benirschke K, Tarzy B. Placental tuberculosis in early and late pregnancy. Am J Obstet Gynecol 1981; 137:858.

Li CK, Chan YF, Har CM. Congenital tuberculosis. Aust Paediatr J 1989; 25:366.

Lowenstein E. Congenital tuberculosis. Am Rev Tuberc 1945; 51:225.

Mathur RP, Ramji S, Cherian S, et al. Congenital tuberculosis. Indian Pediatr 1987; 24:1144.

Mason N. Congenital tuberculosis after pleural effusion in the mother. Br Med J 1954; 1:970.

Miller KS, Miller JM Jr. Tuberculosis in pregnancy: interactions, diagnosis and management. Clin Obstet Gynecol 1996; 39:120.

Nemir RL, O'Hare D. Congenital tuberculosis. Review and diagnostic guidelines. Am J Dis Child 1985; 139:284.

Schaaf HS, Smith J, Donald PR, et al. Tuberculosis presenting in the neonatal period. Clin Pediatr 1989; 28:474.

Stansberry SD. Tuberculosis in infants and children. J Thorac Imaging 1990; 5:17.

Steinhoff MC, Lionel J. Treatment of tuberculosis in newborn infants and their mothers. Indian J Pediatr 1988; 55:240.

Wang JH, Chen WP, Soong WJ, et al. Congenital tuberculosis: a case report. Chung Hua I Hsueh Tsa Chih 1990; 45:266.

Therapy

Atkins JN. Maternal plasma concentration of pyridoxal phosphate during pregnancy: adequacy of vitamin B6 supplementation during isoniazid therapy. Am Rev Respir Dis 1982; 126:714–716.

American Thoracic Society/CDC. Treatment of tuberculosis and tuberculosis infection in adults and children. Am Rev Respir Dis 1986; 134:355.

American Thoracic Society/CDC. Diagnostic standards and classifications of tuberculosis. Am Rev Respir Dis 1990; 142:725.

Aziz S. Therapy in tuberculosis. J Pak Med Assoc 1985; 35:320.

Bothamley G. Drug treatment for tuberculosis during pregnancy: safety considerations. Drug-Saf 2001; 24:553.

Brost BC, Newman RB. The maternal and fetal effects of tuberculosis therapy. Obstet Gynecol 1997; 24:659.

CDC. The use of preventive therapy for tuberculous infection in the United States: recommendations of the Advisory Committee for Elimination of Tuberculosis. MMWR 1990; 39:9.

Lenke RR, Turkel SB, Monsen R. Severe fetal deformities associated with ingestion of excessive isoniazid in early pregnancy. Acta Obstet Gynecol Scand 1985; 64:281.

Powrie RO. Drugs in pregnancy: respiratory disease. Best Pract Res Clin Obstet Gynecol 2001; 15:913.

Snider DE Jr, Cohn DL, Davidson PT, et al. Standard therapy for tuberculosis 1985. Chest 1985; 87:117S.

Tuberculous Mastitis

Alagaratnam TT, Ong GB. Tuberculosis of the breast. Br J Surg 1980; 67:125.

Apps MCP, Harrison NK, Blauth CID. Tuberculosis of the breast. Br Med J 1984; 288:1875.

Bahadur P, Aurora AL, Sibbal RN, et al. Tuberculosis of mammary gland. J Indian Med Assoc 1983; 80:8–12.

Bonnet P, Fastrez J. Breast tuberculosis: apropos of a case. Acta Chir Belg 1987; 87:304.

Cooper AP. Introductory Observations on the Disease of the Breast. London: Longman, Rees, and Co, 1829:73.

Gong TQ. Tuberculosis of the breast. Ho Hu Hsi Tsa Chih 1989; 12:336.

McKeown KC, Wilkinson KW. Tuberculous disease of the breast. Br J Surg 1952; 157:420.

Morgen M. Tuberculosis of the breast. Surg Gynecol Obstet 1931; 53:593.

Mukerjee P, Cohen RV, Niden AH. Tuberculosis of the breast. Am Rev Respir Dis 1971; 104:661.

Symmers W St C. Tuberculosis of the breast. Br Med J 1984; 289:49.

Tuberculosis and HIV

CDC. Tuberculosis and human immunodeficiency virus infection: recommendations of the Advisory Committee for the Elimination of Tuberculosis. MMWR 1989; 38(17):236.

CDC. Purified protein derivative (PPD)-tuberculin anergy and HIV-infection: guidelines for anergy testing and management of anergic persons at risk for tuberculosis. MMWR 1991; 40(RR-5):27.

CDC. Tuberculosis outbreak among persons in a residential facility for HIV infected persons—San Francisco. MMWR 1991; 40:649.

Daley CL, Small PM, Schecter GF, et al. An outbreak of tuberculosis with accelerated progression among person infected with the human immunodeficiency virus. An analysis using restriction-fragment-length polymorphisms. N Engl J Med 1992; 326:231.

Di Perri G, Cruciani M, Danzi MC, et al. Nosocomial epidemic of active tuberculosis among HIV-infected patients. Lancet 1989; 2:1502.

USPHS/IDSA. 1999 USPHS/IDSA guidlines for the prevention of opportunistic infections with human immunodeficiency virus. U.S. Public Health Service (UPHS) and Infectious Disease Society of America (IDSA). Infect Dis Obstet Gynecol 2000; 8:5.

Thillagavathie P. Current issues in maternal and perinatal tuberculosis: impact of the HIV-1 epidemic. Semin Neonatol 2000; 5:189.

Multidrug-Resistant Tuberculosis

CDC. Nosocomial transmission of multidrug-resistant tuberculosis to health-care workers and HIV infected patients in an urban hospital—Florida. MMWR 1990; 39(40):718.

CDC. Nosocomial transmission of multidrug-resistant tuberculosis among HIV-infected persons—Florida and New York, 1988–1991. MMWR 1991; 40(34):585.

CDC. National action plan to combat multidrug-resistant tuberculosis. MMWR 1992; 41(RR-11):5–48.

Advisory Committee for the Elimination of Tuberculosis. A strategic plan for the elimination of tuberculosis in the United States. MMWR 1989; 138(Suppl. No. S3):1–25.

American Thoracic Society/CDC. Treatment of tuberculosis and tuberculosis infection in adults and children. Am Rev Respir Dis 1986; 134:355.

American Thoracic Society/CDC. Diagnostic standards and classification of tuberculosis. Am Rev Respir Dis 1990; 142:725.

CDC. The use of preventive therapy for tuberculous infection in the United States: recommendations of the Advisory Committee for Elimination of Tuberculosis. MMWR 1990; 39(RR-8):9.

CDC. Targeted tuberculin testing and treatment of latent tuberculosis. MMWR 2000; 49/No. RR-6:1.

Comstock GW, Livesay VT, Woolpert SF. The prognosis of a positive tuberculin reaction in childhood and adolescence. Am J Epidemiol 1974; 99:131.

Rieder HL, Cauthen GM, Comstock GW, Snider DE Jr. Epidemiology of tuberculosis in the United States. Epidemiol Rev 1989; 11:79.

Snider DE Jr, Roper WL. The new tuberculosis. N Engl J Med 1992; 326:703.

INTRODUCTION

Chorioamnionitis is more than an inflammatory reaction of the placental tissues in response to organism invasion. In its clinical form, it is a threat to the maternal–fetal unit. The incidence of chorioamnionitis varies between 0.8 and 1.25 per 100 live births. A linear relationship between dissolution of fetal membranes and time selects for the presence of bacteria in amniotic fluid (infection) but not necessarily for disease in a cumulative pattern. The development of chorioamnionitis is not a simple corollary of prolonged rupture of the fetal membranes (PROM).

PATHOGENESIS

The fetal membranes, in conjunction with the cervical plug of pregnancy, constitute a formidable barrier to ascending infection. Nothing more than the extreme rarity of acute gonococcal endometritis/salpingitis disease after the eighth week of gestation despite a 5% to 6% incidence of subclinical gonococcal cervical infection is needed to document the effectiveness of this anatomical–physiological barrier in excluding vaginal commensal and pathogenic bacteria from the privileged sanctuary of the fetus. Once the fetal membranes are ruptured, the potential for ascending infection is great.

Approximately 7% to 12% of gravidas experience prolonged or premature dissolution of the fetal membranes. Of these, approximately 10% to 12% will develop chorioamnionitis. Ninety-six percent of the cases of chorioamnionitis are due to ascending infection.

Hematogenous dissemination to the products of conception as a consequence of extragenital maternal septicemia accounts for 4% of the cases. The bacteria that can induce chorioamnionitis as a consequence of hematogenous dissemination include *Listeria monocytogenes*, *Haemophilus influenzae*, *Streptococcus pneumoniae*, *Salmonella typhi*, and the group A streptococci.

What is not that well appreciated is that with effective labor, the mucous plug of pregnancy is lost. Even though the fetal membranes are intact, selected bacteria including the group B streptococci can infect the amniotic compartment.

Perinatal sepsis as opposed to intra-amniotic fluid infection is predominantly due to aerobic bacteria with augmented virulence that attain fetal/neonatal access as a consequence of ascending infection or of delivery through an infected birth canal. Perinatal sepsis occurs in 1% of neonates whose mothers' membranes are ruptured for more than 24 hours.

With the onset of labor and frank rupture of the fetal membranes, access to the fetus is simplified. The incidence of amniotic fluid infection is almost a direct function of time. When the fetal membranes have been ruptured for 24 hours, cultures of the amniotic fluid taken by the transabdominal route are positive in more than 65% of patients.

Infection of the amniotic fluid does not correlate closely with the successful establishment of infection in the fetus and perinatal sepsis. Amniotic fluid per se constitutes a preferential aerobic microbiological environment. Since exogenous pathogenic bacteria of humans function primarily as aerobes, it is not surprising that there is a reasonable correlation between their presence in amniotic fluid and ensuing disease.

The presence of replicating organisms in amniotic fluid translates itself into neonatal infection in one of two ways:

1. The bacteria are able to multiply sufficiently within the intra-alveolar spaces of the fetal lung so as to overwhelm the host defense mechanisms constituted by the alveolar-lining cells. Being part of the reticuloendothelial system, the alveolar-lining cells relegate this pathway to one of secondary importance.
2. The major pathway for fetal invasion involves direct penetration of the placenta. Once within the chorion, the bacteria gain potential access to fetal vessels. Fetal septicemia is due to arterial vasculitis. If the infection is prolonged, involvement of all three vessels can be demonstrated.

As long as infection is limited to bacterial replication within the amniotic fluid, evidence of maternal involvement is limited. With involvement and penetration into placental arteries and/or the maternal implantation site, bacterial products such as endotoxins, as well as endopyrogens released from lymphocytes and neutrophils, may attain access to the fetal and maternal vascular compartments, respectively (Figs. 1 and 2). At this stage, maternal pyrexia, as well as fetal compromise (reflected primarily by abnormal heart rate changes), may occur. With the progression of the disease process, the fever often rises sharply. Rigors are indicative of significant bacterial penetration into large maternal vascular channels.

MATERNAL INFECTIOUS MORBIDITY

Endometritis and Endomyometritis

The factors that have a positive correlation with an increased incidence of uterine bacterial disease in patients undergoing cesarean section are the following:

1. Presence of selected class II–III anaerobes in amniotic fluid, such as peptostreptococci and/or Bacteroidaceae (particularly in the presence of fresh meconium)
2. Presence of exogenous pathogens such as *Neisseria gonorrhoeae*
3. Presence of endogenous bacteria with enhanced virulence, such as epithelial cell-adherent *Escherichia coli*
4. Absence of intrapartum antibiotic therapy

Patients with clinically overt anaerobic chorioamnionitis who deliver vaginally rarely develop endometritis; however, if the route of delivery is altered, even with prophylactic administration of cephalosporin, a significant incidence of

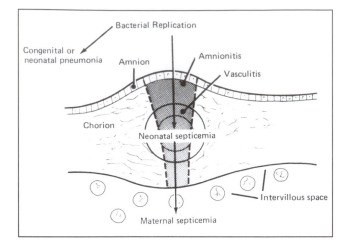

FIGURE 1 Potential infectious consequences of bacterial replication within the amniotic fluid. *Source*: Blanc WA. J Pediatr 1961;59:473.

endomyometritis occurs. Of women who develop chorioamnionitis and receive antibiotic therapy prior to cesarean section, approximately 15% to 30% of economically disadvantaged gravidas develop postpartum endomyometritis in contrast to 60% to 75% who did not receive antibiotics.

Maternal Septicemia

Once significant penetration of the maternal vascular compartment is achieved, the circumstances are almost analogous to an individual's receiving an IV infusion of bacteria owing to
1. inability of the site of penetration to be thrombosed and
2. relatively unlimited substrate represented by the placenta.
Maternal septicemia is an indication for removal of the major nidus of bacterial replication. Therapy is directed at
1. precluding metastatic bacterial complications (e.g., acute bacterial endocarditis) and
2. uncoupling or eradicating the site of bacterial replication to avoid late sequelae such as intravascular coagulopathy and possible adult respiratory distress syndrome.
Analyses of maternal deaths associated with chorioamnionitis reveal two constants:
1. The majority of etiological agents isolated are members of the Enterobacteriaceae.
2. Most, if not all, of the deaths cited in the literature could have been prevented.
The three principal mechanisms for maternal demise in gravidas with chorioamnionitis are
1. septic shock due to the Enterobacteriaceae,
2. *Clostridium* septicemia, and
3. postpartum endomyometritis with septic thrombophlebitis.
In the context of modern day therapeutics, the maternal sequelae of chorioamnionitis are relatively limited. In a prospective study of 251 patients with premature rupture of the fetal membranes between 28 and 34 weeks of gestation, Garite and Freeman (1982) found that while 47 (19%) of the gravidas developed chorioamnionitis, no serious maternal sequelae were observed. Overall the

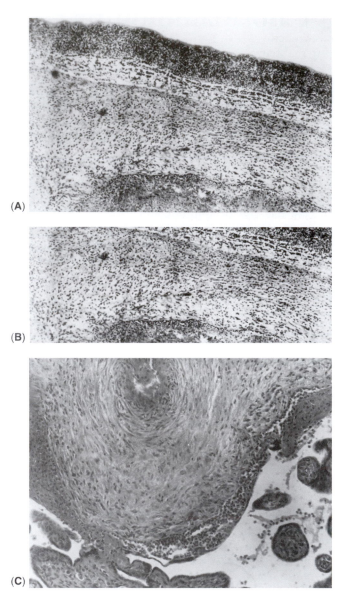

FIGURE 2 Histopathologic changes in chorioamnionitis. (**A**) Destruction of the amnion and an extensive acute inflammatory infiltrate invading the chorion, with transural penetration of the large vascular channels at the lower limits of the photomicrograph (×320). (**B**) Extension of the inflammatory process beyond the interstitium and the cytotrophoblastic layer, resulting in fibrin deposition within the maternal vascular compartment (*arrow*) (×520). (**C**) Large photomicrograph, from which **A** and **B** are taken, is stained with H&E (×65).

incidence of severe complications for the mother with chorioamnionitis has markedly decreased in recent years.

FETAL CONSIDERATIONS

Hyperthermia

Chorioamnionitis is a threat to the fetus by virtue of
1. potential deleterious effects of hyperthermia on the fetal central nervous system and
2. induction of septicemia/pneumonia/meningitis by bacteria of enhanced virulence.

The fetus is in a positive heat-exchange situation with the mother across the maternal implementation site. When the maternal temperature is significantly raised and maternal hyperthermia sustained for any significant period of time, the gradient between fetal core temperature and maternal temperature increases. This increasing disparity between the two temperatures results ultimately in a central nervous system demise of the fetus. A critical point of clinical management is maintenance of a maternal temperature below 38.6°C.

Perinatal Septicemia

Retrospective analyses of 79 perinatal septicemia cases from the Shands Teaching Hospital (Gainesville, FL), University Hospital (Jacksonville, FL), and Saint Joseph's Hospital (Omaha, NE) demonstrate that 21% of neonates with documented septicemia in the first 24 hours of life were born to gravidas with chorioamnionitis and 53% were born to gravidas with PROM. When perinatal septicemia occurs, the bacteria are usually class I aerobic, endogenous organisms, *E. coli*, or the group B streptococci. Exogenous bacteria less frequently associated with perinatal septicemia include *L. monocytogenes*, *H. nfluenzae*, *H. parainfluenzae*, *S. pneumoniae*, group A streptococci, and selected enteric pathogens (e.g., *S. typhi*, *Shigella*).

Fetal morbidity and/or mortality are related not primarily to the causative agent but more directly to

1. the interim between the onset of disease and the institution of appropriate antibiotic therapy and
2. the gestational age of the fetus.

The ensuing morbidity and/or mortality is greater than 50% if therapy is not instituted within three hours of the onset of disease.

Perinatal septicemia due to peptostreptococci and Bacteroidaceae is a rare event and is usually of limited biological significance for the fetus.

In the absence of maternal antibiotic therapy for chorioamnionitis, the anticipated incidence of perinatal septicemia is 19% to 26%. If effective maternal therapy has been instituted for three hours or more prior to delivery, the incidence of perinatal septicemia is markedly reduced (Table 1). When a case of perinatal septicemia occurs despite maternal therapy, it is due to a bacterial strain resistant to the antibiotic regimen used.

DIAGNOSIS

Terminology

In 1980, the term *intra-amniotic fluid infection* was introduced to describe clinically overt maternal–fetal infection.

TABLE 1 Impact of intrapartum maternal antibiotic therapy on perinatal septicemia in patients with chorioamnionitis

	Intrapartum maternal antibiotic therapy	No intrapartum maternal antibiotic therapy
Percentage with perinatal or neonatal septicemia[a]	≥0–2.8%	≥5.7–21%

[a]Collective series of Gibbs et al., Gilstrap et al., Monif et al., and Sperling et al. (total number of cases 425).

Since 1991, the term *intra-amniotic infection* has become interchangeable with clinical amnionitis and clinical chorioamnionitis. These terms, *intra-amniotic fluid infection*, *clinical amnionitis*, and *chorioamnionitis*, are not totally identical clinical entities.

The criteria selected by the San Antonio group for designation of intra-amniotic infection were maternal fever (100.4°F or higher) and rupture of the membranes, plus two or more of the following:

1. Maternal tachycardia
2. Uterine tenderness
3. Purulent, foul-smelling amniotic fluid
4. Fetal tachycardia
5. Maternal leukocytosis

Dorland's Illustrated Medical Dictionary defines infection as a term "most often used to denote the presence of microorganisms within the tissues whether or not they result in detectable pathologic effects." Disease is defined as "a definite morbid process having a characteristic train of symptoms." Chorioamnionitis encompasses intra-amniotic fluid and clinical amnionitis, but intra-amniotic fluid infection is not necessarily chorioamnionitis. Only a minority of cases of intra-amniotic fluid infection progress to chorioamnionitis.

The secondary criteria advocated for the diagnosis of intramniotic infection are expansive and tend to overlap with other disease entities. Case studies using these criteria or components thereof allowed for inclusion of cases whose pathogenesis and ultimate clinical significance diverge significantly. Maternal tachycardia in a gravida with fever, and rupture of the fetal membranes do not equate with clinical chorioamnionitis with a ±1 SD probability.

Clinically overt intra-amniotic fluid infection in the form of anaerobic amnionitis may not have the same maternal and fetal clinical consequences as are observed in cases of chorioamnionitis due to primary class I bacteria. A significant number of infants with anaerobic amnionitis (foul-smelling baby syndrome) are born to gravidas with no systemic manifestations of infectious process. Only a rare neonate in this category ever develops perinatal septicemia, which, when it does occur, is usually of limited biological significance.

Another major problem with the current definition of chorioamnionitis is the prerequisite of rupture of the membranes for the diagnosis. This precludes inclusion of those cases of chorioamnionitis due to *L. monocytogenes*, *H. influenzae*, and *S. pneumoniae*, among others, which occur with intact fetal membranes secondary to hematogenous dissemination from the gravida to the products of conception. Approximately 4% of instances of chorioamnionitis with documented perinatal septicemia are due to these bacteria. Clinical recognition of this subgroup is critical since appropriate antimicrobial therapy can avert an adverse outcome.

In terms of histopathology, the term *chorioamnionitis* defines a demonstrable inflammatory process involving the chorion and amnion of the placenta. In terms of clinical utilization, the term denotes a disease, usually of bacterial etiology, involving the maternal–fetal unit. The clinician is not well served by any significant fusion of these two definitions.

Patients with clinically overt chorioamnionitis almost invariably have a demonstrable inflammatory process within the placenta and membranes. The converse is not necessary or even frequently true. Gravidas who subsequently are demonstrated to have histological evidence of inflammation within the placenta are more often asymptomatic. To avoid confusion, the qualifying adjectives, *histopathological* and *clinical*, should be used to maintain conceptual integrity.

Infection Versus Disease

As long as the fetal membranes are intact and the gravida is not in labor, barring hematogenous involvement, cultures of amniotic fluid do not demonstrate the presence of either aerobic or anaerobic bacteria. With effective labor, despite the presence of intact fetal membranes, bacteria, particularly anaerobic bacteria and the group B streptococci, may gain access to amniotic fluid. Once the fetal membranes are grossly disrupted, the probability of recovering bacteria from amniotic fluid increases almost linearly with time. After 24 hours, one or more bacteria can be recovered from the majority of amniotic fluids obtained by amniocentesis.

Maternal Pyrexia

Although the de novo development of fever in a gravida with ruptured membranes can have a large number of other etiological causes, chorioamnionitis must be the priority diagnosis of exclusion. In chorioamnionitis, maternal pyrexia is a host response to bacterial pyrogens that have reached the maternal intravascular compartment.

Maternal Leukocytosis

The white blood cell count (WBC) tends to be more elevated in the pregnant female than in nonpregnant matched controls at pre- or postpregnancy level. A single elevated WBC is of little diagnostic significance. If serial WBCs are used to monitor a patient with PROM or premature rupture of the fetal membranes, by the time a significant increase in the WBC is demonstrable, other clinical signs indicative of chorioamnionitis (i.e., maternal pyrexia, sustained fetal tachycardia, and/or uterine tenderness) are usually present. A marked increase in the maternal WBC usually indicates that bacteria have attained significant access to a maternal vascular site.

Bacteria in Amniotic Fluid

The presence of bacteria in amniotic fluid documents infection but not necessarily disease. The great majority of cases in which bacteria are recovered from amniotic fluid are from gravidas with no clinical evidence of disease. The number of bacteria present in amniotic fluid is not a good predictor of the probability of ensuing chorioamnionitis. If $\geq 10^4$ cfu of bacteria per milliliter of amniotic fluid is present, it has been contended that these gravidas are more likely to develop chorioamnionitis. Current data indicate that the virulence of the organism, rather than its quantitative presence at a given point in time, is the principal factor selecting for disease.

Presence of White Blood Cells in Amniotic Fluid

Intially the presence of white blood cells in amniotic fluid correlated with the subsequent development of chorioamnionitis. Subsequent studies by Bobbitt and Ledger (1978) have largely put this concept to rest. The numerical scatter in their data is consistent with the concept that infection of the amnion is not uncommon. Infection as well as disease produces an inflammatory response of varying intensity.

Histological Evidence of Chorioamnionitis

There is at best a poor correlation between histological evidence of inflammatory changes involving the amnion, chorion, and/or umbilical cord and clinical disease. Histological evidence of inflammation involving one or more placental components is not uncommon in patients with PROM. False negatives may occur in the histological confirmation of disease.

Chorioamnionitis is a focal disease. Histological analyses of most placental tissue are often limited to a single section of the placenta (often randomly selected) and of the umbilical cord.

Foul-Smelling Amniotic Fluid

The presence of foul-smelling amniotic fluid does not necessarily indicate the presence of chorioamnionitis. What it does indicate is the replication of greater than 10^5 cfu of bacteria per milliliter of amniotic fluid due to polymicrobial bacterial flora in which anaerobic bacteria are dominant. Amniotic fluid is predominantly an aerobic microbiological environment. The presence of anaerobic bacteria in amniotic fluid has more clinical significance in terms of possible postpartum endomyometritis for the mother than in terms of neonatal or maternal septicemia.

Fresh Meconium in Amniotic Fluid

The presence of fresh meconium is a signal of fetal distress and not necessarily of chorioamnionitis. Fetal distress may be the result of chorioamnionitis.

Specific Signs

There are only two signs of chorioamnionitis that, by focusing directly on the maternal–fetal unit, increase the probability of an accurate diagnosis:
1. Uterine tenderness
2. Persistent fetal tachycardia

Uterine Tenderness

Uterine tenderness can be easily confused with uterine irritability and resultant contractions, hence the need for serial observation and early confirmation by a skilled examiner.

Persistent Fetal Tachycardia

Persistent fetal tachycardia is the one criterion almost universally accepted. A point of contention has been what constitutes fetal tachycardia. Fetal tachycardia is defined as a fetal heart rate of 160 beats per minute for five minutes in the absence of maternal medications and maternal pyrexia greater than 38.6°C.

The criteria for the diagnosis of chorioamnionitis are the presence of *two* of the following *three* clinical signs of disease:

1. Maternal pyrexia (nonspecific): a confirmed temperature of greater than 37.8°C
2. Uterine tenderness (specific)
3. Persistent fetal tachycardia (specific): a fetal heart rate greater than or equal to 160 beats per minute for five minutes.

The assessment of all clinical criteria is readily attainable and requires no additional expenditure of healthcare dollars. This potentially can be done under relatively primitive conditions outside of large medical centers.

Cultures

The urinary tract, endocervix, and amniotic fluid should be sampled for the identification of a possible etiological agent. Bacteria that successfully adhere to uroepithelial cells and are present in greater than or equal to 10^5 cfu/mg of urine are bacteria of enhanced virulence and must be effectively covered by the antibiotic regimen selected. Sexually transmitted disease pathogens need to be effectively excluded from diagnostic consideration. To do so, the endocervix must be appropriately sampled for viable organisms or their antigenic equivalents. Unless the amniotic fluid is foul smelling, only aerobic cultures are required. Despite the presence of fever, blood cultures are of limited value.

Locksmith and Duff (1994) reviewed the records of 539 patients with chorioamnionitis who delivered over a three-year period. Thirty-nine of 538 patients (7.2%) had positive blood cultures. In only one of the patients did the blood culture result definitively alter therapy. This patient had a fever of unknown origin, and the blood culture led ultimately to the diagnosis of chorioamnionitis. The mean duration of febrile morbidity was not significantly different in the bacteremic versus nonbacteremic patients, 2.03 versus 1.74 days. None of the repeat blood cultures were positive. The cost of blood cultures in this study population was US$72,759.

THERAPY

Chorioamnionitis is a mandate for maternal and fetal therapy. The antibiotic selected must

1. be broad enough to encompass the aerobic pathogenic spectrum delineated and
2. adequately address the issue of bioavailability to the fetus (be able to traverse the placental barrier in therapeutic concentrations).

The drug of choice for fetal therapy is ampicillin or piperacillin. The reasons for the selection of an aminopenicillin (ampicillin) or a ureidopenicillin (mezlocillin or piperacillin) as the drug of choice are safety for the fetus, bioavailability, and spectrum of efficacy.

Ampicillin lacks coverage for selected Enterobacteriaceae (*Klebsiella pneumoniae*, 20–30% of *E. coli*, *Serratia*, and *Enterobacter* species) and the penicillin-resistant *Bacteroidaceae/ Prevotella* species. Mezlocillin and piperacillin are potentially therapeutic for only 40% to 50% of the strains of *K. pneumoniae* and *Klebsiella* species.

If foul-smelling amniotic fluid is present, an intravenous bolus of metronidazole may be utilized for coverage of the Bacteroidaceae/*Prevotella* species. The relative inability of clindamycin to effectively traverse the placental barrier limits its theoretical efficacy. Although chloramphenicol readily crosses the placental barrier, the inability of the neonate to detoxify the drug with the ensuing clinical corollary, "gray baby syndrome," absolutely contraindicates its administration.

Monoetiological chorioamnionitis due to either hematogenous or ascending infection can be cured in utero. The major problem with fetal therapy is the inability to cover the entire pathogenic spectrum, particularly of the Enterobacteriaceae. Selected third-generation cephalosporins have the ability of attaining therapeutic levels in cord blood and amniotic fluid. These antibiotics may become incorporated into fetal therapy owing to their augmented coverage of the Enterobacteriaceae; however, they lack efficacy for *L. monocytogenes*.

A drug of inclusion for maternal therapy is aminoglycoside. In the majority of gravidas with chorioamnionitis who developed septic shock, an Enterobacteriaceae, usually *E. coli* or *K. pneumoniae*, functioned as the principal causative agent.

The key to therapy is early recognition of chorioamnionitis and the early institution of therapy. The later clinical intervention occurs, the greater the potential for augmented morbidity and possible neonatal and/or maternal demise.

One of the major questions that has yet not been adequately addressed is that of whether or not there is such a thing as in utero therapy. Hematogenously acquired chorioamnionitis due to *L. monocytogenes* has been successfully treated in utero. With premature rupture of the membranes, one has open access to a diverging bacterial flora. Monif (1983) has described a patient with premature rupture of the membranes, recurrent chorioamnionitis, and maternal septicemia due to group G streptococci whose initial episode occurred at 22 weeks. Because of the excellent maternal and fetal response and the inability to abort the fetus, the adoption of a conservative management program was forced. The patient continued to leak amniotic fluid and returned at 29 weeks with renewed evidence of chorioamnionitis and of septicemia due to *E. coli* and *K. pneumoniae*. *E. coli* was also grown from amniotic fluid, placenta, and urine. Because of the inability to reverse fetal signs of chorioamnionitis with antibiotic therapy, the baby was delivered vaginally. The resultant 1090-gram infant survived a stormy neonatal course and, at one year of age, was clinically normal with the exception of oxygen-induced retinopathy.

MONITORING OF PROM FOR INFECTIOUS COMPLICATIONS

One must presume that the majority of gravidas with documented rupture of the fetal membranes greater than 12 hours and a significant number of gravidas who have labored extensively have bacteria present within the amniotic fluid. One must exclude bacteria of enhanced virulence in order to focus tightly on the optimal perinatal plan

for both mother and fetus. Management of these patients involves excluding the presence of the following bacteria:
1. Urinary tract pathogens
2. Groups A, B, C, and G beta-hemolytic streptococci
3. *N. gonorrhoeae*

Bacteriological Screening
Urinary Tract Bacterial Isolates
Any gravida with any of the conditions listed below should have a screening nitrite test and leukocyte esterase analysis, as well as a urine culture done immediately upon admission:
1. Prior documented asymptomatic bacteriuria in pregnancy
2. A history of prior urinary tract infections in pregnancy
3. Frequent urinary tract infections in the pre- and/or postadolescent years
4. No prenatal care

If the nitrite test is positive, the test should be repeated. If again positive, we advocate placing the patient on a third-generation cephalosporin that has Food and Drug Administration approval for gram-negative meningitis. If the nitrite test is negative, but the culture is positive, the choice of antibiotics is predicated upon Gram staining of the urinary sediment. If a gram-positive isolate is identified, ampicillin is administered in lieu of the third-generation cephalosporin.

Beta-hemolytic Streptococci
Gravidas with ruptured fetal membranes and any of the conditions listed below need to be presumed to be infected and managed in accordance with group B *Streptococcus* (GBS) neonatal disease avoidance programs:
1. A beta-hemolytic *Streptococcus* previously isolated
2. Prior neonatal disease or demise due to the GBS
3. An immature or premature gestation
4. An unfavorable cervix
5. No prenatal care

N. gonorrhoeae
At the time of admission to labor and delivery, if the physician is dealing with a term gestation, a more conservative approach can be initiated. If a test is positive for *N. gonorrhoeae*, the mother should receive a cost-effective third-generation drug that is resistant to plasmid-mediated beta-lactamases and capable of traversing th blood–brain and presumably the placental barrier. Although one dose is probably sufficient to eradicate maternal colonization, potential problems in terms of drug bioavailability in therapeutic concentrations within amniotic fluid argues for more than one dose.

Biochemical Testing
The only laboratory value that has been of any assistance in identifying possible disease in evolution has been the C-reactive protein (CRP). The negative predictive value of CRP determination is greater than the positive predictive value. Once the CRP value becomes positive before delivery in a patient with PROM, the test is of limited added value. If chorioamnionitis does develop and a commitment to in utero therapy is made in case of an immature-premature infant, serial CRP determinations again become of value in guiding the duration of therapy. It is our policy to continue antibiotic therapy 24 hours beyond a negative titer.

Once the cultures are obtained under sterile conditions, no further pelvic examination is to be done unless umbilical cord prolapse is suspected.

Presuming that all baseline cultures are negative, we advocate establishing a monitoring regimen that includes temperature, fetal biophysical profile, fetal heart rate, assessment of uterine tenderness, and CRP. These parameters dictate the subsequent clinical management.

Clinical Monitoring
Superimposed upon bacteriological monitoring and/or prophylactic antibiotic administration is careful clinical monitoring.

The patient should be monitored closely every one to four hours for one or more clinical signs of disease:
1. Maternal pyrexia (nonspecific): a confirmed temperature of greater than 37.8°C
2. Uterine tenderness (specific)
3. Persistent fetal tachycardia (specific): a fetal heart rate greater than or equal to 160 beats per minute for five minutes

If one of the above criteria becomes abnormal, the interim of monitoring for all parameters is cut in half or preferably to an hourly occurrence. The appearance of a second abnormal parameter constitutes the basis for the diagnosis of chorioamnionitis.

If the patient has a favorable Bishop score and a viable fetus, delivery by the vaginal route can be attempted. A general rule of thumb is "don't get a failed delivery with induction in a sick baby." Guidelines favoring the prompt termination of pregnancy include
1. a nonresponsive stress test and a positive oxytocin challenge test,
2. fetal bradycardia,
3. fresh appearance of meconium with any concomitant evidence of fetal compromise,
4. evidence of maternal decompensation or worsening of maternal disease, or
5. increasing maternal pyrexia despite antibiotic therapy of 120 minutes duration.

Gravidas with premature rupture of the fetal membranes and PROM who develop chorioamnionitis while under clinical monitoring and who are clinically stable with an immature fetus that is greater than 22 weeks may be candidates for what has been termed an "antibiotic therapeutic challenge."

Aggressive therapy with a ureidopenicillin and an aminoglycoside is instituted. If there is total lysis of fever and documented resolution of all other abnormal parameters within three to four hours of the initiation of antibiotic therapy, subsequent management of the mother and fetus is as if chorioamnionitis had never occurred. Failure of any of the maternal or fetal clinical criteria to respond to antibiotic therapy within four hours, particularly failure of fetal tachycardia to abate or the appearance of variable decelerations with a nonresponsive stress test, argues for prompt termination of pregnancy. This approach is controversial and requires maternal acceptance of the potential grave risks involved including death.

Prevention

Prophylactic use of antibiotic therapy to prevent chorioamnionitis and perinatal septicemia has gained broader acceptance. The criteria developed for GBS early-onset disease prevention have broader applicability. The following settings identify gravidas at risk for more than perinatal GBS sepsis:

1. Preterm rupture of fetal membranes
2. PROM 12 to 18 hours
3. Gravidas with ruptured membranes who have had recurrent asymptomatic bacteriuria or urinary tract infections

SELECTED READING

Premature Rupture of the Membranes

Bobbitt JR, Ledger WJ. Amniotic fluid analysis. Its role in maternal—neonatal infection. Obstet Gynecol 1978; 51:56.

Chaisilwattana P, Monif GRG. Potential use of C-reactive protein determinations in obstetrics and gynecology. Obstet Gynecol Survey 1989; 44:355.

Creatsas G, Pavlatos M, Lolis D, et al. Bacterial contamination of the cervix and premature rupture of the membranes. Am J Obstet Gynecol 1981; 39:522.

Drife JO. Preterm rupture of the membranes. Br Med J Clin Res 1982; 28:583.

Eisenberg E, Krauss AN. Premature rupture of the membranes (PROM): a neonatal approach. Pediatr Ann 1983; 12:110.

Evaldson GR, Malmborg AS, Nord CE. Premature rupture of the membranes and ascending infection. Br J Obstet Gynaecol 1982; 89:793.

Evans MI, Hajj SN, Devide LD, et al. C-reactive protein as a predictor of infectious morbidity with premature rupture of membranes. Am J Obstet Gynecol 1980; 15:648.

Fayez JA, Hasan AA, Jonas HS, Miller GL. Management of PROM. Obstet Gynecol 1978; 52:17.

Garite TJ. Premature rupture of the membranes: the enigma of the obstetrician. Am J Obstet Gynecol 1985; 151:1001.

Garite TJ, Freeman RK, Linzey EM, Braly P. The use of amniocentesis in patients with PROM. Obstet Gynecol 1979; 54:226.

Gibbs RS, Blanco JD, St Clair PJ, Castaneda YS. Quantitative bacteriology of amniotic fluid from women with clinical intra-amniotic infection at term. J Infect Dis 1982; 45:1.

Graham RL, Gilstrap LC, Hauth JC, et al. Conservative management of patients with premature rupture of fetal membranes. Obstet Gynecol 1982; 59:607.

Jagtap PM, Hardas UD. Pathogenic bacteria and premature membrane rupture. Ind J Pathol 1981; 24:267.

Johnson JW, Daikoku NH, Niebyl JR, et al. Premature rupture of the membranes and prolonged latency. Obstet Gynecol 1981; 57:547.

Kurki T, Teramo K, Ylikorkala O, Paavonen J. C-reactive protein in preterm premature rupture of the membranes. Arch Gynecol Obstet 1990; 247:31.

Ledger WJ. Amniocentesis and premature labor. Obstet Gynecol 1981; 58:760.

Newton ER, Prihoda TJ, Gibbs RS. Logistic regression analysis of risk factors for intra-amniotic infection. Obstet Gynecol 1989; 73:571.

Romero R, Scioscia AL, Edberg SC, Hobbins JC. Use of parenteral antibiotic therapy to eradicate bacterial colonization of amniotic fluid in premature rupture of membranes. Obstet Gynecol 1986; 67:15.

Taylor J, Garite TJ. Premature rupture of membranes before fetal viability. Obstet Gynecol 1984; 64:615.

Vintzileos AM, Campbell WA, Nochimson DJ, et al. The fetal biophysical profile in patients with premature rupture of the membranes—an early predictor of fetal infection. Am J Obstet Gynecol 1985; 152:510.

Chorioamnionitis

Arias JW, Saldana LR, Conklin R. Chorioamnionitis due to *Haemophilus parainfluenzae*. Tex Med J 1981; 77:47.

Evaldson GR, Malmborg AS, Nord CE. Premature rupture of the membranes and ascending infection. Br J Obstet Gynaecol 1982; 89:793.

Garite TJ, Freeman RK. Chorioamnionitis in the preterm gestation. Obstet Gynecol 1982; 59:539.

Gibbs RS, Duff P. Progress in pathogenesis and management of clinical intraamniotic infection. Am J Obstet Gynecol 1991; 164:1317.

Gibbs RS, Dinsmoor MJ, Newton ER, Ramamurthy RS. A randomized trial of intrapartum versus immediate postpartum treatment of women with intra-amniotic fluid infection. Obstet Gynecol 1988; 72:823.

Guzick DS, Winn K. The association of chorioamnionitis with preterm delivery. Obstet Gynecol 1985; 65:11.

Kappy KA, Cetrulo CL, Knuppel RA, et al. The changing perinatal and maternal outcome in chorioamnionitis. Obstet Gynecol 1979; 53:731.

Locksmith GJ, Duff P. Assessment of the value of routine blood cultures in the evaluation and treatment of patients with chorioamnionitis. Infect Dis Obstet Gynecol 1994; 2:111.

Lorenz RP, Appelbaum PC, Ward RM, Botti JJ. Chorioamnionitis and possible neonatal infection associated with *Lactobacillus* species. J Clin Microbiol 1982; 16:558.

Monif GRG. Recurrent chorioamnionitis and maternal septicemia. Obstet Gynecol 1983; 146:334.

Petrilli ES, D'Ablaing G, Ledger WJ. *Listeria monocytogenes* chorioamnionitis: diagnosis by transabdominal amniocentesis. Obstet Gynecol 1980; 55:55.

Soper DE, Mayhall CG, Dalton HP. Risk factors for intraamniotic infection: a prospective epidemiologic study. Am J Obstet Gynecol 1989; 161:562.

Sperling RS, Ramamurthy RS, Gibbs RS. A comparison of intrapartum versus immediate postpartum treatment of intra-amniotic infection. Obstet Gynecol 1987; 70:861.

Yoder PR, Gibbs RS, Blanco JD, et al. A prospective, controlled study of maternal and perinatal outcome after intra-amniotic infection at term. Am J Obstet Gynecol 1983; 145:695.

Perinatal Septicemia

Chow AW, Leake RD, Yamauchi T, et al. The significance of anaerobes in neonatal bacteremia. Analysis of 23 cases and review of the literature. Pediatrics 1974; 54:736.

Keffer GL, Monif GRG. Perinatal septicemia due to the *Bacteroidaceae*. Obstet Gynecol 1988; 71:463.

Monif GRG. Maternal risk factors for perinatal septicemia due to the *Enterobacteriaceae*. Am J Perinatol 2000; 17:19.

Monif GRG. Prevention of perinatal septicema. In: Faro, Gibbs, and Mead. Protocols for Infectious Diseases, 2nd ed. Malden, MA: Blackwell Science, 2000.

Monif GRG, Hume R Jr, Goodlin RC. Neonatal considerations in the management of premature rupture of the fetal membranes. Obstet Gynecol Surv 1986; 41:531.

Robinson EN Jr. Pneumococcal endometritis and neonatal sepsis. Rev Infect Dis 1990; 12:799.

Rusin P, Adam RD, Peterson EA, Ryan KJ, et al. *Haemophilus influenzae*: an important cause of maternal and neonatal infections. Obstet Gynecol 1991; 77:92.

61

Infectious Morbidity Associated with Intrauterine Monitoring and Invasive Prenatal Diagnostic Procedures

INTRAUTERINE MONITORING

Intrapartum fetal monitoring has become a standard procedure for the evaluation of fetal well being during labor. The passage of a mechanical conduit through a nonsterile area and the application of a scalp electrode to the fetal head introduce the potential for augmented fetal infectious morbidity. There is no statistically significant increase in the maternal infectious morbidity. The risks to the mother are basically those inherent in the situation, for example, premature rupture of the fetal membranes and labor or the presence of *Neisseria gonorrhoeae* or group A streptococci as part of the vaginal flora. The combination of rupture of the membranes and labor, aside from the presence of exogenous pathogens in the vaginal flora, is the major risk factor for both the frequency and the severity of maternal infection. Once the membranes are ruptured, internal monitoring does not appear to add to the risk for the gravida.

The scalp electrode per se has created a new infectious complication for the fetus: abscess formation at the site of attachment. The incidence of scalp abscess is of the order of 1:200 to 1:400 monitored patients. Although scalp abscesses have been noted with both the clamp-on type and the spiral electrode, spiral electrodes with a barb at the tip may have been associated with a higher incidence. Fortunately, these types of spiral electrodes are no longer clinically employed.

In many instances, there is no correlation between neonatal scalp abscesses and the number of electrode applications, duration of monitoring, or concurrent amnionitis. The pathogenesis of scalp abscesses requires not only a mechanical disruption of the cutaneous barriers but also, presumably, a laceration of an arterial or venous vessel with secondary microhematoma formation. The bacteria isolated from such lesions are predominantly gram-positive cocci. Both the aerobic (coagulase-negative staphylococci, *Staphylococcus aureus*, and group B and D streptococci) and the anaerobic (peptostreptococci) cocci have been recovered from scalp abscesses. An unusual but significant pathogen has been *Haemophilus influenzae* type B. Less frequently, members of the Enterobacteriaceae or Bacteroidaceae (particularly *Bacteroides fragilis*) have been present. The high incidence of so-called "sterile acute scalp abscesses" attests to the important role played by obligate anaerobes in the more advanced lesion and the failure to use appropriate anaerobic technology to isolate and identify these agents.

Specimens for bacteriologic analysis should be obtained by aspiration carefully so as not to draw up any air. If this is not possible, one should submit a fragment of necrotic tissue in a sterile container.

Characteristically, disease is manifested in the first eight days of life. Abscess is usually the clinical presentation. In the absence of septicemia, the infant is afebrile. The treatment of a scalp abscess is basically complete incision and drainage under antibiotic coverage after appropriate cultures have been taken and a representative specimen has been Gram stained. Serious sequelae such as septicemia and osteomyelitis may occur. If osteomyelitis ensues, craniotomy and excision of the area of infection may be required.

In rare instances, a progressive cutaneous gangrene not dissimilar to a Meleney type II ulcer may occur. In such cases, the tissue destruction extends down to the periosteum (Fig. 1). A scalp abscess should not be treated lightly; isolated case reports of neonatal demise are present in the literature in which the site of the scalp electrode provided the portal for lethal infection.

While providing a portal primarily for bacterial infection, scalp electrodes, on rare occasion, may provide a portal of entry for other types of pathogens. Adams et al. (1975) reported scalp infections with *Herpes simplex* type 2 virus at the monitor probe site. Similarly, Golden et al. (1977) reported a case of fatal disseminated neonatal herpetic infection in which the initial clinical manifestation occurred at the site of a fetal scalp electrode.

INVASIVE PRENATAL DIAGNOSTIC PROCEDURES

Intrauterine infection in association with invasive prenatal diagnostic procedures is a rare event. The incidence of maternal/fetal infection increases with the complexity of the diagnostic procedure carried out. The incidence of chorioamnionitis after amniocentesis is estimated to be 3.7 per 1000 cases; that after transcervical chorionic villus sampling is 5 per 1000 cases; and that after cordocentesis is 8.8 per 1000 cases.

The pathogenesis of disease and clinical manifestation vary significantly depending upon the procedure and the functioning pathogen. With transcervical chorionic villus sampling, direct inoculation of vaginocervical bacteria into the uterine cavity is presumed to be the key requisite.

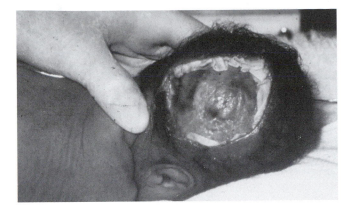

FIGURE 1 Progressive cutaneous gangrene. Cutaneous slough measuring $8 \times 8\,cm^2$ and extending to the periosteum due to necrotizing fasciitis that originated at the site of the fetal scalp electrode. *Source:* Feder et al. (1976).

Transabdominal procedures introduce the potential for the direct inoculati of intestinal pathogens.

The clinical spectrum of disease varies significantly from mild to moderate evidence of intrauterine infection to life-threatening sepsis. The cases that find their way into the literature reflect the latter part of the spectrum. Plachouras et al. (2004) reported a case of fulminant sepsis after multiple invasive procedures due to *Clostridium perfringens*. In their case, cordocentesis was the probable instigating event for disease initiation. Their review of the literature identified 10 additional cases of life-threatening sepsis following transabdominal prenatal diagnostic procedures. Disease was due to primarily *C. perfringens* or *Escherichia coli* functioning individually or in concert.

In its initial stages, the clinical manifestations of disease tend to be those of febrile morbidity with or without abdominal/back discomfort. Progression to life-threatening status can be very rapid. In six of the nine cases in which data are recorded, evidence of uterine infection developed in the first 24 hours following the invasive procedure. The longest interval between diagnostic procedure and disease manifestation was 48 hours. Any evidence of hemolysis and/or clotting abnormalities are mandates for aggressive intervention. Particularly with advanced *clostridium* infection, hysterectomy appears to be a requisite for maternal survival. Of the 11 total cases reported, hysterectomy was deemed necessary in five cases owing to the tendency of *C. perfringens* to invade the myometrium. In every case, removal of the nidus of infection is required. The demarcation between abortion and hysterectomy appears to reside with the speed with which the problem is effectively addressed.

SELECTED READING

Intrauterine Monitoring
Adams G, Puroht D, Bada H, Andrews BF. Neonatal infection by *Herpes virus hominis* Type II: a complication of intrapartum fetal monitoring. Clin Res 1975; 23:69A.
Amann ST, Fagnant RJ, Chartrand SA, Monif GRG. Herpes simplex infection associated with short-term use of a fetal scalp electrode. J Reprod Med 1992; 37:372.

Ashkenazi S, Metzker A, Merlob P, et al. Scalp changes after fetal monitoring. Arch Dis Child 1985; 60:267.
Cordero L, Anderson CW, Zuspan FP. Scalp abscess: a benign and infrequent complication of fetal monitoring. Am J Obstet Gynecol 1983; 146:126.
Feder HM Jr, MacLeon WG Jr, Moxon R. Scalp abscess secondary to fetal scalp electrode. J Pediatr 1976; 89:808.
Fleming AD, Ehrlich DW, Miller NA, Monif GRG. Successful treatment of maternal septicemia due to *Listeria monocytogenes* at 26 weeks gestation. Obstet Gynecol 1985; 66:52.
Gassner CB, Ledger WJ. Relationship of hospital acquired maternal infection to invasive intrapartum monitoring technique. Am J Obstet Gynecol 1976; 126:33.
Gibbs RS, Listwa HM, Read JA. The effect of internal fetal monitoring on maternal infection following cesarean section. Obstet Gynecol 1976; 48:653.
Golden SM, Merenstein GB, Todd WA, Hill JM. Disseminated herpes simplex neonatorum: a complication of fetal monitoring. Am J Obstet Gynecol 1977; 129:917.
Goodin R, Harrod J. Complications of fetal spiral electrodes. Lancet 1975; 1:559.
Hagen D. Maternal febrile morbidity associated with fetal monitoring and cesarean section. Obstet Gynecol 1975; 46:260.
Larsen JW, Goldkrand JW, Hanson TM, et al. Intra-uterine infection on an obstetric service. Obstet Gynecol 1974; 43:838.
Listinsky JL, Wood BP, Ekholm SE. Parietal osteomyelitis and epidural abscess: a delayed complication of fetal monitoring. Pediatr Radiol 1986; 16:150.
Nightingale LM, Eaton CB, Fruehan AE, et al. Cephalohematoma complicated by osteomyelitis presumed due to *Gardnerella vaginalis*. J Am Med Assoc 1986; 256:1936.
Overturf CD, Balfour G. Osteomyelitis and sepsis: severe complications of fetal monitoring. Pediatrics 1975; 55:244.
Plavidal FJ, Werch A. Fetal scalp abscess secondary to intrauterine monitoring. Am J Obstet Gynecol 1976; 125:65.
Sharp DS, Couriel JM. Penetration of the subarachnoid space by fetal scalp electrode. Br Med J 1985; 291:1169.
Siddiqui SF, Taylor PM. Necrotizing fasciitis of the scalp. A complication of fetal monitoring. Am J Dis Child 1982; 136:226.
Thomas G, Blackwell RJ. A hazard associated with the use of spiral fetal scalp electrodes. Am J Obstet Gynecol 1975; 121:1118.
Turbeville DF, Heath RE Jr, Bowen FW Jr, Killiam AP. Complications of fetal scalp electrodes: a case report. Am J Obstet Gynecol 1975; 122:530.
Wiechetck W, Huriguchi T, Dillon TF. Puerperal morbidity and internal fetal monitoring. Am J Obstet Gynecol 1974; 119:230.
Winkel CA, Snyder DL, Schlaerth JB. Scalp abscess: a complication of the spiral fetal electrode. Am J Obstet Gynecol 1976; 126:720.

Invasive Prenatal Diagnostic Procedurers
Ayadi S, Carbillon L, Varlet C, et al. Fatal sepsis due to Escherichia coli after second trimester amniocentesis. Fetal Diagn Ther 1998; 13:98.
Barela AI, Kleinman GE, Golditch IM, et al. Septic shock with renal failure after chorionic villus sampling. Am J Obstet Gynecol 1986; 154:1100.
Cederholm M, Haglund B, Axelsson O. Maternal complications following amniocentesis and chorionic villus sampling. BJOG 2003; 110:392.
Fejgin M, Amiel A, Kaneti H, et al. Fulminating sepsis due to group B streptococci following transcervical chorionic villi sampling. Clin Infect Dis 1993; 17:142.
Hovav Y, Hornstein E, Pollack RN, Yaffe C. Sepsis due to Clostridium perfringens after second-trimester amniocentesis. Clin Infect Dis 1995; 21:235.
Plachouras N, Sotiriadis A, Dalkalitis E, et al. Fulminating sepsis after invasive prenatal diagnosis. Obstet Gynecol 2004; 104:1244.
Tongsong T, Wanapirak C, Kunavkatkul C, et al. Fetal loss rate associated with cordocentesis at midgestation. Am J Obstet Gynecol 2001; 184:719.
Winer N, David A, Leconte P, et al. Amniocentesis and amnioperfusion during pregnancy; report of four complicated cases. Eur J Obstet Gynecol Reprod Biol 2001; 100:108.

Postpartum Endometritis/ Endomyometritis

62

INTRODUCTION

While endometritis following spontaneous vaginal delivery is a relatively rare event, endomyometritis is a common postpartum complication following cesarean section. If prophylactic antibiotics are not used, the incidence of postcesarean endomyometritis varies from a low of 15% to a high of 65%, depending upon the population studied. In general, the lowest incidence of infection occurs in middle- and upper-income women undergoing scheduled elective abdominal delivery; the highest incidence of infection occurs in young, indigent patients having surgery after extended duration of labor and ruptured fetal membranes. The use of prophylactic antibiotics at the time of abdominal delivery usually reduces the number of postoperative infections by approximately 50% to 60%. Approximately 15% of women with endomyometritis will have a documented bacteremia. If disease is not aggressively treated, pelvic abscess, septic thrombophlebitis, septic shock, and adult respiratory distress may ensue.

PATHOGENESIS

The understanding of the pathogenesis of endometritis requires the analysis of selected demographic facts. Following spontaneous vaginal delivery, 1% to 4% of women develop postpartum endometritis. The higher incidence of disease occurs in women from disadvantaged backgrounds or women who have had no antenatal screening for *Neisseria gonorrhoeae*, asymptomatic bacteriuria, or the group B streptococci. If the mode of delivery is changed to an abdominal one, the incidence of disease is 10- to 15-fold that observed in patients delivering vaginally (Fig. 1). The bacteriology of these two groups is significantly different. In the cases of endometritis, more than 90% of the isolates are aerobic pathogens encompassed in groups I and IV of the Gainesville Classification. Included are both exogenous pathogens (e.g., groups A, C, and G streptococci, *N. gonorrhoeae*, *Haemophilus influenzae*) and endogenous pathogens (e.g., group B streptococci and the *Enterobacteriaceae*). Less than 10% of cases involve polymicrobial infection. The latter cases are often associated with retained products of conception or obstetrical trauma. More than 90% of cases of endomyometritis are the consequence of anaerobic progression. Excluding exogenous bacteria with enhanced virulence, the composition of the vaginal bacterial flora and its resultant oxidation–reduction potential partially dictate the risk of endomyometritis following cesarean section. Watts et al. (1990) found a sixfold increase of postcesarean endomyometritis when bacterial vaginosis was present prior to delivery.

Since the advent of modern microbiology, we have asked ourselves the question: "Why do certain women develop postpartum endometritis or endomyometritis?" The introduction of sophisticated anaerobiology has documented the shallowness of our own conceptual thoughts. With appropriate anaerobiological techniques, we can demonstrate the almost universal presence of bacteria in the endometrial cavity of women following spontaneous vaginal delivery. About 70% to 80% of patients can be demonstrated to have moderate ($>10^6$ cfu/g) to heavy growth ($>10^9$ cfu/g) of at least one bacterial species. Whitacre et al. (1946) found that all endometrial cultures will be positive after 24 hours and that this type of endometrial infection persisted for at least five days. Clotted blood and necrotic decidua provide ideal culture media for anaerobic bacteria. An open cervical patulous cervix constitutes an open conduit for the vaginal bacterial flora.

Why do only 1% to 4% of women delivering vaginally and without obstetrical trauma go on to develop endometritis? Why does not every woman develop endometritis in the postpartum period, since bacteriological studies have documented the almost universal presence of bacteria within material obtained by transabdominal aspiration in the immediate postpartum period? Based on a purely qualitative bacteriological assessment of the endometrium, uninfected patients cannot be distinguished from those with postpartum endometritis unless an exogenous pathogen, i.e., group A streptococci or *N. gonorrhoeae*, is present. The mere presence or replication of bacteria within necrotic decidua is not sufficient to produce disease. Underlying the necrotic decidua and clotted blood is a layer of healthy endometrial tissue which usually precludes the penetration of class II and class III anaerobes. Microaerophilic class II and class III anaerobes do not represent a significant cause of postpartum endometritis following spontaneous vaginal delivery; however, if retained products of conception still have continuity with the placental implantation site, the vascular access thus provided circumvents the endometrial basalis barrier. Similarly, when significant obstetrical trauma has occurred and laceration extends through the endocervix, the associated bleeding, coupled with the availability of bacterial flora, creates ideal conditions for the immediate anaerobic syndrome to ensue.

In the course of performing a cesarean section, the basalis layer of the endometrium is iatrogenically disrupted. The devitalized tissue (resulting from clamping, loss of its vascular supply, and coagulation) coupled with microhematoma formation along the line of tissue reapproximation not only creates conditions favorable for anaerobic bacterial replication

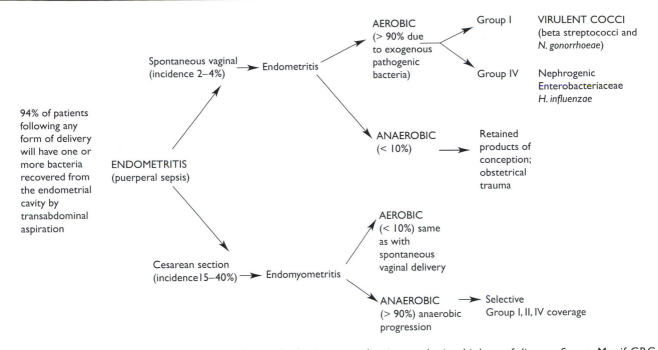

FIGURE 1 Impact of mode of delivery on incidence of infectious complications and microbiology of disease. *Source:* Monif GRG. *Infectious Disease Care Manual—Obstetrics,* 4th ed. Gainesville, FL: IDI, 1988.

but also circumvents the principal anatomical barrier to anaerobic infection. While intra-amniotic fluid infection caused by selected class I aerobes tends to select for chorioamnionitis, the presence of class II anaerobes, i.e., peptostreptococci and Bacteroidaceae, is apparently a partial catalytic factor in the induction of endomyometritis in the absence of virulent class I aerobes.

DIAGNOSIS

The diagnosis of endometritis or endomyometritis is often difficult to make. Fever is the cardinal manifestation of disease. Standard puerperal morbidity is defined by the Joint Committee on Maternal Welfare as "a temperature of 100.4°F (38.0°C) occurring in any two of the first ten days postpartum, exclusive of the first 24 hours." Exclusion of the first 24 hours is predicated upon the observation that, following spontaneous vaginal delivery, 6% to 8% of women will have an isolated febrile spike in the first 24 hours; however, only a quarter to one-third of these individuals will develop overt diseases requiring antibiotic therapy.

The probable reason for the isolated febrile spike is closure of the cervical os by a large necrotic decidual fragment. The reason for the spontaneous resolution of fever is passage of the fragment secondary to uterine contractions and reestablishment of surgical drainage. In patients who have undergone general anesthesia for cesarean section, fever in the first 24 hours is often attributed to "atelectasis." If serial blood gases are done on patients who undergo radical abdominal surgery for four hours, 100% will have evidence of alveolar-perfusion dissociation, and 10% to 12% will have demonstrable linear atelectasis on chest

roentgenogram, yet only a small percentage of these patients will develop fever.

The indications for fever work-up in the postpartum woman are

1. two consecutive temperatures greater than or equal to 38°C taken at least four hours apart, with the second temperature greater than 0.2°C higher than the first,
2. one temperature greater than 38.5°C, or
3. three temperatures greater than or equal to 38°C in any 24 hour period.

The adoption of a policy of aggressive early intervention lessens the likelihood that other corroborating signs, e.g., uterine tenderness or purulent lochia, will be present. A moderate degree of clinical experience is required to distinguish the uterine tenderness engendered by the operative procedure from that associated with endometritis. The presence of a foul-smelling discharge may occur in cases of long-standing duration (often associated with retained products of conception). The primary goal of the physical examination is not to corroborate the diagnosis of endometritis or endomyometritis, but rather to rule out a nonoperative site of infection.

Unless the process is due to documented exogenous pathogens, the bacteriological results engendered by culturing the endometrial cavity flora provide marginal information. To culture the endometrial cavity, a swab must traverse the vagina and endocervix, both of which possess a bacterial flora. The way the swab is used and the way the bacteriological specimen is handled will influence the spectrum of bacteria recovered and the interpretation of data. The real reason for taking an endometrial culture is not to identify the anaerobic bacteria functioning in the anaerobic progression, but to rule out the presence of bacteria of unique virulence (e.g., group A streptococci, *N. gonorrhoeae*) whose identification impacts beyond immediate patient care. Tests to exclude the presence of sexually transmitted pathogens should be done in all cases of endometritis following vaginal delivery.

Utilization of anaerobic methodology does not preclude the identification of aerobic or facultative anaerobic bacteria, whereas the converse is not true. The request for anaerobic culturing of endometrial swab material is a misuse of the microbiological facility. Even if an anaerobic swab is utilized, by being withdrawn back into the vaginal environment, it is exposed to sufficient oxygen to eradicate any class III anaerobes that may be present.

When obtaining a culture that may be expected to yield anaerobic bacteria, it is important to make a Gram stain at the time of the bacteriological sampling and compare it to the Gram stain and bacterial isolate derived from the microbiology laboratory. The demonstration of bacteria on Gram stain that fail to grow on synthetic media indicates the presence of class III anaerobes.

Whether or not blood cultures should be obtained in every case of endometritis or endomyometritis is a point of controversy. The anticipated incidence of positive blood cultures is approximately 4% to 15%, depending upon the number of sets of blood cultures taken. The bacteriological data engendered by positive blood cultures influence therapy in less than 1% of cases. Our policy has been not to obtain blood cultures in a postpartum woman unless

1. her temperature exceeded 39°C or
2. she appeared to be in some degree of clinical difficulty.

It is important that each institution develop its own guidelines.

THERAPY

Endometritis Following Spontaneous Vaginal Delivery

If obstetrical trauma or the presence of retained products of conception can be ruled out, the probable prime etiological agents are exogenous bacterial pathogens: the virulent cocci (groups A, C, and G streptococci or *N. gonorrhoeae*) or the nephrogenic Enterobacteriaceae (*Escherichia coli* or *Klebsiella pneumoniae*). The group B streptococci, though endogenous bacteria, are a frequent etiological agent for early-onset endometritis (disease manifestation in the first 12–18 hours postpartum). Antibiotic coverage for endometritis following spontaneous vaginal delivery can best be achieved by Category I and IV therapy, i.e., ampicillin and an aminoglycoside. If the anticipated therapeutic response fails to develop, a third antibiotic effective against the non–penicillin-sensitive Bacteroidaceae needs to be used.

If obstetrical trauma or retained products of conception are present, greater coverage must be afforded against Category II bacteria capable of functioning in the anaerobic progression.

Endomyometritis Following Abdominal Delivery

The combination of penicillin or one of its semisynthetic analogs with an aminoglycoside leaves an antibiotic gap in Category II of the Gainesville Classification, the penicillin-resistant Bacteroidaceae/*Prevotella* species.

What are the consequences of antibiotic noncoverage of these bacteria? The consequences of a Category II gap in the treatment of endomyometritis following cesarean section are

1. septic thrombophlebitis and
2. pelvic abscesses.

A small percentage (2–4%) of patients develop very serious pelvic infection or septic thrombophlebitis. Gibbs et al. (1975) analyzed 160 patients treated with penicillin and an aminoglycoside. Seventy-eight percent of the 135 patients were cured. Twenty-eight of the 35 therapeutic failures responded to clindamycin or chloramphenicol. Seven patients (4%) developed abscesses or septic thrombophlebitis. Of the 100 patients treated by diZerega et al. (1980) with penicillin and gentamicin, one patient developed a pelvic abscess necessitating hysterectomy, and two responded to heparin challenges. Among the 50 patients treated with penicillin and kanamycin at the Shands Teaching Hospital of the University of Florida, four developed septic thrombophlebitis, and one had a pelvic abscess that required surgical intervention. When antibiotic coverage encompasses the non–penicillin-sensitive Bacteroidaceae/*Prevotella* species, serious complications, specifically pelvic abscess or septic thrombophlebitis, are virtually eliminated.

Endomyometritis, particularly in those cases complicated by septic thrombophlebitis or pelvic abscesses, was once a major cause of maternal mortality and morbidity. With modern day antibiotics, one can anticipate a 93% arrest of disease with literally any antibiotic combination that impacts significantly on Categories I, II, and IV of the Gainesville Classification. When dealing with the early phase of the anaerobic progression, effective therapy will render the temperature less than 37.6°C and result in resolution of local physical findings within 24 hours.

What is important is the physician's ability to deal with the failure to obtain the anticipated therapeutic response in 24 hours. *If the anticipated therapeutic response does not develop within 24 to 36 hours, reexamine the patient.* If the initial clinical diagnosis is still the working diagnosis and retained products of conception are not found on pelvic examination, close the existing bacterial gap of the Gainesville Classification with appropriate antimicrobial therapy.

If then the anticipated therapeutic response does not develop within 24 hours, discontinue all current antibiotics and place the patient on intravenous metronidazole if previously on clindamycin or vice versa. If fever does not lyse in 24 hours, commence heparin challenge unless there are specific localizing signs.

If the fever persists despite metronidazole therapy and heparin challenge, the probability of surgical intervention should be assessed.

The concept of triple therapy coverage plus heparin challenge was developed to cleave medically treatable disease from disease requiring surgical intervention.

Failed Prophylaxis Endomyometritis

The prior antibiotic use in the immediate preoperative or perioperative period influences antibiotic selection. When a cephalosporin has been used, it is impossible to close the remaining categories of the Gainesville Classification with the addition of clindamycin and an aminoglycoside. In this situation, aggressive therapy usually entails "triple therapy" or triple therapy equivalent (e.g., ampicillin–sulbactam, piperacillin– tazobactam acid, or imipenem–cilastatin). If ampicillin is used, the drug effectively impacts on Categories I and III. The gaps in the Gainesville Classification can be effectively closed with clindamycin or metronidazole and an aminoglycoside. If a patient develops endomyometritis following antibiotic prophylaxis, do not incorporate into the subsequent therapy the drug used for prophylaxis or a closely related antibiotic.

CHRONIC ENDOMETRITIS

Endometritis occurring in the absence of parturition or a recent surgical procedure is usually the consequence of ascending infection (i.e., *Chlamydia trachomatis*), endocervicitis associated with an abnormal vaginal flora, foreign body induced [i.e., intrauterine device (IUD)-related] or retrograde spread from the fallopian tubes (*Mycobacterium tuberculosis*, *Actinomyces israelii*).

The earliest manifestation of occult endometritis is the occurrence of so-called "breakthrough" bleeding. Intermenstrual bleeding, especially in a patient previously well regulated on birth control pills, warrants aggressive evaluation to exclude endometritis due to a sexually transmitted disease. Krettek et al. described this syndrome. The predominant cause of this finding in their series was infection with *C. trachomatis*. The second most common etiology was vaginal bacteriosis with or without the concomitant presence of *Trichomonas vaginalis*. As in Burnhill's syndrome (IUD-related bacterial endometritis; Chapter 70), the sudden appearance of inflammatory cells can alert the clinician as to the possibility of an infectious process within the endometrium.

With disease progression, intermenstrual discharge and some degree of cervical motion tenderness will develop well before grossly discernible changes in uterine configuration. What additional signs or symptoms develop is a function of the underlying disease process.

Documentation of the presence of an endocervicitis requires a uterine aspiration biopsy. Such a biopsy can be best obtained using a Pipelle-like apparatus. Part of the specimen, not sent for culture, should be placed in 10% formalin and submitted for histological analysis. When doing a biopsy, it is best to avoid the first few days after a period or those immediately before the onset of menstruation.

An alternate approach, which may suggest the diagnosis, involves obtaining a swab of the uterine cavity using a sheathed swab. The presence of inflammatory and/or plasma cells is presumptive evidence of endometritis. Great care must be given to the manner in which the specimen is collected. A chronic endocervicitis is relatively common.

SELECTED READING

Parturition Endometritis

Cooperman NR, Kasim M, Rajashekaraiah KR. Clinical significance of amniotic fluid, amniotic membranes and endometrial biopsy cultures at the time of cesarean section. Am J Obstet Gynecol 1980; 137:537.

D'Angelo LJ, Sokol RJ. Determinants of postpartum morbidity in laboring monitored patients: a reassessment of the bacteriology of the amniotic fluid during labor. Am J Obstet Gynecol 1980; 136:575.

diZerega GS, Yonekura ML, Keegan K, et al. Bacteremia in post-cesarean section endomyometritis: differential response to therapy. Obstet Gynecol 1980; 55:587.

diZerega G, Yonekura L, Roy S, et al. A comparison of clindamycin-gentamicin and penicillin-gentamicin in the treatment of post-cesarean section endomyometritis. Am J Obstet Gynecol 1979; 134:238.

Eddowes HA, Read MD, Codling BW. Pipelle: a more acceptable technique for outpatient endometrial biopsy. Br J Obstet Gynaecol 1990; 97:961.

Filker R, Monif GRG. The significance of temperature during the first 24 hours postpartum. Obstet Gynecol 1979; 53:358.

Gibbs RS, O'Dell TN, MacGregor RR, et al. Puerperal endometritis: a prospective microbiological study. Am J Obstet Gynecol 1975; 121:919.

Gilstrap LC, Cummingham FG. The bacterial pathogenesis of infection following cesarean section. Obstet Gynecol 1979; 53:545.

Hagglund L, Christensen KV, Christensen P, et al. Risk factors in cesarean section infection. Obstet Gynecol 1983; 62:145.

Hite KE, Hesseltine HC, Goldstein L. A study of the bacterial flora of the normal and pathologic vagina and uterus. Am J Obstet Gynecol 1947; 53:233.

Ledger WJ, Norman M, Gee C, Lewis W. Bacteremia on an obstetric-gynecologic service. Am J Obstet Gynecol 1975; 121:205.

Monif GRG, Baer H. Polymicrobial bacteremia in obstetric patients. Obstet Gynecol 1976; 48:167.

Monif GRG, Hempling RE. Antibiotic therapy for the *Bacteroidaceae* in post-cesarean section infections. Obstet Gynecol 1981; 57:177.

Ott WJ. Primary cesarean section: factors related to postpartum infection. Obstet Gynecol 1981; 57:171.

Roberts S, Maccato M, Faro S, Pinell P. The microbiology of post-cesarean wound morbidity. Obstet Gynecol 1993; 81:383.

Repke JT, Spence MR, Calhoun S. Risk factors in the development of cesarean section infection. Surg Gynecol Obstet 1984; 158:112.

Watts DH, Hillier SL, Eschenbach DA. Upper genital tract isolates at delivery as predictors of post-cesarean infections among women receiving antibiotic prophylaxis. Obstet Gynecol 1992; 77:287.

Watts DH, Krohn MA, Hillier SL, Eschenback DA. Bacterial vaginosis as a risk factor for post-cesarean endometritis. Obstet Gynecol 1990; 75:52.

Whitacre FE, Loeb WM Jr, Loeb L. The time for postpartum sterilization: report of 150 bacteriologic studies on the postpartum uterus. Am J Obstet Gynecol 1946; 51:1041.

Endomyometritis

Apuzzio JJ, Stankiewicz R, Ganesh V, et al. Comparison of parenteral ciprofloxacin with clindamycin-gentamicin in the treatment of pelvic infection. Am J Med 1989; 87:1485.

Azziz R, Cumming J, Naeye R. Acute myometritis and chorioamnionitis during cesarean section of asymptomatic women. Am J Obstet Gynecol 1988; 159:1137.

Cox SM, Gilstrap LC. Postpartum endometritis. Obstet Gynecol Clin North Am 1989; 16:363.

Duff P. Pathophysiology and the management of postcesarean endomyometritis. Obstet Gynecol 1986; 67:269.

Dylewski J, Wiesenfeld H, Latour A. Postpartum uterine infection with *Clostridium perfringens*. Rev Infect Dis 1989; 11:470.

Faro S. Infectious disease relations to cesarean section. Obstet Gynecol Clin North Am 1988; 15:685.

Hillier S, Watts DH, Lee MF, Eschenbach DA. Etiology and treatment of post-cesarean-section endometritis after cephalosporin prophylaxis. J Reprod Med 1990; 35:322.

Martens MG, Faro S, Hammill HA, et al. Ampicillin/sulbactam versus clindamycin in the treatment of postpartum endomyometritis. South Med J 1990; 83:408.

Morales WJ, Collins EM, Angel JL, Knuppel RA. Short course of antibiotic therapy in treatment of postpartum endomyometritis. Am J Obstet Gynecol 1989; 161:568.

Newton ER, Prihoda TJ, Gibbs RS. A clinical and microbiologic analysis of risk factors for puerperal endometritis. Obstet Gynecol 1990; 75:402.

Watts DH, Hillier SL, Eschenbach DA. Upper genital tract isolates at delivery as predictors of post-cesarean infections among women receiving antibiotic prophylaxis. Obstet Gynecol 1991; 77:287.

Watts DH, Krohn MA, Hillier SL. Eschenbach DA: bacterial vaginosis as a risk factor for post-cesarean endometritis. Obstet Gynecol 1990; 75:52.

Chronic Endometritis

Eckert LO, Hawes SE, Wolner-Hanssen Pal K, et al. Endometritis: the clinical-pathologic syndrome. Am J Obstet Gynecol 2002; 186:690.

Hillier SL, Kiviat NA, Hawes SE, et al. Role of bacterial vaginosis-associated microorganisms in endometritis. Am J Obstet Gynecol 1996; 175:435.

Kiviat NB, Paavonen JA, Wolner-Hanssen P, et al. Histopathology of endocervical infection caused by Chlamydia trachomatis, herpes simplex viruses, Trichomonas vaginalis and Neisseria gonorrhoeae. Hum Pathol 1990; 21:831.

Korn AP, Hessol N, Padian N, et al. Commonly used criteria for pelvic inflammatory disease have poor sensitivity for plasma cell endometritis. Sex Transm Dis 1995; 22:335.

Krettek JA, Arkin SI, Chaisilwattania P, Monif GRG. Chlamydia trachomatis in patients who used oral contraceptives and had intermenstrual spotting. Obstet Gynecol 1993; 81:728.

Rotterdam H. Chronic endometritis: a clinicopathologic study. Pathol Annu 1978; (Suppl) 13:209.

Salamonsen LA, Woolley DE. Menstruation: induction by matrix metalloproteinases and inflammatory cells. J Reprod Immunol 1999; 44:1.

Septic Pelvic Thrombophlebitis

Robert J. Fagnant and Gilles R. G. Monif

63

INTRODUCTION

The physiologic changes attending pregnancy fulfill the requisites of Virchow's triad (circulatory stasis, vascular damage, and hypercoagulability of blood). Factors VII, VIII, and X are increased in pregnancy. Postpartum or postoperative infections of the female genital tract caused by the release of thrombin-mediated fibrin may induce septic pelvic thrombophlebitis.

The prevalence, which varies according to the extent of operative trauma, is 10 times more in women who have undergone cesarean section or septic abortion than in women who have delivered vaginally. Aggressive use of antibiotics in infection avoidance schema has rendered its occurrence even less likely. When endomyometritis occurs, failure to cover for the penicillin-resistant Bacteroidaceae/Prevotella species (Category II of the Gainesville Classification) results in an increased prevalence of this postsurgical complication (2–4%). If initial therapy is complete for the anaerobic bacteria, the incidence among cases of endometritis and endomyometritis is less than 0.5%.

Pelvic vein thrombophlebitis occurs once in 2000 spontaneous vaginal deliveries, approximately 10 to 20 times less frequently than after cesarean section.

Septic thrombophlebitis in the obstetric patient occurs in one of three clinical settings:

1. In association with retained products of conception and anaerobic infection
2. After cesarean sections in which endomyometrial bacterial invasion attains vascular access
3. With criminal abortion

In gynecologic patients, septic thrombophlebitis is observed in association with

1. ovarian abscess,
2. tubo-ovarian abscess with involvement of the ovarian parenchyma,
3. ligneous cellulitis, or
4. postoperative gynecologic infections.

PATHOGENESIS

In septic thrombophlebitis, bacterial infection causes an inflammatory process within the vein and ensuing thrombus formation. The process extends from thrombosed sinuses involving continuous uterine and/or ovarian veins. In advanced cases, involvement of the iliac veins, inferior vena cava, and renal vein may occur.

From these foci, septic thromboemboli are sloughed off, resulting in intermittent septicemia, pulmonary emboli, and potential metastatic abscess formation. The bacteria most commonly involved are the peptostreptococci and Bacteroidaceae/Prevotella species, acting singularly or in combination.

CLINICAL PRESENTATIONS

Pelvic vein thrombophlebitis has three characteristic patterns:

1. Pelvic infection with evidence of hematogenous metastatic complications
2. Persistent fever of indemonstrable etiology after therapy for pelvic infection
3. Ovarian vein variant

The most common clinical presentation of pelvic vein thrombophlebitis is fever of unknown origin with no demonstrable focus of infection. Pelvic thrombophlebitis as a cause of fever of obscure etiology was a concept introduced by Michaelis in 1911 (Michaelis's sign).

The diagnosis is difficult because fever is often the only physical finding present unless septic pulmonary infarcts develop as a consequence of peripheral embolization of infected clots.

Rigors (frank chills) are not commonly associated with septic thrombophlebitis in a postpartum patient unless disease is the consequence of retained products of conception at the maternal implantation site.

DIAGNOSIS

The diagnosis of septic thrombophlebitis requires a high index of suspicion: infectious morbidity framed in the appropriate clinical setting. The patient usually has an ongoing infectious process in the pelvis either de novo or in conjunction with parturition or with surgical intervention for benign or malignant disease. The diagnosis is most commonly inferred when a patient continues to have fever despite complete four-category coverage as determined by the Gainesville Classification. A picket-fence fever curve with wide swings from 37.6°C may suggest the diagnosis.

Unless one is dealing with the ovarian vein variant, the pelvic examination is usually unremarkable. In less than 20% of cases can tender, firm wormlike thrombosed veins be identified in the vaginal fornices or in one or both parametrial areas. Not infrequently, a temperature spike occurs within one hour after such an examination (the so-called "pelvic challenge" test).

No consistent laboratory aids are available for making the diagnosis. The white blood cell (WBC) count is usually elevated and shifted to the left. The demonstration of greater than 20,000 leukocytes/mm³ may indicate the concomitant presence of an abscess or conversion of the thrombosed vein into an abscess. Chest X rays, blood gas determinations, and isotopic lung scans, individually or in combination, are of value only when thromboembolic disease to the lungs is suspected. The rarity with which venograms or intravenous pyelograms contribute to establish the diagnosis precludes their routine utilization. Making a definitive diagnosis usually requires the use of one or more of the following: ultrasound, computerized axial tomography (CT), nuclear magnetic resonance imaging, or radiolabeling of WBCs.

Blood cultures obtained at the onset of a fever spike may be positive for one or more anaerobic bacteria.

An alternative, less definitive, but clinically important way to make a presumptive diagnosis of thrombophlebitis is with the heparin challenge test. In this test, the precipitous lysis of fever within 24 to 36 hours after the attainment of effective anticoagulation is presumptive evidence of pelvic septic thrombophlebitis. Persistence of fever and/or tachycardia after effective anticoagulation has been achieved should suggest an erroneous diagnosis. Heparin will not mask the presence of concomitant pelvic disease such as an abscess.

THERAPY

Two therapeutic components, antibiotics and heparinization, must function simultaneously.

Antibiotics

In most cases, patients are already taking antibiotics when septic thrombophlebitis is diagnosed. Complete coverage must be afforded to Categories I and II of the Gainesville Classification. The antibiotic or combination of antibiotics used must provide coverage for the Peptostreptococci and both the penicillin-sensitive and the penicillin-resistant Bacteroidaceae/*Prevotella*.

Heparin

Heparin works by activating antithrombin II to slow the progression of venous thrombosis. Heparin per se does not dissolve the existing clot. Ultimate clot resolution is contingent upon the body's inherent fibrinolytic processes. The secondary effect of heparin in septic pelvic thrombophlehis is to facilitate antibiotic clot penetration.

The goal of heparinization is to maintain the clotting time at two to three times the normal value, four hours after administration. Optimal anticoagulation using unfractionated heparin is obtained with a circulating heparin level of 0.3 U/mL [activated partial thromboplastin time (aPTT) of 1.5 times control value]. To achieve this, unfractionated heparin must be given intravenously in adequate doses. Continuous infusion works best, provided that it is properly monitored and given with strict accuracy. An initial IV bolus of heparin 60 U/kg (4000 U maximum) is given, followed by a 12 U/kg/h (1000 U/hr maximum)

maintenance infusion. Extremely high or low values prior to six hours should not provoke radical dosing changes. After administration of the bolus dose of heparin, the aPTT should be checked every six hours. Heparin dosing is adjusted as follows:

1. If the aPTT is low (less than 1.5 times control value), rebolus with 4000 U and increase the drip by 10%.
2. If the aPTT is high (greater than 2.5 times control value), decrease the intravenous drip by 10%.
3. If the aPTT is extremely high (greater than 100 seconds), hold the heparin drip for one hour and then decrease its administration by 10%.

Once a steady state has been achieved, aPTT should be done daily.

If significant bleeding occurs, the administration of 15 mg of protamine sulfate infused over three minutes usually reverses unfractionated heparin's anticoagulant effect. No more than 50 mg of protamine should be given over any 15-minute period because protamine itself can cause anticoagulation.

Before administering heparin, a complete blood cell count, platelet count, prothrombin time, aPTT, and urinalysis should be obtained.

How long to continue anticoagulation therapy depends in part on the severity of disease. If prompt lysis of fever occurs and there is no prior evidence of thromboembolic phenomena, heparinization for five to seven days is usually adequate. If evidence of pulmonary emboli can be documented by clinical symptomatology or blood gas determinations, heparinization should continue for three days. For the next two or three days, the dosage should be tapered gradually. Oral anticoagulation should be instituted on the third day of anticoagulation therapy and continued for 30 days or more. Warfarin (Coumadin, Dicoumarol, Panwarfin) has no demonstrable effect on the prothrombin time for at least two or three days.

Surgical Intervention

Inferior vena cava ligation carries substantial chronic morbidity. Transient devices achieve the same result with less dangerous effects. Operative intervention is reserved for patients who continue to have pulmonary emboli despite adequate anticoagulation. However, such a procedure does not necessarily preclude continued embolization, which occurs in approximately 7% to 10% of patients.

Hysterectomy and salpingo-oophorectomy may be necessary if ligneous cellulitis is present. In this setting, the procedure is associated with a high degree of morbidity. The involved tissues bleed freely when excised and hold sutures very poorly.

OVARIAN VEIN VARIANT

Signs and Symptoms

Although puerperal ovarian vein thrombophlebitis occurs primarily after delivery, it may also be seen after vaginal or abdominal surgery (Figs. 1 and 2). The clinical characterization of the syndrome is well described in the collected

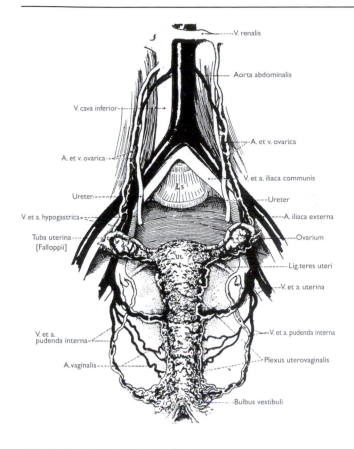

FIGURE 1 Drawing of the inferior vena cava system.

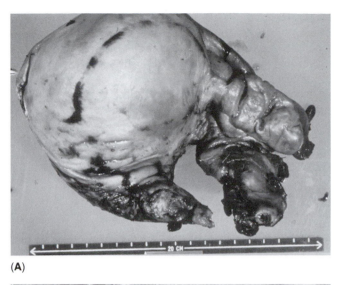

(A)

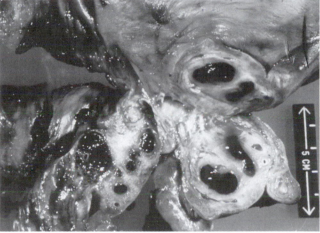

(B)

FIGURE 2 (A) Mass created by a right ovarian vein thrombophlebitis. (B) Close-up of section demonstrating thrombus of the ovarian vein and collateral circulation.

series of Brown and Munsick (1971). The patient may have fever before feeling any pain; nevertheless, pain is the cardinal symptom in nearly all cases. Initially the pain consists of cramps. Once the disease has become established, the pain becomes constant and noncolicky. It may vary in intensity from a dull ache to severe and debilitating pain. The pain may adopt one of several patterns. Most of the time, it resides in the lower abdomen directly over the site of involvement. The clinical presentation is often confused with acute appendicitis. Bilateral pain should alert the physician to the probability of bilateral disease. About 20% of patients may have exclusively costovertebral angle pain. Some patients have both abdominal and flank pain.

Although the onset of symptoms varies greatly, it usually happens on the second or third postpartum or postoperative day. Fever is often low grade at first. If antimicrobial therapy is delayed, the fever may spike in a hectic pattern. When symptoms start, most patients are tachycardic. The pulse rate may be elevated in disproportion to the observed temperature. Some 30% to 40% of patients have nausea, but vomiting is rare. Segmented ileus manifested by local distention without altered bowel sounds is demonstrable in more than 50% of patients.

Although the WBC count may be relatively normal, most patients have leukocytosis with a shift to the left. A WBC count of greater than 20,000 WBC/mm³ suggests the possibility of thrombus conversion into an abscess. Demonstration of an elongated, ropelike, exquisitely tender

mass confirms the diagnosis. The mass, which may be 2 to 8 cm in diameter, extends laterally to the lateral margin of the rectus abdominis muscle and cephalad. On physical examination, direct tenderness usually associated with guarding is almost always found at the site of involvement. Mild distention is common, but bowel sounds are usually normal. Bimanual examination is likely to reveal some tenderness and possible induration involving the parametrium and broad ligament of the site of involvement. In Table 1, considerations for the differential diagnosis are presented. CT can be indicated not only for diagnosis confirmation but also to determine the extent of ovarian vein thrombosis.

TABLE 1 Differential diagnosis for ovarian vein thrombophlebitis

Acute appendicitis
Unilateral right pyelonephritis
Torsion and infarction of right adnexal mass
Ovarian vein thrombophlebitis (bland)
Bowel volvulus

Management

Therapy for ovarian vein thrombophlebitis is the same as for septic thrombophlebitis. When the former converts into an abscess (a rare occurrence), the thrombosed vein must be surgically removed. Witlin et al. (1996) reported a series in patients with ovarian vein thrombosis. Patients responded for an average of 4.7 ± 2.1 days after heparin therapy was started. Unfortunately, the mean time of febrile morbidity to institution of therapy was 5.5 ± 1.9 days. The longer a process has functioned, the longer the time from effective anticoagulation to defervescence.

SELECTED READING

Septic Pelvic Thrombophlebitis

ACOG Educational Bulletin. Thromboembolism in pregnancy. 1997; 3:239.

Barbour LA, Pickard J. Controversies in thromboembolic disease during pregnancy: a critical review. Obstet Gynecol 1995; 86:621.

Cohen MB, Pernoll ML, Gevirtz CM, Kerstein MD. Septic pelvic thrombophlebitis: an update. Obstet Gynecol 1983; 62:83.

Collins CG. Suppurative pelvic thrombophlebitis. Am J Obstet Gynecol 1970; 108:681.

Collins CG, MacCallum EA, Nelson EW, et al. Suppurative pelvic thrombophlebitis. I. Incidence, pathology and etiology. Surgery 1951; 30:298.

Collins CG, Nelson EW, Collins JH, et al. Suppurative pelvic thrombophlebitis. II. Symptomatology and diagnosis. Surgery 1951; 30:311.

Craig F, Handler JA. Thrombophlebits, septic. Medline 2004; topic581.htm.

Duff P, Gibbs RS. Pelvic vein thrombophlebitis: diagnostic dilemma and therapeutic challenges. Obstet Gynecol Surv 1983; 38:365.

Dunn LJ, Van Voorhis LW. Enigmatic fever and pelvic thrombophlebitis: response to anticoagulants. N Engl J Med 1967; 276:265.

Hayden GE. The incidence of unsuspected asymptomatic thrombophlebitis of pelvic veins associated with hysterectomy. Am J Obstet Gynecol 1974; 119:396.

Hirsh J. Heparin. N Engl J Med 1991; 324:1565.

Josey WE, Cook CC. Septic pelvic thrombophlebitis. Obstet Gynecol 1970; 35:891.

Josey WE, Staggers SR. Heparin therapy in septic pelvic thrombophlebitis: a study of 46 cases. Am J Obstet Gynecol 1974; 120:228.

Kapernick PS. Postpartum hemorrhage and the abnormal puerperium. In: Pernoll ML, Benson RC, eds. Current Obstetric and Gynecologic Diagnosis and Treatment 1987. Connecticut: Appleton & Lange Norwalk, 1989.

Ledger WJ, Nakamura RM. Measurement of infectious disease morbidity in obstetrics and gynecology. Clin Obstet Gynecol 1976; 19:195.

Ledger WJ, Peterson EP. The use of heparin in the management of pelvic thrombophlebitis. Surg Gynecol Obstet 1970; 131:1115.

Nageotte MP. When the pregnant patient needs coagulation. Contemp Obstet Gynecol 1982; 20:123.

Pridmore BR, Murray KH, McAllen PM. The management of anticoagulant therapy during and after pregnancy. Br J Obstet Gynaecol 1975; 82:740.

Twickler DM, Setiawan AT, Evans RS et al. Imaging of puerperal septic thrombophlebitis: prospective comparison of MR imaging, CT, and sonography. Am J Roentgenol 1997; 169:1039.

Witlin AG, Mercer BM, Sibai BM. Septic pelvic thrombophlebitis or refractory postpartum fever of undetermined etiology. J Matern Fetal Med 1996; 5:355.

Ovarian Vein Variant

Adkins J, Wilson S. Unusual course of the gonadal vein: a case report of postpartum ovarian vein thrombosis mimicking acute appendicitis clinically and sonographically. J Ultrasound Med 1996; 15:409.

Angel JL, Knuppel RA. Computed tomography in diagnosis of puerperal ovarian vein thrombosis. Obstet Gynecol 1984; 63:61.

Brown TK, Munsick RA. Puerperal ovarian vein thrombophlebitis: a syndrome. Am J Obstet Gynecol 1971; 109:263.

Berlin M. Ovarian vein thrombosis. Am J Obstet Gynecol 1974; 118:880.

Collins CG. Suppurative pelvic thrombophlebitis. A study of 202 cases in which the disease was treated by ligation of the vena cava and ovarian vein. Am J Obstet Gynecol 1970; 108:681.

Janky E, Cambon D, Leng JJ, et al. Thrombophlebitis of the ovarian veins: a case report: review of the literature. Rev Fr Gynecol Obstet 1990; 85:615.

Loos W, von Hugo R, Rath W, et al. Puerperal ovarian vein thrombophlebitis—a rare puerperal complication. Geburtshilfe Frauenheilkd 1986; 48:483.

Maull KI, VanNagell JR, Greenfield LJ. Surgical implications of ovarian vein thrombosis. Am Surg 1978; 44:727.

Munsick RA, Gillanders LA. A review of the syndrome of puerperal ovarian vein thrombophlebitis. Obstet Gynecol Survey 1981; 36:59.

Schulman H. Use of anticoagulants in suspected pelvic infection. Clin Obstet Gynecol 1969; 12:240.

Witlin AG, Sibai BM. Postpartum ovarian vein thrombosis after vaginal delivery: a report of 11 cases. Obstet Gynecol 1995; 85:775.

64

Infectious Complications Associated with Legal Termination of Pregnancy

Revised by William J. Ledger

INTRODUCTION

The legal termination of pregnancy has had a dramatic impact on the severe infectious morbidity associated with criminal abortion, but, in so doing, has introduced its own spectrum of infectious morbidity. The severity of infectious complications increases with gestational age because of the mode of termination of pregnancy that must be utilized. The primary contributing factors are those of omission or commission. The principal error of omission is the failure to monitor the patient for occult infection due to *Neisseria gonorrhoeae* or *Chlamydia trachomatis* prior to the operative procedure. The errors of commission involve primarily technical errors—failure to completely evacuate the uterus or to ensure adequate hemostasis. The infectious morbidity observed is partially dependent on the trimester in which the operative procedure is performed (Table 1).

TRIMESTER I (1–14 WEEKS)

Completed Abortion/Exogenous Pathogens

Acute endometritis/salpingitis/peritonitis due to *N. gonorrhoeae* or the group A or B beta-hemolytic streptococci may occur. In these instances, mechanical disruption of pregnancy has provided the portal of infection. Superinfection by class I and II anaerobes will ultimately occur.

Gonococcal septicemia or arthritis-cutaneous syndrome may ensue. Surgical disruption of mucosal barriers creates not just a portal of infection but also access to the intravascular compartment.

Infection due to *C. trachomatis* may be subtler in clinical presentation, with symptoms so mild, i.e., vaginal discharge, continued spotting, or minimal abdominal discomfort, that the patient may not seek medical care. Too often, the result is fallopian tube damage, which compromises the patient's future obstetrical potential.

TABLE I Infectious morbidity associated with uterine curettage

1. Superimposed due to the presence of exogenous virulent pathogen at the operative site, i.e., groups A, C, and G beta-hemolytic streptococci, *Neisseria gonorrhoeae*, *Haemophilus influenzae*, or *Chlamydia trachomatis*
2. Associated with retained products of conception
3. Surgical trauma to the uterus
    (A) Recognized surgical trauma to uterus
        (i) Midline presentation
        (ii) Lateral uterine perforation
    (B) Unrecognized surgical trauma to uterus

Septic Incomplete Abortion

The patient presents early, within 24 to 48 hours of the operative procedure, because of crampy abdominal pain. In addition to simple technical errors, frequent anatomical variations of the uterus contribute to incomplete septic abortion, e.g., septated uteri favor retained products of conception.

Lateral Wall Perforation/Cervical Tear with Extension

The uterine artery bifurcates approximately 3.8 cm from the endocervix into an ascending and descending (cervical) branch. If an endocervical tear extends to and disrupts this branch of the uterine artery, significant bleeding may occur into the broad ligament with ensuing hematoma formation. Contamination or seeding from the vaginal flora will ultimately lead to abscess formation. The first evidence of febrile morbidity manifests approximately 36 hours after operative intervention.

Central Fundal Perforation

The position of the uterus may predispose to central perforation at the fundus. This probably occurs more frequently than clinically appreciated. Usually fundal perforation is benign because it is sealed by the omentum or small bowel; however, if cesarean section is required at a later date, the operation is likely to be technically more difficult. If the suction curette has devitalized adjacent bowel, severe delayed infectious morbidity may ensue as a consequence of perforation and peritonitis or abscess formation. If the uterus is perforated with a suction curette and omental fat or bowel is observed, a laparotomy must be done to identify or exclude concomitant bowel injury.

TRIMESTER II (14–20 WEEKS)

The hysterotomy incision is comparable to that of classical cesarean section in which serum and blood can leak into the peritoneal cavity. The infectious complications are the same as those for cesarean section:

1. Endometritis/peritonitis/cellulitis septic thrombophlebitis
2. Pyometra (secondary inflammatory closure of the endocervix)
3. Uterine-wall hematoma with abscess formation
4. Abdominal wound infection

If a low vertical incision is used and the operative site is not covered with bladder and chromic gut sutures are used, small bowel obstruction has occurred in rare instances.

The use of PGF2 alpha has markedly diminished in recent years. The triad of unacceptable patient symptomatology prior to evacuation of the uterus, the delivery of a live fetus, and the frequent problems of a retained placenta, which requires operative intervention, has lessened physician enthusiasm for this procedure.

Vaginal evacuation of the unwanted pregnancy of 14 to 24 weeks is associated with fewer problems than are alternative methods, if a few caveats are observed. The physician doing the procedure must be both skilled and experienced. He or she must have access to an operating room with a competent anesthesiologist. The operation area must have competent assistants available, who do not disapprove of the procedure, and the necessary equipment needed to perform the procedures. The procedure requires the preoperative insertion of the laminaria in the cervix to permit slow dilation over time and the availability of instruments to reduce the size of fetal parts so evacuation will be complete.

Infectious problems can occur. They can be due to the presence of virulent exogenous pathogens, such as *Streptococcus pneumoniae*, the group A streptococci, *N. gonorrhoeae*, or *C. trachomatis*. Many of these pathogens can be preoperatively identified and eliminated by appropriate testing.

Most infectious problems are due to immediate tissue damage, uterus perforation with bleeding and subsequent infection, or slowly evolving infection emanating from retained products of conception.

PATHOGENESIS

Exogenous Virulent Pathogens

Infection due to exogenous virulent pathogens usually occurs within eight hours or less of the procedure. Due to the action of the group A, C, or G beta-hemolytic streptococci, the patients get very sick rapidly. The oral temperature is usually greater than 39.6°C. Pelvic examination reveals marked tenderness with little evidence of inflammatory exudate. Gram stains of the uterine swab reveal an abundance of gram-positive cocci in chains and few, if any, concomitant bacteria. Screening for *N. gonorrhoeae* in high-risk populations is advisable. Screening for *C. trachomatis* should be done for all women. If the endocervical culture is positive at the time of curettage, the infection rate for women undergoing operative termination of pregnancy increases threefold. Approximately 15% of women harboring the gonococcus at the endocervix develop postabortal infection. Some centers have addressed this problem by utilizing antibiotic prophylaxis for all women undergoing curettage. Such a policy does obviate the need for screening for *N. gonorrhoeae* in high-risk populations. The gonococcus has epidemiological significance and potential adverse consequences that extend beyond the case of a single patient. When disease is due to a superimposed virulent pathogen concomitantly present at the operative site, the initial drug of choice is a beta-lactamase–resistant third-generation cephalosporin such as ceftizoxime or cefotamine. The rationales for selective use of these antibiotics over a semisynthetic penicillin or a new-generation tetracycline are

1. that very real homage has to be paid to penicillinase-producing strains of *N. gonorrhoeae* and
2. that the tetracyclines are suboptimal antibiotics for both aerobic and anaerobic streptococci.

Antibiotic therapy should be continued until the following sought-for therapeutic response is attained:

1. No temperature equal to or greater than 37.6°C for 24 hours
2. Absence of local physical findings
3. A normal white blood cell count

Toxigenic Clostridial Infection Associated with Medical Pregnancy Termination

A medical method of terminating pregnancy in the first seven weeks' gestation has been associated with maternal death from *Clostridium sordellii* infection. The usual regimen in Europe is oral mifepristone (RU 486) 600 mg, followed by oral misoprostol at 400 or 800 mg. Some European centers have used vaginal misoprostol. This approach has been highly successful, having greater than 95% success rate with no cases of *C. sordellii* infection reported from 12,000,000 pregnancy terminations.

In the United States and Canada in which misoprostol has been administered vaginally, there have been four fatal cases of *C. sordellii* toxigenic infection. There are distinct features of *C. sordellii* toxic shock syndrome with rapid progression to death in a patient who exhibited hemoconcentration, profound leukocytosis, with or without fever. It has been a rare event, occurring in approximately one in every 1,000,000 medical terminations of pregnancy. Mortality data for other modes of pregnancy termination are not accurately recorded. This is not a clinical situation in which a prospective comparative trial can be performed. Observational studies on the use of prophylactic antibiotics with oral misoprostol will probably never provide information as to the best clinical strategies to avoid this problem.

Once these parameters have been attained, parenteral drug therapy is discontinued and the patient is discharged on per oral doxycycline 100 mg b.i.d. for seven days or given azithromycin one-gram bolus dose. One in every three women with gonococcal infection is concomitantly infected with *C. trachomatis*. If disease is due to a beta-hemolytic streptococcus, a simple four- to five-day course (500 mg t.i.d.) of per oral amoxicillin suffices and even this probably represents overkill. Even when the gonococcus is present, it is imperative to document the absence of retained products of conception.

If the patient is polymerase chain reaction positive for *C. trachomatis*, she should receive a 10- to 14-day course of doxycycline, orally.

Retained Products of Conception

The diagnosis of retained products of conception is inferred by the detection of a foul-smelling discharge. The onset of disease is usually delayed for several days. A vaginal ultrasound is helpful in detecting retained secundines within the uterine cavity. Gram stain of the endometrium reveals mixed flora amidst white blood cells. Most patients with postabortion infection due to retained products of conception respond readily to combined medical/surgical therapy. The patient is placed on a combination of antibiotics. A number of parenteral antibiotic combinations have been successful:

1. Penicillin 4 to 8 million units/24 hours and gentamicin 3 mg/kg of body weight/24 hours
2. Ampicillin/sulbactam 6 g/24 hours
3. Gentamicin 3 mg/kg of body weight/24 hours and clindamycin 2400 to 2700 mg/24 hours

A curettage is performed within four to eight hours after admission, irrespective of whether or not the patient has become afebrile from systemic antibiotic therapy. The presence of signs or symptoms following combined therapy should question the validity of the initial diagnosis. The need for continued antibiotic therapy once the anticipated therapeutic response has been attained is questionable. The use of ampicillin 500 mg q.i.d. for four to five days has been used for potential medical-legal rather than serious therapeutic considerations. Once the previously defined therapeutic end-titration points are achieved, no further antibiotic treatment is necessary. Longer courses of antibiotic administration increase the chance of an adverse drug reaction.

Unrecognized Surgical Trauma

Midline perforations of the uterus with the uterine sound in the absence of excessive bleeding in a patient whose vital signs are stable necessitate little more than careful observation. Many physicians will administer antibiotics in this clinical setting. No valid well-controlled studies support or refute the utility of prophylactic antibiotics. If antibiotics are given, the course of therapy should be relatively short. Duration of administration should be governed by temperature curve, vital signs, and physical findings. The presence of unstable vital signs or excessive bleeding warrants immediate operative evaluation. Recognized lateral uterine perforation mandates immediate laparotomy. The patient must be carefully evaluated for damage to the small or large bowel. Prophylactic administration of cefoxitin, if small bowel damage is identified, or metronidazole, if large bowel damage is identified, appears warranted on theoretical grounds. Patients presenting with unrecognized uterine damage at the time of curettage also require operative evaluation. The majority of these patients will be found to have an infected extrauterine hematoma. A rare patient will have an adnexal abscess. The use of two-drug therapy with category designation in Categories I and II is indicated. Duration of therapy postoperatively is dictated by clinical parameters.

MANAGEMENT OF THE PATIENT WITH DELAYED POSTABORTAL INFECTION

The principal differential is distinguishing those patients with retained products of conception from those with unrecognized surgical trauma to the uterus. In both situations, the onset of signs and symptoms of disease is delayed. Both subsets of patients present with fever and tender uterus. The presence of foul-smelling discharge should strongly suggest the possibility of retained products of conception, which can be confirmed by vaginal ultrasound examination. The presence of a tender pelvic mass contiguous to the uterus and an unexplained drop in the hematocrit argues for unrecognized surgical trauma to the uterus. Peritoneal signs (rebound tenderness) are rarely associated with retained products of conception unless infection due to the group A beta-hemolytic streptococci is present. Gram stain of the endometrium or cul-de-sac aspirate can readily sustain or negate this clinical possibility.

If peritoneal signs are present or the patient's condition worsens, a roentgenogram of the pelvis or a CT scan is indicated. The presence of a gas pattern in the uterine wall, the pelvis, or a local ileus is indication for surgical intervention.

If peritoneal signs are present, baseline biopsy cultures of the endometrium and aspiration culture of the cul-de-sac are recommended. Blood cultures should be done in all patients who

1. have advanced disease,
2. have peritoneal signs, and
3. have a history of rigors.

A complete blood count and differential are necessary baselines. The demonstration of asymptomatic bacteriuria warrants the concomitant use of an aminoglycoside, a third-generation cephalosporin, or a fluoroquinolone with optimal anaerobic coverage. The persistence of fever for more than 36 hours after triple therapy and uterine evacuation can be an indication for exploratory laparotomy. Metronidazole should be added to the ongoing antibiotic regimen. If fever persists, laparotomy is indicated.

If the diagnosis is that of surgical trauma, definitive therapy requires surgical intervention under antibiotic coverage. Operative vaginal termination of late pregnancy carries with it the risk of endomyometritis. If tubal ligation is done with hysterotomy, the incidence of infectious complications may be increased.

IMPACT OF THE ABORTION-ASSOCIATED INFECTION ON SUBSEQUENT FERTILITY

The common conception that subsequent fertility is significantly impaired by prior legal termination of pregnancy is difficult to substantiate on statistical grounds. When the issue of ectopic pregnancy in subsequent pregnancies has been looked at, the risk of ectopic pregnancies could not be related to abortion procedures, use of laminara, number of prior induced abortions, or the length of gestation at the time of abortion. Where an association did exist was between the presence of postabortion infection or retained

TABLE 2 Proposed criteria for the prophylactic use of antibiotics in gravidas undergoing voluntary termination of pregnancy[a]

I. Prior documentation of salpingitis or infection with *Neisseria gonorrhoeae* or *Chlamydia trachomatis*
II. Multiple sexual partners
III. Sexual consort with multiple secondary sexual partners
IV. Gravida with mucopurulent cervicitis or a significant vaginal discharge

[a]These patients should be evaluated for gonococcal and chlamydial infections. If documented, appropriate documentation of cure and treatment of sexual consorts are advocated.

secundines and ectopic pregnancies. Women with these complications have a fivefold increased risk of an ectopic pregnancy over those females without these complications within the induced abortion cohort group.

LEGAL TERMINATION OF PREGNANCY

Febrile morbidity involving women who undergo suction curettage abortion is estimated to be between 3–4%. Using a multivariate analysis, prophylactic antibiotics proved to be the most protective factor. Women who received prophylactic antibiotics and women who had previous deliveries were less likely to have febrile complications. Sawaya et al. (1996) performed a literature search of all studies published from January 1966 to September 1, 1994, using Medline, and they manually searched bibliographies of published articles. Using meta-analytic techniques on 12 studies, the authors demonstrated a substantial protective effect of antibiotics in all subgroups of women undergoing therapeutic abortion, even women in low-risk groups. They calculated that routine use of periabortal antibiotics in the United States may prevent up to half of all cases of postabortal infections. In the absence of specific contraindications, the cost of prophylaxis may be justified in high-risk populations (Table 2). Immediate prophylaxis can be achieved readily with any antibiotic with good Category I coverage (Gainesville Classification).

SELECTED READING

Burkman KT, Tonascia JA, Atienza MF, King TM. Untreated endocervical gonorrhea and endometritis following elective abortion. Am J Obstet Gynecol 1976; 126:648–651.
Cates W Jr, Grimes DA. Deaths from second trimester abortion by dilation and evacuation: causes, prevention, facilities. Obstet Gynecol 1981; 58:401.
Centers for Disease Control and Protection. *C. sordelli* toxic shock syndrome after medical abortion with miferpristone and intravaginal misoprostol—United States and Canada, 2001–2005, Morb Mortal Wkly Rep 2005; 54:724.
Cheng M, Andolsek L, Ng A, et al. Complications following induced abortion by vacuum aspiration: patient characteristics and procedures. Stud Fam Plann 1977; 8:125.
Chung CS, Smith RG, Steinhoff PG, Mi MP. Induced abortion and ectopic pregnancy in subsequent pregnancies. Am J Epidemiol 1982; 115:879.
Greene MF. Fatal infections associated with mifepristone-induced abortions. N Engl J Med 2005; 353:2317.
Grimes DA, Schulz KF, Cates W Jr, Tyler CW Jr. Midtrimester abortion by intra-amniotic prostaglandin F2-alpha. Obstet Gynecol 1977; 249:612.
Hakim-Elahi E, Tovell HM, Burnhill MS. Complications of first-trimester abortion: a report of 170,000 cases. Obstet Gynecol 1990; 76:129.
Heisterberg L. Prophylactic antibiotics in women with a history of pelvic inflammatory disease undergoing first-trimester abortion. Acta Obstet Gynecol Scand 1987; 66:15.
Megafu U. Bowel injury in septic abortion: the need for more aggressive management. Int J Gynaecol Obstet 1980; 17:450.
Moberg PJ, Eneroth P, Harlin J, et al. Preoperative cervical microbial flora and postabortion infection. Acta Obstet Gynecol Scand 1978; 57:415.
Querido L, Haspels AA. The incidence of gonorrhea in an abortion population. Contraception 1980; 22:441.
Sabbagha RE, Hayashi TT. Disseminated intravascular coagulation complicating hysterotomy in elderly gravidas. Obstet Gynecol 1971; 38:844.
Sawaya GF, Grady D, Kerlikowske K, Grimes DA. Antibiotics at the time of induced abortion: the case for universal prophylaxis based on a meta-analysis. Obstet Gynecol 1996; 87:884.
Selik RM, Cates W Jr, Tyler CW Jr. Behavioral factors contributing to abortion deaths: a new approach to mortality studies. Obstet Gynecol 1981; 58:631.
Seward PN, Ballard CA, Ulene AL. The effect of legal abortion on the rate of septic abortion at a large county hospital. Am J Obstet Gynecol 1973; 115:335.
Stallworthy JA, Moolgaoker AK, Walsh JJ. Legal abortion: a critical assessment of its risks. Lancet 1971; 2:1245.
Stubblefield PG, Monson RR, Schoenbaum SC, et al. Fertility after induced abortion: a prospective follow-up study. Obstet Gynecol 1984; 63:186.
van der Lugt B, Drogendijk A, Banffer JR. Prevalence of cervical gonorrhoeae in women with unwanted pregnancies. Br J Vener Dis 1980; 56:148.
Westrom L, Svensson L, Wolner HP, et al. A clinical double-blind study on the effect of prophylactically administered single dose tinidazole on the occurrence of endometritis after first trimester legal abortion. Scand J Infect Dis Suppl 1981; 26(Suppl):104.

Infection and Preterm Labor 65

Reinaldo Figueroa

INTRODUCTION

In 2004, 12.5% of all pregnancies in the United States resulted in preterm delivery, most of these as a result of preterm labor. Preterm labor and the resulting preterm delivery continue to be major unsolved problems in obstetrics. Although advances in the fields of obstetrics and neonatology have resulted in significant improvements in perinatal outcomes, preterm delivery is still associated with more perinatal morbidity and mortality than is any other obstetric condition.

Preterm delivery, or delivery occurring before the completion of 37 weeks of gestation, can be indicated or spontaneous. Indicated deliveries account for 20% to 30% of preterm deliveries and include medical or obstetric conditions that increase the risk for a maternal or fetal adverse outcome. Spontaneous preterm delivery includes preterm labor, preterm premature rupture of membranes (PPROM), and related conditions such as cervical incompetence or intra-amniotic infection (amnionitis). Spontaneous deliveries account for approximately 70% to 80% of all preterm deliveries.

In the United States, the preterm delivery rate has increased steadily from 9.4% in 1981 to 12.5% in 2004. Seventy percent of neonatal and infant deaths are associated with preterm birth. In the United States, the total expenditure for maternal hospitalization due to preterm labor with or without delivery has been estimated to be in excess of $820 million. Annual health care costs because of premature births are estimated to be billions of dollars for neonatal intensive care alone. During the last decade, there has been an increase in the survival of the extremely premature infant. Survival rates for neonates at 22 weeks range from 0% to 21%, at 23 weeks range from 5% to 46%, at 24 weeks range from 40% to 59%, at 25 weeks range from 60% to 82%, and at 26 weeks range from 75% to 93%. Among the survivors, 20% to 25% will have at least one major disability. Fifty percent of disabled infants will have more than one major disability. Half of all extremely premature infants will have one or more subtle neurodevelopmental disabilities in the school and teenage years.

RISK FACTORS

Epidemiologic factors that have been associated with preterm delivery include race, age (younger than 17 years or older than 35 years), low socioeconomic status, low prepregnancy weight, occupational exertion, smoking, cocaine use, vaginal bleeding in more than one trimester, uterine anomalies, uterine myomas, cervical conization, and induced abortions.

A history of preterm delivery is a significant risk factor for future preterm delivery, especially if the preterm birth occurred in the second trimester. The risk of delivering prematurely in a subsequent pregnancy is increased six- to eight-fold whether the patient had rupture of membranes or not.

Multiple gestations are responsible for an increase in the incidence of preterm deliveries. Pregnant women with multiple gestations have become an important group at risk for preterm delivery, accounting for 13% of all preterm births. It is possible that the use of assisted reproductive technologies adds to the prematurity risk of multiple gestations, although the reports are inconsistent. In singleton gestations conceived following in vitro fertilization, the risks of preterm delivery and low birth weight neonates are reported to be increased compared with pregnancies conceived spontaneously.

Intrauterine infection has also been associated with preterm labor and preterm delivery, particularly among the subset of women who have progressive labor that is ultimately refractory to tocolysis. Such intrauterine infection may be present even in the absence of clinical maternal infection and has been diagnosed by culturing amniotic fluid obtained by amniocentesis in patients with intact membrane and idiopathic preterm labor and in patients with PPROM. Elevated levels of amniotic fluid cytokines, particularly interleukin 6 (IL-6), tumor necrosis factor (TNF), and IL-1, have been found to be associated with intrauterine infection and preterm delivery.

BIOCHEMICAL MECHANISMS

Many factors are believed to trigger preterm labor. Possible mechanisms for preterm labor may include (*i*) inflammatory responses associated with infection, fevers, flares of systemic lupus erythematosus, inflammatory bowel disease, etc.; (*ii*) tissue ischemia or acidosis associated with placental insufficiency, placental abruption, fetal growth restriction, diabetic ketoacidosis, etc.; (*iii*) uterine stretching or irritation associated with multiple gestations, polyhydramnios, degenerating myomas, abdominal surgery, uterine anomalies, incompetent cervix, etc.; (*iv*) hormonal changes associated with stress, prolonged standing, or other conditions; and (*v*) idiopathic mechanisms (may include racial variation and familial increased incidence of preterm labor).

Term and preterm labor may share a common final pathway composed of uterine contractility, cervical dilatation, and activation of the membranes. Romero and colleagues (1997) have described what they call "the preterm labor syndrome" suggesting that preterm labor is a pathologic condition caused by multiple etiologies. Term labor results from multifactorial physiologic events eventually activating the components of the final common pathway. Preterm labor results from pathologic processes that activate some of the components of the term labor pathway. Both term and preterm labor are associated with an increase in uterine contractility. There is an increase in myometrial gap junction formation and upregulation of myometrial oxytocin receptors. The cervix, composed primarily of connective tissue, undergoes changes in preparation for parturition in both normal and preterm labor. The biochemical events associated with cervical ripening are a decrease in total collagen content, an increase in collagen solubility, and an increase in collagenolytic activity. Another similarity between term labor and preterm labor is activation of the decidua and membranes, which occurs through a series of biochemical and anatomic events. The membranes separate from the decidua, allowing for rupture of membranes and postpartum expulsion of the placenta. Degradation of the extracellular matrix (fibronectin) and the enzymatic activity of the matrix metalloproteinases have been implicated in decidual/membrane activation. These changes seen in human labor at term occur gradually over a period of days to weeks. Once the uterus and the cervix are prepared, endocrine or paracrine factors from the fetoplacental unit switch the irregular uterine contractions to a pattern of regular contractions. This switch in uterine contractility may be coordinated by the fetus through different mechanisms. These mechanisms include the influence of the fetus on placental steroid hormone production, the mechanical distension of the uterus, the secretion of neurohypophyseal hormones, and the stimulation of prostaglandin synthesis.

A number of pathologic conditions have been associated with preterm delivery. At least 25% of preterm births are believed to result from intra-amniotic infection. In this hostile environment to the fetus, the fetoplacental unit would trigger labor prematurely. Elevated levels of lipoxygenase and cyclooxygenase pathway products can be shown in many women with infection. Increased concentrations of cytokines in the amniotic fluid of such women have been found.

Cytokines originate from most nucleated cells and regulate a variety of physiologic functions in humans. Cytokines interact in a complex fashion, influencing the concentrations of many plasma proteins, mediating the immune response to infections, and affecting metabolism and homeostasis. Cytokines are pleiotropic and redundant; while a cytokine can have different and multiple effects depending on the specific stimuli, time, and target, multiple cytokines can have similar effects. In addition, cytokines can have both synergistic and antagonist relationships with other cytokines. Cytokines bind to specific receptors, producing a local or distal response. These receptors may be part of the tissue cell membrane or may be soluble in plasma. The biologic effects are as a result of the interaction of cytokines, cytokine receptors, and cytokine-receptor antagonists. In addition, cytokines may also interact with hormones and other cellular products to produce an effect. Therefore, the actions of cytokines are dependent on the local and systemic conditions of the human body.

Cytokines are known to mediate local and systemic effects in inflammatory responses regardless of the provoking stimuli. Cytokines such as IL-1α, IL-1β, IL-6, IL-8, and TNF have been studied in human pregnancy. Investigators have shown the presence of these cytokines in patients in preterm and term labor, but found great elevation of these cytokines in the presence of intra-amniotic infection. IL-1 has been found to be elevated in the amniotic fluid of women in preterm labor with intra-amniotic infection. IL-1 activity is a response of the host against infection. It is unrelated to preterm labor because in the absence of infection, IL-1 activity is not elevated. Similarly, TNF is not detectable in the amniotic fluid of women without intra-amniotic infection regardless of the success of tocolysis.

Investigators have also studied the presence of IL-6 and IL-8 in patients in preterm labor. Great elevations of these cytokines have been identified in the presence of intra-amniotic infection and in women who failed tocolysis with negative amniotic fluid cultures. It has been proposed that IL-6 and IL-8 are part of the host response to the microbial invasion of the uterine cavity. Higher levels of IL-6 have been found in amniotic fluid of women with severe histologic chorioamnionitis.

Cytokines may serve as mediators of labor in the presence of infection. In cases of negative amniotic fluid culture, the inflammatory reaction as evidenced by cytokine elevation can be explained by an extra-amniotic infection (deciduitis), a noninfectious inflammatory process, or an intrauterine infection that may not be detected with cultures.

INTRAUTERINE INFECTION

Clinical chorioamnionitis has been defined as maternal fever (100.4°F or higher) associated with two or more of the following manifestations: maternal tachycardia (>100 beats per minute), uterine tenderness, leukocytosis (>15,000), fetal tachycardia (>160 beats per minute), or foul-smelling vagina discharge. Clinical signs of chorioamnionitis are insensitive and are present in approximately 12% of patients in preterm labor with intact membranes that have positive amniotic fluid culture.

Intra-amniotic infection (amnionitis) should be suspected in the presence of fever of unknown origin in any patient presenting with threatened preterm labor. The patient may present in preterm labor with intact membranes and maternal symptoms suggestive of intrauterine infection or in preterm labor with intact membranes not responding to tocolysis. This subclinical intra-amniotic infection is identified as a major determinant of maternal and fetal morbidity and mortality.

It has been estimated that approximately 15% of patients presenting in preterm labor and intact membranes (without clinical evidence of infection at presentation) have positive amniotic fluid cultures. These patients are more likely to develop clinical chorioamnionitis, not to respond to tocolytic agents, and to have spontaneous rupture of their membranes than the patients in preterm labor with negative amniotic fluid culture. On the other hand, approximately 49% of patients presenting with PPROM will have positive amniotic fluid cultures.

In twins, interestingly, uterine overdistension is suspected of causing premature activation of the mechanisms responsible for the initiation of labor. Intra-amniotic infection may be a possible cause of preterm labor and delivery, since approximately 12% of twins presenting in preterm labor have had a positive amniotic fluid culture. It is possible that an ascending infection into the intrauterine cavity could result, as there is premature cervical dilatation and effacement in these pregnancies.

Women presenting with acute cervical incompetence in the second trimester have a high rate of intra-amniotic infection (50% or more positive amniotic fluid cultures). Amniocentesis before placement of rescue cerclage has been useful in identifying women who have subclinical intra-amniotic infection. Perinatal loss related to infection and preterm delivery is increased in the setting of rescue cerclage (the internal os of the cervix is dilated at least 2 cm and 50% effaced, with membranes visible at the external os by speculum examination). The chorioamniotic membranes are exposed to the microbial flora of the lower genital tract and an ascending infection may occur. The lingering question is whether intra-amniotic infection is the cause of cervical incompetence or occurs as a consequence of premature cervical dilatation and effacement.

It has been shown that the higher the rates of intra-amniotic infection and histologic chorioamnionitis, the lower the gestational age at which preterm delivery occurs.

Histologic chorioamnionitis is diagnosed based on the demonstration of polymorphonuclear leukocyte infiltration of the intervillous space below the chorionic plate, the amniotic membranes, or umbilical cord vessels. The degree of histologic chorioamnionitis may be graded according to the site of inflammation into chorioamnionitis or funisitis (umbilical cord vessels). Additionally, it may be graded based on the number of polymorphonuclear leukocytes seen per high power field on microscopic examination (significant or sparse), or based on the depth to which polymorphonuclear leukocytes have infiltrated the amnion and chorion (mild through to severe). Histologic chorioamnionitis has been associated with neonatal morbidity and mortality. Pathologic examination of the placenta, membranes, and umbilical cord has several drawbacks; the tissue is available after the event and can only be used as confirmation. Inflammatory responses are common and nonspecific and often occur in the absence of clinically relevant events. Inflammation of the placenta and membranes can be an early event preceding evidence of amniotic fluid or fetal infection; or it can mean that inflammation of the chorion, particularly around the site of membrane rupture, is inevitable. Histologic chorioamnionitis has been associated with abnormal long-term neurologic and developmental outcomes.

Preterm birth may also occur as a result of hematogenous spread of bacteria or cytokines from infected sites distant from the genitourinary tract. Some conditions associated with preterm birth are pneumonia, ruptured appendicitis with peritonitis, shigellosis, rubella, and encephalitis. Periodontal infections (severe or generalized periodontitis) have been recently implicated in the pathogenesis of preterm birth.

Pathways of Intrauterine Infection

It has been postulated that bacteria may reach the amniotic cavity and fetus by ascending from the vagina and cervix, by hematogenous spread through the placenta, by migration from the abdominal cavity through the fallopian tubes, or as a result of invasive medical procedures (amniocentesis, cordocentesis, chorionic villous sampling).

The most common pathway of intrauterine infection is bacteria ascending from the vagina and cervix subsequently colonizing the chorioamniotic membranes and decidua. Initially, there is a change in the lower genital tract microbial flora similar to bacterial vaginosis (overgrowth of facultative organisms or the presence of pathologic organisms) (stage I). Major changes occur in the biochemical properties of the vaginal fluid (pH elevation and increased concentrations of diamides, polyamines, and enzymes such as sialide, mucinases, nonspecific proteases, and phospholipases A_2 and C). During an ascending intrauterine infection, microorganisms may reach the decidua, where they stimulate a local inflammatory reaction (deciduitis) and the production of proinflammatory cytokines (stage II). This infection can extend to the chorion (chorionitis). Moreover, microorganisms may invade the fetal vessels (choriovasculitis) or cross intact fetal membranes (amnionitis) and reach the amniotic cavity, leading to an intra-amniotic infection where they elicit the production of various inflammatory mediators (stage III). Finally, microorganisms gain access to the fetus (pneumonia, otitis, conjunctivitis, omphalitis) and may directly stimulate a systemic inflammatory syndrome, characterized by elevated concentration of IL-6 and other cytokines as well as by cellular evidence of neutrophil and monocyte activation (stage IV). The fetal inflammatory response may result in multiple organ dysfunction, septic shock, and fetal death.

Microbiology of Intrauterine Infection

The bacteria most commonly involved in intrauterine infection are found in the normal vaginal flora. Many infections are polymicrobial. Bacteria cultured from amniotic fluid include *Ureaplasma urealyticum*, *Mycoplasma hominis*, *Bacteroides fragilis*, *Gardnerella vaginalis*, group B streptococcus, *Escherichia coli*, *Peptostreptococcus* species, *Candida* species, and *Lactobacillus* species.

U. urealyticum and *M. hominis* have been implicated in the pathogenesis of PPROM and preterm labor and delivery because they are frequently cultured in the amniotic fluid of women with PPROM and preterm labor with intact membranes. Mycoplasmal species are less likely than other bacterial infections to produce clinical signs of infection.

However, these organisms are important because they cause neonatal pneumonia, meningitis, sepsis, and bronchopulmonary dysplasia. On the other hand, genital colonization of *U. urealyticum* occurs in approximately 70% of pregnant women, but the evidence linking genital colonization and prematurity is inconsistent.

Bacterial vaginosis is a common alteration of the normal vaginal flora in which the normal lactobacilli-predominant flora is replaced by *G. vaginalis*, *Mobiluncus* species, anaerobes, and mycoplasmas. It has been found in 10% to 20% of pregnant women, and more frequently in African American women than in white women. Although the major symptom of bacterial vaginosis is malodorous vaginal discharge, 50% of women with bacterial vaginosis do not have symptoms.

The presence of bacterial vaginosis has been associated with spontaneous preterm delivery, mid-trimester loss, premature rupture of membranes, chorioamnionitis, and amniotic fluid colonization. Bacterial vaginosis has been associated with histologic chorioamnionitis and postpartum endometritis. Varying results have been obtained from a number of trials of screening and treatment for bacterial vaginosis in pregnant women to reduce the incidence of preterm delivery. Initial studies where women at risk for delivering prematurely were screened for bacterial vaginosis and treated with antibiotics (metronidazole/erythromycin or metronidazole alone) showed that there was a reduction in the risk of preterm birth and infectious morbidity, suggesting that treatment was beneficial. More recently, other randomized studies using vaginal clindamycin cream or 2-g doses of metronidazole have not confirmed these findings.

No benefit of treating women with asymptomatic bacterial vaginosis with two 2-g doses of metronidazole at 16 to 24 weeks' gestation and a repeat dose at 24 to 30 weeks' gestation was seen in the most recent and largest double-blinded randomized controlled trial. There was no reduction in the rates of preterm birth or other adverse neonatal outcomes. The treatment did not reduce the occurrence of preterm labor, intra-amniotic or postpartum infections, neonatal sepsis, or admissions to the neonatal intensive care unit.

Currently, the United States Preventive Services Task Force recommends that low-risk women should not be screened for bacterial vaginosis, as there is good evidence that screening and treatment of bacterial vaginosis in asymptomatic women does not improve outcomes such as preterm labor and preterm delivery. On the other hand, there is insufficient evidence to recommend screening and treating high-risk women for bacterial vaginosis because good quality studies have had conflicting results. The conflicting results of these studies could be related to the timing of administration of antibiotics as well as to the route and dosage of antibiotics. Because of the association of bacterial vaginosis with endometritis and first trimester loss, it has been suggested that the risk of preterm labor may be reduced if the women are treated in the first trimester or before conception.

MANAGEMENT OF PRETERM LABOR

Preterm labor is diagnosed between 20 and 37 weeks of gestation and in the presence of uterine contractions when, with intact membranes, cervical change is documented or if the cervix is at least 2 cm dilated or at least 80% effaced on presentation. The diagnosis is also made in the presence of uterine contractions and spontaneous rupture of the membranes.

In a preterm woman presenting with concerns of contractions or labor, monitoring of external fetal heart rate and uterine contraction is instituted. A thorough history is obtained, focusing specifically on duration of symptoms, possibility of membrane rupture, and obstetrical history. Her vital signs are recorded, looking specifically for maternal fever or tachycardia. The heart is evaluated to identify any abnormality that would not allow the use of tocolytics. The lungs are evaluated for evidence of infection or pneumonia. The uterine fundus is palpated, both to discern fetal presentation and to detect the presence of uterine tenderness, which would suggest clinical chorioamnionitis. The woman is also evaluated for pyelonephritis and suprapubic tenderness suggestive of cystitis, both of which are associated with preterm labor.

A sterile speculum examination is performed before digital examination of the cervix in all cases of possible preterm labor. If preterm rupture of the membranes is diagnosed either by grossly evident pooling of fluid in the vaginal vault or by microscopically apparent ferning in secretions obtained via swab from the vaginal vault, digital exam is deferred. In the absence of premature rupture of membranes and persistence of contractions, preterm labor is diagnosed either via initial cervical evaluation or by serial examinations over 6 to 12 hours, preferably by a single examiner. Laboratory studies should include a white blood cell count before corticosteroid administration (preterm labor is associated with a white blood cell count as high as 15,000 to 20,000; however, counts above 18,000 should raise suspicions about the presence of intra-amniotic infection), a urine specimen for microscopic evaluation along with cultures from the genital area for gonorrhea and chlamydia (cervix) and group B streptococcus (rectum and vaginal introitus). In addition, a wet smear can be useful for the diagnosis of bacterial vaginosis or trichomoniasis. If preterm labor is diagnosed, antibiotic chemoprophylaxis for group B streptococcus is administered intrapartum to prevent vertical transmission and early onset neonatal sepsis. In addition, a course of corticosteroid therapy is initiated for acceleration of fetal lung maturity.

The routine use of amniocentesis to guide management of preterm labor is controversial. Amniocentesis may be performed to search for intrauterine infection in the presence of maternal fever, without an obvious localizing source and preterm labor; or in the absence of fever, in women not responding to a first line tocolytic therapy. In addition, amniocentesis may be used for evaluation of fetal lung maturity when the gestational age is in question or when growth restriction is suspected. An amniocentesis should be performed if the results will be used to guide clinical management. The transabdominal procedure is performed in a sterile manner with ultrasonographic guidance. The amniotic fluid is then transported to the microbiology laboratory for gram stain and cultures (aerobic and anaerobic organisms, *M. hominis*, and *U. urealyticum*) and to the chemistry laboratory for determination of the leukocyte count, the glucose and lactate dehydrogenase (LDH) levels, and IL-6.

The standard for the diagnosis of intra-amniotic infection (subclinical chorioamnionitis) has been the documented presence of organisms in the amniotic fluid. The diagnosis of intrauterine infection is made by culture of amniotic fluid, but it takes at least two days before the results of the culture are available for clinical use. In the presence of infection, delivery occurs within a few days of admission to the hospital. Rapid tests have been developed to predict the presence of infection. These rapid tests include gram stain (presence of bacteria), glucose concentration (<15 mg/dL), white cell count (>50 cells/μL), LDH (>400 U/L), and IL-6 (>11.3 ng/mL). When the rapid tests suggest intra-amniotic infection, delivery should be seriously considered and broad spectrum antibiotics should be used during the intrapartum and postpartum period. In gestations less than 28 weeks with documented intra-amniotic infection, appropriate antibiotic therapy without delivery has been attempted with success. This option is considered experimental; the patient should be counseled appropriately before agreeing to accept this treatment plan.

The rapid tests used in the prediction of intra-amniotic infection can be useful but are far from ideal. The gram stain has a high sensitivity (up to 80%) and a low false positive rate in the prediction of intrauterine infection with aerobic or anaerobic organisms. However, the sensitivity of the gram stain is only 20% to 50% in studies where the Mycoplasma species were cultured because the gram stain does not identify them. Many organisms use glucose as a substrate, therefore, in the presence of infection, the amniotic fluid concentration of glucose is often low. However, the sensitivity of this test can be low (60% to 70%) because glucose metabolism may be organism dependent. Intra-amniotic infection in preterm labor produces a significant elevation in amniotic fluid LDH concentration. In the presence of infection, elevation of LDH level in amniotic fluid results from increased leukocyte activity. Noninfectious causes of preterm labor can include small separations of the placenta or degenerating leiomyomata. Separation of the placenta releases erythrocytes rich in cytoplasmic LDH that after lysis elevates amniotic fluid LDH concentrations. Smooth muscle, which also has a high cytoplasmic LDH concentration, increases amniotic fluid LDH if undergoing necrotic degeneration. Noninfectious sources of elevated LDH may explain why this amniotic fluid marker has a sensitivity of 69% in the prediction of preterm delivery. Measurement of the cytokine IL-6, a mediator of the host response to infection and inflammation, has a reported 66% to 100% sensitivity and 83% to 87% specificity in prediction of a positive amniotic fluid culture.

Only when preterm labor is diagnosed is consideration given to the use of tocolytic therapy. Because tocolytic therapy may result in untoward maternal and fetal effects, use of tocolytics should be limited to women in true preterm labor at high risk for spontaneous birth. The risk and benefits of tocolytic therapy must be considered balancing, for example, the negligible improvements in perinatal morbidity and mortality in the face of pulmonary maturity at 34 weeks or more against the side effects of tocolytic agents. Evaluation of the patient for contraindications to the use of tocolytics in general or to the use of specific tocolytic agents is then undertaken. Such contraindications include fetal death, fetal distress when immediate delivery would improve the fetal outcome, or severe fetal malformation. In addition, if maternal infection is present, appropriate antibiotic therapy should be initiated. If the patient is in preterm labor and clinical chorioamnionitis is diagnosed, tocolytic agents should not be started. If the patient is already receiving tocolytic agents, the medication should be discontinued if there is evidence of intra-amniotic infection by amniotic fluid studies (in the case of subclinical intra-amniotic infection) or clinical chorioamnionitis.

Neither the biophysical profile score nor fetal heart rate patterns provide sensitive prediction of intrauterine infection even though studies in patients with PPROM suggest that decreased fetal breathing movements and gross body movements are associated with infection and preterm labor. Similarly, although oligohydramnios in patients with PPROM is associated with a higher incidence of intra-amniotic infection, the assessment of amniotic fluid does not provide a sensitive prediction of intrauterine infection. Additionally, intra-amniotic infection has not been associated with a major degree of vasoconstriction in the uteroplacental or fetoplacental circulation. Therefore, Doppler studies have not provided a clinically useful distinction between infected and noninfected patients. The use of cordocentesis in patients with PPROM or in preterm labor with intact membranes is considered experimental and not clinically useful at this time.

ASSESSMENT OF RISK FACTORS FOR PRETERM LABOR

A significant amount of research has been done, attempting to allow for the early diagnosis of preterm labor and to predict those women who are at the highest risk for developing preterm labor. This could allow the institution of more intensive preterm labor surveillance programs for the pregnancies found to be at increased risk. In predicting whether a woman is at risk of preterm delivery, there is the hope that an intervention will be available to diagnose preterm labor earlier to improve the effectiveness of treatment (delaying delivery) and to improve the neonatal outcome. For example, an important intervention is the opportunity to administer maternal corticosteroid therapy as recommended by the National Institute of Health because it is strongly associated with decreased morbidity and mortality. Tocolytic therapy can be given to the mother to prolong pregnancy so that corticosteroids can be administered.

Risk scoring systems based on historic and epidemiologic information have been designed to determine the risk of preterm delivery. These systems were intended as screening profiles, to stratify women within the general population into high-risk and low-risk groups for preterm delivery, so that high-risk patients could be followed in a more intensive manner during their pregnancies. In general, they have been unable to reliably identify women who will give birth preterm. Since approximately 50% of preterm deliveries occur in a first pregnancy, this single limitation of risk-factor scoring systems renders them particularly ineffective. The low sensitivity of the systems used in these studies shows that up to 70% of women who ultimately deliver before term may not be categorized. The low positive predictive values imply that three-quarters of women categorized "high risk" will eventually have term deliveries and they would not only be categorized incorrectly but also be subjected unnecessarily to potentially costly intervention programs.

Fetal fibronectin is a glycoprotein found in plasma and in the extracellular matrix. It is produced by a variety of cell types including the fetal membranes, and it functions as an adhesion binder of the placenta and membranes to the decidua. It is normally present in cervical and vaginal secretions until 16 to 20 weeks of gestation. It can also be detected in cervicovaginal secretions in term pregnancies with intact membranes suggesting its appearance may be related to the birth process. A number of trials have shown an association with the presence of fetal fibronectin between 20 and 34 weeks and preterm birth. In addition, the risk of preterm birth when the test result is negative is low. It is believed that fetal fibronectin is a marker for the disruption of the chorioamnion and underlying decidua due to inflammation or infection. A positive fetal fibronectin test in the mid-trimester has been associated with subsequently diagnosed chorioamnionitis. A meta-analysis by Leitich, Egarter, and coworkers (1999) concluded that the presence of fetal fibronectin in vaginal or cervical secretions is a moderate predictor of preterm birth with a sensitivity of 61% and a specificity of 83% when the outcome studied is delivery at less than 34 weeks of gestation. When the relationships between fetal fibronectin, a short cervix, presence of bacterial vaginosis, and traditional risk factors for spontaneous preterm birth were analyzed, it was found that the most significant associations with preterm birth were a positive fetal fibronectin test, a cervical length less than 25 mm, and a history of preterm birth. The usefulness of the fetal fibronectin test appears to be lying on its negative predictive value because it helps in reducing unnecessary interventions in symptomatic women. A woman with a negative test result has more than 95% chance of not delivering within the next 14 days. There is no effective intervention available to reduce the preterm birth risk on a woman with a positive fetal fibronectin test. Antibiotic treatment for women with a positive fetal fibronectin test cannot be recommended because the randomized trial of metronidazole and erythromycin or placebo given to asymptomatic patients with a positive fetal fibronectin did not show a difference in preterm delivery.

Transvaginal ultrasound has been shown to be more accurate than transabdominal ultrasound or digital exam in assessing the length of the cervix. In 1996, Lams and colleagues showed an association between cervical length and preterm delivery in a prospective blinded trial. The normal distribution of cervical length in pregnancy after 22 weeks of gestation was established and women with progressively shorter cervices experienced increased rates of preterm delivery. The association of cervical shortening with preterm delivery has been confirmed by other studies. Unfortunately, the performance of the test has varied widely. Leitich, Brunbauer, and coworkers (1999) performed a systematic review of 35 studies using cervical length to predict preterm delivery. The test was found to have sensitivities ranging from 68% to 100% with specificities from 44% to 79%. Guzman and Ananth (2001) reviewed seven major studies in low- and high-risk populations. For deliveries before 32 weeks' gestation, the sensitivities range from 11% to 82% and the positive predictive values from 11% to 52%. Higher sensitivities for the test were obtained in high-risk patients, especially the women with a history of mid-trimester loss. The use of cervical length measurement by transvaginal ultrasound in combination with other methods of screening has been documented. A short cervix defined as less than 25 mm, particularly if associated with a positive fetal fibronectin result, was found to be a strong predictor of preterm birth. The sequential use of cervical length and fetal fibronectin has been tried to stratify risk groups and discern the etiology of preterm birth. The presence of either a cervix less than 25 mm in length at less than 35 weeks of gestation or a positive fetal fibronectin result was strongly associated with preterm birth, especially in women with a history of preterm birth. A short cervix may be the only manifestation of intra-amniotic infection. It has not been established that the detection of a short cervix improves pregnancy outcome, therefore the optimal management of these patients has not been established.

MEASURES IN PREVENTING PRETERM DELIVERIES

Once premature labor has started, several interventions have been used to stop it. Initially, bed rest and hydration are instituted to improve circulation and treat dehydration. When the decision to start tocolytic therapy has been made, different pharmacologic agents may be used. The purpose for the use of tocolytics should be to delay delivery with the hope of improving neonatal outcomes. It has been recognized that tocolytic agents stop contractions and do not treat the condition causing preterm labor. Ideally, in order to prevent preterm delivery the condition initiating the preterm labor must be treated. Specific benefits that may be achieved by delaying the delivery are improvement in neonatal outcome by the administration of corticosteroid therapy, transfer of the mother to a tertiary care facility, and allowing time for other treatments to work (i.e., antibiotics if chorioamnionitis is suspected).

To justify the use of aggressive tocolysis to prolong pregnancy and improve neonatal outcome, the following factors need to be taken into consideration: the likelihood of neonatal survival and morbidity at the initiation of therapy, the likely prolongation of pregnancy from the time of diagnosing preterm labor, and improvement in neonatal outcome at the time delivery is either imminent or permitted. There is a growing body of evidence associating complications of pregnancy such as intrauterine infection, growth restriction, and placental abruption to preterm delivery. Fetal infection has been recognized as an etiologic factor of cerebral palsy. If a suboptimal or hostile environment is associated with preterm delivery, then successful tocolysis might place the fetus at risk for further growth impairment or death.

Underlying infections are treated with antibiotics to decrease the effect of infection as a source of tissue necrosis and cytokine release. Infections of the lower genital tract have been associated with preterm delivery. It is believed that colonization of the lower genital tract may serve as a marker of upper genital tract infection or may lead to direct migration of organisms to the decidua, fetal membranes, and amniotic fluid. During their prenatal care, women should be screened for gonorrhea and chlamydia and treated, if positive, to prevent spread to sexual partners and the newborn. In addition, treatment may improve the pregnancy outcome as it has been shown in nonrandomized trials.

Screening and treatment for asymptomatic bacteriuria has been standard practice to prevent pyelonephritis. An association between asymptomatic bacteriuria and preterm delivery has been shown. Antibiotic treatment of asymptomatic bacteriuria reduces the risk of preterm birth. Trichomoniasis has been shown to increase the risk of preterm birth. There are no randomized studies to support its treatment to prevent preterm birth. Two recent trials found an increased risk of preterm birth in the treated group. Symptomatic patients should be treated for trichomoniasis, but asymptomatic patients should not be screened for trichomoniasis for the purpose of reducing the risk of preterm birth. Bacterial vaginosis (discussed earlier) has been associated with preterm delivery or low birth weight infants. Routine screening of women at high risk for preterm delivery is controversial. The United States Preventive Services Task Force concluded that the evidence was insufficient to recommend for or against routinely screening high-risk pregnant women for bacterial vaginosis. Asymptomatic women at low risk of preterm delivery should not be screened for bacterial vaginosis based on evidence from the literature. Genital tract colonization of mycoplasmas has not been associated with preterm delivery; therefore, treatment for the purpose of decreasing the risk of preterm delivery is not indicated. Finally, genital colonization of group B streptococcus should not be treated during the antepartum period, as it has not been shown to be effective in preventing preterm delivery or decreasing the risk of early neonatal sepsis.

Routine use of antibiotics for pregnancy prolongation in preterm labor with intact membranes is not indicated because published studies have not shown a benefit consistently. In addition, the rates of chorioamnionitis, endometritis, maternal infection, neonatal pneumonia or sepsis, necrotizing enterocolitis, and neonatal death did not decrease by the use of antibiotics. In patients in preterm labor with intact membranes, antibiotics should be given as prophylaxis to prevent neonatal sepsis by group B streptococcus. In patients with premature rupture of membranes, antibiotics may be given, in addition to prevent group B streptococcal sepsis, to prolong pregnancy and decrease complications.

In most cases, antibiotics are ineffective in preventing preterm delivery. It is possible that infections and preterm birth do not share a causal relationship but represent markers of an underlying condition. Alternatively, it is also likely that, once the patient is in preterm labor, the inflammation has progressed too far for antibiotics to be useful.

FETAL INFECTIONS AND NEONATAL OUTCOME

As improvements in neonatal care have made quality survival possible at earlier gestational ages, attention has centered on prolonging preterm gestation at the earlier limits of viability. There appears to be significant neonatal benefit in prolonging pregnancy by as little as one week in the period from 24 to 26 weeks. Even smaller delays in delivery in this period can significantly improve survival. In addition, since infants with very low birth weight appear to do better overall than do those transported to a tertiary neonatal center, it can be argued that even short-term tocolytic success that allows maternal transport to an appropriate center for delivery is warranted by improved neonatal outcome.

Recent information from the Neonatal Research Network of the National Institute of Child Health and Human Development reveals that the neonatal survival rate increases from 0% at 21 weeks of gestation to 75% at 25 weeks of gestation. In addition, neonatal survival increases from 11% at birth weights 401 to 500 g to 75% at birth weights 701 to 800 g. Unfortunately, neonatal morbidity in the form of intraventricular hemorrhage (IVH), periventricular leucomalacia (PVL), chronic lung disease, necrotizing enterocolitis, nosocomial infections, and retinopathy of prematurity contributes to the significant number of extremely premature neonates with disabilities in mental and psychomotor development, neuromotor function, or sensory and communication function.

The prevalence of neonatal sepsis is 4.3 per 1000 live births in premature births compared with 0.8 per 1000 live births for term infants. The lower the birth weight, the higher the prevalence of sepsis. The higher incidence of sepsis in the preterm newborn is partially attributable to the higher incidence of intra-amniotic infection in women in preterm labor with intact membranes and with PPROM.

With improved care in neonatal intensive care units, survival figures for the low birth weight neonate have improved, and long-term neurologic compromise becomes a major concern. PVL is regarded as a reliable predictor of neurologic damage, with estimates ranging from 8% in echodense-persistent lesions to 100% in extensive-cystic lesions. The consequences of IVH are less predictable. IVH grades 1 and 2 are associated with minor deficits, if any; grade 3 and 4 hemorrhages are associated with major sequelae in 30% of cases. Where IVH and PVL coexist, the outcome is dependent on the type of PVL. Chorioamnionitis has been implicated as an obstetrical antecedent of PVL and major IVH. It has been shown that PVL and major IVH occur predominantly in pregnancies delivered prematurely after preterm labor or premature rupture of membranes and rarely in pregnancies delivered prematurely for medical indications. Important neonatal morbidity and mortality have been associated with elevated levels of amniotic fluid IL-6. The significance of amniotic fluid IL-6, umbilical cord plasma IL-6, and neonatal brain injury, represented by PVL, has been described.

Infection has been associated with the development of central nervous system abnormalities in animals and humans. Cytokines have been shown to be produced by brain cells. Whereas normal brain cell growth and differentiation are dependent on production of cytokines in small amounts, higher levels can cause destruction of brain tissue. Endotoxinemia and infection of the central nervous system are known to provoke the formation of TNF and IL-1, which in turn initiate the secretion of IL-6. Hypoxia-reoxygenation of brain tissue and endothelium induces IL-6. High levels of TNF and IL-1 may cause brain damage by their direct neurotoxic and myelotoxic properties. Alternatively, these cytokines cause hypotension and, in the absence of autoregulatory control in the preterm fetus or neonate, would result in hypoperfusion and ischemia of susceptible areas of the periventricular white matter resulting in PVL.

The fetal systemic inflammatory response syndrome is the fetal immune response to intra-amniotic infection resulting in preterm labor, growth restriction, severe neonatal morbidity, brain injury, and chronic lung disease in the neonate. The placental histologic manifestations of this syndrome are funisitis and chorionic vasculitis. This implies that multiple pathologic processes begin before birth in a group of preterm neonates.

SELECTED READING

Allbert JR, Naef RW, Perry KG, et al. Amniotic fluid interleukin-6 and interleukin-8 levels predict the success of tocolysis in patients with preterm labor. J Soc Gynecol Invest 1994; 1:264.

American College of Obstetricians and Gynecologists Committee on Obstetric Practice. Prevention of early-onset group B streptococcal disease in newborns. American College of Obstetricians and Gynecologists Committee Opinion #279, Washington, DC, December 2002. Obstet Gynecol 2002; 100:1405.

American College of Obstetricians and Gynecologists Committee on Practice Bulletins. Perinatal care at the threshold of viability. American College of Obstetricians and Gynecologists Practice Bulletin #38, Washington, DC, September 2002. Obstet Gynecol 2002; 100:617.

Andersen HF. Use of fetal fibronectin in women at risk for preterm delivery. Clin Obstet Gynecol 2000; 43:746.

Arias F, Rodriguez L, Rayne SC, et al. Maternal placental vasculopathy and infection: two distinct subgroups among patients with preterm labor and preterm ruptured membranes. Am J Obstet Gynecol 1993; 160:585.

Bobbit JR, Hayslip CC, Damato JD. Amniotic fluid infection as determined by transabdominal amniocentesis in patients with intact membranes in premature labor. Am J Obstet Gynecol 1981; 140:947.

Bobitt JR, Ledger WJ. Unrecognized amnionitis and prematurity: a preliminary report. J Reprod Med 1977; 19:8.

Bobbitt JR, Ledger WJ. Amniotic fluid analysis: its role in maternal and neonatal infection. Obstet Gynecol 1978; 51:56.

Brocklehurst P, Hannah M, McDonald H. Interventions for treating bacterial vaginosis in pregnancy (Cochrane Review). In: The Cochrane Library, Issue 2, 2001. Oxford: Update Software.

Carey JC, Klebanoff MA, Hauth JC, et al. Metronidazole to prevent preterm delivery in pregnant women with asymptomatic bacterial vaginosis. N Engl J Med 2000; 342:534.

Challis JRG, Gibb W. Control of parturition. Prenat Neonat Med 1996; 1:283.

Colombo DF, Iams JD. Cervical length and preterm labor. Clin Obstet Gynecol 2000; 43:735.

Copper RL, Goldenberg RL, Creasy RK, et al. A multicenter study of preterm birth weight and gestational age-specific neonatal mortality. Am J Obstet Gynecol 1993; 168:78.

Coultrip LL, Lien JM, Gomez R, et al. The value of amniotic fluid interleukin-6 determination patients with preterm labor and intact membranes in the detection of microbial invasion of the amniotic cavity. Am J Obstet Gynecol 1994; 171:901.

Creasy RK, Iams JD. Preterm labor and delivery. In: Creasy RK, Resnik R, eds. Maternal-Fetal Medicine: Principles and Practice. 4th ed. Philadelphia: WB Saunders, 1999.

Dudley DJ. Pre-term labor: an intra-uterine inflammatory response syndrome? J Reprod Immunol 1997; 36:93.

Duff P, Kopelman JN. Subclinical intra-amniotic infection in asymptomatic patients with refractory preterm labor. Obstet Gynecol 1987; 69:756.

Dunlow S, Duff P. Microbiology of the lower genital tract and amniotic fluid in asymptomatic preterm patients with intact membranes and moderate to advanced degrees of cervical effacement and dilatation. Am J Perinatol 1990; 7:235.

Foulon W, Van Liedekerke D, Demanet C, et al. Markers of infection and their relationship to preterm delivery. Am J Perinatol 1995; 12:208.

Garry D, Figueroa R, Aguero-Rosenfeld M, et al. A comparison of rapid amniotic fluid markers in the prediction of microbial invasion of the uterine cavity and preterm delivery. Am J Obstet Gynecol 1996; 175:1336.

Gibbs RS, Romero R, Hillier SL. A review of premature birth and subclinical infection. Am J Obstet Gynecol 1992; 166:1515.

Goldenberg RL, Hauth JC, Andrews WW. Intrauterine infection and preterm delivery. N Engl J Med 2000; 342:1500.

Goldenberg RL, Iams JD, Das A, et al. The preterm prediction study: sequential cervical length and fetal fibronectin testing for the prediction of spontaneous preterm birth. Am J Obstet Gynecol 2000; 182:636.

Goldenberg RL, Mercer BM, Iams JD, et al. The preterm prediction study: patterns of cervicovaginal fetal fibronectin as predictors of spontaneous preterm delivery. Am J Obstet Gynecol 1997; 177:8.

Goldenberg RL, Rouse DJ. Prevention of premature birth. N Engl J Med 1998; 339:313.

Goldenberg RL, Thom E, Moawad AH, et al. The preterm prediction study: fetal fibronectin, bacterial vaginosis, and peripartum infection. Obstet Gynecol 1996; 87:656.

Gomez R, Ghezzi F, Romero, et al. Premature labor and IAI. Clinical aspects and role of the cytokines in diagnosis and pathophysiology. Clin Perinatol 1995; 22:281.

Gomez R, Romero R, Ghezzi F, et al. The fetal inflammatory response syndrome. Am J Obstet Gynecol 1998; 179:194.

Guise JM, Mahon SM, Aickin M, et al. Screening for bacterial vaginosis in pregnancy. Systematic evidence review. Pub No. AHRQ01-S001. Rockville, MD: Agency for Healthcare Research and Quality, 2001.

Guzick D, Winn K. The association of chorioamnionitis with preterm delivery. Obstet Gynecol 1985; 65:11.

Guzman ER, Ananth CV. Cervical length and spontaneous prematurity: laying the foundation for future interventional randomized trials for the short cervix. Ultrasound Obstet Gynecol 2001; 18:195.

Hameed C, Tejani N, Verma UL, et al. Silent chorioamnionitis as a cause of preterm labor refractory to tocolytic therapy. Am J Obstet Gynecol 1984; 149:726.

Hassan SS, Romero R, Berry SM, et al. Patients with an ultrasonographic cervical length < or = 15 mm have nearly a 50% risk of early spontaneous preterm delivery. Am J Obstet Gynecol 2000; 182:1458.

Hassan SS, Romero R, Maymon E, et al. Does cervical cerclage prevent preterm delivery in patients with a short cervix? Am J Obstet Gynecol 2001; 184:1325.

Hauth JC, Goldenberg RL, Andrews WW, et al. Reduced incidence of preterm delivery with metronidazole and erythromycin in women with bacterial vaginosis. N Engl J Med 1995; 333:1732.

Hay PE, Lamont RF, Taylor-Robinson D, et al. Abnormal bacterial colonization of the genital tract and subsequent preterm delivery and late miscarriage. Brit Med J 1994; 308:295.

Hermansen MC, Hermansen MG. Perinatal infection and cerebral palsy. Clin Perinatol 2006; 33:315.

Hillier SL, Nugent RP, Eschenbach DA, et al. Association between bacterial vaginosis and preterm delivery of a low-birth-weight-infant. N Engl J Med 1995; 333:1737.

Hillier SL, Witkin SS, Krohn MA, et al. The relationship of amniotic fluid cytokines and preterm delivery, amniotic fluid infection, histologic chorioamnionitis, and chorioamnion infection. Obstet Gynecol 1993; 81:941.

Hitti J, Tarczy-Hornoch P, Murphy J, et al. Amniotic fluid infection, cytokines, and adverse outcome among infants at 34 weeks' gestation or less. Obstet Gynecol 2001; 98:1080.

Iams JD, Goldenberg RL, Meis PJ, et al. The length of the cervix and the risk of spontaneous premature delivery. N Engl J Med 1996; 334:567.

Ianucci TA, Tomich PG, Gianopoulos JG. Etiology and outcome of extremely low-birth weight infants. Am J Obstet Gynecol 1996; 174:1896.

Inglis SR, Jeremias J, Kuno K, et al. Detection of tumor necrosis factor-alpha, interlukin-6, and fetal fibronectin in the lower genital tract during pregnancy: relation to outcome. Am J Obstet Gynecol 1994; 171:5.

Joesoef MR, Hillier SL, Wiknjosastro G, et al. Intravaginal clindamycin treatment for bacterial vaginosis: effects on preterm delivery and low birth weight. Am J Obstet Gynecol 1995; 173:1527.

Kekki M, Kurki T, Pelkonen J, et al. Vaginal clindamycin in preventing preterm birth and peripartal infections in asymptomatic women with bacterial vaginosis: a randomized, controlled trial. Obstet Gynecol 2001; 97:643.

Kenyon SL, Taylor DJ, Tarnow-Mordi W. Broad-spectrum antibiotics for spontaneous preterm labour: the ORACLE II randomised trial. Lancet 2001; 357:989.

Kirshon B, Rosenfeld B, Mari G, Belfort M. Amniotic fluid glucose and intraamniotic infection. Am J Obstet Gynecol 1991; 164:818.

Klein LL, Gibbs RS. Infection and preterm birth. Obstet Gynecol N Am 2005; 32:397.

Korn AP, Bolan G, Padian N, et al. Plasma cell endometritis in women with symptomatic bacterial vaginosis. Obstet Gynecol 1995; 85:387.

Kurki T, Sivonen A, Renkonen OV, et al. Bacterial vaginosis in early pregnancy and pregnancy outcome. Obstet Gynecol 1992; 80:173.

Kurkinen R, Vuopala S, Koskela M, et al. A randomised controlled trial of vaginal clindamycin for early pregnancy bacterial vaginosis. Br J Obstet Gynaecol 2000; 107:1427.

Leitich H, Brunbauer M, Kaider A, et al. Cervical length and dilatation of the internal cervical os detected by vaginal ultrasonography as markers for preterm delivery: a systematic review. Am J Obstet Gynecol 1999; 181:1465.

Leitich H, Egarter C, Kaider A, et al. Cervicovaginal fetal fibronectin as a marker for preterm delivery: a meta-analysis. Am J Obstet Gynecol 1999; 180:1169.

Lemons JA, Bauer CR, Oh W, et al. Very low birth weight outcomes of the National Institute of Child Health and Human Development Neonatal Research Network, January 1995 through December 1996. Pediatrics 2001; 107:E1.

Llahi-Camp JM, Rai R, Ison C, et al. Association of bacterial vaginosis with a history of second trimester miscarriage. Hum Reprod 1996; 11:1575.

Locksmith G, Duff P. Infection, antibiotics, and preterm delivery. Semin Perinatol 25:295, 2001.

Lockwood CJ, Senyei AE, Dische MR, et al. Fetal fibronectin in cervical and vaginal secretions as predictor of preterm delivery. N Engl J Med 1991; 325:669.

Lorenz JM. The outcome of extreme prematurity. Semin Perinatol 2001; 25:348.

Martinez E, Figueroa R, Garry D, et al. Elevated amniotic fluid interleukin-6 as a predictor of neonatal periventricular leukomalacia and intraventricular hemorrhage. J Matern Fetal Invest 1998; 8:101.

Martius J, Roos T. The role of urogenital tract infections in the etiology of preterm births. A review. Arch Gynecol Obstet 1996; 258:1.

Maymon E, Romero R, Pacora P, et al. Evidence for the participation of interstitial collagenase (matrix metalloproteinase 1) in preterm premature rupture of membranes. Am J Obstet Gynecol 2000; 183:914.

McGregor JA, French JI, Parker R, et al. Prevention of premature birth by screening and treatment for common genital tract infections: result of a prospective controlled evaluation. Am J Obstet Gynecol 1995; 173:157.

Meis PJ, Goldenberg RL, Mercer B, et al. The preterm prediction study: significance of vaginal infections. Am J Obstet Gynecol 1995; 173:1231.

Minkoff H, Grunebaum AN, Schwarz RH, et al. Risk factors for prematurity and premature rupture of membranes: a prospective study of the vaginal flora in pregnancy. Am J Obstet Gynecol 1984; 150:965.

Morales WJ, Schorr S, Albritton J. Effect of metronidazole in patients with preterm birth in preceding pregnancy and bacterial vaginosis: a placebo-controlled, double-blind study. Am J Obstet Gynecol 1994; 171:345.

Negishi H, Yamada H, Mikuni M, et al. Correlation between cytokine levels of amniotic fluid and histological chorioamnionitis in preterm delivery. J Perinatal Med 1996; 24:633.

Newton ER. Preterm labor, preterm premature rupture of membranes, and chorioamnionitis. Clin Perinatol 2005; 32:571.

Nicholson WK, Frick KD, Powe NR. Economic burden of hospitalizations for preterm labor in the United States. Obstet Gynecol 2000; 96:95.

Norwitz ER, Robinson JN. A systematic approach to the management of preterm labor. Semin Perinatol 2001; 25:223.

Norwitz ER, Robinson JN, Challis JR. The control of labor. N Engl J Med 1999; 341:660.

Pacora P, Chaiworapongsa T, Maymon E, et al. Funisitis and chorionic vasculitis: the histological counterpart of the fetal inflammatory response syndrome. J Matern Fetal Med 2002; 11:18.

Potter NT, Kosuda L, Bigazzi PE, et al. Relationships among cytokines (IL-1, TNF, and IL-8) and histologic markers of acute ascending intrauterine infection. J Matern-Fetal Med 1992; 1:142.

Ralph SG, Rutherford AJ, Wilson JD. Influence of bacterial vaginosis on conception and miscarriage in the first trimester: cohort study. Brit Med J 1999; 319:220.

Robinson JN, Regan JA, Norwitz ER. The epidemiology of preterm labor. Sem Perin 2001; 25:204.

Romero R, Avila C, Brekus CA, et al. The role of systemic and intrauterine infection in pre-term parturition. Ann N Y Acad Sci 1991; 662:355.

Romero R, Avila C, Santhanam U, et al. Amniotic fluid interleukin 6 in preterm labor. J Clin Invest 1990; 85:1392.

Romero R, Brody DT, Oyarzun E, et al. Infection and labor. III. Interleukin-1: a signal for the onset of parturition. Am J Obstet Gynecol 1989; 160:1117.

Romero R, Ceska M, Avila C, et al. Neutrophil attractant/activating peptide-1/interleukin-8 in term and preterm parturition. Am J Obstet Gynecol 1991; 165:813.

Romero R, Emamian M, Quintero R, et al. The value and limitations of the Gram stain examination in the diagnosis of intraamniotic infection. Am J Obstet Gynecol 1988; 159:114.

Romero R, Emamian M, Wan M, et al. Prostaglandin concentrations in amniotic fluid of women with intraamniotic infection and preterm labor. Am J Obstet Gynecol 1987; 157:1461.

Romero R, Gomez R, Ghezzi F, et al. A fetal systemic inflammatory response is followed by the spontaneous onset of preterm parturition. Am J Obstet Gynecol 1998; 179:186.

Romero R, Gomez R, Mazor M, et al. The preterm labor syndrome. In: Elder MG, Romero R, Lamont RF, eds. Preterm Labor. New York: Churchill Livingstone, 1997.

Romero R, Jimenez C, Lohda AK, et al. Amniotic fluid glucose concentration: a rapid and simple method for detection of intraamniotic infection in preterm labor. Am J Obstet Gynecol 1990; 163:968.

Romero R, Manogue KR, Mitchell MD, et al. Infection and labor. IV. Cachetin-tumor necrosis factor in the amniotic fluid of women with intraamniotic infection and preterm labor. Am J Obstet Gynecol 1989; 161:336.

Romero R, Mazor M, Sepulveda W, et al. Tumor necrosis factor in term and preterm labor. Am J Obstet Gynecol 1992; 166:1576.

Romero R, Munoz H, Gomez R, et al. Increase in prostaglandin bioavailability precedes the onset of human parturition. Prostaglandins Leukotrienes Essent Fatty Acids 1996; 54:187.

Romero R, Oyarzun E, Mazor M, et al. Meta-analysis of the relationship between asymptomatic bacteriuria and preterm delivery/low birth weight. Obstet Gynecol 1989; 73:576.

Romero R, Sibai B, Caritis S, et al. Antibiotic treatment of preterm labor with intact membranes: a multicenter, randomized, double-blinded, placebo-controlled trial. Am J Obstet Gynecol 1993; 169:764.

Romero R, Sirtori M, Oyarzun E, et al. Infection and labor. V. Prevalence, microbiology, and clinical significance of intraamniotic infection in women with preterm labor and intact membranes. Am J Obstet Gynecol 1989; 161:817.

Romero R, Yoon BH, Mazor M, et al. A comparative study of the diagnostic performance of amniotic fluid glucose, white blood cell count, interleukin-6, and Gram stain in the detection of microbial invasion in patients with preterm premature rupture of membranes. Am J Obstet Gynecol 1993; 169:839.

Romero R, Yoon BH, Mazor M, et al. The diagnostic and prognostic value of amniotic fluid white blood cell count, glucose, interleukin-6, and gram stain in patients with preterm labor and intact membranes. Am J Obstet Gynecol 1993; 169:805.

Sarto S, Kasahara T, Kato Y, et al. Elevation of amniotic fluid interleukin 6 (IL-6), IL-8, and granulocyte colony stimulating factor (G_CSF) in term and preterm parturition. Cytokine 1993; 5:81.

Silver HM, Sperling RS, Gibbs RS. Evidence relating bacterial vaginosis to intraamniotic infection. Am J Obstet Gynecol 1989; 161:808.

Skoll MA, Moretti ML, Sibai BM. The incidence of positive amniotic fluid cultures in patients in preterm labor with intact membranes. Am J Obstet Gynecol 1989; 161:813.

Tsuda A, Ikegami T, Hirano H, et al. The relationship between amniotic fluid interleukin-6 concentration and histologic evidence of chorioamnionitis. Acta Obstet Gynecol Scan 1998; 77:515.

Ugwumadu AHN. Bacterial vaginosis in pregnancy. Curr Opin Obstet Gynecol 2002; 14:115.

Watts DH, Krohn MA, Hillier SL, et al. The association of occult amniotic fluid infection with gestational age and neonatal outcome among women in preterm labor. Obstet Gynecol 1992; 79:351.

Welsh A, Nicolaides K. Cervical screening for preterm delivery. Curr Opin Obstet Gyncol 2002; 14:195.

Yoon BH, Jun JK, Romero R, et al. Amniotic fluid inflammatory cytokines (interleukin-6, interleukin-1β, and tumor necrosis factor-α), neonatal brain white matter lesions, and cerebral palsy. Am J Obstet Gynecol 1997; 177:19.

Yoon BH, Romero R, Kim CJ, et al. Amniotic fluid interleukin-6: a sensitive test for antenatal diagnosis of acute inflammatory lesions of preterm placenta and prediction of perinatal morbidity. Am J Obstet Gynecol 1995; 172:960.

Yoon BH, Romero R, Kim CJ, et al. High expression of tumor necrosis factor-α and interleukin-6 in periventricular leukomalacia. Am J Obstet Gynecol 1997; 177:406.

Yoon BH, Romero R, Moon JB, et al. Clinical significance of intraamniotic inflammation in patients with preterm labor and intact membranes. Am J Obstet Gynecol 2001; 185:1130.

Appendicitis is the most common cause of an acute abdomen pain in women. Its incidence in women of child-bearing age is not altered by pregnancy. The disease appears to be more common in the first two trimesters than in the third. The clinical manifestations of acute appendicitis in pregnancy are more protean owing to the change in both the position and the axis of the appendix during gestation (Fig. 1).

Baer et al. (1932) have demonstrated a gradual shifting in position of the base of the appendix from its normal low-lying position near the iliac fossa to one somewhat above the iliac crest near term. After the seventh month, 88% of all gravidas have their appendix above the iliac crest. The long axis of the appendix also changes from its normal downward and inward direction, first to a horizontal position that points medially, and finally to a vertical position curving around the fundus of the uterus. As a consequence of this gradual outward and upward displacement of the appendix by the growing uterus, the classic localization at McBurney's point is altered.

Were it not for the changing position of the appendix, the symptoms of acute appendicitis in pregnancy would be comparable to those in the nonpregnant female. In the early months of pregnancy, the diagnosis of appendicitis is readily established: the classic combination of a history of right lower quadrant pain, nausea, vomiting, and fever, together with the point of tenderness over McBurney's point, is presumptive evidence of the diagnosis.

In pregnancy, nausea per se is of limited diagnostic significance unless accompanied by other signs and symptoms suggesting appendicitis. The abdominal spasm that is typical in the nonpregnant patient is less pronounced owing to the presumed laxity of the abdominal muscles. The presence of rectal tenderness or the presence of a psoas sign is a valuable diagnostic adjunct.

As gestation progresses, the differential diagnosis is augmented, particularly when the appendix is to be found in the region of the liver or along the right costal margin. It is in these situations that cholecystitis and right-sided pyelonephritis are added to the differential diagnosis, which also includes torsion of an adnexal mass, degenerating leiomyoma, intrinsic gastrointestinal pathology (e.g., regional enteritis, ulcerative colitis), and uterine disease (e.g., abruption). Most laboratory tests are of little use. A diagnostic procedure often neglected in evaluating the gravida for appendicitis is to apply constant pressure over the point of tenderness and then to roll the patient to the opposite side. If the cause of pain is extrauterine, the perception of tenderness persists. A moderate temperature

elevation is consistent with the diagnosis of appendicitis. However, a fever that raises the temperature to greater than 39°C and is accompanied by rigors more often is associated with conditions other than appendicitis unless appendiceal rupture has occurred with resultant peritonitis. The leukocyte count and sedimentation rate may be elevated as a consequence of pregnancy. However, a differential count that is shifted to the left may be the first laboratory indication of significant appendiceal pathology. Urinalysis is helpful in excluding the possibility of right-sided pyelonephritis.

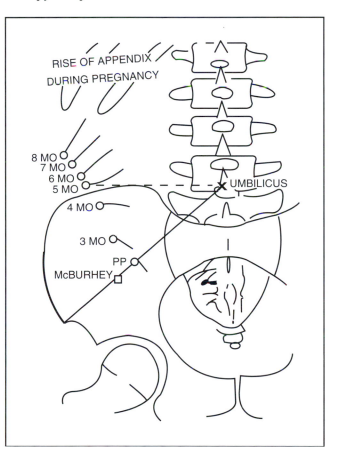

FIGURE I Changes in the position and direction of the appendix during pregnancy. After the fifth month of pregnancy, the appendix lies at the crest level and rises above this level during the last trimester. The postpartum position of the appendix (pp) corresponds to its position in the nonpregnant state. Roentgenologically, the base of the appendix is usually found medial to McBurney's point. The average position of the umbilicus corresponds to the point at which a line extended horizontally from the iliac crest crosses the spine. *Source:* Baer et al. (1932).

Endovaginal and graded compression ultrasonography are potentially valuable diagnostic procedures. Graded compressive ultrasonography is performed by compressing the right lower quadrant with a linear array transducer and is capable of demonstrating an inflamed nonruptured appendix. The criteria for ultrasound diagnosis of acute appendicitis include visualization of a noncompressible aperistaltic appendix with a target-like appearance in transverse view and a diameter greater than or equal to 7 mm. The overall accuracy and specificity of ultrasonography in making the diagnosis of acute appendicitis is over 95% in both instances. Graded compression ultrasound is approximately 98% accurate for disease in the first and second trimesters. With advanced gestation, greater technical difficulties may be encountered. An alternate diagnostic tool potentially applicable to pregnant women is helical computed tomography.

The change in the position of the appendix alters the potential morbid consequences for the gravida. The displacement of the appendix out of the pelvis and into the peritoneal cavity may account for the tendency for maternal morbidity and mortality from appendicitis to be more significant as gestation progresses. Black (1960) demonstrated that, while the overall maternal mortality rate was 4.6%, it increased as gestation progressed to 10.9% in the third trimester and to 16.7% if the disease occurred intrapartum or postpartum. These data were compiled predominantly in the preantibiotic era. More recent studies have demonstrated a collective maternal mortality rate of 2%. However, when the disease was present in the third trimester, the maternal death rate was 7.3%. "The mortality of appendicitis in pregnancy is the mortality of delay." These words were written by Labler in 1908, and unfortunately still have validity today.

There is some increase in fetal wastage and perinatal mortality associated with operative intervention. In most cases, aggressive early intervention and tocolysis minimize the potential adverse fetal impact. Most perinatal complications are related to the severity of disease and operative delay rather than to the operative procedure itself. The incidence of fetal loss is 1.5% or less if appendical perforation has not occurred. Preterm delivery is estimated between 5% and 14%.

The complications of appendicitis are

1. peritonitis,
2. localized periappendicular abscess formation,
3. pylephlebitis with thrombosis of the portal venous drainage,
4. liver abscesses, and
5. septicemia.

The acute vasculitis and inflammatory thrombosis of the blood vessels in the mesoappendix may progress to involve the portal drainage. Septic emboli from such foci of pylephlebitis may result in metastatic hepatic abscess formation and septicemia. The principal bacteria involved are the Bacteroidaceae, peptococci, and peptostreptococci.

The recommendation for therapy is to start intravenous medication with clindamycin and gentamicin; however, prospective data involving nonpregnant patients have shown antibiotic therapy is of limited benefit in cases of nonperforated appendicitis.

There is much individualization in terms of the type of incisions. The major options are a right midtransverse incision and a low midline incision. The latter not only affords adequate exposure for removal of the inflamed appendix but also permits treatment of other conditions that may simulate appendicitis.

Selected cases of appendical abscesses can be managed with ultrasonography-guided fine needle aspiration coupled with aggressive antibiotic therapy.

SUGGESTED READING

Abu-Yousef MM, Franken EA Jr. An overview of graded compression sonography in the diagnosis of acute appendicitis. Semin Ultrasound CT MR 1989; 10:352.

Allen JR, Helling TS, Langenfeld M. Intraabdominal surgery during pregnancy. Am J Surg 1989; 158:567.

Babaknia A, Parsa H, Woodruss JD. Appendicitis during pregnancy. Obstet Gynecol 1977; 50:40.

Baer JL, Reis RA, Arens RA. Appendicitis in pregnancy with changes in position and axis of normal appendix in pregnancy. J Am Med Assoc 1932; 98:1359.

Black WP. Acute appendicitis in pregnancy. Br Med J 1960; 1:1938.

Castro MA, Shipp TD, Castro EE, et al. The use of helical computed tomography in pregnancy. Am J Obstet Gynecol 2001; 184:954.

Dornhoffer JL, Calkins JW. Appendicitis complicating pregnancy. Kans Med 1988; 89:139.

Hunt MG, Martin JN Jr, Martin RW, et al. Perinatal aspects of abdominal surgery for nonobstetric disease. Am J Perinatol 1989; 6:412.

Kurtz GR, Davis RS, Spraul JD. Acute appendicitis in pregnancy and labor. Obstet Gynecol 1964; 23:528.

Lim HK, Bae SH, Seo GS. Diagnosis of acute appendicitis in pregnant women: value of sonography. Am J Roentgenol 1992; 159:539.

Marn CS, Bree RL. Advances in pelvic ultrasound: endovaginal scanning for ectopic gestation and graded compression sonography for appendicitis. Ann Emerg Med 1989; 18:1304.

McCorriston CC. Nonobstetrical abdominal surgery during pregnancy. J Abdom Surg 1973; 15:85.

McGee TM. Acute appendicitis in pregnancy. Aust NZ J Obstet Gynecol 1989; 29:378.

Mourad J, Elliott JP, Erickson L, et al. Appendicitis in pregnancy: new information that contradicts long-held clinical beliefs. Am J Obstet Gynecol 2000; 182:1027.

Sarsonn EL, Bauman S. Acute appendicitis in pregnancy: difficulties in diagnosis. Obstet Gynecol 1963; 22:382.

Schreiber JH. Laparoscopic appendectomy in pregnancy. Surg Endosc 1990; 4:100.

Schwork WB, Witchtrup B, Rothmund M, Ruschoff J. Ultrasonography in the diagnosis of acute appendicitis: a prospective study. Gastroenterology 1989; 97:630.

Sharp HT. The acute abdomen during pregnancy. Clin Obstet Gynecol 2002; 45:405.

Tamir IL, Bongard FS, Klein SR. Acute appendicitis in the pregnant patient. Am J Surg 1990; 160:571.

Taylor JD. Acute appendicitis in pregnancy and puerperium. Aust NZ J Obstet Gynecol 1972; 12:202.

Thomford NR, Patti RW, Teteris NJ. Appendectomy during pregnancy. Surg Gynecol Obstet 1969; 129:489.

INTRODUCTION

Up to 60% of women in the United States initiate breast-feeding after delivery, but only 20% continue for six months or more. Mastitis accounts for 25% of the reasons that women committed to breastfeeding discontinue doing so. Puerperal mastitis usually occurs in the second or third week postpartum. The disease develops in 5% to 30% of women committed to long-term breastfeeding.

Women who have had mastitis in a previous pregnancy are at a threefold risk of puerperal mastitis in a subsequent pregnancy. Nulliparous and multiparous women have the same prevalence.

The portals of infection influence pathogenesis, causative organism, and clinical manifestations. The portal of infection can be either a nipple fissure in the skin leading resulting on cellulitis or ductal obstruction leading to a more occult presentation.

In rare instances, the mastitis occurs due to hematogenous seeding. Puerperal mastitis involves primarily the interlobular connective tissue, causing cellulitis of the breast. Sporadic mastitis is the result of nipple fissuring.

Although staphylococci are the most frequently encountered pathogens in cases of puerperal mastitis, other bacterial species that can cause this clinical entity include beta-hemolytic streptococci of groups B, C, and G and less frequently A, *Streptococcus faecalis, Escherichia coli, Haemophilus influenzae, Klebsiella pneumoniae, Salmonella* species, and *Serratia marcescens*.

With mammary cellulitis, temperature is usually in excess of 38°C and associated with rapid pulse. The febrile response may be associated with malaise, anorexia, headache, and rare chills (Fig. 2). Changes in breast milk constituency may cause the infant to refuse to suckle the infected breast. Marked systemic symptoms are rarely encountered; therefore, when one sees a patient who is breastfeeding with what appears to be an influenza-type syndrome without upper respiratory infection, one must consider the possibility of mastitis.

Ductal mastitis is associated with mammary adenitis or milk stasis. Bacteria are present in breast milk and lactiferous sinuses, secondary to skin colonization. However, the presence of bacteria in lactiferous sinuses does not correlate well with the induction of mastitis.

Ductal mastitis usually occurs in the absence of nipple fissure. In many instances of ductal mastitis, pus can be expressed from the nipple of the infected breast and the symptomatology is similar to that encountered with mammary cellulitis but often less severe. The infectious process is insidious in onset and has a more protracted course than that associated with true mammary cellulitis.

Although mammary adenitis occurs in epidemic forms in hospital settings, it may be encountered two or more weeks after delivery when the mother is at home.

EPIDEMIOLOGY

Both types of mastitis are frequently due to infection by *Staphylococcus aureus*. The epidemiologic pattern of infection is such that the newborn infant becomes colonized within the nursery by a nosocomial penicillin-resistant staphylococcus. Once infection is acquired in the newborn nursery, the nose and throat of the neonate become important reservoirs of colonization from which the bacteria are passed to the mother. The milk of a high proportion of nursing mothers becomes colonized with the strain of *S. aureus* present in the oropharynx of the infant.

Approximately 50% to 75% of nursing personnel are known to be *S. aureus* carriers and a permanent source of penicillin-resistant organisms within the hospital environment. The infant becomes the prime disseminator of the staphylococci to the mother and to its immediate environment. Infection is almost invariably due to a hospital-acquired strain and not to one indigenous to the mother per se, unless maternal staphylococcal cutaneous infection antedated her hospital admission.

The determinants of disease, as opposed to colonization, are difficult to discern. At least one of these appears to be the strain virulence of the organisms. A higher rate of breast infection occurs among nursing mothers when there is a concomitant epidemic of overt *S. aureus* infection in the newborn nursery. Even then, there is not a one-to-one correlation between colonization of a neonate with a virulent strain of *S. aureus* and subsequent maternal puerperal mastitis. Given colonization of the newborn with a virulent strain, some mothers will develop puerperal mastitis but

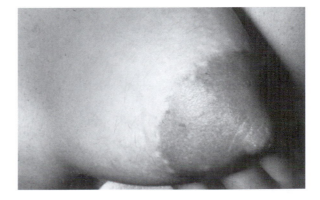

FIGURE 2 Marked erythema characteristic of acute mastitis. *Source*: Marshall (1975).

the majority will not. Colonization of the newborn infant per se is not the sole prerequisite of the disease. Those infants colonized by nonepidemic strains of penicillin-resistant hospital-acquired staphylococci are less likely to be associated with puerperal mastitis in the nursing mother.

DIAGNOSIS

Mastitis presents with localized erythema and tenderness. A low-grade fever is usually present. Accompanying symptoms include sudden onset, generalized malaise, localized pain (usually unilateral), and rejection by the infant of the involved breast. Physical examination may reveal local edema, erythema, and tenderness. The outer quadrants of the breasts are the most frequent site of involvement.

Puerperal mastitis can be distinguished from breast engorgement, which has a gradual onset, is usually bilateral, presents with generalized swelling, heat, and tenderness, and occurs within days of parturition. Women who have sustained a previous episode of mastitis have an increased chance of a recurrence during lactation or a subsequent pregnancy.

It is important to remember that in any type of breast infection, the normal mammary architecture, especially the ligaments of Cooper that support the parenchyma of the breast, acts as a temporary barrier to the extension of the infectious process throughout the breast. Mammary architecture may be maintained despite infection so that the fluctuance that normally accompanies abscess formation and soft tissue infection elsewhere may be masked. Infection may burrow into the breast and be much more extensive than its outward appearance may suggest.

THERAPY

For the treatment of mastitis, penicillin-resistant penicillins or selected cephalosporins have constituted the therapy of choice. Cloxacillin, dicloxacillin, and cephalosporin are the principal antibiotics prescribed in non–penicillin allergic patients. The penicillinase-resistant penicillins are highly active against both penicillinase-producing and non–penicillinase-producing strains of S. aureus and S. epidermidis. More than 90% of hospital-acquired and 70% of community-acquired staphylococci are resistant to penicillin G. In rare instances, disease may be due to a methicillin-resistant strain of S. aureus. If the patient is allergic to penicillin, erythromycin or clindamycin can be used.

Despite symptomatic improvement in 24 to 48 hours, antibiotic therapy should be continued for 10 to 14 days.

The questions may arise as to the desirability or appropriateness of continued breastfeeding in the presence of acute mastitis. If milk stasis is a factor in the pathogenesis of the infection, continued nursing to prevent breast engorgement should be encouraged.

If the infection is diagnosed early and treatment is promptly instituted, resolution is rapid and the symptoms subside over the course of one to two days. If inadequate therapy is prescribed for mastitis and infection becomes firmly established, resolution of the infectious process may not be attained and this may result in suppuration and the formation of a breast abscess. Delay in symptomatic response or increase in local tenderness warrants ultrasonographic or mammogram evaluation to rule out abscess formation.

If a breast abscess is diagnosed, early surgical drainage should be instituted as soon as any evidence of a purulent collection is apparent. Cultures should be obtained from the abscess cavity and antibiotic therapy as prescribed for mastitis instituted. Persistence of infection despite antibiotic therapy without surgical drainage of a breast abscess may result in a chronic indurated breast mass or "antibioma." This indurated honeycomb of small abscess cavities, granulation tissue, and fibrosis may lead to permanent breast deformity. The etiologic agent of the mastitis may induce disease beyond the confines of the breast.

PREVENTION

Postpartum mastitis is a preventable disease. Patient education, direct coaching of mothers, unrestricted access to the baby, and correct positioning of the baby have all been shown to reduce the incidence of mastitis.

NECROTIZING FASCIITIS/ COMPLICATIONS OF MASTITIS

The group A streptococci mastitis if not treated early may progress to what has been termed necrotizing fasciitis. Necrotizing fasciitis initially was termed by Meleney "streptococcal gangrene." The disease was subsequently renamed necrotizing fasciitis in order to reinforce the concept that the disease, although progressively destroys fascia and fat, spares the skin and muscle. Progression of cutaneous erythematous edema to pink and then blue areas of coloration in association with blisters and blebs is characteristic of this type of infection.

The clinical course is rapid, with the patient exhibiting fever (38–39°C) and tachycardia, which occasionally is out of proportion to the fever. With the onset of the disease, the patient usually experiences pain and swelling of the affected part. Chills and tremor are not uncommon. The initial pain is replaced by numbness, which, in conjunction with the toxic metabolic state, usually renders the patient indifferent to her illness. On the second to fourth day of illness, the pathognomonic signs of streptococcal gangrene occur; to quote Meleney, these are dusky hue of the skin, edema with blisters, from which can be expressed a dark serosanguineous fluid. The margins are red, and swelling is neither raised nor clearly demarcated (Fig. 3).

On the fifth to eighth day, the discolored areas become frankly black or gray from gangrenous necrosis. Proportional to the severity of the disease, bacteremia is a common complication, with frequent metastatic involvement of the lung parenchyma. The disease process is one of extensive cellulitis complicated by abscess within fascial planes and widespread superficial fascial necrosis, resulting in separation and infarction of the overlying skin.

The basic pathologic process is a subcutaneous necrosis of the fat and fascia with a secondary occlusion and thrombosis of the dermal vessels, leading to eventual gangrene of the skin.

Diagnosis

Although a presumptive diagnosis can be inferred from the Gram stain, definitive diagnosis is contingent on bacteriologic identification. The organisms are found only in the subcutaneous slough. The surrounding edema is sterile.

Therapy

The primary therapy is aggressive antibiotic therapy and immediate operative debridement in the operating room under anesthesia. High-dose penicillin therapy should be started. All necrotic skin and subcutaneous tissue are removed. Delay to assess the efficacy of antibiotic therapy or local wound care is futile and leads to massive tissue loss with bowel exposure, sepsis, peritonitis, and death.

The wound must be widely opened and the necrotic material removed. Long incisions to the ends of the necrotic areas are necessary to expose the involved tissue adequately. They are generally made in a stellate fashion out from the wound. The viable overlying skin may be left intact. The whole area is irrigated and packed open. Large doses of penicillin, administered intravenously, are also necessary. Because of the nature of the destructive process and the debridement, secondary closure is not possible and healing is by secondary intention. Grafting is sometimes necessary. Once the wound is debrided, local wound care is given as indicated for the more benign infections.

MASTITIS-ASSOCIATED TOXIC SHOCK SYNDROME

Toxic shock syndrome (TSS) can occur in patients whose mastitis is due to TSST-1 producing strain of *S. aureus*. Due primarily to the limited extent of disease before therapeutic intervention, this is a rare event.

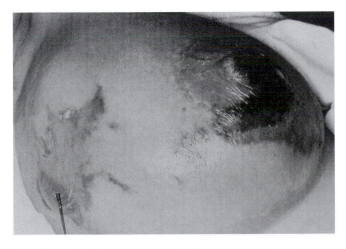

FIGURE 3 Violaceous areas with focal necrosis within an erythematous swollen breast infected with group A streptococci. Note the detachment of the superficial epidermis and the presence of fluid-filled bleb.

TSS is a multisystem illness. A syndrome consisting of malaise, myalgia, low-grade fever, nausea, vomiting, and/or diarrhea may antecede overt disease. In the full-blown, acute systemic illness, the patient presents with fever (>38.9° C or 102° F), sore throat, headache, chills, severe hypotension, myalgia, pharyngitis, conjunctivitis, leukocytosis, and generalized arthralgia. The rash is usually a consistent part of the syndrome and presents as a diffuse "sunburn-like" blanching macular erythema. Neurologic symptomatology, when present, is usually severe. Profound hypotension is one of the characteristic findings of advanced TSS. A number of abnormal laboratory findings may be observed. The white blood cell count is generally elevated but may be normal. A large left shift in the neutrophil series occurs but may not be present on the first day of illness: toxic granulation and Dohle bodies are often found and may be important diagnostic clues. Moderate elevation in liver function tests is common.

The serum amylase may be elevated. Most patients have elevations in the blood urea nitrogen and creatinine. The platelet count often drops below 100,000/mm³ in the first week of illness. Electrocardiogram abnormalities include sinus or supraventricular tachycardia and nonspecific ST segment changes, and first-degree heart block T-wave inversion is sometimes recorded in the precordial leads as are premature atrial and ventricular extrasystole. Patients with TSS may have evidence of pulmonary involvement, which may be mild or progress to frank adult respiratory distress syndrome.

Diagnosis

The diagnosis is inferred by the multiorgan disease (usually with fever, headache, diarrhea, liver, and renal test abnormalities) and a characteristic rash in a patient with focal disease due to *S. aureus*.

Therapy

The initial therapy is that of aggressive volume replacement and initiation of appropriate antibiotic therapy. Because of the large volume of fluids necessary, it is strongly recommended that a Swan-Ganz catheter be placed and anesthesia department be alerted that adult respiratory distress syndrome may develop in this particular patient. Concomitantly, local therapy should be directed to remove as much toxin as possible from the portal of infection. Antimicrobial therapy requires the administration of a beta-lactamase–resistant semisynthetic penicillin such as oxacillin or nafcillin. A single dose of netilmicin is advocated because of its synergistic effect with the semisynthetic penicillins. Because of the probability of underlying renal damage, a second dose is rarely administered. The choice of netilmicin over gentamicin or tobramycin is based on its being the least nephrotoxic of all the aminoglycosides. The patient should be extensively monitored for the development of renal failure and/or adult respiratory distress syndrome.

SELECTED READING

Marshall BR, Hepper JK, Zirbel CC. Sporadic puerperal mastitis—an infection that need not interrupt lactation. J Am Med Assoc 1975; 233: 1377.

C. Breast Abscess

J. Patrick O'Leary / *Revised by* David A. Baker

EPIDEMIOLOGY

Breast abscesses occur in 0.4% to 0.5% of lactating mothers. After the first six weeks, abscess formation rarely occurs. Women with puerperal mastitis have a 5% to 11% risk of developing a breast abscess. The signs and symptoms are similar to those of mastitis with the added finding of a tense, fluctuant mass with erythema in the affected area.

ANATOMY

In the most simplistic terms, the breast is a modified sweat gland that is located on the anterior chest wall and is attached to the chest musculature by suspensory bands of fascia. The glandular structure is surrounded by a layer of fat and the entire organ is encased by an envelope of skin (Fig. 4).

Embryologically, the glandular structure migrates from the area of the axilla, and in the adult a remnant of breast tissue frequently extends superiorly and laterally. This extension is known as the axillary tail of Spence. The glandular lobes, or acini, are connected to the nipple by an arborization of lactiferous ducts. These ducts are specialized and have a surrounding structural stroma that is responsive to hormonal stimuli. An ampullary dilatation of the lactiferous ducts occurs at the apex of the breast before they open onto the surface of the nipple. These areas are known as the lactiferous ampullae, or milk sinuses. Although it appears that each duct is lined by a single layer of epithelial cells, there is a second layer of flat cells of epithelial nature that acts as a basement layer of epidermis.

The nipple is surrounded by a circular area of pigmented skin, which is known as the areola. This area contains contractile smooth muscles that facilitate in nipple contraction.

Fiber septa run throughout the glandular aspect of the breast to support the breast. These suspensory ligaments of Cooper (Fig. 5) attach to the deep fascia of the pectoralis major muscle and to the dermal layer of the skin. This septum provides the breast with a considerable amount of mobility and acts to segment the breast, an important consideration should inflammatory disease occur.

The skin covering the breast is transgressed by minute lines that are circumareolar in location, and then extend out from the nipple in concentric circles much as ripples in a pond. These are known as Langer's lines (Fig. 6), and they help to disguise scars if the incisions are appropriately placed.

CLINICAL DISEASE

Although the vast majority of breast abscesses are associated with lactation, some can occur secondary to ectasia of the lactiferous ducts. If clinical findings suggest inflammation in the nonlactating breast, the primary diagnosis to be excluded is inflammatory carcinoma. Although ectasia of the lactiferous duct would be more common, inflammatory carcinoma can mimic breast abscess and can only be diagnosed with biopsy.

Lactation mastitis has been extensively studied. In the era from the time of availability of penicillin to 1950, this antibiotic was found to be the drug of choice. As studies were continued and as penicillin was used more extensively, the pattern of infection changed. Initially, *Staphylococcus aureus* and beta-hemolytic streptococci were the more common pathogens. Later, staphylococci became the most common pathogen, and this was frequently noted to be of the phage-type 80/81. Prior to the advent of this particular virulent penicillinase-producing strain, the usual duration of a lesion was three to four weeks. With the more common use of antibiotics and the change in infecting organisms, the duration of the illness has lengthened.

It has been shown that there is early colonization with *S. aureus* of babies born in maternity hospitals. The infections

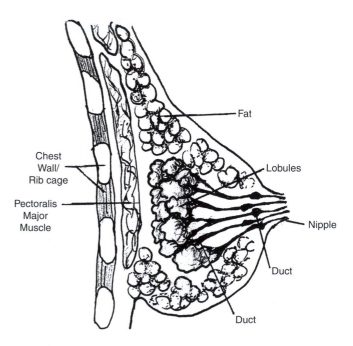

FIGURE 4 A vertical section through the breast, detailing its composite structure. Note the segmentation of the glandular aspect by the ducts and suspensory ligaments. It should also be noted that the lactiferous duct dilates into the lactiferous sinus beneath the nipple and before the glandular structure is reached.

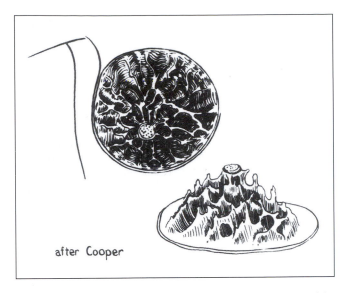

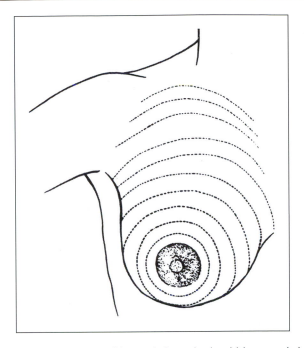

FIGURE 5 A representation of Cooper's original description of the suspensory ligaments that now bear his name. His observations were made at the time from anatomic dissection of the female breast. These suspensory ligaments provide the breast with mobility while at the same time cording the breast off into various smaller subsets.

FIGURE 6 Position of Langer's lines. It should be noted that these small wrinkles in the skin form concentric circles around the nipple. Surgical incisions that are constructed to lie in these miniature crevices are cosmetically pleasing and much less deforming than radial incisions in this part of the body.

of the babies do not seem to be related to contamination by the mothers, as cultures of the nares or vaginas of the mothers do not correlate with cultures from the nares of the infants. This colonization of babies may come from the nursing staff. Cultures taken from the milk of nursing mothers and from the rectum and throats of their babies have shown that *S. aureus* of a similar type can be isolated from both with great regularity. The breast milk is usually infected 24 hours after delivery, but not before delivery.

Although traditionally the microbiology of breast abscess has focused on *S. aureus*, in nonpuerperal breast abscesses, mixed anaerobic bacteria including the Peptostreptococci and *Mobiluncus curtisii* are the more prevalent bacteria. There are two types of breast abscesses: one in which *S. aureus* predominates and one in which class II and III anaerobic bacteria predominate.

The skin flora of the breast plays a relatively minor role in the production of breast abscess. Bacteria gain entry to the breast more commonly through the terminal ducts or through skin fissures in the nipple. Once within the breast, the bacteria proliferate in the milk sinus and throughout the ductal tree. The ensuing inflammatory process occludes the ducts, draining the stimulated glandular tissue. Since milk is an excellent culture medium, the growth of bacteria occurs rapidly.

In patients who have a periareolar abscess, pregnancy is not a common finding. The abnormality in these patients is found in the subareolar space. As the lactiferous ducts approach the surface of the nipple, they dilate to form the lactiferous sinus. This portion of the duct is lined by squamous cells and is normally quite short (less than 2 mm in length). Squamous metaplasia can occur in this area and fill the ductules with keratinous debris. Flow through the ducts is retarded and with stasis, infection is common. The inflammatory process,

though having its origin immediately beneath the areola, can extend into adjacent tissue. The original description of this process by Zuska (1951) identified fistulous tracts around the areola in a small cohort of young women. When the specimens were examined, the lactiferous ducts were found to have been obstructed with desquamated epithelial debris. Although this disease has been demonstrated to be associated with nipple inversion, Haagensen (1971) substantiated an earlier report by showing that the disease could occur in women without nipple inversion. Although there is a positive relationship between nipple inversion and periareolar abscess, the exact relationship is unknown. It is possible that in some patients the nipple inversion is a direct result of retraction of fibrous tissue from chronic inflammation, while in other patients the nipple inversion contributed to the formation of the abscess.

It is unclear whether the ectasia is primary or occurs secondary to obstruction of the ducts by the desquamated epithelium. It is clear, however, that mammary duct ectasia need not always progress to fistula, and it is probable that mammary duct fistulas can occur without ectasia.

Infection of the nonlactating breast is uncommon. If such a condition should arise, the lesion should be suspected of being inflammatory carcinoma. Similarly, the finding of a gram-negative breast infection in a nongravid female warrants abandonment of nonoperative management in favor of tissue confirmation of the disease process.

DIAGNOSIS

The clinical presentation may vary somewhat with respect to time of onset, but most frequently occurs within the first two weeks of the nursing period. The patient generally notices that one breast becomes somewhat tender to the touch, seems to be larger, and may develop some reddening. As the process progresses, the breast becomes exquisitely tender and the patient usually complains of a sensation of heaviness. At this point, systemic symptoms of malaise, weakness, and fever can occur. If aggressive treatment is begun, the maturation of this process to a true abscess can frequently be aborted. If the breast is neglected, or if treatment is inadequate, then gradually the breast becomes less tender and an abscess develops (Fig. 8). Frequently, the abscess will be contained in one section of the breast by the infiltrating septa of Cooper's ligaments. Spontaneous rupture of the abscess can occur either through the nipple or, more commonly, through the dependent part of the breast. Deep sinuses can be produced that may drain for protracted periods if appropriate therapy is not instituted.

Ultrasound studies are valuable in documenting the presence of an abscess. Tiu et al. (2001) analyzed the ultrasound findings of 204 patients in whom a breast abscess had been documented. Most lesions showed grade 1 or grade 2 echogenicity (86%), smooth contours (31%), macrolobulation (31%), irregular contours (16%), and a hypoechoic rim (16%). The combination of a hypoechoic rim surrounding a fluid space and a central area of low-level echoes (grades 1–3) should strongly suggest abscess formation.

The breast abscess must be differentiated from other suppurative processes that can occur in the breast. In the acute state, the diagnosis is usually apparent. The only entity that mimics mastitis is inflammatory carcinoma, and the differentiation between these two pathologic processes is usually self-evident.

In the chronic state, the differentiation between a chronic subareolar breast abscess and a lactation abscess may occur. The chronic subareolar abscess does occur in younger women, but not in those who have recently undergone pregnancy and lactation. The pathophysiology of the chronic subareolar abscess begins with dilated lactiferous sinuses (milk sinuses) just below the nipple. These may become clogged with keratinous debris and thereby produce retention cysts of the milk sinus. Disruption of this distended wall leads to extravasation of material into the subareolar fat and the production of an inflammatory process. Treatment of this lesion requires an appropriate diagnosis and then local resection of the involved milk sinuses.

Neglected lactation mastitis with abscess may be confused with either primary or secondary tuberculosis of the breast. The diagnosis here is made via skin testing, chest X rays, and biopsy of the chronic sinus tracts. The therapy of breast tuberculosis involves specific antituberculous drugs, as well as debridement and adequate drainage.

THERAPY

As in many other disease entities, the optimum therapy is prevention. If prevention is not possible, then early detection and aggressive therapy is the second most desirable

approach. Every woman who nurses her baby is at risk to develop lactation mastitis or abscess. Since the vector to infect the breast is probably the infant, local hygiene at the level of the nipple cannot prevent the inoculation. Since this disease process frequently occurs in epidemics, when one case occurs every attempt should be made to ascertain if a *S. aureus* carrier exists in the nursery. If several cases are reported from one nursery, then all infants should have cultures of their nares prior to discharge. In addition, all employees should be cultured.

When a woman develops the signs and symptoms of lactation mastitis, she should be treated vigorously with adequate hydration, local heat to the breast, cessation of infant suckling, and appropriate antimicrobial therapy. Appropriate therapy dictates an antistaphylococcus antibiotic administered via an appropriate route. Although oral medications may occasionally be indicated, more often the optimal route of therapy is parenteral. In many instances, intravenous administration is the most dependable and ensures the highest serum levels. With this approach, the majority of patients with lactation mastitis will not go on to form a breast abscess.

When a lactation breast abscess occurs, nursing in the involved breast probably should be stopped. Infected serious sequelae (skin infections, staphylococcal pneumonia, staphylococcal empyema, and infant death) have been reported; however, this point of management is controversial.

Aspiration Drainage

Traditional treatment of breast abscesses has involved incision and drainage under antibiotic coverage, with or without ultrasound guidance (Fig. 7). Needle aspiration is

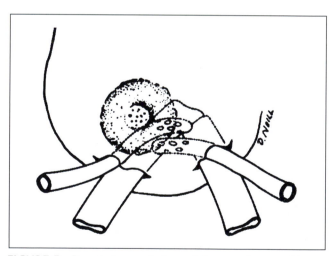

FIGURE 7 Breast abscess drainage. Adequate therapy of breast abscess includes appropriate antistaphylococcal antibiotics as well as adequate drainage. Once an abscess develops, drainage is mandatory. Dependent drainage should be obtained when possible. Although soft, flat, rubber drains are acceptable, in some larger breast abscesses larger catheters will be helpful in irrigating the abscess cavity and providing a larger tract for drainage. When irrigation is used, the irrigating fluid can be infused through one catheter, while the other catheter is used for suction. This sump system will increase patient comfort.

progressively replacing surgical drainage as the first thera-peutic modality of choice for small abscesses.

Schwarz and Shrestha (2001) studied 30 patients with 33 breast abscesses who they treated by needle aspiration, oral antibiotics, and repeated aspiration if indicated. Eighteen patients required only a single aspiration, nine patients required multiple aspiration, and six required incision and drainage. By careful patient selection, good results can be obtained. Imperiale et al. (2001) treated 26 patients with 28 acute abscesses in whom systemic antibiotic therapy had failed with serial ultrasound-guided aspiration and local injection of a broad-spectrum antibiotic. The treatment was repeated weekly until complete resolution was documented. In one case of a relatively large abscess, lesion volume increased at the second evaluation; this patient required sur-gical drainage. There is a need for more precise patient selec-tion criteria to avert prolonged courses of needle aspiration or residual morbidity from delayed intervention. Properly performed, aspiration with local antibiotic installation can be more cost effective than surgical intervention.

Surgical Drainage

If an abscess occurs, then drainage is mandatory. Because of the severe pain associated with the inflammatory process, drainage should be done under light, general anesthesia. This ensures the maximum comfort to the patient and allows the surgeon to adequately decompress the abscess cavity. The incisions in the breast should be curvilinear so that they follow Langer's lines (Fig. 6) and should be in a dependent part of the breast. It is frequently necessary to make two incisions so that maximum drainage is ensured. In most instances, small, flat rubber drains are adequate. In the extensively involved breast, it may be necessary to place hollow rubber tubes so that irrigation can be accom-plished. If tubes are necessary, it is frequently wise to place two tubes. These tubes can then act as an infusion catheter and sump drain, respectively (Fig. 7). The fluid infused should be sterile saline. Antibiotic solutions add little in terms of local control, and blood levels from local absorp-tion are unpredictable, adding another unnecessary vari-able to the treatment regimen. If reaccumulation occurs after the initial drainage, the second area frequently can be entered so that adequate drainage can be provided without taking the patient back to the operating theater. Every attempt should be made to provide adequate drainage at the first procedure.

Dressing should be changed in the beginning every three or four hours, or when saturated. As the disease process is controlled, active granulation tissue may extrude the drains that have been placed. The flat rubber drains should be advanced, beginning with the sixth postsurgical day, so that they are entirely removed on or about the tenth day. If the original incisions were discretely placed, the breast will heal with a reasonably normal configuration and without disfiguring scars.

Treatment of subareolar abscesses depends on the state of the process. In patients with an acute suppurative process, local incision and drainage with antibiotics and

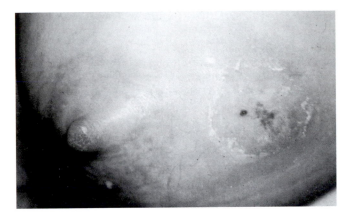

FIGURE 8 Painful erythematous indurated site of a breast abscess. *Source:* Marshall (1975).

local treatment should be instituted. When the breast has become quiescent, a localized core excision of the nipple including the affected lactiferous duct and surrounding granulation tissue should be accomplished. The subareolar space should be inspected closely for ectasia or metaplasia. The site of excision should be drained with a closed suc-tion drainage apparatus that can be removed in 24 hours. At the time of excision, the patient should be given appro-priate antibiotics. Although such infections have classically been caused by *S. aureus*, in recent years, gram-negative aerobic and anaerobic bacteria have been discovered with increasing frequency. Intravenous antibiotic coverage should be directed toward such organisms.

Although the standard management of puerperal abscess by incision, breaking down loculi, and dependent drainage is still the traditional mode of management, an alternative approach—curettage and primary obliteration of the cavity under antibiotic cover—can give equally good results with reduced morbidity.

With the potential for close postoperative care, an alter-native approach to the conventional open drainage pack dressing method is possible. Khanna et al. (1989) studied the effect of incision drainage and primary closure in 50 cases of lactational breast abscess. Their failure rate was 6%. The mean healing time was 7.12 days.

Breast abscesses in the nonlactating breast are not common but may occur. Treatment is generally similar, but biopsies must be taken so that inflammatory or underlying intraductal carcinoma will be appropriately diagnosed, if present.

SELECTED READING

Burry VF, Beezley M. Infant mastitis due to gram-positive bacteria. Am J Dis Child 1972; 124:736.

Carroll L, Osman M, Davies DP, et al. Bacteriologic criteria for feed-ing raw breast milk to babies in neonatal units. Lancet 1979; 2:732.

Fetherston C. Characteristics of lactation mastitis in a Western Australian cohort. Breast Feeding Rev 1997; 5:5.

Gibberd GF. Sporadic and epidemic puerperal breast infections. Am J Obstet Gynecol 1953; 65:1038.

Haagensen CD. Diseases of the Breast. Philadelphia, W.B. Saunders Co. 1971; pp. 337–338.

Imperiale A, Zandrino F, Calabrese M, et al. Abscesses of the breast: US-guided serial peri-cutaneous aspiration and local antibiotic therapy after unsuccessful systemic antibiotic therapy. Acta Radiol 2001; 42:161.

Inch S, Fisher C. Mastitis today: infection or inflammation. Practitioner 1995; 239:472.

Jorrison S, Pulkkinen MO. Mastitis today: incidence, prevention and treatment. Ann Chir Gynaecol Suppl 1994; 208:84.

Kalstone C. Methicillin-resistant staphylococcal mastitis. Am J Obstet Gynecol 1989; 161:120.

Karstrup S, Nolsoc C, Brabrand K, Nielsen KR. Ultrasonically guided pericutaneous drainage of breast abscesses. Acta Radiol 1990; 31:157.

Khanna YK, Khanna A, Arora YK, et al. Primary closure of lactation breast abscesses. J India Med Assoc 1989; 87:118.

Marshall BR, Hepper JK, Zirbel CC. Sporadic puerperal mastitis—an infection that need not interrupt lactation. J Am Med Assoc 1975; 233:1377.

Mass S. Breast pain: engorgement, nipple pain and mastitis. Clin Obstet Gynecol 2004; 47:676.

Michie C, Lockie F, Lynn W. The challenge of mastitis. Arch Dis Child 2003; 88:818.

Prachniak GK. Common breast-feeding problems. Obstet Gynecol Clin North Am 2002; 29:77.

Carroll L, Osman M, Davies DP, et al. Bacteriologic criteria for feeding raw breast milk to babies in neonatal units. Lancet 1979; 2:732.

Rench MA, Baker CJ. Group B streptococcal breast abscess in a mother and mastitis in her infant. Obstet Gynecol 1989; 73:875.

Riordan JM, Nichols FH. A descriptive study of lactation mastitis in long-term breastfeeding women. J Hum Lact 1990; 6:53.

Sabate JM, Clotet M, Gomez A, et al. Radiologic evaluation of uncommon inflammatory and reactive breast disorders. RadioGraphics 2005; 25:411.

Schwarz RJ, Shnestha R. Needle aspiration of breast abscesses. Am J Surg 2001; 182:117.

Sherman AJ. Puerperal breast abscess. I. Report of outbreak at Philadelphia General Hospital. Obstet Gynecol 1956; 7:268.

Smith CO, Varga A. Puerperal breast abscess. Am J Obstet Gynecol 1957; 74:1330.

Tiu CM, Chiou HJ, Chou YH, et al. Sonographic features of breast absecesses with emphasis on "hypoechoic rim sign." Chinese Med J 2001; 64:153.

Thomsen AC, Hansen KB, Moller BR. Leukocyte counts and microbiologic cultivation of diagnosis of puerperal mastitis. Am J Obstet Gynecol 1983; 146:938.

Thomsen AC, Espersen T, Maigaard S. Course and treatment of milk stasis, noninfectious inflammation of the breast and infectious mastitis in nursing women. Am J Obstet Gynecol 1984; 149:492.

Webb JF. Newborn infections and breast abscesses of staphylococcal origin. Can Med Assoc J 1954; 70:382.

Zuska JJ, Crile G, Ayres W. Fistula of the lacterous ducts. Am J Surg 1951; 81:312.

Zylstra S. Office management of benign breast disease. Clin Obstet Gynecol 1999; 42:234.

Vaccination of Women in Pregnancy 67

IMMUNIZATION AND PREGNANCY

Antepartum, intrapartum, or postpartum immunization is modified by virtue of the fact that the risk–benefit balance must be modified to address possible fetal or neonatal adverse consequences. Unfortunately, considerations and recommendations as to whether or not to immunize a gravida or potential gravida are often based on uncontrolled observations or extrapolations from nonpregnant women. Vaccine-induced immunity is distinct from passive immunity, which is the result of the administration of pathogen-specific antibodies.

Vaccines are categorized into two broad groups based on the biologic activity of the immunogen agent or agents and the type of the resultant immunity. A secondary modification is the duration of the immunity induced.

Killed Vaccines

The immunogen, or immunogens, in a killed vaccine is usually an inactive form of the organism, a purified subcellular fragment of the organism, a genetically engineered recombinant protein, or an inactivated exotoxin. In some cases, the immunogenicity of the exciting antigen has been enhanced by conjugation with a carrier protein (Table 1). Antigen-specific antibodies and activation of some elements of cellular immunity result from such vaccination. Detection of antigen-specific antibodies can occur usually within 7 to 10 days; however, the necessary level of immunity to abort or modify infectious challenge may take several weeks to a month to develop after vaccination. If prior vaccination has occurred, the appearance of antigen-specific antibodies is significantly accelerated. Compared with live organism vaccines, the induced immunity is of relatively short duration.

Live Vaccines

The immunogen in a live vaccine is an attenuated form of the infectious agent. Despite attenuation of its pathogenicity, in a number of instances, infection-induced complications or dissemination may occur (Tables 2 and 3). The immunity derived is often life long.

TABLE I Infectious pathogen vaccines potentially impacting on pregnancy (killed vaccines)

Nonviral agents	Viruses
Pneumococcus (polyvalent conjugates)	Hepatitis A
Typhoid (VI polysaccharide)	Hepatitis B
Tetanus	Influenza
Toxoids	Poliomyelitis (inactivated)
	Rabies

Risk from vaccination during pregnancy is largely theoretical. The benefit of vaccination among pregnant women usually outweighs the potential risk when

1. the risk for disease exposure is high,
2. infection would pose a special risk to the mother or fetus, and
3. the vaccine is unlikely to cause harm.

Combined tetanus and diphtheria (Td) toxoids are the only immunobiologic agents routinely indicated for susceptible pregnant women. Previously vaccinated pregnant women who have not received a Td vaccination within the last 10 years should receive a booster dose. Pregnant women who are unimmunized or only partially immunized against tetanus should complete the primary series. Depending on when a woman seeks prenatal care and the required interval between doses, one or two doses of Td can be administered before delivery. Women for whom the vaccine is indicated but who have not completed the required three-dose series during pregnancy should be followed up after delivery to ensure they receive the doses necessary for protection.

There is no convincing evidence of risk from vaccinating pregnant women with other inactivated virus or bacteria vaccines or toxoids. Hepatitis B vaccine (HBV) is recommended for women at risk for hepatitis B infection, and influenza and pneumococcal vaccines are recommended for women at risk for infection and for complications of influenza and pneumococcal disease.

Oral polio vaccine (OPV) can be administered to pregnant women who are at substantial risk of imminent exposure to natural infection. Although OPV is preferred, inactivated polio vaccine (IPV) may be considered if the complete vaccination series can be administered before the anticipated exposure. Pregnant women who must travel to areas where the risk for yellow fever is high should receive yellow fever vaccine. In these circumstances, the small theoretical risk from vaccination is far outweighed by the risk of yellow fever infection. Known pregnancy is a contraindication for rubella, measles, and mumps vaccines. Although of theoretical concern, no cases of congenital rubella syndrome or abnormalities attributable to a rubella vaccine virus infection have been observed in infants born to susceptible mothers who received rubella vaccine during pregnancy.

People who receive measles, mumps, or rubella vaccines can shed these viruses but generally do not transmit them. These vaccines can be administered safely to the children of pregnant women. Although live polio virus is shed by persons recently vaccinated with OPV (particularly after

TABLE 2 Prophylaxis/immunization for viral infections in pregnancy

Virus	Recommendation for risk from disease[a]	Type of exposure
Hepatitis A virus	M: increased severity in third trimester F: potential for abortion or premature delivery, a function of severity of maternal illness; if maternal disease is within 10–14 days of delivery, neonatal hepatitis may occur	Recent exposure: immune serum globulin 0.06 mL/kgh IM; serosusceptible gravida with anticipated exposure: inactivated vaccine 1.0 mL IM, 2 doses given 6 mo apart
Hepatitis B virus	M: severity of maternal disease increases in third trimester F: fetaland neonatal infection possible; greatly increased risk of chronic carrier state	Serosusceptible gravida with anticipated exposure: recombinant vaccine, 1.0 mL IM with repeat dose 4–6 wk later or 1–5 mo later
Influenza virus	M: increased severity of pneumonia in the late second and third trimesters F: very rare congenital disease; questionable nonspecific anomalies	Recent exposure: none; amantadine not recommended in pregnancy; anticipated exposure: killed annual vaccine before influenza season (Nov–April)
Measles virus	M: potential for abortion, stillbirth, preterm delivery a function of severity of maternal disease; F: congenital infection can occur	Recent exposure: immune serum globulin 0.25 mL/kg within 72 hr
Mumps virus	M: unchanged by pregnancy F: adverse fetal outcomes a function of the severity of maternal disease; neonatal parotitis or aseptic meningitis may occur when maternal disease occurs in the periparturitional period	Recent exposure: no active intervention currently recommended
Polio viruses	M: if not previously vaccinated possible aseptic meningitis or poliomyelitis; F: fetal outcomes influenced by the severity of maternal disease	Anticipated exposure: inactivated vaccine 0.5 mL, SC or IM; repeat dose at 4–8 wk and 6–12 mo later; avoid oral vaccine in pregnancy
Rabies virus	M: life-threatening disease F: fetal outcomes influenced by the severity of maternal disease	Known exposure: rabies immune globulin 20 IU/kg; if wounds are present, half infiltrated into puncture site and other half IM; otherwise all IM and vaccine (HDCV) 1.0 mL IM on days 0, 3, 7, 14, and 28
Rubella virus	M: unchanged by pregnancy; F: possible rubella syndrome, rubella embryopathy	Known exposure: immune serum globulin 0.55 mL/kg may mask maternal disease; impact on transplacental transmission questionable; not recommended for routine use
Vaccinia virus	M: unchanged by pregnancy; F: unknown	Anticipated exposure: vaccine not recommended in pregnancy
Varicella-zoster virus	M: increased risk of pneumonia and death; F: possible disseminated varicella, congenital varicella syndrome	Recent exposure: if serosusceptible, varicella-zoster immune globulin 625 IU IM within 96 hr

[a] M=maternal; F=fetal.
Source: Adapted from CDC (1994).

the first dose), this vaccine can also be administered to the children of pregnant women because experience has not revealed any risk of polio vaccine virus to the fetus.

All pregnant women should be evaluated for immunity to rubella and tested for the presence of hepatitis B surface antigen. Women susceptible to rubella should be vaccinated immediately after delivery. A woman infected with HBV should be followed carefully to assure that the infant receives hepatitis B immune globulin and begins the HBV series shortly after birth. There is no known risk to the fetus from passive immunization of pregnant women with immune globulin preparations. Further information regarding immunization of pregnant women is available in the American College of Obstetricians and Gynecologists Technical Bulletin Number 160, October 1991. This publication is available from the American College of Obstetricians and Gynecologists, Attention: Resource Center, 409 12th Street SW, Washington, DC 20024–2188.

TABLE 3   Guide to contraindications and precautions to vaccination situations[a]

True contraindications and precautions	Not contraindications (vaccines may be administered)
General for all vaccines (DTP, DTap, OPV, IPV, MMR, Hib, Hepatitis B)	
Contraindications	*Not contraindications*
Anaphylactic reaction to a vaccine contraindicates further doses of that vaccine or an injectable antigen;[b] anaphylactic reaction to a vaccine constituent contraindicates the use of vaccine containing that substance;[b] moderate or severe illnesses with or without a fever	Mild/moderate local reaction (soreness, redness, swelling) following a dose; mild acute illness with or without a low-grade fever; current antimicrobial therapy; convalescent phase of illnesses; prematurity (same dosage and indications as for normal full-term infants); recent exposure to an infectious disease[b]
DTP/DTaP (diphtheria–tetanus–acellular pertussis)	
Contraindications	*Not contraindications*
Encephalopathy within 7 days of administration of previous dose of DTP	Temperature of ≥40.5°C (105°F) following a previous dose of DTP
Precautions	
Fever of ≥40.5°C (105°F) within 48 hr after vaccination with a prior dose of DTP; collapse or shocklike state (hypnotic-hyporesponsive episode) within 48 hr of receiving a prior dose of DTP; seizures within 3 days of receiving prior dose of DTP	
Family history of convulsions;[c] family history of sudden infant death syndrome; family history of an adverse event following DTP administration	
Persistent, inconsolable crying lasting[c] 3 hr within 48 hr of receiving prior dose of DTP	

Notes: This information is based on the recommendations of the Advisory Committee on Immunization Practices (ACIP) and those of the Committee on Infectious Diseases (Red Book Committee) of the American Academy of Pediatrics (AAP). Sometimes these recommendations vary from those contained in the manufacturer's package inserts. For more detailed information, providers should consult the published recommendations of the ACIP, AAP, and the manufacturer's package inserts.

[a]The events or conditions listed as precautions, although not contraindications, should be carefully reviewed. The benefits and risks of administering a specific vaccine to an individual under the circumstances should be considered. If the risks are believed to outweigh the benefits, the vaccines should be withheld; if the benefits are believed to outweigh the risks (for example, while traveling in a foreign country during an outbreak), the vaccine should be administered. Whether or not to administer DTP to children with proven or suspected underlying neurologic disorders should be decided on an individual basis. It is prudent on theoretical grounds to avoid vaccinating pregnant women. However, if immediate protection against poliomyelitis is needed, OPV is preferred, though IPV may be considered if a full vaccination series can be completed before the anticipated imminent exposure.

[b]Persons with a history of anaphylactic reactions following egg ingestions should be vaccinated with caution. Protocols have been developed for vaccinating such persons and should be consulted (J Pediatr 1993; 102:196–199, J Pediatr 1988; 113:504–506).

[c]Acetaminophen given before administering DTP and thereafter every four hours for 24 hours should be considered for children with personal or family history of convulsions in siblings or parents.

Abbreviations: DTap, diphtheria–tetanus–acellular pertussis; IPV, inactivated polio vaccine; MMR, Measles-mumps-rubella; OPV, oral polio vaccine.

Source: Adapted from CDC (1994).

BREASTFEEDING AND VACCINATION

Neither killed nor live vaccines affect the safety of breast-feeding for mothers or infants. Breastfeeding does not adversely affect immunization and is not a contraindication for any vaccine. Breastfed infants should be vaccinated according to routine recommended schedules.

Inactivated or killed vaccines do not multiply within the body. Therefore, they should pose no special risk for mothers who are breastfeeding or for their infants. Although live vaccines do multiply within the mother's body, most have not been demonstrated to be excreted in breast milk. Although rubella vaccine virus may be transmitted in breast milk, the virus usually does not infect the infant, and if it does, the infection is well tolerated. There is no contraindication for vaccinating breastfeeding mothers with yellow fever vaccine. Breastfeeding mothers can receive OPV without any interruption in the feeding schedule.

ALTERED IMMUNOCOMPETENCE

The statement of Advisory Committee on Immunization Practices (ACIP) on vaccinating immunocompromised persons summarizes recommendations regarding the efficacy, safety, and use of specific vaccines and immune globulin preparations for immunocompromised persons. ACIP statements on individual vaccines or immune globulins also contain additional information regarding these issues.

Severe immunosuppression can be the result of congenital immunodeficiency, HIV infection, leukemia, lymphoma, generalized malignancy or therapy with alkylating agents, antimetabolites, radiation, or large amounts of corticosteroids. Severe complications have followed vaccination with live, attenuated virus vaccines and live bacterial vaccines among immunocompromised patients. In general, these patients should not receive live vaccines except in certain circumstances that are noted below. In addition, OPV should not be administered to any household contact of a severely immunocompromised person. If polio immunization is indicated for immunocompromised patients, their household members, or other close contacts, IPV should be administered. Measles-mumps-rubella (MMR) vaccine is not contraindicated in the close contacts of immunocompromised patients. The degree to which a person is immunocompromised should be determined by a physician.

Limited studies of MMR vaccination in HIV-infected patients have not documented serious or unusual adverse events. Because measles may cause severe illness in persons with HIV infection, MMR vaccine is recommended for all asymptomatic HIV-infected persons and should be considered for all symptomatic HIV-infected persons. HIV-infected persons on regular immunegamma globulin (IGIV) therapy may not respond to MMR or its individual component vaccines because of the continued presence of passively acquired antibody. However, because of the potential benefit, measles vaccination should be considered approximately two weeks before the next monthly dose of IGIV (if not otherwise contraindicated), although an optimal immune response is unlikely to occur. Unless serologic testing indicates that specific antibodies have been produced, vaccination should be repeated (if not otherwise contraindicated) after the recommended interval.

An additional dose of IGIV should be considered for persons on routine IGIV therapy who are exposed to measles more than three weeks after administration of a standard dose (100–400 mg/kg) of IGIV. Killed or inactivated vaccines can be administered to all immunocompromised patients, although response to such vaccines may be suboptimal. All such childhood vaccines are recommended for immunocompromised persons in usual doses and schedules; in addition, certain vaccines such as pneumococcal vaccine or Hib vaccine are recommended specifically for certain groups of immunocompromised patients, including those with functional or anatomic asplenia.

Vaccination during chemotherapy or radiation therapy should be avoided because antibody response is poor. Patients vaccinated while in immunosuppressive therapy or in the two weeks before starting therapy should be considered unimmunized and should be revaccinated at least three months after therapy is discontinued. Patients with leukemia in remission whose chemotherapy has been terminated for three months may receive live-virus vaccines.

The exact amount of systemically absorbed corticosteroids and the duration of administration needed to suppress the immune system of an otherwise healthy child are not well defined. Most experts agree that steroid therapy usually does not contraindicate administration of live-virus vaccine when the steroid therapy treatment is short term (i.e., <2 weeks); low to moderate dose; long-term, alternate-day treatment with short acting preparations; maintenance physiologic doses (replacement therapy); or administered topically (skin or eyes, by aerosol, or by intra-articular, bursal, or tendon injection). Although of recent theoretical concern, no evidence of increased severe reactions to live vaccines has been reported among persons receiving steroid therapy by aerosol and such therapy is not in itself a reason to delay vaccination. The immunosuppressive effects of steroid treatment vary, but many clinicians consider a dose equivalent to either 2 mg/kg of body weight or a total of 20 mg per day prednisone as sufficiently immunosuppressive to raise concern about the safety of a vaccination with live-virus vaccines. Corticosteroids used in greater than physiologic doses can also reduce immune response to vaccines. Physicians should wait at least three months after discontinuation before administering a live-virus vaccine to patients who have received high systemically absorbed doses of corticosteroids for two weeks.

VACCINATION IN THE CONTEXT OF PRIMARY CARE

Traditionally, vaccination has been primarily an issue for obstetricians and gynecologists, as it impacted pregnancy. With the move toward primary care, there are at least two additional vaccines that require both knowledge and appropriate use by obstetricians/gynecologists: the pneumococcal vaccine (23 valent) and the influenza vaccines.

Pneumococcal Vaccine

As obstetricians/gynecologists are called upon to treat elderly patients or patients with immunodeficiency as a consequence of retrovirus infection, pneumococcal vaccination will become an important part of the proactive medical agenda. In the past, uncertainty about local reactions and the duration of protection have limited the use of pneumococcal vaccination. Currently, the use of pneumococcal vaccine should be predicated on (i) the risk to the patient population and (ii) whether a pneumococcal vaccination has been procured six years or more previously.

The pneumococcal vaccine available before 1983 was 14 valent. Since 1983, the vaccine has been 23 valent. Patients recommended for primary or revaccination are listed in Table 4. Immunocompromised individuals with splenic dysfunction, lymphoma, multiple myeloma, chronic renal failure, nephrotic syndrome, transplantation, or hepatitis C virus have an increased risk of pneumococcal disease.

Influenza Vaccine

The aborted swine flu program in 1976 was instrumental in assisting the Centers for Disease Control and Prevention (CDC) to re-evaluate its position regarding pregnancy (Table 5). The position of the CDC is that pregnancy in itself has not been demonstrated as a risk factor for severe influenza infection, except during the largest pandemics during 1918 to 1919 and 1957 to 1958. However, since influenza vaccine is considered safe for pregnant women without a specific severe egg allergy, pregnant women with medical conditions that increase their risk of complications from influenza should be vaccinated.

To minimize any concern over the theoretical possibility of teratogenicity related to the killed vaccine components, vaccine should be given after the first trimester. To date, there is no evidence that the killed influenza vaccines constitute a risk to the developing fetus. However, it may be

TABLE 4 Recommendations for pneumococcal vaccine use

Immunocompromised adults at increased risk for pneumococcal disease include those with
1. chronic cardiovascular disease
2. chronic pulmonary disease
3. diabetes mellitus
4. alcoholism/cirrhosis
5. adults of the age 65 or over

TABLE 5 CDC recommendations for influenza vaccination

Annual vaccination is strongly suggested
- For all older persons, particularly those over 65 yr because the risk of death during influenza outbreaks generally increases with age
- For all persons (children and adults) who are at increased risk of adverse consequences from infections of the lower respiratory tract because of a pre-existing medical condition

Conditions predisposing to such increased risk include
- Acquired or congenital heart disease with actual or potential alterations in circulatory dynamics (e.g., mitral stenosis, congestive heart failure, or pulmonary-vascular overload)
- Any chronic disorder or condition that compromises pulmonary function (e.g., chronic obstructive pulmonary disease, bronchiectasis, heavy smoking, tuberculosis, severe asthma, cystic fibrosis, neuromuscular and orthopedic disorders with impaired ventilation, bronchopulmonary dysplasia following neonatal respiratory distress syndrome)
- Chronic renal disease with azotemia or nephrotic syndrome
- Diabetes mellitus or other metabolic diseases
- Severe chronic anemia, such as sickle cell disease
- Conditions that compromise the immune mechanism, including certain malignancies and immunosuppressive therapy

undesirable to delay vaccinating a pregnant woman who has a high-risk condition and will still be in the first trimester of pregnancy when influenza activity is anticipated.

SELECTED READING

CDC. Disseminated mycobacterium bovis infection from BCG vaccination of a patient with AIDS. Morb Mortal Wkly Rep 1985; 34:227.

CDC. Recommendations of Advisory Committee on Immunization Practices (ACIP): use of vaccines and immune globulins in persons with altered immunocompetence. Morb Mortal Wkly Rep 1993; 42(No. RR-4):1.

CDC. Vaccination in pregnancy: general recommendations or immunization of the Advisory Committee on Immunization Practices (ACIP) as they apply to vaccination during pregnancy. Morb Mortal Wkly Rep 1994; 43:1.

CDC. Prevention of varicella: recommendations of the Advisory Committee on Immunization Practices (ACIP). Morb Mortal Wkly Rep 1996; 45(RR-11):1.

Davidson M, Bulkow LR, Grabman J, et al. Immungenicity of pneumococca revaccination in patients with chronic disease. Arch Intern Med 1994; 156:2209–2214.

Davis LE, Bodian D, Price D, et al. Chronic progressive poliomyelitis secondary to vaccination of an immunodeficient child. N Engl J Med 1977; 297:241.

Gonik B, Jones T, Contreras D, et al. The obstetrician–gynecologist's role in vaccine-preventable diseases and immunization. Obstet Gynecol 2000; 96:81.

Hirschmann JV, Lipsky BA. The pneumococcal vaccine after 15 years of use. Arch Intern Med 1994; 154:373–377.

MMWR. Diphtheria, tetanus and pertussis: guidelines for vaccine prophylaxis and other preventative measures. Immunization Practices Advisory Committee. Morbid Mortal Wkly Rep 1985; 34:405–414, 419–426.

Mufsom MA, Hughey DF, Turner CE, Schiffman G. Revaccination with pneumococcal vaccine of elderly persons 6 years after primary vaccination. Vaccine 1991; 9:403–407.

Ninane J, Gryomonprez A, Burtonboy G, et al. Disseminated BCG in HIV infection. Arch Dis Child 1993; 63:1268.

Redfield RR, Wright DC, James WD, et al. Disseminated vaccinia in a military recruit with human immunodeficiency virus (HIV) disease. N Engl J Med 1987; 316:676.

Yeager DP, Toy EC, Baker B. Influenza vaccination in pregnancy. Obstet Gynecol 1999; 93:33s.

Urinary Tract Infections in Pregnancy 68

PATHOPHYSIOLOGY

The gestational hormones of pregnancy have been demonstrated to have a profound effect on smooth muscle. Loss of tonicity occurs within the uterine musculature in preparation for its enlargement and the accommodation of an expanding intracavitary mass. Comparable changes occur in all smooth muscle organs early in gestation. A significant variation can be demonstrated from individual to individual. The magnitude of the phenomenon is thought to be mediated through the density of hormone receptor sites.

The effect of the gestational hormones on the musculature of the urogenital tract significantly increases the residual volume of urine in the ureters following micturition. The nongravid female will have a residual urine volume of 5 to 15 mL. With gestation, this volume increases to approximately 20 to 60 mL (Fig. 1). Not all individuals exhibit this phenomenon. In some instances, the changes may be limited to a single ureter. Other individuals will maintain a normal ureteral configuration, as determined by intravenous pyelography, throughout the pregnancy.

Because of a second point of fixation involving the right iliac artery, there is a tendency for the right ureter to accommodate for the physiologic elongation by kinking. This phenomenon is thought to be responsible for the predominance of symptoms on the right side when pyelonephritis develops as a consequence of ascending infection.

EPIDEMIOLOGY

The classic work of Edward Kass focused attention on asymptomatic bacteriuria (ABU) as a critical point of intervention.

In the absence of unique factors that predispose to ABU (i.e., sickle cell trait), the incidence of ABU is inversely proportional to the socioeconomic level of a given population. Indigent patient populations have a rate between 6% and 8%, approximately twice that observed in private patients. ABU develops early in the course of pregnancy; 75% of women who will develop ABU during pregnancy have greater than 100,000 colonies of bacteria per milliliter of urine at the first prenatal visit. Statistically, 25% to 30% of gravidas with ABU will progress to pyelonephritis. If ABU is aggressively treated, the incidence of pyelonephritis drops precipitously. ABU reflects either recent infection by a constituent of the vaginal flora or chronic renal parenchymal disease with seeding from above. The ideal point of therapeutic intervention is that of infection (ABU), not that of disease (cystitis, pyelonephritis).

Schieve et al. (1994) examined the effects of antepartum urinary tract infection (UTI) on adverse maternal and perinatal outcomes. Crude and multivariable analyses were performed with a perinatal registry cohort of 25,746 mother/infant pairs. Elevated risks were observed for exposure to UTI and low birthweight, prematurity, preterm low birthweight, premature labor, hypertension/pre-eclampsia, maternal anemia, and amnionitis. UTI was associated with perinatal death only among subjects who are 20 to 29 years of age.

Prior to the 1970s, infections of the urinary bladder or renal parenchyma were designated by the term "-itis," which was applied to the site of organism replication; hence the terms urethritis, cystitis, and pyelonephritis. The perception of the inability to preclude renal parenchymal involvement in patients with ABU and cystitis, coupled with the need to individualize therapy, resulted in the

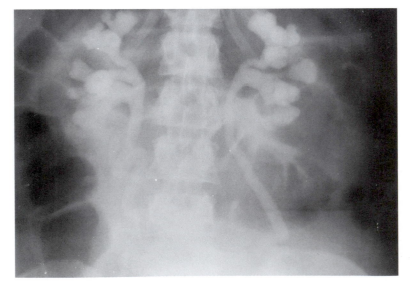

FIGURE 1 Intravenous pyelogram demonstrating a pseudohydronephrosis as a consequence of smooth-muscle relaxation, which is responsible for marked increase in residual volume of urine during pregnancy.

adoption of a broad-label term of UTI to designate a spectrum of involvement that differs significantly in its biologic significance.

Critical in the diagnosis of urinary tract disease is its distinction from infection. Gram-positive and gram-negative aerobic bacteria can replicate in significant quantity in urine without eliciting laboratory or clinical evidence of disease. ABU at a given point of time becomes the cornerstone of therapeutic management. By its diagnosis and therapy, one can frequently abort the progression from infection to disease and, in so doing, implement the pinnacle of therapeutics: preventive medicine.

ASYMPTOMATIC BACTERIURIA

All diagnostic tests except appropriately obtained urine cultures lack either sensitivity or specificity. Bachman et al. (1993) compared the existing rapid screening techniques for detection of asymptomatic UTIs. The results of screening tests of urinalysis, urine dipstick, and Gram staining were compared with the results of standard urine culture at an initial prenatal visit. In follow-up visits, result of urine dipstick testing was compared with that of urinalysis. Rapid screening tests for asymptomatic infection in pregnant women revealed the following: Gram's staining identified 22 of 24 patients (sensitivity, 91.7%; specificity, 89.2%); urine dipstick, 12 of 24 (sensitivity, 50%; specificity, 96.9%); and urinalysis with presence of leukocytes, 6 of 24 (sensitivity, 25%; specificity, 99%). In follow-up visits, urine dipstick tests detected 19 infections and urinalysis detected 3 infections (positive predictive value 5% compared with 3%). Urine dipstick testing for nitrites identified half of all patients with UTIs and was superior to urinalysis on follow-up visits. Although gram's staining is more expensive, it was more accurate than urinalysis or urine dipstick test for nitrites. Urinalysis was never the test of choice because it detected fewer positive cultures. Leukocyte measurement correlated poorly with asymptomatic UTI.

Since there are no clinical signs or symptoms, ABU is diagnosed by prospective culture monitoring of urine. The major problem in diagnosis of ABU is not quantification or bacteriologic identification, but rather proper collection of urine specimens for analysis. With very rare exceptions, UTI is monoetiologic in character. When more than one kind of bacteria exist in a clean midstream voided specimen, it is probable that prior to collection, the urine came in contact with one or both labia minora and majora. For the specimen to have diagnostic validity, the perineum should be cleansed with an antiseptic solution such as povidone-iodine, and the patient should be instructed in the technique required to obtain a valid specimen.

The diagnosis of ABU is predicated on demonstrating more than or equal to 100,000 colonies of a single bacterial genus on two consecutive specimens. A colony count of 50,000 colonies per milliliter of urine obtained from a catheterized specimen should be viewed with suspicion, and additional tests should be undertaken to exclude ABU. ABU may be due to either the de novo acquisition of bacterial replication via ascending urethral infection or seeding of the urine from above due to chronic smoldering pyelonephritis. The distinction is of great therapeutic importance. In the case of the former, eradication of the bacteria can be readily achieved with bolus or short-term administration of an appropriate antibiotic. Chronic smoldering disease requires long-term therapy.

The major diagnostic problem is how to distinguish between these two entities. Localization as to the site of ABU can be achieved by ureteral catheterization, bladder washout techniques, and the analysis of immunoglobulin G (IgG) antibody-coated bacteria. The former are invasive techniques that are of purely academic interest. Only the antibody-coated bacteria determination is a noninvasive technique. It is predicated on the fact that with parenchymal involvement and the elicitation of an inflammatory response, the body responds by elaborating specific antibodies that ultimately adhere to the bacterial surface. Specific bacterial fluorescence can be demonstrated by using an anti-IgG, fluorescence-tagged antibody. Unfortunately, the occurrence of false-positive and false-negative results has limited this test's usefulness.

CYSTITIS

Cystitis is differentiated from ABU by the concomitant presence of clinical symptomatology as well as bacteriuria and pyuria. As with ABU, cystitis, in the absence of mucosal denudation, is rarely a cause of fever. The probability of added maternal urinary tract morbidity is low with uncomplicated cystitis; however, once bacteriuria is documented in a pregnancy, serial monitoring of the urine is advocated to exclude the urinary tract from being a reservoir for bacteria, which may cause perinatal septicemia in the periparturitional period.

DYSURIA

Dysuria occurs because of the loss of urethral or bladder mucosal integrity. The difference in pH between intra- and extracellular fluid (7.47) and urine (4.5–8.0) causes a biophysical reaction that registers as a burning sensation. The timing when dysuria occurs is of diagnostic importance. Dysuria at the beginning of micturition indicates involvement of the outer urethra and is most often caused by a vulvovaginitis or occult infection with *Neisseria gonorrhoeae*. Dysuria associated with urinary bladder infection occurs characteristically at the end of urination. By itself, dysuria correlates with a positive urine culture in approximately 65% of cases.

FREQUENCY

Frequency as a symptom referable to infection is defined as the passage of small amounts of urine. In the simplest sense, the urinary bladder is nothing more than a smooth-muscle sac with peristaltic activity. The submucosal edema and the resultant loss of distensibility induced by the inflammatory response render the urinary bladder less tolerant to volumetric expansion. Frequently, if a significant inflammatory neuritis is present, the patient complains of a suprapubic tenderness or lower midline back pain.

PYURIA

Pyuria in combination with bacteriuria is 99% specific for UTI. The diagnosis of pyuria is established by demonstrating greater than eight white blood cells (WBC) per mm^3 on the viewing of at least 10 high power fields.

Pyuria alone does not correlate well with UTI, owing to problems inherent in specimen collection or distal urethral inflammation due to trauma or a sexually transmitted disease.

Urine dipstick or automated microscopy has been advocated as cost-effective screening modalities for the detection of UTIs.

Demonstration of a positive test for urine leukocyte esterase and/or nitrate is valuable. The problems with this test are its sensitivity and inability to detect bacteriuria in the absence of inflammation. Its minimum threshold is approximately 5 WBC per high power field. This value may vary based on the test strip's manufacturer. A positive leukocyte esterase test warrants evaluation. A number of other conditions not associated with UTI may cause pyuria.

Bacteria possessing nitrate reductase can also be detected using the dipstick test. The test appears to have a low sensitivity for bacteria between 10^3 and 10^5 cfu. A number of urinary tract pathogens, such as *Staphylococcus epidermidis*, *S. aureus*, *Enterococcus* species, and *Pseudomonas* species, lack nitrate reductase. Van Nostrand et al. (2000) found that 78.8% of samples containing a nitrate reductase did not produce a positive reaction with the dipstick. A positive test is a mandate for culture confirmation and therapy in pregnancy.

PYELONEPHRITIS

Whereas ABU and cystitis are very rarely the cause of fever, pyelonephritis is. The diagnosis of pyelonephritis is implied by the recovery of greater than 100,000 colonies of a single bacterial species from a patient with exquisite costo vertebral angle (CVA) tenderness and by the demonstration of clumped WBC and WBC casts in the urinary sediment. The latter are best demonstrated in spun sediment of a fresh urine sample whose specific gravity is greater than 1.020.

CVA tenderness is due to the rapid volumetric expansion of the renal parenchyma due to the inflammatory response and the resultant stretching of the renal capsule. If the capsule of the kidney is stripped away, disease of the renal parenchyma is occult unless it involves major vessels, which carry their own innervation. Unless CVA tenderness is present or a large area of denuded bladder mucosa is present, it would be difficult to ascribe fever to UTI.

In the majority of instances, pyelonephritis is the potential end-titration point for ABU. Parenchymal disease of the kidney (pyelonephritis) is rarely occult. Characteristically, the patients are febrile. Physical examination reveals definite CVA tenderness.

The majority of females who will develop pyelonephritis in pregnancy are readily discernable. Seventy percent of gravidas who have pyelonephritis during gestation will have had an antecedent history of UTI. Smoldering chronic pyelonephritis tends to have an associate pedigree of repeated episodes of UTI in early childhood, honeymoon cystitis, pyelonephritis in a preceding pregnancy, etc.

Pyelonephritis identifies two patient populations: those in whom bacterial infection of the renal parenchyma antedates the acute episodes and those in whom the smooth muscle alterations induced by pregnancy unmask an occult dysfunction of the ureterovesicular junctions. In the case of the former, renal involvement may reflect reactivation of pre-existing disease; in the case of the latter, infection is acquired de novo and parenchymal involvement is the consequence of ascending infection.

In the absence of obstruction, pyelonephritis is a self-limited disease, owing to segmental compartmentalization of the kidney. The demonstration of a true obstruction due to calculi constitutes a medical emergency. Unless the obstruction is relieved, total parenchymal involvement ensues.

LIMITATIONS ON ANTIBIOTIC USE

Pregnancy limits the antibiotic spectrum that can be utilized in the treatment of UTI. The use of fluoroquinolone or the tetracycline class of antibiotics is contraindicated in pregnancy because of either potential for teratogenicity or induction of an embryopathy.

When parturition is imminent, restrictions should be placed on trimethoprim/sulfamethoxazole. Sulfonamides readily traverse the placental barrier and achieve cord drug levels comparable to those in the maternal circulation. The sulfonamides should not be used in the treatment of high-risk pregnancies once fetal viability has been established. Following parturition, the sulfonamides will competitively displace bilirubin from its albumin carrier, and it is the free bilirubin that traverses the blood–brain barrier and induces kernicterus in the neonate. The presence of sulfonamides precludes using total bilirubin levels as a prognostic index of ensuing kernicterus. If an infant is born with significant sulfonamide levels in the cord blood, an exchange transfusion is advocated. The fluoroquinolones have produced permanent lesions in the cartilage of immature dogs.

MANAGEMENT OF UTI IN PREGNANCY

Asymptomatic Bacteriuria

At the time of registration and six weeks prior to the expected date of confinement, all new prenatal patients should be cultured for ABU. Unless the patient has one of the following:

1. history of pyelonephritis or
2. diabetes mellitus or sickle-cell–related disease.

A second specimen should be obtained at 32 to 36 weeks. For patients in the indicated high-risk categories, more frequent monitoring is needed. The documentation of ABU is an indication for therapy (Table 1).

Of all ABU isolates, 90% belong to the Enterobacteriaceae. The therapy of ABU is either a bolus administration with amoxicillin or augmentin or a standard course of an appropriate antibiotic. In the past, the selection of an intermediate semisynthetic penicillin or sulfonamide as first-line therapy had not been predicated on a drug-of-choice concept, but rather on cost–efficacy considerations. Ampicillin will eradicate only 60% of the causative organisms and should be used for empiric therapy only when follow-up cultures are obtained in 24 to 36 hours. The cost difference between ampicillin and an oral cephalosporin may be of such magnitude as to preclude drug purchase by the patients, particularly those from a lower socioeconomic background.

Irrespective of which antibiotic is administered, a test of cure should be obtained 24 to 36 hours after the onset of therapy. If a given antibiotic is effective against the urinary tract pathogen, the urine will be sterile in less than 24 hours. If bacteriuria is still demonstrable after 24 to 36 hours of therapy, the bacterial isolate should be identified and its antibiotic susceptibility pattern established by the Kirby Bauer method. In Table 2 the drugs of choice for the individual urinary tract pathogens are summarized.

Current therapy favors the use of single-dose therapy. There is no convincing evidence that a long course of medication is more effective than a short one. Villar et al. (2000) reviewed the data involving over 400 women as to the duration of treatment for ABU. All studies compared single-dose treatment with four- to seven-day treatments. No differences in "no-cure" rates were detected. Longer duration of therapy was associated with an increase in reports of adverse drug effects.

Cystitis

For premenopausal, nonpregnant women, single-dose antimicrobial therapy is generally less effective than the same antibiotic used for a longer duration. Most antimicrobial agents given for three days are as effective as those given for longer duration and adverse events tend to be found more often with longer therapy. Trimethoprim or co-trimoxazole can be recommended for therapy only in communities when resistance to uropathogens is 10% or less. The fluoroquinolones are the standard drugs of choice in nonpregnant women unless resistance to *Escherichia coli* exceeds 10%. Alternate therapy includes fosfomycin, trometamol, or beta-lactams, such as the second- or third-generation cephalosporins or pivmecillinam.

Single-dose therapy is not recommended for acute cystitis because early pyelonephritis can be mistaken for uncomplicated cystitis. In pregnancy, the use of a fluoroquinolone is to be avoided owing to potential fetal indications.

Pyelonephritis

Pyelonephritis occurs in 1% to 2% of all obstetric patients. It is the most common medical complication

TABLE 1 Therapeutic recommendations for urinary tract infections in pregnancy

Indication	Modifier	Recommended therapy	Follow-up
ABU: due to GBS, *Escherichia coli*, *Proteus mirabilis*, *Staphylococcus saprophyticus*	No history of pyelonephritis. If a history exists, evaluate for L-form variant (presuming one is dealing with a gram-negative isolate)	Least expensive beta-lactam antibiotic	Test of cure
Due to resistant *E. coli*, *Klebsiella pneumoniae*, *Enterobacter* species, etc.	See above	Resistant *E. coli* oral cephalosporin or IM aminoglycoside, *K. pneumoniae* oral cephalosporin	Test of cure
Either of the above	History of pyelonephritis at any time prior to or during pregnancy. Prior episode of ABU or cystitis in this pregnancy	See above. Prophylactic antibiotics either daily or postcoitus	Culture monitored throughout pregnancy. Test of cure
Cystitis	No history of pyelonephritis	Antibiotic selection initially predicated on regional isolation data; ultimate selection by isolate antibiotic sensitivities. Avoid using nitrofurantoins	Test of cure
Pyelonephritis		Third-generation (bid) cephalosporin. Ultimate selection based on isolate antibiotic sensitivity profile (see Table 3)	Culture monitored throughout pregnancy. If recurrent UTI, consider nitrofurantoin prophylaxis. History of pyelonephritis: rule out L-form variant when isolates are identical in each case

Abbreviations: ABU, asymptomatic bacteriuria; GBS, group B streptococci; UTI, urinary tract infection.

TABLE 2 Drugs of choice for urinary tract pathogens in pregnancy

Bacteria	Drug of choice
Gram-positive *Staphylococcus epidermidis*, micrococcus subgroup III, group B beta-hemolytic streptococci, group D streptococci (enterococci)	Ampicillin
Gram-negative (Enterobacteriaceae), *E. coli*, *Klebsiella pneumoniae*, *Enterobacter* spp. (cloacae), *Proteus mirabilis* (indole-negative), *Proteus vulgaris*, etc. (indole-positive)	Determined by sensitivities: 65% susceptible to ampicillin, 80% susceptible to cefazolin, 90% susceptible to cefamandole. Cephalosporin, carbenicillin, ampicillin, an aminoglycoside or cephalosporin (if susceptible in vitro)

during pregnancy requiring hospitalization. The protocol for dealing with pyelonephritis in pregnancy is bed rest, aggressive hydration, and systemic antibiotics (Table 3). The patient should be switched to oral medication after 24 hours and a repeat quantitative urine culture performed. If the repeat urine culture again demonstrates greater than 100,000 colonies per milliliter of urine of the same bacteria, antibiotic therapy should be changed if it can be documented that the patient received the medication initially prescribed.

The critical issues in the therapy of pyelonephritis have been well worked out:

1. Pyelonephritis is a monomicrobial disease process; in less than 1% of cases coinfection between *E. coli* and *Klebsiella pneumoniae* may be present.
2. Urinary tract is an aerobic environment and its pathogenic spectrum is readily identifiable with comparatively simple microbiologic methodology.
3. Urine for valid microbiologic identification of the pathogen is easily attainable.
4. In the absence of obstruction and/or advanced diabetic vascular disease, the anatomical compartmentalization limits the resultant morbid consequences.
5. Most of the drugs effective in this disease process have significant renal elimination, resulting in drug concentrations that are increased in comparison to that of most other organ systems.

Traditionally, when a patient presents with pyelonephritis in pregnancy, urine and blood cultures would be taken and a presumptive commitment to therapy would be implemented. Approximately 90% of all cases of pyelonephritis are due to gram-negative rods, and 10% to 12% of the cases involve gram-positive organisms, i.e., group B streptococci, *S. saprophyticus*, etc.

The selection of the initial antibiotic is often governed not by efficacy but by lower acquisitional cost; i.e., ampicillin versus cephalosporin. One in every three to four cases of pyelonephritis treated with ampicillin will be a therapeutic failure. This is in contrast with an observed failure rate of

one in seven to eight patients for a first-or second-generation cephalosporin. Frequency of administration significantly impacts on the total cost to the patient. When computed, the cost of isolated clinical failures often erases the economies achieved with successful therapeutic interventions in the majority of patients.

Once the diagnosis of pyelonephritis in pregnancy is confirmed, the patient should be placed on broad spectrum second- or third-generation cephalosporins.

Blood cultures are of limited value unless

1. Gram stain of urine reveals gram-positive cocci, suggestive of *S. aureus*;
2. the patient has experienced rigor; or
3. the patient's clinical condition is unstable.

Approximately 20% of patients with pyelonephritis develop occult renal dysfunction similar to acute tubular necrosis. The decrease in renal function is transient, but in isolated instances may persist for three to five weeks after termination of therapy. Baseline evaluation of renal function, including electrolytes, blood urea nitrogen, and creatinine, is deemed advisable.

Another 1% to 4% of women with acute pyelonephritis will manifest septic shock or adult respiratory distress syndrome (ARDS) due to sustained high multiplicity bacteremia due to gram-negative bacteria. Administration of antibiotics can function as a catalytic event that converts the warm-phase of shock into its clinically more significant variant. An increase in respiratory rate in a gravida with pyelonephritis should warrant obtaining blood gases and a chest roentgenogram. Unlike most etiologies of ARDS, the prognosis is good with appropriate therapy.

Confirmation of antibiotic efficacy can be done within hours after the initiation of antimicrobial therapy. Demonstration of continued significant bacteriuria by Gram staining of the urinary sediment or culturing using bacterial culture kits four hours after the initiation of parenteral antibiotic therapy and aggressive hydration should be interpreted as indicative of a therapeutic failure. Under these circumstances, the antimicrobial regimen should be changed to a third-generation cephalosporin and an aminoglycoside with a broader coverage for the *Enterobacteriaceae*.

Once lysis of fever and marked amelioration of CVA tenderness have occurred, conversion from parenteral to oral antibiotics can be implemented. As a rule of thumb, the cost to the patient of intravenously administered antibiotics is 10 to 15 times that of per oral administration. Which antibiotic is chosen is governed by in vitro sensitivity studies and cost of acquisition. If the urinary pathogen is sensitive to ampicillin, conversion from parenteral therapy to an oral cephalosporin cannot be advocated other than for reasons of patient compliance.

Failure of CVA tenderness to respond to therapy as predicted by in vitro antibiotic testing may be due to

1. inaccurate laboratory data;
2. obstructive uropathy; or
3. an independently functioning disease process.

TABLE 3 Sequence for the evaluation and management of pyelonephritis during pregnancy

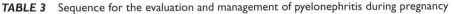

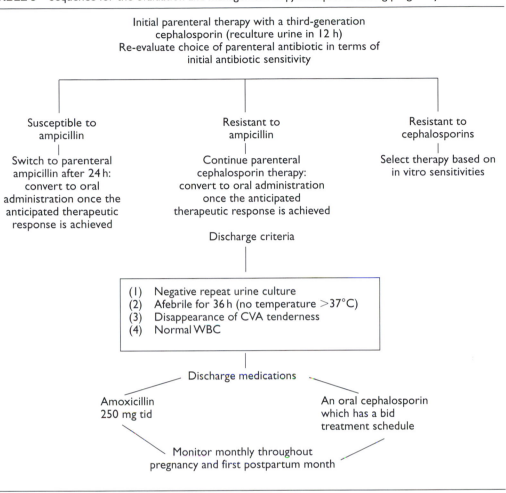

Initial parenteral therapy with a third-generation
cephalosporin (reculture urine in 12 h)
Re-evaluate choice of parenteral antibiotic in terms of
initial antibiotic sensitivity

Susceptible to ampicillin	Resistant to ampicillin	Resistant to cephalosporins
Switch to parenteral ampicillin after 24 h: convert to oral administration once the anticipated therapeutic response is achieved	Continue parenteral cephalosporin therapy: convert to oral administration once the anticipated therapeutic response is achieved	Select therapy based on in vitro sensitivities

Discharge criteria

(1) Negative repeat urine culture
(2) Afebrile for 36 h (no temperature >37°C)
(3) Disappearance of CVA tenderness
(4) Normal WBC

Discharge medications

Amoxicillin 250 mg tid

An oral cephalosporin which has a bid treatment schedule

Monitor monthly throughout pregnancy and first postpartum month

Duration of administration is determined by: (1) history of repeat episodes of pyelonephritis not related to the gestation, or (2) bacteriologic evidence that the patient has had prior infection with the same organism at least once in this pregnancy. If either of these criteria is met, therapy should be extended for a minimum of 21 days; otherwise a 10-day to 14-day course is recommended.
Abbreviations: CVA, costovertebral angle; WBC, white blood cells.

In a gravida with suspected urosepsis on the basis of obstructive uropathy, ultrasonography is the procedure of choice.

Korst et al. (2006) have made a case that the incidence of pyelonephritis in pregnancy is an indicator of the quality of prenatal care. The author strongly agrees with their conclusion.

Ambulatory Treatment of Acute Pyelonephritis
Medical economics have renewed the debate as to whether acute pyelonephritis in pregnancy should be deemed a mandate for hospitalization.

Clinical studies have shown that low-risk gravidas in the first and early second trimesters can, after an initial period of observation and in vitro microbiologic confirmation of effective therapy, be effectively treated on an ambulatory basis.

Millar and Cox (1997) treated 120 pregnant women with acute pyelonephritis at 24 weeks' gestational age or less with either an intramuscular or intravenous cephalosporin. If clinically stable at the end of 24 hours,

the patients chosen for ambulatory care therapy were discharged. The patients then completed a 10-day course of oral cephalexin 500 mg qid. Ten percent of outpatients were rehospitalized because of sepsis, abnormal laboratory tests, or "recurrent pyelonephritis."

Wing (2001) conducted a similar therapeutic study, focusing on gravidas after 24 weeks' gestation. After eliminating 154/256 potential study candidates for reasons that included sepsis, respiratory compromise, recurrent pyelonephritis, urologic abnormalities, allergies to cephalosporins/penicillins, etc., they were left with 92 eligible participants. Among this, 30% of the outpatient subjects had to remain in the hospital because of clinical sepsis, documented bacteremia, or a nonresponsive WBC count. Another 13% failed therapy.

Outpatient therapy for acute pyelonephritis in early pregnancy will require a valid signed informed consent and documentation of bacterial susceptibility to the designated antibiotic. The antibiotic utilized for ambulatory therapy needs to be able to achieve greater than 90% bioavailability with oral administration. Antibiotics meeting this prerequisite include cephalexin, levofloxacin, and trimethoprim-sulfamethoxazole. Extension of hospital-initiated aminoglycoside therapy can be achieved with outpatient parenteral therapy. Owing to their concentration dependency, aminoglycosides can be administered once daily within the context of home care.

FOLLOW-UP OF PATIENTS WITH UTI

Once a UTI is documented in pregnancy, the patient should be screened on a monthly basis, including the first postpartum month.

Whether to place a patient on chronic antimicrobial suppressive therapy versus close monitoring is an issue open to debate. Pfau and Sacks (1989) evaluated the effectiveness of prophylaxis for recurrent UTI during pregnancy. During 39 pregnancies, 33 women with a history of recurrent UTIs (and, in some instances, pyelonephritis) received postcoital prophylaxis consisting of a single oral dose of eithercephalexin (250 mg) or nitrofurantoin macrocrystals (50 mg). While 130 UTIs occurred during a mean observation period of seven months before prophylaxis, only a single UTI occurred during pregnancy after prophylaxis. Problems with compliance with medication stress the need for bacteriologic surveillance in the chronically suppressed group.

Following the initial episode of ABU, culture monitoring of the gravida is advocated. If the urine is sterile after therapy, the preferred choice is to monitor the patient. If ABU or overt disease recurs, culture and sensitivity tests are necessary in order to determine the biologic significance of this event and whether one is dealing with either relapse or reinfection.

The reappearance of greater than 100,000 colonies per milliliter after the bacteriologic evidence of cure (as documented by sterile urine cultures within a week of therapy termination) mandates the differentiation of relapse from reinfection. If the bacteria isolated during the second episode exhibit a different pattern of antibiotic susceptibility from that originally isolated or are of a different genus, the infection is termed a reinfection.If the bacteria isolated are the same in terms of genus and antibiotic sensitivities, the infection is termed a relapse. The distinction is important in terms of pathogenesis and prognosis. Reinfections often represent a problem in terms of hygiene of the female genital tract. Pyelonephritis, when it occurs in this setting, is of limited morbid consequence and no urologic workup is indicated in the postpartum period. If educational steps cannot effectively alter the chain of events producing disease, these patients are good candidates for chronic prophylactic suppression. The most effective drug for long-term, low-dose prophylaxis is nitrofurantoin 100 mg, given at night. More recent studies show that a dose administered on alternate nights, three nights a week, or after intercourse is just as effective. Relapse should alert the physician to the possibility of chronic upper urinary tract disease.

Postcoitus antibiotic prophylaxis with nitrofurantoin (100 mg daily) should be considered for women in whom episodes of UTI are associated with sexual intercourse. Schooff and Hill (2005) looked at recurrent UTIs in non-pregnant women. They found no statistical difference in the rates of microbiologic recurrence between daily use and postcoital use of ciprofloxacin.

Relapse may be indicative of a chronic smoldering form of renal parenchymal disease. Once relapse has occurred, the patient should be closely monitored for renewal of parenchymal bacterial replication. Future therapy should include an antibiotic effective against L-form variants. If the patient has a history of urinary infection at some time other than pregnancy, it is our policy to advocate monthly monitoring for a two-year period and to obtain an intravenous pyelogram approximately 6 to 12 weeks postpartum (Table 4).

POTENTIAL SIGNIFICANCE OF UTI FOR MOTHER AND FETUS

Monitoring for ABU should probably be considered one of the essential components of prenatal care. Traditionally, the potential adverse effects of ABU have been conceptually limited to the development of pyelonephritis. Recent evidence suggests that those species of *Enterobacteriaceae* that are able to establish numerically significant representation in the genitourinary tract by virtue of their augmented ability to adhere to cell surfaces differ from other species of *Enterobacteriaceae* that may be transient constituents of the perineal and vaginal flora. Gravidas with ABU, as opposed to gravidas who have one or more members of the *Enterobacteriaceae* in the perineal or vaginal flora but who do not have ABU, are at augmented risk

TABLE 4 Significance of positive cultures following initial therapy for pyelonephritis

Bacterial species	Follow-up urine specimen	
	24–48 hr after hospitalization	7–10 days after therapy or at any other time during gestation
Same organism	(*i*) Inappropriate antibiotics, (*ii*) failure to receive medication, (*iii*) acquired resistance (R factor)	Relapse: most often indicative of chronic smoldering pyelonephritis and L-phase variant transformation. Rule out possibility of structural abnormalities of the urinary tract
Different organism	Mixed infection unmasked by therapeutic elimination of dominant organism	Reinfection: attempt to rule elimination of dominant organismout mechanized factors or problems with personal hygiene, which may predispose to reinfection. Underlying chronic pyelonephritis not uncommon

for postpartum endometritis and gram-negative septicemia, and their offspring are at augmented risk for perinatal septicemia due to the *Enterobacteriaceae*.

The ability to colonize the urinary tract successfully (ABU) in women is frequently associated with the concomitant appearance of the organism as a constituent of the bacterial flora of the posterior vaginal pool and endocervix. Monif (1982), in a retrospective analysis of *Enterobacteriaceae* septicemia in the immediate postpartum period, revealed that when concomitant blood, urine, and endometrial cultures were available, almost invariably the same genus isolated from the blood could be recovered from the urine and endometrium. In only one case was there with any evidence of renal parenchymal involvement. Minor antibiotic sensitivity differences between the bacterial isolates from blood, urine, and endometrium suggested that not the urinary tract, but rather the maternal implantation site afforded the portal of infection. When gravidas were prospectively monitored, the incidence of postpartum endometritis following spontaneous vaginal delivery was 10 to 20 times greater for those with ABU than for those without.

Preliminary evidence suggests that at least 50% of cases of perinatal septicemia (defined as the onset of disease within the first 24 hours of life) occur in infants born to gravidas who have chorioamnionitis and/or ABU. That bacteria may have access to the fetus in utero has been suggested by the demonstration that lymphocytes of selected neonates born to mothers whose gestation had been complicated by significant UTI would undergo blast transformation when exposed to the specific strain of bacteria responsible for maternal infection.

McDermott et al. (2000) investigated the relative risk for mental retardation or developmental delays among infants of mothers with diagnosed UTI. They compared gravidae who took their antibiotics with those who failed to do so. They found a statistically significant association between maternal UTI without antibiotics and mental retardation or developmental delays within the first and third trimesters.

SELECTED READING

Anderson JD. Single dose treatment of acute urinary infection in women. J Antimicrob Chemother 1980; 6:170.
Andriole VT, Patterson TF. Epidemiology, natural history, and management of urinary tract infections in pregnancy. Med Clin North Am 1991; 75:359.
Bachman JW, Heise RH, Naessens JM, Timmerman MG. A study of various tests to detect asymptomatic urinary tract infections in an obstetric population. JAMA 1993; 270(16):1971.
Bint AJ, Hill D. Bacteriuria of pregnancy—an update on significance, diagnosis and management. J Antimicrob Chemother 1994; 33(Suppl A):93.
Christensen B. Which antibiotics are appropriate for treating bacteriuria in pregnancy? J Antimicrob Chemother 2000; 46(Suppl 1):29.
Dafnis E, Sabatini S. The effect of pregnancy on renal function: physiology and pathophysiology. Am J Med Sci 1992; 303:184.
DeMaio. Outpatient parenteral therapy. Infect Med 2004; 21:496.
Fang LST, Tolkoff-Rubin NE, Runin RH. Efficacy of single-dose and conventional amoxicillin therapy in urinary tract infection localized by antibody-coated bacteria technique. N Engl J Med 1978; 198:413.
Hill JB, Sheddield JS, McIntire DD, Wrndel Jr GD. Acute pyelonephritis and pregnancy. Obstet Gynecol 2005; 105:18.
Kim ED, Schaeffer AJ. Antimicrobial therapy for urinary tract infections. Semin Nephrol 1994; 14:551.
Kiningham RB. Asymptomatic bacteriuria in pregnancy. Am Fam Physician 1993; 47:1232.
Komaroff AL. Urinalysis and urine culture in women with dysuria. Ann Intern Med 1986; 104:212.
Korst LM, Reyes C, Fridman M, et al. Gestational pyelonephritis as an indicator of the quality of ambulatory maternal health care services. Obstet Gynecol 2006; 107:632.
Lucas MJ, Cunningham FG. Urinary infection in pregnancy. Clin Obstet Gynecol 1993; 36:855.
McDermott S, Callaghan W, Szwejbka L, et al. Urinary tract infection during pregnancy and mental retardation and developmental delay. Obstet Gynecol 2000; 96:113.
Mikhail MS, Anyaegbunam A. Lower urinary tract dysfunction in pregnancy: a review. Obstet Gynecol Surv 1995; 50:675.
Millar LK, Cox SM. Urinary tract infections complicating pregnancy. Infect Dis Clin North Am 1997; 11:13.
Monif GRG. Association of enterobacteriaceae septicemia in the immediate postpartum period and asymptomatic bacteriuria. Obstet Gynecol 1982; 60:184.
Monif GRG. Intrapartum bacteriuria and postpartum endometritis. Obstet Gynecol 1991; 78:245.
Naber KG. Treatment options for acute uncomplicated cystitis in adults. J Antimicrob Chemother 2000; 46(Suppl 1): 23.
Patterson TF, Andriole VT. Detection, significance, and therapy of bacteriuria in pregnancy. Infect Dis Clin North Am 1997; 11:593.
Pfau A, Sacks TG: Effective prophylaxis of recurrent urinary tract infections in premenopausal women by postcoital administration of cephalexin. J Urol 1989; 142:1276.
Sanford JP. Urinary tract symptoms and infections. Ann Rev Med 1975; 26:485.
Schieve LA, Handler A, Hershow R, et al. Urinary tract infection during pregnancy: its association with maternal morbidity and perinatal outcome. Am J Public Health 1994; 84:405.
Schooff M, Hill K. Antibiotics for recurrent urinary tract infections. Am Fam Physician 2005; 71:1301.
Semeniuk H, Church D. Evaluation of the leukocyte esterase and nitrite urine dipstick screening tests for detection of bacteriuria in women with suspected uncomplicated urinary tract infections. J Clin Microbiol 1999; 37:3051.
Sheffield JS, Cunningham FG. Urinary tract infections in women. Obstet Gynecol 2005; 106:1085.
Tan JS, File TM Jr. Treatment of bacteriuria in pregnancy. Drugs 1992; 44:972.
Van Nostrand JD, Junkins AD, Bartholdi RK. Poor predictive ability of urinalysis and microscopic examination to detect urinary tract infection. Am J Clin Pathol 2000; 113:709.
Villar J, Lydon-Rochelle MT, Gulmezogla AM, Roganti A. Cochrane Database Syst Rev 2: CD 000491, 2000.
Weissenbacher ER, Reisenberger K. Uncomplicated urinary tract infections in pregnancy and nonpregnant women. Curr Opin Obstet Gynecol 1993; 5:513.
Wing DA. Pyelonephritis in pregnancy: treatment options for optimal outcomes. Drugs 2001; 61:60.
Wisinger DB. Urinary tract infection. Current management strategies. Postgrad Med 1996; 100:229.
Young JL, Soper DE. Urinalysis and urinary tract infection: update for clinicians. Infect Dis Obstet Gynecol 2001; 9:249.
Zinner SH. Management of urinary tract infections in pregnancy: a review with comments on single dose therapy. Infection 1992; 20(Suppl 4):S280.

EPIDEMIOLOGY

Infectious endocarditis superimposed upon pregnancy is a rare condition (Fig. 1). The estimated incidence is 0.005% to 0.015% of pregnancies. The associated maternal mortality is a partial function of therapy. In the preantibiotic era, the maternal and fetal mortalities approached 75% to 100%. With the advent of antibiotic therapy alone, maternal mortality has decreased to an approximate 30%. Maternal mortality for women whose pregnancies are complicated by infectious endocarditis is four times that of women cured of endocarditis prior to pregnancy. Although maternal mortality has dramatically dropped due to more aggressive use of open-heart surgery, fetal mortality continues to be high. Zitnik et al. (1969) reported on 21 patients who underwent cardiac surgery with cardiopulmonary bypass. While their maternal mortality was 5%, fetal mortality was 53%. Technological advances in this area have further reduced the mortality risk for both mother and fetus.

Infectious endocarditis in pregnancy involves three high-risk groups:

1. acute disease in gravidas undergoing abortion and developing subsequent sepsis;
2. gravidas with high velocity flow cardiac lesions, i.e., bicuspid aortic valves, ventricular septal defect, or lesions such as idiopathic hypertropic subaortic stenosis and probably mitral valve prolapse. Atrial septal defects are low pressure cardiac lesions and hence are not at augmented risk for infectious endocarditis; and
3. gravidas who are parenteral drug abusers.

What is done and when are governed primarily by maternal considerations; however, given a reasonably hemodynamically stable gravida, fetal considerations can modify when you do it. A management schema that augments maternal jeopardy to enhance fetal outcome necessitates valid patient participation and consultation. Once the criteria for valve replacement have been met, and if age is consistent with a reasonable probability of a good fetal outcome, the tendency has been to deliver the fetus prematurely in order to avoid intraoperative risks to the fetus. Burstein et al. (1985) have reported successful cardiopulmonary bypass with subsequent aortic valve replacement immediately after an emergency cesarean section in a case of acute gonococcal endocarditis complicated by fetal distress at 30 weeks' gestation as a result of maternal cardiovascular decompensation. When surgery and/or the postoperative course require effective anticoagulation, the risk of internal bleeding to the fetus as well as to the mother is introduced.

The following bacteria have been found to produce endocarditis in pregnancy:

1. Gram-positive cocci
   - *Staphylococcus aureus*
   - Viridans streptococci
   - Group B streptococci
   - *Peptostreptococcus anaerobius*
2. Gram-positive rods
   - *Listeria monocytogenes*
3. Gram-negative cocci
   - *Neisseria gonorrhoeae*
4. Gram-negative rods
   - *Salmonella enteritidis*
   - *Haemophilus aphrophilus*

A single case of polymicrobial endocarditis disease occurred in a heroin addict and was caused by *S. aureus* and a group B streptococcus.

Sexton et al. (1985) reported two fatal cases of acute endocarditis involving the aortic valve, which occurred in a woman after a normal pregnancy and delivery and in the second woman after a second trimester abortion. Both women were thought to have normal heart valves before the onset of their infection. Of the 19 cases of pregnancy-associated group B streptococcal endocarditis, the majority of cases occurred in the preantibiotic stage. The principal site of involvement was the mitral valve, the site of disease being governed by pre-existing valvular disease. When aortic valve involvement occurred, the majority of women had pre-existing congenital cardiovascular anomalies or rheumatic valvular disease. Both of these women with acute aortic valvulitis due to the group B streptococci went on to develop annular abscesses and died.

Prior to the advent of penicillin, *N. gonorrhoeae* was responsible for 6% to 12% of cases of infectious endocarditis. With

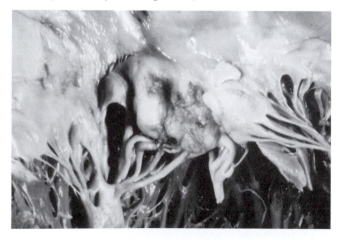

FIGURE I Infectious endocarditis involving the mitral valve of a 23-year-old gravida with mitral valve prolapse.

the introduction of effective antimicrobial therapy, acute gonococcal endocarditis has become an exceedingly rare event. Characteristic of most acute cases of endocarditis in pregnancy, the aortic valve is preferentially involved. Acute valvular perforation and the resultant aortic regurgitation are to be anticipated. The majority of women with postpartum gonococcal endocarditis require valvular replacement.

Infectious endocarditis can be classified into three broad groups based on diverging pathogenesis:

1. naked valve endocarditis (congenital and acquired),
2. prosthetic valve endocarditis, and
3. addict endocarditis.

The subset influences the site of vegetations. In naked valve endocarditis, the vegetations tend to occur on the edge of the valves, whereas in prosthetic valve endocarditis, they occur at the base of the annular rings. In addict endocarditis, there is increased right-sided valvular involvement. The bacteriology is markedly influenced by the categories. With naked valve endocarditis, more than 50% of cases are due to streptococci. With addict endocarditis, more than 50% of the cases are due to staphylococci.

DIAGNOSIS

The major problem confronting obstetricians and gynecologists is recognizing when infectious endocarditis has occurred. The clinical presentations of infectious endocarditis are primarily those of

1. prolonged fever of unknown origins (FUO);
2. FUO and arterial emboli to brain, kidneys, spleen, or extremities; and
3. congestive heart failure with regurgitative murmur and FUO.

A presumptive diagnosis of infectious endocarditis must be entertained when an FUO is documented in high-risk groups such as

1. congenital heart disease except low flow shunts,
2. rheumatic valvular disease,
3. prosthetic heart valves, and/or
4. drug abusers.

Clinical manifestations suggestive of infectious endocarditis and particularly due to *S. aureus* are

1. hemorrhagic infarcts in extremities,
2. presence of pericarditis (indicates extension of abscess through annular ring), and
3. infectious endocarditis in an addict.

On physical examination, one looks for Osler's nodes (painful red nodules on tips of fingers and toes), Janeway's lesions (painless hemorrhagic nodules on palms and soles), Roth's spots (hemorrhagic spots with central white area on funduscopic examination), and splinter hemorrhages under the nail-beds (Fig. 2).

In suspected cases of bacterial endocarditis, at least three sets of blood cultures should be taken at three different

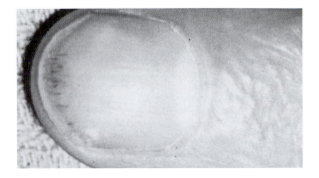

FIGURE 2 Splinter hemorrhages under the nail-bed of a male addict with infectious endocarditis.

intervals (at least 30–60 minutes apart). Additional sets of blood cultures obtained to exclude possible skin contamination are not cost effective. If skin decontamination is done with concern and the syringe needle is changed prior to inoculation of the aerobic and anaerobic blood culture bottles, the probability of contamination is negligible. Multiple sets of blood obtained in a single time frame require clinical clarification if the physician wants all the sets to be processed. Never divide a single sample into multiple sets of blood cultures. It is better to put 10 mL of blood into each culture bottle than to submit two sets of blood cultures with 5 mL in each bottle.

The minimum criteria for presumptive diagnosis of infectious endocarditis include

1. regurgitative murmur or documentation by cardiac catheterization of valvular insufficiency plus positive blood culture,
2. FUO and appropriate murmur,
3. FUO and echocardiographic demonstration of vegetations, and
4. persistently positive blood cultures.

Echocardiography is central to both a presumptive and a definitive diagnosis of bacterial endocarditis. Echocardiographic evidence of an oscillating intracardiac mass or vegetations, an annular abscess, prosthetic valve partial dehiscence, or new valvular regurgitation is deemed highly diagnostic.

Definitive diagnosis of bacterial endocarditis requires fulfilling the criteria requirements within the Duke Diagnostic Schema for infectious endocarditis (Table 1). Clinically definite bacterial endocarditis within this schema requires the presence of two major criteria, one major criterion and three minor criteria, or five minor criteria.

The problem with the Duke Schema is that it is overfocused on certainty. Early therapeutic intervention is a major key to achieving successful outcomes, hence the need to be prepared to act on a high index of suspicion.

THERAPY

Because of changing patterns of antibiotic susceptability *Streptococcus viridans*, enterococci, *S. aureus*, *N. gonorrhoeae*, *Salmonella*, and *Haemophilus* organisms require, once the diagnosis is inferred or established, that patient care be

TABLE 1 Modified Duke diagnostic criteria for infectious endocarditis

Major criteria
1. Documentation at open-heart surgery
2. Documentation at necropsy
3. Well-defined microbiological criteria (high-grade bacteremia or fungemia) plus echocardiographic evidence of mobile, echodense masses attached to valvular leaflets, periannular abscesses, or new dehiscence of a valvular prosthesis

Minor criteria
1. Intermittent bacteremia or fungemia
2. Fever
3. Major embolic events
4. Nonembolic vascular phenomenon
5. Underlying valvular disease
6. Injection drug use
7. Echocardiographic abnormalities that fall short of typical valvular vegetations

transferred to a sophisticated therapeutic interventionist. The choice of antibiotic is dictated by the bacteria's sensitivity profile, absence of contraindications, and bioavailability of drug at the site of disease. When possible, bacterial endocarditis should not be treated in community hospitals. Treatment should be carried out in an institution where bypass surgery can be performed.

The response to antibiotic therapy needs to be monitored with at least two sets of blood cultures obtained every 24 to 48 hours until bloodstream infection is cleared and complete lysis of the fever has occurred (temperature continuously less than 37.6°C).

Bad prognostic signs in bacterial endocarditis are the development of new conduction defects, indicating the possible presence of septal abscess, which may progress to third degree heart block and/or congestive heart failure. The sudden development of congestive heart failure with concomitant cardiomegaly argues strongly for valvular replacement.

The strongest indications that a surgical intervention is or will be required are

1. congestive heart failure or hemodynamically significant mitral regurgitation;
2. suppurative pericarditis;
3. appearance of second- or third-degree atrial-ventricular block;
4. persistence of febrile course after more than one week of effective antibiotic therapy;
5. difficult to eradicate agent, i.e., pseudomonas infectious endocarditis;
6. large vessel embolism with an organism other than viridans streptococci; and
7. presence of large vegetation as documented by echocardiographs associated with significant hemodynamic dysfunction.

SELECTED READING

Atri ML, Cohen DH. Group B streptococcus endocarditis following second-trimester abortion. Arch Intern Med 1990; 150:2579.

Baddor LM, Wilson WR, Bayer AS, et al. Infectious endocarditis. Circulation 2005; 111;e394.

Bayer AS, Bolger AF, Taubert KA, et al. Diagnosis and management of infectious endocarditis and its complications. Circulation 1998; 98:2936.

Bhoola RL, Rajmohamed SE. Acute bacterial endocarditis following criminal abortion. S Afr Med J 1979; 56:85.

Burstein H, Sampson MB, Kohler JP, Levitsky S. Gonococcal endocarditis during pregnancy: simultaneous cesarean section and aortic valve surgery. Obstet Gynecol 1985; 66:485.

Cavalieri RL, Watkins L Jr, Abraham RA, et al. Acute bacterial endocarditis with postpartum aortic valve replacement. Obstet Gynecol 1982; 59:124.

Clinicopathological Conference. Post-abortal fever and shock. S Afr Med J 1983; 63:444.

Cox SM, Leveno KJ. Pregnancy complicated by bacterial endocarditis. Clin Obstet Gynecol 1989; 32:48.

Cox SM, Hankins GD, Leveno KJ, Cunningham FG. Bacterial endocarditis: a serious pregnancy complication. J Reprod Med 1988; 33:671.

Crespo A, Retter AS, Lorber B. Group B streptococcal endocarditis in obstetrics and gynecology. Infect Dis Obstet Gynecol 2003; 11:109.

Dajani AS, Taubert KA, Wilson W, et al. Prevention of bacterial endocarditis: recommendations by the American Heart Association. J Am Med Assoc 1927; 277:1794.

De Swiet M, de Louvois J, Hurley R. Failure of cephalosporins to prevent bacterial endocarditis during labor. Lancet 1975; 2:186.

Everett ED, Hirschmann JV. Transient bacteremia and endocarditis prophylaxis. Medicine 1977; 56:61.

Fry RM. Fatal infections by haemolytic Streptococcus group B. Lancet 1938; 1:199.

Genta PR, Dias MLN, Janiszewki TA, et al. Streptococcus agalactiae endocarditis and giant cell pyomyoma simulating ovarian cancer. South Med J 2001; 94:508.

George J, Lamb JT, Harriman DG. Cerebral embolism due to nonbacterial thrombotic endocarditis following pregnancy. J Neurol Neurosurg Psychiatry 1984; 47:79.

Gill GV. Endocarditis caused by Salmonella enteritidis. Br Heart J 1979; 42:353.

Goodwin JF. Natural history and management of chronic rheumatic endocarditis. Bristol Med Chir J 1969; 84:107.

Hanson GC, Phillips J. A fatal case of subacute bacterial endocarditis in pregnancy: a review of this condition in pregnancy including the incidence, diagnosis and treatment. J Obstet Gynaecol Br Commonw 1965; 72:781.

Hill AM, Butler HM. Haemolytic streptococcal infections following childbirth and abortion. II. Clinical features, with special reference to infections due to streptococci of groups other than A. Med J Aust 1940; 1:293.

Holt S, Hicks DA, Charles RG, Coulshed N. Acute staphylococcal endocarditis in pregnancy. Practitioner 1978; 220:619.

Jemsek JG, Gentry LO, Greenberg SB. Malignant group B streptococcal endocarditis associated with saline-induced abortion. Chest 1979; 76:695.

Kangavari S, Collins J, Cercek B, et al. Tricuspid valve group B streptococcal endocarditis after an elective termination of pregnancy. Clin Cardiol 2000; 23:301.

Koletsky S. Case of acute bacterial endocarditis and septicemia during the puerperium. Ohio State Med J 1941; 37:866.

Lengyel M, Dekov E. Two-dimensional echocardiographic features of Loffler's endocarditis. Acta Cardiol 1982; 37:59.

MacCulloch D. Vancomycin in pregnancy. NZ Med J 1981; 93:93.

Maeland A, Teieh AN, Arnesen H, Garbors I. Cardiobacterium hominis endocarditis. Eur J Clin Microbiol 1983; 2:216.

McComb JM, McNamee PT, Sinnamon DG, Adsey AA. Staphylococcal endocarditis presenting as meningitis in pregnancy. Int J Cardiol 1982; 1:325.

Mooij PN, de Jong PA, Bavinck JH, et al. Aortic valve replacement in the second trimester of pregnancy: a case report. Eur J Obstet Gynecol Reprod Biol 1988; 29:347.

Nazarian M, McCullough GH, Fiedler DL. Bacterial endocarditis in pregnancy: successful surgical correction. J Thorac Cardiovasc Surg 1976; 71:880.

Oakley CM. Cardiovascular disease in pregnancy. Can J Cardiol 1990; 6:3.

O'Donnell D, Gillmer SJ, Mitha AS. Aortic and mitral valve replacement for bacterial endocarditis in pregnancy: a case report. S Afr Med J 1983; 64:1074.

Pastorek JG Jr, Plauche WC, Faro S. Acute bacterial endocarditis in pregnancy: a report of three cases. J Reprod Med 1983; 28:611.

Payne DG, Fishburne JI Jr, Rupty AJ, Johnston FR. Bacterial endocarditis in pregnancy. Obstet Gynecol 1982; 60:247.

Rosenberg K. Subacute bacterial endocarditis complications in pregnancy. Proc Rudolph Virchow Med Soc City NY 1965; 24:132.

Rosenthal AH, Stone FM. Puerperal infection with vegetative endocarditis: report of sulfanilamide therapy in two fatal cases due to streptococcus haemolyticus groups B and C. J Am Med Assoc 1940; 114:840.

Saravolatz LD, Burch KH, Quinn EL, et al. Polymicrobial infective endocarditis: an increasing clinical entity. Am Heart J 1978; 95:163.

Sexton DJ, Rockson SG, Hempling RE, Cathey CW. Pregnancy associated group B streptococcal endocarditis: a report of two fatal cases. Obstet Gynecol 1985; 66:445.

Swift PJ. *Staphylocccus aureus* tricuspid valve endocarditis in young women after gynecological events: a report of 3 cases. S Afr Med J 1984; 66:891.

van der Bel-Kahn JM, Watanakunakorn C, Menefee MG, Long HD, Dicter R. Chlamydia trachomatis endocarditis. Am Heart J 1978; 95:627.

Ward H, Hickman RC. Bacterial endocarditis in pregnancy. Aust NZ J Obstet Gynecol 1971; 11:189.

Windsor HM, Shanahan MX, Golding L. Cardiac surgical emergencies. Med J Aust 1973; 1:476.

Yacoub M, Pennacchio L, Ross D, McDonald L. Replacement of mitral valve in active infective endocarditis. Br Heart J 1972; 34:758.

Zitnik RS, Brandenbury RO, Sheldon R, Wallace RB. Pregnancy and open heart surgery. Circulation 1969; 39:1257.

Infectious Vulvovaginitis

70

Herman L. Gardner   /   *Revised by* Michael S. Burnhill   /
Revised by Gilbert G. Donders

INTRODUCTION

One-third of all women of childbearing age currently have one or more vulvovaginal infections. Despite the discovery of highly effective, specific therapeutic agents against most vulvovaginitis, the overall incidence has not been favorably affected, and patients are inadequately diagnosed and treated by many care-givers all over the world. Indeed, due to the specificity of some complaints, and the avoidance of offering the patient a potentially embarrassing examination, too often patients are not examined well or not at all, and given prescriptions for treatment of a disease that is often thought to be *Candida*. This is a cumbersome evolution, as wrongly or undiagnosed patients are often maltreated or under-treated, and they start complaining after long periods of time without improvement or give up hope that their odyssey of suffering and seeing different care-givers will eventually come to an end. Very often, the answer is hidden in the first clinical encounter, which happens usually during the acute symptomatic phase. Indeed, if one fails to diagnose the disease correctly at first, some patients will develop a long-lasting chronic condition, in which complaints fluctuate, but signs and symptoms, and even laboratory means, become less and less clear and less convincing, further complicating the search for the correct management of an increasingly depressing chronic illness.

Failure of Physician's Accuracy

It is remarkable how many physicians continue to disregard the effects on the general wellness and sexual function such chronic vulvovaginal illnesses can bring along. So every effort has to be put into obtaining a correct and complete diagnosis during the first attack of the disease, in order to make the treatment likely to be successful. In our 20 years of experience in taking care of long-term suffering, mostly desperate patients with long-lasting chronic recurrent vulvovaginal diseases, we discovered three main problems of diagnostic accuracy. The first is that some doctors fail to develop their knowledge and clinical expertise along with the evolving medical advancements. The second is that patients may not recognize that what started as a one disease, for instance *Candida*, may have evolved over time into another disease, let us say chronic vestibulitis posterior (vulvodynia). The third common problem is that doctors fail to realize that women may suffer from two or even more diseases at the same time. A classic example is the long-held belief that *Candida* and bacterial vaginosis (BV) cannot coexist, so treatment is erroneously initiated for only one of them. Also, an infectious condition can fail to be recognized as coexisting with a noninfectious condition, a typical example being candidiasis coexisting with lichen planus or eczema. Therefore, an ideal management regimen has to start with a good history and clinical examination and a clear explanation to the patient of the origin, pathogenesis (risk factors), and treatment possibilities of their disease or diseases. In our experience, patients feel very relieved and thankful if they receive adequate information of what they exactly have, even if immediate or even remote cure is not always achievable. Therefore, more attention to these issues and better pre- and postgraduate education and, perhaps, a better honorarium for doing correct expertise work to solve many of these patient's sufferings and worries, would be desirable.

Failure of Pre- and Postgraduate Training

Unfortunately, and for obscure reasons, obstetrics and gynecology residents and medical students are not receiving adequate training in the diagnosis and management of vulvovaginal infections. We strive to turn every gynecology resident into a super specialist in urogynecology, gynecological oncology, perinatal medicine, endocrinology, etc., but at the same time, we grossly neglect some of the more useful aspects of his/her training. Those in training deserve more instruction in the disorders that affect hundreds of times more women than those afflicted with rare neoplastic diseases or endocrinologic problems, some of which will never be observed in a lifetime of practice.

OFFICE DIAGNOSIS OF VULVOVAGINAL INFECTIONS

Listen to Your Patient

Often, careful listening to your patient and her partner and inquiring with specific questions will help direct your diagnosis in a very fascinating way.

Itching, Burning, and Pain

A first important distinction to be made is that between itching, burning, and pain. Sometimes, patients and inexperienced physicians alike, are very injudicious in the use of these terms. Pruritus or itching is a sensation creating the urge to scratch. Although usually clearly vulvar, it sometimes refers to an itching sensation which is more internal, although from a physiological point of view, "vaginal itching" is less likely to occur because the vagina lacks the nerve endings that convey the sensation. Vulvovaginal itching is usually the result of trichomoniasis or candidiasis, the latter being the leading cause. Pruritus in women of childbearing age suggests candidiasis first and trichomoniasis second, whereas pruritus in postmenopausal women suggests vulvar dystrophy or *Candida* vulvitis in the case of diabetes or hormonal replacement therapy. In young women with small children, pinworms may be present, and in others, vulvar human papilloma virus (HPV) or contact dermatitis may account for other etiologic sources of pruritus.

The sensation of itching is very different from that of burning. This symptom is almost invariably felt from inside the vagina, and is probably more closely related to "vaginal pain" than to "vaginal pruritus." Very often, burning is strongly related to sexual intercourse, which may be the only occasion it occurs, and in rare cases, women complain that the burning sensation is most severe or only present after intravaginal ejaculation of sperm. In contrast to pruritus, the cause of burning may be very difficult to detect, and often a satisfying diagnosis is never found. Burning can accompany candidiasis, but very seldom does treatment of candidiasis result in the disappearance of this annoying symptom. If it is obvious that the symptom is related to sexual intercourse, further inquiry of the time relation with male ejaculation, its occurrence with different partners, and the possible lack of the symptom when condoms are used is warranted. In rare cases, an allergic reaction to sperm can be detected (see later), and a chemical irritation to sperm constituents must be taken into consideration. If large loads of *Ureaplasma urealyticum* are cultured from the vaginal fluid, it may be trysome to initiate treatment to eradicate or lower the load of ureaplasms to decrease the sensation of vaginal burning, especially if it occurs randomly and is not linked to sexual intercourse. In some instances, we have cured women by putting them on continuous progestogens, indicating hormonal influences may also be involved.

Vulvovaginal *pain* can be of infectious or noninfectious origin. Pain can be situated internally, deep in the abdomen, on the introitus, or on the vulva. The pain can be aggravated by attempting sexual intercourse, introduction of tampon, urinating, external touch, or contact with clothing. A typical case is a 16-year-old girl with a sudden attack of increasingly severe vulvar pain over the course of a week, who is avoiding tight-fitting clothing. She tells the physician she refused to use any beverages during the last 24 hours due to the excruciating vulvourethral pain upon urinating. She politely declines to take a seat and prefers to remain standing. Although any care-giver with some common sense would suspect this young girl to be suffering from primary herpes genitalis, it is shameful and disappointing to note that she is generally prescribed miconazole cream by her physician. The physician does not even make a clinical examination, let alone obtain proper viral cultures to confirm and type the herpes strain causing this embarrassing, recurrent disease. Acute eczema, often resulting from external chemical irritants in creams of hygienic pads, also is a common source of vulvar pain. *Candida* is seldom a cause of vulvar pain, except when accompanied by extreme excoriations, fissures, and/or infection. *Trichomonas* can cause painful fissures that rapidly disappear upon treatment with metronidazole.

Dyspareunia

Dyspareunia is a term to indicate pain during sexual intercourse or at the moment of intromission. *Apareunia* may result if intromission is so painful that the attempt to have intercourse is abandoned. Dyspareunia may be primary or secondary. *Primary dyspareunia* refers to painful or impossible intercourse the first time and ever since. Primary dyspareunia is never the result of infection, and can rather be explained as a hymenal anomaly, a vaginal development anomaly, or a chronic vestibulitis posterior (vulvodynia). *Secondary dyspareunia* develops over time, either with the same partner, or as a result of a change of partners. Secondary dyspareunia may be due to a mechanical cause (hymenal fibrosis) or chronic vestibulitis posterior/vulvodynia, but it may also result from vulvovaginal infection. Also cervicitis, cystitis, urethritis, or endometriosis can be the cause of secondary dyspareunia.

Dyspareunia can be divided according to the location of pain: (*i*) *introital* (hymenal, chronic vestibulitis posterior), causing pain on intromission of penis, examining finger, sex toy, or tampon; (*ii*) *vaginal* [*Candida*, *Trichomonas*, aerobic vaginitis (AV)], causing friction pain during the movements of the penile shaft; and (*iii*) *abdominal* (cervicitis, endometriosis, cystitis, ovarian cysts, pelvic infection, etc.), characterized by lower abdominal pain upon deep penetration.

Vaginal Secretion and Vaginal Discharge

The term *discharge*, when used by the patient, is considered a symptom, and is used by the physician to describe a sign. Although discharge has long been used synonymously with leucorrhoea, meaning white discharge, few discharges are, in fact, white. Vaginitis is the primary cause of discharge and not cervicitis. When vulvovaginal secretions are abnormal in volume, color, consistency, or odor, the term *abnormal* or *excessive vaginal secretion* or discharge is applicable.

To classify a vaginal secretion as abnormal discharge, it is first necessary to understand and define the physical characteristics of *normal secretions*. Women with normal estrogen levels may have white or transparent secretions, mainly corresponding to clumps of epithelial cells in serous vaginal transudate, without having any disease. The term "curdy" is sometimes used for these normal secretions, and it should not be confused with thrush patches or curds seen in some patients with candidiasis. A so-called curdy secretion has body, is whitish in color, and does not flow as does a homogeneous secretion, sometimes described as runny, milky, or creamy.

Normal vaginal secretions are usually not malodorous. A few women with apparently normal secretions with a normal pH and a lactobacillus flora will still have some disturbing odor. Such patients may exercise poor hygiene of the vulva, the odor developing from bacterial digestion of smegma and remnants of urine. Also, women with hirsutism and increased apocrine gland activity are more prone to develop such malodor from saprophytic bacterial action on the secretions.

In general, it can be said that any patient without subjective symptoms who has a normal volume of white or clear, curdy vaginal secretion with a pH of 3.8 to 4.2 and no unusual odor has a normal vaginal secretion and not a discharge. The acidific rods, lactobacilli or diphtheroids, usually dominate the flora of the normal vagina.

Abnormal vaginal secretions may be a sign of vaginitis. Although the typical type of secretions can be seen in specific infections, usually these represent only the "tip-of-the-iceberg" cases that are not the most frequently encountered in clinical practice. It may prove difficult to correctly link a discharge to a specific disease, as different grades and types of discharges may coexist, and no infection invariably presents with only one typical discharge. The typical types of discharges for the most frequent causes of vulvovaginitis are summarized in Table 1. A profuse, rotten, malodorous discharge is typically associated with trichomoniasis or severe AV; a moderate-to-profuse, fishy-smelling discharge without irritative symptoms suggests BV; and severe pruritus with cheese-like adherent plaques that can be seen as a "cottage cheese"–like discharge usually suggests candidiasis.

IN-OFFICE CONFIRMATION OF VULVOVAGINAL INFECTIONS

The most meaningful examination of a patient with a vaginal infection or discharge is one made when the patient is experiencing symptoms, when she has not douched for at least two or three days, and when she has not used a vaginal medication, contraceptive jelly, or cream for at least several days. Almost any chemical agent instilled into the vagina shortly before examination distorts the clinical pattern and makes identification or isolation of an infectious agent difficult, if not impossible. Preferably, she must not have menses at the moment of examination, but even if she has, clinical and microscopic examination may still be very rewarding.

Vaginal pH Measurement
Normal Vaginal pH
Normal vaginal flora is characterized by a dynamic balance between lactobacilli and (potential) pathogens. After puberty, increasing levels of estrogens start to circulate, leading to a proliferation of vaginal epithelial cells and the appearance of lactobacilli. Conversion of glycogen to lactate and the formation of hydrogen peroxide (H_2O_2) from the exfoliated intermediate and superficial epithelial cells cause the pH to decrease from 6 to values as low as 3.5 to 4. Therefore, a vaginal pH less than 4.4 is considered normal in premenopausal women.

Abnormal pH and Pathology
When the equilibrium of the vaginal flora is disturbed, the number of lactobacilli can decrease and the acidity diminishes (pH increases). As a consequence, the organisms that are normally suppressed by lactobacilli, will now proliferate. Disturbance of the normal vaginal flora can be seen in infections (BV, AV, *Candida* vaginitis, *Trichomonas vaginalis* infection, cervicitis, etc.), but also in pregnancy, with the use of antibiotics, and at postmenopausal age, and a number of external factors may influence the equilibrium of the vaginal

flora, increasing the likelihood of symptomatic vaginitis occurring (Table 2). In women with BV, the vaginal pH is usually between 4.5 and 5.5; with AV and *Trichomonas* infection, it is between 5 and 7; and with *Candida*, it varies from very acidic (pH < 4) to very basic (up to pH of 7).

During pregnancy, elevated vaginal pH is also associated with an increased risk of preterm rupture of the membranes, preterm birth, and low birth weight. It has been shown that regular testing of the vaginal pH during pregnancy, either by medically trained personnel, or by self-testing, leads to an increased detection of BV and trichomoniasis and that subsequent treatment could decrease the preterm birth rate to half that in controls.

Obtaining a Vaginal Specimen for pH Measurement
To do a pH measurement, fresh vaginal fluid has to be obtained. In older textbooks, it was advised to press the indicator strip or electrode firmly against the upper lateral vaginal wall and let it soak for a few seconds. However elegant this seems, it is far from practical. One has to hold the indicator strip with a long forceps and exert the lateral force with a gloved finger. Through a speculum in an often narrow vagina, this is all but easy to do, requires extra-sterile instruments, and is time consuming, thereby lowering the chances that physicians are going to adapt this method. Therefore, simple adjustments can be made so that the pH can be measured in a much more elegant way by either pressing the strip op the fluid accumulated in the posterior valve op the withdrawn speculum, by directly pressing the cotton swab for culture or wet mount onto the indicator strip, by pressing the gloved finger on the strip or by swirling the strip onto the glass slide with vaginal fluid before using it for microscopic examination (Fig. 1). Care has to be taken to do this before saline is added, as in a comparative study, we have proven that the pH is artificially raised due to the addition of saline, especially in the cases with intermediate pH of 4.4 to 5. It is obvious that addition of KOH is detrimental for the pH and should in any case be prevented.

Methods of pH Measurements
As already mentioned above, vaginal pH can be measured by pH indicator strips or with pH electrodes. The latter provide a more accurate measurement, but are complicated and above all laborious and expensive, and hence they are seldom or never used in routine practice or even in clinical research. Dipstick strips are easy to use, and cheap, need not be calibrated, and only require small amounts of vaginal fluid. Although the strips are less precise (0.1–0.2 pH units compared with 0.001 pH units with electrodes) and need to be interpreted with a subjective eye, this is of minor importance because very small variations in pH, such as measured with electrodes are dramatically influenced by the site of sampling, the moment of the day, the day in the cycle, and by many endogenous and exogenous factors that are always very likely to be present to some extent.

In clinical practice, the ease of use, the low cost, and the opportunity to obtain immediate results are at least as important as the exact numeric values obtained. Therefore,

TABLE 1 Clinical laboratory features of normal vaginal secretions and the most frequent causes of discharge

Features	Normal	Trichomoniasis	Bacterial vaginosis	Aerobic vaginitis	Candidiasis	Atrophic vaginitis	Cervical leucorrhoea	Cytolytic vaginosis
Symptoms								
Discharge	0	+−+++	0−++	++	0−++	0−+	+−+++	0−++
Pruritus	0	0−+++	0−0+	0	+−+++	+−++	0	0
Burning	0−+	0−+	0	0	+	+	0	+
Dysuria	0	0−+	0	+	0−++	++	0	0
Dyspareunia	0	0−+	0	+−++	0−++	++	0	++
Characteristics of discharge								
Amount	0−+	+−+++	0−++	++	0−++	+	+−++	0−++
Consistency	Curdy	Homogeneous	Homogeneous	Serous or mucopurulent	Curdy or thrush patches	Serous or mucopurulent	Mucoid or mucopurulent	Thick white
Color	White or slate	Gray or greenish	Gray	Yellow	White or slate	Variable	Clear/yellow (MPC)	Opaque
Odor	0	+−+++ (rotten)	+−++ (fishy)	+(rotten)	0	0−+	0	0
Frothiness	0	+(10%)	+(7%)	0	0	0	0	0
pH	3.8–4.2	5.5–5.8	5.0–5.5	>6	4.0–5.0	>5	>5	3.8–4.0
Vaginal abnormalities								
Erythema	0	0−+++	0	++	0−++	+	None	0
Swollen papillae	0	+(10%)	0	0−+	0−+	0−+	0	0
Petechiae	0	+(10%)	0	++	0	+(10%)	0	0
Ulcerations	0	0	0	+	0	0−+	0	0
Vulvar abnormalities								
Erythema	0	0−++	0	0−+	+−+++	0−+	0	0
Edema	0	0−++	0	0−+	0−+++	0−+	0	0
Excoriations or ulcers	0	0−+	0	0	0−+	0−+	0	0
Laboratory findings								
Fresh microscopy findings of vaginal fluid (wet mount)								
Lactobacillary grade	I–IIa	IIb–III	III	IIb–III	I–II–III	IIb–III	I–II–III	I
Clue cells	0	0	+	0	0	0	0	0
Trichomonads	0	+	0	(+)	0	0	0	0
Spores and filaments	0	0	0	(+)	+	0	0	0
Leukocytes	0−+	++++	0−+	+−+++	+−+++	+++	0−++	0
Parabasal cells	0	+−+++	0	+−+++	0	+++	0	0
Bacteria	Large rods	Mixed	Small rods	Cocci or small rods	Large rods	Mixed	Lactobacilli	Increased lactobacilli
Laboratory techniques								
Stained smears	Lactobacilli, diphtheroids	Mixed bacteria bacilli	Short, gram-negative diphtheroids	Mixed	Lactobacilli	Mixed	Lactobacilli	Lactobacilli, stripped nuclei
Cultures	Lactobacilli or diphtheroids predominate	Trichomonas vaginalis	Gardnerella vaginalis/anaerobes	Group B streptococci, S. aureus, S. pyogenus, E. coli	Candida species	Mixed bacteria (commensals)	Lactobacilli	Lactobacilli

Abbreviation: MPC: mucopurulent cervicitis.

dipstick tests have been developed for easy use, high stability, quick results, low cost, and wide availability. Two such dipsticks (Merck pH range 4–7, and Macherey-Nagel, pH range 3.8–7) were compared for efficacy and user friendliness. Both tests clearly show increased pH in women with AV and/or BV. Interfering exogenous factors did not seem to influence the pH much in the present study, as both tests measured acid pH, in women with blood, sperm, or cream in the vagina. So, unexpectedly, even during menses or after sexual intercourse pH can be measured, although attention is still placed in circumstances where the vaginal flora is overwhelmed by blood or vaginal medication.

Both the pH tests showed similar results, both in normal healthy circumstances, as in conditions with completely disrupted microflora, or when vaginitis with *Candida* or bacteria was present. Macherey-Nagel indicator strips

TABLE 2 Overview of factors influencing the vaginal pH

Cause	Effect
Microbial factors	
Trichomonas vaginalis	pH > 6
Mucopurulent cervicitis	pH > 6
Aerobic vaginitis	pH > 6
Bacterial vaginosis	pH > 4.7
Candidiasis	pH all types, often pH < 4.5
Cytolytic vaginitis	pH < 4
Intermediate flora	pH 4 tot 6
Dermatologic abnormalities	
Desquamative vaginitis	pH > 6
Bullous vaginal epidermolysis	pH > 6
Endocrinologic factors	
Prepuberty	pH > 4.5
Pregnancy	pH 3.8–4.5
Menopause	Varying, usually pH > 4.5
Exogenous estrogen	pH lowers
Continuous progestogen use	pH increases
Abundant cervical mucus	pH increases
Diabetes mellitus	pH increases
Temporary disturbances	
Intravaginal cremes	Usually pH increases
Vaginal douches	Usually pH increases
Sperm (<24 U)	pH increases
Menstrual blood	pH increases
Use of antibiotics	Usually pH increases
Therapeutic agents	
Exogenous application of lactobacilli	pH decreases
Povidine iodine	pH neutral
Ascorbinic acid	pH decreases
Boric acid	pH decreases
Lactic acid	pH decreases

systematically show lower pH values, although the difference with Merck's test was not significant. A possible explanation is that the color scale of the Macherey-Nagel test permits a lower pH (lowest mark on the color scale is 3.6) than the Merck test (lowest pH is 4.0). Efficacy in detecting abnormal flora was excellent and similar in both tests. However, compared to Merck's test, it was significantly easier and quicker (50% more rapid) to obtain a conclusion of the pH result than when the Macherey-Nagel test was used. Moderate or severe decision-making problems due to difficult reading were 10 times more frequent when the Merck test was used compared to the Macherey-Nagel's test [odds ratio (OR) 10 (4.7 − 22.6), $p = 0.00028$]. Difficult or impossible readings were almost exclusively encountered with the Merck test (16% vs. 1% for Macherey-Nagel test). Furthermore, difficult reading was four times more frequent in the group of women with abnormal flora (for definition of abnormal flora, see below) [lactobacillary grade III (LBG-III): 25%] than in women with normal flora (LBG-I and IIa: 8%). It is concluded that both Merck and Macherey-Nagel are adequate tests for recognizing abnormal bacterial colonization of the vaginal microflora, with no interference of common exogenous or endogenous pH-modulating factors, such as sperm, menses, or recent use of vaginal cream. However, Macherey-Nagel tests seem to be more user friendly than Merck tests, in particular when infections are present.

Microscopy of Fresh Vaginal Fluid

Microscopic examination of the physiologic saline wet mount is the key in-office method for the differential diagnosis of vaginitis or discharge, and it should be made obligatory in the investigation of every single case. It could even be used for screening in almost every gynecologic or obstetric patient, whether she has signs and symptoms or not.

Preparation of a Wet Mount

Preparation of a saline mount requires only a few simple steps: a sample is obtained from the upper vaginal wall with either a spatula, a cervix brush, or a cytobrush [as is used for taking Papanicolaou (Pap) smears], or by a cotton-tipped applicator (as is used for cultures) (Fig. 2).

The cotton swab is less suited for microscopy compared to Pap smear devices, as the cotton may leave behind threads and loose particles on the smear, creating artifacts that may interfere with proper microscopy. Using the device, some vaginal fluid is smeared thinly on a glass slide, and one small (!) droplet of saline is carefully added to the central part of the slide. A coverslip is deposited in the droplet, held perpendicular on top of the glass slide for a few seconds in order to allow the saline to spread over the connecting edge, and dropped slowly in a controlled way so that no air bubbles can form. Excess fluid is removed by soaking it away with a sheet of absorbing paper. Microscopic examination should be performed using both low (100× magnification) and high power (400× magnification). If a delay in examining the slide is anticipated, it is best to prepare the slide the same way, but without adding saline and coverslip, and let it dry on the air and keep it in a plastic holder that permits storage for days or weeks, and even allows easy transportation to experts for a second opinion. The slide can then be rehydrated and read with similar results, with the one exception of trichomonads, which will be missed due to their loss of motility. The older advice to use transport media such as Transcult® is less advisable for delayed reading, as the vaginal flora constituents will have changed too much over time to have a realistic microscopy after reculturing for hours or days.

Phase Contrast Microscopy

The use of phase contrast offers a great advantage in the diagnosis of vulvovaginal infections. Yeast spores are more clearly discernable, and are easier distinguished from sperm heads that lost their tails, as the phase contrast shows better the intracellular organelles that enable to make that difference. Among six international experts, there was a good correlation in the blinded readings of abnormal vaginal flora and the presence of BV in vaginal samples, but not with the two colleagues who used transmission light microscopy without phase contrast. However, when a second reading was allowed with the use of a phase microscope, these investigators also scored high. Phase contrast therefore is ideal to provide a more accurate diagnosis of both bacterial abnormalities and fungal infections.

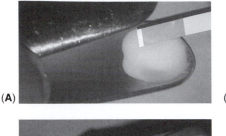

(A)

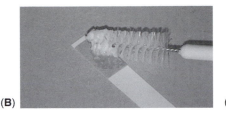

(B)

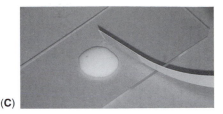

(C)

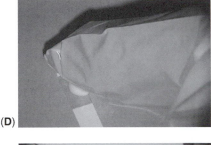

(D)

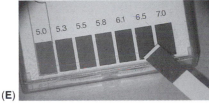

(E)

FIGURE I Vaginal pH can be measured directly by pressing the pH strip against the upper lateral vaginal wall, but this often poses practical problems. Alternative solutions are to measure pH directly from the posterior valve of the withdrawn speculum (care has to be taken not to measure cervical mucus, which is more basic) (**A**); by pressing the spatula or swab onto the pH strip (**B**); by allowing the strip to soak from the smear, best done before adding either saline or KOH solution (**C**); by dipping the gloved finger after examination onto the glass slide (**D**); by comparing with and reading from the visual scale of pH 4 to 7 provided by the manufacturer (**E**).

Comparison with Gram-Stained Specimens

When compared with the diagnosis of BV according to the Nugent score on Gram stains, the presence of clue cells on wet mounts is both highly sensitive (77%) and specific (92%). When experienced microscopists also take the typical granular flora into account, the diagnosis is even more accurate and more rapid as with Gram stains. BV and abnormal LBGs were reliably and with great concordance diagnosed by six international experts, who were blinded to each other's data, especially when phase contrast microscopes were used. There is evidence that the procedure of Gram staining harms part of the lactobacillary flora, and favors the nonlactobacillary flora to become prominent. This leads to a false overemphasis of abnormal flora in Gram stains when compared with wet mounts, wherein normal flora is better visible.

Addition of Potassium Hydroxide (KOH)

Use of 10% KOH is a highly accurate method for diagnosing candidiasis, especially for less-experienced microscopists, as it can detect at least two-thirds of Candida in the hyphal phase. KOH wet mount is prepared by simply dropping a tiny droplet of 10% KOH solution on the slide that has been used for normal microscopy. An excess of solution should be avoided as it may damage the microscope objectives. Upon application, the cellular material on the slide dissolves immediately or becomes transparent, making detection of intact Candida particles more easy. While KOH clears most cells derived from the vagina rapidly, such as epitheliocytes and leucocytes, keratinized cells from the vulva are more resistant and may require the slide to be heated over a gentle flame.

An extra advantage of KOH addition, which is often applied, is its facilitation of the liberation of the typical fishy odor from a specimen with BV, one of the Amsel criteria of the disease. About 5% of patients with clue cell–positive BV have no fishy odor, not even after addition of KOH.

LABORATORY PROCEDURES

Stained Smears
Gram-Stained Smears

Stained smears of vaginal secretions are only occasionally required for the differential diagnosis of vaginitis and discharge. For those unfamiliar with the microscopic diagnosis of BV, however, the Gram-stained smear is very useful for identifying the gram-variable Gardnerella morphotypes, usually outnumbering all other organisms by at least 100 to 1. By assessing such Gardnerella morphotypes, as well as lactobacillary morphotypes and Mobiluncus semiquantitatively, Nugent et al. composed a scoring system that reliably enabled one to recognize full-blown BV (Nugent score of 7 or more), and normal flora (Nugent score less than 4). The score from 4 to 6 is called "intermediate flora," which is really a misnomer, as this condition often does not correspond to a flora that is intermediate between normal flora and BV, but rather is a collection of real transitional flora (intermediate BV) and other types of abnormal flora that are not well defined. For diagnosing full-blown BV, however, the Nugent system is one of the most sensitive and reproducible techniques at the present time, and this technique is used in most studies of the pathogenicity of the BV and the value of treatment. To analyze the intermediate flora, on the other hand, wet preparations allowing additional information about the immune response of the host, may be obligatory (Table 3).

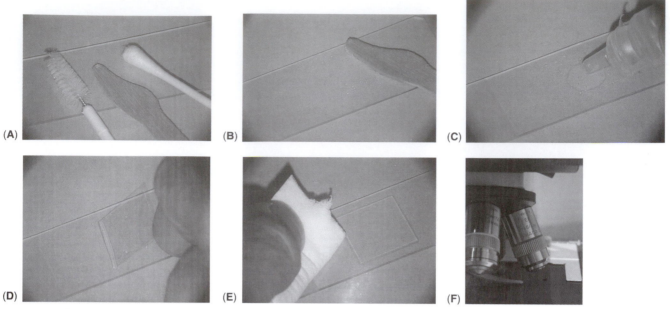

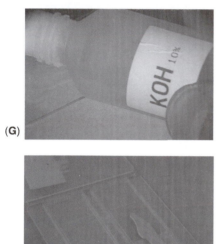

FIGURE 2 Preparation of a wet mount involves four steps, but takes less than one minute and provides an immediate answer to most problems of the differential diagnosis of infectious vulvovaginitis. After sampling, the swab or spatula (**A**) is spread on the glass slide as thin as possible (**B**). The smallest possible droplet of saline is added (**C**), and a coverslip is placed perpendicularly to the droplet in order to allow the fluid to spread from left to right, before it is slowly laid down to avoid air bubbles (**D**). Excessive fluid is absorbed by absorbent paper (**E**) and, without adding KOH, microscopy at 400× phase contrast magnification is performed (**F**). In case of doubt whether *Candida* hyphae or blastospores are being missed, the coverslip can be removed, one droplet of 10% KOH added and covered again before microscoping once more (**G**). This also allows determining whether a fishy smell, typical for BV, is present. It should be noted that this smell will not be released in cases of AV. In case a second opinion is sought, a delayed or remote reading can be organized by putting the smear on the glass slide, let it air dry, and close it, to be kept for later reading after addition of a droplet of saline by an expert (**H**). *Abbreviations*: AV, aerobic vaginitis; BV, bacterial vaginosis;

As *Candida* spores stain efficiently by Gram's method, it is a sensitive method for identifying candidal spores and filaments. For the diagnosis of trichomoniasis, which requires motile parasites for a definitive diagnosis, Gram-stained smears are of limited value. Stained smears and cultures of vaginal secretions may be particularly useful in cases of recurrent vaginitis with negative wet mount microscopy. The technique for making a Gram stain is outlined in Table 4.

Dif-Quick Stain

If you are dealing with a situation in which the discharge has dried or the trichomonads are nonmotile, the use of Dif-Quick stain (dye immunofluorescent stain) will enable the flagella to be seen more readily. However, if you fail to have an appropriate diagnosis after examining the wet mount and Dif-Giemsa–stained smears, preparing a Gram stain is the next step in trying to determine the cause

of recurrent vaginitis. The use of Gram staining allows you to use the oil immersion lens to examine the preparation at 1000× magnification, which in some cases may reveal missed details on gram-positive or gram-negative bacteria (e.g., gram-negative diplococci of *Neisseria gonorrhoeae*).

Pap-Stained Smears

Pap smears can be used for the detection of clue cells and BV flora. The Pap smear was 78% sensitive and 87% specific in the detection of BV in one study and 89% and 90% in another. The problem is that Pap smears are used for the purpose of screening for cervical dysplasia, and not designed as a tool for detecting BV or other genital infections. As a result, pathologists, will be focused mainly on the issue of cervical epithelial disease, and decreasing sensitivity of detection of BV, and treating physicians will have difficulty in tracing and convincing women to get treatment for a

TABLE 3 Nugent criteria to diagnose bacterial vaginosis (score 7 or more), normal flora (score 3 or less), or "intermediate flora" (score 4–6)[a]

	Lactobacilli	Gardnerella	Mobiluncus
0	4+	0	0
1	3+	1+	1–2+
2	2+	2+	3–4+
3	1+	3+	
4	0	4+	

[a]Other flora types such as aerobic vaginitis flora cannot be diagnosed in this system. Intermediate flora is not equal to partial bacterial vaginosis (see text).

benign, asymptomatic disease they did not attend for. Furthermore, it is questionable whether treatment should be initiated for an asymptomatic disease that is harmless in most women. False-positive and false-negative reports of trichomonads are made too often to be reliable.

Cultures and Polymerase Chain Reaction Techniques

Aerobic Routine Cultures

Since an astute clinician can often make a correct diagnosis on the basis of clinical and microscopical features alone, laboratory confirmation is in general useless, but it is still performed for the physician's feeling of comfort, and unfortunately also for a presumed medico-legal back-up.

Clinicians are prone to placing too much confidence on microbiologic cultures. Their use should be reserved to confirm missed diagnoses, to elucidate the etiology of chronic recurrent vaginitis when *Candida* is suspected but not found, or to identify sexually transmitted disease (STD) pathogens.

Routine bacterial cultures as performed in many clinical laboratories are rarely informative for the differential diagnosis of vaginitis. The cultural isolation of a bacterium, even though it might be the predominant agent isolated, does not prove an etiologic relationship with the discharge or vaginitis present. Clinicians must guard against always assigning etiologic significance to bacterial agents enumerated on a laboratory report and certainly not follow the therapeutic advice that may be deduced from the antibiogram provided. Cultures only serve to confirm or deny a presumed diagnosis and require good communication between clinician and microbiologist.

Bacterial quantification has been used by urologists for many years, but it has no significance in the diagnosis of vulvovaginitis, because the great number of bacteria normally

TABLE 4 Technique for preparation of Gram stain

Heat slide briefly
Cover with gentian violet (10 sec)
Wash
Cover with Gram's iodine (10 sec)
Wash
Decolorize with acetone/alcohol (immediately)
Cover with safranin (10 sec)
Wash
Place coverslip on wet, stained surface and examine
Drop saline or mineral oil on the coverslip and reexamine with 100× objective

residing in the vagina constitute a "vaginal zoo" rather than a sterile environment in which positive cultures always have a meaning. Many studies have convincingly shown that essentially the same types and number of bacteria can be recovered from patients with and without vaginitis, except for BV, where 10- to 100-fold, primarily anaerobic, bacteria may be recovered.

Culturing Gardnerella vaginalis

Several excellent culture media for the isolation of *G. vaginalis* have been employed. A number of commercially available broths are suitable for growing *G. vaginalis*, such as Casman's broth with 5% rabbit serum or peptone–starch–dextrose medium. The colonizing morphology with this medium is different from that on Casman's blood agar plates. In most routine laboratories, only Gram stain, showing the so-called typical morphotypes, is used to report on the culture results of *G. vaginalis*.

Cultures of *G. vaginalis* are not useful for diagnosing BV, as up to 50% of healthy women have positive cultures due to low numbers of *G. vaginalis* in the vagina without any sign of BV. However, when no wet mount or Gram stains are done and a clinical diagnosis is doubtful, massive growth of BV or of *Escherichia coli*, group B streptococci, or *Staphylococcus aureus* can help distinguish AV from BV. Also, cultures for *T. vaginalis* and *Candida* may be extremely helpful in doubtful cases, and in cases with mixed infections.

Candida Species

Candida species can be readily identified on most commonly used culture media. When available in screw-capped bottles or vials, they even do not require an incubator to support growth, but growth is faster if an incubator is used. In order to increase sensitivity, a Saborau medium is used. It enables the identification of *C. albicans*, *C. glabrata*, and "other non-*albicans*" strains. If further identification of rare species such as *C. krusei*, *C. paracrusei*, *C. parapsilosis*, or *C. cerevisiae* is required (usually for research purposes), specific chrome agars are applied. In experienced hands, wet mount microscopy may be more sensitive than cultures, as the visualization of spores may not always result in culture-positive findings. On the other hand, when one is not experienced in this type of microscopy, *Candida* spores may be easily missed, resulting in a sensitivity in some studies of only 60%, necessitating cultures in such situations. In chronic recurrent cases of vulvovaginal candidiasis, the detection of low-grade infection may be more troublesome, necessitating cultures with a high grade of suspicion if negative, even with polymerase chain reaction (PCR) techniques.

T. vaginalis

It is extremely important to stress that a normal culture swab on Stuart or Amies medium and grown on a normal blood chocolate agar does not enable the diagnosis of or exclude *Trichomonas*. So even when fresh fluid microscopy and culture results report negative for *Trichomonas*, suspicion of having missed the diagnosis must remain high. Trypticase serum (STS) culture medium, incubated at 37°C for two to three days, containing human serum, provides essential growth factors for *Trichomonas* as well as antibiotics for inhibition of bacterial growth. The Wittington-Fineburg medium has also proved to have satisfactory sensitivity for *Trichomonas* detection. For the near future, specific *Trichomonas* PCR tests are marching in, progressively replacing microscopy as a preferred diagnostic tool, but at the same time losing the opportunity to offer the patients an immediate diagnosis and treatment.

Anaerobic Cultures

Anaerobic cultures require specific and complicated sampling and transport devices (Anaerobic Culturette®), are extremely laborious and expensive and almost never provide information that could not have been obtained by other, simpler techniques such as wet mount microscopy or Gram stain. Hence, there is no place for anaerobic culture techniques in the clinical management of vulvovaginitis outside research projects.

Mycoplasmata Cultures

Specific culture media for *Mycoplasma hominis* and *U. urealyticum* may help to delineate the pathogenicity of certain types of abnormal vaginal flora especially in pregnancy, where there is evidence that the concomitant infection of these organisms with BV may cause a more severe set of complications such as miscarriage or preterm birth.

Enzymology and Immunology

The products of anaerobic infection responsible for the fishy smell, putrescine, cadaverine, diethylamine, and succinate acid, are increased in vaginal washings of BV, and the lactate to succinate ratio has been used as a biochemical marker for BV. Detection of bacterial enzymes such as mucinases, proteinases, *G. vaginalis* hemolysins, and sialidases correlates with BV but not with candidiasis. About 50% of women produce IgA immunoglobulins against *G. vaginalis*, but some women are infected with *G. vaginalis* strains that produce anti-IgA activity by cleaving the immunoglobulins. The presence of enzymes such as sialidase or mucinase may change the pathogenicity of abnormal vaginal flora, while microscopy can by no means detect a difference. Sialidase-positive pregnant women with BV have a higher likelihood of preterm delivery. Interleukins can be measured to assess the host response to vaginal intruders and normal constituents of the vaginal flora. Interleukin 1 (IL-1) is increased in BV, but even more so in AV. IL-8, a proinflammatory cytokine responsible for the attraction of leukocytes, is dramatically increased in AV, but not in BV. All of these tests can be helpful for studying the pathogenicity of abnormal vaginal flora, but are not suitable for diagnosing the different flora types, either because they are too laborious to perform or because they are too aspecific.

CLINICAL TYPES OF VULVOVAGINITIS

Lactobacilli and Normal Vaginal Flora

Lactobacilli are the most well-known markers of normal vaginal flora. Their ability to produce acid vaginal pH, mainly

due to the acidification enzyme hydrogen peroxidase, and bacteriocins that kill off other bacteria makes them prime surveillance candidates of the vaginal health. Many types are present in the vagina, the most frequent being *L. jensenii*, *L. gasseri*, *L. iners*, and *L. crispatus*, and there is a wide variation of species and relative numbers of species according to the population studied. In general, where lactobacilli are predominant, other bacteria and parasites such as *Trichomonas* are not abundant. *Candida* microorganisms are the exception to this rule, as they can thrive as well in a lactobacillus-dominant flora as in a mixed or lactobacillus-deficient flora. In general, lactobacilli-deficient conditions open the door to the development of numerous infectious conditions such as BV and AV and promote the transmission of numerous STDs such as gonorrhea, *Chlamydia*, syphilis, trichomoniasis, and even HIV and HPV, leading to cervical cancer.

Lactobacillary Grades

Normal and abnormal lactobacillary flora are divided into three to four flora types, also depicted as LBGs. LBG-I, corresponding to a "healthy" microflora, has predominantly lactobacillary morphotypes of variable size. LBG-III is a condition wherein the lactobacillary morphotypes are completely replaced by other bacterial morphotypes. LBG-II is an intermediate group, with partial replacement of the lactobacilli by other bacteria. Due to their specific link to the pathology, we refined the three grades, and divided LBG-II into a less severe (LBG-IIa) and a more severe (LBG-IIb) variety (Fig. 3). As LBG-III and, to a lesser extent, LBG-IIb are more likely to be linked to pathological conditions, they are entitled "abnormal vaginal flora." This condition is a screening tool that should not be confused with BV. BV is a condition with abnormal vaginal flora, but abnormal vaginal flora is not always BV.

Some studies demonstrate that the absence of lactobacilli is a more powerful predictor of preterm birth than the presence of BV. In order to diagnose such abnormal LBG, the use of wet mount is preferred above the use of Gram stains due to its superior accuracy and better correlation with lactate in the vaginal content, and it is accepted by most as the best functional test for lactobacillary defense function.

Bacterial Vaginosis
BV as an Ecologic Disorder

BV is an ecological disruption of the normal vaginal flora in which the normal lactobacillus-dominant flora is replaced by 100- to 1000-fold increased numbers of anaerobic bacteria.

Vaginosis is not vaginitis The choice of the suffix "-osis" instead of "-itis" was made to underline the absence of inflammation associated with this disease entity. Symptoms are scarce and most women do not even realize they have the condition. If symptomatic, fishy smell and watery vaginal discharge are most common. These symptoms, together with a pH above 4.5 and typical clue cells on microscopy, compose the clinical diagnosis according to Amsel.

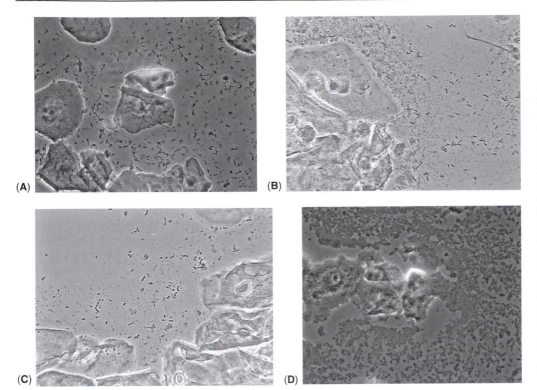

FIGURE 3 Normality of lactobacillary flora can be divided into three or four grades (LBG). Abundant, normal-appearing lactobacilli are designated as LBG-I (**A**), and mixed flora with lactobacilli still outnumbering the other bacteria as LBG-IIa (**B**), both types of flora still being considered normal flora. A mixed flora, but having fewer lactobacilli than other flora, is called LBG-IIb (**C**). LBG-III is devoid of lactobacilli, or contains only very few of them. (**D**) Such abnormal flora can be caused by mucopurulent cervicitis (e.g., gonorrhea, *Chlamydia*), bacterial vaginosis, *Trichomonas*, or aerobic vaginitis. *Abbreviation*: LBG, lactobacillary grades.

G. vaginalis

The etiologic role of *G. vaginalis* as a pathogen was questioned by Herman Gardner himself. These were his historic arguments that led to the experiments to inoculate the vaginas of normal women:

1. *G. vaginalis* is the predominant organism in the vaginas of patients with the described vaginitis.
2. The organism is the only one consistently isolated from the vaginas of patients.
3. The organism is rarely isolated from patients who do not show clinical signs of the disease.
4. The characteristic signs and laboratory findings disappear abruptly upon eradication of *G. vaginalis* from the vagina and reappear upon reinfection.

Experimentally, he successfully inoculated disease-free vaginas with material from the vaginas of patients with proven *G. vaginalis* vaginitis and reproduced signs of BV disease. The recipient subjects were free of all clinical signs of vaginal disease on the day of inoculation, and their vaginal flora consisted predominantly of lactobacilli. Of 15 normal patients inoculated with the infectious vaginal material, 11 developed the clinical disease within 10 days, and *G. vaginalis* became the predominant organism in all 11 vaginas. These induced infections persisted indefinitely in the majority of the subjects. However, when another set of normal women were inoculated with the purified *G. vaginalis* strain obtained from pure pass-over cultures, only one of them developed signs and symptoms of BV, while the others retained a normal flora. It was only later that Gardner's disappointing finding could be explained, when it was recognized that accompanying anaerobes have to be obligatorily present in order to cause symptoms and signs of BV.

Clinical Criteria
Symptoms

Discharge and odor are the principal symptoms of BV. The discharge is characteristically a gray, homogenous, malodorous vaginal discharge. The odor is described as musty or fishy. While many women suffer from these symptoms from the very onset of the infection, other women do not have any complaints at all. However, some of these admit the necessity of frequent douching and notice a positive change when the BV have been successfully treated or the normal vaginal ecology restored. The patient's sexual partner is often conscious of the unpleasant odor, a fact that can cause unsatisfying sexual function. Concomitant presence of pruritus or vaginal itching should alert the clinician to either coinfection or a misdiagnosis. At present, there is insufficient reason to treat a patient for BV if neither she nor her partner has complaints.

Signs

Gross vulvitis and vaginitis are not characteristic of the disease and must initiate a search for other causes. *G. vaginalis* is a surface organism that does not invade the vaginal wall or elaborate toxic substances that provoke reactions in the vulvovaginal epithelia. As a rule, clinical examination, as well as microscopic and histologic preparations, show no more of an inflammatory reaction than does normal vaginal tissue. Based on these facts, the legitimacy of the term *vaginitis* for this entity has been questioned, and *vaginosis* is a better description.

BV produces a varying degree of discharge, from scanty to profuse; its discharge is usually less abundant than in cases of acute trichomoniasis. The consistency of the discharge resembles trichomonal discharge a little; it resembles a thin flour paste, being turbid, homogeneous, and free of grossly visible clumps of epithelial cells that are seen in normal vaginal secretions. In about 95% of the cases, the discharge is gray. Frothiness of the discharge is apparent in about 7% of the cases, but is usually minimal, consisting of only small bubbles. Nevertheless, frothiness should never be considered a diagnostic sign exclusive to trichomoniasis. Its typical fishy odor, different and less offensive than that in the usual case of trichomoniasis or severe AV, is characteristic and of diagnostic value. The pH of the discharge is practically always between 4.7 and 5.5. Patients of child-bearing age who have vaginal secretions of 5.0 or higher, and do not have trichomonads in the vagina, may have an abnormal vaginal flora due to AV as well.

Diagnosis
Clinical Criteria According to Amsel
The great benefit of the clinical diagnosis of Amsel et al. (1983) is that it successfully reverted the former exclusion diagnosis of "nonspecific vaginitis" into a positive, recognizable entity, nowadays known as "bacterial vaginosis." The presence of three of four of the following criteria make the diagnosis: (*i*) homogenous watery discharge, (*ii*) pH greater than 4.5, (*iii*) clue cells present on fresh wet mount, (*iv*) fishy odor after addition of 10% KOH in water. A positive whiff test has a specificity of 87% with a sensitivity of 34%. However, a fishy odor is not always present in BV, not even after the application of KOH. As can be expected, the presence of a thin, homogeneous discharge clinging to vaginal mucosa has the lowest sensitivity (56%) and specificity (49%).

Microscopy of Full-Blown and Partial BV
An experienced microscopist will not only look for clue cells, but is more convinced of the diagnosis of BV if the typical granular vaginal microflora with uncountable coccobacilli (*Gardnerella* morphotypes) are present, so numerous that one cannot see them as separate bacteria. When the normal flora is completely replaced by this typical, granular flora, usually including typical clue cells if this carpet covers the cellular outlines of the epithelial cells, the condition is called "full-blown BV" (Fig. 4A). Fresh fluid microscopy also allows to recognize areas of BV flora in a slide with otherwise predominant flora. This type of flora is called partial BV, i.e., a mixture of normal flora with zones of typical BV flora, as opposed to "intermediate flora," which is seen in Gram-stained specimens scored according to Nugent criteria (Fig. 4B). In this respect, "intermediate flora" is a misnomer and should better be called "undetermined flora," as it corresponds to a flora type that is neither normal, nor BV, and usually not "partial BV" either. Hence this "intermediate flora" is not an entity and gathers as well "partial BV" as other types of abnormal flora such as AV.

Absence of Inflammation
A typical feature of BV is its striking absence of inflammation amidst a world of undesirable bacteria. In BV, there is only a slight increase of IL-1 and an unexpectedly low production of IL-8, thereby preventing massive attraction of inflammatory cells such as macrophages and neutrophils. Hence, if severe inflammation is normally blunted, and if prominently present, e.g., when more than 10 leukocytes are present per epithelial cell, a supplementary diagnosis has to be searched for. Indeed, concomitant cervicitis, trichomoniasis, candidiasis, and/or AV are all known to present with an increased immune response with increased number of monocytes and leukocytes in the vast majority of cases. Therefore, the finding of increased leukocytosis in a vaginal smear with BV must always prompt for an intensive search for another diagnosis.

Microbiology of BV
G. vaginalis, Mycoplasmata, and Anaerobes
The relationship of *G. vaginalis* to disease is not a simple cause-and-effect phenomenon. *G. vaginalis* is a common isolate from the normal female genital tract. The sensitivity of *G. vaginalis* cultures, for instance, is so tremendous that in it can be traced in 70% to 80% of normal women, most of whom have no signs or symptoms of BV. The difference between colonization and disease appears to be a partial function of the magnitude of bacterial replication. It was recognized that BV samples contained 100 to 1000 times more bacteria than normal controls and that this overgrowth became a typical characteristic of anaerobic BV. Quantitative bacteriological studies have shown that disease, when due primarily to *G. vaginalis*, is associated with greater than 10^8 cfu/g of vaginal fluid. *G. vaginalis* is usually the most prominent constituent of a complex polymicrobial anaerobic and aerobic bacterial flora, including *Streptococcus agalactiae*, *E. coli*, *G. vaginalis*, *Peptostreptococcus* species, *Bacteroides* species, *Prevotella* species, *Mobiluncus* species, *Staphylococcus epidermidis*, *Enterococcus faecalis*, and *M. hominis*.

Recently developed PCR techniques can detect genomal DNA or RNA coding for structural proteins, allowing the detection of extremely small numbers of microorganisms. This led to the discovery of several new species linked to the condition.

Mobiluncus
Mobiluncus are small, vibrating, comma-shaped bacteria that are present in about 15% of BV cases (Fig. 4C). Although the presence of *Mobiluncus* establishes an important component of the Nugent score, it has never been related to any sort of pathology and does not cause any symptoms that are different from women without this organism. The prevalence of *Mobiluncus* species within polymicrobial BV varies within the population groups sampled. Royce et al. (1999) demonstrated that *Mobiluncus* species was present in 12% of black gravidas with BV as compared to 1.3% of white gravidas with BV. Quantitatively, 73% of black gravidas, compared to 40% of white gravidas, had high-level replication. Burns et al. (1992) analyzed 299 vaginal swabs by Gram stain and by culture. *Mobiluncus* species were identified in 8.4% of specimens by Gram stain, but only 0.7% by culture.

Atopobium vaginalis and other new discoveries As most women harbor low numbers of potential pathogenic bacteria and yeasts, without being symptomatic, one can question the value of highly sophisticated methods to detect low numbers

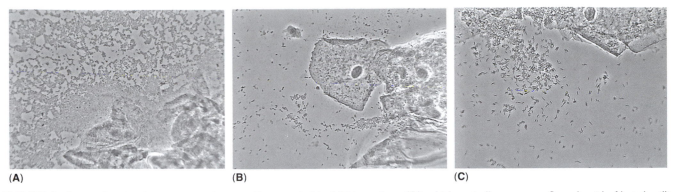

(A)   **(B)**   **(C)**

FIGURE 4 Bacterial vaginosis can present in an easily recognizable, full-blown form (**A**), which typically exposes a flora devoid of lactobacilli and covered with so many small coccoid or coccostaphoid bacteria as if they form a carpet of grains. The bacteria cannot be discerned one from another and are uncountable. In transitional forms (partial BV) area undergoing transition from normal to BV or from BV to normal, such areas with numerous bacteria are mixed with areas where still lactobacillary morphotypes can be found (**B**). *Mobiluncus* morphotypes present as slender, small (smaller than lactobacilli) bacteria that typically vibrate at very high frequency (**C**). *Abbreviation*: BV, bacterial vaginosis.

of such microorganisms. Even more striking is the fact that of some microorganisms often recovered in vaginal fluid, such as the recently discovered *A. vaginalis*, it is not clear whether they constitute a pathogenic risk or are rather a marker of abnormal or even normal vaginal flora. Also, the presence of lactobacilli may not always have the same beneficial influence on vaginal health. Some lactobacilli do not produce H_2O_2 or bacteriocins that contribute to defending the vagina against overgrowth of pathogens, and cause rather than prevent disease. Such lactobacilli often have slender morphotypes and are probably of anaerobic origin (vaginal lactobacillosis).

Pathology of BV
Ascending Infection
The condition has been linked to an increased risk of vaginal cuff infection in women undergoing hysterectomy, and an increased risk of pelvic infection after abortion arte provocatus in women with BV. Women with BV more frequently have intermenstrual bleeding disorders, suggesting a subclinical ascending endometrial infection. There is no question that women with acute salpingitis, ectopic pregnancy, or secondary infertility are more likely than not to have or have had BV; however, one is hard pressed to explain how a noninflammatory process produces disease comparable to *Chlamydia trachomatis* and/or *N. gonorrhoeae*. Bacteria involved in polymicrobial BV can be the same bacteria that can function in the anaerobic progression. In the case of upper tract genital infections, a major STD pathogen usually functions as the initiator of disease.

BV as an STD
In some, but not all, women, BV conforms to the risk factors characteristic of STD. Berger et al. (1995) studied lesbian women who sought gynecologic care at a community center and in a private gynecological clinic. Of 11 index women who had BV, eight (72.2%) had partners who also had BV. The likelihood of a female partner having BV was 19.7 times greater if the index women had BV.

In the Swedish Women's Health Study, Nilsson et al. (1997) compared risk factors associated with BV and

C. trachomatis infection. No significant differences in sexual activity risk factors existed when women with BV were compared with those with chlamydial infection except for a higher frequency of casual sex. Larsson et al. (1991) studied 400 women with and 400 women without BV. Women with BV had a higher number of lifetime sexual partners and exhibited behavior similar to women at risk for STDs.

When the issue of documented, concomitant coinfection is analyzed, a significant portion of women with BV can be demonstrated to have one or more major STDs. Tchoudomirova et al. (1998) found that 37.8% of women attending STDs clinics had BV and were frequently coinfected. In their study, BV correlated with an age less than 25 years, lack of a permanent sexual partner, use of the intrauterine device, other STDs, and smoking. Joesoef et al. (1996) identified a 23.3% prevalence of major STD among pregnant women with BV. Peters et al. (1995) similarly found the presence of BV to be significantly associated with the number of cigarettes smoked per day, age at first intercourse, the lifetime number of sexual partners, and current *C. trachomatis* infection.

Pregnancy Complications
During pregnancy, spontaneous miscarriages seem to occur more often in women with BV, and preterm rupture of membranes, chorioamnionitis, and preterm delivery all seem to be linked to the finding of abnormal vaginal flora or BV early in pregnancy. Furthermore, women with BV may have a completely different risk profile during pregnancy depending on coinfection with *M. hominis*, *Bacteroides* sp., or both. According to other studies, *U. ureaplasma* is a necessary cofactor to induce preterm birth. Some women have immune defense against *G. vaginalis* by means of producing *G. vaginalis*–specific IgA, while in others, vaginal bacteria may produce sialidase and cleavage enzymes that stem this protective action. While all these differences cannot be diagnosed by microscopic appearance alone, other obvious markers, such as the presence of the small vibrating comma-like *Mobiluncus*, do not seem to have any pathogenic meaning. Therefore, BV seems to be a

very heterogeneous condition, and sometimes mixed infections may be very important for explaining some pathogenic effects or treatment results or failures.

Treatment
Metronidazole and Other Imidazoles
The monolithic conceptualization of clinical BV has precluded development of optimal therapeutic efficacy. The current drugs of primary utilization are either per oral or intravaginal metronidazole or clindamycin. The relative efficacy of antibiotics that address the anaerobic constituency of the vaginal bacterial flora lends credence to the concept that eradication of the major anaerobic bacteria tends to abort the disease process. With these drugs, short-term clinical cures can be achieved in 75% to 85% of the cases. Microbiological cures rarely achieve such percentages. The treatment of choice is metronidazole, given orally, either as a single 2 g dose or over 7 to 10 days, 500 mg two times a day. If monitoring is extended to four weeks and beyond, the abnormal bacteria reappear in approximately a third of the previous microbiological cures.

The reasons for therapeutic failures, and to a lesser extent therapeutic successes, have not been well delineated. One of the factors contributing to the former is the fact that individual *G. vaginalis* isolates are resistant to metronidazole. *Mobiluncus* species are resistant to metronidazole and may also be linked to some treatment failures. Depending on whether one is dealing with *M. curtisii* or *M. mulieris*, sensitivity to erythromycin and clindamycin differs. The adequacy of Gram staining alone for the diagnosis of *Mobiluncus* species is debatable.

Another major problem of insufficient treatment may be the fact that the diagnosis of BV with Nugent scores precludes the possibility that some patients with other conditions causing abnormal vaginal flora such as *Trichomonas* and AV will be missed and treated as if they were BV. AV does not respond to metronidazole and is know to be resistant to many other types of antibiotherapy.

Oral metronidazole is frequently followed by a variety of mild-to-severe side effects, such as metallic taste in the mouth, swallowing difficulties, and stomach pains. Drinking alcohol produces severe nausea and vomiting and should be prevented. Currently, the use of either clindamycin or metronidazole vaginal cream for a week has resulted in more or less the same cure rate, but with far fewer side effects.

Clindamycin
During pregnancy, clindamycin, preferably given orally and early in pregnancy, is the preferred treatment of choice, as metronidazole is not able to prevent complications such as preterm rupture of the membranes and preterm birth. Clindamycin given twice 300 mg orally or in an application of 100 mg locally in the vagina at bedtime has been proven to prevent preterm birth in at least four well-designed, prospective randomized studies.

Probiotics and Recurrent BV
Treatment with antibiotics is efficient in eradicating the symptoms and restoring the vaginal flora in up to 85% of the cases, but at the same time, the disease recurs after successful treatment in 75% to 80% in eight months. For these women, BV is a psychologically, socially, and sexually debilitating disease, which is not well managed by recurrent treatment with antibiotics. Furthermore, this approach is not free of side effects and problems with rising resistance of bacteria such as enterococci and *E. coli*. Hence for such recurrent cases, a maintenance therapy with vaginally applied lactobacilli or acidifying products can be tried. In a randomized, double-blinded study we recently performed, treatment with lactobacillus acidophilus has been equally successful in the treatment of BV as intravaginal metronidazole in the short term, but the effect did not last longer than a few weeks. Hence, the ideal prophylactic treatment consists of monthly application of these products for three to five days at the end of the menstrual bleeding period for several months. Other studies have also shown beneficial effects on the restoration of the vaginal flora and pH by using lactobacilli or ascorbinic acid after classic treatment with metronidazole or clindamycin. Still other studies using different types of lactobacilli and other molecules such as dequalinium fluoride to prevent recurrences are ongoing.

Special Treatment Considerations
The question of whether or not to treat women who are unaware of the infection has arisen. Patients who have a habit of frequently douching, and perhaps those habituated to their own odors, are unlikely to complain and seek treatment. Possibly, patients unaware of the disease should be allowed to continue in ignorance if cooperation between them and their consorts is likely to be difficult. However, it should be recognized that even though the woman is unaware of the infection, her consort may be only too conscious of her unpleasant odor.

Since *G. vaginalis* may be sexually transmitted, a woman's sexual consort should be considered and logically treated with the same systemic agent. A difficult therapeutic challenge often develops when a third party or multiple sexual partners are involved. However, treatment of the sexual cohort is of no use in trying to prevent frequent recurrences in women with recurrent BV. Any women with BV should be evaluated for coinfection with major STDs.

The "Intermediate Flora"
Definition and Diagnosis
Intermediate flora on Gram stains   As generally known, a Nugent's score of above 7 on Gram-stained specimens corresponds well with BV, and is nowadays accepted as the golden standard for diagnosing BV in most clinical trials. Compared to this method, wet mount is said to be less sensitive. However, some constraints have to be taken into consideration. First of all, in a continuous scale from 1 to 10, no consensus exists what the intermediate group with a score of 4 to 6 stands for. If Nugent were an ideal scoring system for BV, with scores 1 to 3 being normal and 7 or above being full-blown BV, scores 4 to 6 should be transitional, partial, or intermediate BV, but in reality, it is not. Ideally, this intermediate flora state represents a turning point from a normal state into BV, or

on the opposite, from BV to normal. In reality, however, most of these women with so-called intermediate BV according to Nugent will neither have BV, nor will they become normal. In fact, as they are not having normal flora, nor BV, they rather resemble sort of a "garbage can," but this does not mean that they do not represent important pathology. In fact, in almost all studies addressing the importance of BV and the intermediate group as a separate category, it was clear that the intermediate group was linked to a different and usually more serious scope of complications (e.g., mid-trimester pregnancy loss) than the "classic," full-blown BV.

Concordance in reading difficult slides   In a large international project, many researchers in the field of vaginal infections took the effort to read BV slides, normal slides, and those so-called "difficult slides" to measure the concordance among researchers, and to see whether the diagnosis of BV by use of phase contrast wet mount microscopy concorded well with Nugent's diagnosis on Gram stain. It was confirmed that wet mount, even after later rehydration of air-dried wet mounts, was as accurate in diagnosing BV as Gram stains. But at the same time, it was clear that the most diverse opinions prevailed when the "difficult slides" where studied: some did not read them, and discarded the difficult slides as unreadable or nonclassifiable; others classified them as partial BV; while yet others proposed to classify part of them in a completely different category: AV (see later).

In another study, the interobserver concordance of wet mount reading was tested by six independent vaginal disease specialists in Europe. An excellent kappa index was obtained in the diagnosis of BV and LBGs, reflecting the good interobserver agreement, at least when phase contrast microscopy is used.

Treatment

Intermediate abnormal flora does not respond to treatment as one would expect if it were partial BV. Even full-blown BV (Nugent above 7) does not always respond well to repetitive courses of metronidazole, leaving ca. 15% of cases unchanged, suggesting that a condition other than BV may be involved in such cases (23). Therefore, in the intermediate group, partial BV as well as other abnormal conditions may be present. "Partial BV" is, in our definition, a transient state between normal flora and full-blown BV, as is clearly illustrated in Figure 4. It is obvious that there is a mixed flora, but the strikes of abnormal flora are of the anaerobic, *Gardnerella* morphotype–like microflora. In the full-blown picture of BV, granular flora is omnipresent and covers the epithelial cells, which are called "clue cells." This condition that we call "partial BV" should not be confused with other states of intermediate or abnormal flora such as AV, which is discussed below.

It is not clear whether patients with "intermediate flora" need treatment, and if they do, it is not clear which treatment would be most adequate. It would be our advice to refine the diagnosis first by performing a thorough clinical examination, with extended anamnesis, expert microscopy, and, in some cases, confirmative cultures. Partial BV is treated like BV. In cases with complaints, patients with AV should be told what type of condition they have and that experimental preparations can be tried. In cases without *Trichomonas* or *Candida* infection, antimicrobials should be given.

Aerobic Vaginitis

AV is an entity that was recently introduced in order to get law and order in the group of women who are suffering from vaginal infections with abnormal bacterial microflora, but do not always have anaerobic BV. Due to the unlucky fact that the diagnosis of BV has been displaced out of the office toward the laboratory, and physicians unfortunately often fail to link these findings to the clinical condition of the individual patient, many women formerly diagnosed as suffering from BV were actually having AV or mixed infections.

Symptoms

Like women with BV, those with AV also may have a lactobacillus-deficient syndrome with recurrent symptoms of profuse discharge, foul smell, increased pH, and profound effects on the psychological and sexual well-being (Table 1). However, upon careful analysis of the symptoms, the discharge is often yellowish rather than white-gray, sticky mucorrheic and not watery, and, in severe cases, smells more like rotten meat than like fish, as would be in BV cases. A specific symptom that is notably absent in BV is heavy burning to excruciating pain during sexual intercourse, leading to complete apareunia in severe cases. Some patients suffer for years and break up with their partners before they find a doctor who can elucidate the diagnosis for them and explain the possibilities for improvement.

Signs

The vulvar introitus is often red, but the exterior areas of the vulva and clitoris appear normal, unlike the case of *Candida* vulvovaginitis, where vulva redness and edema are frequent. During speculum examination, the vagina looks red and inflamed, or has very small to confluent dark red ulcerations that typically are found on the upper anterior vaginal wall. Therefore, when doing a speculum examination, it is important to withdraw the speculum slowly, while looking carefully at the anterior vaginal fornix. When rubbing the wall with a cotton swab, small bleeding spots can be revealed. Introducing a speculum or digital examination may cause frictional pain, typical for vaginal dyspareunia. The cotton swab will turn yellow ("yellow swab test"), a sign that leukocytes are abundantly present in the exudates. The vaginal pH can be moderately abnormal, in the range of 4.5 to 5.5, in light or moderate cases, but in severe cases, it goes as high as 6 or 7.

Diagnosis

Diagnosis of AV is solely based on microscopy, and is in that respect comparable to the Nugent's method on Gram stains to diagnose BV (Table 5). LBG are the basis for a composite score to which the four following variables were added: (*i*) proportional number of leukocytes, (*ii*) presence of toxic leukocytes, (*iii*) presence of parabasal epithelial cells, and (*iv*) type of background flora (Fig. 5). Therefore, in this classification, opposite to other infectious conditions such as BV or candidiasis, also the immune reaction of the host is taken into account for the diagnosis (Table 1). Parabasal cells are considered a sign of severe epithelial inflammation usually not seen in uncomplicated BV. They are encountered only in moderate or severe forms of AV, such as in desquamative inflammatory vaginitis. The background flora was allocated a score 0 if the background flora was unremarkable or showed debris and bare nuclei from lysed epithelial cells (cytolysis), score 1 if the lactobacillary morphotypes were very coarse or resembled small bacilli (other than lactobacilli), and 2 if there were prominent cocci or chained cocci visible. Leukocytes were scored according to their proportional number when compared with epitheliocytes. More than 10 per epithelial cell is assigned 2 points, while less than 10 per epithelial cell, but more than 10 per high-power field corresponds to 1 point. Adding these points together comprises a composite score, the "AV" score. A composite score of 1 to 4 corresponds to normal flora, a score of 5 to 6 to moderate AV, and a score above 6 (to maximum 10) to severe AV. In practice, a score of 8 to 10 matches the definition of "desquamative inflammatory vaginitis."

The use of this AV criterion enables us to divide the flora in a more detailed and comprehensive way, avoiding undefined and unclear categories. Bacterial flora is lactobacillary type predominant (normal), or it is abnormal. If abnormal, the flora can be disturbed by anaerobic overgrowth (BV) or by aerobic microorganisms such as *E. coli*, group B streptococci, enterococci, etc. (AV), or it can be a mixture of both (mixed abnormal flora). Therefore one has to be continuously aware that concomitant infections may occur, such as *Candida*, *T. vaginalis*, BV, or cervicitis.

Treatment

The most efficient treatment for AV is not yet well established. The presence of parabasal cells, the fact that the condition is frequently present in women on long-term low-dose contraceptive pills, the prominent abundance of leucocytes in the vaginal exudate, and the high production of vaginal IL-1 and IL-8 seem to suggest that AV may represent an overreaction of the immune system, while the opposite, absence of immune response, is more typical for BV. For that reason, experimental application of high concentrations of estradiol valerate, hydrocortisone, and antibiotics have been tried intravaginally with variable successes. Repetitive application of vaginal lactobacilli has been helpful, but further studies are needed.

T. vaginalis Vulvovaginitis

T. vaginalis (TV) is one of the most frequent sexually transmitted pathogens worldwide. Only about 50% of patients yielding trichomonads complain of irritation at the time the organisms are first discovered. Therefore, sexual transmission often occurs from partners without complaints.

Signs and Symptoms

Vaginal discharge   Discharge is the cardinal symptom of this disease, but practically all women harboring the organism have, have had, or will have irritative symptoms such as itching, burning, and dyspareunia. The color and inflammatory changes seen by the clinician are dependent on the virulence of the strain. High-virulence strains usually present with a profuse, frothy, yellow discharge.

Vulvar symptoms   The medical literature has too long perpetuated the idea that trichomoniasis is practically always associated with a greenish, frothy discharge and a strawberry vagina. About 40% of patients with trichomoniasis have evidence of gross tissue changes of the vulva at the time of the initial examination. There is usually only a mild erythema present and occasionally some edema. Sometimes perineal and perianal fissures, mimicking Candida infection, are present (Fig. 6A).

Vaginal symptoms   One-third of patients with Trichomonas display profuse redness and edema of the vagina, but the typical "strawberry vagina," resulting from swollen papillae projecting through vaginal secretions on the cervix, only present in less than 10% of the acute cases. Also, the typical frothy vaginal secretions occur in less than 10% of infected cases (Fig. 6b); the majority of trichomonal discharges are indeed gray and are often indistinguishable from the discharge of BV or AV, except by microscopy or laboratory methods.

TABLE 5   Criteria for the microscopic diagnosis of AV (400 × magnification, phase contrast microscope)

AV score	LBG	Number of leukocytes	Proportion of toxic leukocytes	Background flora	PBC
0	I and IIa	≤10/hpf	None or sporadic	Unremarkable or cytolysis	None or <1%
I	IIb	>10/hpf and ≤10/epithelial cells	≤50% of leukocytes	Small coliform bacilli	≤10%
2	III	>10/epithelial cells	>50% of leukocytes	Cocci or chains	>10%

ªA composite AV score of <3 corresponds to "no signs of AV"; 3–4 to "light AV"; 5–6 to moderate AV; and any score above 6 to "severe AV." The latter group corresponds well to the entity "desquamative inflammatory vaginitis (45,46)."
Abbreviations: LBG, lactobacillary grades; PBC, proportion of parabasal epitheliocytus; AV, aerobic vaginitis; I, numerous pleiomorph lactobacilli, no other bacteria; IIa, mixed flora, but predominantly lactobacilli; IIb, mixed flora, but proportion of lactobacilli severely decreased due to increased number of other bacteria; III, lactobacilli severely depressed or absent because of overgrowth of other bacteria; hpf, high-power field (400× magnification).

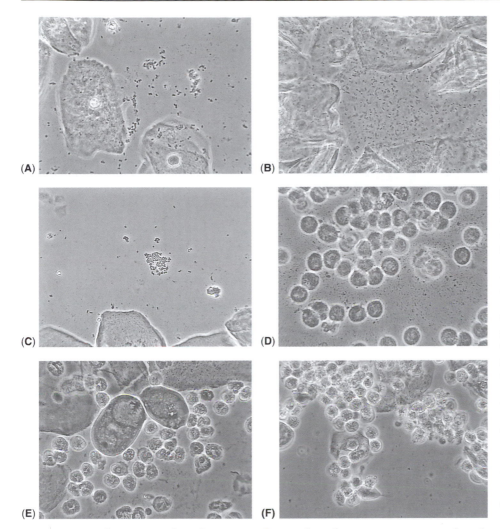

FIGURE 5 AV is characterized by an impaired lactobacillary flora, in which the lactobacilli are replaced by coccoid flora (**A**) or staphoid flora, e.g., *Escherichia coli*, *Klebsiella* sp., *Acinetobacter* sp. (**B**). Unlike BV where the anaerobic bacteria are so numerous that they form a carpet of indistinguishable bacteria, bacteria in AV can be seen separately and could be counted. Sometimes the cocci form clearly visible chains (e.g., group B streptococci) or clusters (e.g., *Staphylococcus aureus*) (**C**). Another characteristic that is frequently encountered is the presence of an increased number of leucocytes (more than 10 leukocytes per epithelial cell are considered abnormal), very often with a toxic appearance due to the activation of phagocytic and lysosomic activity (**D**). Parabasal cells (**E**) may be seen even in young women, and are then a sign of severe AV, with desquamation of the upper epithelial layers of the vagina, exposing the lower parabasal cells to the vaginal content. Coinfection with AV must always be taken into account, as candidiasis and *Trichomonas* infection (**F**) can coexist. *Abbreviation*: AV, aerobic vaginitis, BV, bacterial vaginosis.

An occasional patient with trichomoniasis has a relatively dry vagina with pseudomembrane formation. In fact, some examples are suggestive of the thrush patches of candidiasis. Most cases of the rare occasions of vaginitis emphysematosa, i.e., vaginitis with cystoid spaces filled with gas and lying within the vaginal mucosa, are attributed to trichomoniasis.

Urinary problems Urinary symptoms, suggesting urethritis or cystitis, are reported by some patients with trichomoniasis. Urethrocystitis, caused by Trichomonas infection, is occasionally seen in patients with or without apparent vaginal infection. In other words, a mild, abacteriuric pyuria seen with trichomonads in a clean-voided or catheterized specimen can sometimes be attributed to the organism. An immediate disappearance of a persistent, mild pyuria in such a patient upon administration of metronidazole strongly suggests that she had trichomonal urethrocystitis.

Diagnosis

Wet mount microscopy Because of its simplicity and accuracy (sensitivity of 70% and a specificity of 100%), the microscopic examination of a wet mount preparation using physiologic saline is the laboratory diagnostic method of choice. Identifying actively motile organisms poses no problem. However, immotile, rounded, or "balled-up"

organisms are often discernible only under the high-power objective and are sometimes difficult to discern from toxic leucocytes (loaded with lysozymes) (Fig. 5F). Such organisms may be seen in urinary specimens, in vaginal smears of patients with asymptomatic disease, and occasionally in patients who have recently douched or used vaginal medicaments. An occasional patient is seen who has severe vaginitis, apparent acute trichomoniasis, but with no detectable trichomonads. This phenomenon apparently results from autotoxins within the colony and were observed when studying trichomonads in tissue culture. However, this condition may also be AV.

It is crucial not to delay the examination as the sensitivity drops by 20% if delayed for 10 minutes, the specimen should be diluted with physiologic solution, and the warming effect of the microscopic lamp can be beneficial to seeing the jerky motile parasites with flagellae, which usually are the size of leukocytes. Typically, many leukocytes are present, parabasal epithelial cells and cocci may be seen (AV flora), but also the typical granular flora of BV is frequently present. Usually, the lactobacilli are depressed; in most cases TV is found in a LBG-III flora.

Stained smears The Dif-Quick staining technique often enables trichomonads to be identified easily even after the

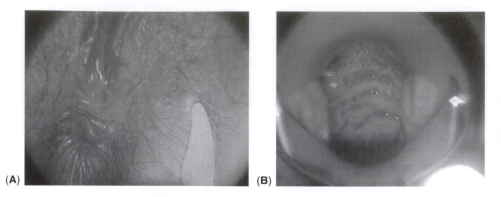

FIGURE 6 *Trichomonas vaginalis* infection may cause vulvar irritation and perineal and perianal fissures (**A**), and typically the vaginal walls are edematous, red, and inflamed, and show a yellowish, profuse discharge that may have a foul smell (**B**). The microscopic appearance is shown in Fig. 5F.

unstained specimen has been nondiagnostic. Gram stains and Pap smears have been tested for use in screening, but the latter are only 57% sensitive. Also, the more modern liquid-based Pap medium does not offer better sensitivity. During menopause, the diagnosis of TV must always be questioned, as the rate of false-positive diagnoses is extremely high.

Cultures   Cultures in a specific medium and PCR have the highest sensitivity for diagnosing Trichomonas (80–85% sensitivity). Rarely, the flagellates identified in the vagina may represent Giardia lambia transmitted from the rectum across the perineum.

Treatment

Metronidazole, treatment of choice   The original therapy recommended by Dr. Gardner, 500 mg bid for five days, taken by both the patient and her consort, is still the treatment of choice. Although most reports on one-day regimens with 2 g metronidazole in a single dose or 1 g twice in one day are extremely encouraging, a safe conjecture might be that in the long run, it will prove considerably less effective than the five-day regimen. Alternative one-day treatments are tinidazole 2 g or ornidazole 1.5 g orally.

Treatment of sexual partners   One study found the same incidence of urogenital trichomoniasis in both sexes. Fewer than 20% of men harboring the organism have symptoms; more have symptoms soon after first contact than subsequently. Other researchers found trichomonads in 68% of men who had been diagnosed as having nongonococcal urethritis. By using proper isolation methods, the organism can be recovered from over 80% of the consorts of infected women. Allegedly, trichomonads die out in the male urethra within a few weeks after the last contact with an infected woman, but this has not been a confirmed observation. LeDuc unequivocally stated that "the current opinion that Trichomonas urethritis is self limited is an error. The concept that the parasites will spontaneously disappear from the urethra of the man who wears a protective sheath to avoid reinfection during coitus is untenable." As a conclusion, since a failure to isolate Trichomonas does not prove that the consort is free of the organism, and treatment is simple, efficient, and safe, it is recommended to treat all male sexual partners regardless of the presence of symptoms and without attempting isolation.

Resistant strains   In the rare instances of Trichomonas infection not responding to five days of treatment with 1 g metronidazole per day, resistance to metronidazole is feared. In such instances, retreatment while ensuring all the partners are treated simultaneously is warranted. If trichomonads are still present, a number of options are possible. Recently, we encountered such an extremely resistant case that persisted even after doubling the dose and prolonging the treatment period to 14 days. We tried paromomycin 250 mg in cream vaginally for 14 days, without cure. Finally, she was cured after a treatment suggested by Dr. Jack Sobel: simultaneous vaginal and oral treatment with tinidazole (1 g orally twice daily and 500 mg vaginally twice daily for two weeks) cures 95% of women and also cured our patient. Other therapies suggested were focusing on the male by performing prostate massage and PCR on his fluid as well as ejaculate, and treatment with local gentian violet and metronidazole gel for two weeks or twice-weekly treatment with 2 g of tinidazole for three to four weeks (G. Monif and R. Weissenbacher).

Vulvovaginal Candidiasis

Candidiasis is the most frequent cause of symptomatic vulvovaginitis, and yet its proper diagnosis and management remains a great challenge for most physicians.

Performing differential cultures on 100 consecutive patients with candidiasis, Dr. C.D. Dukes and Dr. H. Gardner found that 67% of the infections were due to *C. albicans*, followed by *C. glabrata*, *C. tropicalis*, *C. pseudotropicalis*, *C. stellatoidea*, *C. krusei*, and *C. quillermondi*. These findings are probably only of academic interest, since there was no discernible difference in the clinical features of the infections caused by the different species. More recent data from large studies, however, seem to suggest that *C. albicans* remains by far the most frequent cause of vulvovaginal candidiasis, both in acute and in recurrent diseases, with only less than 10% of non-*albicans* strains.

We also found acidific rods (lactobacilli and diphtheroids) to be the predominant vaginal bacteria in patients with candidiasis who yielded no other vaginal pathogens. This should be of no surprise to anyone, as Doderlein, in his historic treatise published in 1892, reported an association between large gram-positive rods and fungi, and stated that the acid medium of the vagina favored both. However, one should be aware that BV and AV are also frequently associated with *Candida*, so that one diagnosis is sometimes not sufficient to explain all complaints or treatment failures (Fig. 7).

Epidemiology

Candida can be recovered from almost any area of the body. It is found in the oral cavity and intestinal tract in a high percentage of women yielding vaginal organisms. Candidiasis is not considered a venereal disease, but men can become infected at the glans penis and develop symptoms and may in this period sexually transfer the organisms from one woman to another. Still, systematic treatment of men is not likely to improve the recurrence rate of candidiasis in most women, showing that the sexual transmission is a rather rare primary cause of infection in women. Furthermore, women without sexual activity present as often with acute and recurrent candidiasis as their sexually active counterparts, and sexual promiscuity does not necessarily lead to more frequent occurrence of candidiasis, unless frequent antibiotics have been prescribed for other infections.

Predisposing Factors

Hormonal influences   Host factors controlling susceptibility are much more important to the development of candidiasis than the chance vaginal contamination with a *Candida* species. Diabetes, obesity, and pregnancy are generally recognized predisposing factors. Most experienced clinicians know that the "pseudopregnancy" produced by contraceptive pills does increase the incidence and intensity of the disease, even though older studies suggest that only older, high-estrogen-content pills seemed to have this side effect. Some of the reasons suggested for this increased susceptibility are (*i*) increased vaginal glycogen from estrogens, (*ii*) vaginal thinning from progestational agents, (*iii*) altered sugar metabolism, and (*iv*) altered sexual habits.

Antibiotics   The wide and at times inappropriate use of antibiotics has produced the greatest increase in candidiasis. Regardless of the exact mode of action, antibiotics play a dual role by increasing candidal colonization by the host and by inducing rapid multiplication of vaginal Candida. The prevailing opinion is that the antibiotics knock out bacterial competition, leaving the door wide open for Candida. Investigators have found other explanations for the effects of antibiotics, including a reduction in phagocytosis of Candida, a reduction of antibodies to Candida, and a direct stimulatory effect on Candida. Especially metronidazole, penicillins, and tetracyclines are prone to increase the relapse rate of candidiasis.

According to Lon and Baker, vaginal colonization with *Candida* may be increased a 1000-fold if also the intestinal gut is colonized. This colonization is long-lasting, difficult or impossible to eradicate, and serves as a continuous source of vaginal reinfection.

Glucose metabolism   Diabetes mellitus, while being a strongly predisposing factor when present, is of little significance to the overall picture of this disease. Patients with diabetes suffering from intractable or recurrent candidiasis are always suspected to have poor regulation of the glucose metabolism. Even if daily profiles are allegedly perfect, it is likely that glycemic bursts at night are present and a pump regulating insulin is able to stem the symptoms. However, most patients with chronic, recurrent candidiasis do not

have diabetes, nor prediabetes. Still, on performing systematic glucose tolerance tests in these patients, a 15% mean increase of plasma glucose levels was found in a recent study. However, despite successes in sporadic cases, it is not entirely clear yet if diet restrictions alone are able to lower the recurrence rate of candidiasis attacks in patients known to have recurrent disease. It is important to recognize that many patients with recurrent candidiasis have an addiction to high-sugar–containing products such as chocolate. This seems to be accentuated just before the onset of the menstrual period and is almost at the level of a severe compulsion or addiction. If the sugar habit cannot be reduced, it is extremely difficult to eliminate candidiasis for any length of time. On the other hand, in selected patients, we were quite successful with the addition of 500 mg metformin daily.

Controlling the diabetes and eliminating all *Candida* organisms does not always result in immediate cure of the long-neglected patient. These patients usually have developed a chronic lichen simplex of the vulva resulting from the scratch–itch reflex. They require prolonged use of topically applied corticosteroids. Even though all three approaches are required, it sometimes takes months to achieve patient relief and some vulvar tissues are never restored to normal.

An interesting observation is the occasional finding of a microscopic diagnosis of vulvar "leukoplakia" (more correctly called hyperplastic dystrophy) in patients with diabetes. The irritative effects of *Candida* on vulvar tissue and the effects of physical trauma from scratching provoke hyperkeratosis, epithelial hyperplasia, and an inflammatory infiltration.

Immune response   Increased susceptibility may also be related to the immune response to Candida species. Some patients with the chronic recurrent disease have lower specific antibody titers to Candida. In patients with chronic recurrent candidiasis, Lourie and Brayton showed diminished candidacidal activity. Increased susceptibility of the vulvar tissues to allergenic or endotoxic substances produced by Candida may be another factor explaining some cases of apparently reduced resistance. It is not easy to explain why an occasional patient with severe tissue reactions yields a minimal number of organisms, whereas another patient may have a red inflamed vagina full of thrush patches without having any symptoms or complaints.

Treatment

There is a big difference between the treatment of acute vulvovaginitis and of chronic recurrent candidiasis, most of which are autogenous reinfections.

Acute infection   Cure of acute candidiasis is almost always complete after treatment with local or oral antimycotics for a few days. There is very little difference in the efficacy of all the products available (Table 6), and the differences in in vivo efficacies of miconazole, terconazole, itraconazole, butoconazole, econazole, and fluconazole are minimal for the acute infections concerned. Oral or vaginal application is not an issue of efficacy but rather of personal preference.

Oral single 150 mg dose fluconazole has been approved as a treatment for acute candidiasis, and so also two times

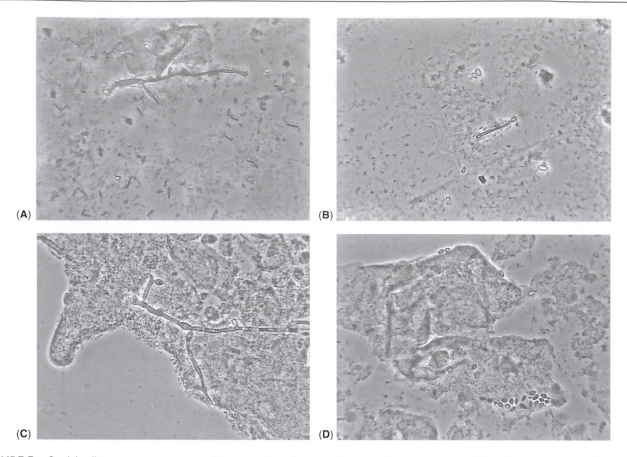

FIGURE 7 *Candida albicans* may present as well in normal lactobacillary dominant flora with hyphae (**A**), or blastospores (in this picture with starting hyphenization) (**B**), or with abnormal flora, such as BV (**C**). In most cases of combined infection with BV and candidiasis, only numerous typical blastospores of *Candida glabrata* are found (**D**). *Abbreviation*: BV, bacterial vaginosis.

100 mg oral ketoconazole. However, in actual practice, especially with recurrent candidiasis, it may require 7 to 30 days of treatment to eradicate a highly pathogenic yeast. Itraconazole is less used nowadays due to the side effect of acute liver toxicity that sometimes occurs. Several authors have found capsules containing 600 mg of boric acid to be useful, especially for non-*albicans* candidiasis.

In resistant cases, one or two applications of gentian violet may offer rapid relief of acute symptoms. This is then followed by the application of the azole cream two or three times daily for a minimum of two weeks. Vaginal medications or oral antifungal drugs can be used simultaneously. Its well-known disadvantage of staining almost everything and the discomfort in attending at the physician's office for its application makes it quite unpopular with patients.

Recurrent infection Chronic, recurrent Candida vulvovaginitis (RCV) is defined as a proven vulvovaginal candidiasis that recurs four times or more per year. Patients suffering from this condition are desperate and frequently wander from doctor to doctor in a search of a definitive cure. The truth is that these patients cannot be promised definitive cure as all the so-called new treatments, except a few, belong to the same family of azoles, and are candidastatic, but not candidacidal. Sometimes treatment with nonazole products such as local amphotericin B, flucytosine,

or oral mepartricin may be worth trying, but in most instances, patients have to be instructed that they suffer from a chronic disease that requires long-term, prophylactic treatment. A few tips to optimize the effect of medication may be tried before engaging in a long-term systematic prophylactic therapy regimen: (*i*) longer therapy not interrupted during menstruation, (*ii*) use of an intravaginal antimycotic once at bedtime for a few days after each menstrual period as a prophylactic measure, (iii) use of mycotic medication during and for several days after a course of antibiotic therapy; and (*iv*) application of nystatin ointment or one of the azole local creams to the patient's preputial folds and to her consort's penis twice daily for 10 days.

Patients should be warned not to lose themselves in the advice of people thinking they understand the problem and manage it properly by using lists of "don't do's," complicated diets, and sophisticated therapies based more on personal beliefs than on medical facts and evidence. In most instances, if you have a chronic recurrent debilitating disease, of which you cannot easily take away the cause, you need preventive treatment. This is not different in the case of RCV.

The principle of suppressive therapy has been tested with repetitive vaginal application of an azole, as well as with oral fluconazole and itraconazole. Weekly treatment

TABLE 6 Treatment of *Candida* vaginitis

Uncomplicated acute VVC
First choice

　Miconazole (Gyno-Dakatarin®): vaginal ovule 200 mg at bedtime for 7 days; vaginal ovule 1.2 g at bedtime once; vaginal cream 2%, 5 g at bedtime for 10–16 days

　Econazole (Gyno-Pevaryl®): vaginal cream 1%, 5 g at bedtime for 15 days

　Butoconazole (Gynomyk®): vaginal ovule 100 mg at bedtime for 3 days; vaginal cream 2%, 5 g at bedtime for 7–14 days

　Clotrimazole (Gyno-Canestene®): vaginal tablets 100 mg at bedtime for 6 days; vaginal tablet 500 mg at bedtime once; vaginal cream 2%, 5 g at bedtime for 3 days

　Omoconazole (Fongarex®): vaginal ovule 900 mg at bedtime once

　Fluconazole (Diflucan®): 150 mg orally once

　Itraconazole (Sporanox®): 200 mg orally bid (in the morning and in the evening the same day) with a meal

Alternative choice

　Mepartricin (Tricandil®): vaginal cream 5 g (5000 U) at bedtime for 15 days; vaginal tablets (25,000 U) at bedtime for 15 days

　Terconazole (Gyno-Terazol®): vaginal ovule 80 mg at bedtime for 3 days

Complicated VVC/recurrent disease
Initial episode: any of the above treatment with a longer duration —7 to 14 days for topical therapy *or* a systemic treatment repeated 3 days later; followed by a 6-mo maintenance regimen (any one of the following):
a) One vaginal ovule treatment once a week (clotrimazole, miconazole, or omoconazole)
b) Fluconazole 150 mg once a week for 6 mo
c) Itraconazole 400 mg once a month
d) Degressive dosage system with 200 mg fluconazole thrice a week, diminished to once a month over the period of 1 yr is being tested and shows very promising first results

VVC due to *Candida* non-*albicans*
Initial episode: fluconazole 200 mg/day for 10 days *or* itraconazole 200 mg (or 2 × 200 mg)/day for 10 days; followed by a 6-mo maintenance regimen

VVC during pregnancy
First choice

　Vaginal miconazole or cotrimoxazole tablets or cream at least for 7 days

Alternative choice

　Mepartricin (Tricandil®): vaginal cream 5 g (5000 U) at bedtime for 15 days; vaginal tablets (25,000 U) at bedtime for 15 days

Side effects, warnings:
- In case of uncontrolled diabetes mellitus, intake of corticosteroids or antibiotics (namely penicillins, nitro imidazoles, tetracyclines), local vulvar application of corticosteroids, and other situations favoring growth of *Candida*, longer treatment (up to 14 days) is usually indicated.
- *Candida krusei* is resistant to fluconazole, but almost never occurs in the vagina.
- Other *Candida* non-*albicans*—resistant strains to azoles are rare but exist in immunocompromised patients, or in patients taking long-duration antibiotic therapy, or in patients chronically applying corticosteroids cream on their vulva.
- Ketoconazole: 1 in 10,000 to 15,000 persons exposed to ketoconazole have severe hepatic toxicity (a few cases of death are described), and it is no more recommended to treat *Candida* infections.
- Itraconazole: rare allergic cutaneous reactions, liver function tests altered; numerous interactions with other drugs; drugs of which intake is contraindicated with itraconazole: terfenadine, astemizole, cisapride, quinidine, pimozide, simvastatin, lovastatin, midazolam, triazolam.
- Fluconazole: rare allergic cutaneous reactions, liver function tests altered; numerous interactions with other drugs; drugs of which intake is contraindicated with fluconazole: terfenadine, astemizole, cisapride.
- Oral azoles: numerous interactions with other drugs, among them: anticoagulants, hypoglycemic sulfamids, hydrochlorothiazides, phenytoin, some oral contraceptives, rifampicin, cyclosporine, theophylline, rifabutin, tacrolimus, zidovudine.
- Terconazole: pyrexia and chills can occur even with a local treatment.
- Oil-based vaginal cream or ovules interact with latex condom and diaphragm, reducing their security.
Abbreviation: VVC, vulvovaginal candidiasis.

with 150 mg of fluconazole for six months was proposed and showed a tremendous advantage with regard to the diminishing number of recurrences of RCV: 91% were still relapse free at the end of the treatment period. After stopping the treatment, half of the patients relapsed in the following six months, although the relapse rate during this period was still significantly less than in patients who had been treated with placebo. In an adapted regimen, using the same amount of medication, we used a system in which the fluconazole treatment was diminished progressively (but only if clinical, microscopic, and culture data were favorable), with very good response rates and satisfaction as a result, even after one year (77% relapse free after one year). As discussed above, it is important to keep on searching during this treatment regimen for possible risk factors that provoke recurrences, in order to enable more

rapid or more definite diminishment or interruption of medication.

Common problems with Candida treatment　Women being treated for yeast infections frequently develop lactobacillus overgrowth syndrome (which will be described in the next section). This pasty, white discharge is frequently misdiagnosed as being a Candida recurrence. This results in an erroneous diagnosis made over the telephone.

Therapy is frequently ordered without a diagnosis being made. Anticandidal therapy does not cure lactobacillus overgrowth syndrome or its symptoms, nor for other conditions that may mimic candidiasis. It is important that the discharge be actually diagnosed in the office or the patient be supplied with culture media to culture her discharge at home. Self-culturing is a simple procedure using sterile cotton tip swabs that can be introduced in the vagina and put in culture medium. It cannot be overemphasized how important it is to actually verify yeast in women with recurrent problems.

The availability of over-the-counter clotrimazole and miconazole vaginal preparations has resulted in an explosive increase of self-treatment of suspected vaginal candidosis. Estimates of incorrect self-diagnosis range as high as 50% to 75%. In cases of recurrent candidiasis, the daily frequency and length of treatment may have to be doubled or tripled.

C. glabrata Vulvovaginitis

According to most authors such as Wickerham, Kerns, Sobel, and Gray and Perju, et al., C. glabrata is a marginal or weak pathogen capable of producing only mild vulvovaginitis in susceptible subjects. The organism can also be present without causing symptoms. Its former name C. torulopsis is now abandoned.

Clinical features The principal clinical feature of infection is a vaginal secretion that resembles a normal secretion, but is more fluid and abundant. The secretion is white or slate colored and is not malodorous. Thrush patches do not form. Vaginal activity is within the range of pH 4.0 to 5.0 in contrast to the 3.8 to 4.2 pH range of normal secretions. Irritative signs such as erythema are only slight, if present at all. The patient may complain of a discharge and mild itching or burning.

Diagnosis Any patient having an increased vaginal secretion with mild irritative signs and symptoms of vulvovaginitis, but whose secretions yield none of the usual vaginal pathogens, might be suspected of having C. glabrata infection. Both wet mount preparations and stained smears reveal tremendous numbers of spores similar to those of Candida, but variable in size and without associated hyphae. The presence of C. glabrata can be confirmed by culture.

Treatment The most effective therapeutic agent for C. glabrata vaginitis has not been determined. Most preparations used for candidiasis are moderately successful and require-long duration of treatment. In vitro differences claimed to make the difference do usually not pay of in clinical results. Boric acid capsules of 600 mg for two to three weeks have been successfully used.

Cytolytic Vaginosis—The Lactobacilli Overgrowth Syndrome

This syndrome is characterized by a pasty discharge with no evidence of vaginal irritation or odor but with low-grade burning or discomfort that is greatly increased during or after sexual activity (Table 1). The smear is characterized by many rod-like lactobacilli of varying lengths, stripped nuclei, cytoplasmic debris, and large numbers of epithelial cells. Few other bacteria or yeast are found on the Gram stain. Cultures are always reported as "normal vaginal flora" or "lactobacilli."

This condition arises in women who have been treated several times for vaginal discharges with an assortment of antibacterial and antifungal medications. The lactobacilli become the dominant vaginal microorganism. It appears that the irritative form of overgrowth contains lactobacilli that are more aggressive than the usual ones found in the vagina. They certainly seem capable of breaking down the vaginal mucosa by producing enough acid to lyse the cytoplasm and strip the nuclei free of the cell (Fig. 8). The condition is easily recognizable on wet mount microscopy, but care has to be taken so that the bare nuclei are not mistaken for leukocytes. Invariably, the pH is more acid than usual and measures 3.8 to 4 or even less.

Treatment

Baking soda douches (NaHCO, one or two tablespoons to a quart of warm water) to raise the vaginal pH can be applied. This remedy is effective if carried out for a considerable length of time, and if no intervening antimicrobial or vaginal therapy is interposed. The aim of therapy is to restore the usual vaginal microflora, and to reduce the excess of lactic acid being secreted.

Viral Vaginitis

It is difficult to ascribe a role to the presence of either HPV, herpes virus, or other viruses in the development of leukorrhea and/or vaginal irritation. Since essentially no specific vaginal lesions have been noted with herpetic infections and the cervical lesions appear not to be associated with profuse discharge, it might be assumed that the herpes viral family is not involved. Papilloma virus, however, is a real problem. One description for the diagnosis of subclinical vaginal HPV infection is elongated vaginal papillae seen with the naked eye but better assessed using the colposcope. Each of these projections contains a central capillary that can be seen with the naked eye but is much clearer when a colposcope is used. A confirmatory diagnosis based on vaginal biopsy sometimes reveals koilocytosis, but in most of the lesions, no HPV infection can be detected. In these women, the chief complaints are related to discomfort after coitus, persistent pain, or burning. Once the diagnosis is made,

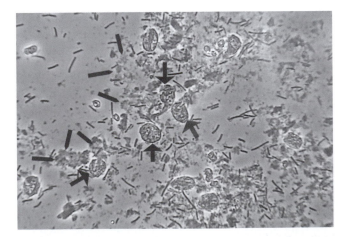

FIGURE 8 Vaginal infectious disease in different flora types.

treatment depends on the extent of the lesions and the persistence of the complaints. In case no complaints are present, no treatment is necessary. Imiquimod cream 5% has not been evaluated or labeled for mucosal use, and usually does not help. If necessary, destructive therapies can be applied, but only in case of persistent symptoms.

Noninfectious Purulent Vaginal Discharge

Occasionally, a profuse leukorrhea persists without any signs of bacterial overgrowth. Here an assumption is made that these represent contact vaginitis or an allergic reaction, but an unknown pathogen may also be involved. In such cases, efforts are redoubled to locate a contact irritant. This search may be rewarded by the discovery of the use of a product, such as talcum powder or deodorant sanitary napkins, that might be the inciting agent. For these contact reactions, non-irritating irrigation douches, such as one or more tablespoons of baking soda to a quart of warm water, is one of the cornerstones of the treatment. A list of possible contact irritants or mechanical irritants is presented in Table 7.

CONCLUDING REMARKS AND OVERVIEW

Office diagnosis is the cornerstone of good clinical practice in the care of women with vulvovaginal symptoms. A careful diagnosis should be made:

1. Listen to your patient. Obtain a complete history including use of possible contact irritants, sexual activities, and associated illnesses.
2. Look at your patient. Note the characteristic appearance of the lesion and satellite lesions, appearance of the vaginal wall, exclude mucopurulent cervicitis, and sometimes examine the partner also.
3. Appropriate diagnostic measures after physical examination include pH measurement, wet smear, potassium hydroxide preparation, Gram stain (possible Dif-Quick stain in the presence of extreme leukocytosis with no visible trichomonads), and the use of culture media for recurrent or mixed infections.

TABLE 7 Chemical and mechanical irritants of the vagina or vulvar area sometimes causing noninfectious leukorrhea and irritation

Mechanical irritants
   Condoms, cervical caps
   Vibrators, frequent and/or vigorous genital manipulation
   Exercise suits, bicycles, etc.
   Tampons, especially with plastic applicators, other vaginal foreign bodies
   Occlusive, nonporous undergarments, tight crotch-hugging jeans, horseback riding
Chemical irritants
   Deodorant soap/spray, perfume, chemically treated toilet paper, talcum powder
   Spermicides, vaginal douches
   Sanitary napkins, tampons, chemically treated permanent-press clothing
   Bubble baths, hot tubs, jacuzzis, chemically treated swimming pool water

Caution has to be taken not to impose all these "don't do's" on every women with vulvovaginal symptoms.

When using wet mounts, the first step should be to grade the lactobacilli. This allows further diagnosis once it is established whether the flora is normal or not. Anaerobic bacteria can be lactobacillary morphotypes (anaerobic lactobacillosis or leptothrix-like) or of the coccoid type (BV). Aerobic conditions can lead to short and coarse lactobacillary types, or aerobic facultative pathogens such as staphylococci, streptococci, and gram-negative rods. Of importance is the point that these flora types are not sharply demarcated, and characteristics of both aerobic and anaerobic type flora can be present (mixed flora types). With this picture in mind, all concurrent infections such as candidiasis, trichomoniasis, and cervicitis can be diagnosed and seen in their respective background flora (Fig. 8).

Candidiasis is sometimes difficult to diagnose, especially if chronically recurrent. Addition of KOH at the wet mount may be of help, as well as cultures or sometimes even PCR. Assessment of the different risk factors influencing the risk of candidiasis is not easy and seldom straightforward. It is advised to single out one risk factor at a time and try for two months whether changing it influences the course of the disease. If so, advice on that risk factor can be implemented, but if not, it should not be added to the long list of "don't do's" of these already desperate patients. Sometimes chronic suppressive therapy is helpful in proven cases where no risk factors can be detected.

Trichomoniasis can also be difficult to diagnose, as in one of three cases, wet mount reveals false-negative results. Use of supplementary Dif-Quick stain, or examination of prostate fluid of the sexual partner, may help document the presumed diagnosis. Metronidazole-resistant cases are rare, but they do exist and must be treated vigorously in both women and their partner(s).

SELECTED READING

Ackerlund M, Mardh P-A. Isolation and identification of *Corynebacterium vaginale* (*Haemophilus vaginalis*) in women with infection of the lower genital tract. Acta Obstet Gynecol Scand 1974; 53:85.

Amsel R, Totten PA, Spiegel CA, et al. Comparison of metronidazole, ampicillin, and amoxicillin for treatment of bacterial vaginosis (nonspecific vaginitis): possible explanation for the greater efficacy of metronidazole. In: Finegold SM, ed. First United States Metronidazole Conference. New York: Biomedia Information Corp, 1982:225–242.

Amsel R, Totten PA, Spiegel CA, et al. Nonspecific vaginitis: diagnostic criteria and microbial and epidemiologic associations. Am J Med 1983; 74:14.

Arevalo MP, Arias A, Andrew A, et al. Fluconazole, itraconazole, and ketoconazole in vitro activity against *Candida* spp. J Chemother 1996; 6:226.

Barbone F, Austin H, Louv WC, Alexander WJ. A follow-up study of methods of contraception, sexual activity, and rates of trichomoniasis, candidiasis, and bacterial vaginosis. Am J Obstet Gynecol 1990; 163:510.

Berger BJ, Kolton S, Zenilman JM, et al. Bacterial vaginosis in lesbians: a sexually transmitted disease. Clin Infect Dis 1995; 21:1402.

Bistoletti P, Fredricsson B, Hagstrom NB, Nord C-E. Comparison of oral and vaginal metronidazole therapy for nonspecific bacterial vaginosis. Gynecol Obstet Invest 1986; 21:144.

Burch TA, Rees CW, Reardon LV. Epidemiological studies on human trichomoniasis. Am J Trop Med Hyg 1959; 8:312.

Burns FM, Gould IM, Patterson A, Wood WJ. Diagnosis of bacterial vaginosis in a routine diagnostic laboratory. Med Lab Sci 1992; 49:8.

Butler BC, Beakley JW. Bacterial flora in vaginitis. A study before and after treatment with pure cultures of Doderlein bacillus. Am J Obstet Gynecol 1960; 79:432.

Carranza-Lira S, Fragoso-Diaz N, Luz A, et al. Vaginal dryness assessment in postmenopausal women using pH test strip. Maturitas 2003; 45:55–58.

Caillouette JC, et al. Vaginal pH as a marker for bacterial pathogens and menopausal status. Am J Obst Gyn 1997; 176: 1270.

Cotch MF, Pastorek JG II, Nugent RP, et al. Demographic and behavioral predictors of *Trichomonas vaginalis* infection among pregnant women. Obstet Gynecol 1991; 78:1087.

Diddle AW. *Trichomonas vaginalis*: resistance to metronidazole. Am J Obstet Gynecol 1967; 98:583.

Donders GGG. Microscopy of the bacterial flora on fresh vaginal smears. Inf Dis Obstet Gynecol 1999; 7:126–127.

Donders GGG, Vereecken A, Dekeersmaecker A, Van Bulck B, Spitz B. Wet mount microscopy reflects functional vaginal lactobacillary flora better than Gram stains. J Clin Pathol 2000; 53:308–314.

Donders GGG, Vereecken A, Bosmans E, Dekeersmaecker A, Salembier G, Spitz. Definition of a type of abnormal vaginal flora that is distinct from bacterial vaginosis: aerobic vaginitis. Br J Obstet Gynecol 2002; 109:1–10.

Donders GGG, De Wet, Hooft P, Desmyter J. Lactobacilli in Pap smears, genital infections and pregnancy. Am J Perinatol 1993; 10:358–361.

Donders GGG, Caeyers, Riphagen I, Van den Bosch T, Bellen G. Comparison of two types of dipsticks to measure vaginal pH in clinical practice. Eur J Obstet Gyn Reprod Biol, 2006; in press.

Donders GGG, Prenen H, Verbeke G, Reybrouck R. Impaired tolerance for glucose in women with recurrent vaginal candidiasis. Am J Obstet Gynaecol 2002; 187:989–993.

Dunkelburg WE Jr. Diagnosis of *Hemophilus vaginalis* vaginitis by Gram-stained smears. Am J Obstet Gynecol 1965; 91:998.

Easmon CS, Ison CA, Kaye CM, et al. Pharmacokinetics of metronidazole and its principal metabolites and their activity against *Gardnerella vaginalis*. Br J Vener Dis 1982; 58:246.

Edelman DA, North BB. Treatment of bacterial vaginosis with intravaginal sponges containing metronidazole. J Reprod Med 1989; 34:341.

Egan ME, Lipsky MS. Diagnosis of Vaginitis. Am Fam Phys 2000; 62:1095–1103.

Eschenbach DA, Hillier S, Critchlow C, et al. Diagnosis and clinical manifestations of bacterial vaginosis. Am J Obstet Gynecol 1988; 158:819.

Evans EG. Diagnostic laboratory techniques in vaginal candidiasis. Br J Clin Pract 1990; 71:70.

Faro S. Vaginitis: diagnosis and management. Int J Fertil 1996; 41:115.

Fouts AC, Kraus SJ. *Trichomonas vaginalis*: reevaluation of its clinical presentation and laboratory diagnosis. J Infect Dis 1980; 141:137.

Fredricsson N, Hagstrom B, Evaldson G, Nord C-E. Gardnerella-associated vaginitis and anaerobic bacteria. Gynecol Obstet Invest 1984; 17:236.

Garcia-Clossas M, Herrero R, Hildesheim A, et al. Epidemiologic determinants of vaginal pH. Am J Obstet Gynecol 1999; 180:1060–1065.

Gardner HL, Dukes CD. *Haemophilus vaginalis* vaginitis. A newly defined specific infection previously classified "nonspecific vaginitis." Am J Obstet Gynecol 1955; 69:962.

Greenwood JR, Pickett MJ. Transfer of *Haemophilus vaginalis* (Gardner and Dukes) to a new genus: Gardnerella. Int J Systemic Bacteriol 1980; 30:170.

Greenwood JR, Pickett MJ, Martin WJ, et al. *Haemophilus vaginalis* (*Corynebacterium vaginale*): method for isolation and rapid biochemical identification. Health Lab Sci 1977; 14:102.

Hardy PH, Hardy JB, Nell EE, et al. Prevalence of six sexually transmitted disease agents among pregnant inner-city adolescents and pregnancy outcome. Lancet 1984; ii:333.

Hay RJ. Risk/benefit ratio of modern antifungal therapy: focus on hepatic reactions. J Am Acad Dermatol 1993; 29:550.

Hill GB. The microbiology of bacterial vaginosis. Am J Obstet Gynecol 1993; 169:430.

Hill GB, Eschenbach DA, Holmes KK. Bacteriology of the vagina. Scand J Urol Nephrol 1984; 86:23.

Hill LVH, Luther ER, Young D, et al. Prevalence of lower genital tract infections in pregnancy. Sex Transm Dis 1988; 15:5.

Hillier S, Krohn MA, Watts H, et al. Microbiologic efficacy of intravaginal clindamycin cream for the treatment of bacterial vaginosis. Obstet Gynecol 1990; 76:407.

Holst E, Wathne B, Hovelius B, Mardh P-A. Bacterial vaginosis: microbiologic and clinical findings. Eur J Clin Microbiol 1987; 6:536.

Horowitz BJ, Giaquinta D, Ito S. Evolving pathogens in vulvovaginal candidiasis: implications for patient care. J Clin Pharmacol 1992; 32:248.

Jirovec O, Petro M. *Trichomonas vaginalis* and trichomoniasis. Adv Parasitol 1968; 6:117.

Joesoef MR, Wiknjosastro G, Norojono W, et al. Co-infection with chlamydia and gonorrhea among pregnant women and bacterial vaginosis. Int J STD AIDS 1996; 7:61.

Khandalavala J, Van Geem TA. Evaluating vaginal pH. Accuracy of two commerciam pH papers in comparison to a hand-held digital pH meter. J Reprod Med 1999; 44:76–80.

Klebanoff SJ, Hillier SL, Eschenbach DA, Waltersdorph AM. Control of the microbial flora of the vagina by H_2O_2-generating lactobacilli. J Infect Dis 1991; 164:94.

Larsson PG, Platz-Christensen JJ. Bacterial vaginosis and vaginal leucocyte/epithelial cell ratio in women attending an outpatient gynecology clinic. Eur J Obstet Gynecol Reprod Biol 1991; 42:217.

Larsson PG, Platz-Christensen JJ, Sundstrom E. Is bacterial vaginosis a sexually transmitted disease? Int J STD AIDS 1991; 2:362.

Livengood CH. Bacterial vaginosis: treatment with topical intravaginal clindamycin phosphate. Obstet Gynecol 1990; 76:118.

Lossick JG. Epidemiology of urogenital trichomoniasis. In: Honiburgh BM, ed. Trichomonads Parasitic in Humans. New York: Springer-Verlag, 1990:311.

Lugo-Miro V, Green M, Mazur L. Comparison of different metronidazole therapeutic regimens for bacterial vaginosis: a meta-analysis. J Am Med Assoc 1992; 258:92.

Mazzuli T, Simor AE, Low DE. Reproducibility of interpretation of Gram-stained vaginal smears for diagnosis of bacterial vaginosis. J Clin Microbiol 1990; 28:1506.

McLellan R, Spence MR, Brockman M, et al. The clinical diagnosis of trichomoniasis. Obstet Gynecol 1982; 60:30.

Monif GRG, Baer H. *Haemophilus* (*Corynebacterium*) *vaginalis* septicemia. Am J Obstet Gynecol 1974; 120:1041.

Naguib SM, Comstock GW, Davis HJ. Epidemiologic study of trichomoniasis in normal women. Obstet Gynecol 1966; 27:607.

Nilsson U, Hellberg D, Shoubnikova M, et al. Sexual behavior risk factors associated with bacterial vaginosis and *Chlamydia trachomatis* infection. Sex Transm Dis 1997; 24:241.

Nugen RP, Krohn MA, Hillier SL. Reliability of diagnosing bacterial vaginosis is improved by a standardized method of Gram stain interpretation. J Clin Microbiol 1991; 29:297.

Nyirjesy P, Seeney SM, Grody MHT, et al. Chronic fungal vaginitis: the value of cultures. Am J Obstet Gynecol 1995; 173:S20.

Paavonen J, Stamm WE. Lower genital tract infections in women. In: Handsfield HH, ed. Sexually Transmitted Diseases. Philadelphia: WB Saunders 1987; 179–98.

Pastorek JG. Bacterial vaginosis: current concepts of diagnosis and management. Infections in Medicine 1992; 48–52.

Peters N, Van Leeuwen Am, Pieters WJ, et al. Bacterial vaginosis is not important in the etiology of cervical neoplasia: a survey on women with dyskaryotic smears. Sex Transm Dis 1995; 22:296.

Pfeiffer TA, Forsyth PS, Durfee MA, et al. Nonspecific vaginitis: role of *Haemophilus vaginalis* and treatment with metronidazole. N Engl J Med 1978; 98:1429.

Phillips RJM, Watson SA, McKay FF. An open multicentre study of the efficacy and safety of a single dose of fluconazole 150 mg in the treatment of vaginal candidiasis in general practice. Br J Clin Pract 1990; 44:219.

Piot P, Van Dyck E, Godts P, Vanderheyden J. The vaginal microbial flora in nonspecific vaginitis. Eur J Clin Microbiol 1982; 1:301.

Rabe LK, Winterscheid KK, Hillier SL. Association of viridans group streptococci from pregnant women with bacterial vaginosis and upper genital tract infection. J Clin Microbiol 1988; 26:1156.

Royce RA, Jackson TP, Thorp JM Jr, et al. Race/ethnicity, vaginal flora patterns and pH during pregnancy. Sex Transm Dis 1999; 26:96.

Schaaf VM, Perez-Stable EJ, Borchardt K. The limited value of symptoms and signs in the diagnosis of vaginal infections. Arch Intern Med 1990; 150:1929.

Skarin A, Sylwan J. Vaginal lactobacilli inhibiting growth of Gardnerella vaginalis, Mobiluncus and other bacterial species cultured from vaginal content of women with bacterial vaginosis. Acta Pathol Microbiol Immunol Scand (Sect B) 1986; 94:399.

Sobel JD. Desquamative inflammatory vaginitis: a new subgroup of purulent vaginitis responsive to topical 2% clindamycin therapy. Am J Obstet Gynecol 1994; 171:1215–1220.

Sobel JD. Candidal vulvovaginitis. Clin Obstet Gynecol 1993; 36:153.

Sobel JD, Cook RL. Lactobacilli: a role in controlling the vaginal microflora? In: Horowitz BJ, Mardh PA, eds. Vaginitis Vaginosis. New York: Wiley-Liss, 1991:46.

Sobel JD, Brooker D, Stein GE, et al. The Fluconazole Vaginitis Study Group: single oral dose fluconazole compared with conventional clotrimazole topical therapy of Candida vaginitis. Am J Obstet Gynecol 1995; 172:1263.

Sobel JD, Weisenfield HC, Martens M, et al. Maintenance fluconazole therapy for recurrent vulvovaginal candidiasis. New Engl J Med 2004; 351(9):876–883.

Somail EH, Kolotila MP, Ruggeri R, Diamond RD. Natural inhibitor from Candida albicans blocks release of azurophil and specific granule contents by chemotactic peptide stimulated human neutrophils. Infect Immunol 1989; 57:689.

Spence MR, Hollander DH, Smith J, et al. The clinical and laboratory diagnosis of Trichomonas vaginalis infection. Sex Transm Dis 1980; 7:168.

Spiegel CA, Amsel R, Eschenbach DA, et al. Anaerobic bacteria in nonspecific vaginitis. N Engl J Med 1980; 303:601.

Spiegel CA, Amsel R, Holmes KK. Diagnosis of bacterial vaginosis by direct Gram stain of vaginal fluid. J Clin Endocrinol Metab 1983; 18:170.

Stein GE, Mummaw N. Placebo controlled trial of itraconazole for treatment of acute vaginal candidiasis. Antimicrob Agents Chemother 1993; 37:89.

Steinhandler LE, Peipert JF, Montagno A, Cruickshank C. Combination of leukorrhea and bacterial vaginosis as a predictor of cervical Chlamydia trachomatis or Neisseria gonorrhoeae infection. Obstet Gynecol 2000; 95:5s.

Swedberg J, Steiner IF, Deiss F, et al. Comparison of single-dose vs one-week course of metronidazole for symptomatic bacterial vaginosis. J Am Med Assoc 1985; 254:1046.

Tchoudomirova K, Stanilova M, Garov V. Clinical manifestation and diagnosis of bacterial vaginosis in a clinic of sexually transmitted diseases. Folia Med Plovdiv 1998; 40:34.

Thomason JL, Gelbard SM, Anderson RJ. Statistical evaluation of diagnostic criteria for bacterial vaginosis. Am J Obstet Gynecol 1990; 162:155.

Thomason JL, Gelbard SM, Broekhuizen FF. Advances in the understanding of bacterial vaginosis. J Reprod Med 1989; 34:581.

Thomason JL, Gelbard SM, Scaglione NJ. Bacterial vaginosis: current review with indications for asymptomatic therapy. Am J Obstet Gynecol 1991; 165:1210.

Thomason JL, Schreckenberger PC, Spellacy WN, et al. Clinical and microbiological characterization of patients with nonspecific vaginosis associated with motile, curved anaerobic rods. J Infect Dis 1984; 149:801.

Totten PA, Amsel R, Hale J, et al. Selective differential human blood bilayer media for isolation of Gardnerella (Haemophilus) vaginalis. J Clin Microbiol 1982; 15:141.

Wolner-Hanssen P, Krieger JN, Stevens CE, et al. Clinical manifestations of vaginal trichomoniasis. J Am Med Assoc 1989; 261:571.

Zinneman K, Turner GC. The taxonomic position of Haemophilus vaginalis (Corynebacterium vaginale). J Pathol Bacteriol 1963; 85:213.

Infectious Complications Associated with Intrauterine Contraceptive Devices

71

INTRODUCTION

The placement of a foreign body within the endometrial cavity for contraception had a partial genesis in Arabic medicine. Dating back to about the 16th century, desert nomads had placed stones in the uterine cavities of camels to prevent conception prior to and during safaris. In the late 1920s and 1930s, a flurry of enthusiasm flourished centering about the Gräfenberg ring as a possible mode of contraception, only to disappear in a relatively short period due to the infectious complications that ensued. The rekindling of interest in the use of foreign bodies as a mode of contraception was predicated on a technologic innovation, namely, the development of inert flexible plastic with a memory from which intrauterine contraceptive devices (IUDs) could be made.

The insertion of an IUD must be viewed as a relatively nonsterile procedure. But even when superficial erosions are produced, the mere introduction of organisms is insufficient to produce disease. The presence of a healthy viable endometrium with its high oxidation–reduction potential is an effective barrier against all organisms except for the virulent cocci. Immediately following the insertion of an IUD, in a significant number of instances, bacteria can be recovered from the endometrial cavity by transuterine aspiration. When resampled within 24 to 72 hours, the endometrial cavity is again sterile.

SIGNIFICANCE OF ENDOMETRIAL BACTERIAL CONTAMINATION

Endometrial contamination is a common event following parturition. It can be demonstrated that 70% to 80% of patients have moderate or heavy growth of at least one bacterium. The incidence of positive cultures is progressive with time. Although only one of every ten endometrial cultures may be positive postpartum, all cultures will be positive after 24 hours and this type of endometrial infection persists for at least five days. Multiple studies have shown no difference between the types of flora in cultures of asymptomatic and clinically infected puerperal uteri. Since an overwhelming number of women are infected during the immediate postpartum period, the obvious question is why do only 1% to 2% of women delivering vaginally and without obstetrical trauma go on to develop disease, more specifically, endometritis? Underlying the necrotic decidua and clotted blood is a layer of healthy endometrial tissue whose oxidation–reduction potential usually precludes the penetration of superficial infection due to Class II and III anaerobes. Microaerophilic Class II and III anaerobes do not represent a significant cause of postpartum endometritis following spontaneous vaginal delivery.

There is a high probability that some contamination of the endometrial cavity occurs at the time of menstruation; however, just as with bacterial contamination associated with parturition, the endometrium is able to rid itself of this inoculum. The transient contaminations that occur at the time of the menses or during sexual intercourse at selected times in the menstrual cycle appear to be of limited biologic significance barring the presence of an exogenous virulent pathogen.

Bacterial contamination of the endometrial cavity can occur at the time of insertion of the IUD. In this setting, infection of the endometrium, unless associated with significant endometrial penetration, is usually of limited clinical significance, and within a short period, the infection is cleared. Relative comparable observations have been observed in the baboon model system. Skangalis et al. (1985) studied a group of 33 female baboons into whose uteri an IUD had been inserted. They observed that bacteria could be present in the uteri of baboons for an extended period and could function in a "benign, almost normal flora fashion" without producing disease.

EFFECTS OF THE IUD

The histologic alterations in the endometrium induced by the presence of an IUD include microscopic erosions of the endometrial surface (particularly at the points of contact), a tendency toward focal predecidual changes, an increase in mononuclear cells, and an increase in local vascularity. Areas with such changes can be shown to have increased glucose and oxygen consumption and presumably an altered oxidation–reduction potential.

With time, the IUD per se is biophysiologically altered. These surface alterations may facilitate bacterial adherence and partially facilitate circumvention of host cell phagocytosis. Marrie and Costerton (1983) studied 10 IUDs by scanning and transmission electron microscopy. All the devices had material adhered to them. The amount of this material varied considerably. Many morphologic types of bacteria were observed adhering to the devices, often buried in a thick biofilm. Electron microprobe analysis revealed the presence of calcium in the biofilm formed by bacterial colonization.

Schmidt et al. (1986) postulated that calcium deposits were apparently vital to the establishment of infection. Calcium is a component of a heterogeneous crust or coating containing both organic and inorganic materials (Fig. 1). The crust appears on the string of an IUD as well as on its body and provides a cozy niche for actinomyces and other anaerobes where they are safe from the body's normal immune defenses. They demonstrated a variety of bacteria, growing both in and under the calcium coating.

The histologic alterations associated with the IUD may not be entirely restricted to the endometrium. Smith and Soderstrom (1976) have demonstrated a lymphocytic infiltration of the fallopian tube segment in less than 1% of non–IUD users undergoing tubal sterilization, as opposed to a 47% incidence in IUD users. Beerthuizen et al. (1982) prospectively analyzed the pathomorphologic changes in the oviducts in 253 women who underwent voluntary sterilization via posterior colpotomy in order to investigate the effect of the intrauterine device. Some form of histologic change was found in 54% of the IUD group and in only 6% of the control group.

Tietze (1973), among others, has documented an increased incidence of ectopic pregnancies in IUD users. This observation focused attention on the hypothesis that these alterations may have, in certain instances, a functional significance in terms of the ovum transport.

MECHANICAL PROBLEMS

Transuterine penetration of the IUD may occur. If both the myometrium and the peritoneal serosal surface are transgressed, depending on the type of device, certain complications can ensue that may ultimately result in infectious morbidity (Table 1). Complications due to the linear-shaped inert plastic IUDs have been relatively few. If an IUD is of a closed configuration, such as a ring, intestinal obstruction can occur when the bowel becomes incarcerated within the enclosed area of the IUD. Copper-containing IUDs, when present in the peritoneal cavity, have been the cause of omental masses. The most significant cause of infectious morbidity is the penetration of a Dalkon Shield into the peritoneal cavity. Unlike the Lippes Loop, the Dalkon Shield, if it becomes entrapped adjacent to the bowel, tends to penetrate into the bowel, causing perforation and subsequent intestinal abscesses or peritonitis.

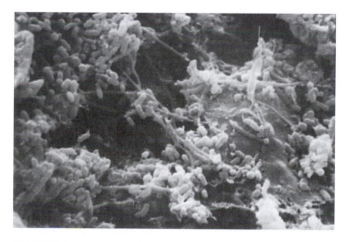

FIGURE I Scanning electron microscopic photomicrograph of the surface of an intrauterine contraceptive device, which demonstrates bacteria interspersed within calcium-coated matter (×5000).

INFECTIOUS COMPLICATIONS ASSOCIATED WITH THE IUD

The infectious morbidity associated with the IUD can be broken down into four major categories:
1. infectious morbidity associated with the insertion of the IUD,
2. induction of a chronic anaerobic endometritis (CAE),
3. superimposition of exogenous sexually transmitted disease (STD), and
4. induction of infectious morbidity in the pregnant patient using the IUD.

Insertional Infectious Morbidity

Infectious morbidity associated with the insertion of the IUD can be broken down into two subcategories:
1. infectious morbidity secondary to incomplete perforation and the resultant trauma to the endomyometrium
2. introduction of exogenous pathogens to the female genital tract and the probable provision of an effective portal of entry.

The insertion of an IUD necessitates the taking of a sterile object, the IUD, traversing a contaminated microbiologic environment, the endocervix, and introducing it into a sterile environment, namely the endometrial cavity. In the course of insertion, bacteria that reside as constituents of the bacterial flora of the endocervical canal are mechanically introduced into the endometrial cavity. Despite the mechanical disruption of the cutaneous barrier and secondary bleeding, there is no ensuing infectious morbidity unless an exogenous pathogen is present or significant myometrial trauma is induced. The reason that the initial contamination of the endometrial cavity does not produce disease is its oxidation–reduction potential. The majority of the constituents of the biologic flora of the female genital tract are by themselves without major pathogenic potential, unless there is a significant alteration in the host defense mechanism that permits their replication and clinical expression. The prime prerequisite for effective anaerobic replication is an alteration in the oxidation–reduction potential. The oxidation–reduction potential of healthy endometrial tissue precludes anything but transient superficial replication of the microaerophilic Class II anaerobes. The normal anaerobic constituents of the female genital tract are usually of little or no biologic significance by themselves.

Data emanating from a multicenter case–control study of the National Institute of Health and Human Development showed that the highest risk of pelvic inflammatory disease (PID) occurred in the first three months following IUD

TABLE I Potential complications secondary to transuterine migration

Copper T or Copper 7	Induction of omental masses
Ring types	Intestinal obstruction
Dalkon Shield	Intestinal perforation and abscess due to peritonitis
Saf-T-Coil or Lippes Loop	Rare uterine perforation
Majzlin Spring	Uterine perforation

insertion (a relative risk of 1.8 compared with women using no contraception).

A significant proportion of infectious morbidity seen in the immediate postinsertion period is due to the presence of exogenous organisms. The two bacteria most consistently associated with postinsertional infectious complications are

1. group A beta-hemolytic streptococci and
2. *Neisseria gonorrhoeae*.

Group A Beta-Hemolytic Streptococci
Given the initial breach in the mucosal integrity, the group A beta-hemolytic streptococci can produce fulminating infection, which, if not quickly checked, can be associated with a lethal outcome. The patient gets sick within the first 24 hours and appears quite toxic. The temperature is markedly elevated (greater than 39°C). The uterus is exquisitely tender, but there is little discharge other than a sparse, salmon-colored, watery exudate.

N. gonorrhoeae
The bleeding induced by trauma of insertion may be of sufficient magnitude to be the catalytic element for the production of disease due to *N. gonorrhoeae*. The onset of disease tends to be delayed, usually beyond 24 hours. Clinical expression of disease is milder in comparison to that induced by the group A (C or G) beta-hemolytic streptococci. The degree of uterine tenderness is markedly less. A purulent discharge can be readily demonstrated.

Irrespective of which bacteria produces disease, a presumptive diagnosis is readily inferred from the Gram stain analysis. A definitive diagnosis is established by bacteriologic culture.

The delayed-onset insertion endometritis appears to be primarily related to myometrial penetration. Insertional trauma creates the opportunity for endogenous organisms to combine and, through the anaerobic progression or a variant thereof, produce disease. If, in the course of the introduction of the IUD, the device is forced through the endometrium and embedded deep into the myometrium, one has effectively circumvented the barrier constituted by the endometrial surface, and contamination by a Class II anaerobe or anaerobes can result. Infectious morbidity due to endogenous organisms may ensue. It is probable that some of the clustering beyond the immediate-onset type of endometritis may be tied to increased probability of contact with a significant STD pathogen. Because there have been no attempts to dissect superimposition of STDs on IUD utilization, the epidemiologic studies concerning the causation of disease in the first 90 days postinsertion have been gravely flawed.

CHRONIC ANAEROBIC ENDOMETRITIS

The presence of a foreign body within the endometrial cavity appears to select for bacterial colonization within the endometrial cavity with time; however, the factors selecting for disease are unique from those that select for infection. The perception of CAE retrospectively emanated from an extremely astute observation that the

Papanicolaou smears of an IUD user who died of disseminated actinomycosis exhibited cytologic evidence of the infection with that organism for a period of years.

The presence of bacteria morphologically consistent with actinomyces on Papanicolaou (Pap) stained smears is a phenomenon seen almost exclusively in women using the IUD as their mode of contraception. When confirmation is attempted with fluorescent isothiocyanate-labeled antisera against *Actinomyces israelii*, approximately 50% exhibit specific immunofluorescence. Part of the explanation is that although *A. israelii* is the most common, *A. naeslundii*, *A. eriksonii*, and *Arachnia propionica* may be the causative agents. No single specific type of IUD predisposes to actinomyces growth. The single most common factor among IUD users with actinomyces infection is the duration of use. Almost 85% of the cases occur in women who had worn an IUD for three or more years.

Pettit et al. carried out a case–control study to determine the factors associated with the presence of actinomyces-like organisms on cervicovaginal Pap smears in users of the IUD. Among about 80,000 Pap smears examined in one year, actinomyces-like organisms were identified on 107 smears; all but three smears were from IUD users. Compared with IUD users who did not have actinomyces-like organisms on Pap smears, those with actinomyces-like organisms had used the IUD for more years. No significant association of actinomyces-like organisms with the type of IUD was found after controlling for differences in duration of use between users of various IUDs. The percentage of women reporting gynecologic symptoms (vaginal discharge, pelvic pain, abnormal bleeding) also did not differ significantly between IUD users with and without actinomyces-like organisms on Pap smear.

Valicenti et al. (1982) prospectively screened the cervical Pap smears from 69,925 women for the presence of *A. israelii*. The organism was not identified in non–IUD wearers. The prevalence of *A. israelii* among IUD wearers ranged from 1.6% (general population) to 5.3% (clinic population). Prolonged IUD use again appeared to predispose to a higher incidence of infection.

In those patients whose IUDs were removed and not replaced, subsequent Pap smears failed to reveal actinomyces. From this type of data, it has been concluded that in the vast majority of cases the organism causes a superficial infection of the endometrium, which can be subsequently shed with the menstrual period. Although uterine actinomyces is usually superficial, the organism is potentially invasive. Systemic actinomyces infection, if it develops, may be fatal.

The low incidence of infectious complications seen with the Progestasert IUD has been postulated to be the result of the regular practice of yearly exchange. Keebler et al. (1983) demonstrated that although first cytologic immunologic evidence of *A. israelii* was noticed after seven months, the risk of infection increased significantly when the IUD had been in place for more than two years.

Van Bogaert (1983) studied a group of 65 IUD users during a period of 165 years of use (with a mean of 2.6 ± 1.7 years per woman). The main complaint that differed significantly from the 120 controls was the occurrence of spotting in 33.8% of IUD users. Normal endometrial mucosa was found in 36.9% of IUD users and 38.7% of controls. Chronic endometritis was evident in 35.4% of IUD users versus 12.5% of controls; the former were asymptomatic in 25% of the cases. Chronic endometritis occurred 2.2 ± 1.3 years after insertion of the device.

Burkman et al. (1982) demonstrated that cytologic evidence of superinfection with CAE was more frequent in women who had used a single IUD for many years than in cytologic preparations obtained from short-term users. The possibility that the tail itself was the mediating factor was suggested by Sparks et al. (1981). They bacteriologically sampled 22 women undergoing hysterectomy using a multiple biopsy technique. All five uteri with tailless IUDs were sterile, but 15 out of 17 tailed devices contained bacteria. Most isolates were constituents of the normal vaginal flora.

Stadel and Schlesselman (1984) from the Contraceptive Evaluation Branch of the National Institute of Health and Human Development had identified in the data from Women's Health Study the fact that continuous use of the same IUD for five or more years appears to increase the risk of PID, requiring extensive surgery, to a greater extent than use for less than five years.

The presence of *A. israelii* in the female genital tract flora is not a critical determinant of disease. Grice and Hafiz (1983) cultured the endocervices of IUD users and non–IUD users. Of 78 users of IUDs, 20 (25.6%) were culture positive. Of the 63 women using various other forms of contraception, 12 (19%) were culture positive. None of these 12 women had an IUD or foreign body in situ. Their data were consistent with the contention that *Actinomyces* species may be a part of the commensal flora of the female genital tract.

Using immunofluorescence, Curtis and Pine (1981) demonstrated the presence of *A. israelii*, *A. naeslundii*, or *Arachnia propionica* in cervicovaginal mucus from 36% of 50 women. One or more of these organisms were found in a surprising 27% of those with neither IUD nor intravaginal foreign bodies. Among those women who harbored actinomyces, the average duration of continuous IUD use was 5.3 years; the comparable figure for those with no infection was 2.1 years.

Most patients who develop unilateral tubo-ovarian complexes have *A. israelii* as a part of a polymicrobial chronic infection of the endometrial cavity. *A. israelii*, when present, enhances the pathogenic potential of the CAE.

What is now understood is that with the use of the IUD, infection of the endometrial cavity is a common phenomenon. The cumulative pattern, with time, strongly infers that some alteration of the microbiologic environment must occur. By changing the biophysical characteristics of the IUD, the endometrium permits bacterial persistence within the endometrial cavity. This infection is able to be present for a prolonged period before producing symptomatology and disease. Although the majority of patients who developed cytologic evidence of actinomyces-like bacteria do not go on to develop disease, a few may develop serious disease. Clinicians have long recognized that after a period of utilization, IUD wearers begin to get into trouble clinically and develop

primarily menstrual irregularities or pain on intercourse. Burnhill (1972) was among the first to describe a specific syndrome that tied chronic infection of the endometrium to selected clinical manifestations (Burnhill's syndrome).

One characteristic pattern of disease associated with CAE is the "unilateral tubo-ovarian complex." The unilateral tubo-ovarian complex is a histologic, not a clinical, diagnosis. What is required is the ability to look at both fallopian tubes and demonstrate clear presence of disease in one fallopian tube and minimal or no disease present in the contralateral tube. This is different from unilateral tubo-ovarian complex seen with the traditional STDs such as gonorrhea or *Chlamydia* infection. In these clinical settings, the bilateralness of the disease, although not clinically overt, is microscopically documentable. Why does unilateral local salpingitis occur? It has been postulated that with time the contact points of the IUD cause pressure necrosis and ultimate penetration of the basialis layer. Once infection extends into the myometrium, it has effectively circumvented a major host defense mechanism that had previously precluded constituents of vaginal flora, which produced the chronic infection of the endometrial cavity, from attaining significant potentially life-threatening proportions.

Clinical recognition of disease takes various forms. The majority of women have little in the way of symptomatology other than minor irregularities with the menstrual period that occur after a prolonged period of normal menses. In its asymptomatic form, CAE is diagnosed by the appearance of gram-positive *A. israelii* (Gupta lesions) present in the Pap smear. Progression of disease may result in menstrual irregularities, foul-smelling intermenstrual discharge, and/or dyspareunia, either singularly or in combination. The full-blown clustering of signs and symptoms is known as Burnhill's syndrome. The incidence of infection/disease appears to be partially governed by the endocervical flora. Women with chronic cervicitis appear to develop IUD-associated CAE more readily than do women whose initial bacterial flora harbored the aerobic lactobacilli. Although their documentation is not well recorded in the literature, a number of forme fruste of Burnhill's syndrome probably exist. There are a significant number of women with IUDs as their mode of contraception, who present their gynecologists with complaints of "difficult periods," characterized by excessive cramping and more profuse bleeding. They are treated with a short course of a new generation tetracycline or semisynthetic penicillin and their symptoms abate for a period. The response to a therapeutic challenge suggests that many of these patients have CAE.

MANAGEMENT OF IUD IN PATIENTS WITH CAE

Once a patient with an IUD develops CAE, how should she be managed? If the patient is asymptomatic and the pelvic examination and cytologic smear are unremarkable, the IUD can probably be pulled out without antimicrobial coverage.

It is advocated that a patient be placed on antibiotic therapy at least one hour prior to the device removal and that the drug be continued for two to three days, when the patient has cytologic evidence of CAE and meets one of the following criteria:

1. IUD use is less than five consecutive months;
2. IUD is in place for more than three years, but there is no evidence of Burnhill's syndrome;
3. elevated erythrocyte sedimentation rate; or
4. mass is evident.

The drug of choice is either doxycycline or amoxicillin. Metronidazole would be an excellent drug, were it not for its relative ineffectiveness against *A. israelii*. If systemic symptoms referable to the female genital tract or Burnhill syndrome (an elevated erythrocyte sedimentation rate, and abnormal pelvic condition) is present, the patient should be evaluated for the possible presence of a tubo-ovarian complex and managed appropriately.

Chatwani and Amin-Hanjani (1993) reported on 173 patients with IUD-associated actinomyces-like organisms detected on Pap smears. The patients were managed by IUD removal with or without antibiotic therapy, antibiotic therapy alone, or no treatment at all. Results were that the success rate as reflected in negative follow-up smear was 100% for IUD removal combined with antibiotics, 97.4% for IUD removal alone, and 36.8% for antibiotics therapy alone.

If a patient with CAE desires to continue that mode of contraception and IUDs are available, what can be done is to remove the IUD under antibiotic coverage, allow two menstrual periods to ensue, and reinsert. It is appropriate to inform the patient as to the signs and symptoms of CAE as well as the potential risks to herself. An appropriate informed consent that clearly documents the fact that the physician has been an agent of the patient and has fulfilled his/her duty as counselor and advocate must be obtained. Monitoring with cytologic smears at least every two months until three sets of postinsertional cytologic smears are negative for the presence of Gupta bodies is advocated. Thereafter, cytologic monitoring can be done on a biannual basis. If cytologic evidence of infection reappears, it is strongly recommended that an alternative mode of contraception be implemented.

Unilateral tubo-ovarian abscess is considered to be the ultimate consequence of IUD-induced CAE. If due to CAE, the induction of tubo-ovarian disease requires transgressions of the endometrium by the IUD in proximity to the orifice of the fallopian tube, particularly when *A. israelii* or *Actinomyces* species are constituents of this polymicrobial anaerobic infection. With a true unilateral tubo-ovarian abscess, there is no evidence of significant disease in the contralateral tube.

The majority of patients present with a prodrome consisting of vague abdominal pains and dyspareunia. Most of these patients have prior symptomatology consistent with Burnhill's syndrome or a forme fruste. When indicated, surgical intervention should be as conservative as possible.

The management of a unilateral tubo-ovarian abscess is not well defined. The two primary therapeutic options are

1. utilization of conservative surgery and
2. commitment to long-term medical therapy and careful monitoring with the intent of allowing the patient the opportunity to conceive without surgical intervention on the contralateral tube.

For the latter approach to be adopted, the patient must have an excellent biologic response to antimicrobial therapy. The criteria used to judge whether or not the patient achieves an excellent clinical response are

1. resolution of fever under antibiotic therapy,
2. loss of mass tenderness, and
3. return to normal of the white blood cell count, erythrocyte sedimentation rate, and the C-reactive protein.

Although initial reduction in size of the tubo-ovarian abscess is not mandatory, the mass should be followed by serial ultrasonographic measurements. Should the mass remain tender and stable in size and the leukocytosis persist, despite adequate and prolonged antibiotic therapy, conservative surgical intervention is probably indicated. If aspiration of the complex is not therapeutic or if there is reactivation of tubal disease at a subsequent point in time following medical management, surgery is often indicated.

For a program of medical management to be implemented, the patient must be willing to accept an incremental increased personal risk: the goal being the preservation to the maximum degree of future fertility. The duration of antimicrobial therapy in these patients is not well established and should be individualized in each case. As a rule of thumb, presuming all other clinical criteria have been met, treatment should be extended until the return of the erythrocyte sedimentation rate to normal.

SURGICAL COMPLICATIONS IN ASSOCIATION WITH IUD-INDUCED ANAEROBIC ENDOMETRITIS

Chronic anaerobic endometritis induced by an IUD may be the cause of serious infectious morbidity in a number of situations.

The presence of CAE with menstrual irregularities and more difficult periods may precipitate the patient's request for a tubal ligation. If the IUD is removed at the time of surgery, subsequent development of a tubal abscess is not an uncommon complication. The presence of chronic anaerobic infection, coupled with that of devitalization of tissue and secondary microhematoma formation, creates ideal conditions for the immediate anaerobic syndrome to ensue. If the patient is suspected of having a forme fruste of Burnhill's syndrome, the IUD should be removed under appropriate antibiotic coverage at some time interval before or after surgery.

ENHANCED CLINICAL EXPRESSION OF OTHER STDS

The IUD causes a leukocytic outpouring in response to the presence of a foreign body in the endometrial cavity. The inflammatory response induced alters the local pH. The rise in pH is hypothesized to potentiate replication of selected venereally acquired exogenous pathogens. The clinical expression of infection due to *N. gonorrhoeae* is governed, in part, by alterations in pH. The IUD does not increase the incidence of gonococcal infection, but it may influence the incidence of gonococcal disease. The incidence of acute salpingitis, Stages I and II, is three times higher in IUD users than in non–IUD users.

A significantly increased risk of PID or tubal infertility among IUD users has been found in 25 reports. These 25 studies, conducted in different countries by different investigators with different diagnostic criteria, have all found an increased risk of PID or its sequelae among IUD users, which argues strongly for a causal relationship. The strength of this association in the most objective studies ranges from a relative risk of 1.5 to 2.6.

Results from analysis of the Women's Health Study data found that women who were using an IUD had a relative risk of PID of 1.9 (95% confidence limits 1.5 to 2.4) compared with women who were using no method of contraception at the time of their hospitalization. However, approximately 20% of this increase in relative risk could be accounted for by the marked increase in risk associated with the use of the Dalkon Shield. Women using the Dalkon Shield had more than eightfold increase in risk of PID, whereas women using other IUD types had a risk of 1.6 (1.2–2.0) compared with women using no method of contraception. The increase in risk associated with Dalkon Shield use did not appear to be explained by confounding effects or by biases such as hospitalization or recall. The Women's Health Study indicated that the Dalkon Shield IUD was different from other IUD types; however, the study provided no indication that other IUD types differed from each other in their risks of PID.

When the impact of women's sexual behavior on the IUD–PID relationship was reanalyzed by the Centers for Disease Control, marital status was demonstrated to be an important variable on the relative risk of PID associated with IUD use. Women reporting only one recent sexual partner, married or cohabiting women, had little increase in risk associated with IUD use, whereas previously or never-married IUD users had at least twice the PID risk as women with similar marital status who used no contraception. Women who were in mutually monogamous sexual relationships, and therefore at low risk for acquiring an STD, probably had little increase in PID risk from IUD use. However, even in this low-risk subgroup of women, PID risk was elevated shortly after IUD insertion, suggesting that the risk associated with IUD use was not entirely related to risk of STD acquisition.

IUDs AND INFERTILITY

Studies published in the late 1970s and 1980s demonstrated a significant risk of PID among IUD users versus nonusers. Unfortunately, many of the studies were poorly designed to control for the unmeasured confounding effect of exposure to STDs and in particular *Chlamydia trachomatis*. When reanalysis was done using better comparison groups and separating results according to the type of IUD, Buchan et al. (1990) could not demonstrate increased risk of PID with medicated devices. In data reported by the World Health Organization, Farley et al. (1992) and Walsh et al. (1998) have cited figures for the incidence of PID among IUD users that are comparable to those cited for the general population. Risk of PID appears to be related to insertion, endometrial penetration, and exposure to STDs. One of the unfortunate consequences of PID is secondary infertility.

Patients using IUDs have a higher prevalence of inflammatory residues than do nonusers. They also have a higher prevalence of chlamydial antibodies. If one examines residue frequency in user versus nonuser groups at the same chlamydial antibody level, no difference exists. This is also true if patients with known causes for residues (explained) are excluded and the remainder (unexplained or silent) are grouped according to antibody titer. Guderian and Trobough (1986) studied the causal relationship between PID and tubal infertility patients (176 patients had not used an IUD and 69 had used one). Chlamydial antibody titers were performed on all patients. Although users had a higher overall prevalence of inflammatory residues than did nonusers, there was no difference in residue prevalence for either group at the same titer levels. No specific type of device appeared to be associated with either an increased or decreased residue frequency. "Silent" chlamydial infections occurred with equal frequency in both users and nonusers.

Gump et al. (1983) studied 204 infertile women for the possible role of *C. trachomatis* and IUD use as factors related to their infertility. A highly statistically significant correlation ($p < 0.001$) was obvious between evidence of prior "PID" as documented by hystero-salpingograms and/or laparoscopy and the prevalence of chlamydial antibody. A significant correlation ($p = 0.01$) could be shown between the prevalence of the antibodies and adnexal adhesions. IUD use could also be shown to correlate significantly with PID. Only about one-third of the patients with PID could ever recall having had an illness consistent with PID.

Recently, Hubacher et al. (2001) reported a large case–control study of 1895 women in order to assess the risk of infertility associated with the use of a copper IUD. They concluded that the previous use of a copper IUD is not associated with an increased risk of tubal occlusion among nulligravid women, whereas infection with *C. trachomatis* is.

To date, a definitive study is yet to be done. What is apparent is that the risk of inflammatory complication leading to secondary infertility is related to exposure to pathogens, insertional trauma, or prolonged utilization.

IUD AND PREGNANCY

When an unplanned pregnancy occurs in an IUD wearer, three problems potentially may develop:

1. ectopic pregnancy,
2. fetal wastage, and
3. septic abortion/maternal septicemia.

Ectopic Pregnancy

A number of investigators have shown that accidental pregnancies occurring in long-term users of an IUD are more likely to be ectopic than those occurring in short-term users. Data reported from the Oxford Family Planning Association contraceptive study show that 6% (17 of 258) of accidental pregnancies occurring in parous women using an IUD were ectopic, while the corresponding figure for those using other methods of contraception was only 0.5% (3 of 632). There is a positive association between the likelihood of an accidental pregnancy being ectopic and the duration of an IUD. Among the pregnancies occurring up to 24 months after insertion of a device, 2.0% (2 of 101) were extrauterine, while the corresponding figure for those pregnancies occurring 49 months or more after insertion was 12.9% (11 of 86). The Oxford Family Planning Association study demonstrated that the absolute risk of ectopic pregnancies remained constant with duration of use at approximately 1.2 per 1000 women per year. A woman who presents with a contraceptive failure after using an IUD for more than three years has about a one in ten chance of having an ectopic gestation.

Studies done in the United States by Ory (1978) and Edelman (1988) have concluded that IUD use was more common in women with ectopic pregnancy than in healthy reproductive-aged women. Approximately 20% of pregnancies occurring in women using IUDs are ectopic. Some of this morbidity is due to concomitant chlamydial infection. Guderian and Trobough (1986) demonstrated a 22.5-fold increase in ectopic pregnancy frequency in IUD users with a titer of >1:512 when compared with their nonuser group. Women who become pregnant while using an IUD should be carefully counseled as to the risk and signs and symptoms of an ectopic pregnancy.

Fetal Wastage

Unplanned pregnancies in women using an IUD are about three times more likely to end in miscarriage than are pregnancies occurring under other circumstances. Approximately half of unplanned pregnancies that occurred among IUD wearers ended in miscarriage, as compared with 17% among women using other methods of birth control at the time of conception. Tatum et al. (1975) demonstrated that when the device (Copper T IUD) was removed or expelled shortly after conception, the incidence of spontaneous fetal loss was 20.3%, a figure similar to the normal incidence of spontaneous abortion in the study population.

Biologically, the most significant problem is second trimester fetal loss. In contrast to first trimester fetal loss, the projected risk of second trimester fetal loss among women beginning the second trimester of pregnancy without an IUD in place is estimated to be 2%. If the IUD was in place at conception, but was removed during the first trimester of pregnancy, the risk of second trimester fetal loss was increased 10-fold. This increase in risk was much greater for septic second trimester fetal loss than for nonseptic fetal loss.

Septic Abortion/Maternal Septicemia and Death

From 1965 to 1982, more than 8 million IUDs have been distributed in the United States. Of the maternal deaths recorded prior to 1977 attributed to IUDs, 16 were attributed to use of the Dalkon Shield, 18 to the Lippes Loop,

four to the Saf-T-Coil, two to the Majzlin Spring, and one to the Bimberg Bow. In two cases, the IUD was not identified.

Analysis of all maternal deaths from spontaneous abortions reported in the period 1972 to 1974 demonstrated that women dying from spontaneous abortions with an IUD in place were more likely to be young, white, and married than those not wearing a device. The risk of death from spontaneous abortion was 50 times greater for women who continued their pregnancy with a device in place than for those who did not. As compared with other devices, the Dalkon Shield carried an added risk of death.

If septic abortion occurs, the importance of complete evacuation of the uterus cannot be overstressed. Hurst reported a case of septic shock and disseminated intravascular coagulopathy in a gravida with an IUD. The patient did not respond to appropriate antibiotic therapy. Her condition improved somewhat following uterine curettage; however, the coagulation abnormalities and evidence of febrile morbidity persisted. Complete resolution did not occur until repeat uterine curettage removed a small amount of residual tissue from the maternal implantation site.

Maternal septicemia and abortion can occur with any of the IUD. The Food and Drug Administration Drug and Device Obstetrical and Gynecological Advisory Committee recommends that patients with an IUD in place who miss their normal menstrual period or who become pregnant seek medical advice as soon as possible for removal of the IUD. Whenever pregnancy coexists with an IUD, irrespective of type, removal is recommended.

THE DALKON SHIELD

The disproportionately large number of cases of septic spontaneous abortions and maternal deaths in women using the Dalkon Shield raised the question of a possible causal relationship between these two events (Fig. 2). Tatum et al. (1975) have demonstrated that in lieu of a single or double strand of plastic monofilament, the tail of the Dalkon Shield consists of a bundle of monofilaments enclosed within a thin plastic sheath (Fig. 3). The standard shield contains approximately 400 separate fibers, whereas the tail of the small shield contains approximately 200 fibers. Bacteria enter the spaces between the fibers within the sheath and are, either by their inherent motility or by capillary action, able to migrate up along the tail (Fig. 4). The tail functions as a wick for the passage of fluid and bacteria throughout its length all the way to the final double knot at the base of the shield but not through it.

The tails of all major devices, by virtue of their intimate contact with the posterior vaginal pool, are contaminated by the vaginal flora. With pregnancy and progressive uterine enlargement, the tail is drawn up through the mucous plug. The latter is normally a lethal barrier to the viruses, fungi, protozoans, mycoplasmas, bacteria, etc., of the vaginal flora. A monofilament or a double-stranded tail is literally wiped clean. The nylon sheath effectively circumvents this protective mechanism. While septic abortion due to a Lippes Loop characteristically occurs in the late first

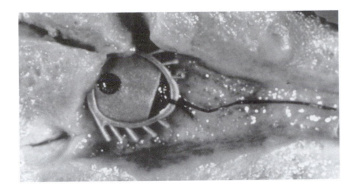

FIGURE 2 Cut section of a uterus containing a Dalkon Shield.

trimester, that observed with the Dalkon Shield is a second- to early third-trimester event. Although the bacteria attain ingress through the tail, the double knot mechanically blocks further migration, and consequently the bacteria must egress by the initial portal of invasion. This accounts for the delayed onset of infectious morbidity and mortality.

When pregnancy occurs in women with an IUD in place, the device should be removed if that can be done without compromising the fetus (Table 2). The presence of the IUD string at the os or in the lower uterine segment usually determines whether or not the IUD will be pulled. There is no question that one runs the theoretic risk of mechanically compromising an established pregnancy; however, maternal considerations and well-being take precedence over those of the fetus. One will do well to counsel the patient that 10% of all pregnancies terminate in abortion. Should abortion then occur, the chances are overwhelming that it is due to a naturally occurring phenomenon and not due to the procedure to which the patient has consented. Such counseling is not only correct in its content, but will go a long way to averting undue guilt on the part of the patient. If the IUD in question is a Dalkon Shield, the course of action should be appropriately aggressive.

IUD AND BACTERIAL ENDOCARDITIS

The patient with congenital valvular disease or a prosthesis in certain instances may be at a high risk for ensuing bacterial endocarditis if the IUD is chosen as the mode of contraception. The insertion of an IUD should be done under antibiotic coverage in a manner similar to that for any surgical procedure. Once the IUD is in place, the patient must be monitored for evidence of intervening anaerobic infection. The best clues are the subsequent development of an intermenstrual, foul-smelling leukorrhea or the appearance of pseudomycelial forms (Gupta lesions) on the Pap smear. Should either develop, it is our policy to advocate removal of the device under antibiotic coverage (specifically, with ampicillin and gentamicin rather than penicillin and streptomycin).

SUMMARY

Much of the infectious morbidity associated with IUD usage can be averted by

1. careful patient selection;
2. prescreening high-risk gravidas for *N. gonorrhoeae* and *C. trachomatis* prior to insertion;
3. prescreening for group A streptococci when disease is in high prevalence in the pediatric population;
4. careful insertion of the IUD;
5. patient education as to the signs of CAE, i.e., (*i*) intramenstrual spotting or de novo menstrual irregularities and (*ii*) intramenstrual discharge;
6. periodic pelvic examination with cytologic evaluation;
7. limiting use of IUD to 24 to 36 months; and
8. removing the IUD in all patients with any significant STD involving the female genital tract.

Women who use the IUD must be carefully counseled as to the fact that they are at augmented risk for the development of CAE and its potential complications as well as being at possible augmented risk for spontaneous first trimester abortions, ectopic pregnancies, and septic abortions should this mode of contraception fail. Should they come in contact with selected STD organisms, the probability of overt destructive disease is enhanced. Women continuing to use the IUD need to be educated as to the early signs and symptoms of clinically significant CAE. Continued use of the IUD should be coupled with a commitment to at least annual cytologic and medical re-evaluation.

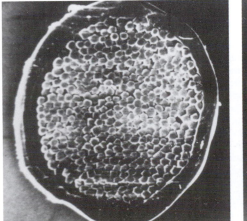

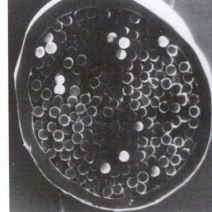

FIGURE 3 Dalkon Shield tails, which are composed of 200–400 monofilaments enclosed in a protective sheath. *Source:* Tatum et al., 1975.

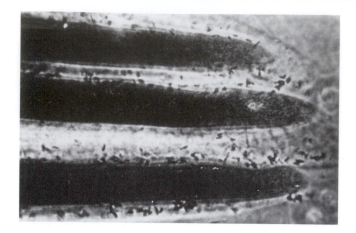

FIGURE 4 Demonstration of bacteria between the individual monofilaments of the Dalkon Shield tail. *Source:* Tatum et al., 1975.

If the problems of CAE are to be circumvented, it is best that women change their form of IUD within a two- but not later than three-year period. If a Dalkon Shield is still the mode of contraception, its removal is strongly urged.

SELECTED READING

Burnhill M. Syndrome of progressive endometritis associated with intrauterine contraceptive devices. Adv Plann Parent 1972; 8:144.

Cates W, Ory HW, Rochat RW, Tyler CW. The intrauterine device and deaths from spontaneous abortion. N Engl J Med 1976; 195:1155.

Grimes DA. Deaths from sexually transmitted diseases: the forgotten component of reproductive mortality. J Am Med Assoc 1986; 255:1727.

Grimes DA. Intrauterine devices and pelvic inflammatory disease: recent developments. Contraception 1987; 36:97.

Kessel E. Pelvic inflammatory disease with intrauterine device use: a reassessment. Fertil Steril 1989; 51:1.

Women's Health Study
Burkman RT and The Women's Health Study. Association between intrauterine device and pelvic inflammatory disease. Obstet Gynecol 1981; 57:269.

Burkman R, Schlesselman S, McCaffrey L, et al. The relationship of genital tract actinomyces and the development of pelvic inflammatory disease. Am J Obstet Gynecol 1982; 143:585.

Kramer RL. The intrauterine device and pelvic inflammatory disease revisited: new results from the Women's Health Study. Obstet Gynecol 1989; 73:300.

Lee NC, Rubin GL, Borucki R. The intrauterine device and pelvic inflammatory disease revisited: new results from the Women's Health Study. Obstet Gynecol 1988; 71:1.

Lee NC, Rubin GL, Ory HW, Burkman RT. Type of intrauterine device and the risk of pelvic inflammatory disease. Obstet Gynecol 1983; 62:1.

Early Onset Postinsertional Infectious Complications
Ledger WJ, Headington JT. Group A beta-hemolytic streptococcus: an important cause of serious infections in obstetrics and gynecology. Obstet Gynecol 1972; 39:474.

Lee NC. IUDs and PID: what have we learned from the Women's Health Study? Infect Med Dis Lett Obstet Gynecol 1989; 11:83.

Marshall BR, Helper JK, Jinguiji MS. Fatal *Streptococcus pyogenes* septicemia associated with an intrauterine device. Obstet Gynecol 1973; 41:83.

Ryden G, Fahraeus L, Molin L, Ahman K. Do contraceptives influence the incidence of acute pelvic inflammatory disease in women with gonorrhea. Contraception 1979; 20:149.

Stathem R, Morton RS. Gonorrhea and the intrauterine contraceptive device. Br Med J 1968; 4:623.

Walsh T, Gromes D, Frezieres R, et al. Randomized controlled trial of prophylactic antibiotics before insertion of intrauterine devices. Lancet 1998; 339:1005.

Significance of Endometrial Bacterial Contamination
Gibbs RS, O'Dell TN, MacGregor RR, et al. Puerperal endometritis: a prospective microbiological study. Am J Obstet Gynecol 1975; 121:919.

Hite KE, Hesseltine HC, Goldstein L. A study of the bacterial flora of the normal and pathologic vagina and uterus. Am J Obstet Gynecol 1947; 53:233.

Ishihama A, Nishjima M, Wada H. Bacteriological study on the users of intrauterine contraceptive devices. Acta Obstet Gynaecol Jap 1970; 17:77.

Marrie TJ, Costerton JW. A scanning and transmission electron microscopic study of the surfaces of intrauterine contraceptive devices. Am J Obstet Gynecol 1983; 146:384.

Mishell DR Jr, Bell JH, Good RG, Moyer DL. The intrauterine device: a bacteriologic study of the endometrial cavity. Am J Obstet Gynecol 1966; 96:119.

Schmidt WA, Schmidt KL. Intrauterine device (IUD) associated pathology; a review of pathogenic mechanisms. Scan Electron Microsc 1986; Pt2:735.

Skangalis M, Mahoney CJ, O'Leary WM. Microbial presence in the uterine cavity as affected by varieties of intrauterine contraceptive devices. Fertil Steril 1985; 37:263.

TABLE 2 Recommendations for the management of the IUD in first trimester

Condition	Recommendations
No history of CAE; string at os	Obtain informed consent delineating risk–benefit ratio. Remove
One or more symptoms suggestive of CAE; string at os	Obtain informed consent. Then, treatment with an antibiotic with good anaerobic coverage for at least 36 hours prior to IUD removal
No string at os	Do not intervene. Instruct patient as to the early signs of infection (tetracyclines contraindicated). Evaluate by ultrasonography as to position with respect to gestational sac. If the string is balled up in lower uterine segment and can be brought down easily, removal is possible but not without some risk

Abbreviation: CAE, chronic anaerobic endometritis.

Smith MR, Soderstrom R. Salpingitis: a frequent response to intrauterine contraception. J Reprod Med 1976; 16:159.

Sparks CA, Purrier BG, Watt PJ, Elstein M. Bacteriological colonization of uterine cavity: role of tailed intrauterine device. Br Med J 1981; 182:1189.

Tatum HJ, Schmidt FH, Phillips D, et al. The Dalkon Shield controversy: structural and bacteriologic study of IUD tails. J Am Med Assoc 1975; 231:711.

Tietze C, Lewit S. Recommended procedures for the statistical evaluation of intrauterine contraception. Stud Fam Plan 1973; 4:35.

Secondary Mechanical IUD-Induced Complications

Chatwani A, Amin-Hanjani S. Management of intrauterine device associated actinomycosis. Infect Dis Obstet Gynecol 1993; 1:130.

Dhall K, Khall GI, Gupta BB. Uterine perforation with the Lippes Loop. Obstet Gynecol 1969; 34:266.

Lippes J. IUD-related hospitalization and mortality. J Am Med Assoc 1976; 235:1001.

Siegler AM, Chen C. Uterine perforation during removal of a broken Majzlin Spring. Fertil Steril 1972; 23:776.

Slaughter L, Morris DJ. Peritoneal-cutaneous fistula secondary to a perforated Dalkon Shield. Am J Obstet Gynecol 1976; 124:201.

Sprague AD, Jenkins VR II. Perforation of the uterus with a shield intrauterine device. Obstet Gynecol 1973; 41:80.

Taylor WW, Martin FG, Pritchard SA, et al. Complications from Majzlin Spring intrauterine device. Obstet Gynecol 1973; 41:404.

Whitson LG, Israel R, Bernstein GS. The extra uterine Dalkon Shield. Obstet Gynecol 1974; 44:418.

IUDs and Infertility

Buchan H, Villard-Mackintosh L, Vessey M, et al. Epidemiology of pelvic inflammatory disease in parous women with special reference to intrauterine device use. Br J Obstet Gynaecol 1990; 97:780.

Cramer DW, Schiff I, Schoenbaum SC, et al. Tubal infertility and the intrauterine device. N Engl J Med 1985; 312:941.

Curtis EM, Pine L. Actinomyces in the vagina of women with and without intrauterine contraceptive devices. Am J Obstet Gynecol 1981; 140:880.

Daling JR, Weiss NS, Metch BJ, et al. Primary tubal infertility in relation to the use of an intrauterine device. N Engl J Med 1985; 312:937.

Grice GC, Hafiz S. Actinomyces in the female genital tract. Brit J Vener Dis 1983; 59:317.

Grimes D. Intrauterine device and upper-genital tract infection. Lancet 2000; 356:1013.

Guderian AM, Trobough GE. Residues of pelvic inflammatory disease in intrauterine device users: a result of the intrauterine device of *Chlamydia trachomatis* infection? Am J Obstet Gynecol 1986; 154:497.

Gump DW, Gibson M, Ashikaga T. Evidence of prior pelvic inflammatory disease and its relationship to *Chlamydia trachomatis* antibody and intrauterine contraceptive device use in infertile women. Am J Obstet Gynecol 1983; 15:146.

Hubacher D, Lara-Ricalde R, Taylor DJ, et al. Use of copper intrauterine devices and the risk of tubal infertility among nulligravid women. N Engl J Med 2001; 345:561.

Keebler C, Chatwani A, Schwartz R. Actinomyces infection associated with intrauterine contraceptive devices. Am J Obstet Gynecol 1983; 145:596.

Moore DE, Spandoni LR, Foy HRM, Want S-P, et al. Increased frequency of serum antibodies to *Chlamydia trachomatis* in infertility due to distal tubal disease. Lancet 1982; 2:574.

Stadel BV, Schlesselman S. Extent of surgery for pelvic inflammatory disease in relation to duration of intrauterine device use. Obstet Gynecol, 1984; 63:171.

Valicenti JF Jr, Pappas AA, Graber CD, et al,: Detection and prevalence of IUD-associated actinomyces colonization and related morbidity: a prospective study of 69,925 cervical smears. JAMA 1982; 247:1149.

Von Bogaert LJ. A clinicopathological study of IUD users with special reference to endometrial patterns and endometritis. Gynecol Obstet Invest 1983; 16:129.

IUD/Endometritis/Salpingitis

Beerthuizen RJ, Van Wijck JA, Eskes TK, et al. IUD and salpingitis: a prospective study of pathomorphological changes in the oviducts in IUD-users. Eur J Obstet Gynecol Reprod Biol 1982; 13:31.

Centers for Disease Control. Elevated risk of pelvic inflammatory disease among women using the Dalkon Shield. Morbid Mortal Wkly Rep 1983; 32:221.

Edelman DA. The use of intrauterine contraceptive devices, pelvic inflammatory disease, and *Chlamydia trachomatis* infection. Am J Obstet Gynecol 1988; 158:956.

Eschenbach DA. IUDs in non-sexually transmitted pelvic inflammatory disease. Infect Med Dis Lttrs Obstet Gynecol 1989; 11:78.

Eschenbach DA, Harnisch JP, Holmes KK. Pathogenesis of acute pelvic inflammatory disease: role of contraception and other risk factors. Am J Obstet Gynecol 1977; 128:838.

Farley TM, Roserberg MJ, Rowe PJ, et al. Intrauterine device and pelvic inflammatory disease: an international perspective. Lancet 1992; 339:785.

Faulkner WL, Ory HW. Intrauterine devices and acute pelvic inflammatory disease. J Am Med Assoc 1976; 235:1851.

Flesh G, Weiner JM, Corlett RC, et al. The intrauterine contraceptive device and acute salpingitis, a multifactorial analysis. Am J Obstet Gynecol 1979; 135:402.

Gareen IF, Greenland S, Morgenstern H. Intrauterine contraceptive device and pelvic inflammatory disease: meta-analysis of published studies, 1974–1990. Epidemiology 2000; 11:589.

Grimes DA. Intrauterine devices and pelvic inflammatory diseases, recent developments. Contraception 1987; 36:97.

Kamwendo F, Forslin L, Danielsson D. Epidemiology and aetiology of acute non-tuberculous salpingitis. A comparison between the early 1970s and the early 1980s with special reference to gonorrhea and use of intrauterine contraceptive device. Genitourin Med 1990; 66:324.

Kaufman DW, Shapiro S, Rosenberg L, et al. Intrauterine contraceptive device use and pelvic inflammatory disease. Am J Obstet Gynecol 1980; 136:159.

Kaufman DW, Watson J, Rosenberg L, et al. The effect of different types of intrauterine devices on the risk of pelvic inflammatory disease. J Am Med Assoc 1983; 250:759.

Lee KC, Rubin GL, Ory HW, Burkman RT. Type of intrauterine device and the risk of pelvic inflammatory disease. Obstet Gynecol 1983; 62:1.

Ory HW. A review of the association between intrauterine devices and acute pelvic inflammatory disease. J Reprod Med 1978; 20:1200.

Osser S, Gullberg B, Liedholm P, Sjoberg N-O. Risk of pelvic inflammatory disease among intrauterine device users irrespective of previous pregnancy. Lancet 1980; 1:386.

Paavonen J, Vesterinen E. Intrauterine contraceptive device use in patients with acute salpingitis. Contraception 1980; 22:107.

Snowden R, Pearsorn B. Pelvic infection: a comparison of the Dalkon Shield and three other intrauterine devices. Br Med J 1984; 288:1570.

INTRODUCTION

Prior to 1979, toxic shock syndrome (TSS) was a rare disease described primarily in children. During the epidemic in 1979 to 1981, TSS became recognized as a disease that occurs primarily in menstruating women using tampons. Tampon users were demonstrated to be more likely to develop menstrual TSS than nonusers. Although recent focus has shifted to nonmenstrual cases, which have occurred in conjunction with wound infections, postpartum endometritis, and vaginitis, the predominance of cases continues to be related to menstruation.

PATHOGENESIS

Staphylococcus aureus can be recovered from the posterior vaginal pool/endocervix in 97% of the cases of TSS. The demographic appearance of numerically significant cases of TSS coincided with the introduction of superabsorbent tampons. The dramatic nature of the presenting symptoms of the illness in otherwise healthy women and its recent incidence largely preclude previous lack of recognition.

The pathogenic mechanism for the association of tampons with TSS has not been adequately explained. Berkley et al. (1987) showed that all users of all brands of tampons have an elevated risk when compared with nonusers. Regardless of the composition of the tampon, absorbency increased the odds ratio for TSS. The chemical composition of the tampons influenced the odds ratio. Polyacrylate-containing tampons had odds ratios that were elevated. Certain materials are superior to unaltered cotton in providing a more absorbent fiber. Nutrients are efficiently drawn in, concentrating protein between fibers, and thereby creating an ideal physiochemical environment for the amplification of TSS-toxin 1 (TSST-1) and other toxins. The greatest stimulation of TSST-1 was observed with, in decreasing order, polyester and carboxymethyl cellulose, polyacrylates, viscose rayon, gelatin foam, polyurethane, and cotton. The use of a low-absorbency tampon appears to reduce the risk of TSS in tampon users (Fig. 1).

TSS SPECIFIC TOXINS

TSST-1 is a protein with a molecular weight of approximately 24,000 daltons and has been proposed as the toxin responsible for TSS. TSST-1 production has been demonstrated in 90% to 100% of *S. aureus* strains recovered from women with menstrual TSS. However, investigators have been able to induce TSS-like illness in 60% of rabbits injected subcutaneously with TSST-1 negative isolates of *S. aureus*. These results suggested that unrecognized toxins

play a role in TSS and that TSST-1 may not be totally responsible for the pathogenesis of toxic shock.

Musser et al. (1990) analyzed the genetic relationships among 315 isolates of the bacterium *S. aureus* expressing TSST-1 recovered primarily from humans with TSS in five countries on two continents. A single clone (ET 41) accounted for 88% of cases of TSS with a female urogenital focus and 53% of TSS cases involving nonurogenital (predominantly wound) infections. With few exceptions, strains representing different phylogenetic lines had a characteristic TSST-1 gene restriction fragment.

The recovery of a single clone from the majority of individuals afflicted with TSS having a urogenital focus and from the genital tract of a large proportion of asymptomatic female carriers strongly suggests that this clone is especially well adapted for colonization of these anatomic sites.

NONENTERIC TOXINS

The ability of extracellular culture filtrates of *S. aureus* to cause inflammatory reactions after inoculation into experimental animals was first reported in 1885. It has subsequently been shown that selected strains of *S. aureus* are capable of elaborating an impressive spectrum of nonenteric toxins. These toxins include exfoliative toxins A and B, alpha, beta, delta, and gamma toxins, and leukocidins. The exfoliative toxins (A and B) are a mixture of two or more products capable of producing intraepidermal cleavage. They are distinct from the other nonenteric toxins. Exfoliative toxin production is not limited to a specific phage group strain of *S. aureus*. The basic mechanism by

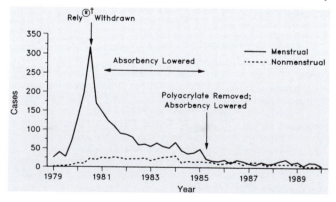

FIGURE I Reported cases of toxic shock syndrome (includes only cases meeting the case definition of Centers for Disease Control) by quarter (United States, 1980–1990). (*Note*: Use of trade names is for identification only and does not imply endorsement by the Public Health Service or the U.S. Department of Health and Human Services). *Source*: From CDC, 1990.

which the alpha toxin works is membrane damage. Although the beta, delta, and gamma toxins all exert profound effects on cell membranes, the importance of alpha toxin is due to its qualitative as well as quantitative effect. Alpha toxin has always been considered to play a significant role in the pathogenesis of staphylococcal disease. The alpha toxin is hemolytic to erythrocytes and cytotoxic and cytolytic to a wide variety of cells. In experimental animal model systems, the principal sites of cytotoxicity are the kidney, where the toxin produces renal necrosis, and the intravascular compartment, where it produces a consumptive coagulopathy. If present in sufficient quantities, alpha toxin causes constriction of the coronary arteries, decreased cardiac output, and ultimately systolic arrest. Beta toxin produces membrane damage via enzymatic activity (sphingomyelinase) and significant degradation of membrane sphingomyelin with secondary effects on membrane permeability.

The ability of the beta toxin to damage cell membrane is directly related to its sphingomyelin content; hence, its effects tend to be more specific than those of the alpha toxin. The delta toxin differs from the other membrane-damaging bacterial toxins elaborated by S. aureus by its relatively hydrophobic nature and low degree of cellular specificity. The delta toxin behaves similarly to cholera toxin. In high doses, it causes histologic damage to the ileum and blocks water absorption. In low doses, it causes significant changes in intestinal iron transport even before cyclic adenosine 3¢5¢ monophosphate levels increase. The gamma toxins have been described only recently. The data concerning specificity of site of cell membrane damage are limited. The clinical manifestation of TSS appears to be the result of the cumulative effect of nonenteric toxin production (Table 1).

Not every strain of S. aureus can produce exfoliative toxins. Approximately 14% of randomly gathered strains of S. aureus can produce the complete spectrum of toxins (exfoliative toxins A and B, alpha, beta, delta, and gamma toxins) incriminated in the pathogenesis of TSS.

The intrigue of TSS is not necessarily why it occurs, but rather why it does not occur more frequently. The Centers for Disease Control (CDC) have estimated that 10% of women harbor S. aureus as a constituent of the vaginal flora. Since superabsorbent tampons once account for 70% of the tampons sold, the recorded incidence of TSS precludes a one-to-one correlation between the presence of S. aureus as a constituent of the bacterial flora of the female genital tract and the use of superabsorbent tampons. These facts suggest that other variables select for disease. Not every strain of S. aureus elaborates either exfoliative toxin A or B. Even when the lack of genetic capability of the majority of S. aureus strains to produce toxin is taken into account, the resultant numbers merely suggest that the genetic endowment of a given strain of S. aureus selects for the potential for disease rather than for the actual disease. The critical event selecting for disease, given a potential TSS strain of S. aureus, is the quantitative increase in toxins produced and secondary to the increased availability of an appropriate growth substrate.

TSS AND CONTRACEPTIVES

Different modes of contraception can also influence the probability of TSS.

Oral Contraceptives
Preliminary data have suggested that the use of oral contraceptives is a protective factor against TSS. The mechanism by which this is achieved is hypothesized to be the reduction in menstrual blood loss, which occurs in users of combined oral contraceptives. This phenomenon may have introduced bias into the prior case–control studies between TSS and tampon use. Women who take oral contraceptives probably require less absorption and menstrual protection because of lighter menstrual blood loss.

TABLE I Potential impact of bacterial toxin production by selected strains of *Staphylococcus aureus* in addition to TSS-toxin I

Clinical evidence of TSS	Proposed mechanism of action	Implicated nonenteric toxin of S. aureus
Fever	Secondary to exogenous pyrogens produced by S. aureus and endogenous pyrogens released from damaged hematopoietic and endothelial cells	Alpha, beta, delta, and gamma toxins
Rash: diffuse, macular erythroderma and hyperemia of mucous membranes	Secondary to membrane damage involving endothelium and smooth muscle	Alpha, beta, and delta toxins
Desquamation of palms and soles	Secondary to intraepithelial cleavage	Exfoliative A and B
Diarrhea	Secondary to inhibition of water absorption from small bowel	Delta toxin
Rising blood urea nitrogen or creatinine (at least twice upper limits of normal)	Secondary to select renal damage	Alpha toxin
Biochemical evidence of hepatocellular dysfunction and central nervous system dysfunction/headache	Combination of secondary vascular and membrane damages	Alpha, beta, delta, and gamma toxins
Hypotension	Secondary to smooth muscle effect and cell membrane damage	Alpha, beta, delta, and gamma toxins

Vaginal Contraceptive Sponge

Faich et al. (1986) described 13 cases of TSS that were thought to be connected with the use of the contraceptive sponge. Three cases evolved during the puerperium or menstrual period. One case occurred in a woman who kept the sponge in place for more than 30 hours. Four cases involved difficulty in removing the sponge, which resulted in its fragmentation. Nine of the 13 cases related to sponge use were not associated with predisposing factors. Using estimates of background of nonmenstrual TSS, these investigators have conjectured that the rate of TSS in sponge users might be elevated above the estimated background but that the risk of this complication is very low. Traumatic manipulation of the sponge, use during menstruation or the puerperium, and prolonged retention of the sponge may increase the risk of occurrence.

Postpartum women and women who have had menstrual TSS previously should avoid using the contraceptive sponge. The sponge should not be used during menstruation and should not be left in place for more than 30 hours. Women who choose to use the sponge should read the package insertion carefully and be aware of the signs and symptoms of TSS.

Contraceptive Diaphragm

A number of cases have been reported of TSS developing in nonmenstruating diaphragm users. In all but one case, the development of TSS was associated with prolonged retention of the diaphragm for 36 hours or more. In the cases described, in addition to the mucosal hyperemia, a significant purulent discharge characterized as being yellowish-green and sometimes foul-smelling was noted. Although a rare occurrence, recognition that TSS can occur in women using barrier contraception is important so that early diagnosis can be implemented.

Prolonged use of a diaphragm is to be avoided, particularly in women who have previously manifested TSS. The appearance of a vaginal discharge occurring in a woman who uses a diaphragm may be sufficient grounds for discontinuation of its use. The rarity of TSS in users of vaginal barrier contraception may be related to the concomitant use of antibacterial spermicides. The use of spermicides retards bacterial growth and may increase the length of time a device can be retained before bacterial replication and toxin production begin. Retention of the diaphragm for 12 to 18 hours may be relatively safe, whereas prolonged use for 36 hours or more without replenishing the spermicide may increase the risk of toxin-mediated disease.

Schwartz et al. (1989) evaluated the use of barrier contraceptives as a risk factor for nonmenstrual TSS. Potential risk factors for nonmenstrual TSS were compared for 28 patients and 100 age-matched controls. Use of barrier contraceptives was associated with a significantly increased risk of nonmenstrual TSS, with matched odds ratios of 10.5 and 11.7 for contraceptive sponge and diaphragm use, respectively. Use of nonbarrier contraceptive methods was unrelated to nonmenstrual TSS. Despite the elevated odds ratio, the incidence of nonmenstrual TSS in barrier contraceptive users and the risk of nonmenstrual TSS attributable to barrier contraceptive use are low.

CLINICAL PRESENTATIONS

TSS is a multisystem illness (Table 2). A syndrome consisting of malaise, myalgia, low-grade fever, nausea, vomiting, and/or diarrhea may antecede overt disease. In the full-blown, acute systemic illness, the patient presents with fever (greater than 38.9°C or 102°F), sore throat, headache, chills, severe hypotension, myalgia, pharyngitis, conjunctivitis, leukocytosis, and generalized arthralgia. The rash is usually a consistent part of the syndrome and presents as a diffuse "sunburn-like" blanching macular erythema. Neurologic symptomatology, when present, is usually severe. Cerebrospinal fluid analyses, when done, are within normal ranges. The patient complains of headache. Disorientation, confusion, agitation, and photophobia are

TABLE 2 Case definition of toxic shock syndrome

Fever: temperature 38.9°C

Rash: diffuse macular erythroderma; desquamation of palms and soles one to two weeks after onset of illness

Hypotension: systolic blood pressure 90 mmHg for adults, below fifth percentile by age for children below 16 years of age, orthostatic drop in diastolic blood pressure 15 mmHg from lying to sitting, or orthostatic syncope

Multisystem involvement: three or more of the following
- Gastrointestinal: vomiting or diarrhea at onset of illness
- Muscular: severe myalgia or creatinine phosphokinase level at least twice the upper limit of normal for laboratory
- Mucous membrane: vaginal, oropharyngeal, or conjunctival hyperemia
- Renal: blood urea nitrogen or creatinine at least twice the upper limit of normal for laboratory or urinary sediment with pyuria (five white cells per high-power field) in the absence of urinary tract infection
- Hepatic: total bilirubin, aspartate aminotransferase, alanine aminotransferase at least twice the upper limit of normal for laboratory
- Hematologic: platelets less than 100,000/mm³
- Central nervous system: disorientation or alterations in consciousness without focal neurologic sign when fever and hypotension are absent

Negative results on the following tests, if obtained:
- Blood, throat (group A beta-hemolytic streptococci), or cerebrospinal fluid cultures
- Rise in titer to Rocky Mountain spotted fever, leptospirosis, or measles
- SGOT, serum aspartate aminotransferase; SGPT, serum alanine aminotransferase

Abbreviations: SGOT, serum glutamic oxaloacetic transaminase; SGPT, serum glutamic pyruvic transaminase.
Source: From CDC. Follow-up on toxic shock syndrome. Morb Mortal Wkly Rep 1980; 29:441.

not uncommon. A small bowel type of watery diarrhea is common in these patients. Diffuse myalgia occurs in the great majority of patients such that they may complain of marked skin and muscle tenderness when touched or moved. Other musculoskeletal symptomatology involves arthralgia of the hands and knees. In rare cases, sterile knee effusions and synovitis of all the metacarpal, phalangeal, and proximal interphalangeal joints may be present.

Profound hypotension is one of the characteristic findings of full-blown TSS. A number of abnormal laboratory findings may be observed. The white blood cell count is generally elevated but may be normal. A large left shift in the neutrophil series occurs but may not be present on the first day of illness; toxic granulation and Dohle bodies are often found and may be an important diagnostic clue. Urinalysis usually shows pyuria (5–10 white blood cells per high-power field) and proteinuria, but cultures (in the absence of an unrelated urinary tract infection) are sterile. Gram stains of vaginal or cervical secretions generally show polymorphonuclear leukocytes and very sparse gram-positive cocci in singlets, doublets, or clumps. Moderate elevations in liver function tests are common, and the serum amylase may be elevated. Most patients have elevations in the blood urea nitrogen and creatinine and a few have required dialysis. Elevation of the creatinine phosphokinase, often dramatic, may occur. Severe illness may be accompanied by other findings. The platelet count often drops below 100,000/mm³ in the first week of illness, and disseminated intravascular coagulation uncommonly occurs.

Electrocardiogram abnormalities include sinus or supraventricular tachycardia, nonspecific ST segment changes, and first-degree heart block. T-wave inversion is sometimes recorded in the precordial leads as are funnel branch, premature atrial, and ventricular extrasystole.

Patients with TSS may have evidence of pulmonary involvement, which may be mild or progress to frank adult respiratory distress syndrome. The development of adult respiratory distress syndrome indicates a poorer prognosis for these patients. On the fifth to the twelfth day following the onset of illness, the patients will experience a danderous-like desquamation involving the face, trunk, and extremities. This is followed by a full-thickness peeling of the palms and soles of the feet (Fig. 2). Despite the extensiveness of the process, healing is without scar formation. Vaginal examination in women with tampon-induced TSS reveals mucosal hyperemia with varying degrees of inflammation. A purulent, malodorous cervical discharge may be observed. Bilateral adnexal tenderness is not an uncommon finding.

NONMENSTRUAL TSS

More and more cases of TSS are occurring in nonmenstruating women. The gravity of illness and the potential for increased mortality are such that obstetricians and gynecologists must be aware of those clinical settings in which disease may potentially occur (Table 3). In obstetrics, the syndrome has been described following vaginal delivery, cesarean section, and spontaneous and therapeutic abortion. In the gynecologic patient, disease has been documented as

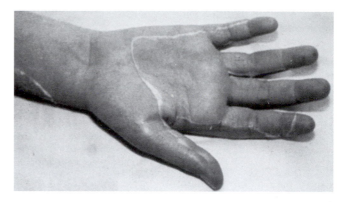

FIGURE 2 Palmar desquamation characteristic of toxic shock syndrome (Courtesy of the CDC)

complicating surgical procedures, such as tubal ligation, vaginal and abdominal hysterectomy, urethral suspension, bladder suspension, exploratory laparotomy, and therapy of extensive condyloma acuminatum. TSS may occur in patients with meatitis, Bartholin's gland abscess, and acute salpingitis. Following abdominal surgery, a unique type of staphylococcal wound infection may occur. In contradistinction to traditional wound infection, where the onset of signs and symptoms is usually about the fourth day, disease usually begins as early as the second day. In the cases reported, local signs of wound infection were minimal or absent. The usual tip-off to the diagnosis of TSS is the development of watery diarrhea and a profuse erythroderma. The absence of local signs of a wound infection does not preclude the existence of staphylococcal infection at the operative site capable of producing TSS. The probability of the diagnosis of TSS is suggested by the development of the sunburn-like rash in conjunction with diarrhea and/or headache. These usually precede full-blown TSS.

DIAGNOSIS

Recognition and definitive documentation of TSS are difficult. The variability of the signs and symptoms of disease (forme fruste) and the large number of clinical conditions on which TSS may be superimposed have been significant impediments to early diagnosis, particularly in the nonmenstruating, nonsuperabsorbent tampon user. There is no definitive early test for TSS.

The diagnosis is based on recognition of a constellation of signs and symptoms indicative of multiorgan involvement that meets the CDC case criteria. Any woman who becomes ill with fever, headache, diarrhea, myalgia, or any combination thereof should be suspected of having TSS. The presence of a rash should greatly heighten the clinician's suspicion of TSS. The diagnosis of TSS early in the clinical course can be quite difficult because the disease can resemble other illnesses.

THERAPY

Proper management of women suspected of having TSS includes a careful vaginal examination, notation of vaginal

TABLE 3 Obstetrical and gynecologic conditions in which toxic shock syndrome has occurred

Category	Conditions
Surgical wound infections	Exploratory laparotomy
	Abdominal hysterectomy
	Urethral suspension
	Bladder suspension
	Dilatation and curettage
	Cesarean section
	Septic abortion
	Surgical removal of condyloma acuminatum
Nonsurgical conditions	Vaginal delivery
	Diaphragm use
	Contraceptive sponge use
	Vaginal infections
	Pelvic inflammatory disease
	Viral influenza

lesions such as ulcerations, and removal of any tampons. A search for focal staphylococcal infections (boils, etc.) should be made. Blood cultures should be obtained. The initial therapy is that of aggressive volume replacement. Because of the large volume of fluids necessary, it is strongly recommended that a Swan-Ganz catheter be placed and anesthesia department be alerted that adult respiratory distress syndrome may develop in this particular patient.

Concomitantly, local therapy should be directed to remove as much toxin as possible from the portal of infection. In cases where the vagina has been the principal portal of infection, it is recommended that the vagina be thoroughly dried out using cotton drumsticks. Extensively irrigating with saline and then cleansing with hydrogen peroxide or betadine iodine are advocated, immediately prior to the institution of antimicrobial therapy.

Antimicrobial therapy requires the administration of a beta-lactamase–resistant semisynthetic penicillin such as oxacillin or nafcillin. A single dose of an aminoglycoside is advocated because of its synergistic effect with the semisynthetic penicillins. Because of the probability of underlying renal damage, a second dose is rarely administered. The choice of the aminoglycosides should take into consideration its potential for renal toxicity.

The patient should be extensively monitored for the development of renal failure and/or adult respiratory distress syndrome. The development of adult respiratory distress syndrome is a poor prognostic sign. Although bacteremia in TSS is a very rare event, when it does occur it has significant therapeutic connotations. Patients with documented bacteremia due to S. aureus should be treated for a minimum of three to four weeks with a combination of parenteral and oral therapy to preclude the delayed development of metastatic complications such as osteomyelitis or brain abscess. If adult respiratory distress develops, mechanical ventilation with a high FI O_2 and positive end-expiratory pressures from 5 to 15 cm of H_2O are often required. Patients who do not respond readily to fluid replacement are at high risk for multiorgan failure and should be immediately transported to centers that can effectively deal with tertiary complications involving lungs, kidneys, and other vital organs.

RECURRENT TSS

Recurrence of TSS in cases related to menstruation has been reported to be as high as 34%. Retrospective data suggest that, with effective antistaphylococcal antibiotic administration, risk of recurrence is decreased to approximately 5%. The incidence of recurrence or relapse in nonmenstruating cases is not known due to an incomplete database. Recurrences have been described in cases of TSS with complicating surgical wound infections. These relapses were associated with recrudescence of the wound infection and incomplete eradication of the TSS strains of S. aureus. Eradication of the causative agent at the site of disease is mandatory to preclude relapse of nonmenstruating TSS.

POSTINFLUENZA TSS

An association between TSS and S. aureus pneumonia was first described in 1985. Pulmonary superinfection in cases of influenza is a well-recognized phenomenon. The decrease in polymorphonuclear leukocyte chemotaxis and tracheobronchial clearance that occurs in viral infection predisposes the organ to bacterial superinfection. With the development of influenza, bacteria tracheitis may on occasion produce TSS symptoms.

Influenza may provide conditions for toxin production that are not ordinarily present for a given staphylococcal strain, which is merely colonizing the respiratory tract. What ensues is a syndrome of unexplained multiorgan failure that develops during the influenza season. The development of rash, disseminated intravascular coagulopathy and multisystem failure are poor prognostic factors. The characteristic pattern of disease is the rapid onset of hypotension, scarlatiniform rash (followed by desquamation and recovery), and other serious manifestations of multiorgan system failure. Since treatment for TSS may be facilitated by drainage of local infection, it becomes imperative to look for pneumonic empyema or sinusitis in all patients who appear to have TSS associated with influenza or upper respiratory tract infections.

TOXIC STREPTOCOCCAL SYNDROME

Close examination of cases of presumed staphylococcal TSS has revealed a multisystem disorder that shares many of the features of staphylococcal TSS, but is caused by toxins elaborated by group A beta-hemolytic streptococcus. Clinically, the nonmenstrual patients fulfill the criteria for the clinical diagnosis of TSS: fever, hypotension, multisystem dysfunction, and diffuse macular erythroderma followed by desquamation.

The TSS-like syndrome usually occurs in patients with severe soft-tissue infections due to S. pyogenes (group A streptococci); however, Herold (1990) reported a case of group A streptococcal toxic shock in a patient with only mild pharyngitis. Lersch et al. (1990) reported a case of a 33-year-old woman suffering from anal erosions who developed severe illness with fever, diarrhea, hypotension, acute abdominal pain, dyspnea, renal and hepatic impairment, myalgia, desquamation of the skin, leukocytosis, anemia, hypocalcemia, and decreased serum albumin and cholesterol levels. Exploratory laparotomy did not reveal pathologic findings. Hemolytic group A streptococci were grown from peritoneal swabs and pleural exudate in bacteriologic cultures. The patient slowly recovered after intensive penicillin and tobramycin therapy.

SELECTED READING

Nonmenstrual TSS
Alcid DV, Kothari N, Quinn EP, et al. Toxic shock syndrome associated with diaphragm use for only nine hours. Lancet 1982; 1:1363.

Baehler EA, Dillon WP, Cumbo TJ, et al. Prolonged use of a diaphragm and toxic shock syndrome. Fertil Steril 1982; 38:248.

Berkley SF, Hightower AW, Broome CV, Reingold AL: The relationship of tampon characteristics to menstrual toxic shock. JAMA 1987; 258:917.

Bowen LW, Sand PK, Ostergard DR. Toxic shock syndrome following carbon dioxide laser treatment of genital tract condyloma acuminatum. Am J Obstet Gynecol 1986; 154:145.

Bracero L, Bowe E. Postpartum toxic shock syndrome. Am J Obstet Gynecol 1982; 143:458.

Bresler MJ. Toxic shock syndrome due to occult postoperative wound infection. West J Med 1983; 139:710.

Bryner CL Jr. Recurrent toxic shock syndrome. Am Fam Physician 1989; 39:157.

CDC. Toxic shock syndrome. Morb Mortal Wkly Rep 1983; 31:136.

CDC. Update. Toxic shock syndrome—United States. Morb Mortal Wkly Rep 1983; 32:398.

CDC. Toxic shock syndrome and the vaginal contraceptive sponge. Morb Mortal Wkly Rep 1984; 33:43.

CDC. Reduced incidence of menstrual toxic shock syndrome—United States, 1980–1990. Morb Mortal Wkly Rep 1990; 39:421.

Chow AW, Wittman BK, Bartless BA, et al. Variant postpartum toxic shock syndrome with probable postpartum transmission to the neonate. Am J Obstet Gynecol 1984; 148:1074.

Demey HE, Hautekeete ML, Buytaert P, et al. Mastitis and toxic shock syndrome. Acta Obstet Gynecol Scand 1989; 68:87.

DeYound P, Martyn J, Wass H, et al. Toxic shock syndrome associated with a contraceptive diaphragm. Can Med Assoc J 1982; 127:611.

Dornan KJ, Thompson DM, Conn AR, et al. Toxic shock syndrome in the postoperative patient. Surg Obstet Gynecol 1982; 154:65.

Dutton AH, Hayes PC, Shepherd AN, et al. Vulvovaginal steroid cream and toxic shock syndrome. Lancet 1983; 1:938.

Faich G, Pearson K. Fleming D, et al. Toxic shock syndrome and the vaginal contraceptive sponge. J Am Med Assoc 1986; 255:216.

Garbe PL, Arko RJ, Reingold AL, et al. *Staphylococcus aureus* isolates from patients with nonmenstrual toxic shock syndrome. J Am Med Assoc 1985; 253:2538.

Green SL, LaPeter KS. Evidence for postpartum toxic shock syndrome in a mother–infant pair. Am J Med 1982; 72:169.

Griffith JE, Perkin RM. Toxic shock syndrome and sinusitis—a hidden site of infection. West J Med 1988; 148:580.

Hyde L. Toxic shock syndrome associated with diaphragm use. J Fam Pract 1983; 16:616.

Hymowitz EE. Toxic shock syndrome and the diaphragm. N Engl J Med 1981; 305:834.

Loomis L, Feder HM Jr. Toxic shock syndrome associated with diaphragm use. Br Med J 1980; 305:1426.

Petitti D, D'Agostino RR, Oldman MJ. Nonmenstrual toxic shock syndrome: methodologic problems in estimating incidence and delineating risk factor. J Reprod Med 1987; 32:10.

Reingold AL. Toxic shock syndrome and the contraceptive sponge. J Am Med Assoc 1986; 255:242.

Reingold AL, Hargrett NT, Dan BB, et al. Nonmenstrual toxic shock syndrome: a review of 130 cases. Ann Intern Med 1982; 96:871.

Reingold AL, Shands KN, Dan BB, et al. Toxic shock syndrome not associated with menstruation: a review of 54 cases. Lancet 1982; 1:1.

Reynolds C. Toxic shock syndrome associated with a contraceptive diaphragm. Can Med Assoc J 1983; 128:1144.

Wager GP. Toxic shock syndrome: a review. Am J Obstet Gynecol 1983; 146:93.

Whitfield JW, Valenti WM, Magnussen CR. Toxic shock in the puerperium. J Am Med Assoc 1981; 246:1806.

Contraception and Toxic Shock Syndrome
Baehler EA, Dillon WP, Cumbo TJ, et al. Prolonged use of a diaphragm and toxic shock syndrome. Fertil Steril 1982; 38:248.

Bowen LW, Sand PK, Ostergard DR. Toxic shock syndrome following carbon dioxide laser treatment of genital tract condyloma acuminatum. Am J Obstet Gynecol 1986; 154:145.

CDC. Toxic shock syndrome—United States, 1970–1980. Morb Mortal Wkly Rep 1981; 30:25.

CDC. Toxic shock syndrome—United States, 1970–1982. Morb Mortal Wkly Rep 1982; 31:201.

Cutler JC. Spermicides as prophylaxis against sexually transmissible diseases (STDs). IPPF Med Bull 1979; 13:3.

Faich G, Pearson K, Fleming D, et al. Toxic shock syndrome and the vaginal contraceptive sponge. J Am Med Assoc 1986; 255:216.

Hymowitz EE. Toxic shock syndrome and the diaphragm. N Engl J Med 1981; 305:834.

Loomis L, Feder HM. Toxic shock syndrome associated with diaphragm use. N Engl J Med 1981; 305:1585.

Reingold AL. Toxic shock syndrome and the contraceptive sponge. J Am Med Assoc 1986; 255:242.

Reingold AL, Hargrett NT, Dan BB, et al. Nonmenstrual toxic shock syndrome: a review of 130 cases. Ann Intern Med 1982; 96:871.

Remington KM, Buller RS, Kelly JR. Effect of the Today contraceptive sponge on growth and toxic shock syndrome toxin-1 production by *Staphylococcus aureus*. Obstet Gynecol 1987; 69:563.

Schwartz B, Gaventa S, Broome CV, et al. Nonmenstrual toxic shock syndrome associated with barrier contraceptives: report of a case–control study. Rev Infect Dis 1989; 11:43.

Shelton JD, Higgins JE. Contraception and toxic shock syndrome: a re-analysis. Contraception 1981; 24:631.

Influenza and Toxic Shock Syndrome
Bonventre PF, Weckbach L, Harth G, et al. Distribution and expression of toxic shock syndrome toxin-1 gene among *Staphylococcus aureus* isolates of toxic shock syndrome and non-toxic shock syndrome origin. Rev Infect Dis 1989; 11:90.

Camner P, Jarstrand C, Philipson K. Tracheobronchial clearance in patients with influenza. Am Rev Respir Dis 1973; 108:131.

CDC. Toxic shock syndrome associated with influenza—Minnesota. Morb Mortal Wkly Rep 1986; 35:143.

Dan BB. Toxic shock syndrome. Back to the future. J Am Med Assoc 1987; 257:1094.

Edwards KM, Dundon MC, Altemeier WA. Bacterial tracheitis as a complication of viral croup. Pediatr Infect Dis 1983; 2:390.

Langmuir AD, Worthen TD, Solomon J, et al. The Thucydides syndrome: a new hypothesis for the cause of the plague of Athens. N Engl J Med 1985; 313:1027.

Larson HE, Parry RP, Tyrrell DAF. Impaired polymorphonuclear leukocytosis after influenza virus infection. Br J Dis Chest 1980; 74:56.

MacDonald KL, Osterholm MT, Hedberg CW, et al. Toxic shock syndrome: a newly recognized complication of influenza and influenza-like illness. J Am Med Assoc 1987; 257:1053.

Roos J. Staphylococcal pneumonia: a review of 18 cases in a Tygerberg Hospital. South Afr Med J 1984; 66:685.

Sperber SJ, Francis JB. Toxic shock syndrome during an influenza outbreak. J Am Med Assoc 1987; 257:1086.

Suhr L, Read SE. Staphylococcal tracheitis and toxic shock syndrome in a young child. J Pediatr 1984; 105:585.

Tashiro M, Ciborowski P, Klenk HD, et al. Role of staphylococcus protease in the development of influenza pneumonia. Nature 1987; 325:536.

Wilkins EGL, Nye F, Roberta C, et al. Probable toxic shock syndrome with primary staphylococcal pneumonia. J Infect 1985; 11:231.

TSS Toxins/Toxic Shock Syndrome

Altemeier WA, Lewis S, Schlievert PM, et al. Studies of the staphylococcal causation of toxic shock syndrome. Surg Obstet Gynecol 1981; 153:481.

Bennett JV. Toxins and toxic shock syndrome. J Infect Dis 1981; 143:631.

Bergdoll MS, Crass BA, Reiser RF, et al. A new staphylococcal enterotoxin, enterotoxin F, associated with toxic shock syndrome S. aureus isolates. Lancet 1981; 1:1017.

CDC. Toxic shock syndrome—United States. Morb Mortal Wkly Rep 1980; 29:229.

CDC. Follow-up on toxic shock syndrome—United States. Morb Mortal Wkly Rep 1980; 29:297.

CDC. Follow-up on toxic shock syndrome. Morb Mortal Wkly Rep 1980; 29:441.

CDC. Toxic shock syndrome—United States, 1970–1982. Morb Mortal Wkly Rep 1982; 31:201.

Chesney PJ, David JP, Purdy WK, et al. Clinical manifestations of toxic shock syndrome. J Am Med Assoc 1981; 246:741.

Fisher RF, Goodpasture HC, Peterie JD, et al. Toxic shock in menstruating women. Ann Intern Med 1981; 94:156.

Fisher CJ, Horowitz BZ, Nolan SM. The clinical spectrum of toxic shock syndrome. West J Med 1981; 135:175.

Helms C, Wintermeyer L. Menstrually-related toxic shock syndrome. Iowa Med 1991; 81:17.

Kehrberg MW, Latham RH, Haslam BT, et al. Risk factors for staphylococcal toxic shock syndrome. Am J Epidemiol 1981; 114:873.

Meeks GR, Lassiter CL. Management of toxic shock syndrome. J Miss State Med Assoc 1990; 31:7.

Musser JM, Schlievert PM, Chow AW, et al. A single clone of Staphylococcus aureus causes the majority of cases of toxic shock syndrome. Proc Natl Acad Sci USA 1990; 87:225.

Novitch M. Menstrual tampons. User labeling. Fed Reg 1980; 45:69840.

Osterholm MT, Davis JP, Gibson RW, et al. Tristate toxic shock syndrome study. I. Epidemiologic findings. J Infect Dis 1982; 145:431.

Reingold AL, Hargrett NT, Shands KN, et al. Toxic shock surveillance in the United States, 1980–1981. Ann Intern Med 1982; 96:875.

Reingold AL, Shands KN, Dan BB, et al. Toxic shock syndrome not associated with menstruation. Lancet 1982; 1:1.

Schlech WF, Shands WN, Reingold AL, et al. Risk factors for development of toxic shock syndrome: association with a tampon brand. J Am Med Assoc 1982; 248:835.

Schlievert PM. Enhancement of host susceptibility to lethal endotoxin shock by staphylococcal pyrogenic exotoxin type C. Infect Immun 1982; 36:123.

Schlossberg D. A possible pathogenesis for recurrent toxic shock syndrome. Am J Obstet Gynecol 1981; 141:348.

Schmid GP, Shands KN, Dan BB, et al. Toxic shock syndrome in menstruating women: its association with tampon use and Staphylococcus aureus and the clinical features in 52 cases. N Engl J Med 1980; 303:1436.

Tieno PM Jr, Hanna BA. Ecology of toxic shock syndrome: amplification of toxic shock syndrome toxin by materials of medical interest. Rev Infect Dis 1989; 11:182.

Todd J, Fishaut M, Kapral F, et al. Toxic shock syndrome associated with phage-group-I staphylococci. Lancet 1978; 2:1116.

Tofte RW, Williams DN. Toxic shock syndrome: evidence of a broad clinical spectrum. J Am Med Assoc 1981; 246:2163.

Wager GP. Toxic shock syndrome: a review. Am J Obstet Gynecol 1983; 146:93.

Toxic Streptococcal Syndrome

Chomarat M, Chapuis C, Lepape A, et al. Two cases of severe infection with beta-haemolytic group A streptococci associated with a toxic-shocklike syndrome. Eur J Clin Microbiol Infect Dis 1990; 9:901.

Gallo UE, Contanarosa PB. Toxic streptococcal syndrome. Ann Emerg Med 1990; 19:1332.

Herold AH. Group A beta-hemolytic streptococcal toxic shock from a mild pharyngitis. J Fam Pract 1990; 31:549.

Jorup-Ronstrom C, Hofling M, Lundberg C, Holm S. Streptococcal toxic shock syndrome in a postpartum woman: case report and review of the literature. Infection 1996; 24:167.

Lersch C, Gain T, von Siemens M, et al. Toxic shock-like syndrome due to severe hemolytic group A streptococcal infection. Klin Wochenschr 1990; 68:523.

Lopez-Zeno JA, Ross E, O'Grady JP. Septic shock complicating drainage of a Bartholin gland abscess. Obstet Gynecol 1990; 76:915.

Noronha S, Yue CT, Sekosan M. Puerperal group A beta-hemolytic streptococcal toxic shock-like syndrome. Obstet Gynecol 1996; 88:728.

Whitted RW, Yeomans ER, Hankins GD. Group A beta-hemolytic streptococcus as a cause of toxic shock syndrome case report. J Reprod Med 1990; 35:558.

Common Nosocomial Problems in Obstetrics and Gynecology

HISTORICAL PERSPECTIVES—PUERPERAL SEPSIS

The genesis of nosocomial infection resides within obstetrics and gynecology; more specifically, with the problem created by the group A beta-hemolytic streptococci—puerperal sepsis.

Hippocrates is reputed to be the first person to recognize the association between puerperal fever and erysipelas:

If erysipelas of the wound seize a woman with child, it will probably prove fatal.

The concept that erysipelas and puerperal sepsis were identical in terms of causative agents was first proposed by Claude Pouteau in 1760; however, its perception was delayed until 1795 when Alexander Gordon and Thomas Denman independently presented the now classic theses whose focal point was the fact that disease was caused by contagion per se and was unrelated to other etiologies. Gordon's paper is the first real epidemiologic study of a nosocomial infection:

The midwife who delivered #1 on the table carried the infection to #2 and to the next woman whom she delivered. The physician who attended #1 and #2 carried the infection to #5 and #6 who were delivered to him and to many others. The midwife who delivered #3 carried the infection to #4 and from #24 to #26 and successively to every woman who she delivered.

Denman wrote,

It is a disagreeable declaration for me to mention that I myself was carrying the infection to a great number of women.

In his second paper appears the following:

There are other consequences of epidemic or even sporadic puerperal fever which would be criminal to be sounded. This is the contagious nature of these fevers: having long been suspected but not fully proven they may be and often have been conveyed by midwives and nurses from one patient to another.

In the realm of therapeutics, the concept later to be advanced by Semmelweis is already to be found in the writings of Robert Collins. Following a long series of epidemics of puerperal fever at the Dublin Lying-In Hospital, Collins in 1729 introduced chlorine disinfection and used the principles of fumigation. This sterile local scouring with chloride of lime (calcium hydrochloride) and sterilization of blankets resulted in the disappearance of puerperal fever. Unfortunately, after Collins's time, his methods were discontinued, and puerperal fever once again returned to Dublin Lying-In Hospital.

Probably the most assertive statement was ultimately to be written by Samuel Kneeland in 1846 in his paper,

The Connection Between Puerperal Fever and Epidemic Erysipelas, Its Origin and Modes of Propagation.

It may be propagated by direct inoculation with fluids of the living and the dead; by the effluvia arising from the bodies of the sick, inhaled in the very chambers of death (as in the wards of the hospital) and carried about by persons, physicians, by clothes, or by bedding floor mites which have been in contact with the diseased person.

Gordon, Denman, and Kneeland are historically overshadowed by Oliver Wendell Holmes and Ignaz Philipp Semmelweis. Their public dominance of the issue has been thought to be in part a function of the fact that they were both extremely young men at a time of intellectual sclerosis. Oliver Wendell Holmes had studied medicine in France and was already familiar with the work of Gordon at the time his essay appeared in 1843 (Fig. 1). While it failed to provide any new insight into the problem of nosocomial puerperal sepsis, it provoked violent outbursts, particularly from Hugh Lenox Hodge and Charles D. Meigs. Meigs in particular attacked the author for wrapping himself in "the gratuitous and illusionary mantle of authority."

Semmelweis's contributions were published over the period of 1847 to 1849 (Fig. 2). A major reason why the life and works of Semmelweis have attracted such wide attention was the result of the violent controversy precipitated in Austria and Germany. Semmelweis's premise emanated from the marked discrepancy in maternal mortality that he observed in two large divisions in Vienna General Lying-In Hospital. In the end, Semmelweis was destined to be his own enemy. He was never one to try honey on bees; an example is an open letter written to Professor Spaeth of the St. Joseph's Academy in Vienna who, in reviewing the obstetric literature of the preceding year for a medical yearbook (published on March 20, 1861), had described the cause of puerperal sepsis as being an inflammation of the fallopian tube. Semmelweis wrote:

From these expressions of opinion Herr Professor has given me the impression that his spirit has not been lit up by the puerperal sun which rose in Vienna in the year 1847, although it shone so near to him.

This stubborn ignoring of my doctrine, the stubborn ruminating over errors, causes me to bestow upon you the following explanation:

I carry with me the consciousness that ever since the year 1847 thousands and thousands of lying-in women and sucklings have died who would not have died if I had not remained silent. But every error concerning puerperal fever which has been spread, the necessary corrections have been made.

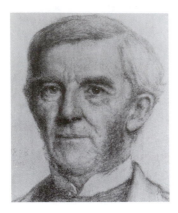

FIGURE 1 Oliver Wendell Holmes, MD. *Source:* Courtesy of National Medical Library, Bethesda, MD.

In this massacre you, Herr Professor, have participated. The homicide must cease, and with this objective of bringing this homicide to an end I will keep watch and every man who dares spread dangerous errors regarding puerperal fever will find in me an active opponent. For me there is no other means of checking the murder than unsparingly to unmask my opponent; and not one whose heart is in the right place will blame me for making use of these means.

The contributions of Holmes and Semmelweis had been sounded before. In reality, they brought no new thoughts to the doctrines which had been developed. Yet we turn with reverence to these individuals. It is a reverence that is a homage in part to the powers of perception and logical thought, but in part to something else. The words of Holmes and Semmelweis were more than those of medical progress; they were the sounds of revolution. As Pasteur has pointed out, all revolutions, even those imposed by scientific demonstration, leave behind them the vanquished who do not forget easily. The something special for which we pay homage to these men is perhaps best expressed in a letter from Oliver Wendell Holmes to a Doctor Chadwich in 1883:

> I shouted my warning louder and longer than any of them and I am pleased to remember that I took my ground on the existing evidence before the little army of microbes was marched up to support my position.

Those well could have been the words of Semmelweis had he not paid the ultimate price for revolution. Confined to a mental sanitarium, Semmelweis died on August 13, 1865, from the same infection that had fostered his intellectual revolution. On the middle finger of the right hand was an

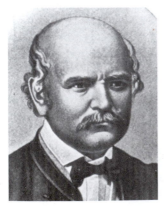

FIGURE 2 Ignaz P. Semmelweis, MD. *Source:* Courtesy of National Medical Library, Bethesda, MD.

infected wound secondary to a gynecologic operation. Metastatic abscesses developed in the right armpit and ultimately invaded the pleura. The day before the death of Semmelweis, Joseph Lister in Glasgow, acting on his interpretation of selected writings of Louis Pasteur, used carbolic acid as an antiseptic in treating a case of compound fracture.

Semmelweis was a mixture of a high sense of morality coupled with the guilt engendered by his unknowing participation in what he had termed "a massacre." He was a man haunted by that knowledge.

The ultimate demonstration of causalities was to be Pasteur's (Fig. 3). The proclamation of this discovery was typical of the man. The date was March 11, 1879. On that day, one of Pasteur's dipoles was expounding on the causes of epidemic puerperal fever in lying-in hospitals. Apparently at a saturation point, Pasteur interrupted him.

> None of these things caused the epidemic. It has been nursing and medical staff who carried the microbe from an infected woman to a healthy one.

In ensuing debate the speaker retorted that the microbes would probably never be found. Pasteur, not replying, merely limped to the blackboard and drew a picture of a chainlike organism. *"There, that is what it is like."* Pasteur had found the streptococci located in the bloodstream of women dying with puerperal sepsis. Thus the page was turned and a new chapter begun.

FACTORS PREDISPOSING TO NOSOCOMIAL INFECTIONS

The concept of nosocomial infections had its genesis in the discovery of the bacterial nature of diseases and the demonstration of the contagiousness of selected diseases, in particular, that due to group A beta-hemolytic streptococci.

The major catalytic event for the perception of nosocomial infections was the creation of hospitals, particularly lying-in hospitals. A prime example is the first series of epidemics of puerperal sepsis that occurred in Great Britain. These were seen in the years 1760 and 1761, shortly after the opening of maternity hospitals. The recognition of the communicability and contagiousness of infections in the hospital environment contributed to the governing concept of cleanliness, sterile surgical techniques, and aseptic wound care.

The advent of effective antimicrobial therapy has had a major effect in redefining nosocomial infections. The initial emphasis placed on exogenous pathogens has progressively shifted in terms of the spectrum from exogenous to endogenous pathogens. The bacterial flora that is dominant within hospital environments results from Darwinian-like pressures induced by antibiotics. A prime example is the problem of the multidrug-resistant *Klebsiella*. When patients are prospectively monitored for the presence of the multiresistant *Klebsiella* organisms, which are responsible for endemic nosocomial infections, 50% of those who become intestinal carriers of the organism during their hospitalization subsequently develop infection, in contrast to approximately 10% of those who do not become intestinal carriers. The prime predisposing factor to intestinal colonization with *Klebsiella* and to exertion of the selective pressure in favor of the multidrug-resistant organism is antibiotic administration. The acquisition of nosocomial strains and their colonization appears to be an important intermediary step in the development of nosocomial infection and serves to perpetuate a significant reservoir of organisms within the hospital.

Augmented technology has radically altered the complex set of circumstances that govern a hospital environment. The newer surgical and anesthetic techniques that have developed now allow for more complex procedures, performed on progressively more debilitated patients. With the introduction of more sophisticated parenteral fluids for hyperalimentation and the necessity for prolonged administration has come a new set of problems. All of these factors have contributed to the changing spectrum of nosocomial infection.

Nosocomial infection is often an interplay between host defense mechanisms and organismal virulence. The patient prone to nosocomial infections is in many instances preselected by an earlier alteration of the host defense mechanisms due to irradiation, antimetabolite therapy, previous antibiotic therapy, or the administration of corticosteroids. What distinguishes obstetric or gynecologic patients from their counterparts in the medical wards, in terms of nosocomial infection, is that with the exception of gynecologic patients undergoing therapy for a malignancy of the female genital tract, they are normal individuals in whom the placement of foreign bodies or iatrogenic surgical disruption of cutaneous or mucosal barriers selects for nosocomial infection.

Unlike many areas in which nosocomial infections function, in obstetrics and gynecology, the immunologic status of patients is rarely a prime selecting factor. The principal problems that obstetricians and gynecologists deal with are those associated with basic procedures such as the use of indwelling intravenous catheters, intra-arterial catheters, intravenous hyperalimentation lines, arteriovenous fistulae (hemodialysis patients), cerebrospinal fluid shunts, presence of urinary catheters or wounds, prior or ongoing antibiotic therapy, and/or the presence of an identifiable cutaneous infection. Since the effect tends to be additive, often, more than one factor is implicated in the pathogenesis of a given infection.

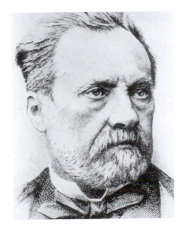

FIGURE 3 Louis Pasteur. *Source:* Courtesy of National Medical Library, Bethesda, MD.

URETHRAL CATHETER-ASSOCIATED INFECTIONS   *Stephen R. Zellner*

Approximately 5% of patients admitted to general hospitals in the United States will develop a nosocomial infection. Infections of the urinary tract account for approximately 40% of these infections, or roughly 3% of all hospital admissions. Usually these infections are the result of catheterization, instrumentation, or urinary tract surgery.

Among the portals of entry by which bacteria may gain access to the catheter system and ascend to the bladder are the urethral meatus and periurethral space, the junction between the catheter and the drainage tube, the junction between the drainage tube and the collection receptacle, and the drainage receptacle. To minimize the infection related to bladder catheterization, special attention has been given to maintaining asepsis of the catheter and drainage system.

Bacteria enter the bladder by migrating through either the periurethral space or the catheter lumen. The sheath of exudate lining the urethra and surrounding the catheter provides an excellent culture medium for bacteria.

The application of antibiotic ointments to the external urethral meatus, catheters impregnated with antibiotics, antibiotic-containing lubricants, and more recently, iodophore-containing lubricants have been used in attempts to decrease bacterial colonization of the periurethral space.

However, double-blinded studies have demonstrated that such lubricants and impregnated catheters had no effect on the subsequent development of urinary tract infection (UTI). Most catheter-associated UTIs occur after the second day of use, by which time the antibiotic–antiseptic combination has been carried away by the flow of urine and mucus and is no longer available.

Closed Urinary Drainage

Much effort has been expended toward developing a system of catheterization that prevents or at least decreases the hazards of infection associated with indwelling urethral catheters.

Once the catheter, tubing, and drainage receptacle have been aseptically placed, the integrity of the system must not be violated. That is, the system should be both initially and permanently a closed one. Several years ago, it was demonstrated that the frequency of catheter-associated infections could be reduced with a closed drainage system. Less than 10% of patients placed on a closed system of drainage developed bacteriuria when catheterized for periods between 1 and 14 days. In contrast, 90% of patients employing this closed system became infected when asepsis and the integrity of the system were broken by disconnecting the drainage tube from the catheter.

Closed systems employing catheters impregnated with antibiotic agents or lubricated with antibacterial-containing gels are of no benefit over a carefully maintained closed drainage system. These antibacterial materials are water soluble and after catheter use for 24 to 48 hours are no longer available or effective. Since most catheter-associated

UTIs develop between the second and fourth day of use, this maneuver adds little to a carefully inserted and maintained closed drainage system.

Use of Antibiotics in Association with Closed Urinary Drainage

Although investigators have been unable to demonstrate any beneficial effect from the systemic administration of prophylactic antibiotics to patients on open catheter drainage, in patients on closed catheter drainage, the therapeutic use of antibiotics has shown some promise. In an open system that permits ready access of organisms to the bladder, the emergence of resistant strains in patients treated with antibiotics frequently occurs. A closed system, however, provides a barrier to reinfection. Using systemic antibiotic agents with demonstrated effectiveness against the infecting organism by in vitro testing, 48% of patients in one study, admitted to the hospital with bacteriuria and placed on a closed system of catheter drainage, were cured. Unfortunately, in only 30% of the group of patients who developed a nosocomial bacteriuria while on catheter drainage was the infection resolved. Removal of the foreign body from the bladder and institution of appropriate antibiotic therapy is of course ideal. In patients in whom this approach is not feasible, systemic antibiotic therapy and careful maintenance of a closed drainage system will be beneficial.

Role of Bladder Irrigation with Closed Urinary Drainage

Techniques of bladder irrigation have been employed in an attempt to decrease the migration of bacteria through the catheter lumen. The ideal irrigation solution should be nontoxic, active against both gram-positive and gram-negative organisms, inexpensive, nonabsorbable, and easy to use, and should have a low incidence of acquired bacterial resistance.

Although such irrigation solutions can decrease the incidence of catheter-associated UTI (Table 1), many physicians do not use this technique as originally described—continuous drip through a triple-lumen Foley catheter. The central lumen drains the bladder contents, the second permits continuous instillation of fluid into the bladder, and the third provides for inflation of the balloon at the proximal end of the catheter.

Recommendations and Techniques

From the preceding discussion, one can only conclude that the insertion of a urethral catheter is not a harmless procedure. Despite sound technique, the insertion and prolonged use of an indwelling urethral catheter, if not properly managed, may result in urinary infection. This iatrogenic infection can predispose patients to the development of acute and chronic pyelonephritis, gram-negative septicemia, and premature labor. Control of infection in patients on catheter drainage is the responsibility of everyone associated with patient care. Previously discussed concepts can be directly applied to techniques of catheter care for use in hospitals:

1. Aseptically inserted sterile closed urinary collection systems can reduce the rate of development of significant

TABLE I Effectiveness of bladder irrigation in preventing bacteriuria in catheterized patients[a]

Catheter group	Protection (%)	Infection (%)
Open drainage	0	100
Open drainage + saline irrigation	0	100
Open drainage + systemic antibiotics	25	75
Closed drainage	77	23
Triple lumen + acetic acid rinse	80	20
Triple lumen + nitrofurazone rinse	80	20
Triple lumen + neomycin–polymyxin B rinse	94	6

[a]Abacteriuric patients requiring indwelling catheter drainage for 10 days or less.
Source: Andriole VT. In: Kaye D, ed. Urinary Tract Infection and Its Management. St. Louis: Mosby, 1972.

bacteriuria from 100% to 21% at seven days of exposure.

2. A sterile three-way closed catheter system employing bladder irrigation with neomycin–polymyxin B solution can further reduce the incidence of bacteriuria to about 6%.

3. Concomitant treatment with systemic antibiotics for patients with indwelling urethral drainage systems does not significantly reduce the incidence of bacteriuria.

Guidelines that can be easily adapted for use by all hospitals are necessary. One possible set of recommendations for the control of catheter-associated bacteriuria is presented for consideration.

(1) The potential risks and attendant morbidity associated with urinary catheterization should always be considered prior to placing the catheter. Indwelling catheters should be avoided unless absolutely necessary for the medical well-being of a patient. They should never be used solely as a matter of nursing convenience and should be discontinued promptly when they are no longer necessary.

(2) Insertion of an indwelling catheter should be done only by trained personnel using sterile techniques.

Materials required to perform the catheterization should be assembled beforehand. Sterile gloves, perineal antiseptic, sterile catheter, closed drainage collecting system, and sterile water-soluble lubricating jelly can be purchased in kit form or assembled by the hospital pharmacy.

Following careful and thorough scrubbing of the hands, sterile gloves are put on. Using one hand, designated as nonsterile, the clinician spreads apart the labia, exposing the urethral meatus. Adequate lighting and having the patient in the correct position greatly facilitate this maneuver. While adequate visualization is maintained, the urethral meatus is cleansed with antiseptic solution. Solutions of 1:1000 aqueous benzalkonium chloride (Zephiran) are not suitable for this purpose because they are frequently contaminated with gram-negative organisms. An iodophore solution should ensure adequate perineal and meatal antisepsis. Cleansing of the perineum should be in the direction of urethra to rectum, never the reverse. The indwelling catheter should be coated with lubricating jelly and slowly threaded through the urethra into the bladder. Lubricants and catheters impregnated with antibiotic compound may be used; however, their efficacy is questionable. The proper-sized catheter should pass easily so as to avoid urethral irritation, yet be of sufficient lumen diameter to permit unimpeded bladder drainage. The catheter should never be forced during insertion since this too causes unnecessary urethral trauma. Following the return of urine through the catheter lumen, the balloon is inflated with sterile saline and the catheter is taped to the patient in order to decrease its motion. The sterile drainage system is connected and attached at the patient's bedside.

(3) A sterile closed drainage system with a disposable clear plastic bag and connecting tubing should be used. The system should permit drainage of urine without disrupting sterile continuity. Currently used collecting bags are fitted with a drain spout at the most dependent portion of the bag to allow evacuation of the container without violating the integrity of the system.

Samples of the urine needed for analysis may be withdrawn from the soft rubber portion of the catheter much as one would perform a venipuncture. The area is prepped with an alcohol sponge, a needle attached to a syringe is inserted, and the urine is aspirated.

Catheters and closed drainage systems that have been inserted aseptically require replacement only if they malfunction. Failure to drain readily or the presence of intraluminal sand or concretions are indications of impending catheter obstruction.

(4) Second only to aseptic insertion of the catheter in importance is a program of daily catheter care:

(a) The junction of the catheter with the drainage tube must not be broken once it is connected.
(b) Collecting bags should be drained at least every eight hours. Care must be taken not to contaminate the mouth of the spigot or permit reflux of urine into the collecting tube.
(c) Bags may be hung at the bedside, on chairs, or on stretchers but must never be raised above the bladder level.
(d) Twice-daily washing of the perineum with soap and water is recommended so as to detect early meatal irritation and catheter malfunction.
(e) When possible, patients with indwelling catheters should be cared for in separate rooms to avoid crowding. Strict attention must be given to handwashing before and after contact with each patient or catheter system.

(5) Catheters should not be irrigated unless this is specifically ordered by the physician.

The sole indication for a single irrigation of a closed drainage system is obstruction of urine flow, usually due to clotted blood. Routine intermittent irrigation is felt by most investigators to be of no value in preventing UTI. Specifically, simple flushing of the system permits only a short contact time between organism and antibacterial agent and does not provide adequate time for killing it. In addition, in order to perform intermittent irrigation of the bladder, the junction of the catheter and drainage tube must be broken, increasing the risk of infection.

Prophylactic continuous irrigation should only be used after the development of an efficient system of sterile closed drainage. Irrigation may then be added to improve bladder care.

(6) All indwelling catheters, regardless of the length of time they are to be used, must be routinely attached to a closed system of drainage.

(7) All patients on bladder drainage must be closely monitored for the development of UTI. Daily routine culturing by either nursing personnel or the hospital epidemiologist is acceptable. Prompt reporting of culture data to physicians is critical if the program is to be effective.

Treatment of Infections in Catheterized Patients

Bacteriuria in a previously abacteriuric patient requiring indwelling closed catheter drainage often reflects breaks in catheter care techniques. Antimicrobial therapy is reported to be effective in about 30% of patients in whom closed catheter drainage is continued. Reinfection and failure to respond to the administered therapeutic agent frequently make removal of the catheter system necessary. Only when antimicrobial therapy is combined with efficient urethral catheter management can UTI in patients with indwelling catheters be resolved.

Antibiotic preparations effective in the treatment of UTI have already been mentioned. In patients requiring long-term catheterization, suppressive therapy with methenamine salts and urine acidification, with nitrofurantoin or with nalidixic acid, may be beneficial once the acute infection is controlled.

Acquired bacteriuria in patients with short-term indwelling urethral catheters can be promptly detected by frequent bacteriologic monitoring. Appropriate antimicrobial therapy can then be selected on the basis of in vitro sensitivity tests, and an antimicrobial agent to which the organism is sensitive can be administered.

INFECTION FROM INTRAVENOUS INFUSIONS OR FEEDINGS

One of the major technologic advances has been the ability to utilize the intravascular compartment. The ease with which fluids and drugs can be given may, on occasion, engender a certain amount of laxity. Often forgotten is the concept that a major host defense mechanism, the cutaneous barrier, has been penetrated iatrogenically and transiently bridged with a foreign body.

With the increasing use of the indwelling intravenous catheter has come a concomitant increase in both local and systemic infectious complications. Intravenous catheters now rank as one of the leading causes of septicemia in hospitalized individuals. The reported incidence of infection ranges from 0.4% to 2%. The principal factor selecting for infection is the duration of time that the catheter is left in place. The longer the time interval a catheter is in place, the greater the risk of catheter-related infection and septicemia. The intravenous catheter should be used only when absolutely necessary—not merely for the convenience of the house-staff and paramedical personnel.

If the catheter tip is serially cultured, it is found to be progressively colonized by bacteria endogenous to the skin flora. There is a very poor correlation between the recovery of organisms from the catheter tip per se and the occurrence of septicemia, and between the incidence of phlebitis and septicemia. The lack of correlation emanates from the fact that in many instances, the solution used is nonphysiologic in terms of pH or that selected antimicrobial agents are extremely sclerosing (e.g., erythromycin, cephalosporins).

While there is little correlation between phlebitis and septicemia (1%), the converse is not true. Patients with catheter-induced septicemia very often have evidence of phlebitis. The prime pathogens are *Staphylococcus aureus* (penicillin resistant) and *Candida albicans*.

When polyethylene and siliconized catheters are used preoperatively in seriously ill patients requiring long-term administration of intravenous fluids, the catheter should be changed 48 hours after insertion. At this time, the choice of cannula becomes important. In patients requiring long-term administration of intravenous fluids, a progressive march up the arm and the initial use of a scalp vein needle is preferable to using a plastic catheter. Scalp vein needles are in general associated with a lower rate of septicemia and phlebitis than plastic catheters (provided they are not subjected to prolonged use). Because the scalp vein needles are not as securely held as plastic catheters, they often require replacement, indirectly contributing to the reduction in iatrogenic infectious morbidity.

Location of Intravenous Site

The arm is the preferred site for short-term intravenous therapy. With patients requiring long-term intravenous therapy, it is advocated that large veins be utilized, particularly when there is the possibility that hypertonic nutrient solutions will be administered. If one uses such a major portal, daily catheter care should include

1. dressing removal,
2. skin cleansing with an antiseptic, and
3. restoration of the sterile dressing.

When antibiotics or other intravenous medications are administered through alimentation lines, great care must be taken in terms of the compatibility of the various solutions being administered. Otherwise, precipitation due to physical or chemical incompatibilities may result. If blood samples are required, they should be taken from separate intravenous sites, not from the catheter.

Preparation of Intravenous Site

The preparation of the site of vena puncture is important and should not be neglected. Guidelines for sterilization of a vena puncture site include vigorously cleansing the site with tincture of iodine, 70% alcohol, or tincture of chlorhexidine (0.5% in alcohol). Allow the area to dry for 30 seconds. Local application of topical antibiotics does not alter the incidence of catheter septicemia but does influence the frequency of local catheter-related infections (Table 2).

TABLE 2 Impact of vascular catheter site antisepsis on local catheter-related infection

Regimen—daily application	Incidence of local catheter-related infection	Catheter septicemia
No topical agent	6.50%	0.70%
Iodophor ointment	3.60%	0.70%
Polymixin, neomycin, and bacitracin[a]	2.20%	0.70%

[a]For antiseptics to exert their maximal benefit on the catheter, the catheter must remain in place over four days.
Source: Maki DG, Band JD. Am J Med 1981; 70:739.

Maintaining the Intravenous Catheter

The intravenous catheter should be fixed to prevent a to-and-fro motion and possible catheter embolization. It is advisable to cover the site with a sterile dressing. The local application of a nonsensitizing local antibiotic cream is of questionable benefit in reducing the incidence of local or systemic infectious complications (Table 2). The intravenous site must be inspected daily. If evidence of local inflammation at the site of penetration or phlebitis is detected, the catheter must be removed. The earliest sign of phlebitis is pain on palpation. Often the patient will be the person who draws the physician's attention to this symptom.

One of the most common mistakes is attempting to reestablish the patency of a catheter that has become occluded or is malfunctioning by manipulation or forced irrigation. Malfunction of a catheter is an indication for its removal. In those instances when the use of sclerosing solutions is anticipated, it is advisable to use small amounts of heparin, unless this is contraindicated, to avoid thrombophlebitis.

The incidence of catheter-related septicemia can be markedly reduced by replacing all catheters within a final time frame. The type of catheter influences the maximum duration of utilization (Table 3).

The rules governing the intravenous administration are the following:
1. Anticipate changing intravenous administration sets.
2. Scalp vein needles rather than short plastic cannulae should be utilized when long-term intravenous administration is required. The risk-per-day of developing phlebitis is significantly greater at all times after the second day.
3. Tenderness at the needle or catheter site and extending up the vein is an indication for immediate discontinuation of the use of that specific site.

Whether or not daily applications of topical polymixin, neomycin, and bacitracin ointment to the catheter site are warranted is still under analysis.

Diagnosis

The diagnosis of nosocomial infection due to multiresistant bacteria (MRB) emanates from the microbiology laboratory. Once such an organism is identified, the problem is twofold:
1. Therapy of the individual patient
2. Eradication of the bacteria from the hospital environment

TABLE 3 Avoidance of catheter-related septicemia by appropriate replacement

Type of intravenous catheter	Maximum duration of utilization
Venous	2–3 days
Arterial	4–5 days
Central	Can use over a prolonged period if daily care provided

Distance from skin to vessel wall influences time sequence for the acquisition of infection.
Source: Maki DG, Band JD. Am J Med 1981; 70:739.

By definition, the antimicrobial therapeutic options are limited. Often the physician is committed to the use of drugs with narrow therapeutic margins. Even more important is the 24 to 36 hour delay incurred by virtue of empiric commitment to an ineffective antimicrobial therapy. Nosocomial infection due to MRB is a precarious situation for both patient and hospital.

The two major areas where MRB function in obstetrics and gynecology are the surgical intensive care unit and the neonatal intensive care unit.

The major bacteria involved are the methicillin-resistant *S. aureus* (MRSA), *Staphylococcus epidermidis*, and the Enterobacteriaceae.

METHICILLIN-RESISTANT *S. AUREUS*

Since the first reports of significant outbreaks of MRSA in hospitals in the United States, the prevalence of MRSA colonization and infection has increased not only in acute and chronic care facilities, but also in outpatient clinics that serve community-based populations.

The emergence of resistance to antibiotics has not been accompanied by an alteration of virulence. MRSA strains cause life-threatening infections, but they are no more pathogenic than methicillin-sensitive strains (MSSA).

The problems posed by MRSA strains are threefold:

1. Incorrect or missed identification of MRSA and, hence, inappropriate or ineffective antibiotic therapy
2. Inappropriate antibiotic use despite adequate identification
3. Nosocomial spread within a health-care unit

MRSA isolates contain what is termed *mecA* gene, a 2130 bp stretch of DNA of nonstaphylococcal origin that, together with a longer block of "foreign" DNA, is incorporated into the staphylococcal chromosome. The *mecA* gene encodes for the 78 KD penicillin-binding protein (PBP) 2A, which has a very low affinity for beta-lactam antibiotics. It is generally assumed that PBP 2A acts as a surrogate enzyme that takes over the task of cell wall synthesis from the normal complement of staphylococcal PBPs.

An intact *mecA* gene component alone does not appear to fully account for phenotype resistance. Additional chromosomal sites outside of the *mecA* determinant locus appear to determine the minimum inhibitory concentration (MIC) value of an MRSA isolate. The auxiliary genes cofunction with the *mecA* gene in bringing about the high level beta-lactam resistance.

Microbiological Identification of MRSA

A number of conditions can affect the results of disk diffusion, broth dilution, and agar screening for MRSA. In the near future, DNA detection methodologies may replace susceptibility testing in identification of MRSA.

Inappropriate Antibiotic Therapy

MRSA strains of the 1990s are significantly different from the MRSA strains that existed in the 1960s and 1970s. The pattern of resistance is significantly broader and encompasses some antibiotics such as clindamycin, imipenem, the newer aminoglycosides, and some of the new-generation tetracyclines. The only antibiotic for which efficacy can be projected with reasonable certainty is vancomycin.

Nosocomial Spread

Once introduced into a health-care unit and allowed to colonize patients, both sporadic and epidemic outbreaks of MRSA may occur. When the units involved are newborn intensive care units, postoperative care units, and intensive care units, the character of the patient population magnifies the morbidity and mortality of MRSA. Traditionally, cases of MRSA infection were due nosocomially to internal antibiotic pressures. Because of the aggressive use of antibiotics in nursing homes, this patient population, when subsequently hospitalized, has proved to be a significant vehicle for unit colonization. MRSA prevalence rates as high as 34% have been reported from long-care settings. Currently, MRSA is in the community.

Management of Wound Sepsis Due to MRSA

Once an MRSA isolate is identified, both active surveillance and control measures need to be implemented. Transmission occurs primarily from colonized or infected patients to others via the hands of health-care personnel. Efforts to prevent the occurrence of new cases center on active surveillance to identify the existing patient reservoirs of MRSA and the institution of control measures to block further transmission from any reservoir. Therapy requires both local wound care and antibiotic therapy.

The following sequence is recommended:

1. Notify infection control of an MRSA isolate.
2. Institute hand care (povidone, iodine, or chlorhexidine) and barrier protection.
3. Isolate the patient from other individuals who may be at potential risk for localized infection.
4. Debride wound and institute appropriate local care.
5. Administer intravenous vancomycin; the end-titration point for parenteral administration should be a patient who is afebrile for 24 to 36 hours and negative wound culture for MRSA.
6. Infection control should
   (a) survey patients in the immediate vicinity and those cared for by nurses involved with the pilot case for nasal MRSA colonization and
   (b) survey all involved health-care personnel for nasal carriage of MRSA.

7. Because the patient has both wound infection and wound sepsis (fever), parenteral vancomycin therapy should be implemented with aggressive wound care.

If multiple patients are colonized, these individuals should be segregated together until all have been discharged. No new additional patients should be admitted to that unit or room. If health-care personnel are nasally colonized, local nasal treatment with mupirocin should be considered. Elimination of nasal carriage is critical to the success of any rational control policy.

Selective screening of "high-risk" groups will miss potential vectors of MRSA. The key to nosocomial control is not waiting until some arbitrary quota of MRSA isolates is identified but using the pilot case to address its existence with the same measures as if one were confronted with a mini-MRSA epidemic.

Mupirocin is a topical antimicrobial that appears to have some promise in dealing with MRSA colonization. The drug has been used to eliminate nasal carriage with local application. In a controlled trial, nasal carriage of S. aureus was eliminated in all subjects and when recolonization eventually took place, only 29% relapse with the pretreatment strain was evidenced. Hill and Casewell (1990) reported an MRSA outbreak at a London hospital. Standard infection control means had failed to prevent colonization and infection of more than 200 patients. They achieved epidemiological control using mupirocin. Of the 40 patients and 32 staff studied, 98.6% and 90.1% respectively were free of nasal MRSA after treatment. With widespread use of nasal mupirocin ointment, resistance develops. Miller et al. (1996) analyzed mupirocin resistance among MRSA over a four-year period in a large teaching hospital. Mupirocin resistance among MRSA increased markedly over this period (1990, 2.7%; 1991, 8.0%; 1991, 61.5%; 1993, 65%) in association with increased use of mupirocin ointment as an adjunct to infection control measures. Mupirocin is a valuable agent in the control of MRSA. The drug must be used judiciously.

Prevention

Monitoring for possible MRSA introduction into the hospital environment is the key to MRSA control. Patients at high risk for colonization with MRSA are listed in Table 4.

Nasal culturing for MRSA needs to be done on these individuals. Multiple studies have shown that nasal carriers of S. aureus are at higher risk for S. aureus bacteremia than are noncarriers in the setting of an MRSA outbreak. Colonization by methicillin-resistant strains represents a greater risk than does colonization by MSSA and strongly predicts the occurrence of MRSA bacteremia. In a prospective cohort study, Pujol et al. (1996) screened with nasal swabs 488 patients admitted to an intensive care unit. Nasal staphylococcal carriers were observed until the development of S. aureus bacteremia, intensive care unit discharge, or death. Of the 488 patients, 147 (30.1%) were nasal S. aureus carriers, 84 (17.2%) harbored

TABLE 4 Patients at high risk for colonization with MRSA

(1)	Patients recently discharged from the hospital requiring antibiotic therapy
(2)	Patients admitted from a nursing home or comparable chronic care facility
(3)	Patients who develop staphylococcal disease while in an intensive care unit
(4)	Patients admitted with obvious staphylococcal disease when MRSA is identified in the community

methicillin-sensitive S. aureus, and 63 (12.9%) harbored MRSA.

Nosocomial S. aureus bacteremia was diagnosed in 38 (7.7%) of 488 patients. Rates of bacteremia were 24 (38%) of the MRSA carriers, eight (9.5%) of the MSSA carriers, and six (1.7%) of noncarriers. After adjusting for other predictors of bacteremia by means of a Cox proportional hazard regression model, the relative risk for S. aureus bacteremia was 3.9 (95% confidence interval, $1.6 - 9.8$; $p = 0.002$) for MRSA carriers compared with MSSA carriers.

Methicillin-Resistant S. epidermidis

The traditional concept of S. epidermidis as a contaminant must be revised. It is now apparent that this bacteria can function as a major nosocomial pathogen. A physician can no longer dismiss the recovery of a coagulase-negative staphylococci as a mere contaminant. In many institutions, S. epidermidis is the most common causative agent of hospital-acquired infection. It is a major pathogen in catheter-related septicemia.

The major problem confronting clinicians is evaluating the significance of recovery of S. epidermidis obtained through central or peripheral venous lines of a patient who is potentially septic and distinguishing bacteremia from superficial cutaneous contamination. The significance of an isolate must be evaluated in the context of the clinical setting, clinical signs, total neutrophil count and, in the neonate, immature neutrophil to total neutrophil count ratio.

Nosocomial infection due to S. epidermidis is associated with clinical situations in which there is a foreign body implanted in the host, i.e., prosthetic cardiac valve, a cerebrospinal fluid shunt, or with prolonged use of an indwelling intravenous line.

The proper procedure for differentiating bacteremia from contamination is to obtain peripheral cultures and evaluate the patient for clinical symptoms or signs of sepsis. In adults, a good correlation exists between repeatedly positive central line cultures, clinical symptoms of sepsis, and positive peripheral blood cultures. Clinical signs of associated coagulase-negative staphylococcal sepsis in infants are relatively nebulous. They include apnea, bradycardia, lethargy, or signs consistent with necrotizing enterocolitis.

The question as to whether removal of the catheter is mandatory for eradication of infection is controversial. If an alternative venous access is available, prompt removal is advocated. The probability of successful therapy without removing the catheter is markedly reduced.

Management

The methicillin-resistant strains of *S. aureus* are uniformly resistant to the semisynthetic penicillinase-resistant penicillins and all the cephalosporins. Strains with this pattern of intrinsic resistance also acquire plasmid-mediated resistance to most other antimicrobials with antistaphylococcal activity. In vitro sensitivity may be demonstrated to rifampin, trimethoprim–sulfamethoxazole, and the new generation tetracyclines. Uniform susceptibility to vancomycin has been demonstrated.

Therapeutic intervention for *S. epidermidis* is complicated by the antibiotic resistance of most nosocomial strains. Between 5% and 40% of septicemic strains are methicillin or oxacillin resistant. Although strains will demonstrate susceptibility to cephalosporins in vitro, the response to this group of drugs is poor. Vancomycin is clearly the drug of clinical choice; however, a few vancomycin-resistant strains have been identified.

Vancomycin is active in a pH range of 6.5 to 8.0. While effective in low concentrations in vitro against most gram-positive cocci and bacilli, the drug is bacteriostatic but not bactericidal for the enterococci in concentrations that can be safely achieved. There is no cross-resistance between vancomycin and other currently available antibiotics.

One of the unique problems associated with vancomycin administration is the so-called "red-neck syndrome." Rapid intravenous administration of vancomycin produces a histamine-like reaction characterized by flushing, tingling, pruritus, tachycardia, and an erythematous macular rash involving the face, neck, upper trunk, back, and arms, with the rest of the body being spared. Systemic arterial hypotension may complicate the whole picture. The syndrome can be avoided by slow intravenous drug administration.

Once a strain of MRSA or methicillin-resistant *S. epidermidis* becomes established as an endemic nosocomial pathogen, its eradication from the hospital environment is difficult.

BACTERIAL COLONIZATION OF NEWBORN INFANTS BY MULTIRESISTANT *ENTEROBACTERIACEAE*

Bacterial colonization with multiresistant *Enterobacteriaceae* or MRS strain, if it occurs, does so within the first three days. Neither the occupancy rate in the unit nor the clinical state of the infant seems to influence the colonization pattern significantly. Barring antibiotic therapy, the bacterial spectrum usually remains essentially the same with increasing age during the stay in the unit. While colonization is a relatively common occurrence, disease is not, which indicates that other factors, such as clinical state of the infant, are of greater importance for major infection than the pattern of bacterial colonization.

ERADICATION OF MRB FROM THE HOSPITAL

Disease due to MRB occurs primarily in intensive care units. Respiratory therapy equipment, fiberoptic bronchoscopes, vascular catheters, arterial pressure monitors, scalp vein needles, and gastrointestinal colonization, rather than environmental sources, constitute the major reservoirs for colonization and potential translation into disease. The rectum is the first and most consistently colonized site. Once a serious nosocomial outbreak has been documented, both personnel and environmental sources must be cultured.

Although colonization occurs within the first few days of admission to the newborn intensive care unit (NICU), disease, if it develops, usually does so late in the second week of hospitalization (10–12 days).

Eradication of MRB from the NICU requires removing all environmental sources of bacteria, cohorting patients and staff into a bacteria-exposed group and a new patient group, giving meticulous care to handwashing between patients, and daily bacteriological surveillance of the new patient group.

The translation from colonization to disease is multifactorial. Factors that select for disease are prematurity, prolonged hospitalization, multiple courses of antibiotic therapy, and the use of vascular catheters and/or central lines.

The primary microbial reservoir is the colonized patient. The major vehicle of dissemination is the hands of the medical personnel among others.

When a previously colonized or infected in-patient is readmitted to the hospital, appropriate microbiological surveillance is indicated.

Management of Nosocomial Clustering of Disease Due to MRB

1. The affected unit should be closed to further admissions.
2. All patients with known or suspected infection must be isolated (glove–gown–stool); their cohort contacts (by common nursing personnel) must also be separated physically from the rest of the noninfected part of the unit and assumed to be infected until proven otherwise.
3. Any nursing personnel who have had contact with known or suspected cases must be restricted from further contact with presumed uninfected infants until the outbreak has been defined and controlled, and they have been proven culture negative. There is no objection to permitting them to care for culture-proven cases; however, they should not, under any circumstances, be assigned to adult outpatient care units.
4. Upon establishment of the above control measures, an epidemiologic investigation, in accordance with the discussion above, seeking the factor or factors responsible for the outbreak should be carried out. This usually will permit the enactment of further, even more specific measures aimed at rapidly curtailing the epidemic. Handwashing before and after administering care to every patient must be strongly reemphasized.
5. Microbiologic surveillance of the patient population should be carried out and environmental culture studies performed after the above activities have been satisfactorily launched.

6. Upon discharge of the affected cohort (and control of the outbreak), a thorough terminal disinfection of the involved area is advocated.

Management of the Individual Patient with MRB

Once a patient is identified as being colonized by a multiresistant gram-negative bacteria, the individual is placed on "antibiotic resistance precaution." The guidelines include the following:

1. Room: one or two beds, no roommate with drainage tubes or Foley catheter.
2. Gowns: not necessary.
3. Masks: not necessary.
4. Hands: must be washed on entering and leaving room, even when gloves are worn.
5. Gloves: must be worn for all patient or secretion contact. Double gloving advocated if it is necessary to do endotracheal suctioning.
6. Articles: must have own urine measuring cup. All sections and contaminated articles should be discarded in plastic bag.

Contemporary strategies to prevent and control multiple drug-resistant nosocomial infections continue to rely on traditional control measures,

1. handwashing,
2. bacterial surveillance,
3. cohortation, and
4. isolation procedures,

to interrupt serial transmission of endemic pathogens in hospitals.

KNOWN OR PRESUMED NEEDLE-STICK EXPOSURE TO HBSAG

There are no prospective studies directly testing the efficacy of a combination of hepatitis B immune globulin (human) (HBIG) and RECOMBIVAX HB® in preventing clinical hepatitis B following percutaneous, ocular, or mucous membrane exposure to hepatitis B virus. However, since most persons with such exposures (e.g., health-care workers) are candidates for RECOMBIVAX HB® and since HBIG (human) plus vaccine is more efficacious than HBIG (human) alone in perinatal exposures, the following guidelines are recommended for persons who have been exposed to hepatitis B virus through

1. percutaneous (needle-stick), ocular, mucous membrane exposure to blood known or presumed to contain hepatitis B surface antigens (HBsAg),
2. human bites by known or presumed HBsAg carriers, that penetrate the skin, or
3. following intimate sexual contact with known or presumed HBsAg carriers.

HBIG (human) (0.06 mL/kg) should be given intramuscularly as soon as possible after exposure and within 24 hours if possible. RECOMBIVAX HB® should be given intramuscularly at a separate site within seven days of exposure, and the second and third doses should be given one and six months, respectively, after the first dose.

RECOMBIVAX HB® is for intramuscular injection. The deltoid muscle is the preferred site for intramuscular injection in adults. Data suggest that injections given in the buttocks frequently are given into fatty tissue instead of into muscle. Such injections have resulted in a lower seroconversion rate than was expected. The anterolateral thigh is the recommended site for intramuscular injection in infants and young children.

Recommendations for Hospital Employees Pricked by Needles

A. For an employee stuck by a needle from a known hepatitis B (HBsAg+) patient:
   1. Draw a sample of the employee's blood for determinations of SGOT, SGPT, HBsAg, and anti-HBs.
   2. If the employee is
      a. negative for both HBsAg and anti-HBs, give HBIG 0.06 mL/kg within seven days after exposure and again 28 to 30 days after exposure;
      b. HBsAg positive or has anti-HBs, there is no need to administer hyperimmune globulin.
   3. Draw follow-up blood samples at two and six months after exposure for retesting of SGOT, SGPT, HBsAg, and anti-HBs.
   4. No tetanus toxoid is necessary.
B. For an employee stuck by a needle from a patient who does not have hepatitis and is known to be HBsAg negative:
   1. Reconfirm the patient's HBsAg status.
   2. If the patient is
      a. reconfirmed to be HBsAg negative, no treatment is necessary for the employee;
      b. HBsAg positive, follow procedure I.
C. For an employee stuck by a needle from a patient with hepatitis or other active liver disease whose HBsAg status is unknown or is known to be negative:
   1. If the patient is HBsAg negative:
      a. Reconfirm the patient's HBsAg status. If negative, continue as listed below in b, c, and d. If the patient is HBsAg positive, follow procedure I.
      b. Draw blood from the employee for baseline SGPT, SGOT, and HBsAg values.
      c. Give standard immune serum globulin 0.02 mL/kg as soon as possible.
      d. Draw blood for follow-up SGOT, SGPT, and HBsAg testing at four to six weeks after exposure.
   2. If the patient's HBsAg status is unknown:
      a. Draw a sample of the patient's blood for HBsAg testing.
      b. If the patient's HBsAg is negative, follow procedure III, 1. If the patient's HBsAg is positive, follow procedure I.
      c. If the patient's HBsAg status cannot be determined, the employee must be treated as though the patient is HBsAg positive. Follow procedure I.
D. For an employee stuck by a needle of unknown origin (e.g., a needle poking through a trash bag):

1. Give tetanus toxoid if the employee has not had a tetanus booster within five to ten years (because of possible soil contamination).
2. Give HBIG as in procedure I. Although the chances are only about 1% to 2% that a needle of unknown origin came from a person who is HBsAg positive the risks associated with the administration of HBIG are so low that it seems prudent to treat the exposed individual. If the employee already has anti-HBs or HBsAg in the serum, treatment with hyperimmune globulin appears to be unnecessary. HBIG costs about $30/mL and its use should be restricted to situations in which it is indicated, as outlined here. The immune globulin should be administered within seven days after exposure.

POST-NEEDLE STICK EXPOSURE PROPHYLAXIS TO HIV

Appropriate exposure management is an important element of workplace safety for preventing occupationally acquired HIV infection.

The average risk for HIV infection from all types of reported percutaneous exposures to HIV-infected blood is approximately 0.3%. In case–control studies, risk is increased for a device previously placed in the source patient's vein or artery (e.g., a needle used for phlebotomy).

Postexposure Prophylaxis

On a global level, triple antiretroviral therapy is becoming standard postexposure prophylaxis (PEP) for HIV needle-stick exposure. Antiretroviral agents from all three classes of drugs currently licensed for first-line therapy of HIV are nucleoside analog reverse transcriptase inhibitors, nonnucleoside reverse transcriptase inhibitors, and proteinase inhibitors. Zidovudine is the only drug for which there is evidence of a reduction in the risk of HIV transmission after occupational exposure. No antiretroviral drugs have been specifically licensed for PEP. Antiretroviral drugs are prescribed for PEP on an "off-label" basis since their use in this context is outside approved indications. In HIV-infected patients, combination drug therapy has been shown to be more effective than zidovudine alone in reducing viral load. In theory, a combination of drugs should increase the potency of PEP and offer increased protection, given the increasing prevalence of resistance to zidovudine and other antiretroviral drugs.

Currently recommended drugs for PEP starter packs are
■ zidovudine 250 mg or 300 mg b.d.
  plus
■ lamivudine 150 mg b.d.
  plus
■ nelfinavir 1250 mg b.d. (or 750 mg t.d.s.).
Other drug combinations can be used predicated upon advances in HIV therapeutics, potential side effects, adverse drug reactions, and/or adverse drug interactions. Any drug regimen should take into account the following:
■ Whether the health-care worker is or may be pregnant
■ Whether the health-care worker has an existing medical condition (i.e., diabetes mellitus)
■ Whether potential drug interaction with other medication is present
■ Whether there is a possibility that the virus may be resistant to one or more of the drugs

As newer antiretroviral drugs develop, it is likely that other drugs will become the preferred regimen for PEP.

Recommendations are provisional because they are based on limited data regarding the efficacy and toxicity of PEP and risk for HIV infection after different types of exposure. Because most occupational exposures to HIV do not result in infection transmission, potential toxicity must be carefully considered when prescribing PEP. When possible, these recommendations should be implemented in consultation with persons having expertise in antiretroviral therapy and HIV transmission. Changes in drug regimens may be appropriate, based on factors such as the probable antiretroviral drug resistance profile of HIV from the source patient, local availability of drugs, and medical conditions, concurrent drug therapy, and drug toxicity in the exposed worker.

1. Chemoprophylaxis should be recommended to exposed workers after occupational exposures associated with the highest risk for HIV transmission. For exposures with a lower, but nonnegligible, risk, PEP should be offered, balancing the lower risk against the use of drugs having uncertain efficacy and toxicity. For exposures with negligible risk, PEP is not justified. Exposed workers should be informed that (a) knowledge about the efficacy and toxicity of PEP is limited; (b) for agents other than zidovudine, data are limited regarding toxicity in persons without HIV infection or who are pregnant; and (c) any or all drugs for PEP may be declined by the exposed worker.
2. PEP should be initiated promptly, preferably within one to two hours postexposure. Although animal studies suggest that PEP probably is not effective when started later than 24 to 36 hours postexposure, the interval after which there is no benefit from PEP for humans is undefined. Initiating therapy after a longer interval (e.g., one to two weeks) may be considered for the highest risk exposures; even if infection is not prevented, early treatment of acute HIV infection may be beneficial. The optimal duration of PEP is unknown. Because four weeks of zidovudine appeared protective, PEP should probably be administered for four weeks, if tolerated.
3. If the source patient or the patient's HIV status is unknown, initiating PEP should be decided on a case-by-case basis, based on the exposure risk and likelihood of HIV infection in known or possible source patients. If additional information becomes available, decisions about PEP can be modified.
4. Workers with occupational exposures to HIV should receive follow-up counseling and medical evaluation,

including HIV antibody tests at baseline and periodically for at least six months postexposure (e.g., 6 weeks, 12 weeks, and 6 months), and should observe precautions to prevent possible secondary transmission. If PEP is used, drug toxicity monitoring should include a complete blood count and renal and hepatic chemical function tests at baseline and two weeks after starting PEP. If subjective or objective toxicity is noted, dose reduction or drug substitution should be considered with expert consultation, and further diagnostic studies may be indicated.

Pregnancy

Pregnancy does not preclude the use of PEP. Expert advice should always be sought if PEP is considered for a female health-care worker who is pregnant. The available evidence is that zidovudine and lamivudine are not contraindicated in the second and third trimesters of pregnancy. A pregnant health-care worker who has experienced an occupational exposure should be counseled about the risks of HIV infection, about the risks for transmission to her baby, and about everything known and not known about the benefits and risks of antiretroviral therapy for her and her baby when offering PEP.

CDC GUIDELINES—UNIVERSAL PRECAUTIONS

Since medical history and examination cannot reliably identify all patients infected with HIV or other blood-borne pathogens, blood and body fluid precautions should be consistently used for all patients (Tables 5–7).

TABLE 5 Blood and body fluid precautions

(1) Blood and other specimens should be labeled prominently with a special warning, such as "Blood and Body Fluid Precautions" along with the lab or specimen sheets. If the outside of the specimen container is visibly contaminated with blood or body fluids, it should be cleansed with household bleach and water (1:10 dilution). Bleach solution should be mixed and labeled for this purpose. All blood specimens should be placed in a second container, such as an impervious bag, for transport. The bag or container should be examined carefully for cracks or leaks

(2) Pap smear slides should be given a "Precaution" label and placed in an empty Pap smear box that is also labeled. The box should then be placed in an impervious bag and taken to the lab. The Pap requisition should be labeled "Blood and Body Fluid Precautions"

(3) Blood spills, body fluids, and secretions should be cleaned up promptly with a disinfectant solution of household bleach and water. Disposable gloves should be worn

(4) Infectious waste hampers should be utilized for disposal of infectious waste (excluding sharps, liquid body wastes, linen, and instruments). Lined infectious waste hampers with infectious waste bags on the inside and clear autoclave bags on the outside are advocated

(5) All contaminated linen should be placed in a water-soluble bag first and then into the nylon linen bag, which is then taken to the area's respective dirty linen room

(6) Examination tables should be wiped down (using the bleach solution) in between patients when soiled with body secretions or fluids

TABLE 6 Contact precautions

(1) Hands should be washed with antimicrobial soap (e.g., Betadine, Hibiclens) and water before entering and leaving room and, if wearing gown and gloves, after removing them

(2) Hands should be washed thoroughly and immediately if they become contaminated with blood or body fluids

(3) Avoid contact of open skin lesions with materials from HIV-positive patients. Wear gloves if lesions are present

(4) Gloves should be worn when handling blood specimens, blood-soiled items, body fluids, excretions, and secretions, as well as all surfaces, materials, and objects exposed to them (e.g., vaginal discharge, amniotic fluid)

(5) Gowns should be worn when clothing may become soiled with body fluids, blood, or excretions

1. All health-care workers should routinely use appropriate barrier precautions to prevent skin and mucous membrane exposure when contact with blood or other body fluids of any patient is anticipated. Gloves should be changed after contact with each patient.

2. Hands and other skin surfaces should be washed immediately and thoroughly if contaminated with blood or other body fluids. Hands should be washed immediately after gloves are removed.

3. All health-care workers should take precautions to prevent injuries caused by needles, scalpels, and other sharp instruments or devices during procedures; when cleaning used instruments; during disposal of used needles; and when handling sharp instruments after procedures.

4. Although saliva has not been implicated in HIV transmission, to minimize the need for emergency mouth-to-mouth resuscitation, mouthpieces or other ventilation devices should be available for use in areas in which the need for resuscitation is predictable.

5. Health-care workers who have exudative lesions or weeping dermatitis should refrain from all direct patient care and from handling patient care equipment until the condition resolves.

6. Pregnant health-care workers are not known to be at greater risk of contracting HIV infection compared to health-care workers who are not pregnant.

TABLE 7 Biosafety policy and procedures for the handling and transportation of blood and biological fluids

(1) All specimens are transported in sealed plastic bags
(2) Leaking specimens are discarded immediately
(3) Needles are never clipped, bent, or recapped after use. Immediately after use, needles and syringes are placed in special puncture-resistant containers
(4) Personnel wear gloves whenever handling blood or body fluid specimens, regardless of the patient's diagnosis. Individuals with cuts or other lesions on the hands must protect the affected areas with finger cots or gloves at all times while working in the laboratory
(5) Masks, gowns, and protective eye coverings are required only in unusual circumstances when splashing is considered likely
(6) Any employee who has had an accidental exposure to blood or other potentially infectious material is referred to the Employee Health Service for examination, further testing, and treatment as needed (e.g., hepatitis B immune globulin)

SELECTED READING

Bridson EY. Iatrogenic epidemics of puerperal fever in the 18th and 19th centuries. Br J Biomed Sci 1996; 53:134.

CDC. Guidelines for prevention of transmission of human immunodeficiency virus and hepatitis B virus to healthcare and public safety workers. MMWR 1989; 38:31.

Craven DE, Steger KA, Barber TW. Preventing nosocomial pneumonia: state-of-the-art perspectives for the 1990's. Am J Med 1991; 91:44s.

Gould D. Nurses' hands as vectors of hospital-acquired infection: a review. J Adv Nurs 1991; 15:1216.

Grosserode MH, Wenzel RP. The continuing importance of staphylococci as major hospital pathogens. J Hosp Infect 1991; 19(Suppl B):p3.

Haley RW. Nosocomial infections in surgical patients: developing valid measures of intrinsic patient risk. Am J Med 1991; 91:145s.

Hershow RC, Khayr WF, Smith NL. A comparison of clinical virulence of nosocomially-acquired methicillin-resistant and methicillin-sensitive Staphylococcus aureus infection in a university hospital. Infect Control Hosp Epidemiol 1992; 13:587.

Howard AJ. Nosocomial spread of Haemophilus influenzae. J Hosp Infect 1991; 19:1.

Hu DJ, Kane MA, Heymann DL. Transmission of HIV, hepatitis B virus, and other blood borne pathogens in health care settings: a review of risk factors and guidelines for prevention. Bull World Health Org 1992; 69:623.

Hudson CN. Nosocomial infection and infection control procedure. Baillieres Clin Obstet Gynecol 1992; 6:137.

Koontz FP. A review of traditional resistance surveillance methodologies and infection control. Diagn Microbial Infect Dis 1992; 15:43s.

Monif GRG. Nosocomial infection due to multiresistant bacteria. Infect Dis Lttrs Obstet Gynecol 1984; 6:53.

Monif GRG. Neonatal nosocomial infection of special importance to obstetrics. Infect Dis Lttrs Obstet Gynecol 1984; 6:59.

Nathens AB, Chu PT, Marshall JC. Nosocomial infection in the surgical intensive care unit. Infect Dis Clin North Am 1992; 6:657.

Polin RA. What's new about newborns? Curr Probl Pediatr 1991; 21:333.

Polin RA, St Geme JW 3rd. Neonatal sepsis. Adv Pediatr Infect Dis 1992; 7:25.

Prutsachativuthi S. Microbiology for surveillance of nosocomial infections. J Med Assn Thai 1992; 75(Suppl 2):48.

Smith PW, Rusnak PG. APIC guideline for infection prevention and control in the long-term care facility. Am J Infect Control 1991; 19:198.

Tenover FC. Novel and emerging mechanisms of antimicrobial resistance in nosocomial pathogens. Am J Med 1991; 91:76s.

Weinstein RA. Epidemiology and control of nosocomial infections in adult care units. Am J Med 1991; 91:179s.

Methicillin-Resistant Staphylococci

Abdo RA, Araj GF, Talhouk RS. Methicillin resistant Staphylococcus aureus (MRSA): disease spectrum, biological characteristics, resistant mechanisms, and typing methods. J Med Liban 1996; 44:21.

Ayliffe GA. The progressive intercontinental spread of methicillin-resistant Staphylococcus aureus. Clin Infect Dis 1997; 24(Suppl 1):S74.

Boyce JM. Should we vigorously try to contain and control methicillin-resistant Staphylococcus aureus? Infect Control Hosp Epidemiol 1991; 12:46.

Boyce JM. Strategies for controlling methicillin-resistant Staphylococcus aureus in hospitals. J Chemother 1995; 7(Suppl 3):81s.

Chambers HF. Detection of methicillin-resistant staphylococci. Infect Dis Clin North Am 1993; 7:425.

de Lencastre H, de Jonge BL, Matthews PR. Molecular aspects of methicillin-resistance in Staphylococcus aureus. J Antimicrob Chemother 1994; 33:7.

Department of Health. Standard principles for preventing hospital acquired infections. J Hosp Infect 2001; 47:21s.

Gould D, Chamberlaine A. Staphylococcus aureus: a review of the literature. J Clin Nurs 1995; 4:5.

Hill RL, Casewell MW. Nasal carriage of MRSA the role of mupirocin and outlook for resistance. Drugs Exp Clin Res 1990; 1(8):397.

Hosein IK. Wound infection. 2. MRSA. J Wound Care 1996; 5:388.

Martln MA. Methicillin-resistant Staphylococcus aureus: the persistent resistant nosocomial pathogen. Curr Clin Top Infect Dis 1994; 14:170.

Miller MA, Dascal A, Portnoy J, et al. Development of mupirocin resistance among methicillin-resistant Staphylococcus aureus after widespread use of nasal mupirocin ointment. Infect Control Hosp Epidemiol 1996; 17:811.

Mulazimoglu L, Drenning SD, Muder RR. Vancomycin-gentamicin synergism revisited: effect of gentamicin susceptibllity of methicllin-resistant. Antimicrob Agents Chemother 1996; 40:1534.

Netto-dos-Santos KR, de-Souza-Fonseca L, Gontijo-Filho PP. Emergence of high-level mupirocin resistance in methicillin-resistant Staphylococcus aureus isolated from Brazilian university hospitals [see comments]. Comment in: Infect Control Hosp Epidemiol 1996; 17:775.

Perry C. Methicillin-resistant Staphylococcus aureus. J Wound Care 1996; 5:31.

Pujol M, Pena C, Pallares R, et al. Nosocomial Staphylococcus aureus bacteremia among nasal carriers of methicillin-resistant and methicillin-susceptible strains. Am J Med 1996; 100:509.

HIV Chemoprophylaxis

Cardo DM, Culver DH, Ciesielski CA, et al. A case-control study of HIV seroconversion in health care workers after percutaneous exposure. N Engl J Med 1997; 337:1485.

CDC. Public Health Service statement on management of occupational exposure to human immunodeficiency virus, including considerations regarding zidovudine postexposure use. MMWR 1990; 39:RR1.

CDC. Case control study of HIV seroconversion in health-care workers after percutaneous exposure to HIV-infected blood—France, United Kingdom, and United States. MMWR 1995; 44:929.

CDC. Update: Provisional Public Health Service recommendations for chemoprophylaxis after occupational exposure to HIV. MMWR 1996; 45:468.

Gerberding JL. Management of occupational exposures to bloodborne viruses. N Engl J Med 1995; 332:444.

Hawkins DA, Asboe D, Barlow K, Evans B. Seroconversion to HIV-1 following a needlestick injury despite combination postexposure prophylaxis. J Infection 2001; 44:12.

HIV post-exposure prophylaxis: guidance from UK Chief Medical Officers' Expert Advisory Group on AIDS. London: Department of Health, February 2004.

Kinloch-de Löess S. Hirschel BJ, Hoen B, et al. A controlled trial of zidovudine in primary human immunodeficiency virus infection. N Engl J Med 1995; 333:408.

Postoperative Infections 74

Mark G. Martens

INTRODUCTION

Pelvic operations are some of the most common procedures performed in the United States today. Surveys have demonstrated that hysterectomy was the second most frequently performed surgical procedure among reproductive-aged women during the past decade. They often require incisions made through contaminated tissue, and thus are at high risk for developing postoperative infections.

The source, the species, and mechanisms whereby infection is established in pelvic surgery has been poorly understood in the past, as many principles are unique to gynecology and do not routinely follow abdominal surgery principles. However, recent research has demonstrated many of the mechanisms whereby infection is established, and with this knowledge, such infection can be more effectively treated or prevented. Despite this knowledge, and because of the often contaminated nature of pelvic surgery (especially vaginal surgery), pelvic postoperative infections are still commonplace and must be addressed if serious postoperative morbidity and mortality are to be avoided. Ledger and Child (1973), and others, have demonstrated that postoperative fever developed in 31% and 38% of abdominal and vaginal hysterectomies, respectively. As a corollary, antibiotics were administered in 45% and 54% of abdominal and vaginal hysterectomies, respectively. Infectious morbidity, defined as postoperative fever plus clinical indications of infection, have been reported following approximately 35% of vaginal and 20% of abdominal hysterectomies. There is infectious morbidity with not only hysterectomy, but also with other pelvic surgery, and these will be discussed as well.

An understanding of the etiology, microbiology, prophylaxis, and treatment of pelvic infections is important to gynecologists. Cesarean section and other obstetric-related infections, while similar in microbiology, have very different etiologic and mechanical considerations and are discussed elsewhere. Also, nonpelvic sources of fever and infections such as pneumonia, urinary tract infections, etc., are similar to other surgical procedures, and thus the main focus in this chapter will be on operative site (pelvic) infections.

ETIOLOGY

Hysterectomy

Hysterectomy, often thought of as one uniform procedure, is actually two or more very different procedures with respect to infectious morbidity. Although abdominal and vaginal hysterectomies have very different routes of access, both eventually entail surgical entry into the vagina. A recently described and more common alternative is the supracervical laparoscopic hysterectomy, which does not enter the vaginal cavity, and holds promise for decreasing infectious morbidity. However, this is a technically more difficult procedure, and thus comparative studies with respect to operative morbidity will need to be conducted.

Abdominal hysterectomy, because of its initial entry through a hopefully uninflamed abdominal incision, is often misclassified as a "clean" procedure. However, the ultimate incision into the vagina for removal of the cervix and uterine specimen generally results in gross contamination of the pelvic cavity by the vaginal flora. Thus, abdominal hysterectomy is now classified as "clean-contaminated," and surgical surveys have demonstrated an infection rate of approximately 10%. However, clean-contaminated procedures exclude cases with "significant spillage," and the amount of contaminated fluid at the vaginal cuff is often times significant in abdominal hysterectomies, and is persistent in vaginal hysterectomies, thereby resulting in higher infection rates.

Such procedures with gross spillage or those performed in an inflamed area are classified "contaminated," and typically have an infection rate of approximately 20%. Surgeries classified as "dirty" procedures are those in which there is a perforated viscus, association with trauma, or purulent material in the operative field. "Dirty" operations with pus present from a tubo-ovarian abscess or pyosalpinx, or reoperations for pelvic abscess, are examples most likely encountered by gynecologists, and the infection rates are 25% or higher, despite antibiotic administration at surgery. Therefore, most abdominal hysterectomies are clean-contaminated or contaminated, and infections such as pelvic inflammatory disease (PID), abscess, etc., are classified as "dirty." In vaginal hysterectomy, the opposite of what occurs in abdominal hysterectomy takes place. Instead of a relatively clean procedure that concludes in a contaminated area (vagina), vaginal hysterectomies begin in a contaminated space, then progress into a sterile environment that is repeatedly contaminated over a period of one or more hours.

After the removal of the uterus, with either hysterectomy route, whether the surgeon should leave the vaginal cuff open, thus allowing drainage, or close the cuff to prevent further vaginal bacterial contamination is a subject of great debate. Although there has been no definitive answer, it is best to look at the immediate outcomes versus late complications in order to decide whether to leave the cuff open. With a closed cuff, continuous drainage is prevented; however, potential bacterial growth media (blood and serous fluid) can accumulate. Contamination from the vagina, if it has not occurred in significant amounts, may not infect such media, and serious infection, such as an abscess, may be avoided.

However, if significant contamination has occurred prior to closure, the developing infection is contained, drainage is prevented, and abscess or an infected hematoma may occur.

If the vaginal cuff is left open, drainage occurs continuously, and exposure of the operative site to persistent bacterial contamination is possible. However, drainage is one of the most important methods to treat or avoid infection, and if an abscess does develop, there is easy access for culture sample collection and further drainage. In a study, Martens et al. (1990) utilized a hysterectomy surgical cuff stapler, which isolated, incised, and closed the vaginal cuff with dissolvable staples simultaneously. The theory behind this strategy was to reduce the contamination of the lower pelvic cavity, decrease necrotic tissue (the staples compress less than 0.5 cm of tissue), and decrease blood loss. The study demonstrated a statistically lower postoperative infection rate; however, adequate exposure was necessary, and difficulty in drainage of abscesses (albeit at a significantly lower incidence) was noted.

Preventing the contamination of the surgical field is also one of the benefits of laparoscopically assisted supracervical hysterectomies (LASH), as the cervix is maintained and the vagina is not entered. Care must be taken to treat or cauterize the remaining endocervical canal without contaminating the pelvic cavity in the process.

Infection rates in laparoscopic supracervical hysterectomies do appear to be lower; however, large studies do not exist to compare other sources of morbidity. There exists the need to distinguish between LASH and laparoscopically assisted vaginal hysterectomies (LAV), wherein the vagina is incised to permit removal of the specimen, and thus contamination can occur at this time. The theoretical benefit, though, is that the entire procedure is not done through the contaminated vagina over one or more hours, and that the potential contamination occurs much later in the procedure. In the LASH procedure, the uterine specimen is morcellated and removed via the laparoscopic trocar, thus never requiring an incision directly into the vagina.

For all postoperative infections, there are three main factors—bacteria, growth media, and host immune responses—that determine infection and its extent. While specific species will be discussed in the microbiology section, the origin and the quantity of bacteria are important and can vary. In abdominal hysterectomy, there are low numbers of organisms on the patient's skin in the abdominal area, and they are the source for the subsequent development of an abdominal wound infection. The rate of abdominal wound infections is generally low, with a threshold set less than 5% by most quality assurance hospital committees. Certain factors are known to increase the rate in larger studies, including shaving of the skin the previous evening, operating in an infected area of the skin, and hypothermia. Additional factors that may increase wound infection rates are excessive use of electrocautery, excessive use of subcutaneous stitches (foreign body), and increased duration of surgery. Factors that have been demonstrated to help in decreasing wound infections include adequate skin decontamination/preparation, maintaining normal body temperature, wound lavage, and, in some studies, intravenous antibiotic prophylaxis.

The next factor relating to infectious morbidity in abdominal hysterectomies is related to the pelvic surgical procedure. Several studies have demonstrated that one of the strongest predictors of low infectious morbidity is good surgical technique. Good surgical technique decreases the second main factor in the development of all infections, that of growth media. Bacteria that gain access to the normally sterile pelvic cavity are maintained by and proliferate in the presence of a nutritional environment suited to their growth requirements. Blood, serum, and necrotic tissue are excellent growth media for all bacteria. The presence or lack of oxygen can determine the species that predominate, either facultative anaerobic (often referred to as aerobes) or obligate anaerobes.

Poor surgical technique can result in increased bleeding. It can also result in excess necrotic tissue from large avascular pedicles, excessively electrocauterized tissue, or excessively large or frequent foreign body use (suture, graft, etc.). Even with excellent surgical technique, there will still be avascular pedicles present, and serous and hematogenous accumulations will be present postoperatively. These sites for potential infections can become contaminated. Although occasionally it may be from bacteria originating from the abdominal incision, it almost always originates from the cervico-vaginal flora that is encountered when the uterus is excised. Since the vagina is not sterile, all vaginal cuffs are therefore contaminated. Also, since all intra-abdominal and pelvic blood and serous fluid will gravitate to the lowest part of the pelvis when the patient is upright and ambulatory, the vaginal cuff almost always has adequate nutrients to sustain bacterial growth. Healing of the vaginal cuff entails a proliferation of all of the inflammatory cells and fibroblasts, which in essence creates a cuff cellulitis. An inflammatory response is actually required for healing, and therefore is a normal response. However, persistent bacterial growth in this area or inadequate immunologic response will lead to worsening cellulitis, resulting in increasingly serious infections such as a pelvic cellulitis or pelvic phlegmon. Extension into thrombosed vessels may also lead to septic pelvic thrombophlebitis. The presence of infected fluid in an enclosed space often created by an extensive inflammatory response and fibroblast proliferation (adhesions) can result in an infected hematoma or vaginal cuff abscess.

The same process occurs in vaginal hysterectomy. However, since the bacterial contamination starts early in the procedure and is often of greater magnitude, a higher incidence of postoperative infection is often seen. Thus, the rate in premenopausal women is generally high enough to warrant routine surgical prophylaxis for vaginal hysterectomy.

Infections in other pelvic surgical procedures depend upon the source of bacterial contamination and the extent and location of the surgical site.

Ovarian Surgery

The ovary is a site for serious infections under certain conditions. The ovaries do not generally become infected if they are left intact following a hysterectomy or other pelvic procedures. However, if the capsule is violated, as with incision or drainage of a cyst or biopsy, any bacteria present may result in an infection. Once the ovary is infected, it is not uncommon for it to progress to abscess formation, causing the need for reoperation and removal. Even pelvic procedures, which do not affect the ovary itself, may result in serious ovarian infection, such as was demonstrated over a half century ago by the development of serious ovarian abscesses following colpotomy tubal ligations. It was determined that ovulation and the subsequent rupture of the ovarian capsule allowed the entrance of bacteria into the ovarian tissue, especially in vaginal surgical procedures.

It is important to attempt to schedule elective surgical procedures, if possible, into the late luteal phase in ovulating women so that the ovaries will be spared. It is also important to avoid penetrating the capsule unless absolutely necessary. Therefore, the practice of needle drainage of small ovarian cysts is not recommended and should be avoided if possible.

Myomectomy

Myomectomy is another pelvic procedure that has a high incidence rate and seriousness of infection. This is a result of the extensive blood supply of the myoma, and the difficulty in achieving hemostasis. The combination of extensive use of foreign body (suture) and necrosis to achieve hemostasis, and the presence of fibroid and serous fluid lead to a fertile area for bacterial contamination to flourish. Fortunately, since the vagina is not entered such as with a hysterectomy, exogenous bacteria from the abdominal incision are few in number and usually do not cause infection. However, if the endometrial cavity is penetrated with the removal of the myoma, contamination from crevice-vaginal flora that has entered the endometrial cavity can occur.

Laparoscopy

Most pelvic operative laparoscopic procedures may leave behind blood and necrotic tissue, but fortunately, bacterial contamination is usually minimal. However, because of the increased difficulty of these procedures, and the limited access for evaluation of the pelvis prior to closing, perforation of a viscus may occur. The bacterial contamination resulting from these procedures is often devastating, as the patient often is an outpatient, and early signs and symptoms of infection are missed with the patient at home. When the patient is rehospitalized, extensive infection and/or abscess formation is often present, requiring extensive debridement, drainage, and repair.

Hysteroscopy

Infections after hysteroscopy are less frequent, due to relatively minimal tissue damage and the presence of endocervical drainage. However, uterine ablation can leave an extensive necrotic area, which can easily get infected if bacteria are present, or perforation into the pelvic cavity can occur incidentally or with large myoma or septum removal. Bacteria present in the hysteroscopic distension fluid or postoperatively from the crevice-vaginal flora can cause uterine or pelvic infection, and need to be considered in a

patient with fever and/or pelvic pain. However, infection from transcervical fluid administration is rare with hysteroscopy, but has been reported with hysterosalpingograms, as the goal of the procedure is to get past the uterine cavity also.

Dilatation and Curettage

Although dilatation and curettage (D&C) is classified as a relatively minor procedure, infections following D&C are not uncommon. These infections are due to the transvaginal nature of the procedures, resulting in contamination by cervico-vaginal flora of the endometrial cavity (now disrupted by curettage) and an increased likelihood of tissue invasion. The resulting infection is an endometritis, which may spread if not recognized early or progress to parametritis or abscess if poor endocervical drainage allows the build-up of blood and necrotic debris.

Tubal Ligation

As mentioned earlier, serious infection can occur with poorly timed colpotomy ligation procedures; however, the rate of infection from the abdominal approach is generally low. Laparoscopic site infections are more common than extensive pelvic procedures, but they can occur and are often associated with a hematoma that may occur at the ligation site or within the broad ligament.

MICROBIOLOGY

Just as the source of the bacteria in gynecologic infections is different from other procedures, the specific species are also different. Therefore, an understanding of the organisms responsible for postoperative infections is important, so that the most appropriate therapy can be utilized. Again, most cases of postoperative pelvic infections originate from the cervico-vaginal flora and are most often polymicrobial in nature. Numerous studies have demonstrated the wide variety of pathogens recovered from patients diagnosed with postoperative pelvic infections. Table 1 is a computation of the antibiotic used in clinical trials done to attain Food and Drug Administration approval for treatment of postoperative gynecological infections. Ohm and Galask (1957) studied the microbiology of 100 patients prior to hysterectomy and found that the most frequent organisms present were gram-positive

TABLE I Recommended parenteral therapy of pelvic infections

	Dose/interval
Piperacillin–tazobactam (Zosyn)	3.75 g q6 h or 4.5 g q8 h
Imipenem–cilastatin (Primaxin)	500 mg q6–8 h
Ampicillin–sulbactam (Unasyn)	3 g q6 h
Ticarcillin–clavulanate (Timentin)	3.1 g q6 h
Levofloxacin (Levaquin)	500 mg q24 h
Clindamycin–gentamicin (Cleocin)	800 mg q8 h plus 5–7 mg/kg q24 h
Meropenem (Merem)	1 g q24 h
Cefoxitin (Mefoxin)	2 g q6 h
Clindamycin–aztreonam (Cleocin–Azactam)	800 mg q8 h admix 500 mg q8 h

cocci, gram-negative rods, and anaerobes, in that order. Microbiological studies of the post-prophylaxis vaginal bacterial flora have demonstrated the preponderance of enterococci and gram-negative bacteria.

The recovery of a variety of organisms in infected patients mimics that in animal studies performed first by Gorbach and then by Martens (1989) and colleagues a decade later. In these studies, inoculums of aerobes, with or without anaerobes, were implanted into rat abdomens and pelvises to ascertain the natural history of abdominal and pelvic infections. Implanted aerobic organisms routinely resulted in severe peritonitis, and a significant increase in abscess development followed in those rats that also had anaerobes implanted. Gorbach's model utilized intra-abdominal pathogens, and Martens' experiments utilized pathogens isolated from female pelvic infections.

This "anaerobic progression" model, whether with pathogens such as the enteric aerobes and Bacteroides fragilis in Gorbach's model or a variety of enterococci or gram-negative rods plus Prevotella bivia and the anaerobic streptococci in the Martens' model, supports the theory of an early aerobic inflammatory response that alters the environment through a change in the pH, redox potential, and reduced oxygenation to create a favorable environment for obligate and facultative anaerobes. This explains in part why prophylactic antibiotics that do not have excellent anaerobic activity still provide adequate prophylaxis, as they interrupt the anaerobic progression at an early stage. However, several studies have demonstrated that when infection is established, using antibiotics that have adequate anaerobic activity is important.

Fortunately, few studies in immunocompetent patients demonstrate the presence of multiply-resistant gram-negatives such as those with extended-spectrum beta-lactamase enzymes (Pseudomonas, Serratia, Halico influenzae) in nononcology gynecology patients. They can be present in patients who have been on long-term antibiotic treatment, especially with cephalosporins, often for urinary tract or skin infections. The most frequently isolated of the multiply-resistant Enterobacteriaceae is Halico Enterobacter cloacae, which is becoming a much more frequent isolate, often after short-course prophylactic regimens with cephazolin or cefoxitin. The enterococci also are becoming much more prevalent, due to the extensive and almost exclusive cephalosporin use for prophylaxis. In most studies, enterococci are recovered in well over 50% to 60% of patients after cephalosporin prophylaxis use. Although the treatment of enterococci may not be essential in all patients when multiple organisms are recovered, it should still be respected as a pathogen and definitely covered if the patient does not respond to adequate broad-spectrum empiric coverage that excludes enterococci activity, such as with clindamycin–gentamicin, cefoxitin, and all other cephalosporins, and even the penicillin–beta-lactamase combination ticarcillin–clavulanate. Adding ampicillin or switching to the beta-lactamase combination of ampicillin–sulbactam or piperacillin–tazobactam provides excellent enterococci coverage.

The anaerobe most studied in intra-abdominal infections, B. fragilis, is a bowel pathogen; however, it is not the most frequent anaerobe found in pelvic infections. The anaerobic streptococci and peptococci are the most frequent gram-positive anaerobes, and P. bivia and P. melaninogenicus are the most frequent gram-negative anaerobes isolated. The Prevotella species were previously classified as Bacteroides species; however, their growth requirements and susceptibility profiles were sufficiently different to justify reclassification. The anaerobic streptococci are highly susceptible to most broad-spectrum cephalosporins and penicillins. However, the gram-negative anaerobes often require specific anaerobic therapy with the penicillin–beta-lactamase combinations, the carbapenems, metronidazole, and then clindamycin, in order of activity.

PROPHYLAXIS

Although much of this discussion will be centered around intravenous antibiotic prophylaxis, other routes or methods have been demonstrated to decrease the incidence of postoperative infection. Swartz and Tanaree in 1976 demonstrated that T-tube suction drainage of the vaginal cuff was as effective as prophylactic antibiotics. Also, endocervical penicillin antibiotics, vaginal metronidazole, and oral trovafloxacin have demonstrated statistically significant efficacies in reducing posthysterectomy infections. However, the most widely utilized prophylactic regimen is intravenous antibiotic administration immediately prior to the gynecologic procedure. Numerous studies have demonstrated the efficacy of dozens of antibiotic regimens. Rather than listing the myriad of options, it is better to review the basic principle of antibiotic prophylaxis initially proposed by Ledger.

The operation should have a significant risk for operative site infection. Although early studies and infectious disease guidelines limited prophylactic antibiotics to premenopausal women undergoing vaginal hysterectomy only, recent large meta-analyses have found that antibiotics benefit both abdominal and vaginal hysterectomy procedures. Also, while the postmenopausal vagina has been found to have a decreased quantity of vaginal flora, hormone therapy and urinary tract conditions have often shown that prophylactic antibiotic usage in this patient population may be helpful. Patients undergoing other procedures that may have significant contamination are administered antibiotic prophylaxis in selected areas. These include D&C, pregnancy termination, myomectomy with penetration into the endometrial cavity, hysterosalpingograms, colpotomy tubal ligations, and intrauterine device removals.

Bacterial contamination by endogenous organisms is to be anticipated. Any procedure whereby the vagina is entered, such as hysterectomy, has a high risk of contamination and should receive prophylaxis. However, abdominal procedures that do not enter the genitourinary tract are usually at low risk of contamination or infection (such as minilaparotomy tubal ligations, endometriosis ablation, or resection, and most laparoscopic procedures) and hence do not require prophylaxis.

The prophylactic antibiotic should have laboratory and clinical evidence of effectiveness against some of the contaminating organisms. Most agents have activity against some, if not many, of the polymicrobial endogenous female flora, and thus have usually shown effectiveness in studies of surgical prophylaxis versus placebo. However, some agents have demonstrated statistical superiority over other antimicrobial agents.

The prophylactic antibiotic should be present in the wound, preferably before incision, and should reach a therapeutic concentration in operative site tissues. Fortunately, most antibiotics are well distributed in the body, and if administered in a timely manner, they reach therapeutic levels. However, some antibiotics do not accumulate in pelvic tissues, such as nitrofurantoin, and thus would not be effective. Also, errors in the time of administration also decrease the antibiotic efficacy. Error in the time of adminsitration due to delays in transportation or induction of anesthesia occurs in up to 50% of cases. Administering the antibiotic once the patient is in the operating room avoids the problem of declining tissue levels, but increases the risk of late administration, resulting in the incision being made before the antibiotic can reach therapeutic levels or is given at all. Several antibiotics have long half-lives and thus delayed time-to-peak levels, and would thereby be poor candidates for prophylaxis. An example is azithromycin, which has a much longer time-to-peak level, and thus would be a poor prophylactic agent. Oral agents used for bowel decontamination and oral vancomycin also are not absorbed significantly enough to be helpful in prophylaxis.

A short course of prophylactic antibiotics should be used. Fortunately, the excessive use of multiple days (sometimes up to several days) of "prophylaxis" administration is found with less frequency. In fact, any prophylaxis with dosage lasting more than 24 hours is technically "treatment" and not prophylaxis. Also, use of repeated smaller doses of prophylaxis makes little sense: why would one expect a subtherapeutic dose that failed to kill a significant number of bacteria initially be of any success at the same subtherapeutic dose several hours later when the bacterial numbers are growing? Most studies have demonstrated that a single dose of antimicrobial prophylaxis is as effective as multiple (usually three) doses. If the operating time is delayed approximately three hours, a second dose of antibiotic should be administered.

Therapeutic agents should be reserved for therapy unless they are demonstrated to be superior to other agents. Antibiotic prophylaxis is not foolproof, and therefore, therapeutic agents to which the patient's pathogenic flora has not been exposed recently would give the patient the best chance of recovery. Few studies have demonstrated superiority, with the exception of the above-mentioned Heinsell study on cefotetan use for hysterectomy prophylaxis. Faro and Martens also demonstrated cefotetan's and piperacillin's superiority over several other prophylactic regimens in cesarean section; however, the use of these agents for prophylaxis, and then treatment of subsequent antibiotic failure, would not be recommended.

The benefits of antibiotic prophylaxis should outweigh the risks. Although in most instances the risk is minimal, the main determinant of choosing a specific antibiotic resides in its efficacy. This efficacy is determined by the factors discussed previously: activity versus pelvic pathogens, tissue penetration, etc. However, there are certain instances where excessive risk for prophylaxis may be present, such as a patient with multiple antibiotic allergies or significant side effects, or such as a rash from sulfa drugs or gentamicin use in a patient with renal failure.

DIAGNOSIS

Once a prophylaxis fails or was not utilized, a postoperative infection must be diagnosed properly before treatment can be chosen. The sign most commonly used by almost all physicians is temperature elevations postoperatively. Postoperative white blood cell (WBC) counts are also often checked. However, they are often mildly elevated, and are rarely acted upon independent of fever. Postoperative pain is an expected sign, and even if present in a heightened fashion, it is not indicative only of infection. Low-grade fevers between 37.5°C and 40°C are often present early in the postoperative course. Following extensive pelvic surgery, such as with hysterectomy, it is usually the result of the inflammatory healing process and vaginal cuff contamination that invariably occurs in all such procedures. This is described by Hemsell and others as "cuff cellulitis," and when it progresses, it rarely causes significant fever or clinical symptoms to warrant antibiotic therapy. In cuff cellulitis, the vaginal cuff is erythematous and mildly edematous, may ooze a slightly purulent or serosanguineous discharge, and will be mildly to moderately tender. However, these signs and symptoms should improve each day and should begin to resolve in two to five days. If cuff cellulitis progresses to a pelvic cellulitis, the extensive inflammatory response will often manifest itself with a fever of at least 38°C and an increasing WBC count. Abdominal symptoms of increasing tenderness to deep palpation and pelvic examination will reveal increased induration. An extensive "balsa-wood" type consistency of the entire vaginal cuff area is consistent with pelvic phlegm or phlegmon, and a tender, fluctuant mass at the vaginal apex is consistent with a hematoma or abscess. Drainage of pus with palpation or probing of the cuff is synonymous with a cuff abscess and requires immediate drainage. Ultrasound or CT evaluation is often performed, but it is not immediately necessary unless a ruptured pelvic abscess or multiple abscesses are suspected, or the patient fails initial drainage and treatment of the cuff mass.

Although a temperature equal to or greater than 38°C is the most sensitive and reliable sign of infection, its absence does not rule out infection, as antipyretics are often used or intermittent readings miss the fever's peak. It is recommended that meperidine or morphine be utilized in the first 24 to 48 hours until the presence or absence of fever can be ascertained. Low-grade fevers (<38°C) do not immediately need to be treated, but should be investigated (i.e., antipyretics stopped, baseline laboratory values obtained, and a physical examination including evaluation of pulmonary status, urinary tract, wound, abdominal examination, pelvic examination, and bloody or vaginal discharges performed). Statistically, almost all temperature elevations greater than or equal to 38°C (100.4°F) represent an infection. If untreated, most will still resolve spontaneously, but a quicker return to normal and a decrease in abdominal and pelvic pain will be accomplished if the patient gets worked up for a pelvic infection and treatment is initiated if confirmed. Atelectasis, a urinary tract infection, or a wound infection rarely causes temperatures greater than 38°C in the first 48 hours. Aspiration pneumonia, pyelonephritis, or bowel perforation will cause a rapid and early rise in temperature and needs to be evaluated immediately. Patients with an early low-grade fever that begins to have a spiking appearance, despite an improvement in the patient's clinical examination, should alert the physician to the possibility of septic pelvic thrombophlebitis. Cultures are often difficult to obtain, but can be helpful if the patient's condition is deteriorating rapidly. Blood and urine cultures for fevers higher than 38.5°C can be obtained, and a transvaginal culture can be obtained if a mass is present. If the cuff has been closed, needle aspiration of the mass after the vaginal cuff is cleaned with betadine is acceptable to get the culture at the time of drainage. If the cuff has been left open, a culture swab, needle, aspirate, or replacement of drain can be utilized to get a sample. A stat Gram stain should be obtained, as culture results will not be available for a few days. Culture results can help direct antimicrobial therapy if the initial empiric choices fail or additional undrained abscesses are suspected.

Infection in pelvic surgery, other than hysterectomy, is more difficult to diagnose. Endometrial sampling by aspirate can be performed in patients with a transmural myomectomy or D&C. However, suspected ovarian masses will need radiologic evaluation of abscess development if the physical examination is suggestive of an intra-abdominal process and the ovarian capsule was violated, making it more likely that contamination of the ovary had occurred.

TREATMENT

Once a pelvic infection has been diagnosed, antimicrobial therapy should be initiated. This initial therapy is invariably empiric in nature and must cover a variety of organisms, as these infections are frequently polymicrobial. However, several factors can help direct therapeutic choices. Prophylaxis with a cephalosporin should lead the physician to consider the enterococci as a possible pathogen, and a penicillin-based broad-spectrum agent such as piperacillin–tazobactam or ampicillin–sulbactam should be considered. The traditional "gold standard" of clindamycin and gentamicin has not been proven in comparative trials to be either superior or inferior. However, administering the two agents separately, and taking into account the potential toxicity of gentamicin, with its suggested peak and trough levels, may not result in significant cost savings, even with these relatively inexpensive drugs. Although costs can be saved by ordering admixing of these drugs and using a once daily large-dose of gentamicin, ampicillin is often added, again raising costs and inconvenience.

The carbapenems, imipenem and meropenem, have been well studied for the treatment of pelvic infections and have demonstrated excellent results. Dosages for antimicrobial agents are listed in Table 1. Ertapenem, a once-a-day intravenous carbapenem, has recently received approval for treatment of pelvic infections. However, usage has been limited and costs may be high. Cost prohibitive when compared to the more widely used carbapenems, the broad-spectrum cephalosporin agents with demonstrated efficacy include cefoxitin, cefotetan, ceftizoxime, and cefotaxime. Anaerobic activity is adequate, and gram-positive aerobic activity is excellent, except for increase in *Enterobacter* species with cefoxitin and the poor *Pseudomonas*-species coverage with most of these agents. Ceftriaxone has poor anaerobic activity and would be a poor choice for polymicrobial coverage of a soft-tissue pelvic infection.

The frequent concern in other specialties regarding the development of resistance with the use of the newer broad-spectrum agents such as piperacillin–tazobactam or imipenem does not apply here, because the alternative clindamycin–gentamicin or the cephalomyins such as cefoxitin or cefotetan have been found to cause increases in *Clostridium difficile* and multiply-resistant enterococci. Also, the use of antimicrobial therapy in gynecology is generally of short duration and usually does not require oral antimicrobial therapy after discharge from the hospital. While on antimicrobial therapy, patients should be monitored for improvement with repeat WBC counts to demonstrate systemic improvement. C-reactive protein (not the high-sensitivity test used for cardiac risk evaluation) has been demonstrated in studies to correlate with improvement. It is important to make certain that the patient is afebrile for at least 24 to 48 hours. Most antibiotics will cause the reduction of fever, which should occur within 48 hours. If the patient is not afebrile in that time period, a therapeutic failure needs to be considered. There are few, if any, reasons why therapy should be continued if a patient remains febrile after two to three days. Causes for failure are varied, but include uncovered bacterial species, abscess, septic pelvic thrombophlebitis, and the development or progression of another infection at a distant site. As most patients will not have had a culture of the operative site and antibiotics were begun empirically, the weaknesses of the treatment antimicrobial should be covered. Although there are no hard and fast rules, clindamycin–gentamicin patients should have ampicillin added to cover enterococci. Cefoxitin or other cephalosporin patients should be switched to agents that cover the enterococci and resistant gram-negative bacteria; piperacillin–tazobactam has the best coverage as a secondary agent. Imipenem and meropenem have equally excellent activities; however, if they have a slight weakness, it is in the area of enterococci. Ticarcillin–clavulanate patients often require a switch to piperacillin–tazobactam or ampicillin–sulbactam to cover enterococci. Ampicillin–sulbactam has some gram-negative weaknesses, and an aminoglycoside or aztreonam provides excellent coverage. If the most active agents, piperacillin–tazobactam or the carbapenems, are not successful as empiric agents, equal consideration should be given to finding another cause for the fever as to expansion of the antimicrobial coverage. Piperacillin–tazobactam has a small number of resistant gram-negative species that would be covered with an aminoglycoside, and meropenem or imipenem misses a few enterococci. However, the activity is so broad that work-up of an undrained collection (abscess or infected hematoma) should be initiated. Pelvic examination with or without radiologic evaluation is strongly suggested. Also, if the patient is clinically improving but has repeated temperature spikes, septic pelvic thrombophlebitis should be considered, as described earlier.

Also, among the treatments mentioned, ofloxacin (and probably levofloxacin) does not kill vaginal lactobacilli, and should have less effect on the promotion of vaginal flora shifts or fungal superinfections. With regard to failure of empiric therapy, a thorough work-up for undrained collections or other sites of infections should be initiated at any time after initial empiric therapy or after secondary treatment coverage is not successful. Detection of an undrained and suspected infected hematoma or radiologic evidence of an abscess necessitates immediate drainage. Percutaneous drainage, guided by ultrasound or CT, has also been demonstrated to be successful. However, if a ruptured abscess is suspected or the patient is septic and unstable, exploration is imperative. If the patient appears to be recovering from the pelvic infection but then becomes febrile again, and it is at least three to four days postoperative, the abdominal wound should be inspected and opened if an abscess or seroma is suspected. Any blackened or necrotic area, or rapidly progressing erythema, should be taken back to the operating room and debrided immediately for fear of the development of necrotizing fasciitis. Other sites to inspect in response to persistent or recurrent fevers, such as the intravenous site and pulmonary or urinary sources, should be evaluated, and they should be treated if found to be source of infection. However, atelectasis or cystitis is not a source of persistent fever, and the search for the actual cause of the fever should continue. Lastly, in a small percentage of patients who receive pelvic instillation of hyaluronate-ferrous adhesion gel (Integel), indicated for adhesion prevention, fever has been known to occur. In cases where the WBC count is not elevated and evidence of a bowel perforation is absent, the fever often resolves spontaneously.

CONCLUSION

Gynecologic procedures are some of the most common operations in the United States today. Their clean-contaminated or contaminated classification means a significant number of postoperative infections can occur. A proper surgical technique and appropriate use of prophylactic antibiotics will help significantly decrease the incidence of postoperative infections, but many will still occur. The most important factor in successful treatment, however, is not antimicrobial choice, but early diagnosis and initiation of appropriate antimicrobial therapy. A delay in diagnosis, often a result of not recognizing or respecting the signs and symptoms of infection such as fever, makes successful treatment increasingly difficult. Also, a thorough history and physical examination is imperative to making the correct diagnosis once fever is present and infection suspected.

A rapid response to therapy should occur, and again, delay in reacting to persistent fever and reexamining the patient will eventually result in serious consequences. Thus a respect for fevers and infections will usually allow you to rapidly cure the patient and give her the favorable outcome for which she came to undertake surgery initially.

SELECTED READING

ACOG Technical Bulletin. Antimicrobial therapy for gynecologic infections. 1986; No. 97.
ACOG Practice Bulletin. Antibiotic Prophylaxis for Gynecologic Procedures 2001; No. 23.
Bennett IL Jr, Petersdorf RG. Alterations in body temperature. In: Wintrobe MM, ed. Harrison's Principles of Internal Medicine. New York: McGraw-Hill, 1970.
Charles D. Value of the erythrocyte sedimentation rate in gynecologic infections. Clin Obstet Gynecol 1976; 19:171.
Cruse P, Foord R. A ten-year prospective study of 62939 surgical wounds. Surg Clin North Am 1980; 60:189.
Gesner BM, Jenkins SR. Production of heparinase by bacteroides. J Bacteriol 1961; 81:595.
Gibb RS, Hunt JE, Schwarz RH. A follow-up study of prophylactic antibiotics in cesarean section. Am J Obstet Gynecol 1973; 117:419.
Gibb RS, O'Dell TN, MacGregor BR, et al. Puerperal endometritis: a prospective microbiologic study. Am J Obstet Gynecol 1975; 121:919.
Gorbach SH, Bartlett JG. Anaerobic infections. N Engl J Med 1974; 190:1177.
Jacoby GA, Swartz MN. Fever of undetermined origin. N Engl J Med 1973; 289:1407.
Josey WE, Stagger SRJ. Herapin therapy in septic pelvic thrombophlebitis: a study of 46 cases. Am J Obstet Gynecol 1974; 120:228.
Kaiser A. Antimicrobial prophylaxis in surgery. N Engl J Med 1986; 35:1129.
Ledger WJ, Child MA. The hospital care of patients undergoing hysterectomy: an analysis of 12026 patients from the professional activity study. Am J Obstet Gynecol 1973; 117:423.
Ledger WJ, Campbell C, Willson JR. Postoperative adnexal infection. Obstet Gynecol 1968; 31:83.
Ledger WJ, Gee C, Lewis WR. Guidelines for antibiotic prophylaxis in gynecology. Am J Obstet Gynecol 1974; 121:1038.
Ledger WJ, Kriewall TJ, Sweet RL, Fekety FR Jr. The use of parenteral clindamycin in the treatment of obstetric–gynecologic patients with severe infections. A comparison if a clindamycin–kanamycin combination with penicillin–kanamycin. Obstet Gynecol 1974; 43:490.
Ledger WJ, Norman M, Gee C, Lewis W. Bacteremia on an obstetric–gynecologic service. Am J Obstet Gynecol 1975; 121:205.
Martens MG. Reduction of infectious morbidity with uterine stapling device. Adv Ther 1990; 7:2.
Martens MG. Evaluation of ticarcillin/clavulanate potassium in the treatment of obstetric and gynecologic infections. Hospital Formulary 1990; 25:2.
Martens MG, Sebastian F. Bacteroides bivius: a major pathogen in Ob/Gyn infections. Infect Surg 1989; 8:294.
Mead PB, Gump DW. Antibiotic therapy in obstetrics and gynecology. Clin Obstet Gynecol 1976; 19:109.
Mondsley RF, Robertson EM. Common complications of hysterectomy. Obstet Gynecol Surv 1968; 20:859.
Ohm MJ, Galask RR. Bacterial flora of the cervix from 100 prehysterectomy patients. Am J Obstet Gynecol 1957; 122:683.
Schulman H, Zatuchni G. Pelvic thrombophlebitis in the puerperal and postoperative gynecologic patient. Am J Obstet Gynecol 1969; 90:293.
Sebastian F, Martens MG, Hunter A, et al. Antibiotic prophylaxis: is there a difference? Am J Obstet Gynecol 1990; 162:4.
Swartz WH, Tanaree P. T-tube suction drainage and/or prophylactic antibiotics—a randomized study of 451 hysterectomies. Obstet Gynecol 1976; 47:665.
Sweet R, Yonekura ML, Hill G, et al. Appropriate use of antibiotics in serious obstetric and gynecologic infections. Am J Obstet Gynecol 1983; 146:719.
Wilkins TD. Antibiotics susceptibility testing of anaerobic bacteria. In: Balows A, DeHaan RM, Dowell VR Jr, Guze LB, eds. Anaerobic Bacteria. Springfield, IL: Charles C Thomas, 1974.
Willson JR, Black JR. Ovarian abscess. Am J Obstet Gynecol 1964; 90:34.

INTRODUCTION

Traditionally, the term "pelvic inflammatory disease" (PID) has been applied to the infectious inflammatory process involving the uterus and/or fallopian tubes. Its broad connotations aggregated various processes of diverging origins. Although it is a convenient categorical term, it does little for the conceptualization of the process within a given patient.

> The term PID does not specify the anatomic distribution of the infectious process or the prognostic consequences for the woman afflicted. Is it not time to replace the diagnosis "pelvic inflammatory disease" with more precise terminology such as endometritis, salpingitis, or pelvic peritonitis.
>
> Lars Westrom
> (*JAMA* 1991; 866:2612)

Certain disease processes require individualization. Early in the course of genital tuberculosis or coccidioidomycosis, salpingitis can occur independently of serosal extension or endometrial spread. Similarly, the group A beta-hemolytic streptococci are more prone to producing combined endometritis and peritonitis rather than endometritis, salpingitis, and peritonitis. The combination of endometritis and peritonitis in the immediate postpartum period differs significantly, bacteriologically and mechanistically, from endometritis–salpingitis with or without peritonitis in a nongravida. The Centers for Disease Control and Prevention's (CDC's) definition of PID has been a significant factor in the failure to achieve precise diagnostic and therapeutic end-points. According to the 1997 MMWR, "PID comprises a spectrum of inflammatory disorders of the female genital tract, including any combination of endometritis, salpingitis, tubo-ovarian abscesses, and pelvic peritonitis. Sexually transmitted organisms, especially *Neisseria gonorrhoeae*, and *Chlamydia trachomatis* complicate most cases. However microorganisms that can be part of the vaginal flora, e.g., anaerobes, *Haemophilus vaginalis*, *H. influenzae*, enteric gram-negative rods and *Streptococcus agalaxtie* can cause PID. In addition, *Mycoplasma hominis*, *Ureaplasma urealyticum* might be etiological agents."

This definition has come under severe criticism by the International Infectious Disease Society for Obstetrics and Gynecology (I-IDSOG). The society reiterated the call previously advanced by other groups within the discipline of obstetrics and gynecology, for terminating the term PID. Recognizing how ingrained PID is in the world literature, it was proposed that if the term PID were to be used instead of upper female genital tract infection, the anatomical sites of inflammation and etiological designation should be clarified.

TheI-IDSOG defines PID thus: "Pelvic inflammatory disease is an inflammatory process of infectious etiology which shares a common epidemiological profile (sexual risk factors), has at least uterine and fallopian tube sites of involvement and which may result in relatively comparable long term sequelae. Diseases due to bacteria not meeting these requirements will be designated upper female genital tract infection (UFGTI or UGTI) and specific or presumed etiology cited."

The ensuing chapter will be restricted to those cases of acute salpingitis that are the consequence of venereal transmission.

PATHOGENESIS OF GONOCOCCAL SALPINGITIS

Initial gonococcal infection involves Skene's and Bartholin's glands and the endocervical and anorectal glandular sites. The predilection of *N. gonorrhoeae* for replicating successfully at these sites is in part a function of the alkaline milieu provided by the glandular secretions.

Beyond organismal virulence factors such as pH, the elements selecting for disease, as opposed to infection, are not fully understood. The increased prevalence of salpingitis due to *N. gonorrhoeae* at the time of menses has fostered the contention that the loss of mucosal integrity and the rich supply of subendolymphatics are important variables in transforming occult glandular infection into clinically recognized disease. Probably more important are the pH changes induced in the vagina as a consequence of the menses. The normal vaginal pH is approximately 4.2 to 4.9. The optimum pH for the replication of *N. gonorrhoeae* is 7.0 to 7.6. The pH of menstrual blood is usually 7.2. The occurrence of acute salpingitis beyond the time of menses, its occurrence in patients several cycles after initial colonization, and its nonoccurrence in other patients despite prolonged endocervical colonization, all focus on the complexity of the variables that combine to produce disease.

Gonococcal salpingitis is a consequence of isolates with the appropriate genetic prerequisites obtaining access to the endometrial cavity by contiguous spread or insertion and the subsequent extension of the disease process to the fallopian tubes. With time, infection may reach the peritoneal cavity either through the fimbriated end of the fallopian tube or as a consequence of transmural penetration in the case of a ruptured tubo-ovarian complex (TOC).

When the disease process is initiated by *N. gonorrhoeae*, there is a progressive alteration in the microbiologic environment within the endometrial cavity (Table 1). This is accomplished by the postulated addition of substances that lower the local oxidation–reduction potential, the removal

TABLE I The development of polymicrobial infections in patients with initial gonococcal infection[a]

Infection	Endocervix	Endometrium–fallopian tubes	Peritoneum–cul-de-sac
Gonococcal	(4+) N. gonorrhoeae	(2+) N. gonorrhoeae	
	(4+) N. gonorrhoeae	(2+) N. gonorrhoeae Class I aerobes	(1+) N. gonorrhoeae
	(3+) N. gonorrhoeae	(2+) N. gonorrhoeae	(1+) N. gonorrhoeae Class I anaerobes
	(2+) N. gonorrhoeae	(1+) N. gonorrhoeae Class II anaerobes	(Trace) N. gonorrhoeae Class I and II anaerobes
	(1+) N. gonorrhoeae	Polymicrobial mixed infection Class II and III anaerobes	Polymicrobial mixed infection Class II aerobes predominate
Nongonococcal	Class I and III anaerobes	Class III anaerobes	Class II and III anaerobes

[a]Diagrammatic sequencing of the anaerobic progression as it applies to uncomplicated, untreated cases of gonococcal ESP (endometritis–salpingitis–peritonitis). The flow, left to right, is the time representation proposed for the endocervix, endometrium–fallopian tubes, and peritoneum cul-de-sac at given stages. *Source*: Monif GRG. *Obstet Gynecol* 1980; 55:1548.

of molecular oxygen, and the progressive reduction of local pH. The fall in pH influences the effectiveness of bacteriocins and bacteriocin-like products of bacteria that regulate strain dominance. This series of events is repeated within the fallopian tubes and the cul-de-sac. With an open portal to the complex endocervical bacterial flora, the alterations induced by *N. gonorrhoeae* initiate the anaerobic progression. The bacteria thus recruited further transform the microbiologic environment. These bacteria are characterized by their progressive ability to replicate within a microbiologic environment characterized by a low redox potential and the relative absence of molecular oxygen. The farther removed the onset of disease is from menses, the more likely the polymicrobial pattern is to be observed.

It is not *N. gonorrhoeae* but rather the superinfecting anaerobic bacteria that appear to be responsible for basement membrane destruction and subsequent healing by fibrosis.

Preexisting damage to the fallopian tube, if present, is thought to be associated with changes in the involved tissue's oxidation–reduction potential that favor earlier conversion to polymicrobial infection.

With time, *N. gonorrhoeae* is also eliminated at the endocervical site of infection through bacterial interference. In gonococcal salpingitis, the endocervix is both the first and the last site of bacterial replication. When the gonococcus is neither demonstrated on Gram staining nor isolated from the endocervix, *N. gonorrhoeae* is rarely isolated from the cul-de-sac. In a very real sense, the way one recovers from gonococcal infection, in the absence of antibiotic therapy, is by bacterial interference engendered by the anaerobic progression. However, the price of bacterial interference is structural damage.

The presence of a foreign body within the endometrial cavity may or may not exert an influence on the sequence of events. The alterations due to mechanical factors (i.e., the induction of predecidual changes, microerosions of the mucosa, the presence of a chronic inflammatory cell infiltrate) and/or concomitant chronic anaerobic bacterial infection may accelerate the anaerobic progression in patients with gonococcal salpingitis. If there is an antedating anaerobic bacterial infection associated with the presence of an intrauterine device (IUD), fallopian tube involvement is more likely to be due to Class II anaerobes, and in particular to members of the Bacteroidaceae/*Prevotella* sp. rather than to *N. gonorrhoeae*.

The anatomic lesions of the fallopian tube are intraluminal as well as interstitial (Fig. 1A and B). Because of the volumetric expansion of the interstitium, owing to edema fluid, hyperemia, and the presence of an inflammatory infiltrate, the finger-like mucosal intraluminal projections are brought into proximity (Fig. 1C and D). While an intense inflammatory exudate is present within the intraluminal space, it is thought that the interstitial microabscesses immediately beneath the mucosal basement membrane are a critical factor in determining whether or not residual damage will ensue (Fig. 1E). These microabscesses are probably not due to *N. gonorrhoeae* but rather to superinfecting anaerobic bacteria from the vaginal flora. As long as the basement membrane is intact, mucosal regeneration is possible. Once the basement membrane is destroyed, the inevitable consequence is healing by fibrosis. The destruction of the basement membrane of two opposed mucosal surfaces leads to the establishment of inflammatory bridges. The ultimate consequence of basement membrane destruction is a permanent structural alteration of the fallopian tube architecture.

Clinically, patients will have a significant endocervical or vaginal discharge owing to the presence of the intense inflammatory response elicited by *N. gonorrhoeae*. With progressive fallopian tube involvement, the patient experiences initially intermittent crampy lower abdominal pain. Secondarily, there is heightened autonomic peristaltic activity of the muscularis in response to a relatively nonflexible submucosal inflammatory edema. The clinical perception of pain may be heightened by the focal inflammatory neuritis. Although there may be a significant extension of the inflammatory process into the muscularis, peritonitis, when it ensues, in most instances is the consequence of purulent material issuing from the fallopian tube. Depending upon the quantity of material reaching the peritoneal surface, the patient may perceive a change in the character of the pain, which is now sharper, more constant, and likely to be exacerbated by positional changes.

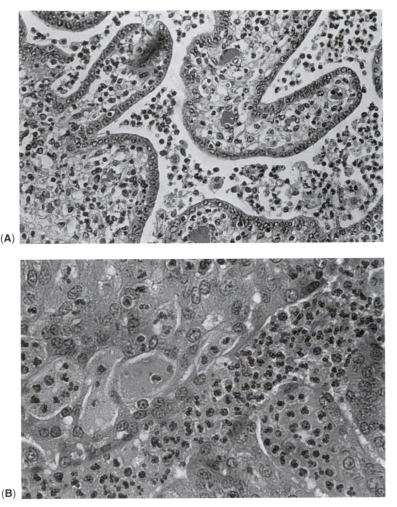

(A)

(B)

FIGURE 1A–E Bacterial replication and the resultant inflammatory response within the fallopian tubes in salpingitis. (**A**) Lesions involve both intraluminal and interstitial sites (H&E, ×175). (**B**) With intensification of the inflammatory process, microabscesses (presumably due to superinfecting anaerobic bacteria) develop at the interstitial site, ultimately resulting in basement membrane destruction (H&E, ×234). (*Continued*)

In the majority of instances, the inflammatory exudate that reaches the peritoneal cavity sequesters within the cul-de-sac. In isolated instances, significant amounts of pus reach the right posterior gutter and ultimately the perihepatic region. The clinical manifestations that ensue depend upon whether the suprahepatic or infrahepatic portion of Glisson's capsule is involved. If intracapsular infection involves the serosal surface of the gallbladder, right upper quadrant pain may ensue, with a pattern of radiation that mimics the one observed in cases of acute cholecystitis. Suprahepatic involvement may produce supraclavicular pain.

CHLAMYDIAL SALPINGITIS

Chlamydial salpingitis has always been part of the sexually transmitted disease (STD) spectrum. In 1732, John Astruc (Fig. 2) wrote, based upon observations of Parisian prostitutes, of a chronic form of salpingitis that

> occurs in women whose uterus is thrown into contractions by lascivious ticklings and by excess of prostitution. Many have no pain, but the infection in time injures the internal surface of the uterus and its tube.

In contrast to gonococcal salpingitis, chlamydial tubal infection can produce a true chronic subclinical infection.

Intracellular chlamydial organisms may persist in the genital tissues for extremely long periods of time and continue to produce silent progressive tubal damage. When infertile patients with chlamydial antibodies are evaluated with laparoscopy, frequently no history of an illness or procedure can be elicited that could explain the presence of postinflammatory tubal damage.

Cultural and serologic data have built an extensive case for *C. trachomatis* as both an etiologic agent and a potential copathogen in acute salpingitis. Chlamydial cervicitis is present in 20% to 40% of patients with acute gonococcal salpingitis.

In contrast to "classical PID" due to *N. gonorrhoeae*, chlamydial disease tends to be more occult (Table 2). Sometimes, only a vague peritoneal pain precipitated by jarring movements motivates the patient to seek medical attention. Characteristically, the temperature is less than 38°C. The principal findings on pelvic examination are cervical motion tenderness and varying degrees of cervicitis.

The role of chlamydia in acute salpingitis is not clearly understood. *C. trachomatis* appears to be able to both initiate infection and pave the way for bacterial superinfection and function as a monoetiological pathogen. Both mechanisms will produce involuntary infertility.

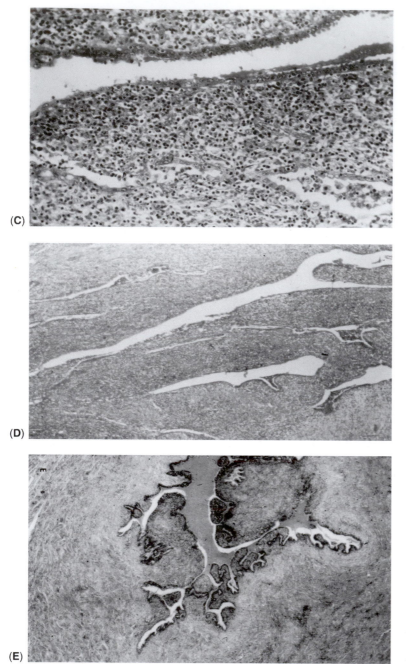

(C)

(D)

(E)

FIGURE 1 (Continued) (**C,D**) With basement membrane destruction (particularly when two such areas are opposed), the potential for the creation of an inflammatory bridge has been achieved (H&E, ×240 and ×110). (**E**) With repeated episodes, the fallopian tube undergoes structural alterations that may significantly alter its functions of transport and nutrition of the fertilized ovum (H&E, ×105).

Although the degree of overlap in the clinical presentation of chlamydial and gonococcal-related salpingitis is extensive, some unique demographic characteristics do exist. Unless preexisting infection with *Trichomonas vaginalis* is present, disease due to *N. gonorrhoeae* characteristically occurs in close proximity to the menstrual period. The occurrence of chlamydial salpingitis is more scattered, with its mean peak incidence delayed by about four to seven days compared to gonococcal salpingitis. Patients with chlamydial disease tend to appear less toxic. The fever elevation and white blood cell count (WBC) characteristically are lower. Patients with Stage I or Stage II salpingitis will have an erythrocyte sedimentation rate below that anticipated for patients with a comparable stage of gonococcal disease.

There is a significantly higher incidence of chlamydial disease among users of oral contraceptives. These patients often have a prior history of Krettek's syndrome ("breakthrough" intramenstrual bleeding that responds to doxycycline therapy).

PROXIMAL STUMP SALPINGITIS

Despite anatomical interruption of the fallopian tubes, the proximal remnants of the fallopian tubes are vulnerable to ascending infection. Proximal stump salpingitis does not present with classical signs and symptoms. Fletcher (1986) reported five cases of disease arising in the proximal remnants of the fallopian tubes. The majority of these patients

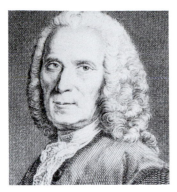

FIGURE 2 John Astruc, MD. *Source*: Courtesy of National Medical Library, Bethesda, MD.

presented with unilateral pain. Physical examination demonstrated exquisite adnexal tenderness. Of note were the relatively normal WBC encountered.

OTHER MONOMICROBIAL ETIOLOGIES

There are at least two organisms capable of producing acute salpingitis in addition to *N. gonorrhoeae*. These are the group A beta-hemolytic streptococci and *Neisseria meningitidis*.

Group A Beta-Hemolytic Streptococci

Monif et al. (1977) have demonstrated that, in isolated instances, *Streptococcus pyogenes* can be a monoetiological cause of acute salpingitis. The recovery of the organism and the ability to exclude the concomitant presence of Class III anaerobes have focused on the probability that the group A streptococci, under selective conditions, can be a rare cause of acute salpingitis in the nonpregnant woman. Although they are bacteria of unique virulence, the group A streptococci require a specific event such as a mechanical disruption of the cutaneous and mucosal barrier to initiate overt infection. The onset of menstruation appears to be an effective initiating event, and consequently, the disease is proximate to the onset of menses in a manner that is not dissimilar to that characteristic of *N. gonorrhoeae*. The clinical manifestations are indistinguishable from those associated with *N. gonorrhoeae*.

The incidence of acute salpingitis due to the group A streptococcus is low. In isolated cases a study of 92 patients with acute salpingitis. Eschenbach et al. (1975), in their study of 241 cases of acute PID, recovered *S. pyogenes* from

the cul-de-sac in a single instance. In their case, as in that reported by Monif et al., a pure culture of group A beta-hemolytic streptococci was recovered from the cul-de-sac.

N. meningitidis

On rare occasions, *N. meningitidis* can be recovered from the endocervix. Epidemiologic delineation of its possible role as a pathogen for the female genital tract has been basically negated. Unlike the case in oropharyngeal infection, carbohydrate fermentation or immunofluorescence is not required for genital tract isolates to establish the diagnosis of *N. gonorrhoeae* infection. The CDC accepts the presumptive criteria for the identification of *N. gonorrhoeae* as being diagnostic in a definitive sense for such isolates. In the course of their studies of the bacteriology of the cul-de-sac isolates in acute salpingitis, Monif et al. (1981) recovered *N. meningitidis* from the cul-de-sac of a patient with presumably gonococcal endocervicitis and polymicrobial peritonitis.

In both group A streptococcal and *N. meningitidis* acute salpingitis, the diagnosis is readily established by cultures of the endometrium and culdocentesis fluid. Neither the group A streptococci nor *N. meningitidis* present therapeutic problems. Both organisms respond readily to penicillin and its semisynthetic analogs. If the new-generation tetracyclines are used, a given isolate of group A streptococci may not respond.

Streptococcus pneumoniae

S. pneumoniae is not a normal constituent of vaginal bacterial flora; however, given the opportunity, *S. pneumoniae* can be a significant pathogen for the female genital tract.

Involvement of the female genital tract as a metastatic process secondary to maternal septicemia due to *S. pneumoniae* was a relatively well-documented phenomenon in the preantibiotic era. The occurrence of cases of chorioamnionitis and/or perinatal septicemia in the absence of pulmonary involvement indicated the possibility of contiguous spread from the vaginal/cervical reservoir and subsequent involvement of the female upper genital tract.

Genital tract disease due to *S. pneumoniae* has been reported in nonpregnant females. Isolated cases of spontaneous pneumococcal peritonitis have been described. Hadfield et al. (1990) reported a case of a 46-year-old woman with bilateral tubo-ovarian masses. Biopsy

TABLE 2 Comparison of gonococcal and chlamydial salpingitis

Parameter	Gonococcal salpingitis	Chlamydial salpingitis
Mode of contraception	More likely to be IUD or none	More likely to be oral contraceptive
Prior history of mid-cycle "break-through bleeding"	Unlikely, unless IUD in place	Occurs in a significant number of cases
Presentation	Acute	Subacute to semiacute
Relationship to menses	Closely associated; if *T. vaginalis* is present, disease may occur later in the menstrual cycle	May occur at any time in the cycle
WBC in Stages I and II	Somewhat elevated	Tends to be more elevated
ESR in Stages I and II		Tends to be normal

Abbreviations: ESR, erythrocyte sedimentation rate; IUD, intrauterine device; WBC, white blood cell count.

specimens from both tubes and from the wall of the abscesses demonstrated gram-positive, lance-shaped diplococci; these were documented to be *S. pneumoniae* by immunoperoxidase staining. Rahav et al. (1991) reported a case of postmenopausal pneumococcal tubo-ovarian abscess (TOA) from which *S. pneumoniae* was recovered. The fallopian tubes in these two cases of spontaneous peritonitis due to *S. pneumoniae* were described as being swollen and hyperemic, with pus emanating from the ends. What was described is not a specific disease entity (spontaneous peritonitis) but more probably a progressive consequence of salpingitis. Patterson et al. (1994) have subsequently reported a case of pneumococcal salpingitis documented by laparoscopy.

Incrimination of *S. pneumoniae* as an etiological agent in cases of acute salpingitis is probably an underreported phenomenon. While *S. pneumoniae* will grow on 5% to 7% sheep blood agar culture when incubated in a CO_2 environment, the recovery of alpha-hemolytic streptococci is usually not worked up any further and is often reported as "mixed vaginal flora." Recovery of alpha-hemolytic streptococci from patients with acute salpingitis needs to be microbiologically evaluated to exclude the possibility that these isolates are *S. pneumoniae*.

Haemophilus influenzae

In rare cases, *H. influenzae* appears to be the causative agent for TOA or salpingitis. Most cases of serious gynecologic infections caused by *H. influenzae* reported previously have occurred in association with an IUD. Recently, Carmeci and Gregg (1997) reported a case of acute salpingitis that was not associated with an IUD or any other predisposing conditions such as *S. pneumoniae*. When *H. influenzae* is a cause of salpingitis, septicemia commonly occurs.

BACTERIOLOGY OF GONOCOCCAL AND NONGONOCOCCAL ACUTE SALPINGITIS

The bacteriologic isolates derived from the cul-de-sacs of 92 patients studied at the University of Florida College of Medicine are listed in Table 3. When the 269 bacterial isolates were grouped in accordance with the Gainesville Classification, 215 aggregated in Category I (gram-positive aerobes and those bacteria with demonstrable susceptibility to penicillin). Since the majority of the group D streptococci (enterococci) are susceptible to penicillin, one can readily appreciate why the majority of patients did well on single-drug penicillin therapy, particularly when the penicillin was given in doses of 10 to 20 million units/day. Bacteriological data derived from the cul-de-sacs of women with acute salpingitis have substantiated well the distribution of bacterial isolates.

One of the major reservations that must be retained when interpreting the significance of a given bacterial isolate from the cul-de-sac is that the data reported are neither qualitative nor quantitative. The critical factor that determines whether or not a bacterial isolate may have potential significance appears to be the oxidation–reduction potential. At any given moment, one organism may be

more significant than another in the presumed bacterial synergism that is postulated in the anaerobic progression. Unless the anaerobic microbiologic environment of the cul-de-sac is in a critical zone, the more aerobic portion of the anaerobic progression is the focus of therapy. If no further alteration is required to achieve the required oxidation/reduction potential, eradication of the total cul-de-sac flora is required in order to achieve the anticipated therapeutic response.

DIAGNOSIS

Traditionally, there are certain physical findings that are typical in acute salpingitis. While the abdominal symptoms are common to a number of disease processes, pelvic examination is often characteristic. Exudate issuing from the endocervix, marked uterine tenderness, and exquisite cervical tenderness to motion are all physical findings characteristic of acute salpingitis. An often neglected differential point in acute salpingitis is the obtaining of serial temperatures. If a temperature is obtained within 20 minutes of doing a bimanual pelvic examination and then retaken every 15 minutes for the next 45 to 60 minutes, a significant number of patients with acute salpingitis are found to exhibit a precipitous elevation in temperature. In these instances, the pelvic examination is a challenge test.

Unfortunately, one has been traditionally geared to the stereotypic picture of acute salpingitis. Our perception of a chronic variant, which is perhaps of greater importance in terms of structural damage, periodically lapses from recognition.

While the diagnosis of acute salpingitis can be made with a high probability of accuracy, the same cannot be said of a subacute or *forme fruste* variant. Making the diagnosis of such upper genital tract infections without resorting to invasive procedures such as an endometrial biopsy or laparoscopy is difficult.

In patients with subacute salpingitis, the onset of symptoms is independent of the menstrual cycle. If febrile temperatures occur, rarely do they exceed 38°C. Not infrequently, there is a history of antibiotic therapy, particularly for urinary tract infection. The patients tend to be more chronically than acutely ill. What is characteristic is that they have had a recent history of lower quadrant pain, which is usually the reason they seek medical consultation. Physical examination often demonstrates little save for cervical tenderness, which may or may not be associated with a discharge. If one does a jar test (which is performed by asking the patient to stand on her tiptoes and then suddenly drop to her heels) and peritoneal pain is apparent, culdocentesis not infrequently will demonstrate the presence of purulent material from which a polymicrobial flora can be isolated.

Up to one-third of patients with laparoscopically confirmed salpingitis neither had an elevation of temperature above 38°C nor had evidence of a leukocytosis. The erythrocyte sedimentation rate (ESR) is of value only if significantly elevated. A markedly elevated ESR should

TABLE 3 Bacteriologic spectrum of isolates from the cul-de-sacs of 64 patients with endometritis–salpingitis–peritonitis

Organism	No. of isolates	Organism	No. of isolates
■ **Group I**		**Total clostridia**	**4**
A. Aerobes and facultative bacteria		*GPNS rods*	
Streptococci, not group D		*Eubacterium* spp.	2
Apha-hemolytic streptococci	16	*Eubacterium lentum*	2
Nonhemolytic streptococci	12	*Eubacterium tenue*	1
Beta-hemolytic streptococci, group B	4	*Eubacterium aureofaciens*	1
		Eubacterium contortum	1
Lactobacilli	2	*Propionibacterium acnes*	1
Microaerophilic streptococci	8	*Propionibacterium avidum*	1
Corynebacteria	12	*Lactobacillus* spp.	1
Staphylococci		*Lactobacillus salivarius*	1
Coagulase negative	8	*Lactobacillus acidophilus*	1
Coagulase positive	3	*Lactobacillus minutus*	1
Micrococci	1	*Lactobacillus fermentum*	1
Eikenella corrodens	1	*Bifidobacterium* spp.	1
Neisseria gonorrhoeae	17	*Bifidobacterium infantis*	3
Total aerobes	**84**	*Bifidobacterium longum*	1
		Bifidobacterium adolescentis	1
B. Anaerobes		Unidentified GPNS rods	12
Peptococci		**Total GPNS**	**32**
Peptococcus spp.	17	**Total anaerobes**	**123**
Peptococcus morbillorum	2	**Total Group I**	**207 (76.9%)**
Peptococcus prevotii	11		
Peptococcus asaccharolyticus	4	■ **Group II** *Bacteroides fragilis*	
Peptococcus variabilis	1	ss. *fragilis*	5
Total Peptococci	**35**	ss. *ovatus*	1
Peptostreptococci		ss. *thetaiotaomicron*	2
Peptostreptococcus spp.	17	ss. *distasonis*	2
Peptostreptococcus anaerobius	9	ss. *vulgatus*	1
Peptostreptococcus productus	1	ss. unknown ("no good fit")	12
Peptostreptococcus micros	2	ss. not determined	2
Total Peptostreptococci	**29**	**Total Group II**	**24 (8.9%)**
Veillonella	6		
Unidentified gram-negative cocci	2	■ **Group III** group D streptococci	
		Enterococci	12 (4.5%)
Bacteroides species other than fragilis			
Bacteroides spp.		■ **Group IV**	
Bacteroides corrodens	1	**A. Enterobacteriaceae**	
Bacteroides pneumosintes	3	*Escherichia coli*	8
Bacteroides nodosus	1	*Serratia marcescens*	2
Bacteroides melaninogenicus ss. *intermedius*	2	*Proteus mirabilis*	1
		Enterobacter cloacae	1
Bacteroides capillosus	4	*Klebsiella pneumoniae*	3
Bacteroides oralis		*Citrobacter diversus*	1
Total bacteroides	**23**	**Total Enterobacteriaceae**	**16**
Fusobacterium spp.		**B. Others**	
Unidentified gram-negative rods	3	*Gardnerella vaginalis*	9
Clostridia		*Gardnerella influenzae*	1
Clostridium spp.	2	**Total others**	**10**
Clostridium malenominatum	1	**Total Group IV**	**26 (9.7%)**
Clostridium haemolyticum	1		
		Total isolates in all four therapy groups	**269**

[a]Bacterial isolates are grouped by the Gainesville Classification.
Abbreviation: GPNS, gram-positive nonsporulating.
Source: Monif et al. Excerpta Medica 1977; 3:26.

suggest the possibility of tubal occlusion or TOC. A normal ESR with a TOC should suggest a chlamydial etiology.

The CDC has developed a clinical case definition that encompasses the majority of these points (Table 4). The major adjunctive diagnostic procedures which are done in cases of acute salpingitis are

1. staging of the disease, and, if signs of peritoneal irritation are present,
2. obtaining Gram stains and cultures of the endocervix and the endometrium for *N. gonorrhoeae* and *C. trachomatis*.

No one laboratory test [serum WBC, vaginal leucocytosis, C-reactive protein (CRP) or ESR] has validity in terms of sensitivity or negative predictive value. Part of the problem is the failure to analyze patients with overt acute salpingitis separately from those individuals with the subacute or chronic variants. Peipert et al. (1996) analyzed 120 women who either met the CDC's minimal criteria for acute PID or had other signs of upper genital tract infection (i.e., atypical pelvic pain, abnormal uterine bleeding, or cervicitis). Sensitivities for elevated WBC, ESR, CRP, and increased vaginal white blood cells were 57%, 70%, 71%, and 78% respectively. If any one test was abnormal, the sensitivity was 100% and specificity 18%. If all four tests were abnormal, sensitivity was 29% and specificity 95%. When all laboratory tests were normal, objective evidence of upper genital tract infection was not found.

Testing for increased vaginal white blood cells was found to be the most sensitive laboratory indicator of upper genital tract infection, whereas serum WBC was the most specific. No one diagnostic laboratory test is pathognomonic for upper genital tract infection. Combinations of positive tests can improve diagnostic specificity and positive predictive value, but with a diminution of sensitivity and negative predictive value.

In a meta-analysis of 12 studies assessing laboratory criteria for the diagnosis of PID, Kahn et al. (1991) found that CRP was significantly predictive in the four studies in which it was part of the data collected. The test displayed good sensitivity (74–93%) with a range of specificity (50–90%). ESR was found to be a significant indicator of upper genital tract infection. When the ESR was greater than 25 mm/hr, its sensitivity was 55% and specificity 84%.

Miettinen et al. (1993) evaluated the ESR and CRP in assessing the severity of acute salpingitis. Separately, they were unacceptable in terms of sensitivity and negative predictive value. When used together (i.e., either test being abnormal), sensitivity and negative predictive value improved to 96% and 97%, respectively, with a decrease in specificity to 61% and maintenance of positive predictive value at 70%. The cut-off levels Miettinen et al. (1993) used were high: ESR > 40 mm/hr and CRP > 60 mg/dL.

In general, CRP determinations are of little diagnostic use; however, when elevated, they are of value in determination of the duration of short-term parenteral antibiotic therapy. In Stage II salpingitis, the mean CRP should be decreased by the third day of treatment. CRP level becomes normal much sooner than does the ESR, and consequently, it becomes a useful predictor of the short-term response to antimicrobial therapy.

The ESR can be normal despite a TOC when the etiological agent is C. trachomatis.

An ESR of greater than 50 mm/hr should alert the clinician to the probable presence of significant tubal occlusion or a definite TOC.

Although the presence of vaginal white blood cells on wet mount analysis increases the probability of genital tract infection, the use of a Q-tip swab sampling of the endometrial cavity is advocated. The sample is a smear on a glass slide and stained. The presence of a significant inflammatory component correlates better with the presence of endometritis and with corroborating physical findings of endometritis/salpingitis.

TABLE 4 CDC PID clinical case definition

A clinical syndrome resulting from the ascending spread of microorganisms from the vagina and endocervix to the endometrium, fallopian tubes, and/or contiguous structures

All of the following clinical criteria must be present:
Abdominal direct tenderness
Tenderness with motion of the cervix
Adnexal tenderness

In addition to all of the above criteria, at least one of the following findings must also be present:
Oral temperature > 38°C
Abnormal cervical or vaginal discharge
Elevated erythrocyte sedimentation rate
Elevated C-reactive protein
Laboratory documentation of cervical infection with *Neisseria gonorrhoeae* or *Chlamydia trachomatis*
Histopathologic evidence of endometritis on endometrial biopsy
Radiologic abnormalities (thickened fluid-filled tubes with or without free pelvic fluid or tubo-ovarian complex) on transvaginal sonography or other radiologic tests
Laparoscopic abnormalities consistent with PID
Leukocytosis > 10,000 WBC/mm³
Purulent material in the peritoneal cavity obtained by culdocentesis or laparoscopy
Pelvic abscess or inflammatory complex on bimanual examination or by sonography

Abbreviations: CDC, Centers for Disease Control and Prevention; PID, pelvic inflammatory disease; WBC, white blood cell count.

Laparoscopic confirmation is the gold standard for diagnosing salpingitis. The use of laparoscopy to attain visual evidence of salpingitis is both expensive and not without risk to the patient. Laparoscopy is best reserved for PID (physical-in-doubt or pretty inadequate diagnosis).

Unless a TOC has ruptured, blood cultures are rarely positive. The use of culdocentesis is largely restricted to situations where clinical ambiguity exists or to obtaining cul-de-sac specimens for research studies.

THERAPY

Acute Salpingitis

Beyond the eradication of disease and infection, therapeutic success for the female must involve preserving fallopian tube structure and function.

In 1917, William Osler was quoted as saying that "the gonococcus is not a great destroyer of life, but as a misery producer Neisser's coccus is king among germs." For Osler, the morbidity of disease was to be found in the "chronic pelvic mischief and unhappiness in sterile marriages." The intervening eight decades have done little to alter the validity of his observation. Therapy in the early 21st century must encompass the preservation of fallopian tube structure and function or, in the cases of advanced disease, preservation of ovarian function by precluding the need for surgical intervention.

In the early 1970s, Westrom demonstrated by laparoscopic evaluation a 12.8% incidence of tubal occlusion following a single episode of acute salpingitis. Following two episodes, the figure increased to 35.5%, and following three episodes, to 75%. When the same investigator reevaluated the impact of an expanded therapeutic armamentarium on fallopian tube morbidity, the observed incidence of tubal occlusion following one, two, and three episodes of acute salpingitis were 11.4%, 23.1%, and 54.3%, respectively (Table 5).

The probability of secondary infertility is statistically linked to age, number of antecedent episodes of acute salpingitis, and severity of disease at the time of institution of appropriate antibiotic therapy. The incidence of infertility was reduced irrespective of the number of prior episodes of acute salpingitis in 15- to 24-year-old women as opposed to 25- to 34-year-old women. In women less than 25 years of age, those who had had gonococcal-associated salpingitis had a significantly better fertility prognosis than those who had had nongonococcal salpingitis.

When the degree of the inflammatory reaction documented by laparoscopy is correlated with subsequent reproductive outcomes, a positive increase in correlation can be demonstrated. Viberg (1964) has demonstrated that early effective antibiotic therapy gives the shortest value of ESR half-time. No involuntary infertility occurred in patients who received early antibiotic therapy and demonstrated a good therapeutic response.

In the treatment of STD, we should be looking for an antimicrobial regimen that provides a cure at least 95% of the time while preserving anatomic structure and function.

The CDC guidelines identify a number of therapies that in clinical trials have been shown to be efficacious. What is wrong in the therapeutic studies in the literature is the aggregation of all stages of acute salpingitis by virtue of nomenclature, but numerical dominance of patients with Stage I and early Stage II in the treatment groups. By the overload of patients who will respond to any regimen effective against all isolates of *N. gonorrhoeae* and *C. trachomatis* (e.g., selected fluoroquinolones), Food and Drug Administration (FDA) approval is achieved for drug regimens that inadequately deal with anaerobic superinfection.

TOC/TOA

The diagnosis of a TOC may be inferred by a physical examination, but it is ultimately contingent on the use of ultrasonography, laparoscopy, or computerized tomography. More recently, magnetic resonance imaging has been successfully used to demonstrate the extent of the disease, characterize the lesion, and demonstrate the involvement of adjacent pelvic organs. This technology has some applicability when attempting to differentiate Stage III (TOC) from Stage IV (ruptured TOC) salpingitis. When attempting to distinguish pelvic masses, transvaginal color Doppler sonography may help diagnostically and prognostically. Fleischer et al. (1995) demonstrated that 72% of masses with a high impedance underwent regression, whereas only 21% of lesions with low impedance did. Only 20% of masses demonstrating low impedance or a morphologically complex structure regressed. Sixty-five percent of lesions that regressed had a significant drop in pulsatility index. The probability of regression was the greatest in young women (less than 40 years of age) and in masses less than 5 cm.

TABLE 5 Incidence of tubal occlusion documented by laparoscopy following one, two, or three episodes of acute salpingitis

Number of episodes of acute salpingitis	Am J Obstet Gynecol	
	1975; 121:707	1980; 131:880
One	12.8%	11.4%
Two	35.5%	23.1%
Three	75%	54.3%

The therapy of women with TOCs or TOAs involves antibiotic therapy that encompasses the STD spectrum of pathogens as well as the bacteria within the anaerobic progression. Large complexes and complexes whose tenderness persists despite 48 hours of appropriate antibiotic therapy should be considered as possible candidates for lesion aspiration under sonographic guidance. Women with ovarian involvement or persisting signs of peritoneal irritation or positive blood cultures for enteric gram-negative rods usually require prompt surgical intervention.

When a TOC has been documented by ultrasonography and the mass remains significantly tender at the end of 48 to 72 hours despite appropriate antibiotic therapy, and no evidence of peritoneal irritation is demonstrable, serious consideration should be given to ultrasound-guided transvaginal drainage of the TOC. Perez-Medina et al. (1996) prospectively compared the outcome after TOC with intensive antibiotic therapy. Patients were assigned to two groups, distributed on a random basis, with a clinical and ultrasound diagnosis of TOA of less than 10 cm maximal diameter. Both groups received an antimicrobial combination of clindamycin and gentamicin. In the study group, they performed early transvaginal drainage of the abscesses. Both short-term (48–72 hours) and medium-term (four weeks) responses to the treatment were evaluated. In the study group, a favorable short-term response was observed in 90% of the cases, whereas this was 65% in the control group. Caspi et al. (1996) used single-step ultrasound-guided aspirations in conjunction with intracavity antibiotic instillation for the treatment of 10 women with TOA who failed to respond to systemic antibiotic therapy. All 10 women improved clinically and none required surgery. The mean time from aspiration to hospital discharge was 3.1 days, with a mean duration of hospitalization of 7.8 days. No major complications were observed. The average time interval between aspiration of the lesion and resolution on sonographic follow-up was 9.5 weeks. In three cases, PID recurred, but none needed surgical intervention.

THERAPEUTIC REQUISITES FOR ANTIBIOTIC SELECTION IN ACUTE SALPINGITIS

For more than three decades, the therapy of acute salpingitis was influenced by the monomicrobial genesis of its counterpart in males and its implied corollary, antimicrobial selection predicated on drug-of-choice concept. The mandate for change came from three sources that ultimately converged to formulate the current basis for therapeutic recommendations:

1. Recognition of diverging mechanisms for disease induction
2. Recognition of polymicrobial superinfection
3. Recognition of polymicrobial etiology

Polymicrobial Superinfection

The utilization of culdocentesis coupled with the application of sophisticated anaerobiology gave investigators the opportunity to look at what could be construed as both the front and the back of the conduit and make a sophisticated guess as to what was happening in the middle. A significant number of women with gonococcal endocervicitis have been shown to have a polymicrobial peritonitis at the other end of the conduit (cul-de-sac).

From bacteriological observations, the concept of polymicrobial superinfection of initial gonococcal salpingitis was developed. *N. gonorrhoeae*, by virtue of its replication, sufficiently lowers the oxidation–reduction potential of the local microbiological environment so as to initiate the anaerobic progression. This process is the mechanism by which a monomicrobial process becomes polymicrobial disease.

As the progressive changes in the microbiological environment select for the more microaerophilic organisms (Class II anaerobes), *N. gonorrhoeae* undergoes autoelimination. This process of autoelimination occurs in the cul-de-sac and also in the fallopian tubes, endometrium, and endocervix. Ultimately, a situation arises wherein the gonococcus cannot be recovered from either end of the conduit. When nonrecovery of *N. gonorrhoeae* can be excluded because of technical problems (delayed plating, use of cold modified Thayer-Martin plates, the absence of initial ambient carbon dioxide, lack of sensitivity to enzyme-linked immunosorbent assay or polymerase chain reaction, etc.), the absence of the gonococcus has come to imply either infection caused by *C. trachomatis* or advanced disease as a result of anaerobic superinfection of initial gonococcal salpingitis. The ability to achieve the anticipated therapeutic response is significantly altered in patients with advanced polymicrobial superinfection.

Ideally, antimicrobial therapy of any infection should be based on the identification of the causative organism in specimens taken from the infected site and the sensitivity of these isolates to the antimicrobial agent. The inability to culture the critical site of organism replication, the fallopian tubes, predicates that the treatment regimens instituted must cover the broad range of the pathogenic spectrum, which participates in the anaerobic progression as well as the primary STD spectrum.

C. trachomatis

The selection of antibiotic therapy for acute salpingitis is complicated by the potential etiologic diversity. *C. trachomatis* is the most common cause of STD in many countries. The frequency of its isolation from the cervix of women with acute salpingitis is between 5% and 40%. In a limited series, the organism has been recovered from the fallopian tubes or peritoneal exudate in up to 30% of cases of acute salpingitis. A significant change in antichlamydial antibody titer can be documented in 18% to 40% of women with acute salpingitis. *C. trachomatis* can be concomitantly isolated with *N. gonorrhoeae* in 20% to 40% of patients with gonococcal infection. Any antimicrobial regimen used to treat women with gonococcal infection should be effective against *C. trachomatis*. Although latency can be induced by penicillin and its semisynthetic analogs, the organism is usually not eradicated by beta-lactam antibiotics. The drug of choice is a tetracycline antibiotic. *C. trachomatis* is an important etiologic agent in acute salpingitis. Irrespective of the agent isolated from the cervix, antichlamydial activity should be an integral part of any therapeutic regimen used.

Polymicrobial Etiology

When polymicrobial infection evolves, if structural damage to the fallopian tubes is to be minimized, it may be imperative to eradicate all bacterial constituents. While it has been shown that, early in the course of the anaerobic progression, partial interruption of the synergism is often effective in aborting the ensuing evolution of strict anaerobic infection, once the polymicrobial infection is established, it may be possible for more than one organism to capitalize on the alteration induced.

Penicillinase-Producing Strains of
N. gonorrhoeae

A third factor that has entered the therapeutic equation is the increasing prevalence of the penicillinase-producing strains of *N. gonorrhoeae* (PPNG). Chromosomal mutation has accounted for the stepwise increase in the resistance of *N. gonorrhoeae* to penicillin observed since 1943. Plasmid-mediated resistance is directly related to the production of beta-lactamase, which is coded for by either a 3.3 megadalton plasmid (West African origin) or a 4.4 megadalton plasmid (Southeast Asian origin). The spread of the PPNG strains has forced a major reformulation of our current therapeutic recommendations.

The critical issue in the therapy of acute salpingitis goes beyond the treatment of the complexity of monomicrobial disease or infection; it involves the prevention or eradication of bacterial superinfection. A growing body of data indicates that the secondary anaerobic invaders and not *N. gonorrhoeae* are the principal agents responsible for basement membrane destruction and resultant healing by fibrosis.

Antibiotic selection is governed by the need to accommodate polymicrobial etiology, polymicrobial superinfection, and PPNG, when possible, into a single therapeutic regimen. Since the ultimate goal of the therapy of acute salpingitis is preservation of fallopian tube structure and function, a regimen cannot be instituted and subsequently corrected if the anticipated therapeutic response does not materialize within a specific time. It is quite probable that appropriate antibiotic therapy in the first 24 hours is the critical determinant in preserving fallopian tube structure and function.

THERAPEUTIC STAGING OF ACUTE SALPINGITIS

The intent of nomenclature or classification is to render meaning or clarity to a given set of facts or concepts. Without individualization of treatment and delineation of appropriate stages of disease, the consequences for women have been unwanted secondary infertility, ectopic pregnancies, increased occurrence of TOCs, and possible surgical removal of the genital organs. Each state of disease can be differentiated by virtue of its major therapeutic goal and the means by which this goal can be achieved (Table 6). Although an inverse therapeutic correlation is documentable between achieving the anticipated therapeutic response with single-drug therapy effective against both *N. gonorrhoeae* and *C. trachomatis* and increased stage of disease, the ability to achieve the anticipated therapeutic response with the recommended therapy of the Gainesville staging has been demonstrated for Stages I and II.

Papavarnavas et al. (1990) compared the accuracy of the Gainesville staging with laparoscopic findings. The clinical staging of acute salpingitis correlated with laparoscopic findings in 82.6% of cases, and when the diagnosis was correct, the severity of the clinical staging correlated with that of laparoscopic staging as the probability increased of polymicrobial superinfection. Staging is a guideline for the initiation of therapy and setting of priorities. Failure to achieve the anticipated therapeutic response requires aggressive reassessment of clinical management.

Stage I—Acute Salpingitis without Peritonitis

In Stage I disease, barring the presence of PPNG, patients without peritonitis or an IUD who have no underlying structural damage to the fallopian tubes show excellent response to the penicillins or the tetracyclines. When patient compliance can be assured, these patients can be treated on an outpatient basis; however, we prefer to hospitalize all patients for whom future fertility is an important issue. The presence of an IUD in a patient with Stage I disease warrants hospitalization.

TABLE 6 Gainesville staging of acute salpingitis

Stage	Therapeutic goal
I: Acute salpingitis without peritonitis (ES)	Eradication of symptomatology and infectivity
II: Acute salpingitis with peritonitis (ESP)	Preservation of fallopian tube structure and function
III: Acute salpingitis with evidence of tubal occlusion or tubo-ovarian complex	Primary therapeutic goal: preservation of ovarian function
IV: Ruptured tubo-ovarian complex	Primary therapeutic goal: preservation of life

Abbreviations: ES, endometritis–salpingitis; ESP, endometritis–salpingitis–peritonitis.

Stage II—Acute Salpingitis with Peritonitis

A patient with Stage II disease is clinically similar to one with Stage I disease, except that bilateral lower quadrant rebound tenderness is demonstrable. The therapeutic goal for Stage II disease is the preservation of fallopian tube structure and function. Stage II is documented by the demonstration of peritonitis by physical examination; if the gonococcus is a constituent of the polymicrobial bacterial flora, the probability of achieving the anticipated therapeutic response is approximately 60%. If the gonococcus is not present, the probability drops to 30%. In Stage II disease, the gonococcus, although important in the induction of the anaerobic progression, becomes more a biologic marker of the status of the microbiologic environment induced by the anaerobic progression than the primary functioning pathogen. If therapy is broadened significantly to encompass etiologic diversity and the anaerobic progress, i.e., by the addition of cefoxitin, these figures become 90% and 80%, respectively.

The selection of antibiotic therapy for Stage II disease is one of the rare situations in which knowledge of the spectrum of organisms that can function in this type of polymicrobial infection is insufficient. Initial monomicrobial disease may be due to three entities that potentially influence antibiotic selection: *N. gonorrhoeae*, the PPNG, and *C. trachomatis*. Polymicrobial bacterial superinfection requires the traditional four-category coverage of the Gainesville Classification. The therapy of choice for Stage I or Stage II disease is cefoxitin 2 g IV every six hours *plus* doxycycline 100 mg IV or PO, every 12 hours (Table 7).

Because of the pain associated with infusion, doxycycline should be administered orally when possible, even when the patient is hospitalized. If intravenous administration is warranted, use of lidocaine or other short-acting local anesthetics, heparin, or steroids with a steel needle or extension of the infusion time may reduce infusion problems. Parenteral therapy may be discontinued 24 hours after a patient shows clinical improvement, and oral therapy with doxycycline 100 mg two times a day should continue for a total of 14 days. The rationale for the antibiotic combination of cefoxitin and doxycycline is to achieve the best coverage for the maximal numbers of these seven categories (Table 8). Cefoxitin and doxycycline offset each other's relative deficiencies. The principal shortcoming of this drug combination is its inadequacy for enterococci.

If the presence of tubal occlusion or a TOC is suspected, the disease should be staged upward in terms of a presumptive Stage II to Stage III, and antibiotic therapy with penicillin, clindamycin, and an aminoglycoside (triple therapy) should be implemented. Once signs of peritoneal irritation have abated, ultrasonography should be performed to stage the disease accurately (peritoneal irritation precludes earlier use of ultrasonography because of the inability to fill the bladder). If ultrasonography reveals merely tubal occlusion, aminoglycoside therapy can be discontinued. If a TOC is identified, aminoglycoside therapy is continued for a total of 72 hours.

TABLE 7 Therapeutic recommendations for acute salpingitis within a hospital setting

Regimen A
Cefotetan[a] 2 g IV every 12 hr, or cefoxitin 2 g IV every 6 hr *plus* doxycycline 100 mg IV or PO every 12 hr

Regimen B
Clindamycin 900 mg IV every 8 hr *plus* gentamicin loading dose IV or IM (2 mg/kg of body weight) followed by a maintenance dose (1.5 mg/kg) every 8 hr. Single daily dosing may be substituted

Alternative parenteral regimen
Limited data support the use of other parenteral regimens, but three regimens have undergone at least one clinical trial and have broad spectrum coverage

Ofloxacin 400 mg IV every 12 hr *plus* metronidazole 500 mg IV every 8 hr

Ampicillin/sulbactam 3 g IV every 6 hr *plus* doxycycline 100 mg orally or IV every 12 hr

Ciprofloxacin 200 mg IV every 12 hr *plus* doxycycline 100 mg IV or PO every 12 hr, *plus* metronidazole 500 mg IV or PO every 8 hr

[a]Cefotetan does not have an anaerobic coverage total comparable to cefoxitin. The anaerobic coverage of selected second-generation cephalosporins is the reason they have not been supplanted by third-generation cephalosporins (ceftizoxime, cefotaxime, and ceftriaxone).

Stage III—Suspected Tubal Occlusion or TOC

In selected instances, the interstitial inflammation and secondary edema result in focal tubal occlusion at a proximal and distal part. The inflammatory exudate, denied access to the peritoneum and cul-de-sac or retrograde drainage into the endometrial cavity, exerts volumetric intraluminal pressure, thus increasing the local diameter of the fallopian tube. Prior structural damage with focal submucosal fibrosis predisposes to the evolution of this type of clinical presentation. The distinction between transitory tubal occlusion and TOA is determined by the permanency of the occlusions.

Stage III (tubal occlusion or a TOC) represents the anatomic progression of disease. The probability of preserving fallopian tube function is diminished. The major goal becomes the preservation of ovarian function by negating the need for surgical intervention. We use triple therapy (penicillin, clindamycin, and an aminoglycoside) in this setting. Why the need for an aminoglycoside? In our experience, when rupture has occurred, Enterobacteriaceae frequently are present. The therapy of Stage III is primarily a therapeutic assault on the anaerobic progression. The duration of aminoglycoside therapy rarely needs to exceed

72 hours. It is our policy to discontinue parenteral therapy 24 hours after rectification of monitored parameters.

A major advance in the therapy of Stage III disease will be the use of percutaneous and transvaginal aspiration drainage under ultrasonographic guidance. Use of this technique in TOCs that remain tender after 48 hours lessens morbidity and shortens hospital stays.

Stage IV—Ruptured TOC

In Stage IV, rupture of a TOC has occurred. The therapeutic goal for Stage IV disease is the preservation of life. The distinction between tubal and ovarian sites is predicated on the observation that occasionally, patients with tubal sites of rupture may respond to medical therapy. In these cases, closure of the site of rupture is probably provided by the mating of omentum or bowel to the site of rupture. When the infection directly involves the ovary, the probability of associated concomitant septic thrombophlebitis is markedly increased. Unless surgical intervention is implemented, mortality is the anticipated outcome for patients with a ruptured ovarian abscess. Therapy for Stage IV disease is surgical removal of the site of rupture under appropriate antibiotic coverage. Triple therapy (penicillin, clindamycin, and an aminoglycoside) is administered to minimize or abort metastatic infectious complications. Definitive therapy involves the surgical removal of the diseased organ and effective peritoneal lavage. If an ovarian abscess is found at the time of surgery, care must be given to ruling out concomitant septic thrombophlebitis.

DURATION OF ANTIMICROBIAL THERAPY FOR ACUTE SALPINGITIS

What constitutes a good therapeutic response is a controversial issue. The duration of antibiotic therapy for acute salpingitis is not known. Determination of the length of antibiotic administration requires identification of therapeutic titration points. For many, including the CDC, organismal eradication, resolution of the signs and symptoms of disease within a four-day period, and nonprogression to a TOC equated with a good therapeutic response. Once it was documented that, in the absence of complicating factors such as the use of an IUD, significant prior structural damage, or tubal ligation, monomicrobial disease had an anticipated therapeutic response [lysis of

TABLE 8 Rational use of cefoxitin and doxycycline in acute salpingitis (stage II)

Antibiotic	Neisseria gonorrhoeae	Chlamydia trachomatis	Penicillinase-producing N. gonorrhoeae	Categories of the Gainesville Classification			
				I	II	III	IV
Doxycycline[a]	+++— ++++	++++	+—++[a]	++1/2	++1/2— +++ (75–85%)	+—	++
Cefoxitin[a]	+++— ++++	—	+++— ++++	+++	++1/2	—(75–85%)	+++
Combined coverage	+++— ++++	++++	+++— ++++	+++	+++–+++[b] (85–90%)	+—	+++

+++ = ≥85% efficiency; ++++ = ≥94% efficiency.
[a]Effectiveness of doxycycline and cefoxitin limited to African strain of *N. gonorrhoeae*.
[b]Effectiveness is additive for the penicillin-resistant Bacteroidaceae (Category II).

fever within 36 hours, disappearance of signs of peritoneal irritation and marked amelioration of deep organ tenderness within 36 to 48 hours, and a WBC below 10,000/mm³ within 48 hours after the onset of therapy), the questions changed to how long therapy needed to be continued and which antibiotics were to be utilized. One way to evaluate therapy is to use multiple parameters: patient's sense of well-being, serial WBCs, abdominal and pelvic physical findings, and temperature. This permits the establishment of an end-point for Stage II and Stage III disease. The ESR should be followed in Stage III disease to decide on the duration of therapy. The ESR should be declining before the discontinuation of multiple drug therapy. Once the therapeutic end-points have been documented, our policy is to continue parenteral antimicrobial therapy for 24 hours and then discharge the patient to continue with oral medication.

Outpatient therapy for Stage I and Stage II disease is that required for complete eradication of C. trachomatis. Our drug of choice is doxycycline. Five days of oral therapy is the upper limit of patient compliance that we can achieve in a primarily poorly educated, low socioeconomic population without again seeing the patient in the gynecologic clinic. Outpatient therapy for Stage III acute salpingitis involves the administration of metronidazole and doxycycline. The duration of doxycycline therapy is governed by the time of administration required to eradicate C. trachomatis. Duration of metronidazole therapy is based on the CRP or ESR changes.

The real answers as to appropriate antimicrobial therapy for each of the Gainesville stages of acute salpingitis and for the corresponding duration of therapy ultimately need to be assessed longitudinally through detailed studies of subsequent fertility.

CRITERIA FOR THE SELECTION OF PATIENTS FOR AMBULATORY THERAPY OF ACUTE GONOCOCCAL SALPINGITIS

No firm criteria exist that delineate which patients with acute gonococcal salpingitis can be successfully managed on an outpatient basis and which patients would be best handled by hospitalization. The following segment represents personal guidelines that govern the selection of candidates for ambulatory therapy of acute salpingitis.

The criteria governing patient selection for ambulatory care of women with acute salpingitis are listed in Table 9.

Unless the issue of future fertility is not a consideration, first and foremost, my personal policy is to offer and counsel hospitalization for all women with acute gonococcal salpingitis. Even when all other ambulatory care criteria are met, hospitalization is most adamantly advocated for all adolescents and nulligravidas. Hospitalization should be used as an educational as well as a therapeutic vehicle.

Gram Stain Demonstration of Gram-Negative Intracellular Diplococci in Endocervical Smear
Demonstration of gram-negative intracellular diplococci correlates with greater than or equal to 10⁴ cfu/mL of bacteria in the sample fluid. The visual demonstration of a high multiplicity of N. gonorrhoeae argues against significant

alteration of the microbiological environment so as to favor the replication of Class II anaerobes that will in turn lead ultimately to the autoelimination of the gonococcus. The Gainesville studies of acute salpingitis documented that the demonstration of gram-negative intracellular diplococci in smears from the endocervix was associated with a statistically significant increased probability that one was dealing with monoetiological bacterial disease.

Erythrocyte Sedimentation Rate
ESR has been a valuable adjunctive laboratory aid. The ESR was used primarily in staging patients with significant peritoneal irritation in the interim prior to ultrasonographic evaluation. A value of 60 mm or greater correlated in a statistically significant manner with the probability of a tubal occlusion or TOC as demonstrated by ultrasonography. Most patients with acute gonococcal salpingitis tend to have ESRs in the 20s and low 30s. The use of ESR in chlamydia salpingitis is nearly worthless. Patients with laparoscopically documented TOCs may have normal ESRs.

The choice of an ESR of 30 mm as a demarcation point in deciding whether or not to hospitalize a patient is arbitrary, predicated on a desire to err on the side of patient welfare.

Prior or Advanced Disease Presentations
The "therapeutic window" (that interval in which effective antibiotic therapy against monoetiological disease due to N. gonorrhoeae will preclude alteration of fallopian tube structure and function) may be as short as 24 hours. Prior structural damage may, through the acceleration of the anaerobic progression as a consequence of adverse impact on local host defense mechanisms, reduce the time frame of the therapeutic window. Based on theoretical considerations, hospitalization for all patients with disease beyond Stage I acute salpingitis is recommended. The issue of therapeutic window for C. trachomatis cannot be defined based on current experience or data.

Prior History of Chlamydial Infection
Since prior or concurrent structural damage to the fallopian tubes cannot be ruled out, asymptomatic or minimally symptomatic chlamydial infection, for management purposes, is deemed equivalent to prior salpingitis. Thirty-four percent of individuals with endocervical chlamydial infection will have the presence of lymphocytic plasma cell infiltration in their

TABLE 9 Omaha criteria for possible ambulatory care of acute gonococcal salpingitis

(1)	Nonadolescent/nonnulligravida women
(2)	Ability to demonstrate presence of gram-negative intracellular diplococci on Gram stain of endocervix
(3)	ESR<30 mm
(4)	Absence of signs of peritoneal irritation (rebound tenderness)
(5)	High probability of follow-up in 24–48 hr
(6)	No prior history of documented salpingitis or chlamydial infection
(7)	Absence of pregnancy

Abbreviation: ESR, erythrocyte sedimentation rate.

endometrial biopsy. What percentage of these have concomitant fallopian tube involvement and whether the process identified by histology is due to *C. trachomatis* are issues for continued analysis.

Absence of Peritoneal Signs

Patients whose clinical findings go beyond the criteria of lower abdominal pain, cervical motion tenderness, adnexal tenderness, and two or more of the minor diagnostic criteria and who have demonstrable rebound tenderness represent individuals with a more advanced stage of disease, in which the probability of polymicrobial superinfection is markedly augmented. The option for possible ambulatory therapy should be restricted to those patients with monoetiological disease due to *N. gonorrhoeae* or coinfection due to *N. gonorrhoeae* and *C. trachomatis*.

Pregnancy

When acute salpingitis occurs in a gravida, it does so within the first eight weeks of gestation. The pathogenesis of disease partially embraces the same mechanisms that result in superinfection. An exceedingly rare case may occur at 12 weeks of gestation. Intrauterine disease places the pregnancy at risk. For maximum fetal support, hospitalization is strongly recommended. Despite effective maternal therapy, 30% to 40% of patients will abort either in association with maternal disease or within two to three weeks posttherapy.

In 2001, the International Infectious Disease Society published its recommendation for ambulatory care (Table 10).

The PID Evaluation and Clinical Health (PEACH) randomized trial is the most recent attempt to compare the efficacy of outpatient versus inpatient therapy for PID. Unfortunately the study was fundamentally flawed by reliance on the CDC's definition of PID. The inclusion of a large number of patients who were not documented to have gonococcal or chlamydial disease diluted the validity of conclusions, which centered on the occurrence of long-term sequelae.

AMBULATORY CARE MANAGEMENT

Patients receiving oral therapy should show substantial clinical improvement (e.g., defervescence, reduction in direct or rebound abdominal tenderness, and reduction in uterine, adnexal, and cervical motion tenderness) within 36 hours of initiation of therapy (Table 11).

If the provider elects to prescribe oral or parenteral outpatient therapy, follow-up examination should be performed within 36 to 48 hours using the criteria for clinical improvement previously described.

Because of the risk of persistent infection, particularly with *C. trachomatis*, patients should have a microbiologic reexamination 7 to 10 days after completing therapy. Some experts also recommend rescreening for *C. trachomatis* and *N. gonorrhoeae* four to six weeks after completing therapy. If polymerase chain reaction or ligase chain reaction is used to document the test of cure, rescreening should be delayed one month following completion of therapy.

Data emanating from the PEACH Randomized Trial provide the basis for wider utilization of outpatient therapy. In this study, there was only a nonstatistically significant difference in terms of therapeutic response, fertility rate, and risk of PID sequelae between women treated with hospitalization and broad-spectrum intravenous antibiotics compared to women treated on an ambulatory basis with oral antibiotics. The PEACH study effectively addresses a societal need to validate ambulatory therapy for women with acute salpingitis, but in itself, it is a less than definitive study. Rather than dealing with laparoscopically verified diseases, the investigators pooled together a large number of patients who met the minimum set of diagnostic criteria. The study focused upon women with what they termed mild PID. Analyses of the end therapeutic titration points revealed the need to change therapy in 26 patients due to overt therapeutic failure. Persistent organ tenderness was present in 132 of the 841 study participants at the 30 day examination. Repeat endometrial biopsy reveal evidence of inflammation in 187 of the 458 women in whom a second endometrial biopsy was obtained.

As long as disease processes of diverging etiology, but sharing clinical manifestation, are grouped under the term "PID" and are subject to a limited spectrum of therapeutic options, the net result will not be clarity.

By using antibiotics with greater than 90% bioavailability via oral administration and appropriate for the offending organism or organisms, therapeutic responses comparable to those with intravenous administration can be achieved. The problem is proper staging of etiologically specific disease. Unfortunately, staging is a less than perfect art. The transition time between Stage I and Stage II salpingitis in the Gainesville Classification can be relative short. Monif (1995) reports two cases that he contends demonstrated the therapeutic window of time between Stage I and Stage II. One of the cases reported was that of a 21-year-old, married female who presented with a 10-hour history of fever and bilateral lower quadrant pain. Four months prior to admission, she had delivered a term infant. Her physical examination revealed rebound tenderness, a significant vaginal discharge, purulent material coming from the endocervix, and cervical motion tenderness. A Gram stain of the endocervical exudate revealed the presence of gram-negative diplococci. A culdocentesis yielded 3 to 4 cc of pus. A Gram stain of the fluid revealed the rare presence of gram-negative intracellular diplococci. She was deemed to have monoetiological gonococcal salpingitis and she was started on intravenous minocycline therapy. She had initial short-term lysis of her temperature.

TABLE 10 Ambulatory care for acute salpingitis

Only women with clinically documentable Stage I disease, with the following exceptions:
- Pregnant women
- Women and teenaged girls
- Any nulligravida female who desires future pregnancy
- Any female who is unable to take oral medication or unable to be seen in follow-up

Source: From Guidelines for PID, CID 2001:32(1 Jan).

TABLE II 1998 CDC therapeutic recommendations for ambulatory therapy of acute salpingitis

Regimen A
Either ceftriaxone 250 mg IM once, *or* cefoxitin 2 g IM *plus* probenecid, 1 g orally in a single dose concurrently once, *or* other parenteral third-generation cephalosporin (e.g., ceftizoxime, cefotaxime), *plus* doxycycline 100 mg orally bid for 14 days, *plus* metronidazole 500 mg PO tid for 7 days

Regimen B
Ofloxacin 400 mg orally bid for 14 days *plus* metronidazole 500 mg orally bid for 14 days

Alternative oral regimens
Amoxicillin/clavulanic acid 250/125 mg orally every day for 14 days *plus* doxycycline 100 mg orally every 12 hr for 14 days

Abbreviation: CDC, Centers for Disease Control and Prevention.

Because of a progressive increase in her temperature, a repeat culdocentesis was performed, and it demonstrated the presence of small gram-positive cocci. The antibiotic therapy was changed and the temperature returned to normal within four to six hours. By CDC criteria, this was deemed a successful intervention. The STD pathogen and superinfecting organisms were eradicated. Clinical normality was established in less than three days. In the following 27 months in which she was monitored, she and her husband practiced unprotected coitus without achieving a conception. In the second case reported, serial culdocentesis documented the raid conversion of monoetiological disease to polymicrobial disease. If one is to do ambulatory therapy for acute salpingitis, one needs to be able to confirm therapeutic responsiveness in the first 24 hours if reproductive morbidity is to be avoided.

MANAGEMENT OF SEX PARTNERS

Evaluation and treatment of sex partners of women who have PID is imperative because of the risk for reinfection and the high likelihood of urethral, gonococcal, or chlamydial infection of the partner.

Sex partners should be treated empirically with regimens effective against both of these infections.

Salpingitis and HIV Infection
Acute salpingitis is two to seven times more prevalent among HIV-infected women than matched counterparts attending prenatal clinics. The question initially posed was whether compromised cell-mediated immunity influenced the clinical response to disease. Cohen et al. (1998) looked at the effect HIV-1 infection had on the treatment outcome of laparoscopically verified salpingitis. They found that HIV-seropositive and HIV-seronegative women had comparable median lengths of hospitalization and duration of antibiotic therapy; however, women with CD4 counts less than 14% required longer hospitalization and longer administration of antibiotics. The same group redid a comparable study eight years later. They again found that although HIV-1 infection may prolong hospitalization in women with severe salpingitis, the norm for women hospitalized with acute salpingitis is to respond appropriately to therapy and surgical drainage regardless of HIV-1 infection status. The key issues to achieve a good therapeutic outcome are proper staging and correspondingly appropriate therapy.

Prior to the publication of the 2002 Centers for Disease Control Treatment Guidelines, hospitalization and intravenous antibiotics were the recommended standard of care for HIV-infected women with acute salpingitis. Most HIV infections occur in, what has been termed, third-world countries in which universal hospitalization and intravenous administration of antibiotics is not pragmatically possible.

Salpingitis and Douching
A positive relationship exists between douching and PID. This association has been the basis for postulating a causal relation between the two entities. The association is sufficiently strong such that the FDA has given serious consideration to the banning of commercial douching preparations. The studies postulating a causal relationship have been primarily static-group comparison and/or pseudo- or quasi-experimental designs. Many of these studies contained potentially invalidating demographic variables. The postulated mechanism by which douching is reputed to cause disease involves two steps. It is theorized that douching disrupts the normal vaginal flora and selects for the inducing of bacterial vaginosis. Bacterial vaginosis, through some unidentified mechanism, causes salpingitis.

The problem with the first component of the proposed pathogenesis is that it lacks microbiological foundation. Two studies have used quantitative and qualitative microbiological techniques in assessing the effects of douching on the bacterial flora of the female genital tract. Onderdonk et al. (1992) studied the effects of 0.04% acetic acid and 0.30% povidone–iodine preparations. Acetic acid douches induced a transient reduction in the total bacterial count, which was attributed to a wash-out effect. Povidone–iodine caused a statistically significant reduction in the total bacterial count when compared to physiological saline in the same individual. Monif et al. (1977) have demonstrated that povidone–iodine gel causes a dramatic, transient elimination of bacterial isolates from the female genital tract. They noted that the first bacteria to demonstrate logarithmic growth were the aerobic natural constituents of the female genital tract and not the so-called bacterial vaginosis (BV) flora.

Povidone–iodine gel has been used therapeutically to achieve both clinical and less frequently microbiological cures in patients with BV. Of interest in the Ness et al. (2002) paper that postulated a causal relationship between BV and PID was the observation that women who douched before or after sex did not have an increased risk of BV. This group had reported a statistically higher frequency of sexual intercourse on an average than other women in the study.

The postulate that BV causes salpingitis has to overcome the fact that both BV and STDs share common demographic profiles. The three most common characteristics of women who douch are lower socioeconomic status, greater risk for STDs, and symptoms suggestive of vaginal infections.

Multiple studies of women with BV have revealed a high incidence of coinfection with STD pathogens. No mechanism showing how douching or BV causes PID has been demonstrated. Such data exist for *C. trachomatis*.

Finally, Ness et al. (2005) did a more appropriate longitudinal, rather than vertical, study that better controlled for invalidating confounding factors. They studied the incidence of PID in a cohort of high-risk women. After adjusting for confounding factors, douching two times or more per month at baseline was associated with neither PID nor gonococcal/chlamydial genital infection. They interpreted their data as not supporting an association between douching and development of PID or gonococcal/chlamydial genital infection among predominantly young, African American women.

SELECTED READING

Barbosa C, Macasaet M, Brockmann S, et al. Pelvic inflammatory disease and human immunodeficiency virus infection. Obstet Gynecol 1997; 89:65.

Barrett S, Taylor C. A review of pelvic inflammatory disease. Int J STD AIDS 2005; 16:715.

Cacciatore B, Leminen A, Ingman-Friberg S, et al. Transvaginal sonographic findings in ambulatory patients with suspected pelvic inflammatory disease. Obstet Gynecol 1992; 80:912.

Chow AW, Malkasian KL, Marshall JR, et al. The bacteriology of acute pelvic inflammatory disease: value of cul-de-sac cultures and relative importance of gonococcal and other aerobic or anaerobic bacteria. Am J Obstet Gynecol 1975; 123:876.

Chow AW, Patten V, Marshall JR. Bacteriology of acute pelvic inflammatory disease. Am J Obstet Gynecol 1979; 133:362.

Cunningham FG, Hauth JC, Gilstrap LC, et al. The bacterial pathogenesis of acute pelvic inflammatory disease. Obstet Gynecol 1978; 52:161.

Curtis AH. Bacteriology and pathology of fallopian tubes removed at operation. Surg Gynecol Obstet 1921; 33:621.

Eschenbach DA, Buchanan TM, Pollock HM, et al. Polymicrobial etiology of acute pelvic inflammatory disease. N Engl J Med 1975; 293:166.

Faro S, Martens M, Maccato M, et al. Vaginal flora and pelvic inflammatory disease. Am J Obstet Gynecol 1993; 169:470.

Greaves WL, Whittington WL. Penicillinase-producing *Neisseria gonorrhoeae* infections. Infect Dis Lett Obstet Gynecol 1983; 5:31.

Hemila M, Henriksson L, Ylikorkala O. Serum CRP in the diagnosis and treatment of pelvic inflammatory disease. Arch Gynecol Obstet 1987; 241:177.

Hemsell DL, Ledger WJ, Martens M, et al. Concerns regarding the Centers for Disease Control's published guidelines for pelvic inflammatory disease. Clin Infect Dis 2001; 32:103.

Hemsell DL, Nobles BJ, Heard MC, et al. Upper and lower reproductive tract bacteria in 126 women with acute pelvic inflammatory disease. Microbial susceptibility and clinical response to four therapeutic regimens. J Reprod Med 1988; 33:799.

Jaffe HW, Biddle JW, Johnson SR, et al. Infections due to penicillinase-producing *Neisseria gonorrhoeae* in the United States: 1976–1980. J Infect Dis 1981; 144:191.

Lip J, Burgoyne X. Cervical and peritoneal bacterial flora associated with salpingitis. Obstet Gynecol 1966; 28:461.

Livengood CH, Hill GB, Addison WA. Pelvic inflammatory disease: findings during inpatient treatment of clinically severe, laparoscopy-documented disease. Am J Obstet Gynecol 1992; 166:519.

Monif GRG. Significance of polymicrobial bacterial superinfection in the therapy of gonococcal endometritis-salpingitis-peritonitis. Obstet Gynecol 1980; 55:154s.

Monif GRG. Clinical staging of acute bacterial salpingitis and its therapeutic ramifications. Am J Obstet Gynecol 1982; 143:489.

Monif GRG, Welkos SL, Baer H, et al. Cul-de-sac isolates from patients with endometritis-salpingitis-peritonitis and gonococcal endocervicitis. Am J Obstet Gynecol 1976; 124:838.

Monif GRG, Welkos SL, Baer H. The bacteriological spectrum of isolates obtained from the cul-de-sac of patients with endometritis-salpingitis-peritonitis. Excerpta Medica 1977; 3:26.

Monif GRG. Hospitalization versus ambulatory therapy for women with acute salpingitis. Infect Med 2002; 19:346.

Ness RB, Hillier SL, Kip KE et al. Bacterial vaginosis and risk of pelvic inflammatory disease. Am J Obstet Gynecol 2004; 104:761.

Nilsson U, Hellberg D, Shoubnikova M, et al.: Sexual risk factors associated with bacterial vaginosis and *Chlamydia trachomatis* infection. Sex Trans Dis 1997; 24:241.

Soper DE, Brockwell NJ, Dalton HP, et al. Observations concerning the microbial etiology of acute salpingitis. Am J Obstet Gynecol 1994; 170:1008.

Spence MR, Adler J, McLellan R. Pelvic inflammatory disease in the adolescent. J Adolesc Health Care 1990; 11:304.

Thompson S III, Hater WD, Wong KH. The microbiology and therapy of acute pelvic inflammatory disease in hospitalized patients. Am J Obstet Gynecol 1980; 136:179.

Viberg L. Acute inflammatory conditions of the uterine adnexa. Acta Obstet Gynecol Scand 1964; (Suppl) 5:43.

Walker CK, Workowski KA, Washington AE, et al. Anaerobes in pelvic inflammatory disease: implications for the Centers for Disease Control and Prevention's guidelines for the treatment of sexually transmitted diseases. Clin Infect Dis 1999; 28:s29.

Westrom L. Effects of acute pelvic inflammatory disease on fertility. Am J Obstet Gynecol 1975; 121:707.

Diagnosis

Fleischer AC, Cullinan JA, Jones HW, et al. Serial assessment of adnexal masses with transvaginal color Doppler sonography. Ultrasound Med Biol 1995; 21:435.

Ha HK, Lim GY, Cha ES, et al. MR imaging of tubo-ovarian abscess. Acta Radiol 1995; 36:510.

Hagdu A, Westrom L, Brooks C, et al. Predicting acute pelvic inflammatory disease: a multivariate analysis. Am J Obstet Gynecol 1986; 155:954.

Hemila M, Henriksson L, Ylikorkala O. Serum CRP in the diagnosis and treatment of pelvic inflammatory disease. Arch Gynecol Obstet 1987; 241:177.

Hemsell DL, Ledger WJ, Martens M, et al. Concerns regarding the Centers for Disease Control's published guidelines for Pelvic Inflammatory Disease. Clin Infect Dis 2001; 32:103–107.

Jacobson L. Laparoscopy in the diagnosis of acute salpingitis. Acta Obstet Gynecol Scand 1964; 43:160.

Jacobson L, Westrom L. Objectivized diagnosis of acute pelvic inflammatory disease. Am J Obstet Gynecol 1969; 105:1088.

Kahn JG, Walker CK, Washington AE, et al. Diagnosing pelvic inflammatory disease: a comprehensive analysis and considerations for developing a new model. J Am Med Assoc 1991; 266:2594.

Lehtinen M, Laine S, Heinonen PK, et al. Serum C-reactive protein determination in acute pelvic inflammatory disease. Am J Obstet Gynecol 1986; 154:158.

Miettinen AK, Heinonen PK, Laippala P, et al. Test performance of erythrocyte sedimentation rate and C-reactive protein in assessing the severity of acute pelvic inflammatory disease. Am J Obstet Gynecol 1993; 169:1143.

Papavarnavas CP, Venter PF, van Staden MJ. Acute salpingitis—laparoscopic and microbiological evaluation. S Afr Med J 1990; 77:403.

Peipert JF, Soper DE. Diagnostic evaluation of pelvic inflammatory disease. Infect Dis Obstet Gynecol 1994; 2:38.

Peipert JF, Sweeney PJ. Diagnostic testing in obstetrics and gynecology: a clinician's guide. Obstet Gynecol 1993; 169:1143.

Peipert JF, Boardman L, Hogan JW, et al. Laboratory evaluation of acute upper genital tract infection. Obstet Gynecol 1996; 87:730.

Sellors J, Mahony J, Goldsmith C, et al. The accuracy of clinical findings and laparoscopy in pelvic inflammatory disease. Am J Obstet Gynecol 1991; 164:113.

Teisala K, Heinonen PK. C-reactive protein in assessing antimicrobial treatment of acute pelvic inflammatory disease. J Reprod Med 1990; 35:955.

Teisala K, Heinonen PK, Punnonen R. Laparoscopic diagnosis and treatment of acute pyosalpinx. J Reprod Med 1990; 35:19.

Terry J, Forrest T. Sonographic demonstration of salpingitis. Potential confusion with appendicitis. J Ultrasound Med 1989; 8:39.

Thompson S III, Holcomb G, Change S, et al. Antibiotic therapy of outpatient pelvic inflammatory disease. Presented at the Twentieth International Interscience Conference on Antimicrobial Agents and Chemotherapy, New Orleans, Louisiana, September 22, 1980, p. 671.

Therapy

Apuzzio JJ, Stankiewicz R, Ganesh V, et al. Comparison of parenteral ciprofloxacin with clindamycin-gentamicin in the treatment of pelvic infection. Am J Med 1989; 87:148.

Barrett S, Taylor C. A review of pelvic inflammatory disease. Int J STD AIDS 2005; 16:715.

Brihmer C, Kallings I, Nord CE, et al. Second look laparoscopy: evaluation of two different antibiotic regimens after treatment of acute salpingitis. Eur J Obstet Gynecol Reprod Biol 1989; 30:263.

Bruhat MA, LeBouedec G, Pouly JL, et al. Treatment of acute salpingitis with sulbactam/ampicillin. Int J Gynecol Obstet 1989; 2:41.

CDC, 1995 Guidelines for Treatment of Sexually Transmitted Diseases. January 1995; 47 No. RR-1.

Hemsell DL, Nobles BJ, Heard MC, Hemsell PG. Upper and lower reproductive tract bacteria in 126 women with acute pelvic inflammatory disease: microbial susceptibility and clinical response to four therapeutic regimens. J Reprod Med 1988; 33:799.

Hemsell DL, Wendel GD, Gall SA, et al. Multicenter comparison of cefotetan and cefoxitin in the treatment of acute obstetric and gynecologic infections. Am J Obstet Gynecol 1988; 158:722.

Hemsell DL, Wendel GD, Hemsell PG, et al. Inpatient treatment for uncomplicated and complicated acute pelvic inflammatory disease: ampicillin/subactam vs. cefoxitin. Infect Dis Obstet Gynecol 1993; 1:123.

Hillis SD, Joesof R, Marchbanks PW, et al. Delayed care of pelvic inflammatory disease as a risk factor for impaired fertility. Am J Obstet Gynecol 1993; 168:1503.

Kousseim M, Ronald A, Plummer FA, et al. Treatment of acute pelvic inflammatory disease in the ambulatory setting: trial of cefoxitin and doxycycline versus ampicillin-sulbactam. Antimicrob Agents Chemother 1991; 35:1651.

Monif GRG. Choice of antibiotics and length of therapy in the treatment of acute salpingitis. Am J Med 1985; 78:188.

Monif GRG. Requisites of therapy for acute salpingitis. Infect Dis Lett Obstet Gynecol 1986; 9:15s.

Monif GRG. Combination of bacteriostatic and bacteriocidal antibiotics in the treatment of acute salpingitis. Neb Med J 1987; 71:394.

Monif GRG. Hospitalization versus ambulatory therapy for women with acute salpingitis. Infect Med 2002; 19:346.

Monif GRG. Regarding the PEACH randomized trial. Am J Obstet Gynecol 2003; 187:1067.

Monif GRG. "Therapeutic Window" in acute salpingitis. Infect Dis Obstet Gynecol 1995; 3:45.

Ness RB, Soper DE, Holley RL, et al. Effectiveness of inpatient and outpatient treatment strategies for women with pelvic inflammatory diseases: results from the Pelvic Inflammatory Disease Evaluation and Clinical Health (PEACH) Randomized Trial. Am J Obstet Gynecol 2002; 186; 929.

Obwegeser J, Kunz J, Wust J, et al. Clinical efficacy of amoxycillin/clavulanate in laparoscopically confirmed salpingitis. J Antimicrob Chemother 1989; 24:165.

Pastorek JG. Antibiotic therapy for pelvic inflammatory disease. J Reprod Med 1990; 35:329.

Chlamydial Salpingitis

Cates W Jr, Wasserheit JN. Genital chlamydial infections: epidemiology and reproductive sequelae. Am J Obstet Gynecol 1991; 164:1771.

Cates W Jr, Joesoef R, Goldman MB. Atypical pelvic inflammatory disease: can we identify clinical predictors? Am J Obstet Gynecol 1993; 169:341.

Kiviat NB, Wolner-Hanssen P, Peterson M, et al. Localization of *Chlamydia trachomatis* infection by indirect immunofluorescence and culture in pelvic inflammatory disease. Am J Obstet Gynecol 1986; 154:865.

Mardh P-A, Moller BR, Paavonen J. Chlamydial infection of the female genital tract with emphasis on pelvic inflammatory disease. A review of Scandinavian studies. Sex Transm Dis 1981; 8:140.

Mardh P-A, Ripe T, Svensson L, et al. *Chlamydia trachomatis* infection in patients with acute salpingitis. N Engl J Med 1977; 296:1377.

Paavonen J. Chlamydial infections of the female genital tract and neonate. Part I. Infect Dis Lett Obstet Gynecol 1982; 4:19.

Paavonen J, Vesterinen E, Meyer B, et al. Genital *Chlamydia trachomatis* infections in patients with cervical atypia. Obstet Gynecol 1979; 54:289.

Ripa KT, Svensson L, Tracharne JD, et al. *Chlamydia trachomatis* infection in patients with laparoscopically verified acute salpingitis: results of isolation and antibody determinations. Am J Obstet Gynecol 1980; 138:960.

Svensson L, Mardh PA, Westron L. Infertility after acute salpingitis with special reference to *Chlamydia trachomatis*. Fertil Steril 1985; 40:322.

Tubo-Ovarian Complexes

Caspi B, Zalel Y, Or Y, et al. Sonographically guided aspiration: an alternative therapy for tubo-ovarian abscess. Ultrasound Obstet Gynecol 1996; 7: 439.

Hsu YL, Yang JM, Wang KG. Transvaginal ultrasound-guided aspiration in the treatment and follow-up of tubo-ovarian abscess: a report of two cases. Chung Hua I Hsueh Tsa Chih Taipei 1995; 56:211.

Murthy JH, Hiremagalur SR. Differentiation of tubo-ovarian abscess from pelvic inflammatory disease, and recent trends in the management of tubo-ovarian abscess. J Tenn Med Assoc 1995; 88:136.

Perez-Medina T, Huertas MA, Bajo JM. Early ultrasound-guided transvaginal drainage of tubo-ovarian abscesses: a randomized study. Ultrasound Obstet Gynecol 1996; 7:435.

Slap GB, Forke CM, Cnaan A, et al. Recognition of tubo-ovarian abscess in adolescents with pelvic inflammatory disease. J Adolesc Health 1996; 18:397.

H. influenzae Salpingitis

Carmeci C, Gregg D. *Haemophilus influenzae* salpingitis and septicemia in an adult. Obstet Gynecol 1997; 89:863.

Kragsbjerg P, Nilsson K, Persson L, et al. Deep obstetrical and gynecological infections caused by non-typeable *Haemophilus influenzae*. Scand J Infect Dis 1993; 25:341.

Kristensen K. *Haemophilus influenzae* type b infections in adults. Scand J Infect Dis 1989; 21:651.

N. meningtides Salpingitis

Monif GRG. Recovery of *Neisseria meningitidis* from the cul-de-sac of a woman with endometritis-salpingitis-peritonitis. Am J Obstet Gynecol 1981; 139:108.

S. pneumoniae Salpingitis

Austrian R, Gold J. Pneumococcal bacteremia with special reference to bacteremia pneumococcal pneumonia. Ann Intern Med 1964; 60:759.

Gomez RJ, Padilla B, Delgado IA, et al. *Streptococcus pneumoniae* peritonitis secondary to genital tract infection in a previously healthy woman. Clin Infect Dis 1992; 15:1060.

Hadfield TL, Neafie R, Lanoie LO. Tubo-ovarian abscess caused by *Streptococcus pneumoniae*. Hum Pathol 1990; 21:1288.

Jensen LS. Primary pneumococcal peritonitis. Ann Chir Gynaecol 1984; 73:9.

Patterson D, Johnson CM, Monif GRG. *Streptococcus pneumoniae* as a cause of salpingitis. Infect Dis Obstet Gynecol 1994; 1:290.

Rahav G, Ben DL, Persitz E. Postmenopausal pneumonococcal tubo-ovarian abscess. Rev Infect Dis 1991; 13:896.

Group A Streptococcal Salpingitis

Eschenbach DA, Buchanan TM, Pollock HM, et al. Polymicrobial etiology of acute pelvic inflammatory disease. N Engl J Med 1975; 293:166.

Fikrig E, Worthington MT, Lefkowitz LB Jr. Septic shock and acute respiratory distress syndrome after salpingitis caused by *Streptococcus pyogenes* group A. South Med J 1989; 82:634.

Monif GRG, Williams BT, Dase DF. Group A streptococcus as a cause of endometritis/salpingitis/peritonitis in a nongravid female. Obstet Gynecol 1977; 50:509.

Proximal Stump Salpingitis

Fletcher V Jr. Proximal stump salpingitis. Am J Obstet Gynecol 1986; 155:496.

Semchyshyn S. Fallopian tube stump perforation. Can Med Assoc J 1975; 113:275.

Salpingitis and Pregnancy

Acosta AA, Mabray CR, Kaufman RH. Intrauterine pregnancy and co-existent pelvic inflammatory disease. Obstet Gynecol 1971; 37:282.

Blanchard AC, Pastorek JG 2nd, Weeks T. Pelvic inflammatory disease during pregnancy. South Med J 1987; 80:1363.

Friedman S, Bobrow ML. Pelvic inflammatory disease in pregnancy: a review of the literature and report of 5 cases. Obstet Gynecol 1959; 14:417.

Hemsell DL, Ledger WJ, Martens M, et al. Concerns regarding the Centers for Disease Control's published guidelines for pelvic inflammatory disease. Clin Infect Dis 2001; 32:103.

Hunt SM, Kinchelow BW, Schreier PC. Tubo-ovarian abscess in pregnancy. Obstet Gynecol 1974; 43:57.

Lowrie RJ, Kron WL. Ruptured tubo-ovarian abscess at the seventh month of utero-gestation. Am J Obstet Gynecol 1951; 62:454.

McCord M, Simmons CM. Acute purulent salpingitis during pregnancy. Am J Obstet Gynecol 1953; 65:1136.

Odendaal H, Dekock M. Acute salpingitis in pregnancy. S Afr Med J 1973; 47:21.

Sarrel PM, Pruett KA. Symptomatic gonorrhea during pregnancy. Obstet Gynecol 1968; 32:670.

Salpingitis and Immunodeficiency Virus Infection

Barbosa C, Macasset M, Brockmann S, et al. Pelvic inflammatory disease and immunodeficiency virus infection. Obstet Gynecol 1997; 89:65.

Cohen CR, Sinei S, Reilly M, et al. Effect of human immunodeficiency virus type 1 infection upon acute salpingitis. J Infect Dis 1998; 178:1352.

Mugo NR, Kiehlbauch JA, Nguti R, et al. Effect of human immunodeficiency virus-1 on treatment of acute salpinitis. Obstet Gynecol 2006; 107:807.

Ness RB, Hillier SL, Richter HE, et al. Douching in relation to bacterial vaginosis, lactobacilli, and facultative bacteria in the vagina. Obstet Gynecol 2002; 100:765.

Ness RB, Hillier SL, Kip KE, et al. Douching, pelvic inflammatory disease and incident gonococcal and chlamydial genital infection in a cohort of high-risk women. Am J Epidemiol 2005; 161:186.

Salpingitis and Douching

Martens M, Monif GRG. Douching: a risk to women's healthcare? Infect Dis Obstet Gynecol 2003; 11:1.

Monif GRG, Thompson JL, Stephens HD, Baer H. Quantitative and qualitative effects of povidone-iodine liquid and gel on the aerobic and anaerobic flora of the female genital tract. Am J Obstet Gynecol 1980; 137:432.

Ness RB, Hillier SL, Richter HE, et al. Douching in relation to bacterial vaginosis, lactobacilli, and facultative bacteria in the vagina. Obstet Gynecol 2002; 100:765.

Ness RB, Hillier SL, Kip KE, et al. Douching, pelvic inflammatory disease and incident gonococcal and chlamydial genital infection in a cohort of high-risk women. Am J Epidemiol 2005; 161:186.

Onderdonk AB, Delaney ML, Hinkson PL, Dubois AM. Quantitative and qualitative effects of douching preparations on vaginal microflora. Obstet Gynecol 199280:33.

ANATOMICAL CONSIDERATIONS

In the majority of instances, the term "tubo-ovarian abscess" (TOA) is a misnomer. An abscess indicates the collection of purulent exudate within a newly created tissue space. The majority of so-called tubo-ovarian "abscesses" are nothing more than collections of pus within an anatomically distinct space created by two-point closure. A superior term to "abscess" is "tubo-ovarian complex" (TOC). Although the ovaries are frequently involved in the resultant inflammatory mass, the ovarian capsule is an effective barrier to parenchymal involvement. Consequently, a perioophoritis rather than intraparenchymal disease occurs. If a fresh corpus hemorrhagica is present to provide the critical portal of infection, a true ovarian abscess may develop.

Isolated ovarian abscesses can occur. They usually evolve in association with vaginal hysterectomy or with ovarian biopsies (particularly if done concomitantly with an incidental appendectomy or an invasive procedure on the gastrointestinal tract). Any break in the ovarian capsule introduces the potential for contamination and subsequent development of an abscess. Isolated ovarian abscesses are far more dangerous than an ovarian abscess within a TOC. Because of its anatomical positioning, when rupture occurs from an ovarian abscess, spillage tends to be into the peritoneal rather than the pelvic cavity. Significant spillage into the peritoneal cavity is often associated with clinically overt septic shock.

In contrast, TOCs tend to be bound down into the pelvis. The pelvis does not have the same absorptive capacity as does the peritoneal cavity. Consequently, the inductions of hypotension, disseminated intravascular coagulopathy, etc., are far less frequent events for patients with ruptured TOCs. Any time the ovary is the site of abscess formation, the potential for subsequent development of septic thrombophlebitis is present. The induction of unrecognized thrombophlebitis and its metastatic complications secondary to septic thromboemboli can be the deciding factors determining the outcome in a critically ill patient. TOCs must be distinguished from a pelvic abscess. The latter may coexist with a TOC. The most common pelvic abscess is that which occurs in and around the adnexa where one wall is the broad ligament and the other, the adnexa. Another type is that where the anterior abdominal wall and the posterior wall are the bowel and omentum. The large pelvic abscesses occur in the posterior cul-de-sac and rarely in the anterior cul-de-sac.

PATHOGENESIS OF RUPTURED TOA

A significant number of etiological agents are capable of altering the anatomy of the fallopian tubes, ovaries, and uterus; yet the events that combine to produce a ruptured TOC are basically limited to endogenous anaerobic bacteria. *Mycobacterium tuberculosis*, *Coccidioides immitis*, and schistosoma can all produce significant disease involving the fallopian tubes, but not abscess formation. Although *Neisseria gonorrhoeae* and *Chlamydia trachomatis* are the catalytic agents for the induction of disease, they do not per se cause abscess formation. The gonococcus, by virtue of its replication, alters the microbiological environment and, in so doing, induces the anaerobic progression. *N. gonorrhoeae* cannot replicate or survive in the intra-abscess environment. Superinfecting anaerobic bacteria in conjunction with Enterobacteriaceae are the most frequent microbial combinations associated with rupture of a previously anatomically altered fallopian tube.

There is a tendency for rupture of a TOC to occur on the left side. The close anatomic relationship between the descending sigmoid colon and the adnexa on the left side has been cited as being etiologically significant.

Although the fallopian tube is commonly regarded as the prime site of rupture, the involvement of the ovarian parenchyma is the most important factor that selects for rupture. The fimbriated end of the tube becomes attached to the ovarian cortex, and infected material within the tube may gain access to the ovary either through the site of follicular rupture or, under rare conditions, by direct penetration of the ovarian tunic. An ovarian abscess is a true abscess and not an entrapped loculation of purulent material. Pedowitz and Bloomfield (1964), in their report of 44 cases of ruptured TOA, found that in 28 cases, the site of rupture was the ovary. Once an ovarian abscess develops, lack of an overlapping distensible muscularis mucosae renders the ovary more vulnerable than adnexal structures to rupture. With appropriate antibiotic therapy, the interstitial and submucosal edema elicited recedes, permitting effective drainage of the loculated purulent material either through the uterus or into the pelvic cavity. Whether resolution, entrapment, or rupture ensues is determined by the effectiveness of antimicrobial therapy and the ability of the muscularis to accommodate the engendered intraluminal pressure.

Although the sexually transmitted diseases (STDs) are the prime disease entity capable of producing fallopian tube complexes that rupture, they do not represent the sole mechanism. A chronic anaerobic endometritis (CAE) may develop as a consequence of prolonged use of an intrauterine contraceptive device (IUD). If superimposition of an STD or myometrial penetration occurs, the CAE appears to accelerate the anaerobic progression. If the device has mechanically penetrated the endometrium, it will effectively circumvent the uterine barrier to anaerobic infection. An important distinction between these two mechanisms is that in the case of STD-induced disease, more bilateral disease is likely to develop, whereas, with myometrial penetration, there is usually almost complete sparing of the contralateral fallopian tube.

DEMOGRAPHIC CHARACTERISTICS OF HIGH-RISK PATIENTS

Patients who experience rupture of a TOC exhibit two distinct demographic profiles.

One group is usually from a disadvantaged background. A TOC that ruptures tends to occur in older women, in the third or fourth decade. Frequently, there is an antecedent history of acute inflammatory disease or documented secondary infertility.

The second group tends to have a history of fertility that has been interrupting prolonged use of the IUD. Not infrequently, a prior history of foul-smelling intramenstrual discharges or menstrual irregularities can be elicited. The prodromal signs and symptoms leading up to rupture tend to be more like those of subacute disease in contrast to the relatively acute onset observed when an STD is the principal catalyst.

CLINICAL MANIFESTATIONS OF PATIENTS WITH RUPTURED TOC

There are two basic presentations for patients with ruptured TOCs. They present as being hemodynamically compromised or in shock.

Hemodynamically Compromised Patients

Those individuals who have had significant peritoneal spillage will present with evidence of septic shock or of an intra-abdominal catastrophe. The recognition of an adnexal mass is instrumental in formulating the differential diagnosis.

Rupture is usually heralded by a sudden, severe thrust of pain at the site of rupture. The predilection of rupture for the left side may be significant in the differential diagnosis of a woman complaining of acute abdominal pain. The clinical pattern depends primarily on the degree of rupture sustained. Although the predominant pain pattern involves the lower abdomen with localization to the rupture site, it may occasionally be that of upper abdominal pain, especially marked in the right upper quadrant. Spread of exudate up the colonic gutters and under the liver and diaphragm may so accentuate the signs and symptoms in the upper abdomen as to mask the clinical features of pelvic disease. However, pelvic pain and tenderness are almost always present. With rupture of a TOA in a bedridden patient, it is not uncommon for the patient to experience shoulder pain indicative of diaphragmatic irritation. If a concomitant pelvic abscess is present, diarrhea is a prominent symptom. Once a generalized peritonitis has developed, bowel function ceases.

For those patients who present with shock, the onset of pain is frequently followed by chills, less often by vomiting, in conjunction with the signs of generalized peritonitis and

progressive vasomotor collapse. The degree of rupture and peritoneal cavity involvement determine the rapidity with which shock becomes manifest. Shock grossly correlates with the amount of inflammatory exudate liberated into the intraperitoneal cavity.

In contrast to most inflammatory conditions, the patient's temperature is so variable as to be of little or no diagnostic significance. Not infrequently, patients with ruptured TOAs have temperatures between 38°C and 38.6°C. A common clinical finding in these patients is a tachycardia far beyond that expected with the temperature observed. Leukocytosis in excess of 20,000 is characteristic; however, patients with marked leukopenia (which is usually a poor prognostic indicator) have been seen.

Hemodynamically Stable Patients

More commonly, the patient presents with signs and symptoms that are almost indistinguishable from those of unruptured TOC.

The major diagnostic dilemma is distinguishing the ruptured from the unruptured TOC (Tables 1 and 2). Most patients with unruptured TOA respond within 72 hours to aggressive systemic administration of antibiotics and fluid replacement. The development of rectal tenesmus, diarrhea, progressive tachycardia, or prolonged fever, or the persistence of peritoneal signs should suggest the possibility of a ruptured TOA. Such patients require operative intervention. Even in the acute phase of abscess, aggressive surgical therapy has been done in a controlled situation without undue serious difficulties in the postoperative period.

In many cases of ruptured unilateral TOA associated with prolonged IUD use, there appears to be a prodromal syndrome before abscess formation during which the patient complains of vague lower abdominal pain, pelvic tenderness, and dyspareunia. Although most patients are symptomatic weeks to months prior to the detection of an adnexal mass, a few may have a rather rapid course, which, if not aggressively treated, may result in perforation, peritonitis, and death. This sequence is particularly true when *Actinomyces israelii* is the predominant anaerobic bacterium.

BACTERIOLOGY

Although it is generally conceded that infection with *N. gonorrhoeae* is of overwhelming importance in the initial alterations of tubal and ovarian architecture, cultures of a ruptured TOA rarely yield the gonococcus. The conditions of abscess are not conducive to multiplication of *N. gonorrhoeae*. The principal bacteria isolated include members of the Enterobacteriaceae, coagulase-positive *Staphylococcus aureus*, the Peptostreptococci, enterococci, and the Bacteroidaceae/*Prevotella*. The incidence of recoveries of Enterobacteriaceae, particularly *Escherichia coli* and *Klebsiella pneumoniae*, is disproportionately high when compared to the incidence of their recovery from the cul-de-sac of women with acute salpingitis. The presence of Enterobacteriaceae is postulated to be one of the catalytic

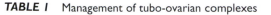

TABLE 1 Management of tubo-ovarian complexes

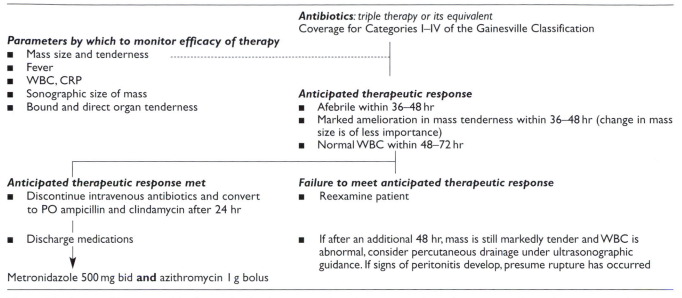

Antibiotics: *triple therapy or its equivalent*
Coverage for Categories I–IV of the Gainesville Classification

Parameters by which to monitor efficacy of therapy
- Mass size and tenderness
- Fever
- WBC, CRP
- Sonographic size of mass
- Bound and direct organ tenderness

Anticipated therapeutic response
- Afebrile within 36–48 hr
- Marked amelioration in mass tenderness within 36–48 hr (change in mass size is of less importance)
- Normal WBC within 48–72 hr

Anticipated therapeutic response met
- Discontinue intravenous antibiotics and convert to PO ampicillin and clindamycin after 24 hr
- Discharge medications

Metronidazole 500 mg bid **and** azithromycin 1 g bolus

Failure to meet anticipated therapeutic response
- Reexamine patient

- If after an additional 48 hr, mass is still markedly tender and WBC is abnormal, consider percutaneous drainage under ultrasonographic guidance. If signs of peritonitis develop, presume rupture has occurred

The need for Category IV coverage of the Gainesville Classification stems from the perception that in those patients whose tubo-ovarian complexes rupture, members of the Enterobacteriaceae, particularly *E. coli* and *K. pneumoniae*, may function as lead organisms.
Abbreviations: WBC, white blood cell count; CRP, C-reactive protein.

ingredients necessary for rupture to occur. When rupture occurs in the setting of prolonged IUD usage and associate CAE, the presence of *A. israelii* and/or Bacteroidaceae/*Prevotella* within the polymicrobial anaerobic infection appear to be factors selecting for rupture.

RUPTURED TOC IN PREGNANCY

The development of a TOC in a pregnant woman can reputedly evolve through four mechanisms:

1. Formation following abortion or attempted interruption of pregnancy
2. Intrapartum formation due to acute salpingitis in the first 8 to 12 weeks of gestation
3. Preexistent tubo-ovarian salpingitis antedating pregnancy wherein disease was localized primarily to one of the adnexa and developed prior to the establishment of conception
4. Unilateral ovarian abscess unassociated with tubal involvement

The pathogenesis of TOAs in the context of pregnancy has been an area of broad speculation. Salpingitis/pelvic inflammatory disease usually occurs in the first trimester. Ovarian and/or TOAs are distributed throughout pregnancy. This observation coupled with the barrier to ascending infection constituted by the cervical plug of the cervix and intact fetal membranes has fostered the concept that some, if not most, abscesses have a different pathogenesis than that associated with gonococcal infection in the nonpregnant female.

Once pregnancy is established, ascending infection due to *N. gonorrhoeae* is a rare event, and after the first 8 to 16 weeks of gestation, it virtually never occurs. Access

to the endometrial cavity in this time frame may occur because of continued ovulation. Ovulation induces changes in the endocervical mucus that facilitate bacterial and sperm penetration. The progressively diminishing incidence of superinfection and acute gonococcal salpingitis with time indicates that this phenomenon is time limited. Development of a TOC in association with gonococcal infection is due primarily to polymicrobial superinfection. *N. gonorrhoeae*, through its impact on the local microbiological environment, permits Class II and III anaerobic bacteria to govern the subsequent course of disease. Reported cases of TOCs in pregnancy are relatively few. The earliest case in the English literature was reported in 1869. A ruptured TOC was found at the autopsy of a pregnant woman who died on the tenth postpartum day of a generalized peritonitis. Subsequent cases have been sporadically reported. Jafari et al. (1977) reviewed 19 cases that were documented by laparoscopy. The identification of disease was scattered throughout the gestational period. Six were diagnosed in the first trimester, eight in the second, and five in the third. Only two TOCs were found at term. Of these 19 cases, in only one instance was the diagnosis made preoperatively.

Dudley et al. (1970), in reviewing the literature, noted certain factors peculiar to ovarian abscesses and TOCs in pregnancy. All previous cases of TOCs were unilateral, and more importantly, all occurred on the right side. In all of the cases, the opposite adnexa was found to be normal. This observation has been cited as evidence that the etiology of TOC in pregnancy is different than in the absence of pregnancy.

RUPTURED TOA AFTER MENOPAUSE

TOAs are considered a problem of women of childbearing age. When they occur in postmenopausal women, they

TABLE 2 Sequence management of ruptured tubo-ovarian complex

Diagnostic findings
- Demonstration of a pelvic mass (either by bimanual examination or by sonography)
- Elevated ESR (>60 mm)
- Tachycardia out of proportion to fever
- Signs of pelvic or abdominal peritonitis
- Pus demonstrable on culdocentesis
- Progression of disease despite triple therapy

↓

Management sequence
- Central venous monitor — preferably utilizing wedge pressure
- Aggressive IV therapy to reexpand contracted intravascular compartment (may require RBCs) and correct electrolyte imbalances
- Antibiotics — triple therapy or triple therapy equivalent
- Cross-match and type
- Vasogastric suction for decompression and insertion of urinary catheters

↓

Laparotomy
- Magnitude of operative procedure directed by the findings at the time of surgery
- Drainage of the lower pelvis using soft rubber clamp drains through vaginal vault plus abdominal drains is advocated

Abbreviations: ESR, erythrocyte sedimentation rate; RBCs, red blood cells.

present formidable problems in both diagnosis and therapy. In contradistinction to the history in premenopausal women, a prior history of salpingitis is uncommon. The most frequent presenting symptom is postmenopausal bleeding or lower abdominal pain. As is characteristic of other infectious disease processes in older patients, systemic signs of infectious morbidity are often depressed. *Only 50% to 60% of patients will have concomitant fever and leukocytosis.* Not infrequently, individuals show few or no signs and come to laparotomy without invoking any preoperative suspicion of the possibility of a ruptured TOA.

The pathogenesis of this entity involves multiple factors and may be distinct from that in the premenopausal woman. A significant percentage of cases have either primary disease in the gastrointestinal tract with apparent secondary involvement of the female genital tract or an associated genital tract malignancy: invasive carcinoma of the cervix or adenocarcinoma of the fallopian tubes. At laparotomy, the finding of bilateral TOA is more common than unilateral disease. The bacteriology of this disease entity is poorly defined. Most laboratories do not resort to the use of appropriate anaerobic technology. Aerobically, the most significant organisms isolated are members of the *Enterobacteriaceae* (*E. coli*, *K. pneumoniae*, etc.). The most common bacteria isolated from the intravascular compartment have been the Bacteroidaceae/ *Prevotella* and/or the Peptostreptococci.

The patients in whom rupture has occurred differ by virtue of evidence of infectious morbidity. Almost invariably they present with fever, lower abdominal pain, and

tachycardia. Abdominal distention associated with decreased bowel sounds ensues. Less frequent is the development of rebound tenderness.

DIAGNOSIS

The diagnosis of a TOC in pregnancy is seldom made prior to actual rupture; even then, inconsistencies of the signs of peritonitis in pregnancy render the diagnosis difficult. The clinical presentation varies significantly. Ultimately, however, the patient manifests the signs of peritoneal irritation or overt peritonitis followed by impending vasomotor collapse. The differential diagnosis is that which is classic for pregnancy, namely, appendicitis, ectopic pregnancy, hemorrhagic pancreatitis, and torsion and infarction of an ovarian mass (e.g., a dermoid cyst). The only clinical clue that points to the probability of a ruptured TOC in pregnancy is documentation of PID prior to the establishment of pregnancy. The augmented technology achieved through ultrasonography and computed tomography (CT) scan has impacted primarily on the ability to make the diagnosis of TOC rather than that of a rupture. Spirts et al. (1982) have demonstrated that over 50% of cases with TOA will have significant fluid collections in the cul-de-sac. Its presence may not correlate with the apparent severity of disease. When bilateral TOCs are present, they may fill the pelvis and imperceptibly blend with the uterus. The concomitant presence of a significant amount of fluid in the cul-de-sac of a patient with a TOC and slowly resolving physical findings should bias clinical thought to the possibility that rupture has occurred. The demonstration of an abscess within the ovary is a mandate for operative intervention. CT in the series reported by Knochel et al. (1980) is the more accurate of the two modalities and has better predictive value. The correlation between anatomical findings at surgery and diagnostic CT scan was 96% compared to 90% with ultrasonography. However, because of the cost differential and the need to respect the intents of diagnosis-related groups, ultrasonography is preferentially used.

The presumptive diagnosis of ruptured TOC is made by clinical evaluation. Basically, you have a patient who has clinical findings that are inconsistent with anatomically limited disease and that have persisted despite appropriate medical therapy (Table 1). Under careful questioning, about a third of the cases of ruptured TOCs will give a characteristic history. Initial pain is in the lower quadrant and is crampy in nature. A sudden exacerbation and/or change in the character of the lower abdominal pain will then occur. The pain not infrequently gets transiently better only to return within hours. At this time, the pain becomes more constant and is sharp rather than colicky in character. The magnitude of temperature elevation does not tend to mirror the severity of disease. The white blood cell count (WBC) is usually elevated and shifted to the left. Almost invariably, the erythrocyte sedimentation rate (ESR) is above 60 mm/hr when disease is associated with or initiated by *N. gonorrhoeae*. The most significant clinical clue is the presence of four-quadrant abdominal tenderness.

Three-quadrant *rebound tenderness* can develop when the Curtis–Fitz Hugh variant of gonococcal or chlamydial peritonitis is present, but rarely does it involve *all four quadrants*. The presence of four-quadrant tenderness is a clinical red light.

In many instances, the diagnosis of rupture is in dispute. When dealing with a medically stable patient, it is not inappropriate to treat such an individual with triple therapy and monitor closely the titration points. Patients with both ruptured and unruptured TOCs will initially respond to triple therapy or its equivalent. The persistence of peritoneal signs, a WBC > 15,000, and tachycardia inappropriate for temperature beyond four days in association with persistent mass tenderness should reinforce the concept that one may be dealing with a ruptured TOC that is partially sealed by an overlay of bowel and omentum.

MANAGEMENT OF A RUPTURED TOC

Therapy requires an understanding of the potential lethal complications that can ensue (Table 2). Women with rupture can die due to

1. adult respiratory distress syndrome (ARDS),
2. septic shock,
3. inappropriate management of intravascular volume, and
4. septic thrombophlebitis and metastatic complications.

Physicians must anticipate that their patient may

1. become hypovolemic,
2. develop ARDS,
3. exhibit some evidence of acute tubular necrosis,
4. develop local (loop-to-loop or subphrenic) or distant (pulmonary) abscesses, or
5. develop wound infection and/or wound dehiscence.

The prerequisites for a good outcome are the following:

1. A good anesthesiologist
2. Use of a Swan-Ganz catheter
3. Aggressive antibiotic therapy
4. Therapy of ARDS
5. Surgical removal of diseased organ
6. Retention sutures
7. Secondary closure

Swan-Ganz Catheter

An anesthesiologist should be used for the placement of a Swan-Ganz catheter. This permits reexpansion of the intravascular volume by using the pulmonary artery wedge pressure as the guiding parameter.

Antibiotics

The patient is placed on a fourth-generation semisynthetic penicillin and metronidazole. This combination gives excellent I, II, and III coverage in terms of the Gainesville Classification. The Category IV weakness is covered by the bolus aminoglycoside therapy, which is usually maintained at therapeutic levels by the induced alterations in renal function. The appropriate dosage of an aminoglycoside

(adjusted for body weight) is given. Thereafter, the drug is usually stopped. Continued use of an aminoglycoside is contingent upon assessment of the patient's renal status.

Some form of tubular necrosis is to be anticipated, and hence the necessity to limit the prolonged administration of nephrotoxic drugs.

Adult Respiratory Distress Syndrome

ARDS is an extreme form of noncardiogenic pulmonary edema associated with alveolar-capillary damage. Clinical features include acute respiratory distress, dyspnea and tachypnea, severe hypoxemia refractory to oxygen therapy, and diffuse bilateral pulmonary infiltrates. Pulmonary capillary hydrostatic pressure is usually normal. Filling or closure of alveoli leads to reduced functional residual capacity, decreased pulmonary compliance, and intrapulmonary right-to-left shunting. Shock or sepsis, functioning separately or in consort, can cause ARDS, but the processes leading to the alveolar permeability defect are not understood. Therefore, therapy remains nonspecific and supportive. Treatment includes positive end-expiratory pressure, careful fluid management, steroid therapy, and adequate nutrition. Unfortunately, even with the most sophisticated intensive care, the mortality of ARDS is greater than 50%.

Surgical Intervention

Increased morbidity and mortality are directly related to the degree of procrastination prior to operative procedure. Many clinicians consider 12 hours the upper limit of safety. The importance of close observation, early diagnosis, and prompt surgical intervention cannot be emphasized enough. Next to the general condition of the patient, the time interval before surgery takes prognostic precedence over all other factors. In the series reported by Lardaro (1954), only one of the seven patients brought to surgical repair within 12 hours after rupture died, whereas 7 of the 12 patients operated on after 12 hours died. In general, if surgical treatment is performed within the first 12 hours, 70% of patients recover and 30% die. If surgery is performed after 48 hours, 20% recover and 80% die. Death approaches 100% if patients do not have the abscess removed.

The surgical procedure depends partly on the patient's clinical status. The procedure of choice is hysterectomy and bilateral salpingo-oophorectomy. Since the most difficult part of the procedure is mobilization of the adnexa from the uterus prior to their removal, the uterus can be extirpated with relative ease without excessive prolongation of the operation. If the patient is premoribund at the time of operative intervention, simple salpingo-oophorectomy should be performed.

It is important to explore the entire abdomen and to search out purulent loculations between loops of bowel and beneath the diaphragm. Copious irrigation of the entire abdomen with physiologic saline solution containing a potassium supplement is mandatory.

When possible, it is valuable to evaluate the pelvic veins carefully in all cases of TOA for suppurative pelvic thrombophlebitis due to Bacteroidaceae/*Prevotella* or the anaerobic streptococci. Unless extensive, this complication is best treated with anticoagulants.

The possibility of preserving ovarian function should be explored; however, when a limited procedure is done, additional surgical treatment is not infrequently required. The effects of previous laparotomy and generalized peritonitis render such an operative procedure difficult, if not potentially hazardous.

In the total hysterectomy, peritonealization is often impossible; the vaginal vault is left open except for the hemostatic angle sutures. If subtotal hysterectomy is done, drainage can be achieved by splitting the cervix or by entering the vagina through the cul-de-sac. In most patients, adequate drainage of the peritoneal cavity cannot be achieved. In general, no drain is left in the place of the vaginal cuff.

Wound Closure

Closure of the peritoneum and fascial layers of the abdominal wall is best achieved with Tom Jones wire sutures and leaving the skin and subcutaneous area open, to be closed at a later date (Table 3). It should be noted that surgical rupture of a large ovarian abscess during the operation is relatively benign compared with rupture within the enclosed abdomen. The impact of a good diagnosis can be negated by an inadequate surgical exposure. A ruptured TOC should never be handled through a vertical incision. Be sure that the vertical incision extends sufficiently above the umbilicus to permit exploration of the bowel and upper abdomen. Since anatomical relationships are often obscured or distorted, the operating physician must be experienced. The extent of surgery is that which is required to save an individual's life. When dealing with unilateral disease, if possible, residual ovarian function should be preserved.

The prior presence of generalized peritonitis and ileus negates any consideration of primary closure. It is best to use a permanent suture such as prolene or wire in the Smead-Jones fashion, closing the perineum muscle and fascia in one layer and then leaving the subcutaneous tissue and skin open. This can usually be closed in four or five days or it can be left to granulate, but closing the subcutaneous tissue in the skin almost always results in a wound infection and leaving it open to be closed by secondary intention almost always results in healing without wound infection.

No one wants to deal with a major wound dehiscence in a previously severely stressed individual. Secondary closure is an important surgical adjunct. What we specifically recommend is summarized in Table 3.

TABLE 3 Management of the contaminated wound associated with ruptured tubo-ovarian abscess

- Close the fascia and peritoneum but leave the subcutaneous tissue and cutis open
- Pack with moist gauze 4–5 times/day
- Close secondarily on the fifth or sixth day; prior to closing the wound, scrape both surfaces of the granulation tissue so that they ooze. If one attempts to oppose two surfaces composed of granulation tissue by secondary closure, infrequently a serosoma forms

Potential Use of Ultrasound-Guided Drainage of TOA

Most TOAs are not true abscesses, but rather TOCs. With appropriate antibiotic therapy, point-specific inflammatory edema ameliorates, permitting the inflammatory exudates to drain into either the uterine or pelvic cavity. The potential for rupture under therapy resides with the large TOAs that remain constant in size and tender, with concomitant evidence of a continuing inflammatory response.

In the absence of evidence of rupture, serious consideration should be given for ultrasound-guided drainage or operative laparoscopic incision and lavage. Transabdominal drainage under ultrasound guidance should be considered for any large TOC that remains tender after 48 hours of appropriate antibiotic therapy.

LIGNEOUS CELLULITIS

This indolent cellulitis is another complication of chronic and repeated pelvic infections. Bacteriologic studies in terms of causative agents and pathogenesis are poorly delineated at the present time.

Symptoms are nonspecific; postoperatively or posttherapy, the patient may complain of fatigue, anorexia, vague pelvic discomfort, and/or weight loss. She may or may not be febrile. Not infrequently, abnormal or prolonged uterine bleeding may be the main reason the patient seeks medical care.

Bimanual examination reveals fixation of the pelvis. The pelvic floor has a characteristic woody-hard, smooth texture. It is not difficult to comprehend how the physician may misdiagnose the lesion as pelvic cancer. Biopsy of the endometrium and cervix reveals extensive inflammatory debris, and chronic infection rather than cancer. The WBC may be elevated but usually is normal. The patient is frequently anemic, with a hemoglobin level of 10 g or less. The ESR, a useful indicator of response to therapy, is elevated.

Once the diagnosis is made, the patient should be hospitalized, treated initially with antibiotics having Category I and II designation, and kept at bed rest. Attention should be given to nutrition. Some clinicians have advocated simultaneous administration of cortisone or other antiinflammatory agents with the antibiotic in order to speed resolution of the inflammatory process. However, this is rarely necessary.

When the patient's temperature has returned to normal and she is eating well, she may be discharged from the hospital with instructions to continue treatment at home by resting, adhering to a well-balanced diet, and taking an appropriate antibiotic.

Within 6 to 12 weeks, the cellulitis should clear. When the pelvic examination is normal, the patient should have a hysterectomy and bilateral salpingo-oophorectomy. Some patients with ligneous cellulitis develop septic pelvic thrombophlebitis heralded by spiking temperature, shaking chills, and (sometimes) pelvic or abdominal pain. Intravenous administration of heparin and more aggressive antibiotic therapy should be instituted.

OVARIAN ABSCESS

Ovarian abscess is a distinct clinical entity that should not be confused with TOA. These disease entities differ significantly both in their pathogenesis and in the clinical circumstances under which they occur. The overriding distinction is that TOA develops from a naturally occurring disease process, whereas isolated bacterial ovarian abscess is almost always an iatrogenic phenomenon.

Pathogenesis

The epithelial covering of the ovary exhibits a remarkable degree of resistance to bacterial penetration and involvement of the underlying stroma. What is required for bacterial penetration is either

1. a natural disruption of the ovarian surface epithelium and the subsequent creation of a new tissue space (as might be constituted by a hemorrhagic corpus luteum cyst),
2. intentional or unintentional surgical incision into the ovarian parenchyma, subsequent hematoma formation, and bacterial contamination during a surgical procedure, or
3. hematogenous seeding of a hemorrhagic corpus luteum cyst.

Most commonly, an ovarian abscess occurs after rupture of a follicular ovarian cyst, with subsequent seeding of bacteria into the stigmata or colonization of the ovarian stroma. The onset of an ovarian abscess is insidious and usually presents as pain and low-grade fever with acute peritonitis occurring from one week to six months following initial contamination.

The suturing of the ovarian pedicle to the angle of the vaginal cuff places the adnexa in close proximity to any area containing devitalized tissue, which in turn is in contact with the vaginal flora (Fig. 1). The surgical alteration of the natural barriers to infection permits penetration by the more aggressive bacterial organisms. In those circumstances in which a surgical procedure produces significant tissue damage, this process selects for a specific group of pathogens by creating an environment conducive to anaerobic growth. The pathogens cultured from an ovarian abscess are almost invariably those indigenous to the patient's own flora.

Natural History of Ovarian Abscesses

Bacteria capable of septicemic disease from the gastrointestinal tract on occasion may seed a recently ruptured follicular site and create a metastatic abscess. *Nontyphoidal salmonella* and *Pasturella multocida* have been recovered from ovarian abscesses and/or previously established TOA.

Ovarian abscess is primarily a disease of women of childbearing age. Some operative procedure precedes the establishment of infection; the great majority of cases occur following vaginal or gastrointestinal surgical procedures. Willison and Black (1964) note that the majority of their patients were in the secretory phase of the menstrual cycle and implied that the hemorrhagic corpus luteum cyst acted as the portal of infection for the ovary. However, this contention was not later substantiated by Ledger et al. (1968), in whose study, only 5 of the 17 patients with isolated ovarian abscesses were known to be in the luteal phase. In the author's experience, patients with an isolated ovarian abscess have had either hemorrhagic corpus luteum cysts at the time of surgery or surgical penetration of the ovarian surface.

The interval between initial operative intervention and clinical manifestations of disease varies considerably, depending on

1. the dose of the bacterial inoculum,
2. whether infection was due to direct contamination at the time of operation or to spread through devitalized tissue to a new tissue space, and
3. the type of bacterium and its relative virulence.

In the characteristic case, the patient becomes febrile postoperatively. There may be an initial clinical response to

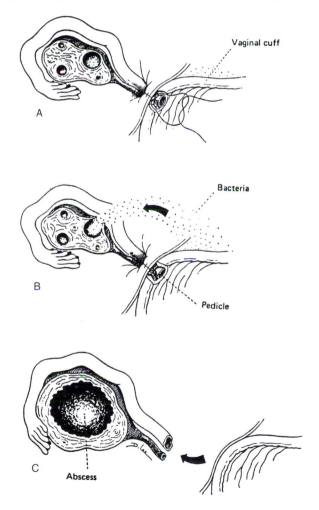

FIGURE 1 Proposed mechanism for development of an ovarian abscess after vaginal hysterectomy. (**A**) The proximity of adnexal structures to the vaginal cuff following vaginal hysterectomy is shown. (**B**) Postoperative ovulation estroma of the ovary to bacterial invasion from the infected vaginal cuff. (**C**) Disintegration of the suture holding the pedicle to the vaginal cuff permits retraction of the adnexal abscess high into the pelvis. *Source*: Ledger W et al. Surg Gynecol Obstet 1969; 129:973.

antibiotics; however, it is usually transient, the patient again becoming septic (often before the termination of antibiotic therapy). It is not uncommon for there to be a prolonged delay of 6 to 45 days between operative procedure and clinical manifestation of abscess. In at least one instance, 133 days elapsed between the two events. Bacteriologic analysis commonly reveals a single pathogen. In approximately one-third of the cases, two or more genera of bacteria have been isolated. The principal pathogens are the obligatory anaerobes.

Once abscess formation is well established, the patient develops the characteristic hectic spiking temperature curve. The WBC count is often in excess of 20,000. Septicemia, clinically manifested by shaking chills, may occur and is often indicative of ovarian vein thrombophlebitis.

Therapy

The long interval between initial seeding of the ovary and clinical recognition of disease is often of sufficient duration to permit disintegration of the sutures holding the ovarian pedicle to the vaginal cuff, thus allowing retraction of the adnexal mass into the pelvis. When the ovarian pedicle still adheres to the vaginal cuff, the abscess may dissect through adjacent tissue and drain through the vaginal vault. However, when a sufficient interval occurs to permit retraction of the adnexal mass into the pelvis or when abscess has formed secondary to surgical disruption of the ovarian capsules at the time of elective appendectomy, and the site of abscess is high in the pelvis, it is unlikely that such an abscess is amenable to simple surgical drainage.

Conservative management runs the risk of intraperitoneal abscess rupture. If this occurs, it is associated with high mortality (comparable to that seen with ruptured TOA). The treatment of ovarian abscess is abdominal excision within hours following institution of antibiotic therapy. Antibiotic therapy should be directed primarily against anaerobic organisms. Large doses of penicillin in conjunction with metronidazole or clindamycin and an aminoglycoside antibiotic are deemed suitable combinations. Antibiotics are primarily administered to prevent systemic or metastatic complications. The definitive therapy of ovarian abscess is surgical, not medical.

OVARIAN ABSCESS FOLLOWING THERAPEUTIC INSEMINATION

Serious bacterial infections associated with therapeutic insemination are rare. Sable et al. (1993) reported the first case of a ruptured TOA following intrauterine insemination. Kolb et al. (1994) have described a case of ovarian abscess following intrauterine insemination with the husband's semen. The patient became symptomatic within five days of insemination. Despite treatment with triple antibiotics, an oophorectomy was required. Violation of the natural cervical barrier that occurs with therapeutic insemination can, in rare instances, theoretically place the patient at increased risk for infectious morbidity.

SELECTED READING

Tubo-Ovarian Abscess

Bamberger DM. Outcome of medical treatment of bacterial abscesses without therapeutic drainage: review of cases reported in the literature. Clin Infect Dis 1996; 23:592.

Buchweitz O, Malik E, Kressin P, et al. Laparoscopic management of TOA: retrospective analysis. Surg Endosc 2000; 14:948.

Ginsburg DS, Stern JL, Hamod KA, et al. Tubo-ovarian abscess: a retrospective review. Am J Obstet Gynecol 1980; 138:1055.

Hemsell DL, Hemsell PG, Heard ML, Nobles BJ. Piperacillin and a combination of clindamycin and gentamicin for hospital and community acquired acute pelvic infections including pelvic abscess. Surg Gynecol Obstet 1987; 165:223.

Hemsell DL, Wendel GD, Hemsell PG, et al. Inpatient treatment for uncomplicated and complicated acute pelvic inflammatory disease: Ampicillin/Sulbactin vs. Cefoxitin. Infect Dis Obstet Gynecol 1993; 1:123.

Henry-Suchet J, Soler A, Loffredo V. The laparoscopic treatment of tubal ovarian abscesses. J Reprod Med 1984; 29:579.

Hoffman M, Molpus K, Roberts WS, et al. Tubovarian abscess in postmenopausal women. J Reprod Med 1990; 35:525.

Landers DV, Sweet RL. Tubo-ovarian abscess: contemporary approach to management. Rev Infect Dis 1983; 5:876.

Landers DV, Sweet RL. Current trends in the diagnosis and treatment of tubal ovarian abscess. Am J Obstet Gynecol 1985; 151:1098.

Manara LR. Management of tubo-ovarian abscess. J Am Osteopath Assoc 1982; 81:476.

Monif GRG. Clinical staging of acute bacterial salpingitis and its therapeutic ramifications. Am J Obstet Gynecol 1982; 143:489.

Nebel WA, Lucas WE. Management of tubo-ovarian abscess. Obstet Gynecol 1968; 32:382.

Paik CK, Waetjen LE, Xing G, et al. Hospitalizations for pelvic inflammatory disease and tuboovarian abscess. Obstet Gynecol 2006; 107:611.

Perez-Medinia T, Huertas MA, Bajo JM. Early ultrasound-guided vaginal drainage of TOA: a randomized study. Ultrasound Obstet Gynecol 1996; 7:435.

Roberts W, Dockery JL. Operative and conservative treatment of tubo-ovarian abscess due to pelvic inflammatory disease. South Med J 1984; 77:860.

Schreier PC, Adams JO, Everett BE. Optimum time for surgery in pelvic inflammatory disease. South Med J 1957; 50:1473.

Ruptured TOA

Anderson G, Buchlwe WB. Abdominal surgery and tubo-ovarian abscess. West J Obstet Gynecol 1962; 70:67.

Clark JFJ, Moore-Hines S. A study of tubo-ovarian abscess at Howard University Hospital (1965 through 1975). J Nat Med Assoc 1979; 71:1109.

Franklin EW, Hevron JE, Thompson JD. Management of the pelvic abscess. Clin Obstet Gynecol 1973; 16:66.

Ginsburg DS, Stern JL, Hamond KA, et al. Tubo-ovarian abscess: a retrospective review. Am J Obstet Gynecol 1980; 138:1055.

Landers DV, Sweet RL. Tubo-ovarian abscess: contemporary approach to management. Rev Infect Dis 1983; 5:876.

Lardaro HH. Spontaneous rupture of the tubo-ovarian abscess into the free peritoneal cavity. J Am Med Assoc 1954; 156:699.

Mickal A, Sellmann AH, Beebe JL. Ruptured tubo-ovarian abscess. Am J Obstet Gynecol 1969; 100:432.

Shittu OS, Ifenne DI, Ekwempu CC. A simple mass-closure technique compared with layered technique in the closure of high-risk abdominal wounds. West Afr J Med 1995; 14:11.

Pedowitz P, Bloonfield RD. Ruptured adnexal abscess (tuboovarian) with generalized peritonitis. Am J Obstet Gunecol 1964; 88:721.

Wetchler SJ, Dunn LJ. Ovarian abscess. Report of a case and review of the literature. Obstet Gynecol Surv 1985; 40:476.

Ruptured TOC in Pregnancy

Baydoun AB, Sarram M. Ovarian abscess in pregnancy. Obstet Gynecol 1961; 18:739.

Cron RS. Three month's pregnancy complicated by tubo-ovarian abscess. Wisc Med J 1924; 23:194.

Cummin RC. Ovarian abscess during pregnancy. Br J Obstet Gynaecol 1951; 58:1025.

Dashow EE, Cotterill R, BeMiller D. Ruptured tubo-ovarian abscess in early gestation. A case report. J Reprod Med 1990; 35:418.

Dudley AG, Lee F, Barclay D. Ovarian and tubo-ovarian abscess in pregnancy: report of a case and a review of the literature. Milit Med 1970; 135:403.

Friedman S, Kinchelde BW, Schreier RC. Tubo-ovarian abscess in pregnancy. Obstet Gynecol 1974; 43:57.

Jafari K, Vilovick KDS, Webster A, Stepto RC. Tubo-ovarian abscess in pregnancy. Acta Obstet Gynecol Scand 1977; 56:1.

Knochel JQ, Koehler PR, Lee TG: Diagnosis of abdominal abscesses with computed tomography, ultrasound and 111-In leukocyte scans. Radiology 1980; 137:425.

Spirtos NJ, Bernstine RL, Crawford WL, Fayle J: Sonography in acute pelvic inflammatory disease. J Reprod Med 1982; 27:312.

Stubbs RE, Monif GRG. Ruptured tubo-ovarian abscess in pregnancy: recovery of a penicillinase-producing strain of Neiseeria gonorrhoeae. Sex Trans Dis 1985; 12:235.

Postmenopausal Ruptured TOC

Heaton FC, Ledger WJ. Postmenopausal tubo-ovarian abscess. Obstet Gynecol 1976; 47:90.

Mann LI, Rommey SL. Postmenopausal ruptured adnexal abscess. Obstet Gynecol 1966; 28:707.

Ovarian Abscess

Black WR. Abscess of the ovary. Am J Obstet Gynecol 1936; 31:487.

Hall WL, Sobel AI, Jones CP. Anaerobic postoperative pelvic infections. Obstet Gynecol 1967; 30:1.

Kolb BA, Mercer L, Peters AJ, Kazer R. Ovarian abscess following therapeutic insemination. Infect Dis Obstet Gynecol 1994; 1:249.

Ledger WJ, Campbell C, Taylor D, Willison JR. Adnexal abscess as a late complication of pelvic operatory. Surg Gynecol 1968; 129:973.

Ledger WJ, Campbell C, Willison JR. Postoperative adnexal infection. Obstet Gynecol 1968; 31:83.

Sable DB, Yanushpolsky EH, Fox JH. Ruptured pelvic abscess after intrauterine insemination: a case report. Fertil Steril 1993; 59:679.

Willison JR, Black WT. Ovarian abscess. Am J Obstet Gynecol 1964; 90:34

Pelvic Abscess

James W. Daly

INTRODUCTION

The pelvic abscess may have a multiplicity of etiologies. Although most pelvic abscesses are complications of sexually transmitted diseases (STDs), they may also be due to complications of pregnancy, chronic anaerobic endometritis associated with prolonged intrauterine device usage, ruptured appendix, diverticulitis, or endomyometritis. A certain number of pelvic abscesses will be due to primary operations in the pelvis or in the upper abdomen. The discussion here focuses on those pelvic abscesses that are the consequences of STDs or pelvic surgery.

BACTERIOLOGY

Neisseria gonorrhoeae and/or *Chlamydia trachomatis* are the prime initiators of diseases that ultimately produce a pelvic abscess; however, cultures of a pelvic abscess rarely yield these organisms. The principal bacteria isolated from pelvic abscesses include members of the Enterobacteriaceae, the Peptostreptococci, the Peptococci, and the Bacteroidaceae. The high incidence of negative cultures or so-called "sterile abscesses" primarily tends to reflect the lack of skill in taking anaerobic cultures and/or suboptimal microbiology.

ANATOMICAL CONSIDERATIONS

Pelvic abscesses are often casually referred to as "tubo-ovarian" abscesses. Actually, tubo-ovarian abscesses are not common and are a distinct entity in which the process has also extended into the ovarian parenchyma. Primary ovarian abscesses are quite uncommon and are usually seen postoperatively as complications following vaginal surgery.

The most common pelvic abscess is that which occurs in and around the adnexa where one wall is the broad ligament, the other the adnexa. The uterus is usually anatomically involved. This type of abscess is generally small and easily resolves with medical therapy. The larger abscesses usually occur in the posterior cul-de-sac and rarely in the anterior cul-de-sac. Posterior cul-de-sac abscesses are the most prone to peritoneal leakage. The lid is imperfect, being formed of the colon, small intestine, and omentum.

CLINICAL PRESENTATION

A pelvic abscess may occur at any age. It is most prevalent during the middle of the reproductive age span (the third and fourth decade); however, it may also occur at or after menopause.

The patient with a pelvic abscess usually has been sick for some period of time and may not be able to document or give an exact description of the time or circumstances of the onset of a process. Eventually the patient will have regional pain, fever, or lower abdominal tenderness. In some patients, there is a poor correlation between abscess size and symptomatology. On physical examination, the patient's lower abdomen is usually tender. Rebound tenderness may be present depending upon etiology and extent of disease. The pelvis is usually quite tender. Masses may or may not be identified depending upon their location and the patient's tenderness. Occasionally, the abscess may be rather high on the pelvic wall and the examiner will have difficulty feeling it from below. Usually, a sense of fullness or induration can be identified.

Cul-de-sac abscesses present posteriorly; but occasionally, they may be quite high, which allows for their detection on rectal examination. When a posterior cul-de-sac abscess has been present for some time, it can dissect into the rectovaginal septum. On bimanual examination, the examining finger and/or speculum run immediately into a posterior mass with the uterus and cervix displaced upward and anteriorly out of clear view.

Some, but not all, of the patients will have an elevated temperature and tachycardia. In general, the more acute the process, the more likely the patient is to have rapid pulse and fever. The presence of hypotension or shock is usually indicative of significant spillage into the peritoneal cavity.

Not all the patients will have elevated white blood cell counts (WBC) comparable to those encountered in acute phases of disease. As the process becomes subacute or indolent, the WBC returns toward normal, but the erythrocyte sedimentation rate (ESR) will be markedly elevated. The patients frequently have anorexia, nausea, sometimes vomiting, and very often diarrhea. *Diarrhea is often one of the prime symptoms of the pelvic abscess.*

It is important to consider in the initial survey of the patient whether or not the abscess is localized to the pelvis or if the whole abdomen is contaminated. Those patients who have tenderness confined to the lower abdomen can be assumed, at least initially, to have a confined abscess. Those patients who have tenderness and/or rebound in the upper abdomen should be suspected of having a leaking or ruptured process with generalized peritoneal contamination. Persistent signs of peritoneal irritation, despite hydration and antibiotic therapy, dictate an aggressive evaluation of the patient. The patient who is initially seen with shock should be resuscitated, started on antibiotics and, once stabilized, operated on.

There has been an off and on debate over the years as to whether all patients with abscesses should have immediate surgery under antibiotic coverage. Somewhere between 10% and 30% of patients who are admitted to the hospital with a diagnosis of pelvic abscess will require surgery during the initial hospitalization. Approximately one-third of these require operative intervention because the abscess has ruptured or is leaking. The rest come to surgery because they have failed to respond.

CLINICAL EVALUATION

Noninvasive imaging procedures increase our ability to be more specific in our diagnosis of pelvic abscesses. In addition, radionuclide scanning can be highly site specific. Computed tomography (CT) is sensitive but is expensive. Combined abdominal/transvaginal ultrasound examination is quick, relatively inexpensive, and reasonably sensitive and specific. The patient with pelvic infection and a mass or suspected abscess should have an ultrasound examination to document and measure the mass. Subsequent examinations can be useful in measuring response. Clinical evaluation includes an ESR, WBC and platelets, serum electrolytes, blood urea nitrogen, creatinine, blood culture, and chest X ray, and in the severely ill, an arterial blood gas for PO_2, PCO_2, pH, and central monitoring.

DIAGNOSIS

The techniques available to a clinician for identifying the source of infection have been divided into those that detect anatomical abnormalities (CT, ultrasonography, and magnetic resonance imaging) and those that detect inflammation (radionuclide scans) (Table 1).

When the normal anatomy has been altered by prior surgery, damage, or trauma, a combination of techniques that demonstrate anatomical abnormality and those that detect information is required. The overall accuracy for CT and sonography in detecting an abdominal abscess is in the order of 90% to 95%.

Ultrasonography is preferably used for diagnosing right upper quadrant and pelvic abscesses. In these areas, there is no intervening bowel gas that potentially could impede sonography visualization. In patients with poorly localized abscess or with postoperative open surgical wounds and drains, CT is with the superior of the two methods for abscess localization.

With CT or ultrasonography, abscesses appear as complex fluid collections. However, these imaging findings are nonspecific and can be mimicked by hematomas, seromas, lymphoceles, etc. X ray may be used to demonstrate gas within the mass.

THERAPY

Once the diagnosis of a pelvic abscess is made, antibiotic therapy is instituted with penicillin, clindamycin, or metronidazole, and an aminoglycoside. The parameters used to monitor response to therapy should include the following:

1. Fever
2. WBC
3. Physical findings
4. Patient's sense of well-being
5. ESR
6. Ultrasound or CT finding

Once the therapeutic titration points have been achieved, parenteral antibiotics can be discontinued. The patient should be treated for a minimum of 10 days, but not all of this needs to be with triple antibiotics. Most patients respond within 72 hours to aggressive systemic administration of antibiotics and fluid replacement. If therapy has been effective, the WBC count should be normal or near normal. Patients who do not improve on triple antibiotic therapy, who continue to have fever, who continue to have pain, whose mass is growing, who have persistent ileus, and/or who are definitely not thriving, should be operated upon and the abscess removed and/or drained.

Those patients who do not respond to medical therapy or who deteriorate should have surgical intervention. Response equates with normalization of temperature, a normal WBC, and subjective and objective improvement in the patient's condition and physical findings.

Surgical therapy has traditionally been hysterectomy and bilateral salpingo-oophorectomy. Recent experience indicates that removing only the diseased area, for instance, a unilateral salpingo-oophorectomy, can be effective. It seems clear that the standard operation of removing the uterus and both adnexa has no advantage over a more conservative surgical approach preserving potential fertility. Landers and Sweet (1985) identified a 14% subsequent pregnancy rate in patients treated with a unilateral adnexectomy for pelvic abscess. However, the incidence of ensuing ectopic pregnancies will be high in this group of patients.

Imaging techniques permit percutaneous or vaginal abscess drainage. Transvaginal drainage guided by real-time ultrasonography has been shown to be an effective mode of therapy in selected cases (Fig. 1).

The patient treated conservatively with antibiotics should have a pelvic examination several times a week to determine if the abscess is pointing into the cul-de-sac. If it does, then drainage may be achieved by a simple colpotomy. To be safe and successful in this approach, the abscess must be fluctuant, mid-line, and dissecting into the rectovaginal septum. "It is ready when you cannot put a speculum in the vagina because there is a mass there."

TABLE I Noninvasive diagnostic technique

Detection of anatomical abnormalities
(1) Computed tomography, radionuclides
(2) Ultrasonography, human serum albumin
(3) Magnetic resonance imaging

Detection of inflammation
(1) Technetium 99m
(2) 67 gallium-citrate
(3) White blood cell counts—indium
(4) Immunoglobulin G—indium

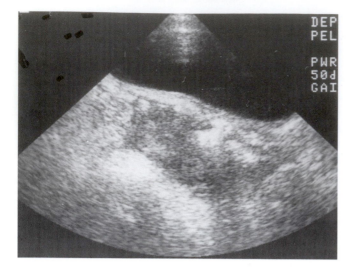

FIGURE 1 Ultrasonographic demonstration of a postoperative pelvic abscess that has the potential for fine-needle aspiration. *Source:* Courtesy of Susanne Granger, MD.

However, it is a mistake to try to drain a pelvic abscess that has not pointed. Once a surgeon starts dissecting posteriorly in the pelvis, injury to the ureters and intestine becomes a very real possibility. If the abscess is successfully drained posteriorly and the patient thrives, it is usually enough; nothing else may need to be done.

There are some patients who will develop upper abdominal tenderness, shoulder pain, and/or shock, which is evidence of a leaking or ruptured abscess. These should be operated within hours of the diagnosis. In these cases, it is usually difficult to preserve either adnexa or the uterus. The wisest course is to remove the infected pelvic structures and to irrigate the abdomen copiously to remove all the pus from the entire abdomen. The latter may take liters of Ringer's lactate. The surgeon who undertakes to operate on these patients should be quite experienced with the pelvis and with complicated surgical cases because this is often a very difficult operation technically. While inspecting the abdomen in these cases, it is important to seek out intraloop abscesses should they exist and abscesses between the diaphragm and liver. The pelvis needs to be appropriately drained. Some surgeons advocate draining the pelvis through the vagina. Having had little experience and no success with this method, I prefer to drain the abdomen in these infected cases with some type of sump drainage in the pelvis, both gutters, and through the abdominal wall.

Operation intervention can be a very bloody procedure. Because of the possibility of adult respiratory distress syndrome, secondary to infection and/or shock, expert anesthesia backup is necessary. It is wise to have an ample supply of blood available. All patients should have preoperative blood gases available. Patients exhibiting any evidence of shock need a Swan-Ganz catheter. Postoperative care must be in an intensive care unit manned by an experienced team. There are a few patients whose abscesses can be drained vaginally. This is a worthwhile endeavor, quite easy to do, and in some patients, this is all that is necessary from a surgical standpoint.

Operative Considerations

Since the anatomy is often, if not always, distorted, we found that the best place to start the procedure is retroperitoneally over each pelvic wall. By opening the lateral pelvic peritoneum, the common and external iliac vessels can be observed and palpated along with the hypogastric artery and ureter. The abscess is almost always involved with the side wall of the pelvis. The ureter, being attached to the inferior position, is quite susceptible to injury unless it is visualized continually throughout the case. I might add that I have been called to the operating room a number of times to help surgeons deal with pelvic infection and almost invariably they had difficulty identifying anatomy and almost universally they were operating through a small incision and sometimes a transverse incision. If you are going to operate on a pelvic abscess, I recommend a midline incision that goes above the umbilicus. Adequate exposure is absolutely necessary.

The uses of gamma radionuclides however need to be understood. Iridium 111 conjugated to human immunoglobulin G is suboptimal when dealing with subphrenic abscesses owing to the concentration of radionuclide in liver, spleen, and kidney, which interferes with detection. When dealing with gallium 67 citrate, this type of nuclear type cannot be utilized in areas in close proximity to bowels.

The presence of gas within a fluid collection is the most suggestive feature of an abscess; however, only approximately one-third of abdominal abscesses will demonstrate this finding.

On CT, abscesses are often well defined or encapsulated areas of decreased attention (CT numbers from 0 to 20 Hounsfield units). Not infrequently, these areas exhibit mass effects and displace bowel loops or impinge on adjacent structures. The sonographic features of an abscess are relatively protean. They can be anything from a complex fluid collection with fluid degree level to sonolucent masses.

Percutaneous Abscess Drainage

Percutaneous abscess drainage (PAD) of pelvic abscesses is an established radiologic procedure. The procedure has gained wide acceptance as an adjunct in the management of patients with pelvic abscesses. The procedure involves minimal trauma, is well tolerated, and produces early relief of symptoms. In many instances, it may shorten the length of the hospital stay, reduce costs, and often eliminate the need for surgical intervention. In selected patients, PAD may serve as a temporizing measure in a critically ill or endstage patient.

Patient Selection

Selection of patients is predicated primarily on three criteria (Table 2).

Radiologically guided percutaneous drainage generally avoids the need for anesthesia in critical ill patients and can be accomplished with a relatively minimum amount of morbidity and at a fraction of the medical cost.

The decision to attempt percutaneous drainage should be a joint decision by the therapeutic physician and the intervening radiologist. CT is the procedure of choice to

TABLE 2 Patient criteria for percutaneous drainage

(1) Presence of liquefied pus that is potentially accessible by a drainage catheter
(2) Well-encapsulated abscess or an abscess within an indiscrete anatomical department
(3) The absence of intestinal, pleural, or vascular structures that would impede safe access for catheter insertion

stage the extent of the abscess and to determine the safety of percutaneous drainage based on imaging criteria. It affords more precise visualization of the adjacent anatomy and is not handicapped by the presence of overlying bowel, surgical drainage, etc.

Procedure
CT or ultrasound-guided needle aspiration is performed with a 20 gauge needle. If no free flowing fluid is obtained, then a larger gauge needle is inserted into the collection. Unless fluid can be aspirated from an 18 gauge needle, it is unlikely that the abscess is sufficiently liquefied to be drained percutaneously.

Significant debate still exists over the suitability of multilocular abscesses for percutaneous drainage. Many multisynaptic or multilocular abscesses in fact intercommunicate with a single dominant cavity and do lend themselves to this technique. When a true multioculative abscess exists, more than one catheter can be inserted. By and large, the overriding contraindication to attempted percutaneous drainage is the lack of safe access because of intervening major vessels.

Management of Drainage Catheter
Once an abscess has been evacuated, care should be taken to ensure catheter patency. This can be achieved by injecting 10 to 20 mL saline through the catheter t.i.d. The parameters used to evaluate the effectiveness of percutaneous drainage include the disappearance of fever, decreased leukocytosis, and disappearance of C-reactive protein and decrease in drainage volume. In most cases, these parameters are anticipated to respond within 48 hours and definitely within 72 hours. Once the volume of drainage has decreased to 1020 mL/day, the catheter can be slowly advanced over several days and ultimately removed. Patients who do not respond within 72 hours need to be reevaluated.

Complications
If one restricts observations to abdominal abscesses involving the lower pelvis, the major complications are the induction of transient septicemia with hypotension and surgical wound infections. In the lower abdomen, the major complication is perforation or laceration of one of the mesenteric vessels.

The overall success rate for percutaneous drainage of abscesses is in the order of 85%. Recurrence rates have been as high as 8%. The key to successful percutaneous drainage of lower abdominal abscesses is a close working cooperation between the intervention radiologist and the obstetrician gynecologist.

Transvaginal Abscess Drainage
Endovaginal ultrasonographically directed transvaginal drainage of pelvic abscesses has been utilized to treat patients who failed intravenous antibiotic therapies and whose abscesses were not amenable to percutaneous or colpotomy drainage.

The ultrasound-guided transvaginal approach offers a direct, nonsurgical means of drainage of deep pelvic abscesses. It is often difficult, however, to place drainage catheters through the vaginal wall by using the Seldinger technique. The drainage procedure can be facilitated by the use of a Colapinto needle as a dilator. The Colapinto needle may also serve as a stiffening cannula for the passage of a fascial dilator.

Sonographically guided drainage is an effective treatment of pelvic abscess, being either completely curative or temporizing in 78% of patients. Catheter treatment was unsuccessful and surgery was necessary in 22% of patients.

SELECTED READING

Abbitt PL, Goldwag S, Urbanski S. Endovaginal sonography for guidance in draining pelvic fluid collections. Am J Roentgenol 1990; 154:849.

Acholonu F, Minkoff H, Delke I. Percutaneous drainage of fluid collections in the bladder flap of febrile post cesarean patients. J Reprod Med 1987; 32:140.

Burton EM, Boulden TF, Magill HL, et al. Case of the day. Appendicitis with appendiceal rupture and pelvic abscess. Radiographics 1990; 10:372.

Eschelman DJ, Sullivan KL. Use of a Colapinto needle in US-guided transvaginal drainage of pelvic abscesses. Radiology 1993; 186:893.

Fabiszewski NL, Sumkin JH, Johns CM. Contemporary radiologic percutaneous abscess drainage in the pelvis. Clin Obstet Gynecol 1993; 36:445.

Feld R, Eschelman DJ, Sagerman JE, et al. Treatment of pelvic abscesses and other fluid collections: efficacy of transvaginal sonographically guided aspiration and drainage. Am J Roentgenol 1994; 163:1141.

Fribourg S: Definition of pelvic abscess—complex or not? Am J Obstet Gynecol 1994; 171:1164.

Gagliardi PD, Hoffer PB, Rosenfield AT. Correlative imaging in abdominal wound infection: an algorithmic approach using nuclear medicine, ultrasound and computed imaging. Sem Nucl Med 1988; 13:330–334.

Knochel JQ, Koehler PR, Lee TG, Welch DM. Diagnostic of abdominal abscess with computed tomography, ultrasound, and 111 Indium leukocyte scans. Radiology 1980; 137:425.

Kuligowska E, Keller E, Ferrucci JT. Treatment of pelvic abscesses: value of one-step sonographically guided transrectal needle aspiration and lavage. Am J Roentgenol 1995; 164:201.

Landers DV, Sweet RL: Current trends in the diagnosis and treatment of tubal ovarian abscess. Am J Obstet Gynecol 1985; 151:1098.

Loy RA, Gallup DG, Hill JA, et al. Pelvic abscess: examination and transvaginal drainage guided by real-time ultrasonography. South Med J 1989; 82:788.

Mecke H, Semm K, Freys I, et al. Pelvic abscesses: pelviscopy or laparotomy. Gynecol Obstet Invest 1991; 31:231.

Nelson GH. Definition of pelvic abscess. Am J Obstet Gynecol 1994; 170:257.

Nelson AL, Sinow RM, Rensio R, et al. Endovaginal ultrasonographically guided transvaginal drainage for treatment of pelvic abscesses. Am J Obstet Gynecol 1995; 172:1926.

Stubblefield PG. Intraovarian abscess treated with laparoscopic aspiration and povidone-iodine lavage. A case report. J Reprod Med 1991; 36:407.

Walker CK, Landers DV. Pelvic abscesses: new trends in management. Obstet Gynecol Surv 1991; 46:615

Wound Infections 78

James W. Daly and Gilles R. G. Monif

If I had the HONOR of being a surgeon, since I am convinced of the dangerous conditions which can be caused by the germs of microbes which are to be found everywhere, especially in hospitals, not only would I use only instruments in a perfect state of cleanliness, but also after having cleaned my hands with the greatest of care, I would flame them rapidly, a practice not much more dangerous than a smoker passing a hot charcoal from one hand to the other, and I would only use bandages, cloths and sponges which would have been exposed to air heated at 130° to 150°. I would use only water which would have been heated to 110° to 120°.

L. Pasteur, 1878

HISTORICAL DEVELOPMENT

Wound infection is a problem as old as mankind. It was only in the latter half of the nineteenth century that wound infection was recognized as a disease process in itself. Until that time, infection and inflammation seemed inevitably to go hand in hand and were generally considered a single process in wound healing. Various salves, ointments, noxious concoctions, incantations, and prayers all have had their place in the art of promoting wound healing or preventing certain types of infections or inflammations. The physician or surgeon, until quite recently, has anxiously awaited the appearance of "laudable pus."

Galen, the famous Greek physician, was appointed surgeon to the gladiators of the city of Pergamon early in his career. He found that, when treating the wounds of gladiators (especially the incised wounds), if he washed them with wine, removed the blood clots and foreign material, and sutured them, many healed without suppuration. For some unknown reason, this observation was neither disseminated nor practiced, and he later advised the introduction of ointments and drugs that favored the formation of laudable pus and healing by secondary intention. Because Galen became the infallible authority in medicine and surgery, this doctrine of healing by suppuration became the accepted one until the time of Lister. Perhaps Galen observed that some wounds rapidly proved fatal before pus appeared, for example, wounds infected with virulent streptococci or gas bacilli, but that wounds left open, with pus formation, healed, although the healing process was dilatory. Whatever the reason, Galen's conclusion was that suppuration is an essential part of wound healing. Some of his observations are accurate. We have found that leaving the contaminated wound open is the best method of management but that suppuration is not necessary for healing.

Several military surgeons in the thirteenth and sixteenth centuries advocated primary wound healing and wound closure. But the doctrine of laudable pus and healing by secondary intention remained the basic doctrine of wound care. Such diverse objects as unicorn's horn, mummy's skin, boiling oil, and a hot cautery were recommended not only to decontaminate wounds but to promote healing. One of the most successful methods of wound treatment in the fifteenth and sixteenth centuries was the use of weapon salve. This melange consisted of various noxious and magical ingredients and was carefully applied to the weapon that caused the wound. The weapon dressing was changed every third day until the patient's wound was healed. Meanwhile, the wound itself was covered with a linen dressing and forgotten. During the same period, bandaging of wounds became important, and one of the bandages devised by a German surgeon, Scultetus, is still in use today.

It was not until the nineteenth century, following the development of the microscope, when Koch, Pasteur, and Lister established the bacterial etiology of wound purulence, that the principles of healing, inflammation, and bacterial infection were separated and incorporated into medical practice. According to current concepts, we expect the cleanly incised surgical wound to heal by primary intention, and we go to extraordinary lengths to prevent infection. However, since the acquisition of an armamentarium of antibiotics, we sometimes forget that infection is a surgical threat. We have delegated much of the responsibility for the prevention of infection to others, such as the ward nurse and the operating room personnel; as physicians, we forget that this facet of management of the patient is primarily our responsibility.

DEFINITION OF WOUND INFECTION

A wound infection can be defined, after Ljungquist, as a collection of pus that empties itself spontaneously or after incision; it is usually associated with intense redness, infiltration, and elevated temperature of the wound. Traditionally, wounds have been classified by the degree of contamination (Table 1).

EPIDEMIOLOGY

The source of bacteria recovered postoperatively from a wound infection is most commonly the patient herself,

TABLE I Classification of wounds based on the degree of contamination

Degree of contamination	Type of wound
Clean	Elective surgery, noncontaminated No drain
Clean contaminated	Operations on the gastrointestinal tract Cholecystectomy Hysterectomy
Contaminated	Operations in an area with acute inflammation but no pus Spillage from the gastrointestinal tract Major breaks in technique
Dirty	Operations in an area with pus Peritonitis Perforated viscus

Source: National Academy of Sciences, National Research Council Cooperative Study Ad Hoc Committee on Trauma, Division of Medical Sciences. Ann Surg 1964; 160(Suppl 2):11.

either from the skin surface, from adjacent mucosal surfaces, or as a contaminant from the gastrointestinal tract or an abscess cavity.

A second, less likely source of contamination is the skin of the surgeon and assistants, particularly as it comes in contact with the wound through frequently torn gloves. It has been estimated that in 50% of operative cases, the surgeon's or assistant's gloves are torn. Bacteria can traverse a blood- or sweat-soaked surgical gown, another potential source of wound contamination. Many modern gowns are therefore waterproof in the arms and front. For several years, we have worn plastic aprons under our gowns, which may have contributed to a lessened wound infection rate. On occasion, the nasopharynx of the people present in the operating room can be a source of wound sepsis, but the modern paper mask is 90% efficient. Cloth masks are less so, and tend to be worn longer. The air and environment in the modern operative suite is rarely implicated in surgical infection. The traditional preoperative shave may be a source of wound infection, particularly if done the day before surgery. The inevitable small nicks and scratches become infected and may provide the nidus of future infection. Shaving the area immediately before surgery or simply not attempting to remove the hair are all associated with a lessened wound infection rate.

INCIDENCE

The incidence of wound infection in clean operative cases varies from 2% to 5% and generally remains constant from hospital to hospital. Most abdominal gynecologic procedures are in the clean-contaminated category and occasionally are grossly contaminated. Any time the vagina is opened from above, the area must be considered as contaminated. Historically, the rate of postoperative wound sepsis in abdominal hysterectomy usually ranges between 3% and 6%, while cesarean section is somewhat higher—ranging between 4% and 8%. With the aggressive and proper use of preoperative antibiotic prophylaxis, these rates have been significantly reduced.

PATHOGENESIS

Healthy tissues have a remarkable resistance to bacterial contamination. For infection to occur, it requires one of four conditions to be met:

1. The bacterial pathogen has a unique ability to circumvent or negate local host resistance, e.g., group A beta-hemolytic streptococci.
2. The amount of contamination is overwhelming in terms of both the number of organisms and lowering the local redox potential, e.g., feces.
3. Two or more bacteria function in a synergistic manner, e.g., Meleny Type II ulcer–progressive synergistic bacterial gangrene.
4. A foreign body is placed; e.g., suture or drains (*Staphylococcus aureus*).

Until granulation tissue has formed, the surgical wound is a spectrum, from healthy to devitalized tissues. Dead and devitalized tissue has little, if any, ability to impede significant bacterial replication. It is a major key to the anaerobic component of wound infection. The low oxidation–reduction potential of dead or devitalized tissue allows for the preferential recruitment of organisms that have the ability to grow at a low redox potential and in the diminished presence of molecular oxygen.

The presence of dead or devitalized tissue within the wound environment is the consequence of one or more of the following mechanisms:

1. Crushing injury or trauma caused by a clamp or tie
2. Iatrogenic impairment of the regional blood supply by ligation or compromise of relatively large vessels or suturing under tension
3. Creation of anatomical dead spaces, e.g., hematomas and seromas via incomplete hemostasis

MICROBIOLOGY

The microbiological data derived from studies of wound infections prior to the late 1970s are flawed due to the use of inappropriate culture techniques that impeded the isolation of class II and class III anaerobic bacteria.

A postoperative wound infection is caused by bacteria that gain entrance to the incision—admittedly a simplistic statement, but it is only since the turn of the century that this has been universally recognized. The source of the bacteria is most commonly the patient: from the skin surface, the adjacent mucous membrane, the gastrointestinal tract, an abscess cavity, the vagina, or the endocervix. A second, but much less frequent source of wound contamination is the skin or nasopharyngeal tract of the surgeon and/or assistants.

Wound infection may also be due to a concomitant infection in a distant site such as the kidney or respiratory tract and an associated bacteremia contaminating the incised wound.

Most postoperative wound infections are polymicrobial in nature rather than being due to a single bacterium.

Admittedly, the bacteriology of wound infections is poorly delineated if inappropriate sampling techniques are applied. The literature would indicate that the most common organisms in wound infection are *S. aureus*, *Staphylococcus epidermidis*, *Escherichia coli*, Bacteroidaceae/Prevotella, *Proteus mirabilis*, and *Pseudomonas*.

The simple swab culture technique is biased toward predominantly aerobic bacteria. However, if the tissue biopsy technique is used or if anaerobic methods are used to culture the wound, the percentage of anaerobic bacteria in the given wound rises. The best method for culturing a wound infection is to debride a small amount of necrotic tissue and use it as the culture specimen. If a significant amount of pus is present, an aspirated sample submitted in a syringe without air inclusion is the preferred method of culturing.

S. aureus and the beta-hemolytic streptococci can function as monoetiologic agents. *S. aureus* is one of the few bacteria in wound infections that may be monomicrobial or polymicrobial. Monomicrobial disease involves aerobic bacteria of enhanced virulence or the staphylococci. Polymicrobial wound infections are a function of synergistic bacterial coupling or the anaerobic progression.

Monomicrobial Wound Infections

The prime monomicrobial bacteria causatively associated with abdominal wound infections are listed in Table 2.

With iatrogenic disruption of the cutaneous barrier, exogenous and endogenous bacteria with enhanced virulence gain potential access to subcutaneous tissue planes and their endolymphatics. These anatomical structures provide the avenues for lateral spread. A prime example is necrotizing fasciitis and erysipelas-like disease emanating from wound margins due to the group A or B streptococci.

Polymicrobial Wound Infections

The oxidation–reduction potential of healthy tissues constitutes a primary barrier to most bacteria lacking augmented virulence factors.

For polymicrobial wound infection to evolve, some critical change in the microbiological environment must occur. Given the appropriate microbiological environment at the operative site, synergistic interfacing of bacteria may result in the induction of disease. The majority of abdominal wound infections occurring after cesarean section are observed in women who had prolonged rupture of the fetal membranes and/or prolonged stimulated labor, owing to a quantitative augmentation of the associated amnionitis.

When bacterial coupling involves an aerobic bacterium of augmented virulence with an anaerobic bacterium, e.g., *S. aureus*, and a microaerophilic streptococcus, *Streptococcus millerii*, with a Bacteroidaceae (progressive synergistic bacterial gangrene) or an Enterobacteriaceae with a Bacteroidaceae/Prevotella (Daly's syndrome), a significant gangrenous wound infection may ensue.

The majority of abdominal wound infections are the consequence of some variant of the anaerobic progression. Necrotic tissue and/or microhematoma formation in conjunction with

TABLE 2 Principal bacteria that may produce monomicrobial abdominal wound infections

Clostridium perfringens
Clostridium sordellii
Haemophilus influenzae
Streptococcus groups A, B, C, F, and G
Staphylococcus aureus
Staphylococcus epidermidis

bacterial contamination are the prime catalytic factors initiating disease.

Toxin-Related Wound Infections

Both *Clostridium perfringens* and *Clostridium sordellii* have the capability of producing a unique type of wound infection. The syndromes produced by both *C. perfringens* and *C. sordellii* are mediated primarily through exotoxins and require only the establishment of infection. Neither case appears to require the initiation of the anaerobic progression for disease to evolve. Given the proper microbiological environment, exotoxin-mediated disease with the induction of systemic symptomatology as well as lateral and vertical spread through tissue planes occurs. The microbiological environment is a critical factor in initiating disease. Both of these species of *Clostridium* are relatively common in nature in contrast to the rarity of disease they cause.

CONTRIBUTING FACTORS

The Patient

A large number of factors are thought to increase the probability of ensuing abdominal wound infections. These factors are summarized in Table 3.

In addition, clinical experience indicates that cancer, even remote from the surgical area, enhances the risk of infection. This may be related to a depressed immune mechanism, malnutrition, and hypovolemia as well as the type and length of the operation. Prior radiation to the abdominal wall can also facilitate wound infection (Daly's syndrome). Radiation injury to the stroma is primarily one of vascular obliteration with time. Initially, the endothelial cells are damaged; they become edematous and eventually are destroyed and replaced with fibrous tissue. During radiation therapy, and for the first four to six weeks afterwards, there is actually a net increase in tissue perfusion because of the inflammatory changes associated with the initial radiation insult. However, over time, the inflammatory response subsides and an eventual loss of vascular supply to the area results. Therefore, the wound that has been irradiated in the distant past has a relative lack of tissue perfusion, which is an important determinant of wound infection.

The Surgeon

Perhaps this section should be entitled "Trauma," but the surgeon creates it and must be responsible for the result. Each wound infection is iatrogenic—the ultimate goal is perfect healing with a 0% wound infection rate. Therefore, part of the surgeon's attention should be directed to this

TABLE 3 Factors contributing to wound infections

Obesity	Adipose tissue is relatively avascular and consequently less likely to overcome even a small bacterial inoculum
Malnutrition	Protein deprivation significantly retards wound healing
Hypoxia	Both chronic (anemia) and acute (shock) as well as excessive pressure on the side of the wound due to retractors
Impairment to host defense mechanism	Diabetes mellitus (insulin dependent) Prior radiation to operative site Chemotherapy Corticosteroids
Shaving operative site	Shaving of indicated area should be done just prior to the operation and *not* the night before surgery
Incomplete hemostasis	Enhances anaerobic replication and provides a potential site for abscess formation
Length of operation	In contaminated cases, the incidence of infection begins to rise steeply if the operation lasts more than 2 hr
Foreign bodies	Highest incidence of wound infection is associated with cotton and silk sutures (plain catgut promotes the most inflammation)
Drains	Particularly if the drains come out through the incision

goal before, during, and after the operation. He (or more often now, she) must be cognizant of local wound factors.

A cleanly incised wound offers less damaged tissue than a terraced incision (the neophyte will make multiple strokes of varying depth and pull the knife toward himself, producing a terraced slope resembling an Austrian vineyard—this produces bleeding, and the surgeon, losing his way, produces another valley, the bottom of which is not the abdominal fascia, but a cavern excavated beneath the skin on his side of the table). Large bites of the hemostat or vigorous cauterizing of bleeders produces an abundance of necrotic tissue, a happy commune for opportunistic bacteria. There continues to be a low-key debate regarding ligature or cautery of wound bleeders. This author favors ligature but either method used with precision and delicacy is suitable. The point is to control bleeding, leaving a minimum of necrotic and foreign material in the wound. Historically, Halstead demonstrated that staphylococci could be injected into the leg muscle of a dog without causing infection, yet when the same bacteria were injected into a previously crushed muscle, an abscess invariably resulted. He was an early proponent of fine technique and gentle handling of tissue. Foreign bodies in wounds have been known for centuries to be promoters of suppuration. In the twentieth century, the military surgeon has taught us to debride dirty wounds, remove the foreign material, and leave the wound open for secondary closure. In civilian practice, the most common foreign body in the

incision is suture material. The degree of inflammatory response (an attempt at rejection) to different types of sutures is greatest for chromic and plain catgut, least for steel, and intermediate for cotton, silk, and synthetic material. The finer the suture, the less the total tissue reaction.

Decreased local wound perfusion is associated with an increased incidence of wound sepsis. This may be associated with a decreased circulatory blood volume, shock, anemia, or local factors; for instance, adrenalin infused locally causes vascular spasm, a dramatic drop in local perfusion, and, on an experimental basis at least, an enhanced infection rate. The general and nonspecific inflammatory response of a wound is dependent on local circulation. Excessive pressure on the sides of the wound by metal retractors can cause not only decreased local perfusion but actual crushing and damage to the tissue. Anesthesia plays a part here in that a properly placed retractor can suddenly produce an excessive pressure on the side of the wound if the patient's level of anesthesia changes and the abdominal musculature becomes tight. Therefore, good anesthesia with adequate relaxation throughout the procedure can prevent wound infections.

Drains and bowel stomas entering the primary operative site act as foreign bodies in the wound and as carriers of bacteria from the inner and outer sides of the wound. Therefore, drains and stomas should not be brought through the primary operative site if at all possible, but through a separate opening. Drains in the subcutaneous space really drain very little, but do act as a foreign body and as a portal of entry for bacteria from the skin and environment into the subcutaneous tissue.

It is particularly important to preserve fine-vesseled areolar connective tissue about the fascia since it nourishes and vascularizes the fascia. The fascia itself has no blood vessels.

Vigorous stripping or cleaning of the fascia retards healing and promotes infection. Likewise, grasping the fascial edges with a crushing clamp, such as a Kocher, will crush the tissue and may act as a site for bacterial growth.

COURSE AND DIAGNOSIS

Local infection manifests with intense redness, induration, and elevated temperature of the surrounding skin with or without the presence of pus. What distinguishes local infection from its more systemic counterpart is the presence of fever.

The majority of patients with a postoperative wound infection will have an elevated temperature, which begins on the day of surgery or the day after. The temperature curve is such that the bottom never reaches normal. Early in the process, examination will show little, and other causes are frequently thought to be responsible for the fever, such as pulmonary complications or a urinary tract infection. As the infection advances, the temperature, on the third, fourth, or fifth day, will reach higher levels. By this time, all or part of the wound becomes tender and inflamed, and eventually pus will escape. This may occur prior to or during removal of the skin sutures. When the wound is inflamed and tender, it is useful to put warm, moist packs on the incision; this often speeds up the process of bringing pus to the surface.

Some abscesses, however, are subfascial and due to anaerobic bacteria, which grow slowly. The patient may have an intermittent fever that lasts for days or weeks without any local sign until pus finally escapes through the fascia into the subcutaneous tissue. This is followed by the rapid development of a tender, inflamed area in the abdominal wall. We refer to this as a collar-button abscess (Fig. 1).

Wound infection due to the coagulase-positive beta-hemolytic streptococcus manifests itself quite early by severe temperature elevation, toxicity, and extreme inflammation in the area of the incision. This picture will give a clinical indication of the organism even before the cultures have been returned. In all cases of wound infection, aerobic and anaerobic cultures should be obtained as soon as pus is present. The necrotizing wound infections usually begin in the same way as the more common wound infections but later show an undermining and purple discoloration of the surrounding skin. There is also a loss of considerable amounts of tissue from the abdominal wall.

TREATMENT

Local wound infections rarely require antibiotic therapy. Aggressive local care usually suffices.

Antibiotics alone are generally ineffective in treating an established wound infection. When the diagnosis is suspected owing to swelling, redness, and tenderness of the area, heat frequently will accelerate the process and bring the pus to the surface. Once the purulent material has begun to escape from the wound, it should be cultured aerobically and anaerobically, and if there is anything more than a very superficial abscess under the skin margins, the entire wound, or at least that part of the wound involved, should be opened wide. We prefer to do this in the operating room under anesthesia. It is much more comfortable for the patient, and the wound can be thoroughly investigated and adequately debrided. Occasionally an infection is associated with a dehiscence, and it is embarrassing and dangerous to open the patient's wound in the hospital ward and to have the bowel pour out from the abdominal cavity along with the pus.

With the wound opened, the area is generally irrigated with normal saline solution and the necrotic material is then debrided. Fascial defects are sought out and subfascial abscesses opened. The peritoneum is usually found to be

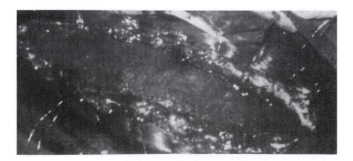

FIGURE I Subfascial collar-button abscess.

quite thickened in these cases. Once the patient's wound is debrided and cleaned, it is packed with moistened sponges. If the fascia has been opened, it is wise to keep the patient at bedrest until the base of the wound has become thoroughly granulated. During the active phase of treatment, when pus is present, we like to use hydrogen peroxide as well as saline to irrigate the wound. Some physicians pack the wound with iodoform gauze, but the iodine crystals may be toxic to tissues and seriously interfere with the establishment of the local circulation and granulation tissue. This may also be true of hydrogen peroxide, so that once pus is absent from the wound, only saline should be used for irrigations.

The wound ablutions and packings are repeated four to five times each day. It is necessary to have the gauze sponges packed into all the crevices of the wound so that they adhere to the surface; when they are removed, they will remove surface debris and mechanically stimulate the granulation tissue.

If, on the other hand, the surgeon chooses to let the wound heal secondarily, this can be cared for at home. The rate of wound contracture and healing depends to a large extent upon the patient's nutrition, general health, and age. However, the wounds generally close rapidly. The resulting scar is somewhat broader than that produced by a primarily healed incision but is usually much more satisfactory than either the patient or the physician anticipates.

Evisceration

When evisceration occurs through an infected wound, surgical intervention must be immediate. With the patient anesthetized, the abdominal cavity is copiously irrigated with saline and the wound debrided and closed in one layer with wire-retention sutures. We have found that heavy silver wires that are twisted rather than tied are useful. This type of suture creates a minimum of local tissue reaction and can be easily loosened as the wound swells. On occasion, definite layers in the abdominal wall can be ascertained, and then it is possible to close the fascia and the peritoneum together, using the Smead-Jones technique with the skin left open. As we have indicated above, systemic antibiotics should be administered, based on the cultures, since peritoneal contamination is inevitable. If, however, culture information is not available, it is best to start the patient on triple antibiotic therapy.

When tissue destruction is extensive, the bowel may be exposed but not actually eviscerated. The necrotic tissue should be debrided under anesthesia and either the wound is closed primarily or, if this is not possible, Marlex mesh is sewn to the fascial edges with nylon or wire suture, the Marlex is covered with moistened sponges and abdominal pads, and it is held in place with Montgomery straps. Once the wound is clean and the infection has subsided, the Marlex can be removed and the wound closed primarily (Fig. 2).

NECROTIZING WOUND INFECTIONS

Necrotizing infections include the monobacterial, "clostridial," and the multibacterial synergistic infections,

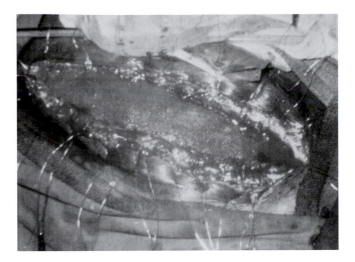

FIGURE 2 Closure of an abdominal wound defect with Marlex mesh that is sewn to the fascial edges with wire sutures.

which the literature addresses as necrotizing fasciitis, synergistic bacterial gangrene, and Daly's syndrome.

The synergistic infections usually appear in a predisposed host, such as the diabetic, the malnourished, or the immunosuppressed patient, and in the area of radiation injury. The necrotizing infections of interest to the gynecologist include those that occur after episiotomy and operations through the abdominal wall. The destructive process can occur spontaneously in both of these areas.

Necrotizing Fasciitis (Acute Hemolytic Streptococcal Gangrene Wound Erysipelas)

Necrotizing fasciitis, now a relatively rare disease, was recognized during the American Civil War as "hospital gangrene" and was associated with a high mortality rate (46%). By 1918, Pfanner identified the beta-hemolytic streptococcus as the causal agent and called the disease process "necrotizing erysipelas." In 1924, Meleney reported 20 cases and called the process "acute hemolytic streptococcal gangrene." He confirmed the beta-hemolytic streptococcus as the cause. The present term, "necrotizing fasciitis," is from a 1952 report by Wilson, who found other organisms in his cases.

Nevertheless, the basic pathologic process is a subcutaneous necrosis of the fat and fascia, with a secondary occlusion and thrombosis of the dermal vessels, leading to eventual gangrene of the skin. In the classic case (due to beta-hemolytic streptococci), the local toxin is a macromolecular complex of mucopolypeptides and polysaccharides. The bacterium also produces hyaluronidase, which may account for the rapidly spreading cellulitis. As the pathologic process continues, areas of necrosis offer a favorable medium for the growth of secondary invaders, both aerobes and anaerobes, which may overgrow the beta-hemolytic streptococci in vitro. The beta-hemolytic streptococcus was the predominant organism in the preantibiotic era. More recently, other causative organisms, usually in mixed cultures, have been incriminated. At times it is difficult to differentiate necrotizing fasciitis from synergistic bacterial gangrene on bacterial and clinical grounds. With the exception of the

pure beta-hemolytic streptococcal gangrene, they are probably the same entity. The majority of cases (80%) occur after minor trauma or insignificant injuries, usually involving the extremities. Although diabetes, atherosclerosis, and a suppressed immune status (from cancer, chemotherapy, etc.) seem to be common factors, disease also occurs in previously healthy individuals. Necrotizing fasciitis has been described after spontaneous vaginal delivery (where episiotomy provides the portal of infection), postcesarean delivery, postlaparoscopic surgery, and a variety of minor surgical procedures involving the vulva. The incidence of disease fluctuates with the prevalence of the group A streptococcus in the community. Attack rates of 1.8 per 1000 women undergoing cesarean section have been identified. Often, infection initially presents as what appears to be mild, innocuous cellulitis. Delays in recognition of the rapidly progressing infection and in the institution of aggressive surgical management results in increased morbidity and mortality. A delay greater than 48 hours between initial recognition and treatment may result in up to 60% to 70% mortality.

The acute fulminating postoperative case does occur, but, fortunately, rarely. Within 24 to 48 hours after the operation, the patient will have a high temperature and be acutely ill to the point of disorientation. The wound and surrounding tissue is fiery red, swollen, and very tender. Blebs or blisters eventually appear, surrounded by blue or black areas of necrosis. Streptococci can often be cultured from the blebs. Over half of the patients will have positive blood cultures. Early in the disease process, there is extensive subcutaneous and fascial necrosis with undermining of the skin (thus the blotches of necrotic skin). In the classic case, gray or serosanguineous fluid exudes from the wound. The cases with mixed infections frequently have pus present. The muscle tissue is usually spared. During this time of fever, toxemia, and massive destruction, fluid may shift into the involved area at the expense of the vascular compartment, with associated electrolyte imbalance. Serious serum calcium deficits have been reported due to sequestration into the area of fat necrosis.

In most instances, C-reactive protein values will be markedly elevated, with values often exceeding 200 mg/L. Biochemical markers of disseminated intravascular coagulopathy may be present. Cases of a toxic shock-like syndrome characterized by a generalized maculopapular rash, hypotension, respiratory distress, and renal hepatic abnormalities have been described in patients with necrotizing fasciitis involving the female genital tract. The diagnosis of necrotizing fasciitis is usually made by a combination of clinical features and recovery of an M-serotype isolate of the group A beta-hemolytic streptococci. The demonstration of asymmetric fascial thickening and soft-tissue gas are supportive of the diagnosis.

Hyperintense T2-weighted signals within deep fascial planes on MRI is supportive of the diagnosis; however, abnormally high-signal intensity is not specific for necrotizing soft-tissue infection. A variety of nonnecrotizing conditions can produce similar findings.

The primary therapy is immediate operative debridement in the operating room under anesthesia. The incision is opened and all necrotic skin and subcutaneous tissue is removed (Fig. 3).

Aerobic and anaerobic cultures of wound (pus and tissue) and blood are important. High-dose penicillin therapy (20 million units/day IV) should be started when there is marked cellulitis, severe toxicity, or a positive blood culture. In cases with mixed infection (foul pus), antibiotics are not effective unless the patient is septic or has a positive blood culture.

The immediate need is surgical debridement; these are emergency cases. Delay caused by waiting for culture reports or trying antibiotic therapy or local wound care is futile and leads to massive tissue loss with bowel exposure, sepsis, peritonitis, and death.

Once the wound is debrided, local wound care is given as indicated for the more benign infections. Since there is usually considerable fascial loss, postoperative hernias are common. If a full-thickness debridement is necessary, a Marlex graft can be placed and removed later with secondary wound closure.

Progressive Synergistic Bacterial Gangrene

This gangrenous wound infection was reported by Cullen in 1924 and reaffirmed by Brewer and Meleney in 1926. The majority of cases have followed operations involving abdominal abscesses or bowel procedures and closure by retention sutures (Fig. 4).

The earlier cases were all associated with a microaerophilic or anaerobic streptococcus in the outer rim of induration and a hemolytic staphylococcus in the central area of slough. Animal experiments indicate that either organism alone does not produce the clinical picture, but when acting together in the same wound, they apparently work synergistically even though, or perhaps because, they have very different oxygen requirements. More recently, similar wound problems have been described with anaerobic streptococci and various gram-negative organisms (*E. coli, Proteus, Pseudomonas, Klebsiella*) as the aerobe, and some with *Bacteroides* as the anaerobe coupled with gram-negative aerobes. It would appear that the presence of aerobic and anaerobic organisms in the infected area is the

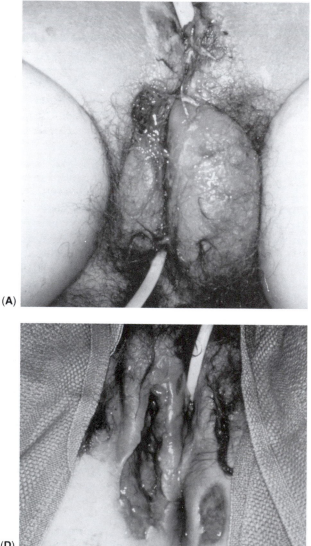

(A)

(D)

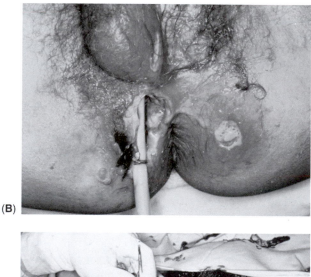

(B)

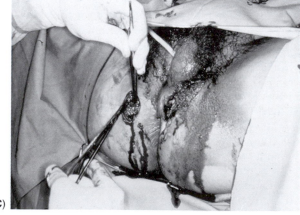

(C)

FIGURE 3 Necrotizing fasciitis. (**A**) Patient with necrotizing fasciitis. (**B**) Degree of resolution achieved with antibiotic therapy. (**C**) Operative debridement. (**D**) Lesions postsurgical debridement.

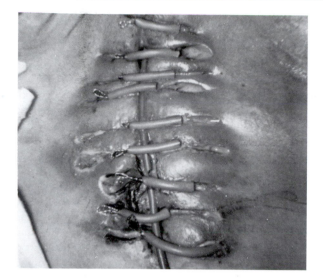

FIGURE 4 Progressive synergistic bacterial gangrene. Abdominal wound 14 days after secondary closure with stainless steel wire. Note the marked edema at the wound's margins and gangrenous areas around the sutures. *Source:* de Longh et al. (1967).

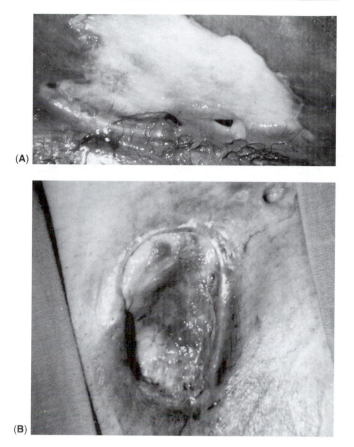

FIGURE 5 Spontaneous synergistic wound infections. **(A)** Occurrence in the abdominal wall. **(B)** Occurrence in the inguinal groin area. Note in both cases the presence of a fistulous tract. *Source:* Daley et al. (1978).

requirement for synergism rather than the species of bacteria. As opposed to necrotizing fasciitis, the course in progressive synergistic bacterial gangrene is indolent ("chronic gangrene") and usually not associated with marked systemic toxicity. Initially, the wound is quite painful, with an outer erythematous indurated rim surrounding an ever-enlarging area of necrosis. There is undermining and gangrene of the skin and eventual destruction of the underlying fascia and muscle. The process becomes clinically apparent on the fourth or fifth postoperative day, but only after 10 to 12 days is it obvious that a gangrenous synergistic process is present. The classic case enlarges at the rate of 1 to 2 cm/wk. However, some of the infections populated by *Bacteroides* and gram-negative aerobes can be very rapid and aggressive, with invasive tissue destruction in width and depth associated with more systemic toxicity. These infections are difficult to separate from necrotizing fasciitis except that synergistic bacterial gangrene of the aggressive variety involves the full thickness of the abdominal wall, with destruction of all tissues at an even rate. Although the majority of these infections follow surgery, they have been noted to occur spontaneously in Bartholin's gland and the abdominal wall.

Treatment is based on wide surgical removal of the infected area, including the erythematous outer margin. The excision must be deep enough as well as wide enough to remove the entire infected area. This may leave a large defect in the abdominal wall, which can be closed with Marlex and the wound closed primarily several weeks later. Antibiotics are probably not useful or necessary unless the patient is septic. Cases have been treated with hyperbaric oxygen. Although not effective in cases of necrotizing fasciitis, hypertonic oxygenation therapy is a potentially valuable adjunct in patients with progressive synergistic bacterial gangrene and *C. perfringens*–induced necrotic infections.

Daily et al. (1978) have described the counterpart of Fournier's disease (spontaneous occurrence of progressive synergistic bacterial gangrene) in women. This disease entity occurs primarily in diabetic patients in the areas of Bartholin's gland or the abdominal wall. These patients are treated by wide surgical excision of the area of involvement. Of interest is that in the cases involving the abdominal wall, the fascia is usually not involved (Fig. 5).

Postirradiation Necrotizing Wound Infection

We have noted a third type of destructive wound process in patients who have received radiation therapy for cancer. We have called it "postirradiation necrotizing wound infection." These infections occurred in the irradiated field at least six weeks after the radiation therapy. The wound dissolution was apparent by the third or fourth day following abdominal surgery although the patients had no fever, pain, or systemic toxicity. The loss of tissue from the full thickness of the abdominal wall was from 1 to 3 cm/24 hours. That portion of the incision that extended beyond the irradiated field was not involved. The wounds were not purulent. In all cases, the bowel was exposed. In several earlier patients, the process proceeded to rapid destruction of all of the abdominal wall within the radiation port, then stopped. These patients developed bowel fistulas and peritonitis, and died.

The bacteriology of these wounds (derived from central and marginal tissue samples) revealed *Bacteroides fragilis* and *E. coli* in each case, together with a variety of other aerobes and anaerobes such as *Pseudomonas*, anaerobic streptococci, *Klebsiella*, and *P. mirabilis*.

This wound infection, like the other gangrenous infections, must be excised widely to bleeding, well-vascularized margins. Since a full-thickness excision is done, closure is usually not possible, so a Marlex mesh is sewn to the fascial edges of the wound. This allows the patient to ambulate and serves as a prosthetic fascia. The Marlex is covered with sponges and pads. Eventually, the epithelium will migrate from the edges, or the area, when granulated, can be grafted. In one case, relaxing incisions were made outside the irradiated field and the wound was successfully closed secondarily. This is not usually possible because of the rigidity of the irradiated area.

As in all other gangrenous wound infections, rapid recognition and immediate (at night if necessary) and bold excision results in less loss of abdominal wall, a better cosmetic result, and less mortality. The ability to replace the excised abdominal wall with Marlex mesh allows one to be bold (Fig. 6).

GENERAL CONSIDERATIONS

In preventing wound infection, a number of things should be taken into consideration and should become part of the surgeon's plan and technique.

Do not use a lot of force in scrubbing the operative site in the operating room. This local irritation is associated with a dilatation of the vessels under the skin. This in turn causes more bleeding. *Do not clean off* the fascial layers, since the blood supply to this area will be decreased. In the excessively obese and certainly in contaminated cases, it is wise to close the fascia and peritoneum and leave the skin open for closure in four or five days. *No free space* should be left in the wound and hematomas are to be prevented. The best type of closure for the abdominal incision, particularly in

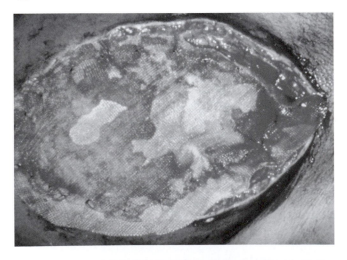

FIGURE 6 Replacing the excised abdominal wall with Marlex mesh. A large abdominal wall defect created by full-thickness resection of necrotic tissue back to bleeding margins in a case of postirradiation necrotizing wound infection.

disadvantaged patients, is the far-and-near or Smead-Jones type closure, where the peritoneum and fascia are closed in one layer, or mass closure with running technique.

Prophylactic Antibiotics
Local
Irrigating the incision with saline may wash out material such as blood clots and other foreign matter, but the bacteria are unaffected and saline irrigations do not influence wound infection rates. Experimental and clinical data indicate that povidone–iodine, ampicillin, neomycin, tetracycline, and kanamycin sulfate are all effective in lowering infection rates, particularly in those patients who are at high risk. One must be cautious, however, in using these agents, particularly neomycin, since they are absorbed from the tissue. Specifically, in the case of neomycin, toxicity and nephrotoxicity have been reported secondary to local wound irrigation.

Systemic Agents
In recent years, a number of studies with regard to prophylactic antibiotics have been and are being published, but the data with respect to wound infection rate are mixed. To be effective, the prophylactic antimicrobial should be administered long before bacterial lodgment has occurred. Animal data indicate that the effective period of preventive antimicrobial action in the wound is quite short, beginning the moment the bacteria gains access to the wound and ending within about three hours. The presence in the wound of a suture or other foreign material considerably limits the activity of the antibiotics. Penicillin, ampicillin, and the cephalosporins diffuse slowly into the wound and are present in the wound fluid within one hour. Clindamycin, on the other hand, takes two to four hours to show an appreciable level in the wound fluid, while carbenicillin, nafcillin, amoxicillin, gentamicin, and erythromycin have very little concentration even five hours after administration.

Operative Field
It is our practice to have the patient shower, or at least have the operative area washed, with an iodophor soap on the night before surgery. We have given up the surgical shave on the night before. For a time, we were using depilatories and found this to be a suitable method of hair removal, but some patients reacted to the depilatory with local dermatitis. Therefore, at the present time, we do not have patients shaved at all, and have not seen any increase in wound infections.

In the surgical suite, the operative area should be scrubbed for three to five minutes with iodophor soap. Numerous studies have indicated that the traditional 10-minute scrub is not necessary. The area should be scrubbed not with vigor but with thoroughness. If one presses hard on the skin, it produces a local inflammatory response that, on cutting the skin, leads to numerous bleeders in the superficial area of the incision. This in turn leads to either postoperative hematomas or increased amounts of foreign material in the wound in the way of sutures or cauterized tissue. If the patient is impregnated with dirt and grease, this should be removed well before the actual operation. The soap should be removed and the area painted with an iodophor solution, which is left to dry. Povidone–iodine acts relatively quickly but requires several minutes to achieve its local bactericidal effect, so it must be left in place and not wiped away. Placing plastic sheets over the exposed skin does not prevent infection but we find them practical to use since they hold towels in place without clips and keep the towels under them dry. If the patient has a stoma in the intra-abdominal wall, such as a urinary conduit or colostomy, the plastic adhesive drape is placed so as to exclude the stoma from the incision.

Good Technique

The incision should be cleanly made and should be carried down to the fascia quickly in one line without terracing. It is unwise to clean off the fascial layers since this will greatly decrease the blood supply to the fascia. Bleeders should be appropriately clamped and tied or cauterized, using delicate technique. It is our preference to use a clamp on the vessel and a polyglycolic acid suture tie. Once the abdomen is open, we suture towels to the peritoneum and the fascia so that the wound is excluded from the operative area. Using adhesive tapes rather than sutures to close the skin does not alter the infection rate and often results in a wider scar.

In contaminated cases, it is best to close the fascia and peritoneum with either nylon or stainless steel sutures. If sutures are put in the subcutaneous tissue, polyglycolic acid suture should be used, as this is the least reactive material. No free space should be left in the incision. In patients who have pulmonary or cardiac problems, are malnourished, or are expected to show a prolonged recovery phase with ileus, it is wise to use a running mass closure with permanent sutures. We have found through experience that the retention suture that comes to the outside leads to many infections. Over the last eight years, we have used the Smead-Jones far-and-near closure (Fig. 7) and have had no eviscerations. We feel that this technique leads to fewer infections and gives a strong, permanent closure.

In heavily contaminated cases with abscesses or peritonitis, and where there is bowel surgery with fecal spillage, it is best to close the anterior abdominal fascia and the peritoneum with Smead-Jones sutures and leave the skin open (Table 4). At some time between the fourth and the sixth day, the skin can be closed with previously placed sutures,

TABLE 4 Correlation of wound classification system for elective surgical cases and corresponding reported wound infection rates for penetrating abdominal wound and bite wounds

Wound classification	Risk of postoperative wound infection
Clear	1–3%
Clear-contaminated	7–10%
Contaminated	20–25%
Dirty	40%

Source: Adapted from the National Research Council. Weigelt JA. Infect Dis Clin Pract 1996; 5:S92–S95.

a procedure done on the ward under local anesthesia. Rarely do these secondarily closed wounds become infected, and the postoperative stay is not prolonged.

The cosmetic result is as good as in those cases closed primarily. A study of delayed primary wound closure in Canada indicated that the authors decreased their wound infection rate from 24% to 3% by leaving the wound open and closing it on the fourth day. Other studies have confirmed these results. If fewer than 105 bacteria per gram of tissue are found in the open wound, the wound, when closed secondarily, will heal 98% of the time. If the bacterial contamination is greater than this, the infection rate is much higher. However, most of us are not able to do bacterial counts and depend on the time and the appearance of the wound; generally by the fourth or fifth day, the surface granulations are healthy and delayed closure is possible.

PROPHYLACTIC MEASURES FOR INJURIES AND WOUNDS

Management of traumatic wounds involves three major principles:

1. Immediate wound care
2. evaluation of the need for prophylactic antibiotic therapy
3. Evaluation of the need for prophylactic vaccination

Immediate Wound Care

Therapy begins with careful cleansing of the wound in order to remove any organic contamination created by abrasion, deep puncture, or bite wound injury. Sterile saline followed by the use of hydrogen peroxide coupled with debridement

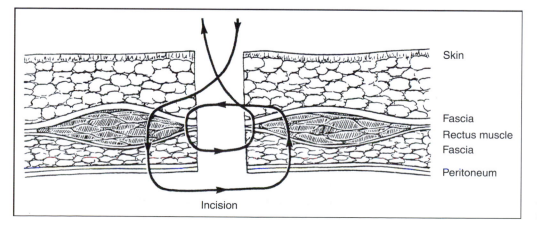

Incision

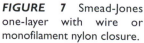

FIGURE 7 Smead-Jones one-layer with wire or monofilament nylon closure.

Skin

Fascia
Rectus muscle
Fascia

Peritoneum

TABLE 5 Tetanus prophylaxis guidelines

Situation	Recommendations
Clean, minor wounds: No prior history of tetanus immunization	Primary immunization consisting of two doses (0.5 mL each) of tetanus (combined tetanus/diphtheria toxoid) vaccine intramuscularly 4 wk apart followed by a third dose 6 to 12 mo later
Prior tetanus immunization, but >10 yr	Tetanus vaccine booster (0.5 mL) intramuscularly
Prior tetanus immunization <3 yr	Optional
Status unknown	Primary vaccinations (three doses)
All wounds contaminated with dirt, feces, soil, saliva, punctures, crush, burns, or frostbite.	Combined tetanus and diphtheria toxoids absorbed *plus* TIG 200 IU intramuscularly. TIG provides immediate immunity for 25–28 days during which time the patient is developing active immunity. Injection should be given at a separate site

Abbreviation: TIG, tetanus immune globulin.
Source: Modified from MMWR 1985; 34:405–414; 419–426.

of any necrotic tissue and documented hemostasis achieves the first level of care. When evaluating a wound that occurred at a time more remote, careful examination for pus, foreign bodies, and the presence of gas in the adjacent tissues is imperative.

Antibiotic Therapy

Prophylactic antibiotic therapy is usually advocated in the following conditions:

1. Heavily contaminated wounds
2. Cat bites
3. Human bites
4. Wounds in diabetic or immunocompromised individuals

A combination of a beta-lactam antibiotic such as amoxicillin/clavulanate (Augmentin) 250 to 500 mg q8h for three to five days and a fluoroquinolone with extended anaerobic coverage is effective prophylactically. Greater anaerobic coverage is required when dealing with supportive or dirty wounds. If there is any evidence of a systemic response such as fever, tachycardia, cellulitis/lymphangitis or fasciitis, systemic antibiotic therapy becomes the standard of care. If a puncture wound results from a nail or similar object going through the bottom of a sneaker, coverage against *Pseudomonas aeruginosa* is mandatory. *P. aeruginosa* colonizes the inner layers of athletic shoes. The presence of gas in adjacent tissue should alert the clinician to the possibility of clostridial infection. In diabetics and patients with vascular insufficiency, selected *Enterobacteriaceae* such as *Escherichia* may produce this phenomenon.

Prophylactic Vaccination

Tetanus prophylaxis must be considered in all wound cases. The recommended guidelines for the administration of tetanus toxoids and tetanus immune globulin are listed in Table 5.

Factors that increase probability include active infection at the operative site, fecal contamination, site of fecal contamination, presence or absence of shock, hemostasis.

In cases of fecal contamination of operative site, prophylactic antibiotic combinations that did not include anaerobic coverage resulted in greater than 20% wound infection rates, whereas rates of 10% to 14% were documented when the antibiotic coverage effectively included anaerobic agents. Studies with cefoxitin, cefotetan, and ampicillin/sulbactam have documented infection rates of approximately 10% or less.

Should bowel penetration involve the stomach or small bowel due to the shift toward class I antibiotic coverage and particularly the Enterobacteriaceae, consideration should be given to the use of a prophylactic combination whose primary coverage encompasses both the anaerobic spectrum of bacteria and the Enterobacteriaceae, e.g., trovafloxacin, clinafloxacin, clindamycin/aminoglycoside. Timing of dosing is critical. Tissue levels need to be established and in optimal range at the time of surgery. Redosing is currently based on the known antibiotic half-life; however, fluid volume distribution and blood loss should be taken into account.

SELECTED READING

Gangrenous Wound Infections
Addison WA, Livengood CH III, Hill GB, et al. Necrotizing fasciitis of vulvar origin in diabetic patients. Obstet Gynecol 1984; 63:473.
Borkow HI. Bacterial gangrene associated with pelvic surgery. Clin Obstet Gynecol 1973; 16(2):40.
Brewer GE, Meleney FC. Progressive gangrenous infection of the skin and subcutaneous tissues, following operation for acute perforative appendicitis. Ann Surg 1926; 84:438.
Chelsom J, Halstensen A, Haga T, Hoidby EA. Necrotising fasciitis due to group A streptococci in western Norway: incidence and clinical features (see comments). Lancet 1994; 344:1111.
Daly JW, King CR, Monif GRG. Progressive necrotizing wound infections in postirradiated patients. Obstet Gynecol 1978; 52(Suppl):5S.
Daly JW, Lukowski MJ, Monif GRG. The spontaneous occurrence of progressive synergistic bacterial gangrene on the abdominal wall. Am J Obstet Gynecol 1978; 1131:624.
de Longh DS, Smith IP, Thomas GW. Post-operative synergistic gangrene. J Am Med Assoc 1967; 200:227.

Dellinger EP. Antibiotic prophylaxis in trauma: penetrating abdominal injuries and open fractures. Rev Infect Dis 1991; 13:s847.

Donaldson PM, Naylor B, Lowe JW, Gouldesbrough DR. Rapidly fatal necrotising fasciitis caused by *Streptococcus pyogenes*. J Clin Pathol 1993; 46:617.

Fabian TC, Croce MA, Payne LW, et al. Duration of antibiotic therapy for penetrating abdominal trauma: a prospective trial. Surgery 1992; 112:788.

Farley DE, Katz VL, Dotters DJ. Toxic shock syndrome associated with vulvar necrotizing fasciitis. Obstet Gynecol 1993; 82:660.

Goepfert AR, Guinn DA, Andrews WW, et al. Necrotizing fasciitis after cesarean delivery. Obstet Gynecol 1997; 89:409.

Golshani S, Simons AJ, Der R, Ortega AE. Necrotizing fasciitis following laparoscopic surgery. Case report and review of the literature. Surg Endosc 1996; 10:751.

Hirn M. Hyperbaric oxygen in the treatment of gas gangrene and perineal necrotizing fasciitis. A clinical and experimental study. Eur J Surg 1993; Suppl 570:1.

Hooker KD, DiPiro JT, Wynn JJ. Aminoglycoside combinations vs. β-lactams alone for penetrating abdominal trauma: a meta-analysis. J Trauma 1991; 31:1155.

Jarrett P, Rademaker M, Duffill M. The clinical spectrum of necrotising fasciitis. A review of 15 cases. Aust NZ J Med 1997; 27:29.

Lille ST, Sato TT, Engrav LH, et al. Necrotizing soft tissue infections: obstacles in diagnosis. J Am Coll Surg 1996; 182:7.

Loh NN, Ch'en IY, Cheung LP, et al. Deep fascial hyperintensity in soft tissue abnormalities as revealed by T2-weighted MR imaging. Am J Roentgenol 1997; 168:1301.

Macias MA, Sariol O Jr, Ramos-Jimenez J. Necrotizing fasciitis secondary to vulvar infection. Infect Surg 1989; 8:432.

Meade JW, Mueller CB. Necrotizing infections of subcutaneous tissue and fascia. Ann Surg 1968; 168:274.

Meleny FL. Bacterial syngergism in disease processes. Ann Surg 1931; 94:961.

Meleny FL. Hemolytic streptococcal gangrene. Arch Surg 1924; 9:317.

Meltzer RM. Necrotizing fasciitis and progressive bacterial synergistic gangrene of the vulva. Obstet Gynecol 1983; 61:757.

McHenry CR, Azar T, Ramahi AJ. Monomicrobial necrotizing fasciitis complicating pregnancy and puerperium. Obstet Gynecol 1996; 87:823.

Moore FA, Moore EE, Ammons LA, et al. Presumptive antibiotics for penetrating abdominal wounds. Surg Gynecol Obstet 989; 169:99.

Nolan TE, King LA, Smith RP. Necrotizing surgical infections and necrotizing fasciitis in obstetric and gynecologic patients. South Med J 1993; 86:1363.

Pauzner D, Wolman I, Abramov L, et al. Post-cesarean section necrotizing fasciitis: report of a case and review of the literature. Gynecol Obstet Invest 1994; 37:59.

Roberts DB, Hester LL Jr. Progressive synergistic bacterial gangrene arising from abscesses of the vulva and Bartholin's gland duct. Am J Obstet Gynecol 1972; 114:285.

Roberts DB. Necrotizing fasciitis of the vulva. Am J Obstet Gynecol 1987; 157:568.

Rowan JA, North RA. Necrotizing fasciitis in the puerperium. Am J Obstet Gynecol 1995; 173:241.

Sellers BJ, Woods ML, Morris SE, et al. Necrotizing group A streptococcal infections associated with streptococcal toxic shock syndrome. Am J Surg 1996; 172:523.

Shupak A, Shoshani O, Goldenberg I, et al. Necrotizing fasciitis: an indication for hyperbaric oxygenations therapy? Surgery 1995; 118:873.

Stephenson H, Dotters DJ, Katz V. Necrotizing fasciitis of the vulva (see comments). Am J Obstet Gynecol 1992; 166:1324.

Sutton GP, Smirz LR, Clark DH, Bennett JE. Group B streptococcal necrotizing fasciitis arising from an episiotomy. Obstet Gynecol 1985; 66:733.

Wysoki MG, Santora TA, Shah RM, et al. Necrotizing fasciitis: CT characteristics. Radiology 1997; 203:859.

Prophylactic Antibiotics—Local and Systemic

Alexander IW, Altmeier WA. Penicillin prophylaxis of experimental staphylococcal wound infections. Surg Gynecol Obstet 1965; 120:243.

Branemork P. Local tissue effects of wound disinfectants. Acta Chir Scand Suppl 1965; 166:166.

Burdon LGW, Morris PL, Hunt P, Watts IM. A trial of cephalothin sodium in colon surgery to prevent wound infection. Arch Surg 1977; 112:1169.

Burke IF. The effective period of preventive antibiotic action in experimental incisions and dermal lesions. Surgery 1961; 50:161.

Edlich RF, Custer J, Madden L. Studies in management of the contaminated wound: assessment of the effectiveness of irrigation with antiseptic agents. Am J Surg 1969; 118:21.

Foster PD, O'Toole RD. Primary appendectomy: the effect of prophylactic cephaloridine on post-operative wound infection. J Am Med Assoc 1978; 239:1411.

Gilmore OIA, Sanderson PI. Prophylactic interparietal povidone-iodine in abdominal surgery. Br J Surg 1975; 62:792.

Halasz NA. Wound infection and topical antibiotics. Arch Surg 1977; 112:1240.

Hunt TK, Alexander IW, Burke IF, MacLean LD. Antibiotics in surgery. Arch Surg 1975; 110:148.

King CR, Daly JW, Monif GRG. Topical kanamycin in the prevention of abdominal wound infections. J Abdom Surg 1974; 19:156.

Motolo NM, Sheldon EC, Wolfman EF. Effects of antibiotics on prevention of infection in contaminated abdominal operations. Am Surg 1976; 42:123.

Noon GP, Beall AC, Jordan GL, et al. Clinical evaluation of peritoneal irrigation with antibiotic solution. Surgery 1967; 62:73.

Parker TH, O'Leary IP. Effect of preparation of the small intestine on micro flora and post-operative wound infection. Surg Gynecol Obstet 1978; 146:379.

Rodeheaver G, Ederton MT, Smith S, et al. Antimicrobial prophylaxis of contaminated tissues containing suture implants. Am J Surg 1977; 133:609.

Waterman NG, Howell RS, Batrich M. The effect of a prophylactic topical antibiotic on the incidence of wound infection. Arch Surg 1968; 97:365.

Weinstein AJ, McHenry MC, Gavan TL. Systemic absorption of neomycin irrigating solution. J Am Med Assoc 1977; 238:152.

Management of Wound Infections

Alexander LW, Kaplen IZ, Altmeier WA. Role of suture materials in the development of wound infection. Ann Surg 1967; 165:192.

Baggish MS, Lee WK. Abdominal wound disruption. Obstet Gynecol 1975; 46:530.

Bernard HR, Cole WR. The epidemiology of post-operative surgical infection. Surg Clin N Am 1965; 45:509.

Bierens dr Haan R, Ellis H, Wilks M. The role of infection on wound healing. Surg Gynecol Obstet 1974; 138:693.

Brooks S. Civil War Medicine. Springfield: Charles C. Thomas, 1966:84.

Brote L. Wound infections in clean and potentially contaminated surgery. Acta Chir Scand 1976; 142:191.

Brown SE, Allen HH, Robins RN. The use of delayed primary wound closure in preventing wound infections. Am J Obstet Gynecol 1977; 127:713.

Charmley J, Eftekhor N. Penetration of gown material by organisms from the surgeon's body. Lancet 1969; 1:172.

Conolly WB, Hunt TK, Dunply JE. Management of contaminated surgical wounds. Surg Gynecol Obstet 1969; 129:593.

Daly JW, Rutledge F. Experience with wound dehiscence in patients treated for pelvic malignancy. South Med J 1965; 58:308.

Davidson AIG, Smylie HG. A bacteriological study of the immediate environment of a surgical wound. Br J Surg 1971; 58:326.

Disseen P. An evaluation of the duration of the surgical scrub. Surg Gynecol Obstet 1969; 129:1181.

Edlich RF, Panek PA. Physical and chemical configuration of sutures in the development of surgical infection. Ann Surg 1973; 177:679.

Edlich RF, Rogers W, Kaspar G, et al. Studies in the management of the contaminated wound. Am J Surg 1969; 117:323.

Findlay GM. Histamine and infection. J Pathol Bact 1928; 31:633.

Galle PC, Homesley HD, Rhyne AL. Reassessment of the surgical scrub. Surg Gynecol Obstet 1978; 147:215.

Herfretz CJ, Richards FO, Lawrence MS. Comparison of wound healing with and without dressings. Arch Surg 1952; 65:746.

Hohn DC, Granelli SG, Burton RW, Hunt TK. Antimicrobial systems of the surgical wound: detection of antimicrobial protein in cell free wound fluid. Am J Surg 1977; 133:601.

Kronberg O. Polyglycolic acid (dexon) versus silk for fascial closure of abdominal incisions. Act Chir Scand 1976; 142:9.

Leissner KH. Post-operative wound infection in 32,000 clean operations. Acta Chir Scand 1976; 142:433.

Ljungquist U. Wound sepsis after clean operations. Lancet 1964; May:1095.

May J, Chalmers JP, Lowenthal J, Rountree PM. Factors in the patient contributing to surgical sepsis. Surg Gynecol Obstet 1966; 122:28.

Polk HC, Lopez-Mayor LF. Post-operative wound infection: a prospective study of determinant factors and prevention. Surgery 1969; 66:97.

Robson MC, Krizek TJ, Heggers JP. Biology of surgical infection. Curr Prob Surg 1973; March:1.

Robson MC, Lea CE, Dalton JB, Heggars JP. Quantitative bacteriology and delayed wound closure. S Forum 1968; 19:501.

Rollins RA, Corcoran JL, Gibbs CE. Treatment of gynecologic wound complications. Obstet Gynecol 1966; 28:268.

Strauss RJ, Wise L. Operative risks of obesity. Surg Gynecol Obstet 1978; 146:286.

Tucci VJ, Stone AM, Thompson C, et al. Studies of the surgical scrub. Surg Gynecol Obstet 1977; 145:415.

Usher FC, Wallace SA. Tissue reaction to plastics. Arch Surg 1958; 76:997.

Webster FJT, Davis PW. Closure of abdominal wounds by adhesive strips: a clinical trial. Br Med J 1975; 3:696.

Wenzel RP, Hunting KI, Osterman CA. Post-operative wound infection rates. Surg Gynecol Obstet 1977; 144:749.

Williams IA, Oates GD, Brown PP, et al. Abdominal wound infections and plastic wound guards. Br J Surg 1972; 59:142.

Collection and Handling of Bacteriological and Viral Obstetrics and Gynecology Specimens

I

DIRECT EXAMINATION

Gram Stains

The Gram stain is used to determine morphological bacterial types, aid in the selection of culture media, and assess specimen quality (Table A.1). Smears should be examined for both microorganisms and cells. It is important to assess the morphology and quantity of microorganisms present. Microorganisms are seen on smears only if present in the specimen at a concentration of greater than or equal to 10^4 organisms/mL.

The character and relative quantity of epithelial cells and leukocytes should be determined. The presence of leukocytes generally indicates a good-quality specimen has been obtained from the area of inflammation. The presence of squamous epithelial cells in sputa and other specimens correlates with a poor-quality specimen. Squamous epithelial cells should not be confused with ciliated epithelial cells. In the case of a sputum sample, the latter cells indicate that the specimen is of a lower respiratory tract origin.

Some bacteria do not stain well with the Gram stain and require tissue stains such as the Giemsa/Wright stain (for *Calymmatobacterium granulomatis*, *Borrelia*, *Rickettsia*, and *Chlamydia*) or Giemsa (for *Rickettsia*, *Chlamydia*, and *Legionella pneumophila*). The physician must indicate to the microbiologist the possibility that one or more of these agents may be present in order to assure proper staining of the specimen.

Gram-Staining Technique

The thinly smeared sample should be allowed to dry, and is then gently heat-fixed by passing it quickly over a Bunsen burner flame or microbiologic incinerator a few times. The slide should be handheld and not allowed to become more than warm to the touch. Excessive heating will lead to a disruption of cellular elements and may sometimes obscure microorganisms by causing clumping of proteinaceous material. Then, while holding the slide over a sink with a soft flow of tap water, the staining reagents are added in the following fashion:

1. Crystal violet: cover the smear and swirl gently for a few seconds, then pour off and wash in tap water.
2. Gram's iodine: same procedure as for crystal violet, then rinse gently with water.
3. Decolorizer: carefully cover the smear while holding it horizontally and allow blue stain to elute for a second or two. Then tilt it gently and continue to add decolorizer. As the blue begins to fade noticeably, wash quickly but gently in water. In a thinly smeared sample,

approximately three to five seconds is adequate, using acetone–alcohol decolorizer. This step is most critical and requires careful attention.

4. Safranin: same procedure as for crystal violet. After pouring off the counter-stain (safranin), wash gently with water. Then blot the slide carefully between clean filter paper and allow it to air-dry before microscopic examination. Residual moisture may interfere with oil-immersion microscopy.

BACTERIOLOGICAL CULTURES

Skin Cultures

Abscesses

Material from a previously undrained wound abscess should be aspirated with a needle and syringe after appropriate decontamination of the overlying skin. Fluid thus obtained should be forwarded to the microbiological facility in a needleless, capped syringe with all of the air expressed out, or in an anaerobic transport vial (see section titled Anaerobic Cultures).

Ulcers

Ulcers should be carefully debrided and proper samples collected from the base or progressive edge where bacteria actively multiply. Unremoved crust or surface pus should not be collected since it is often contaminated by other bacteria, thus not reflecting the true infecting flora.

Vesiculopustules

This type of lesion should be unroofed with a sterile needle before obtaining the specimen. Rub the base of the lesion with a Dacron swab to obtain cellular material. For viral cultures, place the swab in a transport media. A touch preparation should also be made using a separate swab and clean microscope slide (see section titled Laboratory Detection of Viruses).

Anaerobic Cultures

Specimen Collection and Transport

Good anaerobic bacteriology starts with proper collection of the specimen (Table A.2).

TABLE A.1 Bacteriological specimens which require concomitant Gram staining

Sputum
Abscess material
Infected peritoneal fluid
Endocervical/endometrial cultures
Cerebrospinal fluid
Other body fluids (except urine)

Sites normally inhabited by a rich indigenous flora, such as the intestinal tract or vagina, should not be sampled for anaerobes except under special circumstances and in special ways (e.g., for quantitative study of upper, small-bowel flora in the blind loop syndrome) or should be done using specialized techniques that minimize contamination from the sites to be sampled. Using a double lumen catheter, bronchial brushings, and bronchoalveolar lavage fluid allows the lower respiratory tract to be sampled. An endometrial suction curette biopsy can be used to obtain endometrial samples.

Specimen Selection

Good anaerobic bacteriology is time consuming and expensive. Therefore, it is important that only specimens that have been selected and collected properly be submitted for anaerobic culture. A poor specimen will not only give useless or misleading results, but will also prevent the laboratory personnel from devoting sufficient attention to valid specimens.

Pus, when present, is best aspirated into a syringe through a needle and injected into an anaerobic (oxygen-free) transport vial containing an oxidation–reduction indicator. Great care must be taken to exclude air. Even transient contact with molecular oxygen is as lethal as an autoclave for strict anaerobes. Syringes used for aspiration should not be used as transporters (with the needles attached) because of the potential danger of needle-stick injuries. Anaerobic vials are commercially available from several manufacturers.

In selected instances (i.e., ruptured tubo-ovarian abscess or gangrenous wound infections), it is not possible to obtain a specimen for bacteriological analysis by aspiration. In these circumstances, *pieces of infected tissue* obtained by excision or biopsy are best transported in loosely capped containers sealed in anaerobic gas-impermeable bags.

Conditions of transport do affect the viability and/or relative proportions of bacteria present. Rapid delivery at room temperature is best for transportation of specimens. Oxygen diffuses better at lower temperatures. The gross appearance (purulence, necrotic tissue) and odor of the specimen can give the laboratory valuable clues to the presence of anaerobes.

Gram Stain for Anaerobic Infections

Next to the physician's ability to anticipate when the anaerobic infection is present on clinical grounds, the most important diagnostic tool is the Gram stain. When dealing with a well-established abscess, the ocular-cerebral reflex is almost as accurate as an anaerobic diagnostic facility. *Whenever you take an anaerobic culture, make a Gram stain!*

The morphotypes and relative quantities of both the host and the bacterial cells present in the preparation will provide information on the specimen quality and may give clues to the presence of particular bacterial species and suggest the need for special selective media (Table A.3). Furthermore, the Gram stain information provides quality control for specimen transport and isolation efficiency.

Blood Cultures

Site Selection and Preparation

Venipuncture sites involved with dermatologic disease will often yield a higher rate of contamination. Arterial blood provides no higher yield than does venous blood.

Site preparation for the withdrawal of blood is one of the most important aspects of culturing blood for bacterial pathogens. The recommended procedure involves decontamination with 70% isopropyl or ethyl alcohol for one minute followed by povidone iodine for one minute. If the patient exhibits or has a known allergy to iodine, only 70% alcohol should be used.

The antiseptic solution is applied concentrically, starting at the center. The disinfectant should be allowed to dry completely before the vein is punctured. After disinfection, the vein should not be repalpated. Sterile gloves should be used throughout this process, in accordance with current infection-control guidelines for universal precautions. The site should be prepared with a double applicator of alcohol. Do not change the needle after venipuncture and before inoculation of blood into the culture media. Intravascular catheters are most acceptable as alternatives to cutaneous venipuncture.

Volume of Blood Per Culture

One of the most important variables in the detection of bacteremia is the volume of blood cultured. The minimum volume that should be collected is 10 mL. Collecting 20 or 30 mL of blood increases the yield of isolates over 25% and 50% respectively. Because the magnitude of bacteremia is greater in children than in adults, cultures of 1 to 5 mL are reasonable. Blood contains complement antibodies and enzymes that are potentially bactericidal.

To counter these naturally occurring systems, a blood-to-broth ratio of 1:5 to 1:10 should be achieved. In addition, most commercial blood culture broths contain sodium polyanetholsulfonate, which neutralizes the antibacterial activity of blood.

Never divide a single sample into multiple sets of blood cultures. In other words, each blood sample drawn equals one blood culture (one aerobic and one anaerobic bottle).

As shown in Table A.3, the percentage of bacteremias detected is optimal if three separate blood cultures are

TABLE A.2 Acceptable specimens for anaerobic culture

(1)	Normally sterile fluids (i.e. blood)
(2)	Normally sterile area (i.e. peritoneal and pleural cavities)
(3)	Deep abscesses
(4)	Deep aspiration of wounds and tissue specimens
(5)	Transtracheal, cul-de-sac aspirates

TABLE A.3 Probability of documenting bacteremia with increasing numbers of blood culture

Percentage of bacteremia detected	Number of 20 ml blood cultures
80	1
88	2
99	3

Source: Washington J-II. *Mayo Clinic Proc* 1975;50:91.

obtained. A single blood culture lacks sensitivity (80%) and thus should be avoided. On the other hand, more than three blood cultures adds little to the sensitivity and should also be avoided.

Types of Blood Culture Bottles

A routine blood culture involves the use of two blood culture bottles (referred to as a set). One is for aerobic blood culturing, the other for anaerobic blood culturing. There are a number of different types and brands available.

If antibiotic therapy has already been initiated prior to collection of the blood specimen, this diminishes the probability of obtaining an isolate, but does not totally invalidate the culture. Some blood culture bottles contain antibiotic removal resins. These nonspecifically bind and remove many antibiotics.

In some instances, the physician may suspect an L-form or cell-wall–deficient organism. A blood culture bottle containing a hypertonic medium with 10% sucrose should be used in these cases.

Timing and Spacing of Blood Cultures

There are little data on the optimal time to collect blood for culture in humans. Animal data suggest that the optimal time for collection of blood for culture is immediately prior to a fever spike. Since this is somewhat impractical, it is generally recommended that blood be collected at the fever spike. The spacing of blood cultures is somewhat dependent upon the clinical situation and the need to initiate antimicrobial therapy. When possible, separate blood cultures should be spaced 30 to 60 minutes apart and should be collected before the initiation of antibiotic therapy.

Urine Cultures

Obtain early morning specimens whenever possible. Bacterial counts will be higher at this time. Care must be taken to avoid contamination of the specimen with organisms from perineum, distal urethra, vaginal secretions, hands, skin, and clothing. Cleansing procedures must remove contaminating organisms from the vulva, urethral meatus, and perineal area.

Urine must be obtained properly, and transported and processed as soon as possible. No more than one hour should elapse between specimen collection and incubation. If this time schedule cannot be followed, the urine specimen must be refrigerated immediately.

ENDOCERVICAL CULTURES

Endocervial and/or anal mucosal cultures are done to identify the presence of sexually transmitted disease pathogens, primarily *Neisseria gonorrhoeae* and *Chlamydia trachomatis*. The tests available are discussed in detail in Appendix V; recommendation for appropriate specimen selection and collection techniques are summarized in Tables A.5 and A.6.

Neisseria gonorrhoeae

The principal reason for obtaining an endocervical culture is to document *N. gonorrhoeae* in cases of presumed rape

TABLE A.4 Do's and don'ts of culturing for *Neisseria gonorrhoeae*

(1)	Never inoculate a culture plate which is not at least at room temperature.
(2)	Be sure to roll (not merely streak) a cotton swab in a Z or W pattern.
(3)	Assure a source of CO_2 – JEMBEC uses a $NaHCO_3$ tablet. – modified Thayer Martin method uses a candle jar or a CO_2 incubator.
(4)	Be sure to incubate 12–18 hours before transporting to a diagnostic facility.

(Table A.4). If a culture is to be performed, it should be obtained before any other procedures.

In obtaining bacteriological specimens for identification, it is important to moisten the speculum only with warm water. Do not use any other lubricants, as the majority of lubricants have been shown to be partially bacteriocidal for *N. gonorrhoeae* and may mask detection of occult infection.

1. Never culture a specimen on a plate that is not at least at room temperature. *N. gonorrhoeae* has an extremely limited thermal tolerance. Preferential growth occurs between 30°C and 38°C. Temperatures below room temperature will rarely sustain the replication of *N. gonorrhoeae* and often account for nonrecovery of the organism.

2. Incubate cultures immediately. Again, the thermal lability of the organism is such that maintaining cultures at room temperature for more than one hour will have a deleterious effect.

3. Be sure to provide a source of carbon dioxide. In dealing with the Thayer-Martin or Martin-Lewis plates, it is not only imperative that they be incubated, but also that candle jars be utilized to provide the critical 5% CO_2 atmosphere required for the initiation of bacterial replication.

4. *N. gonorrhoeae* is extremely temperature liable and will not grow, or does so only poorly, on culture plates recently taken from the ice box.

Probably the single greatest factor contributing to falsely negative cultures is the failure of the physician to roll the swab in a "Z" or "W" manner. The endocervical swab samples 360°, yet if the swab is not rolled on the culture medium, a maximum of only 33% to 50% of the swab sample is obtained. Total (100%) sampling is especially important when *N. gonorrhoeae* is present in quantities that are numerically reduced (e.g., the asymptomatic carrier or the patient with initial gonococcal salpingitis who is now undergoing a competitive elimination of *N. gonorrhoeae* at the endocervix).

If these conditions cannot be met, consideration should be given to the potential consequences emanating from a false-negative culture report.

LABORATORY DETECTION OF VIRUSES

The number of infectious particles and the temperature of incubation in an appropriate culture line are the prime determinants of how quickly cytopathic effects will be observed.

TABLE A.5 Recommendations for collection of specimens for isolation of viruses

Vesicles/pustules: Rupture vesicles or pustules with a sterile needle and proceed as follows:

Ulcers:
(1) Vigorously touch the underlying ulcer with a dacron swab.[a]
(2) Place the swab in an unfrozen viral transport media.
(3) Confirm all patient care data for label.
(4) Place the viral transport at 4°C as quickly as possible. If the culture cannot be inoculated into appropriate tissue culture lines within 72 hours, freeze specimen at −60°C.

[a] A swab gently touched on a lesion collects a small fraction of the virus present, compared to a firm and complete rolling of the swab.

TABLE A.6 Specimen collection for *Chlamydia* cultures

A. Acceptable specimens:

Disease	Specimen
Urethritis	urethral swab
Cervicitis	endocervical swab
Conjunctivitis	conjuctival swab
Trachoma	conjuctival swab
Infant pneumonitis	nasopharyngeal swab
Lymphogranuloma venereum[a]	bubo aspirate
Fitz-Hugh-Curtis syndrome (perihepatitis)	peritonmeal fluid, endocervical swab
Pelvic inflammatory disease (PID)	peritoneal fluid, tissue, endocervical swab
Psittacosis[a]	sputum, lung tissue
Pneumonitis, upper respiratory tract infection of adults[a] and older children	nasopharyngeal or throat swab, endotracheal aspirate or wash, bronchoalveolar lavage fluid, lung tissue
Sexual abuse (prepubescent female)	vaginal, rectal, throat, urethral swab
Sexual abuse (male)	rectal, throat, urethral swab

B. Unacceptable specimens:
- Saliva
- Semen
- Urine
- Blood
- Vaginal specimens (except for prepubescent females or women with a previous history of hysterectomy)

C. Specimen collection:
(1) Collect swab specimens using a dacron tipped plastic shafted swab. Do not use wooden shaft swabs or calgiswabs, as they are toxic to the *Chlamydia*.
(2) After collection, place the swab in a thawed tube of *Chlamydia* transport media, cut the plastic shaft leaving the swab in the tube, and recap the tube.
(3) Other specimens, such as tissue and fluids, can be added directly to a tube of *Chlamydia* transport media.
(4) Place the specimen in a water-crushed ice bath (wet ice), at 4°C.
(5) Transport to the laboratory on wet ice.

[a] Serum for acute and convalescent titers should be collected for diagnosis of lymphogranuloma venereum, psittacosis, and *Chlamydia pneumoniae* infections.

Virus Identification
Nucleic Amplification Testing
The development of nucleic acid amplification tests for all the major viruses relevant to obstetrics and gynecology has

TABLE A.7 Specimen collection for *Chlamydia* DNA and/or *Neisseria gonorrhoeae* DNA probe tests

A. For specimen collection use only the Gen-Probe collection swabs

B. Urethral specimens:
(1) The patient should not have urinated for at least one hour prior to sampling.
(2) Insert the male swab into urethra and rotate for 3–5 seconds.
(3) Immediately insert swab into the Gen-Probe transport tube.
(4) Transport as soon as possible to the microbiology laboratory.

C. Endocervical specimens:
(1) Remove mucus from the exocervix with one of the large swabs. Discard the swab.
(2) Rotate the second large swab in the endocervix 15–30 seconds. Avoid touching the vaginal walls when inserting and removing the swab.
(3) Immediately insert swab into the Gen-Probe transport tube.
(4) Transport as soon as possible to the microbiology laboratory.

D. Conjunctival specimens (for *Chlamydia* DNA test ONLY):
(1) Using the male swab, firmly stroke the lower conjunctiva 2–3 times.
(2) Immediately insert swab into the Gen-Probe transport tube.
(3) Transport as soon as possible to the microbiology laboratory.

E. *Chlamydia* DNA specimens are not acceptable from suspected cases of sexual assault or abuse.

replaced the use of tissue culture as the prime diagnostic vehicle for the identification of viral isolates from either specimen samples or tissue culture fluid (Appendix V). This technology is extremely sensitive. Primary emphasis is on proper specimen collection and handling. When dealing with mucosal lesions, the recommendations for specimen collection are those previously advocated for virus culture (Table A.7).

Virus Isolation
Viurs Tissue Culture Isolation Media
A number of viral transport media are available. The media can be kept at 4°C for two weeks (and several months if kept frozen). When using frozen transport media, the media need to adequately thaw prior to insertion of the Dacron-tipped swab.

Specimen Handling and Storage
The specimen should be maintained at 4°C until it can be inoculated onto an appropriate tissue culture line. Most cultures remain stable in transport media at 4°C for periods of 48 to 72 hours. Freezing a specimen, even at −60°C, will result in a reduction in the number of infectious viral particles present.

Cytological Techniques
The cytomegaloviruses cause cytoplasmatic giantism. This finding, coupled with the presence of a single large Fuelgen-positive intranuclear inclusion body, is highly suggestive. Urine specimens for cytology should have a high specific gravity (e.g., early morning specimens).

Diagnostic Procedures Following Careful Physical Examination and Graphic Delineation of Lesions

II

Revised by Paul Summers

VULVAR ULCERS OF POSSIBLY INFECTIOUS ETIOLOGY

Perhaps one of the most challenging problems confronting the obstetrician–gynecologist is obtaining a definitive diagnosis in a patient with a vulvar ulcer. The frequency with which infectious agents produce such a lesion and the multiplicity of etiologies necessitate the clear-cut delineation of pragmatic steps that will lead to the ultimate diagnosis in most instances.

Physical Examination

When confronted with a lesion for which the diagnosis is in doubt, a defined procedure is helpful.

1. Draw a diagram of the lesion and its relationship to the surrounding architecture. At this time, note the number of lesions and determine whether the lesion is in the field of inguinal lymphatic drainage or in that of the anorectal lymph nodes. *Example:*

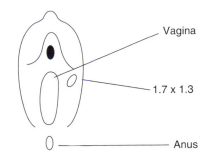

2. Carefully examine the margin and base of the lesion (a cut-edge diagram is often helpful in determining whether the edges are heaped up and rolled, well defined, shaggy, undermined, etc.). Record the character of the exudate.

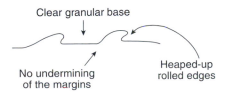

3. Note the presence of pain.
4. Determine the presence of adenopathy.
5. Record any associated clinical features.

By utilizing this stepwise procedure, one has not only defined the characteristics of the lesions, but also availed oneself of certain broad categories that have a relatively specific differential diagnosis. Painless lesions or lesions with well-defined margins have distinct differential diagnoses (Table A.1).

Diagnostic Procedures

Following careful physical examination and graphic delineation of the lesion:

1. The most useful diagnostic procedure is direct examination of the exudate or transudate taken from such a lesion (Table A.2); e.g., touch preparations, cytologic smears, and wet mounted preparations (dark-field examination where indicated) are an integral part of the initial differential. *Example*: motile spirochetes on dark-field examination.
2. Biopsy of the margin and a portion of the base of the lesion is probably the second most valuable diagnostic procedure, after microscopic observation, in establishing a definitive diagnosis. *Example:* plasmacytic lymphocytic infiltrate; spirochetes demonstrable with Levaditi stain.
3. Culturing for bacteria, mycobacteria, and protozoa is often a costly procedure with a low yield and should be avoided unless indicated on clinical or histologic grounds. Suspicion of one sexually transmitted disease should intensify monitoring for a second agent at other sites.
4. In certain instances, such as lymphogranuloma venereum, additional procedures may be necessary. The diagnostic work-up for the individual organisms listed in Table A.1 is described in Table A.2.

The procedures listed should all be performed in the same visit.

GRANULOMA INGUINALE (*KLEBSIELLA GRANULOMATIS*)

Granuloma inguinale is a disease due to an intracellular gram-negative rod, *K. granulomatis* (*Calymmatobacterium granulomatis*), which is usually endemic in areas with both high temperatures and humidity. In the United States, disease occurs primarily in port cities in the southern part.

The disease is apparently not very contagious even though a significant mode of transmission involves sexual

TABLE A.I Differential diagnosis of vulvar ulcers

Pathogen	Lesions	Pain	Characteristics of lesion	Clinical features	Diagnostic procedure
Herpes simplex types I & 2 or multiple	Single	Yes	Vesiculopustules; shallow ulcers with secondary infection		Virus isolation (any tissue culture line)
Vaccinia virus	Single or multiple	Yes	Vesiculopustules; shallow ulcers with secondary infection	History of recent vaccination or intimate contact with recently vaccinated person; VDRL may be +, but FTA –	Virus isolation (any tissue culture line)
Behcet's syndrome (causative agent unknown)	Multiple	Yes	Shallow-based ulcers with secondary infection	Concomitant oral apthous lesions; possible uveitis or iridocyclitis	None
Treponema pallidum (syphilis)	Single	No	Well-defined margins; rolled; clean	Tender inguinal adenopathy	Darkfield examination or VDRL and FTA
Chlamydia trachomatis (lymphomogranuloma venereum)	Single	No	Granular base; shallow ulcer with secondary infection	Anorectal proctitis possible	Complement fixation F test or Frei intradermal skin test for LGV
Squamous cell carcinoma	Single	No	Firm lesion with rolled margins		Biopsy
Mycobacterium tuberculosis	Single	No	Well-defined borders; granular base	Systemic disease; PPD +	Culture; touch prep or biopsy with Zieh-Neelsen staining
Calymmatobacterium (Donovania) granulomatis (donovanosis)	Single; may be several	Yes	Well-defined borders; clean, granular base	Inguinal adenopathy; pseudobubo formation	Donovan bodies; touch prep of lesion or biopsy
Hemophilus ducreyi (chancroid)	Single	Yes	Shaggy borders surrounding necrotic exudate		Culture; response to therapy
Entamoeba histolytica (amebiasis)	Single	Yes	Shaggy undermined edges; exudate similar to "anchovy paste"	Possible history or presence of acute diarrhea	Amebas on touch prep biopsy
Trauma with secondary bacterial infection	Pattern of involvement depends on bacterial pathogens				
a) Microaerophilic B-streptococci and coagulase+ staphylococci (Meleney's ulcer type II)	Single	Yes		Fulminating pattern of spread and tissue destruction	Culture
b) *Bacteroides* (Anaerobic organism)	Single	Yes	Ulcer with underlying abscess	Deep traumatic penetration with foul-smelling exudate	Culture

contact. The disease does not invariably affect conjugal partners despite repeated contact.

Natural History of the Disease

The predilection of lesions for the genital areas and the occasional occurrence of disease in sexual partners of infected individuals constitute the prime evidence to support the concept of granuloma inguinale as a venereal disease.

The prevalence of the disease among pederasts and the predominant anal and perianal predilection of the lesions strongly suggest that rectal coitus is the prime means of transmission of infection, either by contamination of the skin directly through anal intercourse (whether it be heterosexual or homosexual) or indirectly by faulty hygiene. Further evidence supporting the inferred thesis of venereal disease transfer, secondary to rectal coitus, can be drawn from the observations that the disease process is infrequent among prostitutes. In the preantibiotic era, individuals in the florid stage of the disease only occasionally transmitted infection to their sexual partners. From clinical studies, an incubation period of 17.4 days has been calculated; however, experimental infection of human volunteers has produced disease in 50 days.

The disease is only mildly contagious. In most cases, lesions cannot be demonstrated in sexual consorts. Evidence

TABLE A.2 Value of diagnostic procedures for specific organisms

Pathogen	Touch preparation and darkfield examination	Biopsy	Culturing or serologic analysis
Herpes simplex virus	Multinucleated giant cells with intranuclear clear inclusion bodies	Intranuclear inclusion bodies in parabasilar cells of epidermis	Virologic culture
Vaccinia virus	Intracytoplasmic inclusion bodies	Intracytoplasmic inclusion bodies	Virologic culture
Behcet's syndrome	—	—	—
Treponema pallidum	Motile spirochetes demonstrable on darkfield examination of tissue transudate	Mixed plasmacytic-lymphocytic infiltrate with small-vessel endarteritis; using silver-impregnated Levaditi stain, spirochetes may demonstrate	VDRL and FTA-ABS tests may be +
Chlamydia trachomatis (Lymphogranuloma venereum)	—	Central necrosis surrounded by epithelial cells and infected granulation tissue	Diagnosis inferred from CF antibody titer of 1:40 or higher, or + Frei test with 1 cm papule in 48–72 h
Squamous cell carcinoma	Diagnosis suggested by cytologic atypia	Definitive diagnosis based on histopathology	—
Mycobacterium tuberculosis	Demonstrable with Ziehl-Neelsen staining	Diagnosis inferred on finding epithelial and Langhans giant cells	Negative PPD aids in excluding diagnosis Culture
Calymmatobacterium (Donovania) granulomatis	Donovan bodies with macrophages	Donovan bodies within macrophages	—
Haemophilus ducreyi	"School of fish" pattern	—	Bacteriologic culture
Entamoeba histolytica	Trophozoites on wet mounts	Trophozoites with PAS stain	—
Secondary bacterial infections	Gram staining may give presumptive diagnosis	—	Bacteriologic culture

of infection as opposed to disease is detected in 12% to 52% of marital or steady sexual partners.

The common sites for lesions, in women, are the labia minora, fourchette, and labia majora. The perianal region also can be affected. Another site that may occasionally be affected by this disease is the oral cavity.

The initial lesion usually begins as a reddish brown, flat-topped papule, which often spreads and then ulcerates in the center. Not infrequently, other papules appear at about the same time. When they ulcerate, the lesions eventually coalesce.

The ulcer may show variation in its morphology:

1. The ulcerative or ulcerogranulomatous form—the fleshy, exuberant lesion—presents as a beefy-red granulomatous ulcer, usually single, which is nontender, non-indurated, and bleeds profusely on touch.
2. The hypertrophic or verrucous form consists of an ulcer or growth with a raised, irregular edge or surface, drier than the ulcerative variety, with an elevated, granulomatous base.
3. The necrotic type gives rise to extensive destruction of genitalia with profuse, foul-smelling exudate.
4. The sclerotic or cicatrical variety presents as a band-like scar in and around the genitalia.

As a rule, the ulcer tends to have a clean base composed of fresh granulation tissue and well-defined borders. The advancing edge of the lesion exhibits a scrolled appearance owing to epithelial hyperplasia and acanthosis of the squamous epithelium. The degree of hyperplasia (and not infrequently dysplasia) in response to infection may cause an erroneous diagnosis of low-grade squamous cell carcinoma.

Spread of the disease may be by contiguous contact, autoinoculation, or lymphatic extension. The histologic demonstration of lymph node involvement and the development of pseudobubo in males stress the role of lymphatic dissemination from the superficial genital lesion. In females, the regional lymph nodes enlarge somewhat and are occasionally tender, but they do not suppurate unless gross secondary infection of the initial lesion is present.

Biopsy of the initial lesion reveals, in addition to the secondary epithelial change, a granulomatous proliferative response and a secondary connective tissue attempt at repair. The histopathologic feature of the ulcer of donovanosis is that of a dense granulomatous tissue reaction consisting mainly of small lymphocytes, with a scattering of the typically large mononuclear cells that may contain the pathognomonic Donovan bodies. Small collections of polymorphonuclear neutrophils (microabscesses) secondary to superimposed bacterial infection are typical. In the absence of secondary infection, neutrophils are conspicuously absent. Within the granulation tissue, the capillaries tend to be prominent, owing to reactive hyperplasia of their endothelial cells. Even in the absence of Donovan bodies, the histopathology of infection due to *K. granulomatis* (*C. granulomatis*) is sufficiently characteristic to warrant a presumptive diagnosis.

The more advanced lesions represent a composite of the two processes of exuberant granulomatous proliferation and fibroblastic repair. With partial resolution of infection, isolated foci of plasma cells and lymphocytes appear, as well as occasional macrophages within the interstices of connective tissue. With arrest of the disease process, the granulation tissue is replaced by newly grown connective tissue.

One of the less commonly seen features of the disease is a gross local swelling of the affected area. It may develop before treatment or during the phase when the ulcers are healing. These hard, knobby swellings are due to obliteration of predominantly efferent lymphatics. Biopsy of such a lesion reveals grossly dilated lymphatics.

With secondary infection of the initial ulcers, the gross appearance of the lesions changes, owing to extension of the area of ulceration deep into the underlying dermis, with excavation and undermining of the margins. With appropriate therapy, the fibroblastic component predominates, leaving scar formation as the end-stage lesion of genital involvement. In 6% of the cases, extragenital lesions are observed. Metastatic hematogenous infection as well as involvement of the oral cavity has been described. The infection, particularly after delivery or abortion, infrequently extends from the cervix and may involve the uterus, fallopian tubes, and ovaries.

With extensive disease and secondary infection, systemic signs such as fever, anemia, weight loss, malaise, and leukocytosis may occur. Although the diagnosis may be inferred because of the clinical presentation and the exclusion of other disease processes, a definitive diagnosis is still contingent upon the demonstration of Donovan bodies.

Some of the lesions are separate. Multiple lesions may become confluent. The margin of a lesion is raised and scrolled. The base is granular and covered imperfectly by a thin gray slough.

Diagnosis

Many clinicians examining their first case of donovanosis think it is carcinoma, regardless of whether the lesion is of the vulva or the cervix. Adequate biopsies must be taken and carefully studied. Pathologists can also be misled. The hyperplasia and dysplasia of squamous epithelium at the edge of an ulcer can easily be mistaken for low-grade squamous cell carcinoma. Occasionally, however, the diagnosis is carcinoma.

The clinical diagnosis is suggested by the clinical appearance of the lesion or lesions. A diagnosis can be made from a stained crush preparation from the lesion. A piece of clear granulation tissue from a lesion is spread against the slide which is then air-dried and stained with Wright or Giemsa stain.

The diagnosis of granuloma inguinale is almost invariably based on the identification of classic Donovan bodies in biopsy material. Donovan bodies appear as clusters of blue or black staining with an organism's "safety pin" appearance (from bipolar chromatin) in the cytoplasm of large

mononuclear cells. Biopsies should be taken radially through the edge of the ulcer and include some of its base. The affinity of the intracysts of *K. granulomatis* for silver salts facilitates the recognition of the Donovan bodies. Because Donovan bodies are very hard to find, they may be more readily demonstrated in tissue spreads stained with Giemsa's stain than in histologic sections stained with either hematoxylin and eosin or silver stains. In either case, success in their identification depends on the sharp eyes and persistence of the pathologist, who often has to search many slides in order to establish the diagnosis of donovanosis.

Therapy

K. granulomatis is susceptible to a wide number of antibiotic preparations that interfere with protein synthesis. The tetracyclines (0.5 g every six hours orally) are the drug of choice. Trimethoprim–sulfamethoxazole (two tablets every 12 hours) has been effective. Chloramphenicol (0.5 g every eight hours orally) is reserved for resistant cases. Ampicillin and erythromycin to be somewhat erratic in efficiency, the combination of ampicillin and erythromycin has been found to be satisfactory in the treatment of pregnant patients. Treatment should be continued until the lesions have healed completely, which usually takes three weeks. Long-standing lesions may be so mutilating that adjunctive surgical care may be necessary. The elimination of secondary infection by topical cleansing and antimicrobial therapy accelerates healing. Relapses are frequent; some cases require prolonged courses of antibiotic therapy. It is wise to treat infection vigorously and to insist on compulsive follow-up even after apparent cure.

The local areas of "elephantiasis" remaining after effective treatment of active infection are often uncomfortable and cause cosmetic embarrassment. Once infection is cured, local excision of such focal swelling can be carried out.

CHANCROID (HAEMOPHILUS DUCREYI)

Chancroid is a superficial infection of the external genital tract caused by *H. ducreyi*. *H. ducreyi* has a worldwide distribution but is found more frequently in tropical and subtropical countries. Within the United States, disease is more prevalent in the southern states.

The infection is disseminated venereally. Genital lesions appear 3 to 14 days after sexual contact and may be single or multiple. The initial lesion is usually one or more small erythematous macules that rapidly become vesicular pustules. The lesion ruptures, leaving behind a small circumscribed ulcer with an erythematous base (Table A.3). The ulcer is painful and tender to palpation and is characterized by a nonindurated base, painful overhanging edges, and ragged margins. The lesion frequently has an erythematous halo. The base of the ulcer is covered with a dirty-looking, necrotic, grayish exudate. Lymphadenitis occurs in approximately 30% of the cases. The lymphadenopathy is regional and is often unilateral (generally on the same side as the lesion). Without adequate therapy, there may be extension of the process from the lymph nodes to the overlying skin, resulting in draining sinuses.

TABLE A.3 Clinical characteristics of chancroid ulcer

Number	Usually multiple but may occur as an isolated lesion
Shape	Irregular
Depth	Deep
Purulence	Present
Tenderness	Present
Induration	None

Superinfection of the ulcer or ulcers, especially by fusospirochetes, may lead to extensive destruction of the external genitalia (phagedenic chancroid).

Diagnosis

Diagnosis is inferred by the demonstration of small gram-negative rods, often with bipolar staining.

The bacteria are often seen in short chains or parallel arrays ("school of fish" or "fingerprint" patterns). They may be cultivated with difficulty. A presumptive diagnosis can be inferred from the identification of short gram-negative rods in strands on smears stained with Gram or Wright stain, and an ulcer characterized by noninduration of the base and painful, ragged, overhanging margins. Specific fluorescent antibody staining of bacteria in smears from suspected lesions provides a means for substantiation of the diagnosis; unfortunately, the availability of this diagnostic procedure is limited. Biopsy of the lesion is useful since it eliminates granuloma inguinale, syphilitic chancre, and herpetic ulcer from diagnostic consideration.

A definitive diagnosis established with isolation of the organism in gonococcal agar supplemented with bovine hemoglobin and fetal calf serum or Mueller-Hinton agar supplemented with chocolatized horse blood is required to maximize recovery on primary isolation.

Therapy

The emergence of *H. ducreyi* that is multiply resistant to antibiotics has limited the effectiveness of many antimicrobials for therapy of chancroid. Trimethoprim–sulfamethoxazole (160/800 mg twice a day for seven days) and erythromycin (500 mg four times a day for seven days) have been the drugs of choice.

Current therapeutic regimens include the following:

- Erythromycin: 500 mg four times a day until the ulcers and/or adenopathy have resolved.
- Ceftriaxone: 250 mg intramuscularly once.
- Trimethoprim–sulfamethoxazole: 800 mg/1600 mg orally twice a day for seven days.
- Ciprofloxacin: 500 mg twice daily for three days.

Erythromycin-resistant strains of *H. ducreyi* have been reported from Singapore. Erythromycin is highly effective in treating chancroid in dosages of 500 mg four times a day for at least seven days. Because this dosage of erythromycin can cause gastrointestinal discomfort, physicians should be alerted to poor patient compliance. Shorter courses may be effective, but such data are lacking.

Ceftriaxone appears to be as effective as erythromycin and has the advantage of being administered as a single intramuscular dose of 250 mg. The drug is extremely active against *H. ducreyi* in vitro and no strains resistant to it, or to cefotaxime, have been reported.

The efficacy of trimethoprim–sulfamethoxazole appears to be less than that of erythromycin or ceftriaxone, particularly in areas where trimethoprim resistance is common. Ciprofloxacin (500 mg twice daily for three days) is highly effective. A bolus dose of 750 to 1000 mg can achieve almost comparable results.

With effective therapy, a clinical response, first subjective and then objective, should be apparent within several days of instituting therapy. A subjective response (diminished tenderness and pain) occurs within 48 hours of institution of antimicrobials. An objective response generally occurs within 72 hours and almost always within seven days. Healing takes 10 to 11 days after institution of therapy. Large ulcers may require relatively longer time periods to heal. Patients should be seen seven days after beginning therapy, when objective signs of ulcer healing will be present in virtually all successfully treated patients, and adenopathy should be less painful and usually smaller. Some nodes may progress to fluctuation despite adequate therapy and require needle aspiration through normal skin to prevent spontaneous drainage.

While ulcers in successfully treated patients respond to therapy quickly, adenopathy may not, and progression to fluctuation is not necessarily a sign of treatment failure.

If by day 7, a clinical response has occurred and therapy has been taken as directed, therapy need not be continued. If a clinical response is not apparent, the clinician should reconsider the clinical diagnosis of chancroid or, if it has been confirmed by a culture, consider a mixed infection, e.g., herpes and chancroid.

Sexual contacts of patients with chancroid should be examined and treated with an effective antimicrobial regimen, whether lesions are present or not. Asymptomatic carriage of *H. ducreyi* appears to be uncommon, but colonization of the vagina, penis, and mouth in the absence of lesions has been described. Initial treatment guidelines recommended that therapy be continued for at least 10 days and until clinical resolution of ulcer(s) and adenopathy. Subsequent studies have shown the high efficacy of one- to seven-day courses of therapy and indicate that antimicrobial courses of 10 days offer no therapeutic advantage over shorter courses, even though ulcers have not completely healed and adenopathy is persistent.

Inguinal adenopathy will occur in 30% of patients with chancroid. Because of the possibility of concomitant syphilitic infection, dark-field analysis of all lesions should be performed. Serologic tests for syphilis should be obtained during therapy. If the antimicrobial agent utilized will not eradicate incubating syphilis, the serological test should be repeated six to eight weeks after its termination.

HERPETIC GENITAL ULCERS (HERPES SIMPLEX VIRUSES)

Initial contact with herpes simplex viruses usually occurs early in childhood and involves herpes simplex virus type-1

(HSV-1). About 10% of primary infections with HSV-1 are clinically overt.

HSV-1 is the causative agent for most nongenital herpetic lesions: herpes labialis, gingivostomatitis, and keratoconjunctivitis. Infection of the female genital tract by HSV-1 may occur at this time; however, the virus can often be simultaneously cultured from nongenital sites, suggesting that genital involvement is most often a secondary phenomenon.

Herpetic vulvovaginitis due to HSV-1 is observed primarily at the time of initial herpetic infection in infancy or early adolescence; subsequently, type 2 becomes increasingly more prevalent. Type 2 antibodies usually appear first about the time of puberty and exhibit a significant increase during the prime reproductive years. The greatest incidence of overt type 2 infection occurs in women in their late teens and early twenties.

HSV-2 is recovered predominantly from the female genital tract. Epidemiologic data strongly support the thesis that dissemination of the type 2 strain is primarily but not exclusively contingent on venereal transmission. The incidence of specific antibody approaches 100% among prostitutes. Following exposure to males with active herpetic lesions of the genitalia, 50% to 90% of susceptible sexual partners develop infection.

HERPETIC VULVOVAGINITIS

Primary Infection

Primary genital infection due to HSV-2 may be asymptomatic or may be associated with severe symptoms. In primary vulvovaginitis, the genital lesions on the vulva, vagina, and cervix occur between two and seven days following exposure to infectious virus. Like those in primary herpes labialis, the lesions are multiple and larger than those observed in recurrent disease or in those who have had prior infection with HSV-1. At this time, patients usually experience vaginal discharge, discomfort, and pain. The mucocutaneous lesions are prone to trauma. The initial vesicles rupture and tend to become secondarily infected. They subsequently appear as shallow, eroded, painful ulcers covered by a shaggy white membrane. Regional lymphadenopathy is readily demonstrated as the consequence of virus replication in the sites of lymphatic drainage as well as nodal stimulation by secondary bacterial infection.

Whereas local symptoms of dysuria, soreness of the vulva and vagina, dyspareunia, and a sudden increase of discharge are common in both primary and recurrent infection, systemic symptoms (malaise, myalgia, and fever) are virtually restricted to primary herpetic infection (Table A.4). These symptoms reflect the viremia engendered during primary infection. Whether a systemic response to infection occurs is dependent upon the presence or absence of heterologous antibodies to HSV-1.

The lesions tend to persist for 7 to 10 days. However, when secondary bacterial, mycotic, or protozoan infection is not treated, the lesions may persist for two to four weeks.

Primary herpetic infection may occur on the cervix. The appearance of extensive cervical involvement may mimic that observed with squamous cell carcinoma of the cervix.

Recurrent Infection

Confinement of the ulcers to one area of the vulva, vagina, or cervix is more common in recurrent forms of the disease. The ulcers tend to be limited in size and number. Cervical involvement may occur as a diffuse cervicitis or as a single large ulcer. Local symptoms predominate over systemic symptoms, with increased vaginal discharge or pain being the usual presenting complaint.

In certain women, it can be demonstrated that once it is involved, the genital tract is the site of intermittent virus replication. Virus shedding, particularly from the cervix, may be demonstrated intermittently for two weeks. The titer of virus is significantly reduced compared to the level of recoverable virus when clinically overt lesions are present.

Random sampling of a female population by cytologic examination of routine cervical smears reveals a 0.3% to 5% incidence of herpes infection, depending upon the patient population studied. The higher figure is derived from patients attending venereal disease clinics. If careful virologic screening is superimposed, an additional 1% to 2% may be identified. The total figure is roughly comparable to the incidence of recovery of HSV-1 from the oropharynx in a random sample study.

Diagnosis

Infection may be documented in several ways. Being DNA viruses, the HSV produce histologic stigmata indicative of

TABLE A.4 Clinical differences between primary and recurrent vulvovaginitis due to herpes simples virus type 2

Signs or symptoms	Primary	Recurrent
Number of lesions	Multiple	Scattered 1 to 3
Location of lesions	Tend to involve both labia and vagina; cervix may be concomitantly involved	Limited involvement of vulva, vagina, or cervix
Size of lesions	Variable; tend to be larger than those observed in recurrent disease	Tend to be smaller
Inguinal adenopathy	Present	Usually absent
Viremia	Occurs	Absent
Systemic symptoms (malaise, myalgia, fever)	Present*	Absent
Local symptoms (dysuria, itching, dyspareunia)	Present	Present
Specific antibody titer	Greater than fourfold rise observed between pre- and postconvalescent sera	Usually no significant change

*Only in the absence of preexisting antibodies to herpes simplex type I.

virus replication. Papanicolaou smears of a given lesion may demonstrate large multinucleated cells containing eosinophilic intranuclear inclusion bodies. Cytological tests have a maximum sensitivity of 60% to 70% when dealing with overt clinical disease. Both the Papanicolaou and Zanck smears are poor screening procedures. The presence of multinucleated giant cells is predominantly a phenomenon of herpetic involvement at free surfaces, as opposed to the single intranuclear inclusion body observed within organ tissues. Biopsy in conjunction with cytologic analysis of a cell preparation from the lesion very often leads to a diagnosis, even in the absence of virus isolation studies.

The recent introduction of enzyme-linked immunoabsorbent assays and DNA probes gives clinicians additional diagnostic tools. Overt lesions that are not in the ulcerated state should be unroofed and the fluid sampled.

Serologic testing is of relatively limited value because of the frequent presence of cross-reacting antibodies to the heterologous virus. Only if the acute-phase serum had a nondetectable or very low titer and the convalescent serum obtained 10 to 14 days after the onset of clinical disease demonstrated a fourfold or greater rise in the complement titer or the presence of immunoglobulin M (IgM)–specific antibodies could one serologically distinguish between primary and recurrent infections. The presence of an antibody titer in the initial specimen obtained at the onset of disease, and the failure of the titer to exhibit a fourfold or greater rise in the convalescent specimen or the presence of IgM-specific antibodies argues strongly for recurrent infection with HSV-2 or prior infection with HSV-1. The distinction between primary and recurrent infection (Table A.4) is of more than just academic interest when a gravida is concerned. Primary infection with either virus, in the absence of cross-protecting antibodies, exposes the fetus to the small risk of transplacental infection.

Management

Currently, most nondrug therapeutic measures are directed toward providing the patient with symptomatic relief from pain and vaginal discomfort. Almost invariably, the ulcers are secondarily infected by either bacterial or mycotic organisms, or both. If one aggressively treats the superinfection, the patient will be markedly improved within 24 hours and relatively symptom free in 72 hours.

The inflammatory process renders the perineum exquisitely tender in primary herpetic vulvovaginitis. Therapy requires the ability to do a pelvic examination. Not infrequently, parenteral analgesia is required. The therapeutic regimen at Creighton University is as follows: The perineum is cleansed with a 4×4 sterile gauze pad or with cotton drumsticks. A wet mount and KOH preparation are obtained and the major lesions are then selected for documenting the herpetic etiology. If the lesions are still in the vesiculopustular stage of the disease, they are unroofed. Scrapings of the base and margins of either the unroofed vesicles or ulcerated lesions are obtained with a wooden spatula and smeared onto a clean slide for cytologic analysis. The diagnosis of herpes is made by the finding of the characteristic giant cells with intranuclear inclusion bodies. Where facilities exist, cultures for herpes simplex virus should be obtained.

At this point, one can introduce a speculum to see if there are intravaginal or cervical lesions. A patient with one sexually transmitted disease should be considered to be at high risk for another sexually transmitted disease. It is imperative that tests be taken at this time for *Neisseria gonorrhoeae* and *Chlamydia trachomatis*, and that serology be done for *Treponema pallidum*, prior to the institution of systemic therapy.

The vaginal canal is dried with sterile drumsticks, and an intravaginal medication (determined by results of the KOH preparation and wet mounts) is instilled. If neither *Trichomonas vaginalis* nor *Candida albicans* is identified, 2% clindamycin intravaginal cream or povidone iodine is applied intravaginally; otherwise, intravaginal medications should be specific for the major superinfecting organism. To avert the problems of local maceration, one should use either Sultran® in a zinc oxide base or simple white petroleum jelly as a lubricant. With this aggressive regimen, the lesions tend to clear in two to five days.

Failure to eradicate secondary mycotic or pyogenic infection results in prolongation of the inflammatory vulvar edema and retardation of healing. The edema associated with the ulcerative stage of the disease is an important contribution to the patient's overall pain and discomfort. Local analgesic ointments are effective not only in eliminating the pain associated with the vesicular-ulcerative stage of infection, but also, if dispensed in an appropriate ointment base, in protecting the skin from further maceration and bacterial overgrowth.

Topical or systemic administration of steroids has no place in the treatment of herpetic vulvovaginitis. Corticosteroids, by their ability to stabilize lysosome membranes and inhibit the production of interferon, exert a deleterious effect in experimental viral and mycotic infections. Although the exact mechanism for the immune elimination of viruses from a host is not yet completely defined, current data confer the central role to interferon. Although effective in combating the associated inflammatory edema, the corticosteroids enhance virus replication.

Antiviral Therapy
Zovir

Zovir (acyclovir) is the prototype antiviral drug for human use in the treatment of acute herpetic infection. Efficacy depends on the way the drug is administered. Topical acyclovir (5% ointment) is effective only in selected clinical situations. Oral acyclovir can be highly effective in aborting recurrent episodes of genital herpes.

Mechanism of action   Acyclovir itself is not active against the herpes virus. It is selectively converted to another form in the body, triphosphate, by herpes virus–infected cells. This conversion does not occur to any significant degree in normal cells. Acyclovir triphosphate interferes with herpes simplex viral enzymes and in so doing inhibits viral replication.

Topical Acyclovir

Topical acyclovir is currently available only as a 5% ointment and is supplied in 15 g tubes. It is recommended that a sufficient quantity should be applied to adequately cover all lesions every three hours, six times per day, for seven days. A finger cot or rubber glove should be worn when applying the drug to prevent autoinoculation of other body sites and transmission of infection to other persons.

Timing of therapy To be effective, drug application should be initiated as early as possible following the onset of signs and symptoms.

Impact of infectivity Acyclovir will diminish the amount of virus present and its duration of shedding; hence, theoretically, it should alter infectivity.

Valtrex

Valtrex (valacyclovir) is the L-valyl ester of acyclovir. The formulation allows for greater drug absorption. Once absorbed, valacyclovir is almost completely converted to acyclovir after oral administration. The higher oral bioavailability of valacyclovir results in greater or comparable drug concentration, which can be achieved by taking the medicine less frequently. To date, the clinical results and safety profile achieved with valacyclovir and acyclovir in acute outbreaks are comparable. The recommended dosage is 500 mg twice a day for five days.

Famvir

Famvir (famciclovir), an oral prodrug of the antiviral agent penciclovir, has been recently introduced. Like valacyclovir, famciclovir is selectively absorbed and rapidly converted into its active ingredient. It has a long intracellular half-life. The recommended dosage is 125 mg bid for five days. Initial therapy should be within the first three to five hours from the onset of signs or symptoms. Neither valacyclovir nor famciclovir have been adequately studied as to their ability to suppress recurrent episodes.

The therapeutic efficacy of topical acyclovir and oral acyclovir in the treatment of active infections has been disappointing. The recommended regimen for the first episode of disease in an immunocompetent host is acyclovir 200 mg PO five times per day for 10 days. The drug is a purine analog and is a substrate for the viral enzyme thymidine kinase; this converts the compound to acyclovir triphosphate, which then inhibits viral DNA synthesis. Acyclovir reduces the virus titer present and shortens the duration of disease against placebo but is not superior to aggressive local therapy. To have efficacy, the drug must be administered at the time of prodromal symptomatology, i.e., cutaneus tingling, etc. There is a subgroup of patients with frequent recurrent disease who appear to benefit from prophylactic longer-term use of the medication. Because the long-term risks are not fully assessed, prophylactic therapy with the drug should be limited to less than six months. The current treatment schedule for suppression of recurrent genital herpetic infection is acyclovir 200 to 400 mg PO two times daily for up to six months. This regimen is advocated for women with more than six symptomatic recurrences per year.

C. TRACHOMATIS LYMPHOGRANULOMA VENEREUM (L) STRAINS

Although its distribution is worldwide, lymphogranuloma venereum is more common in tropical and semitropical climates. The mode of transmission is believed to be through coitus or intimate physical contact. A number of small endemic foci have been traced to a specific prostitute. The disease may also be disseminated by close nonsexual contact as well as by autoinoculation. Disease has occurred in laboratory workers. Although a grippe-like syndrome characterized by fever, malaise, headache, and anorexia may occur, it is rarely the chief presenting complaint in patients with lymphogranuloma venereum. Fever is present in over 50% of the cases and tends to correlate primarily with the severity of illness. When lymphogranuloma venereum involves the vulva, it is as part of its inguinal syndrome.

Genital Lesions

The initial genital lesion that develops varies from a slight erosion to a small cutaneous herpetiform lesion. It may either disappear or develop into an ulcer. The lesion is painless and only slightly tender to palpation. It exhibits ill-defined shallow margins and a fibrogranular base. The fourchette, urethral meatus, and medial surface of the labia are the usual sites of primary lesions. Clinical recognition of infection at this stage is the exception, not the rule. When multiple lesions are present, the adjacent labia or clitoris are often edematous. In the absence of secondary infection, most of the lesions will have healed prior to the onset of lymph node enlargement.

More than 50% of infected patients manifest no clinical symptoms. Although most male patients develop inguinal adenopathy during the course of disease, this manifestation is relatively unusual in females. The adenopathy may vary from shoddy nodes to fluctuant masses often associated with draining sinuses. Lymph node involvement is indicative of lymphatic drainage from the primary lesions, and consequently, unilateral adenopathy is not uncommon. The regional glands draining the primary site of infection, particularly in the male, enlarge dramatically and may appear as a series of buboes. Sixty percent of the buboes rupture, discharging a copious watery-to-purulent granular exudate.

The early histologic appearance of lymph nodes is that of diffuse reticular and lymphocytic hyperplasia. In the more advanced lesion, macrophages appear in significant numbers prior to the development of central necrosis. The macrophages assume a palisade-like arrangement around the central focus of necrotic cellular debris. Plasmacytosis is one of the important supplementary criteria in the histologic diagnosis of lymphogranuloma venereum. Healing is associated with fibroblastic proliferation and (ultimately) with the replacement of the diseased foci by fibrous connective tissue. Extensive cutaneous scarring may suggest the diagnosis in a patient seen for the first time late in the course of the disease.

If urethral involvement occurs, it exhibits the same sequential pattern—first ulceration and then destructive lesions with healing by fibrosis. Patients with partial urethral destruction may remain continent as long as the distal portion of the urethra is intact. Partial obstruction may cause difficulty in voiding. The resultant symptoms are those of urethral obstruction. Complete urethral destruction represents a difficult therapeutic challenge, necessitating surgical reconstruction.

Diagnosis

The disease is difficult to diagnose since the female patient is more likely to present with the genitorectal than with the inguinal syndrome or with inguinal adenopathy in a subclinical form. With primary infection, she may complain of a small boil on the vagina or a slight discharge or irritation. Most often, the small shallow red ulcers with flat margins due to lymphogranuloma venereum escape clinical detection. The second stage of disease, in which adenitis predominates, may pass unnoticed until a late phase in which fibrosis or tissue destruction has developed. The patient may complain of discomfort. Lymphogranuloma venereum must be considered in the differential diagnosis of any fistulous tract involving the perineum or inguinal adenopathy (Table A.5).

Laboratory results, with the exception of complement fixation or microimmunofluorescent tests for lymphogranuloma venereum, are inconclusive. Abnormalities in the white blood cell count include mild-to-marked leukocytosis with a relative lymphocytosis. Biologically false-positive serologic tests for syphilis not infrequently occur. In longstanding disease, the albumin–globulin ratio is inverted.

Serologic confirmation of prior and/or concurrent antigenic experience with *Chlamydia* organisms coupled with a characteristic disease clustering makes for the diagnosis of lymphogranuloma venereum. Aspiration of fluctuant nodes can be implemented as a therapeutic adjunct in adenitis. Aspiration of suppurative nodes in lieu of spontaneous rupture has been advocated and appears to be free of significant complications. Aspiration is best achieved with a number 20 gauge needle. Insert the needle through adjacent noninvolved skin rather than aspirating the lesion directly through skin overlying the node. A patient with significant disease must be monitored for possible development of vulvar carcinoma. Biopsy of any suspicious lesion is mandatory.

T. PALLIDUM (SYPHILIS)

A vulvoulcerative disease due to *T. pallidum* is the consequence of primary syphilis. The time required for development of the primary lesion is partly a function of the number of organisms establishing the initial infection and their subsequent replication at the portal of entry. Infections with a large inoculum (e.g., 10^7 organisms) may cause a chancre in five to seven days. The inoculation of 50 to 100 organisms is followed by an incubation period of about three weeks. The longest incubation period appears to be approximately five weeks.

The primary lesion consists of a small papule that breaks down to form a superficial, painless ulcer with a clean granular base and firm scrolled margins. Classical chancres are solitary lesions. However, multiple chancres have been identified in up to 40% of individuals with primary syphilis. Histologic analysis reveals, in the absence of secondary infection, an extensive plasma cell and lymphocytic infiltration. Characteristic of the lesion is the effect of *T. pallidum* on the small blood vessels. Extensive endothelial proliferation in association with a significant plasma cell infiltrate should suggest a diagnosis of primary syphilis on histologic grounds alone.

When dissemination from the portal of infection to the regional lymph nodes occurs during the primary phase of the disease, the result is "satellite" buboes (Table A.5). Regional adenopathy normally accompanies the chancre of primary syphilis. The adenopathy usually develops a week after the appearance of the initial lesions. Untreated, a chancre will persist for two to eight weeks and then spontaneously disappear.

Physical examination reveals enlarged, firm but tender lymph nodes, reflecting both organismal replication and reticular and lymphocytic cellular proliferation.

Irrespective of the subsequent clinical course, the chancre heals spontaneously. In approximately 30% of cases, disease is limited to replication at the portal of entry, and even without therapy, eradication of the infection may occur in

---

TABLE A.5 Differential diagnosis of inguinal adenopathy associated with a presumed venereal disease

Disease	Genital lesion	Nodal involvement	Cutaneous lesions
Granuloma inguinale	Extensive in males; less evident in females	Involvement of lymph nodes; draining cutaneous sinuses; late in the course of the disease, nodes become tender	Primary skin infection with superficial ulceration
Lymphogranuloma venereum	Occurs but is extremely transient in nature	Bilateral node involvement is determined by site of primary lesion	Multiple sinus tracts draining a thick, creamy exudate
Chancroid	Usually present	Primarily unilateral with limited involvement of lymph nodes	Acute, with crater-like slough
Genital tuberculosis	None	Bilateral inguinal adenopathy	Pleomorphic, often with sinus tract draining, scanty but thick exudate
Syphilis	Usually present	Bilateral; firm, rubbery nodes	Protean in its clinical manifestations

conjunction with the disappearance of serologic evidence of syphilitic infection as measured by nontreponemal tests.

From regional lymph node drainage of the portal of infection, hematogenous dissemination characteristic of the secondary phase of the disease occurs.

Diagnosis

Confirmation of a syphilitic chancre depends on the demonstration of *T. pallidum* on dark-field microscopic examination. The lesion should be cleansed and abraded with gauze to induce superficial bleeding, and the blood blotted away. Once the serum begins to ooze, a small aliquot is placed on a glass slide and a cover slide applied. Dark-field analysis should be completed before the slide dries. If a serum specimen must be transported a short distance, it should be collected in a relatively large-bore capillary tube. One end of the tube should be sealed with clay.

An alternate means of diagnosis confirmation entails the use of biopsy taken from the rim of the lesion. Spirochetes are not detectable by conventional staining techniques. Demonstration of the organism requires utilization of the ability of silver salts to delineate the organisms' contours.

By the time the primary lesion is detected, both humoral and cell-mediated immune mechanisms have been activated.

The serologic tests for the detection of *T. pallidum* can be broken down into two broad categories: nontreponemal (flocculation and complement-fixation tests) and treponemal (*T. pallidum* immobilization, *T. pallidum* microhemagglutination, and fluorescent treponemal antibody tests). The former are serologic assays for antibodies that react with cardiolipin, a nonspecific antigen; the latter, by using *T. pallidum* or an avirulent strain of *T. pallidum*—known as the Reiter treponeme—as the test antigen, detect specific antibodies.

Therapy

The therapeutic recommendations of the Centers for Disease Control and Prevention are listed in Table A.6.

GENITAL APHTHOUS ULCERS OF BEHCET'S DISEASE AND VULVAR CROHN'S DISEASE

Natural History

Deep, extremely painful recurrent genital ulcers of uncertain etiology are generally termed aphthous ulcers. Genital aphthous ulcers are the most frequently encountered cause for recurrent painful nonherpetic vulvar ulceration. Similar ulcers may occasionally concomitantly develop in the oral cavity. Aphthous ulcers may appear in two forms: aphthous major (over 10 mm in diameter) and aphthous minor (3–8 mm in diameter).

Genital aphthous ulcers can be a metastatic expression of underlying disease due to either Crohn's disease or Behcet's disease. Genital aphthous ulcer disorders due to these two entities are most prevalent in Asia, the Middle East, and the Mediterranean. Turkey reports the highest rate: over 300 cases per 100,000. Prevalence among women in the United States is unknown, and is possibly in the range of 5 to 10 cases per 100,000.

Crohn's disease is a chronic granulomatous disease of the gastrointestinal tract due possibly to *Mycobacterium avium* subspecies paratuberculosis. Fecal contamination and a resultant immediate type of hypersensitivity reaction is postulated to account for its association with recurrent painful vulvar ulcers.

Behcet's disease is a disease entity of unknown etiology that affects the eyes, bowel, and vascular and muscular organ systems. The uvitis associated with Behcet's disease is the leading cause of blindness in the areas of the world where this order is prevalent.

TABLE A.6 Preliminary 1997 therapeutic recommendations of the Centers for Disease Control

PRIMARY AND SECONDARY SYPHILIS

Recommended regimen for non-pregnant women

Non-allergic patients with primary or secondary syphilis should be treated with the following regimen*:

- Benzathine penicillin G, 2.4 million units IM in a single dose

Penicillin allergy

Non-pregnant penicillin-allergic women who have primary or secondary syphilis should be treated with the following regimen:

- Doxycycline 100 mg orally 2 times a day for 2 weeks or
- Tetracycline 500 mg orally 4 times a day for 2 weeks

RECOMMENDED REGIMEN FOR PREGNANT WOMEN

Treatment during pregnancy should be the penicillin regimen appropriate for the woman's stage of syphilis.[a]

Penicillin allergy

- There are no proven alternatives to penicillin. A pregnant woman with a history of penicillin allergy or positive skin test should be treated with penicillin after desensitization.
- Tetracycline and doxycycline are both FDA Pregnancy Category D and usually not used during pregnancy. Erythromycin (FDA Category B) should not be used, because it does not reliably cure an infected fetus.

---

[a]Parenteral penicillin G is effective in achieving local cure (healing of lesions and prevention of sexual transmission) and in preventing late sequelae. However, no adequately conducted comparative trials have been performed to guide the selection of an optimal penicillin regimen (i.e., dose, duration, and preparation). Penicillin regimens should be used to treat all stages of syphilis among HIV-infected patients. Some experts recommend additional therapy in some settings. A second dose of benzathine penicillin 2.4 million units IM may be given 1 week after the initial dose for women with primary, secondary, or early latent syphilis. Ultrasongraphic signs of fetal syphilis (i.e., hepatomegaly and hydrops) indicate a higher risk for fetal treatment failure.

Diagnosis

Women with recurrent painful genital ulcers must be evaluated for sexually transmitted diseases (STD) such as herpes. If the STD work-up is negative, biopsy of the lesion's margin is advocated; however, no diagnostic tests exist for these two entities. The diagnosis is inferred by recurrence of characteristic ulcers, country of origin, and/or nonvulvar evidence of findings indicative of either Crohn's or Behcet's disease. An ophthalmological evaluation is advocated for all women with recurrent painful genital aphthous ulcers to check for early uvitis. If the ophthalmologic examination is negative and there is no history of gastrointestinal dysfunction, one may presume that the patent has isolated aphthous vulvar ulcer disease.

Therapy

If the diagnosis of Behcet's or Crohn's disease is established, therapy is that required to achieve systemic amelioration. Local ulcer therapy is directed at lessening any superinfection and pain symptomology.

SELECTED READING

Foster D. Vulvar disease. Obstet Gynecol 2002; 100:145.
McBride DR. Management of aphthous ulcers. Am Fam Physician 2000; 62:149.
Mertz KJ, Trees D, Levine WC, et al. Etiology of genital ulcers and prevalence of human immunodeficiency virus coinfection in 10 US cities. J Infect Dis 1998; 178:1795.
Sakane T, Takeno M, Suzuki N, Inaba G. Current concepts: Behcet's disease. N Eng J Med 1999; 341:1284.
Scully C. Aphthous ulcerations. N Eng J Med 2006; 355:165.

Understanding Abdominal Pain of Gastrointestinal Etiology

III

INTRODUCTION

As obstetricians and gynecologists move into the area of primary care, they need to understand the significance of abdominal pain beyond that associated with acute salpingitis, pyelonephritis, ectopic pregnancy, and torsion of adrenal masses. This segment deals with the principal pain patterns encountered in the common care of women, and in doing so, assists physicians in identifying when abdominal pain is of infectious etiology.

William Olser once said, "let me take the history and let anyone do the physical examination and I will give you the correct diagnosis in 80% of the cases." One of the problems with our technology is our growing dependence on it. Too often, we abort a detailed history because of the ability of X rays or fiberoptic technology to establish a probable or definitive diagnosis. Although a good history can only imply what the probable etiology is, it will tell you exactly where that technology needs to be applied. The principal laboratory modalities that are valuable in the analysis of acute abdomen are white blood cell count, its differential count, and an erythrocyte sedimentation rate. A problem associated in dealing with the gastrointestinal tract is the difficulty in differentiating between the pain associated with organic disease and that caused by functional disturbances.

The perception or description of a pain's character arising from the same lesion in the gastrointestinal tract will vary depending upon the type of person involved (e.g., two patients with comparable duodenal ulcers may complain of agonizing pain or of a slight gnawing sensation). Differences in intensity at different points in time may similarly alter the perception of the character of pain. The threshold for pain varies at different times in the same person. One day, a patient may complain of burning epigastric pain, whereas on another day, the sensation arising from the same source may be described as a vague discomfort. Although there is potential variation in the character of sensation, localization of pain caused by a disturbance in a given part of the gastrointestinal tract tends to be referred to a specific site on the abdomen (indirect visceral pain/somatic referral).

This type of pain is distinct from direct splenic visceral pain. Somatic pain is usually a deep, heavy pain felt in the region of the diseased organ. With somatic pain, the area of cutaneous referral is often accompanied by cutaneous hypersensitivity within the same segment of distribution.

The principal tools in diagnosing acute abdominal pain emanating from one of the five cardinal organ systems: gastrointestinal tract, urinary tract, female genital tract, biliary tract, and blood vessels are

(a) character of pain,
(b) pain localization,
(c) pain radiation, and
(d) factors that ameliorate or exacerbate the pain.

This segment focuses on the first two aspects of abdominal pain.

CHARACTER OF PAIN

The character of the pain can assist the physician in focusing on the probable diagnosis. Crampy or gripping, intermittent pain (colic) is indicative of a smooth muscle site of disease.

PAIN LOCALIZATION

Potential Diagnostic Significance of Localized Abdominal Pain

The initial localization of pain begins using the simple four-quadrant localization. A superior system places pain in the context of right and left hypogastric and periumbilical and right and left iliac areas and then focuses on midline (central) pain.

Pain Emanating from the Gastrointestinal Tract (Figs. A.1 to A.7)

Pain involving the substernal region, the upper portions of the sternum, tends to be primarily of esophageal etiology. Lesions involving the upper one-third of the esophagus are usually referred to the episternal notch and the first portion of the manubrium. On rare occasions, this pain sometimes is referred to the back of the throat.

Esophageal pain is always in the midline under the sternum. Lesions in the midesophageal area are referred to the middle portion of the sternum corresponding to C3–C4 distribution. Disease in the inferior portion, the cardiac portion of the esophagus, will be referred to the infrasternal notch.

Stomach

Prior abdominal diseases, particularly those that result in operative procedures, may modify pain in such a way that it is no longer referred to the usual site. Pain from these two sites are referred to the epigastrium. With involvement of cardiac portions of the stomach, pain is referred to the epigastrium near the xyphoid while that from the pyloric end of the stomach is felt lower in the epigastrium. Pain may be referred through to the back or to the left side in the T6–T7 distribution.

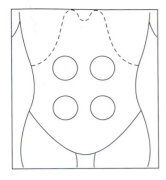

FIGURE A.1 Infectious diseases eliciting abdominal pain involving one or more quadrants. Four-quadrant pain. Potential etiologies: (1) ruptured TOA into the peritoneum; (2) perforated viscus, especially peptic ulcer; (3) peritonitis due to other causes. *Abbreviation*: TOA, tubo-ovarian abscess.

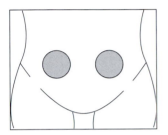

FIGURE A.2 Bilateral lower-quadrant pain. Potential etiologies: (1) acute appendicitis; (2) acute salpingitis; (3) ruptured TOA; (4) infected ruptured ectopic pregnancy. *Abbreviation*: TOA, tubo-ovarian abscess.

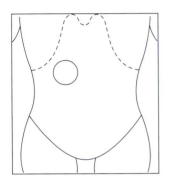

FIGURE A.3 Tenderness and rigidity in the right hypogastrium. Potential etiologies: (1) leaking duodenal ulcer; (2) acute cholecystitis; (3) appendicitis (high appendix); (4) right basilar segment pleurisy.

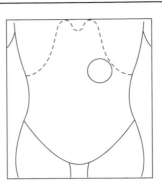

FIGURE A.4 Tenderness and rigidity in the left hypogastrium. Potential etiologies: (1) perforated gastric ulcer (subphrenic abscess); (2) jejunal diverticulitis.

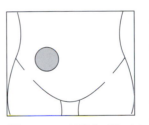

FIGURE A.5 Tenderness and rigidity in the periumbilical area. Potential etiologies: (1) earliest stage of acute appendicitis; (2) small bowel obstruction; (3) acute pancreatitis; (4) acute gastritis; (5) coronary occlusion.

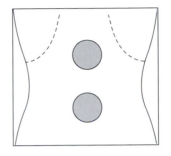

FIGURE A.6 Tenderness and rigidity in the right iliac region. Potential etiologies: (1) below the epigastrium is obstruction of the transverse colon; (2) appendicitis, late stage; (3) ileocecal colitis; (4) Meckel's diverticulum; (5) acute cholecystis (low gallbladder); (6) biliary peritonitis; (7) ruptured TOA; (8) right annexal torsion. *Abbreviation*: TOA, tubo-ovarian abscess.

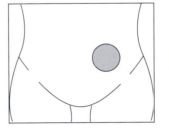

FIGURE A.7 Tenderness and rigidity in the left iliac region. Potential etiologies: (1) diverticulitis; (2) ruptured TOA; (3) left annexal torsion; (4) obstruction of transverse colon. *Abbreviation*: TOA, tubo-ovarian abscess.

Duodenum

Duodenal pain is referred to the midline and mid-epigastrium. When referred to the back, localization tends to be under the scapula or the right of the midclavicular line at the level of the seventh rib. Lesions in the second portion of the duodenum may result in pain referred straight through to the back or around the right costal margin to the back at the same level as the pain is noted anteriorly.

Jejunal Ileum

Pain from the jejunal/ileum tends to locate near the midline in the region of the umbilicus. Referred pain from the large bowel is primarily below the umbilicus, halfway between the umbilicus and the pubic symphysis.

Cecum

Disease located in the cecum, just below the ileocecal valve, will produce pain at McBurney's point. Disease involving the hepatic or splenic flexure results in a more lateral displacement to the midclavicular line. Fixation of the flexures is thought to be responsible for this modification of referred pain.

Colon

When disease is located in the descending colon, the pain tends to occur more on the left side between the umbilicus and toward the left lower quadrant. There is a closer correlation between somatic pain and its splenic cutaneous referral. When disease involves the rectosigmoid or rectum, the pain is again in the midline just above the pubis. Disease of the terminal ileum and ascending colon may radiate from the periumbilical area laterally; however, maximum symptomatology will be midline.

Significance of Posterior Radiation of Abdominal Pain

Back pain is not common with diseases of the gastrointestinal tract and female genital tract.

However, when it does occur, it may have marked significance (Table A.1 and Fig. A.8).

TABLE A.1   Importance of referral back pain

Posterior back pain in the region of the tenth dorsal vertebra is seen with duodenal peptic ulcer disease and posterior penetration
Gallbladder occlusive disease
Cancer of the rectum
Disease of the hepatic flexture
Disease of the body and tail of the pancreas

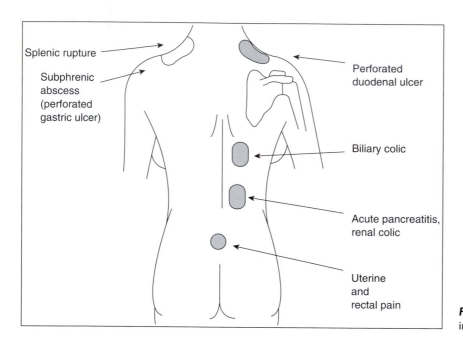

Splenic rupture

Subphrenic abscess (perforated gastric ulcer)

Perforated duodenal ulcer

Biliary colic

Acute pancreatitis, renal colic

Uterine and rectal pain

FIGURE A.8   Patterns of referred-back pain in acute abdominal situations.

Antibiotics: Parenteral and Oral   IV

Mark Martens

ORAL ANTIBIOTICS

Antibiotics have proven to be essential in the battle to prevent and treat postoperative infections. This is especially crucial for the obstetrician and gynecologist. The most frequently performed major surgical procedures in the United States are cesarean section and hysterectomy. Because these surgeries are generally classified as clean-contaminated procedures, they not infrequently result in postoperative infections. Obstetricians and gynecologists have therefore become quite familiar with many of the intravenous antibiotics utilized in the treatment of these infections. However, with the recent emphasis on primary care, the obstetrician–gynecologist has needed to become well versed in a variety of ambulatory infections such as sinusitis, bronchitis, skin and soft tissue infections, etc., and the oral antibiotics that are often utilized to treat them.

The number of new antibiotics and new classes of antimicrobials has rapidly proliferated in the past decade (Tables A.1 and A.2).

Principles of Oral Antibiotic Therapy

1. *The most site-specific agent should be utilized*: Women, more so than men, may have several additional adverse effects from the disruption of the normal balance of bacteria in their bodies. Although both men and women may demonstrate unwanted effects of antibiotics on intestinal flora, such as diarrhea and pseudomembranous colitis, only women will have a disturbance of vaginal flora, which may result in vaginitis or disruption of their gut flora, which, in turn, may alter their absorption of contraceptive or postmenopausal hormones. Therefore, site specificity, whether as a result of the pharmacokinetic properties of the antibiotic or the local application of topical agents, should be considered before the prescription of any antimicrobial agent to a female patient.

2. *The most narrow-spectrum agent is preferred if effective for the diagnosed infection*: Using an agent with the most narrow spectrum is different from, but just as important as, site specificity in antibiotic selection. Using broad-spectrum agents has a very important place in the treatment of infections that are polymicrobial in nature or are as yet undiagnosed and thus empirical. However, broad-spectrum agents should not be utilized if more narrow-spectrum agents are available and have been demonstrated to be effective against a specific pathogen. Unnecessary use of broad-spectrum agents may lead to selection pressures for resistant species or strains of pathogens. Examples include the overuse of beta-lactam agents for urinary tract infections, which has resulted in greater than 50% resistance of *E. coli* to inexpensive penicillin agents. This is despite the availability of more narrow-spectrum agents specific for the most common etiologic agent *E. coli*. Also, the overuse of fluoroquinolone agents in the Far East for the treatment of *N. gonorrhoeae* has led to a more rapid distribution of resistance to fluoroquinolones in those areas of the world.

3. *Oral antimicrobial agents should demonstrate in vitro activity versus the offending agent and should have been demonstrated to be effective in the treatment of the specific infectious disorder*: Newly released agents should not be utilized just because they are newer agents within a specific class. Newer is not necessarily better. Examples include the decreasing gram-positive antimicrobial activity with the higher generations of cephalosporins, and some of the newer fluoroquinolones with respect to *C. trachomatis*. Antibiotic selection should be predicated upon superior coverage for the implied or determined pathogen or pathogenic spectrum.

4. *The benefit of any specific agent should outweigh the risks of its use*: Again, this recommendation is of greater importance in the treatment of infections in pregnant women. It must be safe not only for the women, but also for the fetus.

ANTIBIOTIC ANALYSIS

As new antibiotics are introduced, evaluation of whether or not a drug can penetrate an individual's clinical armamentarium can benefit from the following analysis:

1. *Specific-use designations*: Is the antibiotic proposed as a "drug-of-choice" for a given monoetiological disease or is it a drug with a singular or multicategory coverage?

2. *Safety profile*: Is it a safe drug for your patient?

TABLE A.1   Parenteral antibiotics commonly used in obstetrics and gynecology

Antibiotic	Dosage range[a]	Route of administration	Dosing interval
Category I Antibiotics			
First generation penicillins			
Beta lactamase-sensitive			
Crystalline G	1–4 Mu	IV	q4–6 h
Benzathine syphilis:	2.4 Mu/d × 1–3 doses	0.6–1.2 Mu IM	q12 h
Procaine			
Beta lactamase-resistant			
Methicillin	1–2 g	IV or IM	q4–6 h
Nafcillin NA	500 mg–2 g	IV or IM	q6 h
Oxacillin	1–2 g	IV or IM	q4–6 h
Second generation penicillins			
Ampicillin	1–2 g	IV	q4–6 h
Third generation penicillins			
Ticarcillin	3 g	IV	q4–6 h
Fourth generation penicillins			
Mezlocillin	3 g	IV	q4–6 h
Piperacillin	3–4 g	IV	q4–6 h
Fifth generation penicillins/carbapenems			
Ampicillin and Sulbactam	1–2 g	IV or IM	q6 h
Ertapenem	1 g	IV	qd
Imipenem and Cilastatin	500 mg	IV	q6 h
Meropenem	1 g	IV	q8–12 h
Piperacillin and Tazobactam	3.375–4.5 g	IV	6–8 h
Ticarcillin and Clavulanic acid	3.1 g	IV	q6 h
Cephalosporins			
First generation cephalosporins			
Cefazolin	1 g	IV or IM	q8 h
Cephalothin	500 mg– 2 g	IV	q8 h
Cephapirin	0.5–2 g	IV	q4–6 h
Second generation cephalosporins			
Cefamandole	0.5–2 g	IM or IV	q4–8 h
Cefmetazole	2 g	IV	q6–12 h
Cefonicid	0.5–2 g	IV or IM	q24 h
Cefotetan	2 g	IV or IM	q12 h
Cefoxitin	2 g	IV or IM	q6–8 h
Cefuroxime	75–1.5 g	IV or IM	q8 h
Third generation cephalosporins			
Cefoperozone	1–2 g	IV or IM	q6–12 h
Cefotaxime	1–2 g	IV or IM	q6–8 h
Ceftizoxime	1–3 g	IV or IM	q6–8 h
Ceftriaxone	0.5–1 g	IV or IM	q24 h
■ gonorrhea: bolus 250 mg IM			
Fourth generation cephalosporins			
Ceftazidine	1–2 g	IV or IM	q8–12 h
Vancomycin	15 mg/kg	IV	q12 h
Category II Antibiotics			
Clindamycin PO₄	300–900 mg	IV	q6–8 h
Metronidazole	0.5 g	IV	q6 h
Ampicillin and Sulbactam	3 g	IV or IM	q6 h
Ticarcillin and Clavulanic acid	3.1 g	4–6 h	IV
Imipenem/Cilastatin	500 mg	IV	q6 h
Category III Antibiotics			
Trimethoprim–Sulfamethoxazole	3–5 mg/kg	IV	6–12 h
All penicillins are effective as Category III antibiotics (especially if therapy is coupled with the use of an aminoglycoside)			
Category IV Antibiotics			
Aminoglycosides			
Gentamicin	1.7 mg/kg	IV or IM	q8 h
Netilmicin	2 mg/kg	IV or IM	q8 h
Fluoroquinolones			
Ciprofloxacin	400 mg	IV	q12 h
Trovofloxacin	300 mg IV followed by 200 mg	oral	

[a]For moderately severe infection.

TABLE A.2 Orally and intramuscularly administered antibiotics commonly used in obstetrics and gynecology

Antibiotic	Formulations	Daily dosage	Dosing
Ampicillin	250 mg, 500 mg caps	1–2 g/day	q6 h
Amoxicillin	250, 500 mg caps	0.75–2 g/day	q6–8 h
Amoxicillin and Clavulanate	250/125 mg tab; 500/125 mg tab;	0.75–1.5 g day 1	q8 h
Azithromycin ■ chlamydia: 1 g bolus ■ gonorrhea: 2 g bolus	250 mg tab; 500 mg day 1 then 250 mg qd		
Carbenicillin	382 mg tab;	382–764 mg	q6 h
Cefaclor	250–500 mg cap		q8 h
Cefadroxil	500 mg or 1 g tab		q12 h
Cefuroxime	125 mg, 250 mg	500 mg cap	q12 h
Cephalexin	250 mg, 500 mg caps;	250 mg q6 h or 500 mg q12 h	
Cefixime	200, 400 mg tab;	200 mg q12 h or	400 mg q24 h
Clarithromycin	250, 500 mg tab;	500–1000 mg/day	q12 h
Clindamycin	150, 300 mg cap;	0.6–1.2 g/day	q6 h
Ciprofloxacin	100 mg, 250 mg;	500 mg, 75 mg tabs	0.2–1.5 g/day
Dicloxacillin	125, 250, 500 mg tab	125–250 mg q6 h	q6 h
Doxycycline	50,100 mg tab or cap	200 mg/day	q12 h
Erythromycin	250 mg	333mg 500 mg tab	q6 h
Ofloxacin	200, 300,4 00 mg	400–800 mg/day	q12 h
Penicillin V	250, 500 mg		q6–8 h
Trovofloxacin	100, 200 mg	200 mg/day	q24 h

3. *Cost*: In evaluating cost, cost of acquisition should not be confused with cost of utilization. The latter includes the costs of
   a. acquisition,
   b. administration,
   c. adverse reactions,
   d. failure, and
   e. toxicity monitoring,

For example, gentamicin is an inexpensive antibiotic to purchase; however, it is an expensive antibiotic to use when the cost of monitoring drug serum concentrations is included.

ORAL ANTIFUNGAL DRUGS

The principal uses of the azoles have been in the treatment of cutaneous, vaginal, and oral mycotic infections. The azoles are active against the major endemic mycoses (histoplasmosis, blastomycosis, and coccidioidomycosis) as well as most yeast and many filamentous fungi. Only itraconazole possesses in vitro activity against *Aspergillus* species.

Pharmacokinetics
Fluconazole
Owing to its water solubility, fluconazole is readily absorbed from the stomach and does not require gastric acidity for absorption (Table A.3). The drug is minimally bound and consequently achieves excellent penetration into cerebrospinal fluid (CSF) and other sites often inaccessible to drugs. Fluconazole is excreted unchanged primarily by the kidneys. The dosage must be reduced in patients with compromised renal function. For many forms of Cryptococcus and candidiasis, fluconazole is the drug of choice.

Itraconazole and Ketoconazole
Pharmacokinetically, itraconazole and ketoconazole are similar. Both are poorly soluble in water, require low gastric pH for absorption, are highly protein bound, and do not penetrate in CSF and intraocular fluids well. Itraconazole exhibits a saturation phenomenon. Doses above 200 mg do not increase appreciably its serum level.

Adverse Drug Reactions
All of the azoles have the potential to cause or exacerbate hepatitis. The risk is most significant for ketoconazole (estimate at 1:15,000 courses of therapy). Serum liver function test should be done on patients receiving azole therapy for greater than one week. Because of its superior efficacy and diminished toxicity, itraconazole has become the drug of choice in treating endemic mycosis. Some of the most serious problems encountered with the azoles are their potential drug interactions (Table A.4). Both ketoconazole and itraconazole interact with the antihistamines terfenadine (Seldane®), astemizole (Hismanal®), cisapride (Propulsid®), and probably digoxin. Increased levels of these drugs may lead to ventricular arrhythmia. Phenytoin toxicity and bleeding secondary to increased warfarin levels may occur with fluconazole therapy. Cyclosporine toxicity has occurred with all three azoles. Concomitant administration of rifampin or isoniazid may lower serum azole concentration and induce a therapeutic failure.

TABLE A .3 Pharmacological comparison of azoles commonly used in ambulatory settings

Pharmacological properties	Fluconazole	Itraconazole	Ketoconazole
Absorption	Excellent; not affected by anti-acids	Requires acid pH decreased by antacids, H_2 blockers etc.	Requires acid pH decreased by antacids, H_2 blockers etc.
Distribution	Excellent in CSF, eye and other sites	Minimal in CSF, eye and other and other sites	Minimal in CSF, eye and other sites
Dosing frequency	Once daily	Once daily	Once daily
Excretion in urine	>80%	Little	Little
Formulation	100,150 mg	100 mg	200 mg
Metabolism	>80 % renal excretion	Almost completely hepatic metabolism	Almost completely hepatic metabolism

THIRD-WORLD USE OF ANTIBIOTICS WITHIN THE CONCEPT OF THE GAINESVILLE CLASSIFICATION

In many underprivileged countries, therapy is limited to oral administration. The following is an integration of orally administered antibiotics into the Gainesville Classification.

TABLE A.4 Dosing of fluconazole for candidiasis

Disease	Dosing regimen
Vulvovaginal candidiasis	150 mg – one dose
Oropharyngeal candidiasis in HIV positive individuals	100 mg daily for 7–14 days
Candidal esophagitis	200 mg daily for 7–14 days
Candidal urinary tract infections	200 mg daily for 14 days

Triple Therapy Equivalence

It is possible to approach the four-category coverage required for the anaerobic progression of the Gainesville Classification with oral antibiotics. Total coverage of the anaerobic progression would require

1. penicillin, amoxicillin, or ampicillin for Categories I and III;
2. metronidazole or thiamphenicol[1] for Category II; and
3. a fluoroquinolone for Category IV.

An alternate approach would be trimethoprim/sulfamethoxazole plus metronidazole. This combination would be less optimal. In the penicillin-hypersensitive individual, erythromycin would be substituted for penicillin. The use of trimethoprim/sulfamethoxazole and a fluoroquinolone is restricted to the nongravid individual. For a gravida, the closest approximation to a triple therapy would be amoxicillin/clavulanate (Augmentin®) plus metronidazole and a fluoroquinolone.

---

[1]Contradicted in pregnancy.

Molecular Diagnostic Tests for Sexually Transmitted Infections in Women

V

Craig S. Hill

INTRODUCTION

Over the past decade, molecular diagnostic technology has revolutionized the laboratory detection of pathogens associated with sexually transmitted infections (STIs). Nucleic acid amplification tests (NAATs) are now routinely performed in many clinical diagnostic laboratories for the detection of infectious diseases. These tests have become particularly important for such diseases as HIV-1, human papillomavirus (HPV), *Chlamydia trachomatis* (CT), and *Neisseria gonorrhoeae* (GC). NAATs are increasingly being applied toward the detection of pathogens associated with other STIs, such as *Trichomonas vaginalis* (TV). This review will focus on the most widely used commercial NAATs for detecting pathogens associated with STIs in women. Topics included will be NAAT technology, comparative test performance, STI screening guidelines, interpretation of NAAT results, and how these results can be applied to clinical diagnosis of STIs in women.

OVERVIEW OF MOLECULAR DIAGNOSTIC TECHNOLOGIES

Molecular diagnostic technologies have evolved from home-brew assays to commercial, Food and Drug Administration (FDA)–cleared NAATs that are widely used in clinical laboratories. Home-brew assays are still used in some molecular diagnostic laboratories, but there has been a major shift over the last decade to the use of commercial FDA-cleared kit assays for the detection of pathogens responsible for STIs. There are two main types of nucleic acid–based molecular diagnostic tests used in clinical laboratories: nonamplified DNA probe tests and NAATs.

Nonamplified DNA Probe Tests

Commercially available nonamplified DNA probe tests utilize nucleic acid probes that are specific for a unique nucleic acid sequence ("target sequence") present in the organism to be detected ("target organism"). First, the sample is treated to release nucleic acids. If the target organism is present, the DNA probe (usually labeled with fluorescent or chemiluminescent molecules) hybridizes with the target sequence. Once a stable probe:target sequence hybrid is formed, the labeled DNA probe emits a signal (fluorescence or chemiluminescence; Fig. A.1) that discriminates the hybridized probe from a nonhybridized probe. The signal is then measured.

The first nonamplified DNA probe assays were not sensitive enough to be used as clinical diagnostic tests. Several strategies were developed to increase the analytical sensitivity of the nonamplified tests for direct detection of microorganisms in clinical specimens. One strategy to increase sensitivity is to target ribosomal RNA (rRNA), of which thousands of copies exist in a single cell for most bacteria. For example, up to 2000 copies of CT rRNA are present in a single cell, in contrast to target sequences in genomic DNA, of which there are only one to a few copies per cell. The use of rRNA as a target greatly increases the sensitivity of the assay because there are so many more target sequences available to form hybrids. Examples of this technology include the PACE®2 assays (Gen-Probe Incorporated, San Diego, CA) for the detection of CT and GC. These assays were some of the first FDA-cleared nonamplified DNA probe tests widely used in clinical laboratories for direct detection of pathogens associated with STIs in clinical specimens (Table A.1).

A second strategy used to increase the sensitivity of DNA probe assays is signal amplification. An example of this is the Hybrid Capture® assay technology (Digene Corporation). Antibodies labeled with an enzyme that generates a signal bind to RNA:DNA hybrids. Multiple antibodies bind to a target hybrid to produce enough signal to be detected.

Nucleic Acid Amplification Tests

Nonamplified DNA probe assays are increasingly being replaced by NAATs because NAATs are more sensitive. NAATs are more sensitive because they utilize target-amplification technologies to produce millions of copies of RNA or DNA targets from as little as one target sequence from a single microorganism. NAAT procedures are usually divided into three main steps: sample processing, amplification, and detection. The replicated sequences from the amplification reaction (amplicons) are usually detected using labeled DNA probes. Some NAATs combine the amplification and detection steps into a single reaction that is termed "real-time amplification."

Three target-amplification methods are currently used in commercial FDA-cleared NAATs for the detection of pathogens associated with STIs: polymerase chain reaction (PCR), transcription-mediated amplification (TMA), and strand displacement amplification (SDA) (Table A.1).

PCR technology was the first target-amplification technology developed. It has been used extensively for both research and clinical diagnostic purposes (Fig. A.2A). In most FDA-cleared PCR tests, detection of amplicons is performed using a colorimetric reaction. The Roche PCR test uses an avidin-biotin-HRP system to capture amplicons generated in

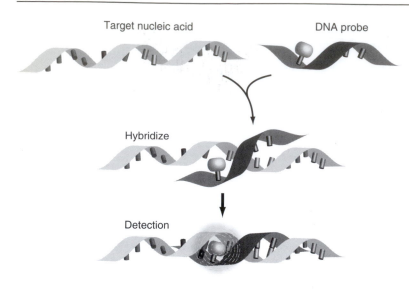

Target nucleic acid   DNA probe

Hybridize

Detection

FIGURE A.1 DNA probe test. DNA probes are oligonucleotides labeled with a detector molecule. The DNA probes are specific to a unique sequence on the DNA or RNA of the target microorganism to be identified. If this sequence is present in the specimen, the probe will hybridize specifically to the target nucleic acid of the organism. The hybridization reaction is detected by the signal emitted by the detector molecule on the DNA probe.

the PCR reaction to the bottom of microtiter plate wells. The colorimetric reaction is detected with a spectrophotometer.

TMA is an isothermal process that amplifies RNA or DNA sequences using primers and two enzymes: reverse transcriptase and RNA polymerase (Fig. A.2B). Detection of the amplicon is performed using the hybridization protection assay (HPA) method. HPA uses acridinium ester-labeled probes, which hybridize specifically with the amplicons. After hybridization, a reagent is added to hydrolyze the acridinium ester on the unhybridized probes to a nonchemiluminescent form. The hybridized probes remain chemiluminescent because the acridinium ester label is protected within the hybrid structure. Detection is achieved by adding reagents, which results in the emission of signal (chemiluminescent light) by the acridinium ester label on the hybridized probes. The signal is then measured with a special instrument called a "luminometer."

SDA is also an isothermal method that uses DNA polymerases to initiate DNA replication. Instead of using heat denaturation like PCR to separate double-stranded DNA, a restriction endonuclease enzyme is used to cleave the primer of the newly synthesized DNA. DNA polymerase recognizes the break and reinitiates DNA synthesis at that point, displacing the previously made strand as it proceeds

to copy the DNA once more. In this way, multiple DNA copies are generated and can reenter the SDA process. Detection is performed using a fluorescent probe called a molecular beacon and is measured by a fluorimeter instrument. This probe produces signal when it hybridizes to the amplicon. This is termed "real-time amplification," because the signal is generated as the amplification reaction proceeds. Real-time detection technologies have also been applied to both PCR and TMA technologies for certain research and diagnostic applications. Real-time amplification offers some advantages such as shortened assay times and increased precision when quantitation of target sequences is required.

All of the NAAT technologies are capable of producing billion-fold amplification of nucleic acids from very small quantities of target nucleic acids. The actual clinical performance of commercial assays is often more dependent on the specimen processing and detection technologies used with the amplification method. Sample processing is critical for reducing the effects of inhibitory factors in some samples that can cause false-negative results in some NAATs. Second-generation NAATs increasingly use sample purification methods such as target capture to purify target nucleic acids prior to amplification to remove potential inhibitory factors.

TABLE A.1 Examples of molecular diagnostic technologies used in commercially available, FDA-cleared assays for the detection of pathogens associated with STIs

Test type	Technology	Nucleic acid target	Label type	Commercial source
DNA probe tests	HPA	rRNA	Chemiluminescent	Gen-Probe Inc.
	Solid phase capture	rRNA	Colorimetric	Becton-Dickinson
	Hybrid capture	DNA	Chemiluminescent	Digene Corp.
Target-amplified NAATs	PCR	DNA	Colorimetric	Roche
	TMA	rRNA	Chemiluminescent	Gen-Probe Inc.
	SDA	DNA	Fluorescent	Becton-Dickinson

Abbreviations: FDA, Food and Drug Administration; HPA, hybridization protection assay; NAAT, nucleic acid amplification test; PCR, polymerase chain reaction; SDA, strand displacement amplification; STI, sexually transmitted infection; TMA, transcription-mediated amplification.

Target DNA

Heat Denaturation

Cool
Primers Hybridize
to Target

Primer Extension by
DNA Polymerase

DNA Pol

DNA Pol

Two New DNA
Hybrids Formed

(A)

Cycle Repeats

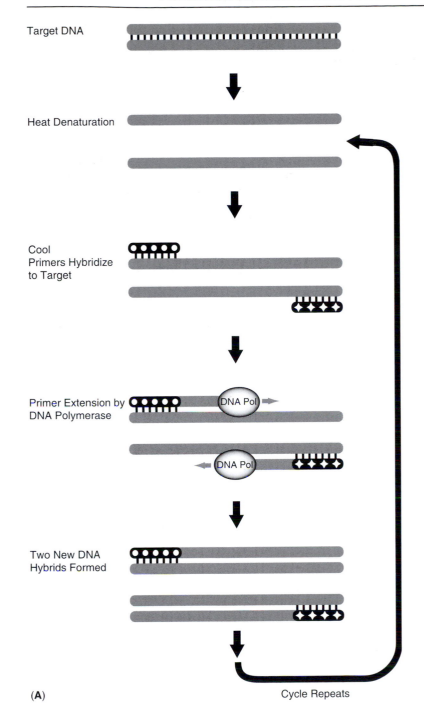

FIGURE A.2 (A) PCR technology. The first step of the PCR procedure is to heat-denature the DNA target sequence from the microorganism and amplify using a DNA polymerase enzyme. Primers bind specifically to the ends of the target sequence and direct the DNA polymerase to copy only that sequence. Each round of DNA synthesis is followed by a heat-denaturation step to separate the newly synthesized DNA strand from the strand from which it was copied. A special instrument called a thermocycler is needed to carry out the PCR process. The number of target molecules doubles with each cycle and results in a million-fold production of amplicon in less than two hours. PCR copies only DNA; therefore, if the target sequence is RNA, the RNA must first be converted to DNA using a separate enzymatic reaction.

Comparison of NAATs with Culture and Immunological Methods

The advantages of NAATs over traditional culture and immunological methods include the following:

- Rapid turnaround time (three to six hours). Although this is similar to the turnaround time for enzyme immunoassays (EIA), it represents a significant improvement over culture, which can take anywhere from 10 hours to several weeks depending on the organism. Rapid assays allow for timely patient treatment.
- Detection of unculturable organisms. Many microorganisms cannot be cultured (e.g., hepatitis C virus) or are

very difficult to culture (e.g., HIV-1), but they are readily identified by molecular diagnostic tests.

- High sensitivity of NAATs. NAATs can theoretically detect as little as one organism per sample, while the detection threshold of other methods such as EIA and nonamplified probes is often more than 1000 organisms per sample. With clinical sensitivities generally greater than 90%, NAATs are usually more sensitive than standard culture methods, especially with certain specimen types (e.g., detection of CT in urine specimens).
- Increased specimen stability. Specimen stability is usually much improved for molecular diagnostic tests compared to culture since viable organisms are not required

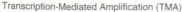

Transcription-Mediated Amplification (TMA)

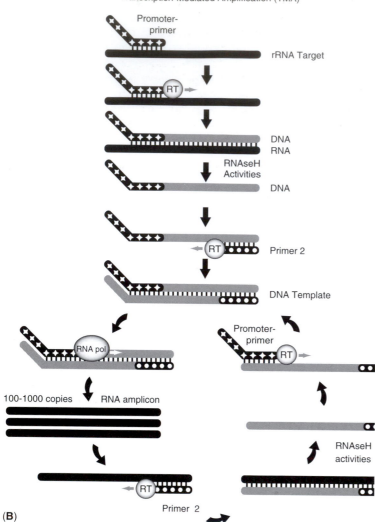

(B)

FIGURE A.2 (B) TMA technology. TMA uses two primers and two enzymes: RNA polymerase and reverse transcriptase. One of the primers contains a promoter sequence for RNA polymerase. In the first step of amplification, the promoter-primer hybridizes to the target rRNA at a defined site. Reverse transcriptase creates a DNA copy of the target rRNA by extension from the 3' end of the promoter-primer. The RNA in the resulting RNA:DNA duplex is degraded by the RNAse H activities of the reverse transcriptase. A second primer then binds to the DNA copy. A new strand of DNA is synthesized from the end of the primer by reverse transcriptase, creating a double-stranded DNA molecule. RNA polymerase recognizes the promoter sequence in the DNA template and initiates transcription. Each of the newly synthesized RNA amplicons reenters the TMA process and serves as a template for a new round of replication, leading to an exponential expansion of the RNA amplicon. Since each of the DNA templates can make 100 to 1000 copies of RNA amplicon, this expansion can result in the production of 10 billion amplicons in less than one hour. The entire process is autocatalytic and is performed at a single temperature.

for detection. Specimens can be stored for longer periods of time and at greater temperature ranges than are possible with culture specimens.

- Wide variety of specimen types. NAATs can often use a wider variety of specimen types, including those that may be difficult or impossible to use with culture or EIAs.

The potential limitations of NAATs include the following:

- Amplification inhibition. In the case of some first-generation NAATs, amplification inhibition may decrease the sensitivity of the assays. Inhibition is usually sample specific and may cause false-negative results. Inhibition can be monitored by using internal amplification controls or it can be eliminated by special sample-processing techniques, such as target capture. Despite occasional inhibition, most NAATs still have higher clinical sensitivities compared to nonamplified DNA probe tests, culture, and EIAs, which are not usually susceptible to inhibition.
- Carry-over contamination of amplicon between samples. Carry-over contamination occurs when amplicon from a previous reaction contaminates another sample. The

NAAT technology amplifies the amplicon, resulting in a false-positive result that can lead to decreased clinical specificity. This is rarely a problem with most of the FDA-cleared NAATs if the test procedure is performed carefully in accordance with good laboratory practices.

- Current FDA-cleared NAATs do not test for drug resistance. In cases where drug resistance data is desirable, both NAAT and culture may be performed.
- Increased costs. The costs of NAATs are often higher than those of culture and EIA. Some notable exceptions are CT and HIV-1 culture, which are typically difficult to perform and more costly than NAATs.

MOLECULAR DIAGNOSTIC ASSAYS FOR STIs

Molecular Diagnostic Tests for CT and GC

CT is the most common bacterial STI in women. Its prevalence in the United States has been increasing despite the implementation of improved detection and public health control programs. GC prevalence is about one-quarter the prevalence of CT, and coinfection with both pathogens is common.

Up to 27% of sexually active adolescent females are infected with CT, and 50% to 70% of infected females may be asymptomatic. GC may also be asymptomatic in about half of the infected women. Undiagnosed and untreated CT and GC infections can lead to pelvic inflammatory disease (PID) in 10% to 50% of infected women, which can result in ectopic pregnancy, infertility, and chronic pelvic pain. The asymptomatic nature of these infections together with the potential severe morbidity has led to the increased demand for highly sensitive tests to screen for CT and GC.

Nonmolecular diagnostic tests for CT and GC detection include culture, EIAs, and direct fluorescence assays. Most of these tests are being replaced by molecular diagnostic tests. In addition to their increased sensitivity, many of the molecular diagnostic tests have the advantage of the ability to detect both CT and GC from the same sample. This is important since coinfection is common; up to 50% of patients infected with GC also have a CT infection.

The first molecular diagnostic tests made commercially available for CT and GC testing were the PACE 2 assays (Gen-Probe Incorporated), which are nonamplified DNA probe assays. These assays were cleared by the FDA for the detection of CT and/or GC in endocervical and male urethral swab specimens and conjunctival swab specimens (CT only). Using a single swab specimen, the PACE 2 assays detect either organism individually (PACE 2 System for CT or GC, respectively), or both together (PACE 2C System for CT and GC). The sensitivity and specificity of the PACE 2 assays are similar to those of culture. The sensitivity of the PACE 2 GC assay is similar to the sensitivities of NAATs, but the PACE 2 CT assay is less sensitive than NAATs (Table A.2).

Cell culture for CT is no longer used in most clinical laboratories due to the technical difficulty of the procedure, slow turnaround time, and low sensitivity compared to NAATs. Culture for GC is still performed in many laboratories, but it is also being replaced due to the lower sensitivity of culture, which can result from delays in delivering viable specimens to the lab in a timely manner. CT and GC NAATs have higher clinical sensitivities than conventional microbiology techniques and allow the use of alternative, less-invasive specimen types. Many studies have demonstrated that the performance of NAATs in urine and vaginal swab specimens (both physician- andpatient-collected) is comparable to the performance of NAATs using the traditional endocervical swab specimens.

There are currently three commercial, FDA-cleared CT and GC NAATs in widespread use in clinical laboratories (Table A.2). The PCR-based Amplicor® CT/NG tests (Roche Diagnostics, Pleasanton, CA) for CT and GC and the SDA-based BD ProbeTec™ ET CT and GC amplified DNA assays (Becton, Dickinson and Company, Franklin Lakes, NJ) are both first-generation NAATs. These assays target sequences present in genomic DNA or in plasmids that are usually present in the organisms. The most recently introduced CT and GC NAAT is the TMA-based APTIMA COMBO 2® assay (Gen-Probe Incorporated). This is a second-generation multiplex NAAT using TMA, which detects and identifies both CT and GC in a single specimen by targeting CT and GC rRNA molecules simultaneously.

The assay includes a target capture method of sample preparation that purifies the target molecules by removing inhibitors that may be present. The target capture method uses specific capture probes to capture target rRNA molecules onto magnetic particles, allowing unwanted sample components to be washed away. The purified and concentrated target is then amplified by TMA. The combination of target capture and rRNA targeting has been reported in several studies to increase the analytical sensitivity of the assay up to 100 times that of the first-generation PCR and SDA tests.

The clinical sensitivity and specificity of NAATs for CT and GC detection are generally excellent (Table A.2). NAATs for CT are more sensitive than nonamplified DNA probe tests, EIA, and culture. NAATs for GC are similar in sensitivity to both nonamplified DNA probe tests and culture. The ProbeTec and Amplicor NAATs generally have a high sensitivity for CT detection with endocervical swab specimens. The APTIMA assay has been reported in many comparative studies to have the highest sensitivity (>95%) for CT detection and is now used by many clinical researchers as the reference standard for CT and GC testing.

Testing with NAATs can be performed not only using endocervical or male urethral swab specimens, but also using urine specimens. Urine collection is noninvasive and results in better patient acceptance, reduced staff workload, and decreased cost of testing. However, the sensitivity of first-generation NAATs is typically 5% to 20% lower with urine specimens (especially urine specimens from women) than with swab specimens, due to high levels of inhibitory substances in the urine specimens. The Amplicor PCR assay is not cleared for GC detection in urine specimens from women. The BD ProbeTec assay is cleared for testing urine specimens (from both men and women), but the assay sensitivity in urine specimens from women is typically lower than with endocervical swab specimens. The target capture specimen processing method of the APTIMA Combo 2 assay decreases inhibition, therefore ensuring a consistently high sensitivity of the assay with urine specimens. Some studies of the APTIMA Combo 2 assay have shown the sensitivity for CT detection to be equivalent for swab and urine specimens from women.

The APTIMA Combo 2 assay was recently cleared by the FDA for use with physician- and patient-collected vaginal swab specimens. Recent studies have suggested that assay sensitivity may be even higher using vaginal swab specimens compared to endocervical swabs, and that performance in physician-collected specimen is equivalent to that in patient-collected vaginal swab specimens. This may be due to the shedding of CT organisms from both endocervical and urethral infections into the vagina.

The Amplicor and APTIMA assays are also FDA cleared for use with ThinPrep® Pap test (Cytyc Corporation, Marlborough, MA) liquid-based cytology (LBC) specimens obtained for Pap testing. Studies have demonstrated that assay performance using LBC specimens is similar to performance when using endocervical swab specimens. Use of LBC specimens offers greater convenience to physicians

TABLE A.2 Comparison of the Four FDA-cleared molecular diagnostic tests for the detection of CT in women[a]

Assay	Technology	Target nucleic acid	Sensitivity for CT detection	
			Endocervical swab specimens	Urine specimens
PACE 2 for CT (nonamplified)	HPA	rRNA	50–80%	Not applicable
Amplicor CT/NG test	PCR	DNA	>70%	60–90%
BD ProbeTec ET CT and GC assays	SDA	DNA	>80%	70–90%
APTIMA COMBO 2 assay	TMA	rRNA	>95%	>90%

[a] Sensitivity ranges were estimated using published results, reviews, and comparative studies using a patient-infected status as the gold standard.
Abbreviations: CT, Chlamydia trachomatis; FDA, Food and Drug Administration; GC, Neisseria gonorrhoeae; HPA, hybridization protection assay; PCR, polymerase chain reaction; SDA, strand displacement amplification; TMA, transcription-mediated amplification.

and laboratories since Pap, HPV testing, and CT/GC testing can be performed from the same LBC specimen.

Several studies have shown that NAATs can also be used with rectal and pharyngeal swab samples to detect CT and GC. These studies have suggested that NAATs have a higher sensitivity than culture, but none of the NAATs are FDA cleared for these sample types.

Several professional and public health organizations, including the Centers for Disease Prevention and Control (CDC), advocate routine yearly CT screening for sexually active women under the age of 25 and for women over 25 who have certain risk factors (Table A.3). Despite these recommendations, the compliance rate for screening has been relatively low, with as few as one-third of physicians routinely screening women at high risk for CT infections. Survey studies have shown that many physicians are unaware that NAATs can detect the presence of CT and GC with high sensitivity when noninvasive specimens such as urine and vaginal swab specimens are used. Many of these physicians indicated they would screen more often if they had access to NAATs and could use noninvasive specimens. Greater use of these specimens in the future may drive an increase in overall screening of women at high risk for STIs.

Studies have consistently shown that screening at-risk women for CT with NAATs is cost effective despite the higher cost of NAATs compared to DNA probe tests or other nonmolecular diagnostic technologies. Screening sexually active women under the age of 25 once per year for CT prevents many cases of PID, ectopic pregnancy, and infertility. The costs saved by disease prevention outweigh the screening costs. Recent studies have shown that noninvasive samples such as urine samples can additionally increase the cost effectiveness of the assays. Yearly screening of men at risk for CT infection has not been shown to be cost effective but can help decrease the spread of disease.

Molecular Diagnostic Tests for TV

Trichomoniasis, caused by infection with TV, is the most prevalent nonviral STI in the United States, with approximately 5 million new infections per year. TV infection is considered to be underdiagnosed partly due to the low sensitivity

(approximately 40–50% sensitivity) of the commonly used wet mount procedure. Culture for TV is considered the gold standard and has a sensitivity of 70% to 90%. Many infections are also not diagnosed because physicians often rely on signs and symptoms for diagnosis. Reliance solely on classic signs and symptoms has been shown to result in up to 88% of infections not being diagnosed. Untreated TV has been associated with atypical PID, preterm birth, and tubal infertility, and is a risk factor for transmission of HIV.

Molecular diagnostic tests are available for the detection of TV. The BD Affirm™ VPIII Microbial Identification Test (Becton, Dickinson and Company) is an FDA-cleared, nonamplified DNA probe assay that detects TV, *Gardnerella vaginalis*, and *Candida* (yeast) species in the same assay. The test uses two probes for each organism: a capture probe and a detection probe. The rRNA target sequence first hybridizes with the capture probe, which is immobilized onto a bead, and then with the detection probe. The BD Affirm VPIII test is capable of consistently detecting all three organisms with good sensitivity compared to culture (sensitivity vs. culture is 81% for *Candida*, 89% for *Gardnerella*, and 92% for TV).

NAATs using PCR or TMA technologies have also been developed for the detection of TV. The TMA-based APTIMA® TV analyte specific reagent (ASR, Gen-Probe Incorporated) has been used to detect TV in clinical specimens. ASRs are reagents that are manufactured under FDA Good Manufacturing Practice guidelines for use by clinical laboratories as home-brew assays but have not been clinically tested by the manufacturer and cleared by the FDA. Laboratories using ASRs must complete extensive validation testing and generate their own performance data before reporting assay results. Several studies that tested clinical specimens with the home-brew TMA or PCR assays have suggested that these assays are about 60% more sensitive than wet mount and about 40% to 50% more sensitive than culture or the nonamplified DNA probe assay and can be used with vaginal swab or urine specimens. These studies also demonstrated that a large percentage of TV infections were asymptomatic in both women and men and that TV prevalence was much higher than expected in many of the population groups examined.

TABLE A.3 Screening guidelines for CT/GC

Professional organization	Guideline	Source
AAP	All sexually active patients should be screened for STIs	http://www.aap.org/policy/ re9939.html
ACOG	Screen all pregnant women for common STIs such as chlamydia All sexually active adolescents should be screened for CT and GC infections routinely. The National Committee on Quality Assurance's Health Plan Employer Data and Information Set defines routinely to be annually	http://www.acog.org
American College of Preventative Medicine	All sexually active women 25 yr of age or younger as well as sexually active women with other risk factors should be screened annually for CT	http://www.scienceblog.com/ community/article1535.html
AMA	All sexually active adolescents should be screened for STIs	http://www.ama-assn.org/ama/ upload/mm/39/gapsmono.pdf women should be screened for
CDC	Sexually active adolescent women Treatment Guidelines, p. 32 Annual screening of all sexually active women 20 to 25 yr of age is recommended Screening of women 25 yr of age or older if risk factors are present (e.g., new or multiple sex partners)	2002 Sexually Transmitted Disease should be screened for CT at least annually, even if asymptomatic
USPSTF	Screen all sexually active women up to age of 25 yr for CT (and older women if risk factors are present) Screen all pregnant women up to age of 25 yr for CT	http://www.ahrq.gov/clinic/ uspstf/uspschlm.htm

Abbreviations: AAP, American Academy of Pediatrics; ACOG, American College of Obstetricians and Gynecologists; AMA, American Medical Association; CDC, Centers for Disease Control and Prevention; CT, Chlamydia trachomatis; GC, Neisseria gonorrhoeae; STI, sexually transmitted infection; USPSTF, US Preventative Services Task Force.

Molecular Diagnostic Tests for HIV-1

Over the last decade in the United States, HIV-1 infections have evolved from being primarily an infection of homosexual men to an infection of heterosexual adults, particularly women. HIV-1 infection can lead to severe and fatal complications. In addition, infected pregnant women are at risk of passing the virus to the baby. Early detection of HIV-1 in pregnant women can lead to appropriate therapy to treat the mother and help prevent the spread of the infection to the baby.

Although the diagnosis of HIV-1 infections is usually made using serological tests, molecular diagnostic testing plays a major role in helping to diagnose and monitor HIV-1 infections. Most of the molecular diagnostic testing for HIV-1 is performed with quantitative viral load tests for monitoring patients undergoing treatment for HIV-1 infection. The Amplicor HIV-1 Monitor® test (Roche Molecular Diagnostics) was the first molecular HIV-1 test to be FDA cleared for monitoring disease and is now the primary test used by most laboratories for viral load testing.

In addition to the monitoring of HIV-1 infections, HIV-1 NAATs are sometimes used as diagnostic tests together with EIAs to detect new infections. HIV-1 NAATs are often used to test newborn babies from mothers infected

with HIV-1. HIV-1 NAATs can also be used in conjunction with other confirmatory tests such as Western blot to confirm reactive results from HIV-1 EIA tests.

HIV-1 NAATs are particularly useful for testing people with acute HIV-1 infections before they have developed an immune response to HIV-1. Studies have shown that HIV-1 NAATs can detect acute infections approximately 16 days earlier than EIAs on average (Fig. A.3). People who have potentially been exposed to HIV-1 (e.g., through rape, needle-stick injury, unprotected sex with an HIV-1 infected individual) can be tested with an HIV-1 NAAT to determine more quickly if they are infected with the virus.

Several studies have shown that HIV-1 NAATs can be used in high-risk populations to detect HIV-1 infections that were undetected in individuals recently tested by EIA. EIA-negative samples from these individuals were pooled and tested with HIV-1 NAATs. Up to 10% more infections were detected. These additional cases represent recently infected individuals who were in the acute phase of HIV-1 infection and had not yet developed an immune response.

The identification of HIV-1 infection in the acute stage is particularly important because extremely high concentrations of virus are present in the blood stream during the acute stage. It is estimated by some studies that up to 50%

of all new HIV-1 infections are transmitted by individuals in the acute stage of infection. Pregnant women with acute HIV-1 infections are also more likely to transmit the virus to their newborns. Earlier detection allows infected individuals to be treated sooner and may decrease the spread of HIV-1 by limiting high-risk behaviors in individuals who have been recently infected with HIV-1.

Most of the current molecular diagnostic testing for HIV-1 is performed with the Amplicor HIV-1 MONITOR test, even though it is not FDA approved for diagnostic use. The qualitative APTIMA HIV-1 RNA Qualitative assay (Gen-Probe Incorporated) was recently approved by the FDA for HIV-1 diagnostic testing and is the only NAAT currently approved for diagnostic purposes. This test has been used for several years by blood-testing centers to detect HIV-1 RNA in donated blood and has been shown to have a very high sensitivity.

Molecular Diagnostic Tests for HPV

HPV is the most prevalent STI, with over 5.5 million new cases occurring per year in the United States. Most sexually active men and women will be infected with the virus sometime during their lifetime, and latent genital HPV infection can be detected in 5% to 40% of sexually active women of reproductive age.

There are more than 100 HPV types, of which at least 30 are sexually transmitted. Most sexually transmitted HPV infections are asymptomatic, do not cause disease, and are eventually cleared. Some HPV infections of the genital tract may persist and lead to warts or cervical disease. Fourteen types of HPV have been demonstrated to be the causal factor for cervical cancer ("high-risk types"). These types are associated with 99.7% of all cervical cancers. HPV types 16 and 18 cause 70% of cervical cancers; the 12 other high-risk types cause the remaining 30% of cervical cancers. The vast majority of women infected with these high-risk types will eventually clear the virus and will experience no symptoms or adverse health consequences. However, a small minority of women will have a persistent cervical infection, putting them at greater risk of developing cervical disease, including cervical cancer.

The HPV E6 and E7 genes are thought to be the oncogenes responsible for progression to and maintenance of cervical neoplasia. The E6 protein causes degradation of the tumor suppressor protein p53. The E7 protein affects the retinoblastoma gene product (pRB) by releasing it from the E2F-1 type transcriptional control, leading to unchecked cell cycle progression. The relative expression levels of E6 and E7 have been found to increase in tandem with increasing severity of cervical disease.

Molecular diagnostic tests for HPV have been incorporated into Pap test screening programs in the United States and many other countries. Screening programs based only on Pap testing have limitations, primarily due to sampling problems and the subjective interpretation of cytology results. An audit of a U.K. program found that 47% of the fully invasive cancers in women younger than 70 years of age occurred in individuals with an adequate Pap testing history. Pap testing is particularly unsuccessful in low-resource regions where the incidence of cervical cancer is unchanged or increasing. Use of molecular diagnostic HPV tests together with Pap testing can increase the overall sensitivity of screening programs.

There are currently several commercial HPV molecular diagnostic tests including the Hybrid Capture 2 High-Risk HPV DNA test (Digene Corporation) and the PCR-based Amplicor HPV test (Roche Diagnostics). The Hybrid Capture test is the only molecular diagnostic test currently cleared by the FDA for HPV screening. The test was originally cleared for the management of women with atypical squamous cells of undetermined significance (ASC-US). Since then, the test has also been cleared in combination with a Pap test for primary screening of women over the age of 30 years (Table A.4).

The Digene HPV test is a DNA probe test that uses Hybrid Capture signal amplification technology to detect DNA from high-risk HPV types in LBC specimens. The Hybrid Capture test can detect the presence of one or more of 13 high-risk HPV types with a sensitivity of greater than 90%. A low-risk panel is also available. Studies have shown that Pap tests alone have a sensitivity of 50% to 85% for the detection of high-grade cervical disease or cancer. Combining the Hybrid Capture test with Pap testing can increase the sensitivity to approximately 96% to 99%. With a negative predictive value of 99% to 100%, the risk of developing high-grade cervical disease or cancer would be very low in women with negative HPV DNA and Pap test

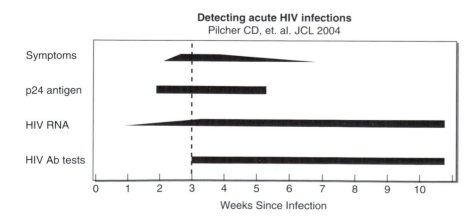

Detecting acute HIV infections
Pilcher CD, et. al. JCL 2004

Symptoms

p24 antigen

HIV RNA

HIV Ab tests

0 1 2 3 4 5 6 7 8 9 10
Weeks Since Infection

FIGURE A.3 Detection of acute HIV infections. Patients newly infected with HIV typically cannot be detected with antibody-based tests until approximately three weeks after infection. HIV NAATs can detect HIV RNA about 16 days earlier than the EIA tests on average and allow the earlier detection of HIV-infected patients during the acute phase of infection.

results. This could potentially permit the use of longer screening intervals in women who have high-risk HPV DNA negative results and normal Pap test results. The Hybrid Capture test does have some cross-reactivity with low-risk HPV types. The Hybrid Capture test has relatively low specificity for predicting the progression toward cervical cancer when used together with Pap test results.

The PCR-based Amplicor HPV test detects the same high-risk HPV types as the Hybrid Capture test. Several studies have suggested that the sensitivity and specificity of the PCR test is similar to the Hybrid Capture test. Roche also has a genotyping test (Linear Array) that individually identifies 37 HPV types (both high- and low-risk types) using a solid phase probe hybridization reaction. The Linear Array test is mostly used for research purposes. Neither of the Roche tests is FDA cleared.

Most women with high-risk HPV DNA positive results and normal Pap test results have transient HPV infections (80%) that will not progress to high-grade cervical disease or cancer. These high-risk HPV DNA positive results are considered to be false positives in relation to morbidity, which decreases the clinical specificity and positive predictive value of the test. The challenge becomes how to discriminate between transient and persistent infections, thereby improving the specificity of HPV testing. The possibilities that have been suggested are the following:

1. Restrict screening to older women. Although peak prevalence of genital HPV infections occurs among women in their teens and 20s, these HPV infections and associated mild lesions tend to clear spontaneously. HPV prevalence declines with age, but viral persistence tends to increase. The incidence of severe cervical dysplasia starts rising as women reach their late 20s to early 30s, and the incidence of cervical cancer rises as women reach their late 30s. HPV screening at a young age is inefficient, as it results in many positive HPV results that have no clinical significance. Because of this, the ACS has developed guidelines suggesting that HPV DNA screening with the Pap test be restricted to women aged 30 years and older, as they are most at risk for cervical disease. The FDA has allowed this indication for Hybrid Capture 2 high-risk HPV DNA test. Restricting screening to this older population helps decrease the detection of transient infections and improve specificity and PPV by screening only those women at highest risk for the development of cervical disease. The American College of Obstetricians and Gynecologists (ACOG) has also recommended the following: "Because HPV DNA testing is more sensitive than cervical cytology in detecting CIN 2 and CIN 3, women with negative concurrent test results can be reassured that their risk of unidentified CIN 2 and CIN 3 or cervical cancer is approximately 1 in 1000" (Level A, ACOG Practice Bulletin, 2005, HPV) The NCI-ASCCP interim guidance has suggested that women who have negative Pap test and high-risk HPV DNA test results do not need to be screened for three years.
2. Specimens from women who have positive high-risk HPV DNA test results could be further tested with a

TABLE A.4 ASCCP and ACOG guidelines for the management of women with ASC-US who have positive results for high-risk HPV types

Testing for high-risk types of HPV should be performed using a sensitive molecular test, and all women who are HPV positive should be referred for colposcopic evaluation

Women with ASC-US who are high-risk HPV negative can be followed-up with repeat cytology at 12 mo

Acceptable management options for women who are positive for high-risk types of HPV, but who do not have biopsy-confirmed CIN, include follow-up with repeat cytology at 6 and 12 mo with referral back to colposcopy if a result of ≥ASC-US is obtained, or HPV testing at 12 mo with referral back to colposcopy of all HPV-positive women

Women with HPV-positive ASC-US who are referred to colposcopy and found to have biopsy-confirmed CIN should be managed according to the appropriate ASCCP or ACOG guidelines for the management of histological abnormalities

Because of the potential for overtreatment, diagnostic excisional procedures such as loop electrosurgical excision should not be routinely used to treat women with HPV-positive ASC in the absence of biopsy–confirmed CIN

Abbreviations: ACOG, American College of Obstetricians and Gynecologists; ASC, atypical squamous cells; ASCCP, American Society for Colposcopy and Cervical Pathology; ASC-US, atypical squamous cells of undetermined significance; CIN; HPA, hybridization protection assay. *Source:* Adapted from Cox JT. HPV testing in patient management: atypical squamous cells of undetermined significance and low-grade squamous intraepithelial lesion. In: Monsonego J, ed. Emerging Issues on HPV Infections. Basel: Karger, 2006.

genotyping test to determine if the woman is infected with HPV types 16 or 18. Since these two high-risk types are responsible for up to 70% of cervical cancers, a woman with a positive genotype test would be referred to colposcopy. Use of the genotyping tests is limited because there are currently no FDA-cleared HPV 16 and 18 genotyping tests.

3. Use tests that detect HPV mRNA expressed from the E6 and E7 viral oncogenes. New technologies and tests are being developed to detect HPV mRNA oncogene products rather than DNA. Expression of HPV mRNA is essential to lesion development, and detection of these mRNA targets could possibly result in a test that is more specific and able to predict which women will progress toward CIN2+ or greater. There are currently two NAATs that detect HPV mRNA. The PreTect® HPV-Proofer assay (NorChip AS, Klokkarstua, Norway) is available in Europe and detects mRNA transcripts from high-risk HPV types 16, 18, 31, 33, and 45. The APTIMA HPV assay (in development, Gen-Probe Incorporated) uses TMA to detect E6 and E7 mRNA from all 14 high-risk types. Preliminary studies have suggested that the mRNA tests will be at least as sensitive as and potentially more specific than the Hybrid Capture test and other DNA tests.

Recent proposals have suggested that primary screening for cervical disease should initially be performed with HPV NAATs, with reflex to Pap testing only when high-risk types are detected. This algorithm would take advantage of the superior sensitivity of the HPV NAAT and the high specificity of Pap testing. Women with high-risk HPV DNA positive results and abnormal Pap test results would undergo colposcopy. This algorithm would be particularly appropriate for low-resource settings where HPV screening might be easier to implement and less expensive than Pap testing. Further studies will be needed to validate these proposals, but it is likely that primary screening using HPV NAATs will become the standard of care in the future, with Pap testing playing a secondary role as a reflex test.

Molecular Diagnostic Tests for Other STIs

There are currently many home-brewed NAATs for pathogens associated with other STIs such as *Treponema pallidum*, herpes simplex virus, and *Mycoplasma genitalium* (Mgen). None of these tests are FDA cleared, and the performance characteristics of the tests are not well characterized. The tests are not widely used and are mainly restricted to esoteric clinical laboratories and research laboratories.

In the case of poorly characterized STIs such as Mgen infection, molecular diagnostic tests are needed to identify and characterize the organisms and link them to disease in humans. Mgen has been of particular interest in recent years because of its link to urethritis, cervicitis, and other urogenital disease. This organism is very difficult to culture and can only be reliably detected by NAATs. Some researchers have suggested that Mgen infection may be "the next chlamydia" and is potentially responsible for a significant amount of undiagnosed urogenital disease. Further clinical research will be needed to determine the etiology of this organism and whether there is a need for a clinical diagnostic test.

CONCLUSION AND FUTURE TRENDS

Molecular diagnostic tests, in particular NAATs, have played a major role in increasing the quality and performance of laboratory testing for STIs. Molecular diagnostic technology has not only increased the sensitivity of STI testing overall, but has also linked some of these microorganisms, such as HPV, to significant morbidity and mortality. This contributes to earlier detection and management of infections to prevent serious disease. Molecular diagnostic testing has led to the development of effective screening programs for detection of asymptomatic CT and GC infections to prevent serious complications in women. The asymptomatic natures of these infections, with their potential for significant downstream morbidity, were not widely recognized until the widespread implementation of CT/GC molecular diagnostic testing. Molecular diagnostic testing also has the potential to identify STIs that are currently underdiagnosed, such as TV and Mgen infections.

Universal swab and transport devices will become more common in the future. These will allow for the more convenient testing for multiple organisms from a single sampling vial. This is already occurring with LBC specimens, such as the ThinPrep Pap test vial, which can be used to test for HPV, CT, and GC, in addition to Pap testing. It is expected that the intended uses of other STI NAATs will be expanded for use with this or similar universal transport devices.

Molecular diagnostic technology is rapidly evolving. New molecular array technologies are being developed that will detect many organisms in a single specimen in a cost-effective manner. Molecular diagnostic tests will become simpler and cheaper to run and molecular point-of-care tests will become more common. Molecular diagnostic tests will eventually replace many of the nonmolecular diagnostic tests. New molecular diagnostic tests will also be developed for microbial susceptibility testing. Multiplex tests are being developed that will be capable of identifying specific microorganisms and test for drug susceptibility at the same time. These new advances in molecular diagnostic technology will increasingly change the way medicine is practiced and continue to improve overall healthcare.

SELECTED READING

Centers for Disease Control and Prevention 2002. Screening tests to detect Chlamydia trachomatis and Neisseria gonorrhoeae infections, 2002. Morb Mortal Wkly Rep 51:1–40.
Hill CS. Molecular diagnostic testing for infectious diseases using TMA technology. Expert Rev Mol Diagn 2001; 1(4):445–455.
Holmes K, Stamm WE. Lower genital tract infection syndromes in women. In: Homes KK, Sparling F, Mardh PA, Lemon SM, Stamm WE, Piot P, Wassherheit JN, eds. Sexually Transmitted Diseases, 3rd ed. New York: McGraw-Hill, 1999:761–781.
Paavonen J, Critchlow CW, DeRouen T, et al. Etiology of cervical inflammation. Am J Obstet Gynecol 1986; 154:556–564.
Weinstock, H, Berman S, Cates W Jr. Sexually transmitted diseases among American youth: incidence and prevalence estimates, 2000. Perspect Sex Reprod Health 2004; 36:6–10.

Chlamydia/Gonorrhoeae
Bouadzhyan B, Yashina T, Yatable JH, Patnaik M, Hill CS. Comparison of the APTIMA CT and GC assays with the APTIMA Combo 2 assay, the Abbott LCx assay, and direct fluorescent-antibody and culture assays for detection of Chlamydia trachomatis and Neisseria gonorrhoeae. J Clin Microbiol 2004; 42:3089–3093.
Chernesky M, Jang, D, Luinstra K, et al. High analytical sensitivity and low rates of inhibition may contribute to detection of Chlamydia trachomatis in significantly more women by the APTIMA Combo 2 assay. J Clin Microbiol 2006; 44:400–405.
Chernesky MA III, Hook EW, Martin DH, et al. Women find it easy and prefer to collect their own vaginal swabs to diagnose Chlamydia trachomatis or Neisseria gonorrhoeae infections. Sex Trans Dis 2005; 32:729–733.
Chernesky MA, Jang DE. APTIMA transcription-mediated amplification assays for Chlamydia trachomatis and Neisseria gonorrhoeae. Expert Rev Mol Diag 2006; 6(4):519–525.
Chernesky MA, Martin DH, Hook EW, et al. Ability of new APTIMA CT and APTIMA GC assays to detect Chlamydia trachomatis and Neisseria gonorrhoeae in male urine and urethral swabs. J Clin Microbiol 2005; 43:127–131.
Chernesky MA. Chlamydia trachomatis diagnostics. Sex Trans Infect 2002; 78:232–234.
Chong S, Jang D, Song X, et al. Specimen processing and concentration of Chlamydia trachomatis added can influence false-negative rates in the LCx assay but not in the APTIMA Combo 2 assay when testing for inhibitors. J Clin Microbiol 2003; 41:778–782.
Chong S, Jang D, Song, X et al. Specimen processing and concentration of Chlamydia trachomatis added can influence false-negative rates in the LCx assay but not in the APTIMA Combo 2 assay when testing for inhibitors. J Clin Microbiol 2003; 41:778–782.
Gaydos CA, Quinn TC, Willis D, et al. Performance of the APTIMA Combo 2 assay for detection of Chlamydia trachomatis and Neisseria gonorrhoeae in female urine and endocervical swab specimens. J Clin Microbiol 2003; 41:304–309.

Gaydos CA, Theodore M, Dalesio N, Wood BJ, Quinn TC. Comparison of three nucleic acid amplification tests for detection of *Chlamydia trachomatis* in urine specimens. J Clin Microbiol 2004; 42:3041–3045.

Hook III EW, Handsfield HH. Gonococcal infections in the adult. In: Holmes KK, Mårdh P-A, Sparling FP, et al. eds. Sexually Transmitted Diseases, 3rd edn. McGraw Hill Companies, Inc. USA, 1999, 451–466.

Johnson RE, Newhall WJ, Papp JR, et al. Screening tests to detect *Chlamydia trachomatis* and *Neisseria gonorrhoeae* infections—2002. MMWR Recomm Rep 2002; 51:1–38.

Marrazzo JM, Celum CL, Hillis SD, Fine D, DeLisle S, Handsfield HH. Performance and cost-effectiveness of selective screening criteria for *Chlamydia trachomatis* infection in women. Implications for a national *Chlamydia* control strategy. Sex Transm Dis 1997; 24:131–141.

Østergaard L, Anderson B, Møller JK, Olesen F. Home sampling versus conventional swab sampling for screening of *Chlamydia trachomatis* in women: a cluster-randomized 1-year follow-up study. Clin Infect Dis 2000; 31:951–957.

Schachter J, Chernesky MA, Willis DE, et al. Vaginal swabs are the specimens of choice when screening for *Chlamydia trachomatis* and *Neisseria gonorrhoeae*: results from a multicenter evaluation of the APTIMA assays for both infections. Sex Trans Dis 2005; 32:725–728.

Schachter J, Chernesky MA, Willis DE, Fine PM, Martin DH, Fuller D, Jordan JA, Janda W, Hook EW III. Vaginal swabs are the specimens of choice when screening for *Chlamydia trachomatis* and *Neisseria gonorrhoeae*: results from a multicentre evaluation of the APTIMA assays for both inflections. Sex Trans Dis 2005; 32(12):725–728.

Schachter J, Hook EW, Martin DH, et al. Confirming positive results of nucleic acid amplification tests (NAATs) for *Chlamydia trachomatis*: all NAATs are not created equal. J Clin Microbiol 2005; 43:1372–1373.

Stamm WE. *Chlamydia trachomatis* infections of the adult. In: Holmes KK, Sparling FP, Mardh P, Lemon SM, Stamm WE, Piot P, Wasserheit JN, eds. Sexually Transmitted Diseases, 3rd edn. New York: McGraw Hill, 1999:407–422.

US Preventive Services Task Force. Screening for chlamydial infection: recommendations and rationale. Am J Prev Med 2001; 20(3 Suppl):90–94.

T. vaginalis

Hardick AJH, Miller R, Wood BJ, Quinn TC, Gaydos CA. Comparison between the Gen-Probe TMA *Trichomonas vaginalis* assay and a real-time PCR, B-TUB FRET, for the detection of *Trichomonas vaginalis*. ISSTDR. The Netherlands, Amsterdam, July 10–13, 2005.

Hardick J, Yang S, Lin S, Duncan D, Gaydos C. Use of the Roche LightCycler instrument in a real-time PCR for *Trichomonas vaginalis* in urine samples from females and males. J Clin Microbiol 2003; 41:5619–5622.

Kaydos SC, Swygard H, Wise SL, et al. Development and validation of a PCR-based enzyme-linked immunosorbent assay with urine for use in clinical research settings to detect *Trichomonas vaginalis* in women. J Clin Microbiol 2002; 40:89–95.

Madico G, Quinn TC, Rompalo A, McKee KT Jr, Gaydos CA. Diagnosis of *Trichomonas vaginalis* infection by PCR using vaginal swab samples. J Clin Microbiol 1998; 36:3205–3210.

Soper D. Trichomoniasis: under control or undercontrolled? Am J Obstet Gynecol 2004; 190:281–290.

Wendel KA, Erbelding EJ, Gaydos CA, Rompalo AM. *Trichomonas vaginalis* polymerase chain reaction compared with standard diagnostic and therapeutic protocols for detection and treatment of vaginal trichomonasis. Clin Infect Dis 2002; 35:576–580.

Wendel KA, Erbelding EJ, Gaydos CA, Rompalo AM. Use of urine polymerase chain reaction to define the prevalence and clinical presentation of *Trichomonas vaginalis* in men attending an STD clinic. Sex Transm Infect 2003; 79:151–153.

HIV-1

Cohen M, Pilcher C. Amplified HIV transmission and new approaches to HIV prevention. J Infect Dis 2005; 191:1391–1393.

Cohen M. Preventing transmission of HIV: a biological and medical perspective. AIDS Patient Care STDS 2001; 15:427–429.

Klausner JD, Grant RM, Kent CK. Detection of acute infections. New Engl J Med 2005; 353:631.

Pilcher C, Eron J, Vernazza P, et al. Sexual transmission during the incubation period of primary HIV infection. JAMA 2001; 286:1713–1714.

Pilcher C, Tien H, Eron J, et al. Brief but efficient: acute HIV infection and the sexual transmission of HIV. J Infect Dis 2004; 189:1785–1792.

HPV

Castle PE, Sadorra M, Garcia F, Holladay EB, Kornegay J. Pilot study of a commericalized human papillomavirus (HPV) genotyping assay: comparison of HPV risk group to cytology and histology. J Clin Microbiol 2006; 44:3915–3917.

Castle PE, Schiffman M, Burk RD, et al. Restricted cross-reactivity of hybrid capture 2 with nononcogenic human papillomavirus types. Cancer Epidemiol Biomarkers Prev 2002; 11:1394–1399.

Cuzick J, Clavel C, Petry KU, et al. Overview of the European and North American studies on HPV testing in primary cervical cancer screening. Int J Cancer 2006; 119:1095–1101.

Cuzick J, Szarewski A, Cubie H, et al. Management of women who test positive for high-risk types of human papillomavirus: the HART study. Lancet 2003; 362:1871–1876.

Monsonego J, Karger B, Lorincz AT, Richart RM. Human papillomavirus DNA testing as an adjuct to cytology in cervical screening programmes. Arch Pathol Lab Med 2003; 127:959–968.

Gravitt PE, Peyton CL, Apple RJ, Wheeler CM. Genotyping of 17 human papillomavirus types by using L1 consensus PCR products by a single-hybridization, reverse line blot detection method. J Clin Microbiol 1998; 36:3020–3027.

Herrero R, Castle PE, Schiffman M, et al. Epidemiologic profile of type-specific human papillomavirus infection and cervical neoplasia in Guanacaste, Costa Rica. J Infect Dis 2005; 191:1796–1807.

Kraus I, Molden T, Enro LE, Skomedal H, Karlsen F, Hagmar B. Human papillomavirus onocogenic expression in the dysplastic portio; an investigation of biopsies from 190 cervical cones. Br J Cancer 2004; 90:1407–1413.

Kraus I, Molden T, Holm R, et al. Presence of E6 and E7 mRNA from human papillomavirus types 16, 18, 31, 33, and 45 in the majority of cervical carcinomas. J Clin Microbiol 2006; 44:1310–1317.

Kulasingam SL, Hughes JP, Kiviat NB, et al. Evaluation of human papillomavirus testing in primary screening for cervical abnormalities: comparison of sensitivity, specificity, and frequency of referral. JAMA 2002; 288:1749–1757.

Molden T, Kraus I, Karlsen F, Sckomedal H, Nygard JF, Hagmar B. Comparison of human papillomavirus messenger RNA and DNA detection: a cross-sectional study of 4,136 women >30 years of age with a 2-year follow-up of high-grade squamous intraepithelial lesion. Cancer Epidemiol Biomarkers Pre 2005; 14:367–372.

Molden T, Kraus I, Karlsen F, Skomedal H, Hagmar B. Human papillomavirus E6/E7 mRNA expression in women younger than 30 years of age. Gynecol Oncol 2006; 100:95–100.

Molden T, Nygard JF, Kraus I, et al. Predicting CIN2+ when detecting HPV mRNA and DNA by PreTect HPV-proofer and consensus PCR: a 2-year follow-up on women with ASCUS or LSIL Pap smear. Int J Cancer 2005; 114:973–976.

Munoz N, Bosch FX, de Sanjose S, et al. Epidemiologic classification of human papillomavirus types associated with cervical cancer. N Engl J Med 2003; 348:518–527.

Peyton CL, Gravitt PE, Hunt WC, et al. Determinants of genital human papillomavirus detection in a US population. J Infect Dis 2001; 183:1554–1564.

Schiffman M, Herrero R, Desalle R, et al. The carcinogenicity of human papillomarvius types reflects viral evolution. Virology 2005; 337:76–84.

Schiffman MH, Bauer HM, Hoover RN, et al. Epidemiologic evidence showing that human papillomavirus infection causes most cervical intraepithelial neoplasia. J Natl Cancer Inst 1993; 85:958–964.

Sherman ME, Lorincz AT, Scott DR, et al. Baseline cytology, human papillomavirus testing, and risk for cervical neoplasia: a 10-year cohort analysis. J Natl Cancer Inst 2003; 95:46–52.

Stoler MH. HPV testing in cervical cytology practice—It's all about choice. Acta Cytol 2005; 49:117–119.

Walboomers JM, Jacobs MV, Manos MM, et al. Human papillomavirus is a necessary cause of invasive cervical cancer worldwide. J Pathol 1999; 189:12–19.

Wright TC Jr, Schiffman M, Solomon D, et al. Interim guidance for the use of human papillomavirus DNA testing as an adjunct to cervical cytology for screening. Obstet Gynecol 2004; 103:304–309.

Wright TC Jr, Schiffman M. Adding a test for human papillomavirus DNA to cervical-cancer screening. N Engl J Med 2003; 348:489–490.

Other STIs

Cohen CR, Manhart LE, Bukusi EA, et al. Association between *Mycoplasma genitalium* and acute endometritis. Lancet 2002; 359:765–766.

Cohen CR, Mugo NR, Astete SG, et al. Detection of *Mycoplasma genitalium* in women with laparoscopically diagnosed acute salpingitis. Sex Transm Infect 2005; 81:463–466.

Hardick J, Giles J, Hardick A, Hsieh YH, Quinn T, Gaydos C. Performance of the Gen-Probe transcripton-mediated amplification research assay compared to that of a multitarget real-time PCR for *Mycoplasma genitalium* detection. J Clin Microbiol 2006; 44:1236–1240.

Manhart LE, Critchlow CW, Holmes KK, et al. Mucopurulent cervicitis and *Mycoplasma genitalium*. J Infect Dis 2003; 187:650–657.

Schlicht MJ, Lovrich SD, Sartin JS, Karpinsky P, Callister SM, Agger WA. High prevalence of genital mycoplasmas among sexually active young adults with urethritis or cervicitis symptoms in La Crosse, Wisconsin. J Clin Microbiol 2004; 42:4636–4640.

Index

Dot blots, 101
Douching, 465–466
Doxycycline, 25, 147, 251, 264
Duke diagnostic criteria for infectious
endocarditis, 388
Duodenum, 511
Dyspareunia, 391
Dysuria, 303, 379

Early-onset neonatal infection, 221
Eberhart-Phillips' series, 124
Econazole, 409
Ectopic pregnancy, 242, 419
Efavirenz and neural tube defects, 92
Elephantiasis, 147
Embryopathy, mumps, 127
Endocarditis, 36–37, 165. See also Bacterial
endocarditis
Endocervical cultures, 497
Endometrial bacterial contamination, 414
Endometritis, 153, 207, 241–242, 331–332,
342–343. See also Postpartum
Endometritis/endomyometritis
Endomyometritis, 331–332.
See also Postpartum
endometritis/endomyometritis
endomyometritis–septic
thrombophlebitis–septicemia, 185
failed prophylaxis endomyometritis, 343
following abdominal delivery, 342
ENGERIX-B®, 63
Entamoeba histolytica (amebiasis), 277–279.
See also Amebiasis
Enterobacter, 201–202
Enterobacter cloacae, 14
Enterococcus, 230–235
antimicrobial resistance and therapy,
234–235
Enterococcus faecium, 234
in lower female genital tract, 232–233
major clinical processes, 232
microbiology and taxonomy, 230
obstetrical and gynecologic implications,
233–234
pathogenic attributes of, 230–231
peritoneal infections and intra-abdominal
abscess, 234
Enteroviruses, 45–49
congenital and neonatal infection/disease
congenital echovirus infection, 47
congenital poliovirus infection/disease, 48
live virus and inactivated virus vaccines,
48–49
management, 45
maternal enterovirus infection/disease, 45
neonatal poliomyelitis, 48
poliovirus, 47–48
Enzyme immunoassay (EIA), 83
Chlamydial infection, 245
Enzyme-linked immunosorbent assay
(ELISA), 45, 83, 111, 138, 258,
260, 278
Epithelial cells in the vagina, 6
Epizootic listeriosis, 156
Erythema chronicum migrans (ECM), 260
Erythema infectiosum (EI), 109
Erythrocyte Sedimentation Rate (ESR), 463
Erythromycin, 22, 147, 251, 503
Escherichia coli, 14, 193–194
Ethionamide, 24
Evisceration, 486

Exogenous virulent pathogens, 350
Exposed gravid, management, 125
Extraintestinal infection, 277
Extremely oxygen sensitive (EOS) organism, 9

Facilitating flora, 35
Facultative anaerobes, 9–10
False-positive VDRL test, Syphilis, 269
Famciclovir, 72–73, 139
Famvir (famciclovir), 506
Female genital tract involvement
antibody production, 7
Amebiasis, 278
Actinomyces israelii, 181
bacteriology of, 1–3
diseases, 1. See also Bacterial diseases
normal female genital tract flora, 1–2.
See also Vaginal flora
Chlamydia trachomatis, 239–241
Coccidioides immitis and Coccidioides
posadasii, 314–315
Escherichia coli, 193
in HSV, 68–73
immunological defense mechanisms in,
5–8. See also Immunological
defense mechanisms
mycoplasma, 258
Neisseria gonorrhoeae, 159–163
Peptostreptococci, 207–208
Proteus group, 209–210
Salmonella typhi, 170
Streptococcus pyogenes, 176–179
Streptococcus pneumonia, 173–174
Fetal candidiasis, 307–308
Fetal fibronectin, 358
Fetal impact, 193
Fetal indications, therapy for, 291–292
Fetal infection, 177, 359–360
Fetal wastage, 139, 419
Fetus, antibiotics for, 19
Fever, 28, 387
First trimester congenital infection, 43–44
Flat warts, 97
Flocculation tests, 269
Fluconazole, 309, 409, 515
Flucytosine, 408
Fluorescent antibody, 245
Fluorescent treponemal antibody (FTA)
tests, 269
Fluoroquinolones, 19, 22
5-Fluorouracil, 104, 105
Formes frustes of rubella, 130
Foscarnet, 46
Funguria evaluation, 306–307
Fused papillae, 100
Fusidic acid, 31

Gainesville classification, 11, 12, 15, 16,
35, 516
Ganciclovir, 46
Gardnerella vaginalis, 33, 196–200, 400
Genital aphthous ulcers, 508–509
Genital herpes, 70
Genital lesions, 506–507
Genital listeriosis, 155
Genital strains, 252
Genital tract, female, 79, 220. See also
Female genital tract involvement
Genital tuberculosis, 326–327
Genital warts, 97
Genitorectal syndrome, 249–250

Genitourinary tract procedures, 37
Gentamicin, 351
Gestation, exposure to rubella during, 134
Glucose metabolism, 407
Glutathione S-transferase, 18
Gonococcal acute salpingitis, 456
Gonococcal arthritis, 161
Gonococcal chorioamnionitis, 162
Gonococcal endocarditis, 161–162
Gonococcal endometritis, 162
Gonococcal infections, 166
Gonococcal ophthalmia in neonates, 165
Gonococcal ophthalmia neonatorum, 162
Gonococcal perihepatitis (Stajano–Curtis–
Fitz-Hugh Syndrome), 163
Gonococcal pharyngitis, 163
Gonococcal salpingitis, 451–453
Gonococcal septicemia, 160–161
Gonorrheal endometritis, 160
Gram's iodine, 495
Gram-stained smears, vaginal secretions, 395
Gram-staining technique, 495, 496
Granuloma inguinale (Klebsiella
granulomatis), 145, 499–502.
See also Donovanosis
Granulomatosis infantiseptica, 155–157
Gray zone, temperature, 28
Gray-baby syndrome, 21
Gross vulvitis, 399
Group A beta-hemolytic streptococcus
(streptococcus pyogenes), 176–179,
416, 455
Group B streptococci (GBS), 219–225
Group C beta-hemolytic streptococci
(Streptococcus milleri), 228
Group F streptococci, 237
Group G beta-hemolytic streptococci, 237
Gynecological infection, 253–254

Haemophilus ducreyi, 149–151.
See also Chancroid ulcer
Haemophilus influenza, 152–153, 456
HAVRIX®, 63
HCV antibody–positive gravida, 59
Heat shock proteins, 5
Hemagglutination inhibition (HAI), 253
Hemodynamically compromised patients, 470
Hemodynamically stable patients, 470
Hemolytic streptococcal gangrene, 178
Hemophilus influenza, 86
Heparin, 346
Hepatitis A virus (HAV), 51–64
Hepatitis B vaccine (HBV), 51–53, 373
chronic hepatitis B infection, 52–53
hepatitis B core antigen (HBcAg), 51–52
hepatitis B surface antigen (HBsAg),
51–52
Hepatitis C virus (HCV) infection, 53–55
chronic hepatitis C, 55
cirrhosis of the liver, 55
configuration, 54
mode of transmission, 54
primary infection, 54–55
RNA virus, 54
serologic response, 54
Hepatitis viruses/Hepatitis virus infection,
51–64
active immunization, 63
clinical manifestations of, 56–57
congenital hepatitis, 57–58
diagnosis, 60–61